DIAGNOSTIC OPHTHALMOLOGY

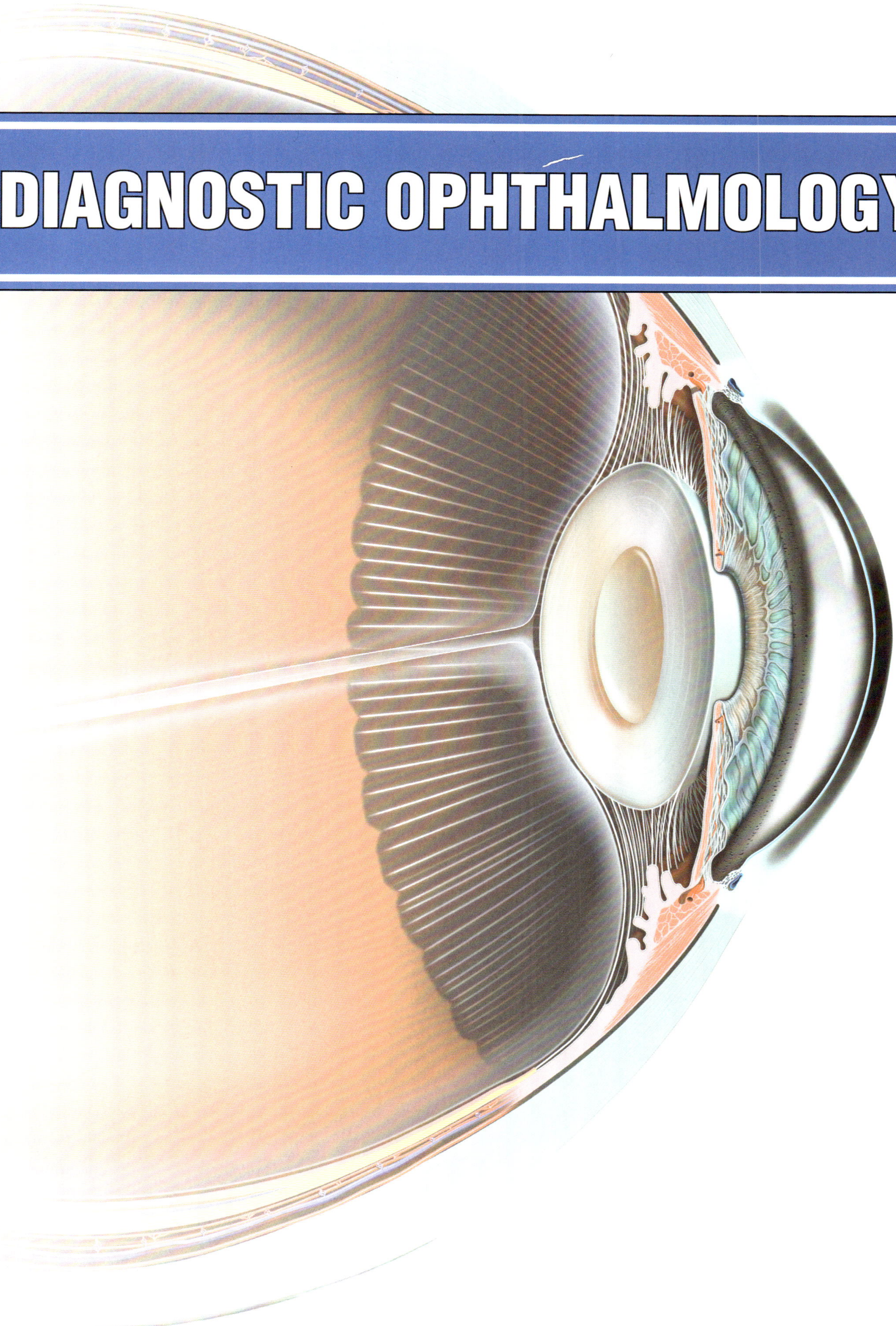

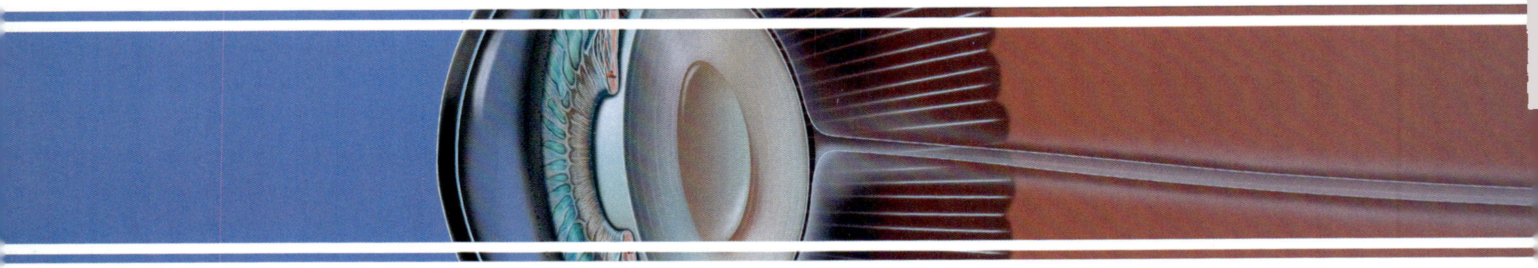

DIAGNOSTIC OPHTHALMOLOGY

Brian Stagg, MD
Editor-in-Chief
Ophthalmology Resident
Department of Ophthalmology
Moran Eye Center
University of Utah School of Medicine
Salt Lake City, Utah

Balamurali K. Ambati, MD, PhD, MBA
Editor-in-Chief
Professor of Ophthalmology
Director, Cornea Research
Moran Eye Center
University of Utah School of Medicine
Salt Lake City, Utah

James Gilman, CRA, FOPS
Image Editor
Project Administrator
Moran Eye Center
University of Utah Hospitals and Clinics
Salt Lake City, Utah

AMIRSYS®
Names you know. Content you trust.®

First Edition

Printed in Canada by Friesens, Altona, Manitoba, Canada

ISBN: 978-1-931884-94-5

Notice and Disclaimer

Library of Congress Cataloging-in-Publication Data

Diagnostic ophthalmology / editor-in-chief, Balamurali K. Ambati, editor-in-chief, Brian Stagg. -- First edition.
p. ; cm.
Includes bibliographical references.
ISBN 978-1-931884-94-5
I. Ambati, Balamurali K., editor of compilation. II. Stagg, Brian, editor of compilation.
[DNLM: 1. Eye Diseases--diagnosis--Handbooks. 2. Diagnosis, Differential--Handbooks. WW 39]
RE75
617.7'15--dc23

2013035877

Dedicated to our families, mentors, and patients for their inspiration, insight, confidence, and challenge.

We must gladly acknowledge that this undertaking would not have taken place without the invaluable assistance of many. Our coauthors and image contributors have worked incredibly hard in gathering the content of this endeavor, and they are the best "posse" we could have ever asked for. We would like to give special thanks to Dave Chance, Kellie Heap, Ashley Renlund, Katherine Riser, and Mike Hasson of Amirsys whose editorial guidance, good humor, encouragement, and patient yet persistent shepherding were essential to bringing this endeavor to fruition. Derick Holt, Evandro Lucena, Lloyd Williams, Gustave Alberti, and Mariam Rachid deserve great recognition for their Thorough medical editing and countless suggestions. The photographers who obtained the beautiful pictures of various pathologies and the artists who drew the clarifying artwork that adorn the chapters merit special commendation. To all the others who helped and assisted, a very big thank you.

BS and BKA

CONTRIBUTORS

Allison R. Jarstad, DO
Ophthalmology Resident
SUNY Upstate
Syracuse, New York

David DeMill, MD
Ophthalmology Resident
Department of Ophthalmology and Visual Sciences
Kellogg Eye Center
University of Michigan
Ann Arbor, Michigan

Gustave N. Alberti, MD
Chief, Department of Ophthalmology
MacDill Air Force Base
Tampa, Florida

Adam Jorgensen, MD
Ophthalmology Resident
Moran Eye Center
University of Utah School of Medicine
Salt Lake City, Utah

Russell Swan, MD
Ophthalmology Resident
Department of Ophthalmology
Moran Eye Center
Salt Lake City, Utah

Maximilian R. Padilla, BS
Medical Student
University of Utah School of Medicine
Salt Lake City, Utah

Pooja D. Jani, MD
Postdoctoral Research Fellow
Department of Ophthalmology
Kittner Eye Center
University of North Carolina at Chapel Hill School of Medicine
Chapel Hill, North Carolina

Steven M. Christiansen, MD
Ophthalmology Resident
University of Iowa
Iowa City, Iowa

M. Aabid Farukhi, BA
Medical Student
University of Utah School of Medicine
Salt Lake City, Utah

Bryce Radmall, MD
Transitional Year Intern
Intermountain Medical Center
Salt Lake City, Utah

Erica Liu, MD
Ophthalmic Pathology and Research Fellow
Moran Eye Center
Salt Lake City, Utah

Nicholas Behunin, MD
Ophthalmology Resident
Penn State Hershey Eye Center
Hershey, Pennsylvania

Jerica Johnson, BS
Medical Student
University of Utah School of Medicine
Salt Lake City, Utah

Nathan Lambert, BS
Medical Student
University of Utah School of Medicine
Salt Lake City, Utah

Anne Margaret Floyd, MD, MS
Ophthalmic Pathology and Research Fellow
Moran Eye Center
University of Utah School of Medicine
Salt Lake City, Utah

Joshua R. Ford, MD
Ophthalmic Pathology and Research Fellow
Moran Eye Center
University of Utah School of Medicine
Salt Lake City, Utah

Christopher B. Smith, MD
Resident Physician
Saint Louis University Eye Institute
Saint Louis, Missouri

James Tucker, PhD
Medical Student
University of Utah School of Medicine
Salt Lake City, Utah

Cecinio Ronquillo, Jr., PhD
Medical Student, MD/PhD Program
University of Utah School of Medicine
Salt Lake City, Utah

Ashlie Bernhisel, BA
Medical Student
University of Utah School of Medicine
Salt Lake City, Utah

Isha Gupta, BS
Medical Student
University of Utah School of Medicine
Salt Lake City, Utah

Jason Jensen, BS
Medical Student
University of Utah School of Medicine
Salt Lake City, Utah

Shannon L. Stallings, MD
Ophthalmic Pathology Fellow
Moran Eye Center
University of Utah School of Medicine
Salt Lake City, Utah

Justin C. Kohl, MD
Ophthalmic Pathology and Research Fellow
Moran Eye Center
University of Utah School of Medicine
Salt Lake City, Utah

Nathan Eshenroder, BS
Medical Student
University of Utah School of Medicine
Salt Lake City, UT

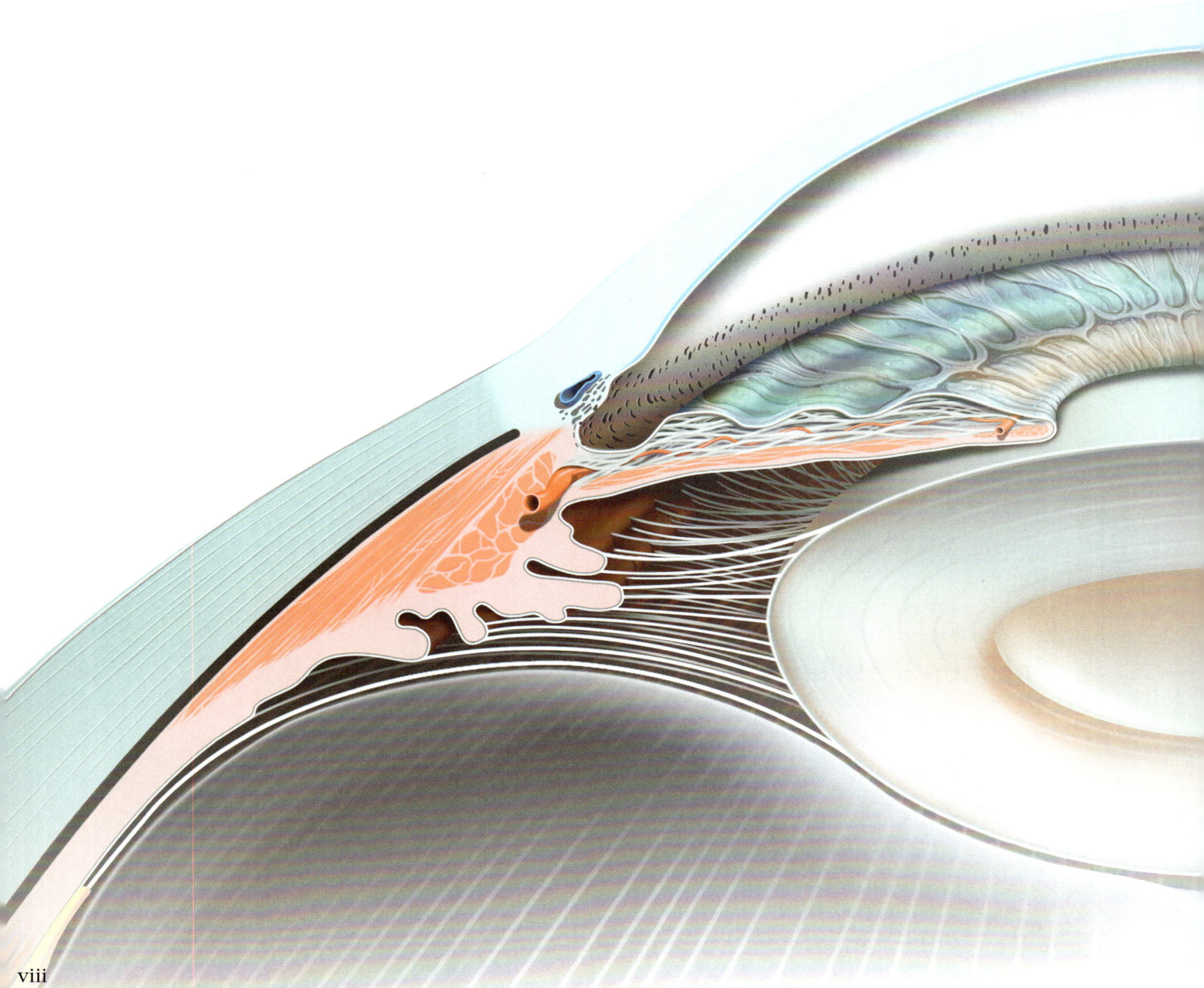

IMAGE CONTRIBUTORS

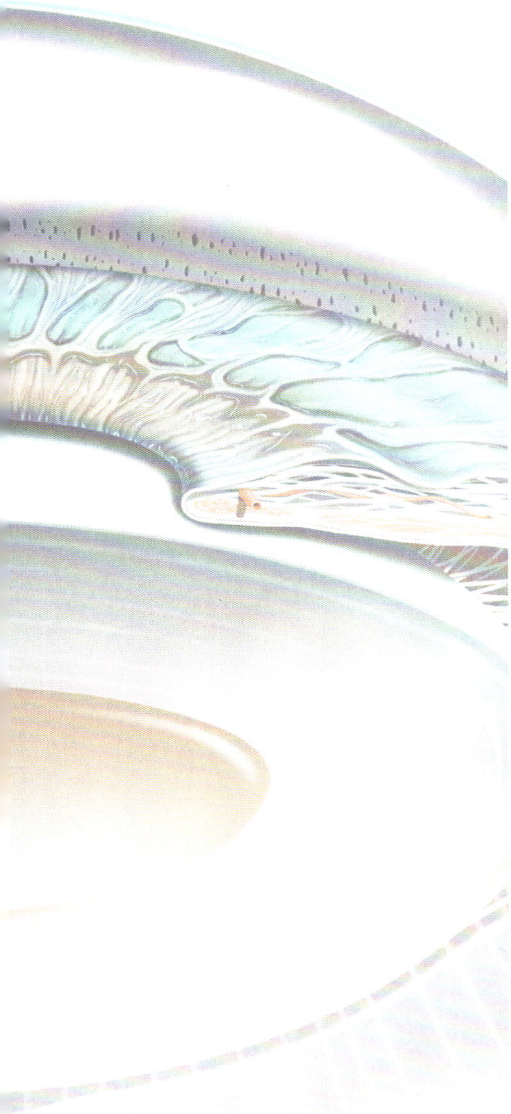

Erin E. Anstadt, BA

Jacob K. Barney, BS

Jefferson R. Brown, BS

Stephen J. Campbell, BS

Edward B. Feinberg, MD, MPH

Bradley S. Henriksen, BS

Stephen Craig Morris, BS

Henry Daniel Perry, MD

Christopher E. Starr, MD, FACS

Amith C. Subhash, BS

Noelle M. Teske, MSc, BA

Albert Y. Wu, MD, PhD

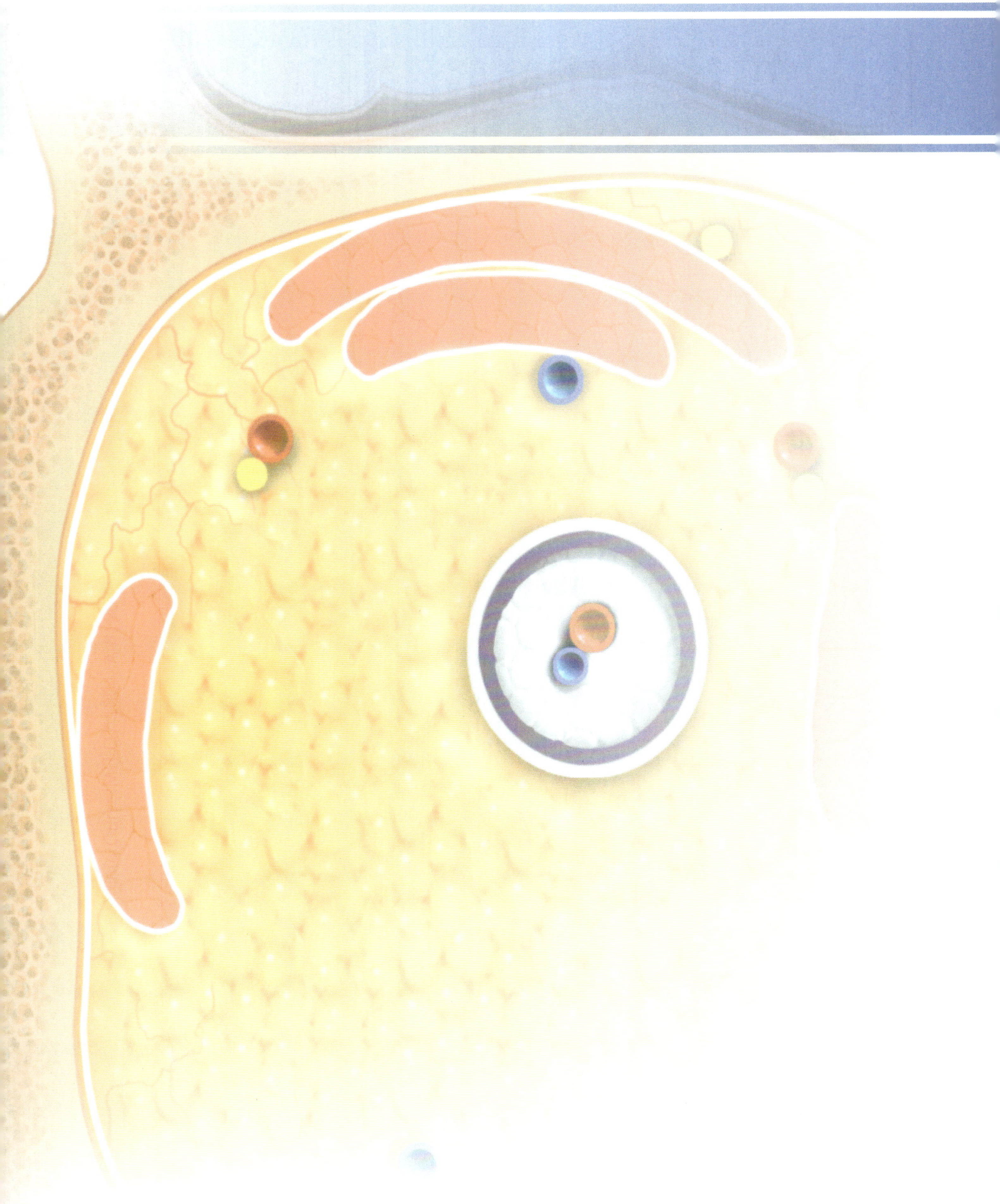

FOREWORD

In our harried world, we have never had such a great need for knowledge. The paradox is that finding the knowledge we need takes exactly what we are often short on– time. This is even more true for the busy ophthalmologist who has increasing demands from insurers, CMS, regulators, administrators, EMR, and most importantly, patients, all of whom want and expect immediate answers.

Yes, we have the Internet, but trying to find obscure subjects in one helpful snippet can be daunting. Periodicals? Though filled with cutting edge material, they are not a speedy source of all the core facts nor are they an easy read. Besides, few have the time to look there during the rush of the day. We can perhaps turn to our recall. But what if this is a corneal question and we are retinal specialists? Or we simply want to refresh our memory? Once again, we are faced with the problem of time.

There are always textbooks, but are they too low tech? We may be able to find a tome that includes every esoteric substance, but do we always need 750 pages on every aspect of a single specialty? The answer is no, and this is why *Diagnostic Ophthalmology* by Dr. Balamurali Ambati and team is a boon in the hectic and modern diagnostic world. This book lays out all of the facts in a crisp, short summary on essentially every diagnostic category. In a minute, which is often all the time we have, the latest information can be at our fingertips to refresh our memories on subjects we only distantly remember from residency. This collective but succinct knowledge is truly vital in our day of super-specialization.

Even still, there's more. While this title is a godsend to the busy practicing ophthalmologist, it can supply vital knowledge to the residents in training or the ER physicians who are seeing cases of ophthalmic problems they never encountered in medical school. The text rapidly ties interesting patient cases to core facts and images on all diagnoses of importance in our field.

So, congratulations to Dr. Ambati and his fine gang of coauthors for bringing this timely book to the fore. To save all ophthalmologists the time we often feel short on, they have sacrificed their own to get it right for the rest of us. Please read and enjoy!

Randall J. Olson, MD
Professor and Chair
Department of Ophthalmology and Visual Sciences
CEO, Moran Eye Center
Director of the Vision Institute
University of Utah School of Medicine
Salt Lake City, Utah

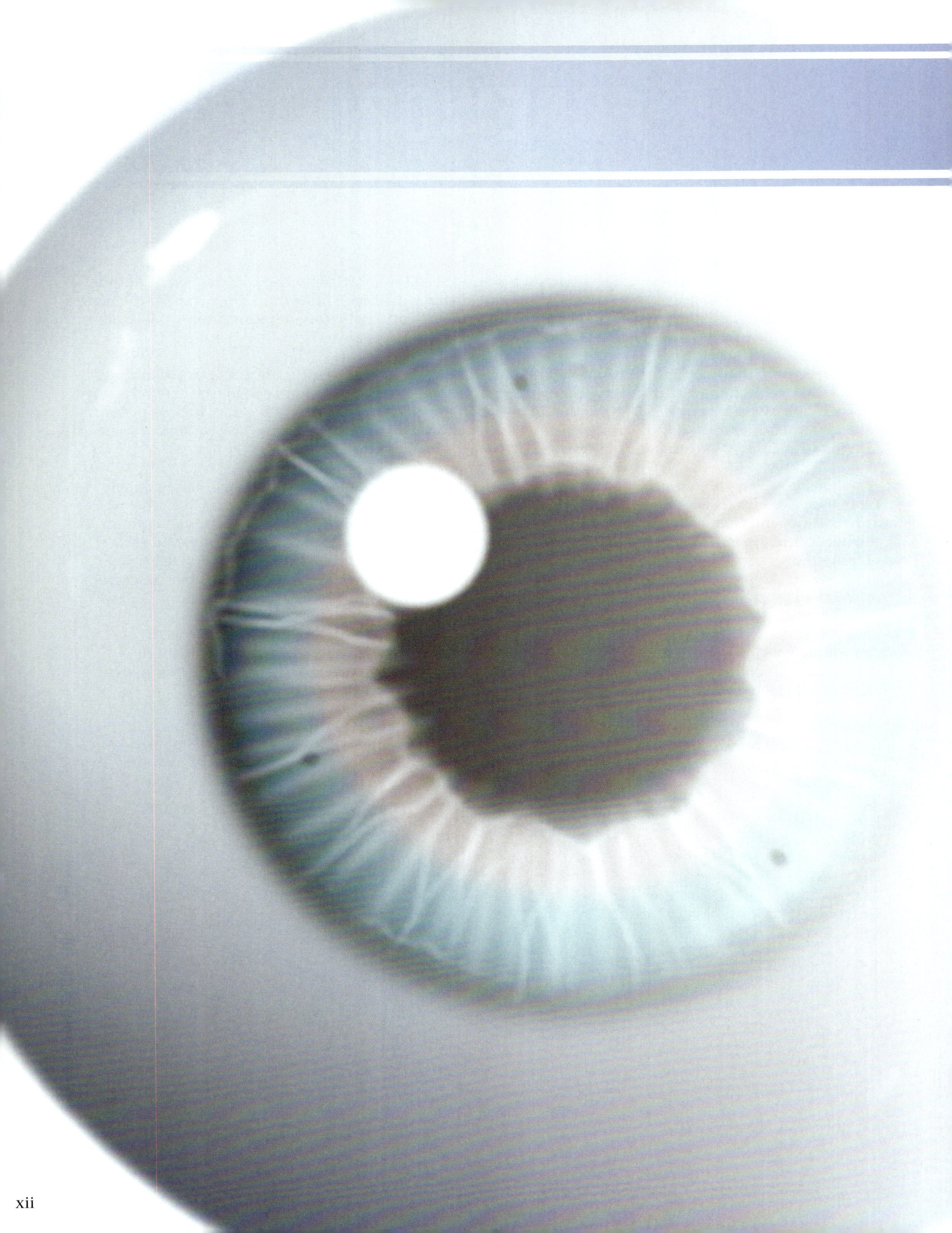

PREFACE

One man cannot summon the future. – Spock
But one man can change the present. – Kirk, in "Mirror, Mirror"

Ophthalmology is a rare mix of medicine and surgery, pediatrics and geriatrics, with opportunities to diagnose life-threatening conditions and offer life-ennobling treatments and cures. We all entered this field that we love and care about with the desire to make a difference and give back to our community. Our team of coauthors and image contributors have come together to do precisely that.

The reader would be fully justified in asking, "Is another book in ophthalmology really necessary?" Does any practitioner, with a multitude of centrifugal demands of time and energy, have enough "bandwidth" to read another tome? We approached this book with the mission to save ophthalmologists and trainees time by bringing together a structure of rapid overviews, concise facts on diagnosis and treatments, clarifying photographs and images, and a central resource of current clinical trials in ophthalmology, which was last done over 15 years ago. This crystallized distillate of clinical basics, insights, and protocols is accessible and contains the breadth and depth to be helpful in a variety of situations — patient care, general background, review, and test preparation. We have borne in mind the old saying that brevity is the soul of wit but have tried not to sacrifice essential knowledge on the altar of concision.

This book was written primarily by young trainees; this should provide freshness of perspective and pith in prose. We hope that our efforts in selectively strategic streamlining have navigated the waters between redundancy and disconnectedness so as to keep each chapter whole but the book brief. It is inevitable that we have made errors of omission and commission; for those, we ask your forgiveness and trust that the readership will bring these to our attention. We look forward to your comments, compliments, and criticisms in the months and years to come.

We genuinely hope that this book aids in ophthalmic care and training in the United States and abroad and that physicians of all stages find value in it. If it assists the treatment of patients and the growth of trainees, then we will have succeeded.

Balamurali K. Ambati, MD, PhD, MBA
Editor-in-Chief
Professor of Ophthalmology
Director, Cornea Research
Moran Eye Center
University of Utah School of Medicine
Salt Lake City, Utah

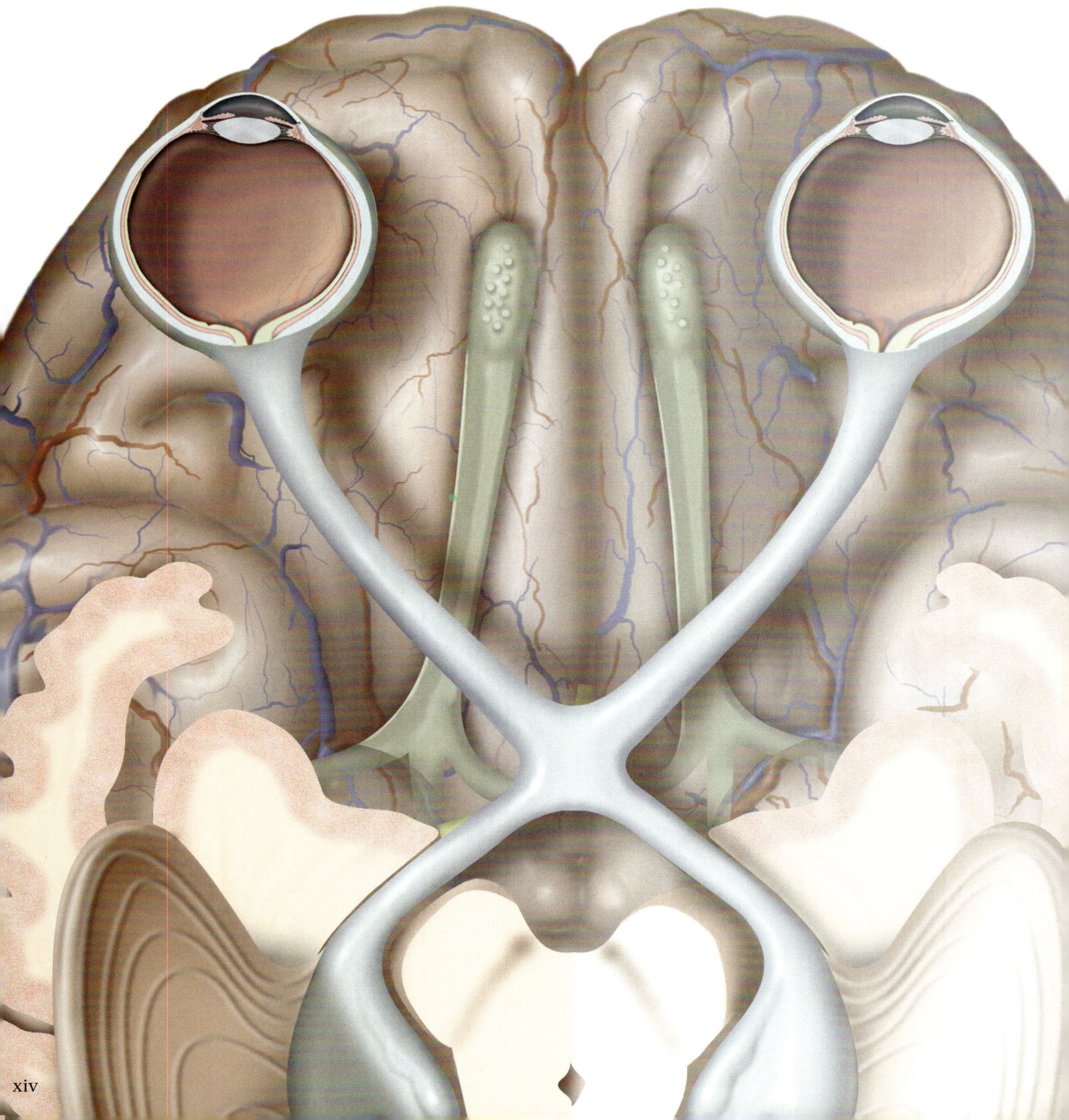

ACKNOWLEDGMENTS

Text Editing
Arthur G. Gelsinger, MA
Lorna Kennington, MS
Rebecca L. Hutchinson, BA
Angela M. Green Terry, BA
Kalina K. Lowery, MS
Sarah J. Conner, BA

Image Editing
Jeffrey J. Marmorstone, BS
Lisa A. M. Steadman, BS

Medical Editing
Derick G. Holt, MD, PhD
Lloyd B. Williams, MD, PhD
Evandro Lucena, MD
Mariam Rachid, MD

Illustrations
Lane R. Bennion, MS
Richard Coombs, MS
Laura C. Sesto, MA

Art Direction and Design
Laura C. Sesto, MA
Lane R. Bennion, MS

Lead Editor
Dave L. Chance, MA, ELS

Publishing Lead
Katherine L. Riser, MA

AMIRSYS®
Names you know. Content you trust.®

TABLE OF CONTENTS

PART I
Cornea and External Disease

SECTION 1
Conjunctiva

Degenerations

Malignant Neoplasms

Treatment-Related Disorders

Miscellaneous

PART VI
Ophthalmic Plastic Surgery

SECTION 1
Eyelids

Introduction and Overview

Autoimmune and Inflammatory Disorders

Trauma

Nonneoplastic Cysts

Malignant Neoplasms

Miscellaneous

SECTION 2
Lacrimal System

SECTION 3
Orbit

PART VII
Neuroophthalmology

SECTION 1
Optic Nerve

Infectious Disorders

Trauma

Vascular Disorders

Benign Neoplasms

Malignant Neoplasms

Miscellaneous

SECTION 2
Strabismus

Introduction and Overview

Congenital Disorders

SECTION 1
Conjunctiva

Introduction and Overview

Normal Variants

Congenital Disorders

Infectious Disorders

Autoimmune and Inflammatory Disorders

Trauma

Vascular Disorders

Degenerations

Nonneoplastic Masses

Benign Neoplasms

Malignant Neoplasms

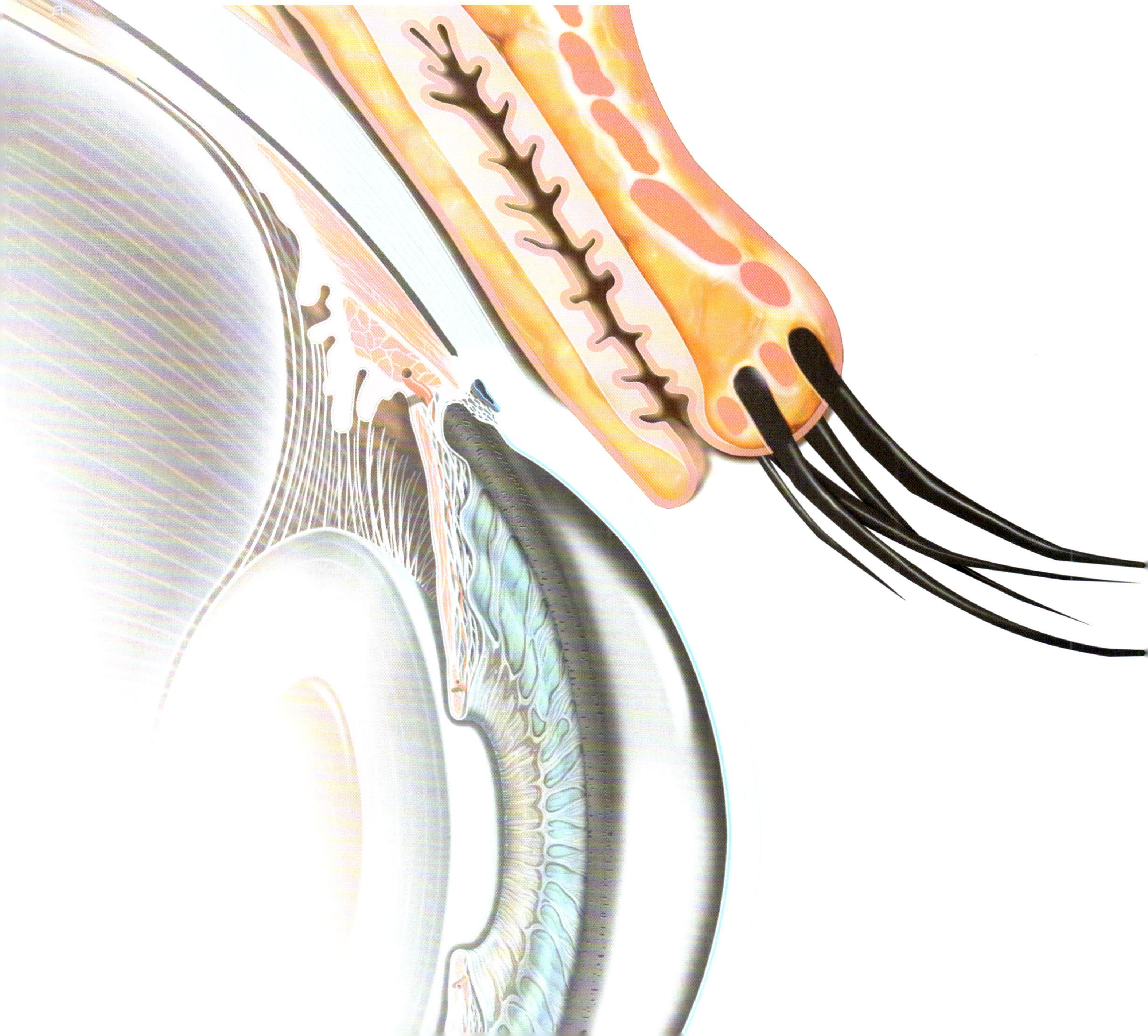

CONJUNCTIVA OVERVIEW

TERMINOLOGY

Definitions

- Conjunctiva
  - Thin, translucent mucous membrane lining inner surfaces of eyelids
  - Reflected onto the exterior surface of the eye to extend from the anterior episclera and sclera to the limbus of the cornea, where it becomes continuous with corneal epithelium

CONJUNCTIVAL FUNCTION

Clinical Importance

- Allows for unrestricted movement of the globe and eyelids
- Forms inner mucous layer of the tear film and part of the aqueous layer
  - Secretes antibacterial proteins, electrolytes, and water to protect the cornea and anterior globe from external environment; goblet cells secrete mucins
  - Tear film is composed of 3 layers
    - Mucous layer = innermost layer; secreted by conjunctival goblet cells
    - Aqueous layer = middle layer; secreted by main and accessory lacrimal glands
    - Lipid layer = outermost layer; secreted by meibomian glands
- Provides reservoir for tear meniscus
- Provides a barrier to infection and foreign bodies
- Provides immunologic protection to ocular surface

EMBRYOLOGY

Development

- Conjunctival epithelium originates from ectoderm and mesoderm overlying the optic vesicle when the eyelids fuse together at 8 weeks of intrauterine development
- Lacrimal glands (glands of Wolfring and Krause) form from invaginations of conjunctival epithelium in the fornices
- Caruncle forms from conjunctival and skin tissues during development of nasolacrimal duct

GROSS ANATOMY

Anatomical Features

- Conjunctiva extends continuously from the mucocutaneous junction at the palpebral margins of the eyelids to the palisades of Vogt at the corneoscleral limbus
  - Palisades of Vogt contain corneal stem cells
- 3 conjunctival subdivisions
  - Palpebral or tarsal = tightly adherent conjunctiva lining inner surface of upper and lower eyelids
  - Forniceal = conjunctiva lining upper and lower fornices
  - Bulbar = conjunctiva covering anterior sclera; loosely adherent to Tenon capsule
- Mucous membrane-lined conjunctival sac is composed of superior, inferior, and temporal fornices, an extendible semilunar fold medially, and the bulbar and palpebral conjunctiva
  - Plica semilunaris: Small fold of bulbar conjunctiva that lies between the caruncle and globe at medial canthus of the eye
    - Plica facilitates tear drainage into the nasolacrimal duct and allows for unrestricted movement and rotation of the ocular globe and eyelids
- Extraocular muscles and tendons attach to the conjunctiva to create and maintain the shape of the fornices
  - Superior fornix = levator palpebrae smooth muscle fibers
  - Temporal fornix = lateral rectus tendon
  - Medial fornix = medial rectus tendon
    - Created during globe adduction, when a cul-de-sac is formed as the eye moves into medial gaze
  - Inferior fornix = inferior rectus tendon

HISTOLOGY

Layers

- Conjunctival epithelium is composed of 6-9 layers of irregularly arranged nonkeratinized stratified squamous epithelium with mucin-secreting goblet cells and mucous glands dispersed throughout
  - Large number of goblet cells are located in the tarsal and inferonasal bulbar conjunctiva
- Thickness and histological appearance of conjunctiva varies from eyelid margin to limbus
  - Palpebral conjunctiva = stratified cuboidal epithelium
  - Forniceal conjunctiva = columnar epithelium
  - Bulbar conjunctiva = irregularly arranged nonkeratinized stratified squamous epithelium (in contrast to more regular arrangement of corneal epithelium)
- Conjunctival epithelium does not have an organized basement membrane; rather, it rests on the vascularized stromal bed of the substantia propria
  - Superficial layer of substantia propria is composed of loose connective tissue and adenoid tissue
  - Deep layer of substantia propria is composed of fibrovascular tissue containing vessels, nerves, and lymphatics
- Conjunctival epithelium is more permeable than corneal tissue
  - Stratified squamous and goblet epithelial cells are attached to each other by tight junctions and desmosomes, allowing for greater permeability
- Corneal epithelial stem cells inhabit the limbal area where conjunctival stratified squamous epithelium becomes contiguous with corneal epithelium

CONJUNCTIVAL VASCULATURE

Vessels and Lymphatics

- Conjunctival blood supply is mostly derived from muscular, medial palpebral, and lacrimal branches of the ophthalmic artery, which is derived from the internal carotid artery
  - Additional blood supply comes from facial artery branches
- Anterior ciliary arteries branching from the muscular arteries that supply the rectus muscles supply blood to the perilimbal conjunctiva and palisades of Vogt by forming a superficial marginal plexus at the limbus

CONJUNCTIVA OVERVIEW

- Conjunctival vessels branching from anterior ciliary arteries remain superficial; deeper circulation feeds the anterior segment (cornea, iris, and ciliary body)
  - Inflammation of the conjunctiva usually occurs peripherally and involves the superficial vessels
  - Inflammation of the cornea, iris, and ciliary body leads to dilation and engorgement of deep vessels around the limbus, leading to ciliary flush
- Conjunctival capillaries are fenestrated, allowing for vascular permeability and more rapid passage of immunologic factors during inflammation
  - Conjunctival infection or inflammation causes plasma leakage from conjunctival capillaries faster than absorption by lymphatic channels or diversion to the eye surface
    - Leads to conjunctival edema or chemosis
- Conjunctiva contains extensive subepithelial lymphatic channels and circumlimbal channels
  - Limbal lymph channels join large stromal collecting channels and drain into the tarsal lymphatic system

CONJUNCTIVAL INNERVATION

Nerve Supply

- Sensory innervation from numerous free nerve endings supplying the conjunctiva from the lacrimal, supraorbital, supratrochlear, and infraorbital branches of the ophthalmic division of the trigeminal nerve
  - Inferior portion of the conjunctiva also receives some innervation from branches of the maxillary division of the trigeminal nerve
- Pain either increases or decreases when nerve endings are damaged by inflammation, hypoxia, &/or injury
- Inflammatory proteins can also stimulate nerve endings and cause pain sensation

NORMAL OCULAR FLORA

Organisms and Defense

- Consists of *Staphylococcus epidermidis*, *Propionibacterium acnes*, and diphtheroids
- Defense mechanisms protecting the conjunctiva from infectious organisms include
  - Mechanical sweeping of eyelids over ocular surface
  - Lysozyme and lactoferrin in tear film
  - Other antimicrobial factors in tears (IgA)

CONJUNCTIVAL INFLAMMATION

Common Signs

- Discharge
  - May be watery, mucous, mucopurulent, or purulent depending on cause of inflammation
- Papillae
  - Palpebral conjunctival inflammation creates small, dome-shaped nodules of conjunctival epithelium with a central vascular core surrounded by edema and mixed inflammatory infiltrate
  - Fibrous septa separate papillae and prevent conjunctival tissue from swelling diffusely
- Follicles
  - Larger, dome-shaped elevations of palpebral conjunctiva without a vascular core; normal vessels are pushed up along the surface of each follicle
  - Contain mixed inflammatory infiltrate and occur secondary to chronic irritation
- Chemosis
  - Edema and diffuse swelling of conjunctiva
- Hyperemia
  - Engorgement of conjunctival blood vessels leading to eye redness; nonspecific clinical finding that occurs secondary to various conditions
    - Bulbar, palpebral, forniceal, limbal vessels = superficial, winding conjunctival vessels
    - Episcleral vessels = fine, linear vessels that are deep to the conjunctiva
    - Scleral vessels = large vessels that are deep to the episclera
  - Vasodilation and inflammatory response
    - Vasodilation increases blood flow, causing fluid and protein leakage from capillaries
    - Leakage increases inflammatory cells and mediators and causes edema
    - Inflammatory response creates a characteristic pattern of vessel dilation depending on the etiology of conjunctival hyperemia
- Involvement of conjunctival, episcleral, and ciliary vasculature varies in hue, location, and degree of intensity with different conditions; recognizing patterns helps in diagnosis
  - Allergic conjunctivitis
    - Mild, diffuse pink coloration without scleral vessel involvement
  - Bacterial conjunctivitis
    - Superficial vasodilation of bulbar conjunctiva may start unilaterally and worsen progressively; mucopurulent discharge differentiates bacterial from viral conjunctivitis
  - Dry eye
    - Mild red hyperemia with horizontal, fine vessel dilation in the interpalpebral fissure
  - Contact lens-related inflammation
    - Variable hyperemia around limbus
  - Ophthalmic drug-induced allergic reaction
    - Hyperemia of lower 1/2 of conjunctiva, inferior cul-de-sac, and lower eyelid
  - Iritis and anterior uveitis
    - Pink, circumlimbal flush of dilated ciliary vessels
  - Severe ocular infection
    - Deep and intense red or purple hue with deep scleral vessel involvement

RELATED REFERENCES

1. Dartt DA: The conjunctiva: structure and function. In Tasman W: Duane's Foundations of Clinical Ophthalmology. Philadelphia: Lippincott Williams & Wilkins, 2006. http://oculist.net/downaton502/prof/ebook/duanes/pages/v8/v8c002.html. Accessed May 11, 2013
2. Abelson MB et al: Code red: The key features of hyperemia. Review of ophthalmology. 17(4):92-94, 2010
3. Kanski JJ. Clinical Ophthalmology: A Systematic Approach. 6th ed. Oxford: Butterworth-Heinemann. 215-18, 2007
4. Spalton DJ et al: The normal conjunctiva. In Spalton DJ et al: Atlas of Clinical Ophthalmology. 3rd ed. Philadelphia: Elsevier. 61-86, 2006
5. Krachmer JH et al: The conjunctiva: Anatomy and physiology. In Krachmer JH et al: Cornea: Fundamentals, Diagnosis, and Management. Vol 1. 2nd ed. Philadelphia: Elsevier. 37-43, 2005

CONJUNCTIVAL ANATOMY

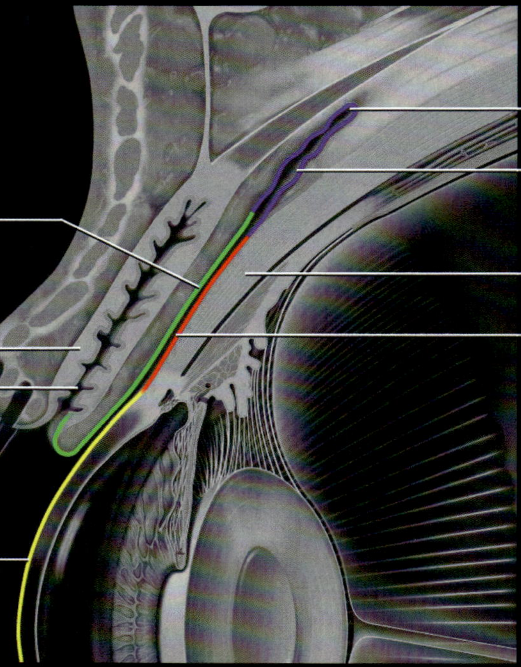

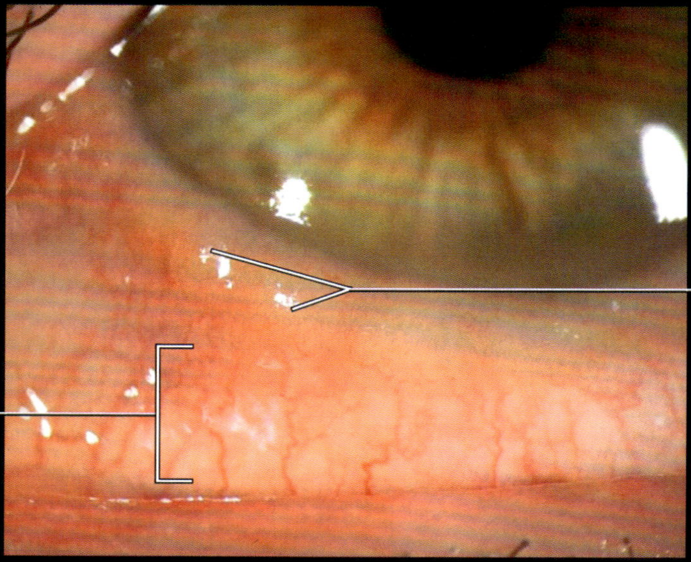

(Top) The thin, translucent mucous membrane of the conjunctiva lines the posterior surfaces of the superior and inferior tarsi and is reflected onto the exterior surface of the eye at the point of the superior, inferior, temporal, and medial fornices. The conjunctiva then extends from the anterior surface of the episclera and sclera to the limbus, where it becomes continuous with corneal epithelium. The extendible plica at the medial canthus creates the cul-de-sac of the medial fornix during eye adduction. The fornices allow for full rotation of the ocular globe and for movement of the eyelids. ***(Bottom)*** *Conjunctival hyperemia varies in hue, location, and degree of intensity based on the etiology of ocular inflammation. This photo shows circumlimbal chemosis and the diffuse, peripheral, pink-red hue of vasodilated bulbar conjunctival vessels secondary to viral conjunctivitis. Watery discharge is typical of viral conjunctivitis whereas bacterial conjunctivitis demonstrates mucopurulent discharge.*

CONJUNCTIVAL HISTOLOGY

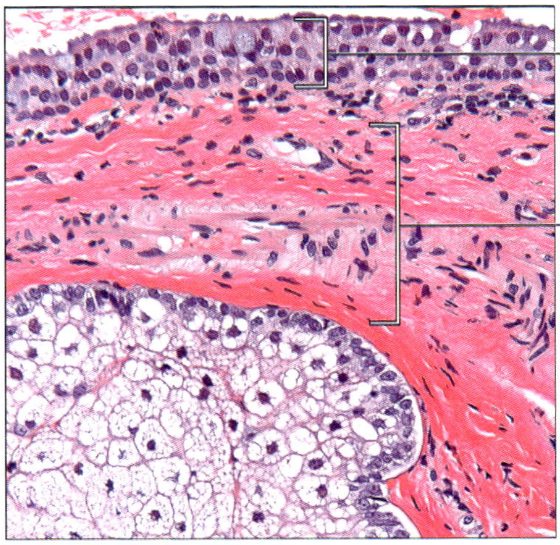

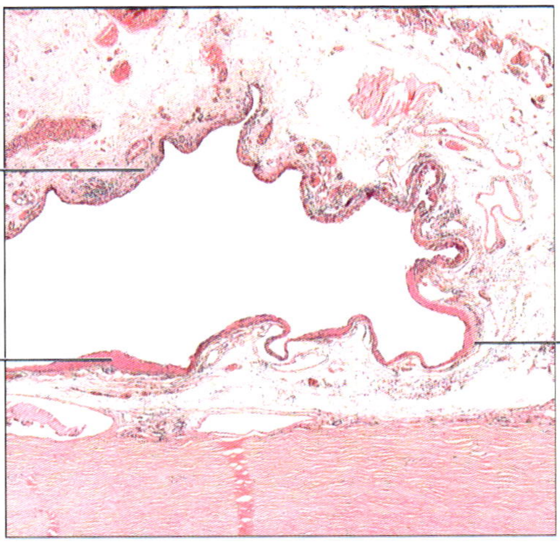

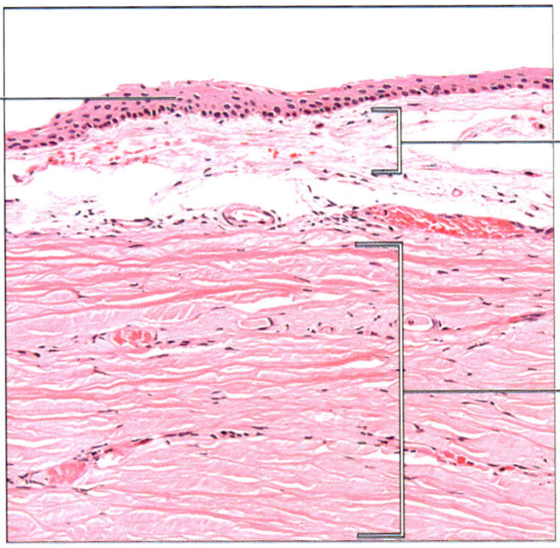

(Top) *The palpebral conjunctiva begins at the mucocutaneous junction along the palpebral margin of the eyelid, where meibomian gland openings are located. This region marks the junction where dry, keratinized stratified squamous epithelium of the eyelid transitions to nonkeratinized stratified squamous epithelium of the conjunctival mucous membrane. The palpebral conjunctiva allows the eyelid to slide smoothly over the globe. (Courtesy H. Brown, MD.)* ***(Middle)*** *Lymphoid aggregates and mucin-secreting goblet cells are abundant in the superior and inferior fornices. These cells produce the mucous layer of the tear film, which helps spread the tear film evenly over the cornea to create a smooth optical surface. (Courtesy H. Brown, MD.)* ***(Bottom)*** *The stroma of the bulbar conjunctiva is composed of loose connective tissue and fibrovascular tissue containing vessels, nerves, and lymphatics. This arrangement allows for the bulbar conjunctiva to remain loosely adherent to Tenon capsule. (Courtesy H. Brown, MD.)*

CONJUNCTIVAL NEVI

Key Facts

Introduction
- Hamartoma that arises due to a benign proliferation of melanocytic cells
- Subtypes
  - ○ Junctional
  - ○ Compound (most common type)
  - ○ Subepithelial

Demographics
- Most common melanocytic conjunctival tumors
- < 1% of conjunctival nevi become malignant

Presentation
- Usually arise as a discrete, mobile lesion before adulthood
- Typically flat near limbus and elevated elsewhere
- Most common location is bulbar conjunctiva, followed by caruncle and plica semilunaris
- Pigmentation varies from dark brown to amelanotic
- Small epithelial inclusion cysts are found in majority of nevi
- Potential signs of malignancy
  - ○ Rapid growth or increase in pigmentation
  - ○ Development after adolescence
  - ○ Nevi in unusual location (e.g., palpebral conjunctiva)
  - ○ Heavy vascularization with large nutrient vessels

Treatment
- Initial management for a typical conjunctival nevus is observation with serial photographs
- Surgical excision may be indicated for cosmetic purposes or if malignant transformation is suspected
- Due to rarity of palpebral conjunctival nevi, pigmented lesions in fornix or on tarsus should be excised
- Benign lesions that rarely become malignant

*(**Left**) This slit-lamp photo shows a pigmented conjunctival nevus near the temporal limbus ⇾. Nevi are most often found on the bulbar conjunctiva and are typically flat near the limbus and elevated elsewhere. (**Right**) This slit-lamp photo displays a flat, almost amelanotic conjunctival nevus at the temporal juxtalimbal area ⇾. A slit-lamp exam is necessary to differentiate this from other non-pigmented conjunctival lesions, and histopathology can be analyzed if the diagnosis is still uncertain.*

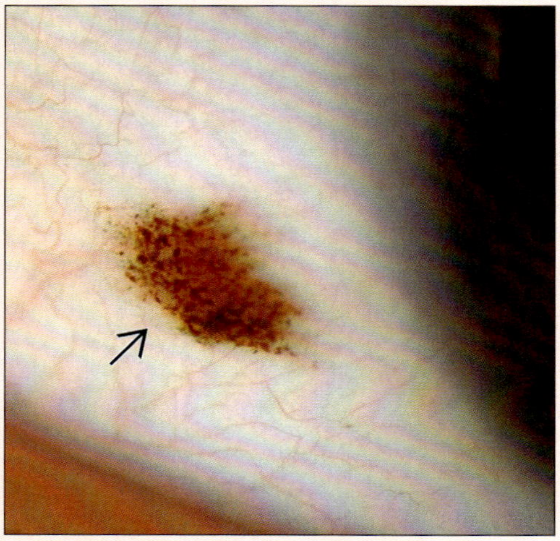

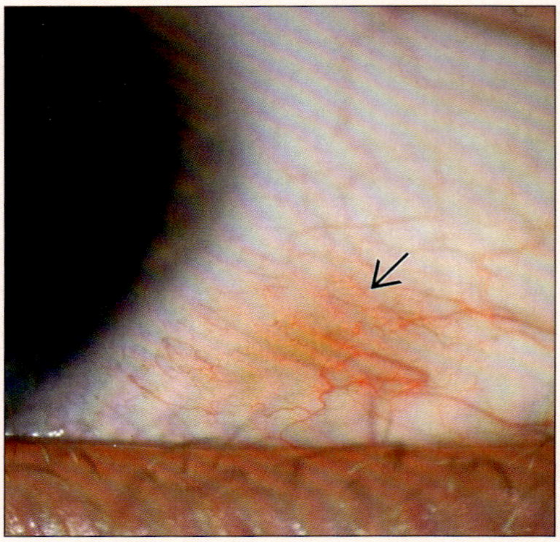

*(**Left**) This slit-lamp photo demonstrates a pigmented conjunctival nevus at the superior limbus ⇾. No signs of malignancy, including rapid growth, increase in pigmentation, late development, unusual location, or heavy vascularization, were noted in this patient. Cysts also indicate benignity. (**Right**) This slit-lamp photo shows a darkly pigmented caruncular conjunctival nevus ⇨. Lesions at the caruncle are diverse and uncommon, with the majority of pigmented lesions being benign conjunctival nevi.*

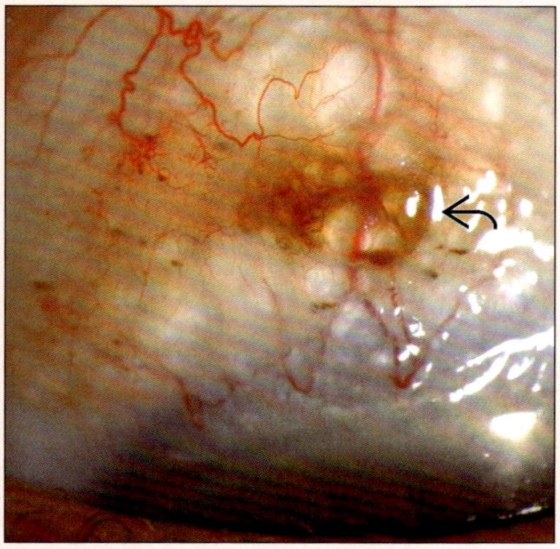

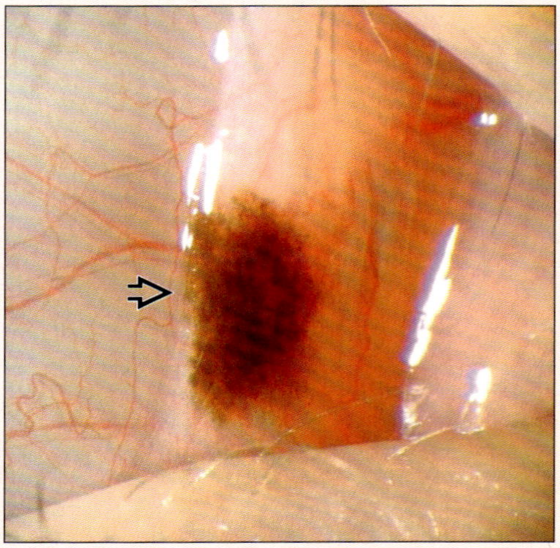

CONJUNCTIVAL NEVI

INTRODUCTION

Definitions

- Hamartoma that arises due to a benign proliferation of melanocytic cells

Subtypes

- Junctional (or intraepithelial)
- Compound
- Subepithelial
- A variety of unusual nevi may be identified in the conjunctiva
  - Balloon cell nevi, Spitz nevi, epithelioid cell nevi, dysplastic nevi, recurrent nevi, episcleral melanosis and the nevus of Ota, blue and cellular blue nevi, melanocytoma, and composite or mixed nevi

DEMOGRAPHICS

Etiology/Risk Factors

- Unknown etiology
  - Usually sporadic but can rarely be associated with dysplastic nevus syndrome or Carney complex

Epidemiology

- Nevi are the most common melanocytic conjunctival tumors
- < 1% of conjunctival nevi become malignant (more common in Caucasians)

PRESENTATION

Symptoms

- Arises as a discrete, mobile lesion during childhood or adolescence
- Often accelerated growth at puberty or pregnancy
- Large nevus can disrupt hydration of ocular surface and cause irritation and secondary inflammation

Exam Findings

- Typically flat near limbus and elevated elsewhere
  - Subepithelial and compound nevi, unlike junctional nevi, usually cause conjunctival surface elevation
- Variable size
- Most common anatomic location is bulbar conjunctiva, followed by the caruncle and plica semilunaris
  - Rare on palpebral conjunctiva
- Pigmentation varies from dark brown to amelanotic
- Small epithelial inclusion cysts are found in majority of nevi (indicating benignity)
  - Mucin secretion by cells within these cysts can cause a nevus to enlarge
- Potential signs of malignancy
  - Rapid growth or increase in pigmentation
    - Sudden changes in size or color in children are more likely due to inflammation
  - Development after adolescence
  - Nevi in unusual location (e.g., palpebral conjunctiva)
  - Heavy vascularization with large nutrient vessels
  - Large lesions that contain no cysts
  - Recurrence of a previously excised nevus

DIFFERENTIAL DIAGNOSIS

Primary Acquired Melanosis

- Typically acquired and appears during middle age, while conjunctival nevi appear during childhood

Conjunctival Melanoma

- Signs of a melanoma include lesions with rapid growth, increase in pigmentation, late development, unusual location, &/or heavy vascularization

Papilloma, Lymphoma, Amelanotic Melanoma

- These diagnoses generally do not have inclusion cysts, which helps differentiate them from amelanotic nevi

EVALUATION/WORK-UP

Pathology

- Classified based on relationship of nevus cells to conjunctival layers
  - Junctional nevi
    - Located at epithelial-subepithelial junction
    - Rare, except in children
  - Compound nevi
    - Most common type of conjunctival nevi
    - Have features of both junctional and subepithelial nevi, with cells at the epithelial-subepithelial junction and in subepithelial stroma
  - Subepithelial nevi
    - Located completely underneath epithelium
    - Often have a cobblestone appearance

TREATMENT

Medical

- Initial management for a typical conjunctival nevus is observation with serial photographs

Surgical

- Surgical excision may be indicated for cosmetic purposes or if malignant transformation is suspected
  - Excisional biopsy is preferred over incisional biopsy for lesions that can be entirely removed in 1 procedure
- Due to rarity of palpebral conjunctival nevi, pigmented lesions in fornix or on tarsus should be excised

Prognosis

- Benign lesions that rarely become malignant

SELECTED REFERENCES

1. Harooni H et al: Current appraisal of conjunctival melanocytic tumors: classification and treatment. Future Oncol. 7(3):435-46, 2011
2. Zembowicz A et al: Melanocytic lesions of the conjunctiva. Arch Pathol Lab Med. 134(12):1785-92, 2010
3. Shields CL et al: Conjunctival nevi: clinical features and natural course in 410 consecutive patients. Arch Ophthalmol. 122(2):167-75, 2004
4. Folberg R et al: Benign conjunctival melanocytic lesions. Clinicopathologic features. Ophthalmology. 96(4):436-61, 1989
5. McDonnell JM et al: Conjunctival melanocytic lesions in children. Ophthalmology. 96(7):986-93, 1989

LIMBAL DERMOIDS AND OTHER CHORISTOMAS

Key Facts

Introduction

- Tumor-like growth composed of elements not normally present at involved site
- Subtypes
  - Dermoids and dermolipomas
  - Ectopic lacrimal gland
  - Epibulbar osseous and neuroglial choristomas

Demographics

- Typically sporadic congenital lesions
- Make up ~ 3% of conjunctival and corneal tumors

Presentation

- Small choristomas are usually asymptomatic, but larger choristomas can cause irritation, inadequate eyelid closure, astigmatism, and amblyopia
- Dermoids are round, soft, white masses located in the inferotemporal limbus, often with a protruding hair
- Dermolipomas are similar to dermoids but are yellow, contain more fat, and occur superotemporally with possible posterior orbital extension
- Ectopic lacrimal glands appear as well-vascularized, pink nodules
- Epibulbar osseous choristomas appear superotemporally as hard, yellow nodules
- Neuroglial choristomas are diffuse, solid tumors

Treatment

- Smaller, asymptomatic choristomas can be observed
- Surgical excision is warranted for amblyopia, astigmatism, visual axis encroachment, chronic irritation, &/or cosmetic purposes
- Surgery not recommended for dermolipomas because of frequent posterior orbital extension of tumor
- Typically benign tumors that grow slowly, if at all, and do not progress to cancer

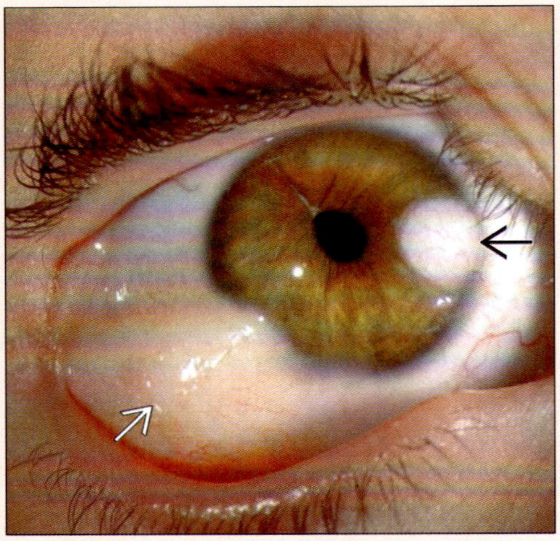

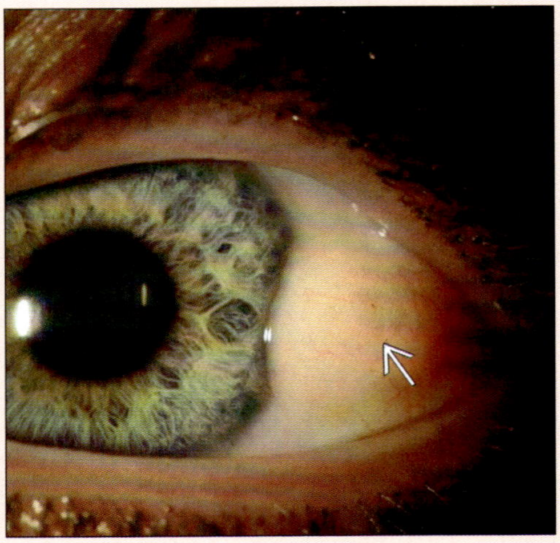

(Left) *This is a slit-lamp photo of a patient with multiple dermoids. The large temporal dermoid ➡ has a tan appearance, while the smaller nasal dermoid → is more white in color. The smaller nasal dermoid has encroached into part of the visual axis.* ***(Right)*** *This slit-lamp photo demonstrates a typical temporal limbal dermoid with a fine hair ➡ protruding from its surface. Large lesions can cause inadequate eyelid closure, astigmatism, amblyopia, and irritation.*

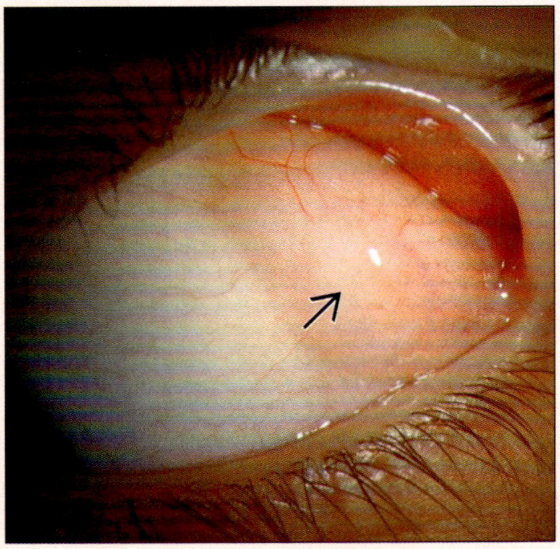

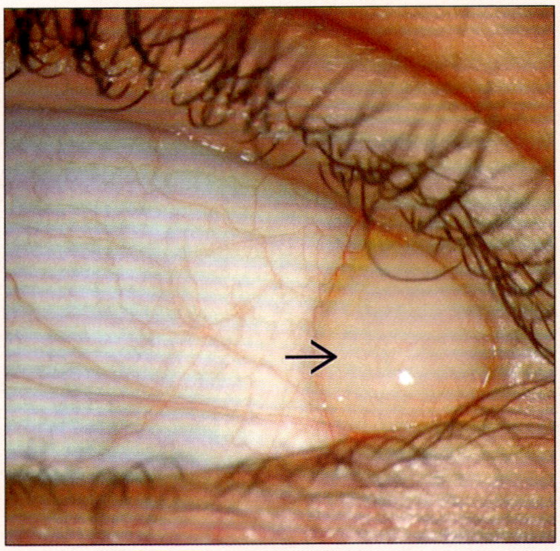

(Left) *This slit-lamp photo demonstrates a typical supertemporal dermolipoma →. Prolapsed orbital fat, lymphomas, and prolapse of the palpebral lobe of the lacrimal gland are all similar in appearance but freely mobile, unlike the more stationary dermolipoma. Surgical excision of a dermolipoma is not recommended because of possible posterior extension into the orbit.* ***(Right)*** *This is a slit-lamp photo of a temporal, flesh-colored dermolipoma → that contains adipose tissue.*

LIMBAL DERMOIDS AND OTHER CHORISTOMAS

INTRODUCTION

Definitions

- Tumor-like growth composed of elements not normally present at involved site
  - Simple choristoma: Consists of 1 tissue type
  - Complex choristoma: Consists of multiple tissue types including adipose, cartilage, bone, smooth muscle, lacrimal gland, and pilosebaceous units

Subtypes

- Limbal dermoids and dermolipomas
- Ectopic lacrimal gland
- Epibulbar osseous and neuroglial choristomas

DEMOGRAPHICS

Etiology/Risk Factors

- Typically sporadic congenital lesions
- Limbal dermoids and dermolipomas can be associated with other systemic malformations, including Goldenhar syndrome, Treacher Collins syndrome, and linear nevus sebaceus of Jadassohn

Epidemiology

- Choristomas make up ~ 3% of conjunctival and corneal tumors
  - Dermolipomas are the most common type, followed by dermoids and ectopic lacrimal glands
  - Epibulbar osseous and neuroglial choristomas are rare
- Choristomas are the most common epibulbar and orbital tumors in children
- Epibulbar dermoids occur in ~ 1 in 10,000 people

PRESENTATION

Symptoms

- Small choristomas are usually asymptomatic, but large choristomas can cause irritation, inadequate eyelid closure, astigmatism, and amblyopia
- Usually present in childhood with exception of dermolipomas, which present early in adult life

Exam Findings

- Dermoid
  - Round, well-circumscribed, elevated, smooth, soft, white or tan mass, often with a hair protruding from it
  - Typically occurs in inferotemporal limbal corneal and epibulbar region
    - An unusual variant (ring dermoid syndrome) may bilaterally encircle the entire limbus
- Dermolipoma
  - Similar to a dermoid but is often yellow in color and contains adipose tissue
  - Typically occurs superotemporally with possible posterior extension into orbit
- Ectopic lacrimal gland
  - Appears as a well-vascularized, pink nodule
- Epibulbar osseous choristoma
  - Hard, yellow nodule typically occurring superotemporally on bulbar surface
- Neuroglial choristoma
  - Diffuse, solid tumor most often found on eyelid

DIFFERENTIAL DIAGNOSIS

Prolapsed Orbital Fat, Lymphoma, and Prolapse of Palpebral Lobe of Lacrimal Gland

- Can be confused with dermolipomas, but in contrast to dermolipomas, they are all freely mobile

EVALUATION/WORK-UP

Pathology

- Dermoid
  - Solid, placoid tumors lined by epidermoid epithelium
  - Deep to epithelium is dense collagenous tissue, within which fat lobules, sebaceous glands, and hair follicles can be found
- Dermolipoma
  - Similar to dermoids but with more fat and fewer, if any, pilosebaceous units
- Ectopic lacrimal gland
  - May contain only lacrimal gland tissue (simple) or multiple tissue types (complex)
- Epibulbar osseous choristoma
  - Composed of mature, compact bone often surrounded by connective tissue
- Neuroglial choristoma
  - Likely composed of ectopic neural tissue from anterior lip of optic cup or vesicle

Imaging

- Ultrasound biomicroscopy to determine lesion depth

TREATMENT

Surgical

- Smaller, asymptomatic choristomas can be observed
- Surgical excision is warranted for amblyopia, astigmatism, visual axis encroachment, chronic irritation, &/or cosmetic purposes
  - Large nodules may require lamellar keratosclerectomy
- Surgery not recommended for dermolipomas because of frequent posterior orbital extension of tumor
  - Debulking anterior portion of a dermolipoma can be performed for cosmetic reasons

Prognosis

- Typically benign tumors that grow slowly, if at all, and do not progress to cancer

SELECTED REFERENCES

1. Shields CL et al: Tumors of the conjunctiva and cornea. Surv Ophthalmol. 49(1):3-24, 2004
2. Panda A et al: Surgical outcomes of Epibulbar dermoids. J Pediatr Ophthalmol Strabismus. 39(1):20-5, 2002
3. Cunha RP et al: Epibulbar tumors in children: a survey of 282 biopsies. J Pediatr Ophthalmol Strabismus. 24(5):249-54, 1987
4. Grossniklaus HE et al: Conjunctival lesions in adults. A clinical and histopathologic review. Cornea. 6(2):78-116, 1987
5. Pokorny KS et al: Epibulbar choristomas containing lacrimal tissue. Clinical distinction from dermoids and histologic evidence of an origin from the palpebral lobe. Ophthalmology. 94(10):1249-57, 1987

EPITHELIAL CYSTS

Key Facts

Introduction
- Benign conjunctival cysts lined by normal conjunctival epithelium

Demographics
- Can be congential or acquired
- Smaller cysts are formed by apposition of conjunctival folds
- Larger, single cysts typically develop because of epithelium implantation into substantia propria due to
  - Nonsurgical trauma
  - Inflammation
  - Surgery

Presentation
- Do not typically cause discomfort
- Appearance
  - Thin walled
  - Smooth
  - Filled with clear or turbid fluid
  - Often contain desquamated cellular debris
- Patients often concerned about cosmetic appearance

Evaluation/Work-Up
- Lined by conjunctival epithelium (nonkeratinized stratified squamous) and filled with clear fluid

Treatment
- Observation is generally recommended
- Surgery is recommended if
  - There is concern for malignancy
  - Cyst is symptomatic
  - Desired for cosmetic purposes
- Cysts commonly recur after simple incision due to remaining inner epithelial cells
  - Complete excision is preferred to avoid recurrence
- These benign cysts have an excellent prognosis

*(**Left**) This slit-lamp photo demonstrates a temporal conjunctival cyst ➔. Smaller conjunctival cysts are caused by the apposition of conjunctival folds, whereas larger conjunctival cysts develop due to epithelial implantation into the substantia propria. (**Right**) This slit-lamp photo depicts a typical temporal conjunctival cyst →. These thin-walled cysts, lined by conjunctival epithelium, are generally smooth and contain a clear or turbid fluid.*

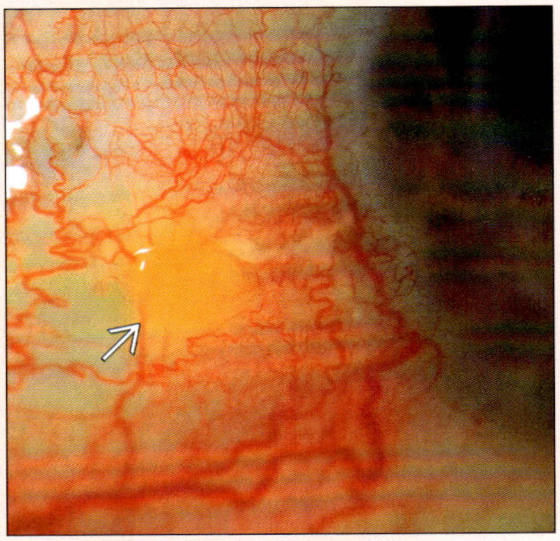

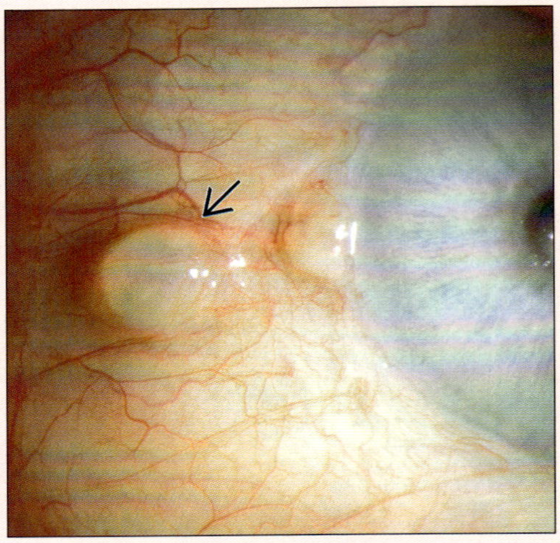

*(**Left**) This slit-lamp photo is of a large temporal conjunctival cyst ➔. Observation is the recommended therapy unless there is concern for malignancy, the patient is symptomatic, or surgery is desired for cosmetic purposes. Cysts commonly recur after simple excision, necessitating a complete excision if surgical therapy is warranted. (**Right**) This slit-lamp photo shows a more subtle temporal conjunctival cyst →. Cysts of this nature are typically asymptomatic.*

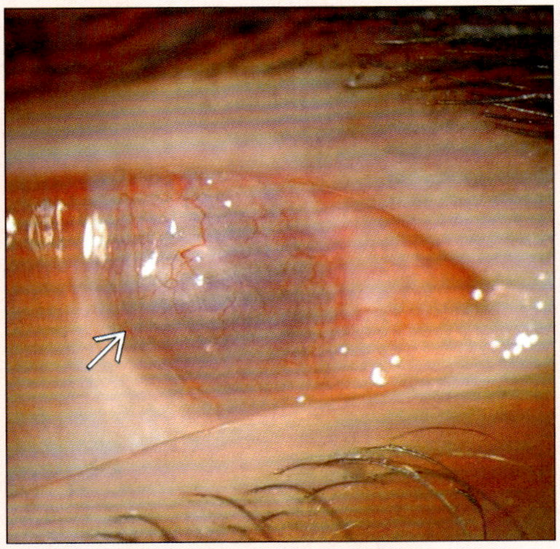

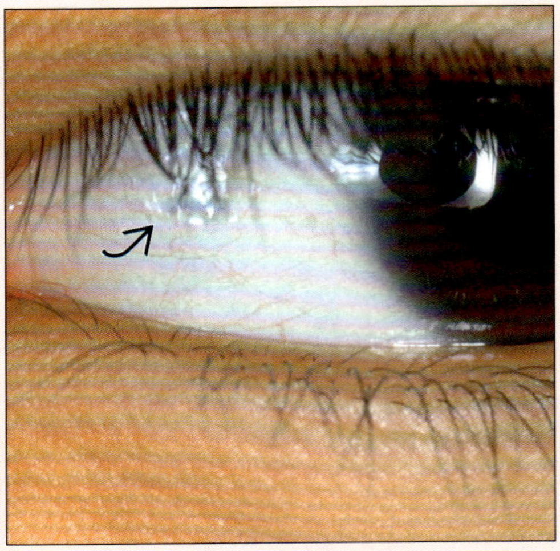

EPITHELIAL CYSTS

INTRODUCTION

Definitions

- Frequently encountered, benign conjunctival cysts lined by normal conjunctival epithelium

DEMOGRAPHICS

Etiology/Risk Factors

- Can be congenital or acquired
  - Smaller cysts are formed by apposition of conjunctival folds
  - Larger, single cysts typically develop because of epithelium implantation into substantia propria due to
    - Nonsurgical trauma
    - Inflammation
    - Surgery
      - Strabismus surgery
      - Pars plana vitrectomy
      - Scleral buckle surgery
- Can be associated with Stevens-Johnson syndrome
- Can occur spontaneously over a pterygium and secondarily affect cornea

Epidemiology

- Very common
  - Small cysts often seen in fornix of healthy individuals
  - Account for ~ 80% of all conjunctival cystic lesions
  - No gender predilection
  - Average patient age at diagnosis is 47 years

PRESENTATION

Symptoms

- Do not typically cause discomfort
  - Larger cysts can
    - Extend into orbit and become symptomatic
    - Cause astigmatism
    - Lead to dry eye or foreign body sensation
- Patients often concerned about cosmetic appearance

Exam Findings

- Appearance
  - Thin walled
    - Wall can be lined with pigment, leading to suspicion of malignant melanoma
  - Smooth
  - Filled with clear or turbid fluid
  - Often contain desquamated cellular debris
    - Debris can deposit inferiorly and give a pseudohypopyon appearance
- Often found in tumors
  - Conjunctival nevi
  - Lymphangiomas
    - Can have intralesional bleeding, causing cysts of blood ("chocolate" cysts)
- Can appear on eyelids
- Corneal epithelial inclusion cysts are rare unless surgery or trauma displaces epithelium into stroma

DIFFERENTIAL DIAGNOSIS

Lymphangiectasia

- Can mimic a conjunctival inclusion cyst
- Often appear as multiple, small epibulbar bumps
- Contain irregularly dilated lymphatic channels
  - Channels may fill with blood if an anomalous communication with a venule is present

Parasitic Cyst

- Often due to cysticercosis (pork tapeworm)
  - Ask patient about travel to endemic region
  - If suspected, perform ultrasound to look for a central echogenic scolex
  - Can be found in conjunctiva or globe

EVALUATION/WORK-UP

Pathology

- Lined by conjunctival epithelium (nonkeratinized stratified squamous) and filled with clear fluid
  - May contain desquamated cellular debris, mucinous material, &/or keratin

TREATMENT

Medical

- Observation is generally recommended
  - Lesion may disappear over time

Surgical

- Surgery is recommended if
  - There is concern for malignancy
  - Cyst is symptomatic
  - Desired for cosmetic purposes
- Cysts commonly recur after simple incision due to remaining inner epithelial cells
  - Complete excision is preferred to avoid cyst recurrence
- Visualization of cyst during surgery can be facilitated by using trypan blue and 2.3% sodium hyaluronate
- Nd:Yag laser has been shown to be effective for acquired inclusion cysts of the conjunctiva

Prognosis

- These benign cysts have an excellent prognosis

SELECTED REFERENCES

1. Kobayashi A et al: Successful removal of a large conjunctival cyst using colored 2.3% sodium hyaluronate. Ophthalmic Surg Lasers Imaging. 38(1):81-3, 2007
2. Shields CL et al: Tumors of the conjunctiva and cornea. Surv Ophthalmol. 49(1):3-24, 2004
3. Başar E et al: Subconjunctival cyst extending into the orbit. Int Ophthalmol. 22(6):341-3, 1998
4. Grossniklaus HE et al: Conjunctival lesions in adults. A clinical and histopathologic review. Cornea. 6(2):78-116, 1987
5. Panda A et al: Cystic lesions of conjunctiva. Ann Ophthalmol. 19(2):60-2, 1987
6. de Bustros S et al: Treatment of acquired epithelial inclusion cyst of the conjunctiva using the YAG laser. Am J Ophthalmol. 98(6):807-8, 1984

ACUTE BACTERIAL CONJUNCTIVITIS

Key Facts

Introduction
- Conjunctival inflammation due to bacterial infection

Demographics
- Caused by either direct eye contact with infected secretions or invasion and proliferation of indigenous organism
- Most common pathogens
  - *Staphylococcus aureus*, *Haemophilus influenzae*, and *Streptococcus pneumoniae*

Presentation
- Usually bilateral involvement, with 1 eye often becoming infected 1-2 days before other eye
- Diffuse conjunctival injection
- Mucopurulent discharge
  - Thick, globular, and yellow, white, or green in color
- Papillary reaction of palpebral conjunctiva
- Burning, tearing, &/or foreign body sensation

Evaluation/Work-Up
- Uncomplicated cases do not require lab investigation
- Gram-stained smears and cultures of a conjunctival swab are indicated in the following situations
  - Severe cases
  - Immunocompromised patients (including neonates)
  - Conjunctivitis refractive to treatment

Treatment
- Initial medical therapy includes topical antibiotics, usually dosed 4x daily for 5-7 days
  - Topical antibiotics improve rate of clinical and microbiological remission
- Common topical agents
  - Fluoroquinolone, aminoglycoside, macrolide, and polymyxin combination drops
  - Bacitracin, ciprofloxacin, and other ointments
- Follow-up initially every 2-3 days, then every 5-7 days until resolution of symptoms

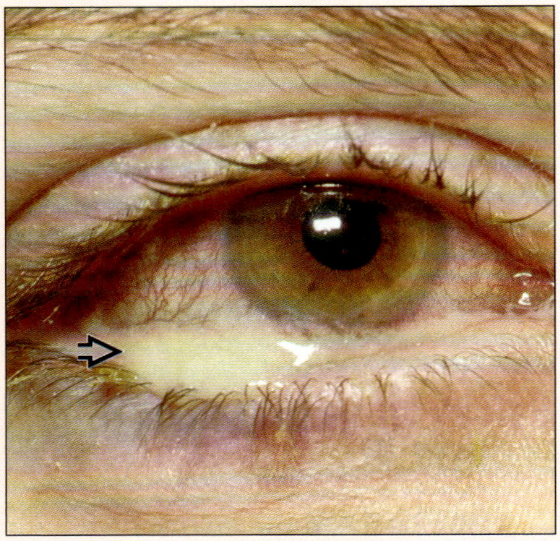
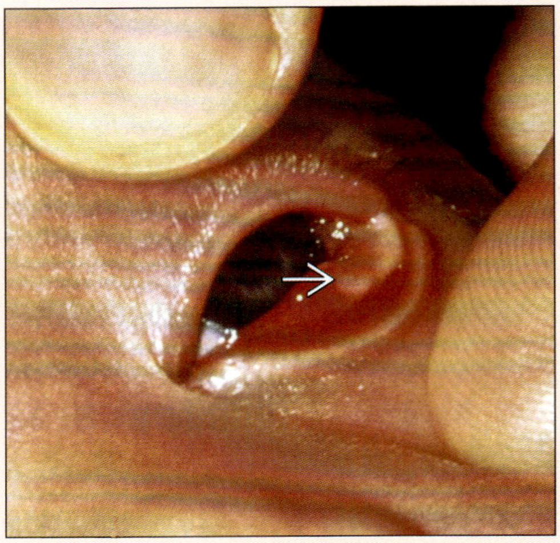

(Left) *This slit-lamp photo shows a patient with acute bacterial conjunctivitis with prominent mucopurulent discharge ⇨, which is typically thick, globular, and yellow, white, or green in color. (Courtesy C. Miller, MD.)* ***(Right)*** *This external photo depicts the left eye of a patient with acute bacterial conjunctivitis that also has a pseudomembrane ➡. Membranes/ pseudomembranes are most often seen in Corynebacterium diphtheriae and Streptococcus pyogenes infections. (Courtesy C. Miller, MD.)*

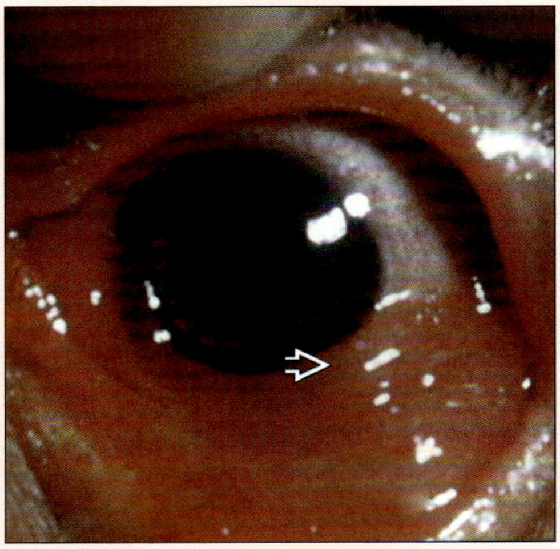
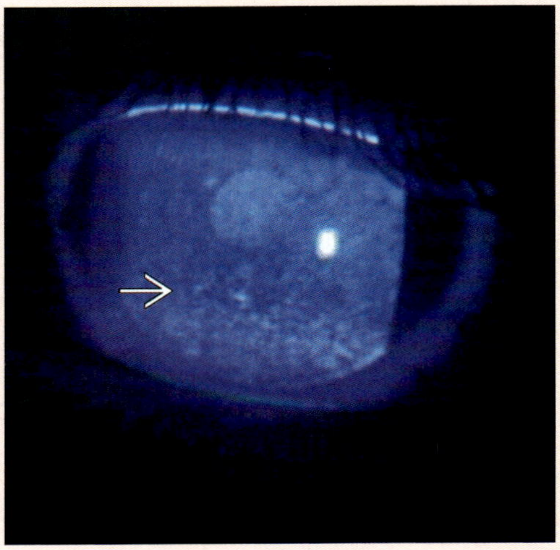

(Left) *This slit-lamp photo demonstrates a patient with acute bacterial conjunctivitis with diffuse conjunctival injection and chemosis ⇨. Bilateral involvement is most common. (Courtesy C. Miller, MD.)* ***(Right)*** *This slit-lamp photo shows punctate epithelial keratitis ➡ in a patient with acute bacterial conjunctivitis. Staphylococcus aureus is the most common causative pathogen in adults (MRSA is increasing in frequency) and Haemophilus influenzae is the most common pathogen in children.*

ACUTE BACTERIAL CONJUNCTIVITIS

INTRODUCTION

Definitions
- Conjunctival inflammation due to bacterial infection

DEMOGRAPHICS

Etiology/Risk Factors
- Caused by either direct eye contact with infected secretions or invasion and proliferation of indigenous organism
- Predisposing conditions include dry eye, blepharitis, anatomic ocular abnormalities, crowded living or social conditions, immunosuppression, and poor hygiene
- Most common pathogens
  - *Staphylococcus aureus* (most common in adults)
    - MRSA increasing in frequency
  - *Haemophilus influenzae* (most common in children)
  - *Streptococcus pneumoniae*
  - *Moraxella catarrhalis*

Epidemiology
- Annual incidence in USA is ~ 135 in 10,000 people

PRESENTATION

Symptoms
- Conjunctival discharge, burning, tearing, foreign body sensation
- Mattering of eyelids upon awakening
- Usually bilateral involvement, with 1 eye often becoming infected 1-2 days before other eye
  - If unilateral involvement, examine nasolacrimal system for abnormalities

Exam Findings
- Diffuse conjunctival injection
- Mucopurulent discharge
  - Thick, globular, and yellow, white, or green in color
- Conjunctival papillae
- Eyelid edema and erythema (in severe infections)
- Chemosis
- Punctate epithelial keratitis
- Membranes and pseudomembranes
  - Most often seen in *Corynebacterium diphtheriae* and *Streptococcus pyogenes* infections

DIFFERENTIAL DIAGNOSIS

Viral Conjunctivitis
- Signs that suggest viral over bacterial
  - Watery discharge, preauricular lymphadenopathy, follicular reaction, itchy eyes (signs are controversial)

Hyperacute Bacterial Conjunctivitis
- Severe, hyperpurulent discharge with onset < 24 hours

EVALUATION/WORK-UP

Labs
- Uncomplicated cases do not require lab investigation
- Gram-stained smears and cultures of a conjunctival swab are indicated in the following situations
  - Severe cases, to differentiate from hyperacute conjunctivitis
    - Culture on chocolate or Thayer-Martin agar if *Neisseria gonorrhoeae* is suspected
  - Immunocompromised patients (including neonates)
  - Conjunctivitis refractive to treatment

TREATMENT

Medical
- Initial medical therapy includes topical antibiotics, usually dosed 4x daily for 5-7 days
- Common topical agents
  - Fluoroquinolone drops (ciprofloxacin, ofloxacin, levofloxacin, moxifloxacin, gatifloxacin)
  - Aminoglycoside drops (gentamicin and neomycin)
  - Polymyxin combo drops (polymyxin B + TMP-SMX)
  - Macrolide drops (azithromycin)
  - Bacitracin, ciprofloxacin, and various other ointments
    - Eyedrops generally preferred in adults because ointments blur vision
    - Ointments are preferred in children because drops are diluted by tearing and squeezed out
  - In general, no apparent significant difference in clinical response or cure between different antibiotics
    - Take into account local microbial resistance patterns, cost, dosing regimens, and other patient factors when selecting antibiotics
- Systemic antibiotics are used in
  - Hyperacute bacterial conjunctivitis
  - Association with dacryocystitis, preseptal cellulitis, or orbital cellulitis
  - *H. influenzae* infection, particularly in children, due to risk of extraocular involvement
    - Treat with oral amoxicillin/clavulanate

Follow-Up
- Initially every 2-3 days, then every 5-7 days until resolution of symptoms
  - Antibiotic therapy should be tailored based upon culture and sensitivity results

Prognosis
- Excellent prognosis, mild cases are usually self limited
  - *S. aureus* and *M. catarrhalis* are exceptions and without treatment can become chronic
- Topical antibiotics improve rate of clinical and microbiological remission
- Reduce risk of transmission by washing hands and avoiding towel sharing

SELECTED REFERENCES

1. Cavuoto K et al: Update on bacterial conjunctivitis in South Florida. Ophthalmology. 115(1):51-6, 2008
2. Høvding G: Acute bacterial conjunctivitis. Acta Ophthalmol. 86(1):5-17, 2008
3. Sheikh A et al: Antibiotics versus placebo for acute bacterial conjunctivitis. Cochrane Database Syst Rev. (2):CD001211, 2006
4. Sheikh A et al: Topical antibiotics for acute bacterial conjunctivitis: Cochrane systematic review and meta-analysis update. Br J Gen Pract. 55(521):962-4, 2005
5. Jackson WB: Differentiating conjunctivitis of diverse origins. Surv Ophthalmol. 38 Suppl:91-104, 1993

ADENOVIRAL CONJUNCTIVITIS

Key Facts

Demographics
- Transmissible by personal contact with fomites, ocular or respiratory secretions, and small bodies of water
- Highly contagious for ~ 10-14 days after onset of symptoms

Presentation
- Itching, irritation, foreign body sensation, watery discharge, usually bilateral involvement
- Variable timing, but most patients present with symptoms 6-9 days after exposure
- General exam findings for all subtypes include tender preauricular lymphadenopathy, eyelid edema and erythema, conjunctival follicles, and hyperemia
- 53 adenoviral serotypes and 6 subgroups (A-F), but infections classically present as 1 of 4 syndromes
- Acute nonspecific simple follicular conjunctivitis
  - Mild ocular signs and symptoms
- Pharyngoconjunctival fever (serotypes 3, 4, 5, and 7)
  - Presents with fever, pharyngitis, and conjunctivitis
- Epidemic keratoconjunctivitis (serotypes 8, 19, and 37)
  - Epithelial keratitis occurs in 80% of cases
  - Subepithelial infiltrates (SEIs) can blur vision
- Chronic keratoconjuctivitis

Evaluation/Work-Up
- Laboratory confirmation (from conjunctival scrapings, swabs, and cultures) is typically unnecessary
- RPS Adeno Detector, a relatively new test, makes an inexpensive, rapid (10 minutes), in-office, sensitive, and specific diagnosis of infection

Treatment
- Self-limited condition; provide symptomatic relief
- Discuss precautions to reduce risk of transmission
- Topical steroids can be used in specific situations
- Usually resolves in 1-2 weeks
  - SEIs can persist for months and cause scarring

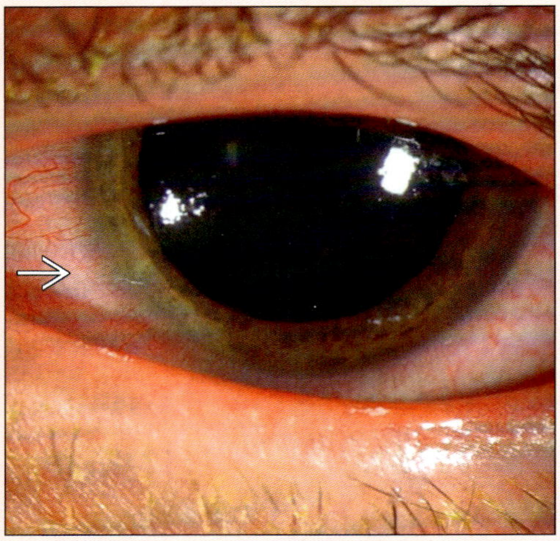
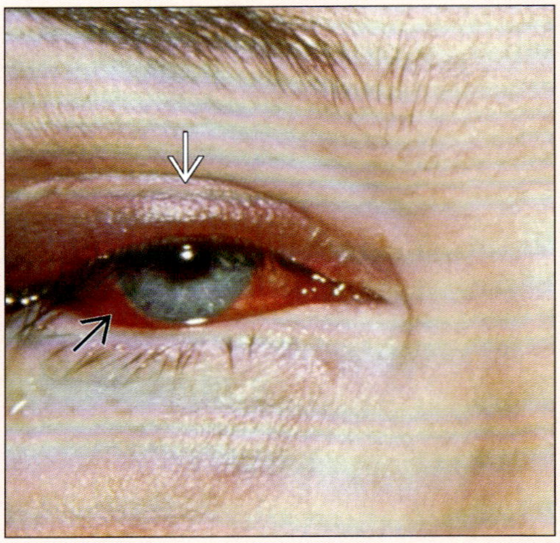

(Left) *This slit-lamp photo demonstrates adenoviral conjunctivitis with a classic finding of prominent conjunctival hyperemia. Patients also tend to have a watery, nonpurulent discharge and tender preauricular lymphadenopathy.* ***(Right)*** *This external photo depicts a patient with adenoviral conjunctivitis with eyelid edema and erythema. Again, prominent conjunctival hyperemia can be noted. This disease is highly contagious for 10-14 days after symptom onset. (Courtesy C. Miller, MD.)*

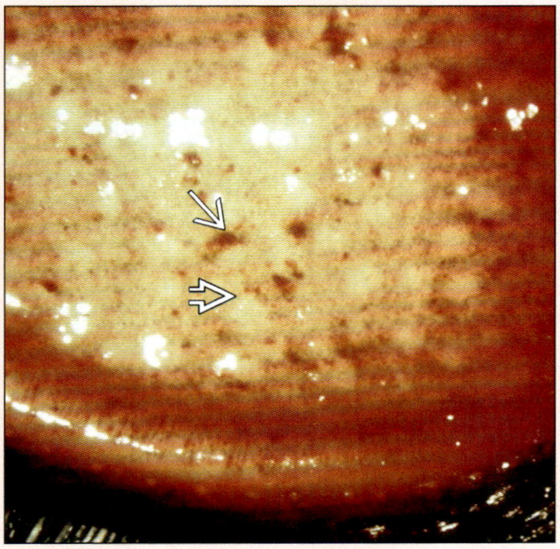
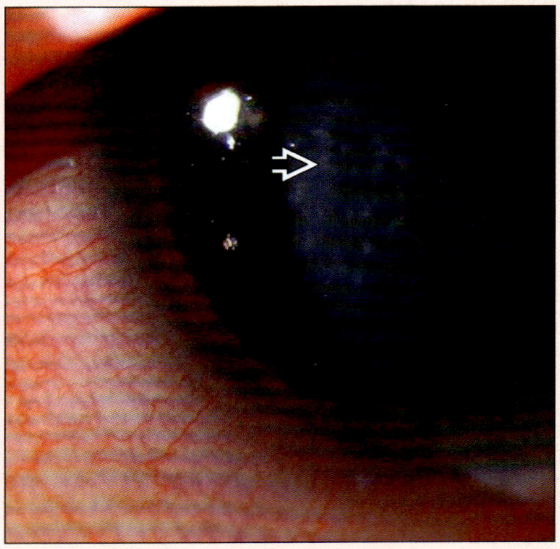

(Left) *This slit-lamp photo shows palpebral conjunctival follicles, some of which are petechial, in a patient with adenoviral conjunctivitis. (Courtesy C. Miller, MD.)* ***(Right)*** *This slit-lamp photo depicts epidemic keratoconjunctivitis (EKC) with subepithelial infiltrates (SEIs). Adenoviral conjunctivitis classically presents as 1 of 4 syndromes: Acute nonspecific follicular conjunctivitis, pharyngoconjunctival fever (PCF), EKC (most severe form), and chronic keratoconjunctivitis.*

ADENOVIRAL CONJUNCTIVITIS

INTRODUCTION

Definitions

- Conjunctival inflammation due to adenoviral infection
  - Adenovirus is a double-stranded DNA virus

Subtypes

- 53 adenoviral serotypes and 6 subgroups (A-F)
- Classically presents as 1 of 4 syndromes
  - Acute nonspecific simple follicular conjunctivitis (associated with serotypes 1-11, 19)
  - Pharyngoconjunctival fever (PCF) (associated with serotypes 3, 4, 5, and 7)
  - Epidemic keratoconjunctivitis (EKC) (associated with serotypes 8, 19, and 37)
  - Chronic keratoconjuctivitis

DEMOGRAPHICS

Etiology/Risk Factors

- May occur sporadically or as an epidemic
- Transmissible by personal contact with
  - Fomites
    - Live virus survives up to 5 weeks on plastic surfaces
  - Ocular or respiratory secretions
  - Contaminated small bodies of water
    - Swimming pools, ponds
- Highly contagious for ~ 10-14 days after onset of symptoms
  - Spreads rapidly in crowded conditions, including nursing homes, schools, and military housing

Epidemiology

- Most common cause of conjunctivitis
  - Accounts for 5-20% of cases of acute conjunctivitis

PRESENTATION

Symptoms

- Itching
- Irritation
- Foreign body sensation
- Watery discharge
- Photosensitivity
- Variable timing, but most patients present with symptoms 6-9 days after exposure
- Usually bilateral involvement, with 1 eye often becoming infected 1-2 days before the other
- May have nonocular viral symptoms (e.g., upper respiratory tract infection)

Exam Findings

- General findings for all subtypes include
  - Tender preauricular lymphadenopathy
  - Eyelid edema and erythema
  - Palpebral conjunctival follicles
  - Conjunctival hyperemia
  - Watery, nonpurulent discharge
- Unique findings for each classic syndrome
  - Acute nonspecific simple follicular conjunctivitis
    - Mild ocular signs and symptoms with no, or mild, epithelial keratitis
    - Self-limited; usually resolves in days to weeks
    - Often accompanied by mild systemic sequelae (e.g., pharyngitis)
  - PCF
    - Presents with fever, pharyngitis (mild or severe), and acute follicular conjunctivitis
    - Mild punctate keratitis is found in 30% of cases
    - Usually resolves within 2 weeks
  - EKC
    - Most severe ocular adenoviral disease
    - Significant corneal involvement
    - Higher prevalence (~ 1/2) of unilateral disease than other types
    - Conjunctival follicles and papillae are common, most often located in lower fornix
    - Epithelial keratitis occurs in 80% of cases
      - Fine punctate epithelial keratitis arises after 2-4 days and progresses into coarse punctate epithelial keratitis that resolves within 2 weeks
      - At 2 weeks, multifocal subepithelial infiltrates (SEIs) appear under the epithelial lesions and can persist for months
      - SEIs can blur vision and may eventually lead to scarring
      - Graded from stage 0 to stage V
    - Chemosis, petechial or subconjunctival hemorrhages, membranes, pseudomembranes, epithelial microcysts, large central corneal erosions, and anterior uveitis can also be found
  - Chronic keratoconjuctivitis
    - Patient has intermittent conjunctivitis with SEIs that come and go
    - Rare, but can persist for years

DIFFERENTIAL DIAGNOSIS

Acute Hemorrhagic Conjunctivitis

- Normally caused by enterovirus type 70 and coxsackievirus A24 variant
- Dramatic, sudden onset of painful follicular conjunctivitis with subconjunctival hemorrhages
  - Hemorrhages progress from petechial to confluent
  - Normally a highly contagious tropical disease that occurs in epidemics and resolves after 1-2 weeks

Herpes Simplex Virus

- Often causes a unilateral follicular conjunctivitis
  - Associated with skin or eyelid margin vesicles and dendritic epithelial keratitis

Epstein-Barr Conjunctivitis

- Most common causative agent of infectious mononucleosis syndrome, which can occasionally include follicular conjunctivitis, often membranous
- Dacryoadenitis, keratitis, subconjunctival hemorrhages, episcleritis, uveitis, and discrete subepithelial infiltrates can also be seen
- Generally resolves without treatment

Other Systemic Viral Diseases

- Including measles, mumps, rubella, and influenza
- Can cause nonspecific follicular conjunctivitis
- Treat underlying disease
- Topical lubrication if patient needs symptomatic relief

ADENOVIRAL CONJUNCTIVITIS

EVALUATION/WORK-UP

Labs

- Laboratory confirmation (from conjunctival scrapings, swabs, and cultures) is typically unnecessary unless disease is severe or chronic
  - Previous techniques, including direct immunofluorescence and viral cultures with specific fluorescent antibody, were valuable but not required
    - Special equipment
    - Adequate operator experience
    - Significant time
      - Disease typically resolves before results become available
  - PCR has increased sensitivity and same specificity when compared to viral cultures
    - However, PCR also requires special equipment, specially trained personnel, and significant time
    - Results not available during office visit
  - RPS Adeno Detector, a relatively new test, has the following advantages
    - Makes a rapid (10 minutes), sensitive, and specific diagnosis of adenoviral infection
    - Inexpensive, can be performed in office without special equipment or specially trained personnel
    - As accurate as culture and fluorescent detection methods
    - Testing with this device is societally cost effective because it promotes more timely and accurate diagnosis of infection

Pathology

- Giemsa stain would demonstrate
  - Predominant lymphocytosis in viral conjunctivitis
  - Predominant neutrophilia in bacterial conjunctivitis
  - Eosinophils in allergic conjunctivitis

TREATMENT

Medical

- Self-limited condition
- Symptomatic relief can be found with the following
  - Single-vial, preservative-free artificial tears instilled 4-8x a day
    - Multiuse eyedrop bottles can be a vector for transmission and should be avoided, if possible
  - Cool (or warm) compresses multiple times a day
  - Sunglasses for photophobia
  - Antihistamines for severe itching
- Reduce risk of transmission by
  - Appropriate hand hygiene
  - Avoiding eye rubbing
  - Not sharing towels, pillows, and other personal items
  - Physicians need to clean and disinfect all equipment and instruments handled during patient visit
    - Use a hypochlorite solution, povidone-iodine solution, or 70% ethyl alcohol
- Patients with significant exposure to others, both adults and children, should avoid school and work while symptomatic
  - Patients with hyperemia and tearing are still considered to be infectious
- Physicians and other healthcare workers who contract the disease should spend 2 weeks isolated from patient care to prevent spread of the disease
- Remove detectable membranes or pseudomembranes with forceps or a cotton swab every 2-3 days if needed
- Topical steroids are normally warranted only for severe membranes or pseudomembranes, severe keratitis, or symptomatic SEIs
  - Use a higher potency steroid for pseudomembranes or membranes (e.g., 0.5% loteprednol 4x a day)
  - Use a lower potency steroid for SEIs (e.g., 0.2% loteprednol 2x a day)
  - Treat for 1-3 weeks, followed by a gradual taper
    - SEIs often recur after steroid cessation; topical cyclosporine may be useful if long-term immunosuppression for SEIs is needed
    - NSAIDs, while not useful as an initial therapy for SEIs, may help prevent recurrence after steroid taper
  - Steroids can reduce symptoms, but they may enhance viral replication and increase duration of viral shedding, prolonging infectious period
- Povidone-iodine is not helpful in already established viral infections but may be useful in preventing transmission of disease
  - Topical dexamethasone 0.1%/povidone-iodine 0.4% drops provide symptomatic relief while reducing viral infectious titers
- Antiviral drugs are commonly used in herpesvirus infections and are being further investigated for use in adenoviral infections
  - Cidofovir has been successfully used to treat adenoviral conjunctivitis, but use is limited by toxicity
  - Ganciclovir (Zirgan) gel has recently shown some efficacy
- Prescribe antibiotics for a secondary bacterial infection, which is rare in adenoviral conjunctivitis

Follow-Up

- In 2-3 weeks or if clinical picture significantly worsens

Prognosis

- Usually resolves in 1-2 weeks with no residual problems
  - However, SEIs can persist for months and occasionally cause scarring

SELECTED REFERENCES

1. Clement C et al: Clinical and antiviral efficacy of an ophthalmic formulation of dexamethasone povidone-iodine in a rabbit model of adenoviral keratoconjunctivitis. Invest Ophthalmol Vis Sci. 52(1):339-44, 2011
2. Kaufman HE: Adenovirus advances: new diagnostic and therapeutic options. Curr Opin Ophthalmol. 22(4):290-3, 2011
3. Skevaki CL et al: Treatment of viral conjunctivitis with antiviral drugs. Drugs. 71(3):331-47, 2011
4. O'Brien TP et al: Acute conjunctivitis: truth and misconceptions. Curr Med Res Opin. 25(8):1953-61, 2009
5. Udeh BL et al: Cost effectiveness of a point-of-care test for adenoviral conjunctivitis. Am J Med Sci. 336(3):254-64, 2008
6. Sambursky R et al: The RPS adeno detector for diagnosing adenoviral conjunctivitis. Ophthalmology. 113(10):1758-64, 2006
7. Nauheim RC et al: Prolonged recoverability of desiccated adenovirus type 19 from various surfaces. Ophthalmology. 97(11):1450-3, 1990

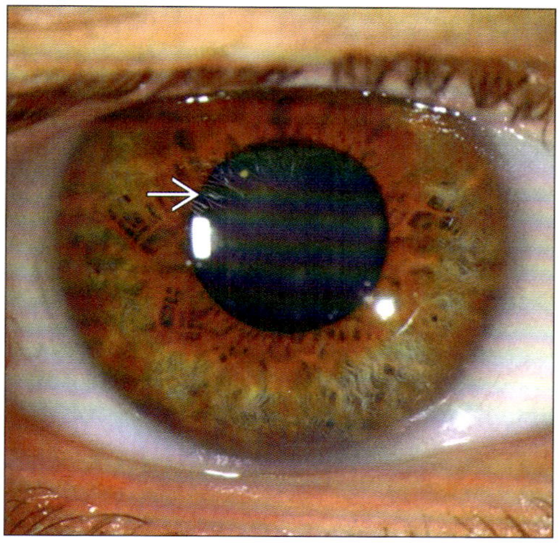

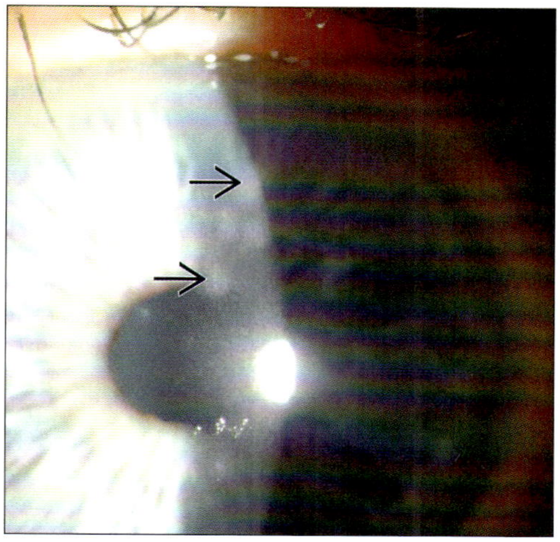

(Left) *This slit-lamp photo shows a patient with adenoviral conjunctivitis with epithelial keratitis ➔. In some cases, this viral keratitis is self-limited, and in other cases, it may progress and lead to multifocal subepithelial infiltrates (SEIs) that appear under the epithelial lesions. These SEIs can persist for months.* ***(Right)*** *This slit-lamp photo is of a patient with epidemic keratoconjunctivitis (EKC) and SEIs →, which can blur vision and may eventually lead to scarring.*

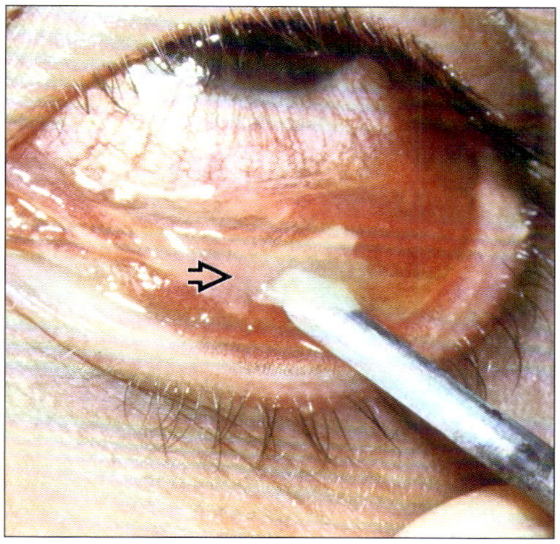

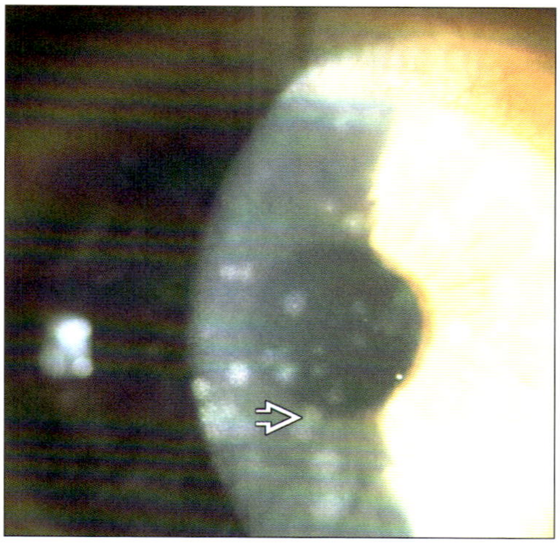

(Left) *This slit-lamp photo depicts pseudomembranes, which can be seen in patients with EKC ⇨. Pseudomembranes, as opposed to true membranes, are typically not integrated with the conjunctival epithelium and can be removed. (Courtesy C. Miller, MD.)* ***(Right)*** *This slit-lamp photo demonstrates multiple SEIs ➔ in the anterior stroma of a patient with EKC. Topical steroids can be used for symptomatic SEIs, but they can reoccur after steroid cessation. (Courtesy C. Miller, MD.)*

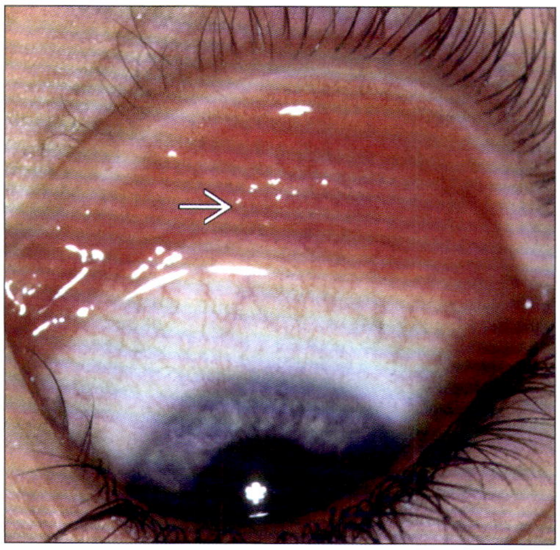

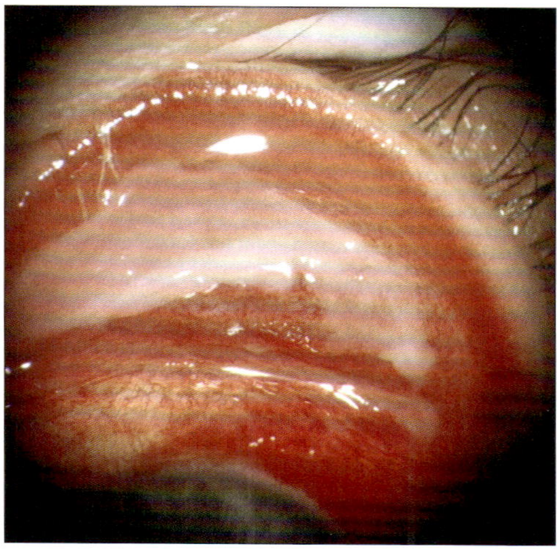

(Left) *This slit-lamp photo again demonstrates a patient with adenoviral conjunctivitis. Conjunctival hyperemia and palpebral conjunctival follicles can be seen ➔. (Courtesy C. Miller, MD.)* ***(Right)*** *This slit-lamp photo demonstrates a pseudomembrane in a patient with EKC. Diagnosis of EKC is normally made by physical exam findings, and laboratory confirmation is typically unnecessary, but new, inexpensive, in-office tests are available that can aid in making the diagnosis. (Courtesy C. Miller, MD.)*

CHRONIC BACTERIAL CONJUNCTIVITIS

Key Facts

Introduction
- Bacterial conjunctivitis with a duration > 4 weeks

Demographics
- Etiology
  - *Staphylococcus aureus* (most common pathogen), *Moraxella lacunata*, enteric gram-negative bacteria

Presentation
- Symptoms
  - Similar to acute bacterial conjunctivitis but milder
  - Foreign body sensation, burning, tearing, conjunctival discharge, and mattering of the eyelids upon awakening
- General exam findings
  - Diffuse conjunctival hyperemia, mucopurulent discharge, conjunctival papillae

Evaluation/Work-Up
- Uncomplicated cases do not require lab investigation
  - Refractory cases merit gram-stained smears and cultures of conjunctival and lid margin swabs

Treatment
- Initial therapy is similar to that of acute bacterial conjunctivitis, with the following topical agents used
  - Fluoroquinolone, aminoglycoside, polymyxin combo, or macrolide drops and various ointments, including ciprofloxacin and bacitracin
  - 5-7 day course employed in acute bacterial conjunctivitis is not always effective (longer topical antibiotic course is often needed)
- If associated with blepharitis, recommend the following in addition to topical antibiotic drops
  - Good lid hygiene (hot compresses and eyelid scrubs)
  - Application of topical antibiotic ointment to eyelid margins at night
  - If refractory, consider adding oral doxycycline or tetracycline to the regimen

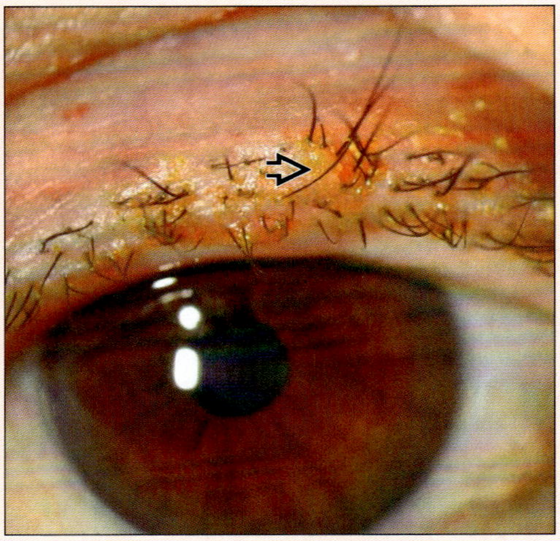
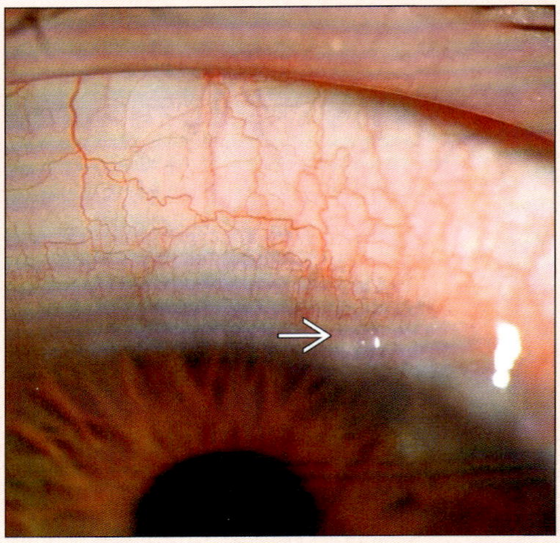

(Left) *This slit-lamp photo shows a patient with the golden yellow eyelid crusting seen in blepharitis, which can be found in patients with chronic bacterial conjunctivitis. Staphylococcus aureus is the most common cause of chronic bacterial conjunctivitis and is associated with blepharoconjunctivitis.* ***(Right)*** *This slit-lamp photo is of a patient with chronic bacterial conjunctivitis (duration > 4 weeks) with diffuse conjunctival injection and staphylococcal marginal keratitis.*

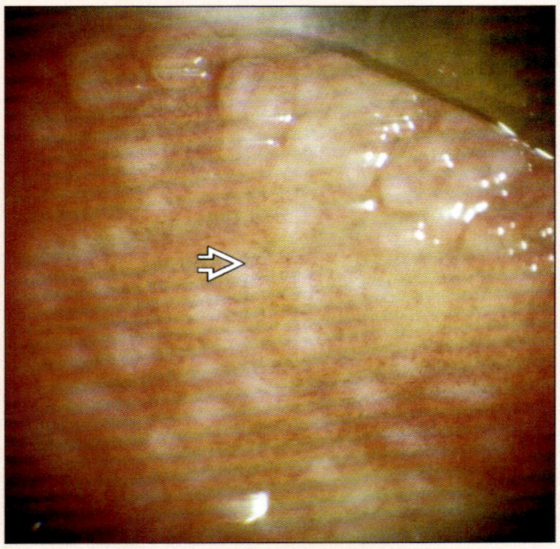
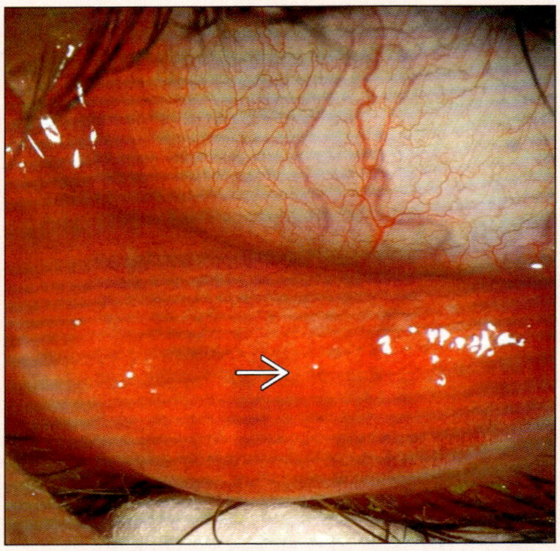

(Left) *This slit-lamp photo depicts conjunctival papillae that can be seen in bacterial conjunctivitis. In contrast to centrally avascular follicles seen in viral conjunctivitis, papillae have vascular cores and are typically larger. (Courtesy C. Miller, MD.)* ***(Right)*** *This slit-lamp photo demonstrates a patient with adenoviral conjunctivitis. Conjunctival hyperemia and palpebral conjunctival follicles, not the papillae most often seen in bacterial conjunctivitis, are visible.*

CHRONIC BACTERIAL CONJUNCTIVITIS

INTRODUCTION

Definitions

- Bacterial conjunctivitis with a duration > 4 weeks

DEMOGRAPHICS

Etiology/Risk Factors

- *Staphylococcus aureus*
  - Most common pathogen
- *Moraxella lacunata*
  - Alcohol abuse is a common risk factor
- Enteric gram-negative bacteria
  - *Proteus mirabilis, Klebsiella pneumoniae, Escherichia coli, Serratia marcescens, Moraxella catarrhalis*
    - Often associated with previously compromised ocular surfaces
- Unilateral ocular involvement is often caused by an abnormality in the nasolacrimal system, including
  - Chronic dacryocystitis and canaliculitis
    - Typically caused by *Actinomyces israelii*
- *Chlamydia trachomatis* is in differential diagnosis (tends to have superior follicles, can progress to reticular scarring)

Epidemiology

- Incidence of *Moraxella* has significantly decreased over recent years

PRESENTATION

Symptoms

- Similar to acute bacterial conjunctivitis but milder
  - Foreign body sensation, burning, &/or tearing
  - Conjunctival discharge
  - Mattering of the eyelids upon awakening

Exam Findings

- General exam findings include diffuse conjunctival hyperemia, mucopurulent discharge, and conjunctival papillae
- Exam findings associated with specific pathogens
  - *S. aureus*
    - Associated with blepharoconjunctivitis
    - Conjunctival thickening
    - Matted golden crusts and ulcers on anterior eyelid margin
    - Superficial punctate keratopathy, typically inferior
    - Conjunctival or corneal phlyctenules
    - Marginal corneal infiltrates and ulcerations
  - *M. lacunata*
    - Often associated with chronic angular blepharoconjunctivitis
    - Crusts and ulcers of the skin in the medial and lateral canthal angles
    - Conjunctival follicles
    - Punctate keratitis and subepithelial infiltrates

DIFFERENTIAL DIAGNOSIS

Dacryocystitis

- Presents with punctal discharge and erythematous, painful swelling over the nasal part of the lower eyelid

Parinaud Oculoglandular Conjunctivitis

- Presents with conjunctival granulomatous nodules and ipsilateral preauricular lymphadenopathy

EVALUATION/WORK-UP

Labs

- Uncomplicated cases do not require lab investigation
  - Refractory cases merit gram-stained smears and cultures of conjunctival and lid margin swabs and *Chlamydia* culture (typically sent in red tube with red viral culture medium)
    - Keep in mind that *S. aureus* may be found in the lid margin of normal eyes

TREATMENT

Medical

- Initial therapy is similar to that of acute bacterial conjunctivitis, with the following topical agents used
  - Fluoroquinolone drops (ciprofloxacin, ofloxacin, levofloxacin, moxifloxacin, gatifloxacin)
  - Aminoglycoside drops (gentamicin and neomycin)
  - Polymyxin combo drops (Polymyxin B + TMP-SMX)
  - Macrolide drops (azithromycin)
  - Bacitracin, ciprofloxacin, and various other ointments
  - 5-7 day course employed in acute bacterial conjunctivitis is not always effective
    - Longer topical antibiotic course (e.g., 2 weeks) is often needed
- If associated with blepharitis, recommend the following in addition to topical antibiotic drops
  - Good lid hygiene, including hot compresses and eyelid scrubs
  - Application of topical antibiotic ointment to eyelid margins at night
    - Erythromycin, bacitracin, or other antibiotic with gram-positive coverage
- If refractory, consider adding oral doxycycline or tetracycline to the regimen
- If severe eyelid inflammation is present, consider applying corticosteroid ointment to lid margins after eyelid scrubs

Follow-Up

- Initially, every 2-3 days, then every 5-7 days until resolution of symptoms
  - Antibiotic therapy should be tailored based upon culture and sensitivity results

Prognosis

- Generally, excellent prognosis

SELECTED REFERENCES

1. Hay-Smith G et al: Lacrimal gland ductulitis caused by probable Actinomyces infection. Ophthalmology. 119(1):193-6, 2012
2. Kowalski RP et al: Incidence of Moraxella conjunctival infection. Am J Ophthalmol. 101(4):437-40, 1986
3. McCulley JP: Blepharoconjunctivitis. Int Ophthalmol Clin. 24(2):65-77, 1984
4. Thygeson P et al: Chronic Conjunctivitis. Trans Am Acad Ophthalmol Otolaryngol. 67:494-517, 1963

HERPES SIMPLEX VIRUS CONJUNCTIVITIS

Key Facts

Introduction
- Conjunctival inflammation caused by herpes simplex virus (HSV), which is double-stranded DNA virus

Demographics
- Transmission of HSV occurs by contaminated secretions, direct contact with lesions, or exposure to asymptomatically shed viruses
- Most often contracted in adolescence and childhood

Presentation
- Unilateral ocular irritation, lacrimation, watery discharge, foreign body sensation, and itching
- Exam findings include
  - Conjunctival hyperemia
  - Conjunctival follicles, most often in fornices
  - Tender, palpable preauricular lymph node
  - Eyelid and conjunctival edema
  - Single or grouped vesicles on skin or eyelid margin; however, nearly 25% of patients with HSV conjunctivitis have no cutaneous lesions
  - Epithelial keratitis or dendritic ulcers can be present

Evaluation/Work-Up
- Laboratory investigation is needed only in atypical cases of HSV conjunctivitis
- Vesicular lesion samples, conjunctival scrapings, and impression cytology specimens can be tested by numerous methods

Treatment
- Treat with topical antiviral medications, such as
  - Trifluridine 1% drops 5-8x per day for 10 days
  - Vidarabine 3% or ganciclovir ophthalmic ointment 5x per day for 10 days
- Uncomplicated HSV conjunctivitis typically resolves without treatment in 7-14 days

__(Left)__ This slit-lamp photo illustrates superior lid margin ulcers that are often seen in patients with herpes simplex virus (HSV) conjunctivitis. It is important to remember, however, that nearly 25% of patients with HSV conjunctivitis have no cutaneous lesions. __(Right)__ This slit-lamp photo of an eye stained with fluorescein shows a dendrite in a patient with a primary HSV infection. Primary HSV typically presents as blepharoconjunctivitis, but patients can develop epithelial keratitis and dendritic ulcers.

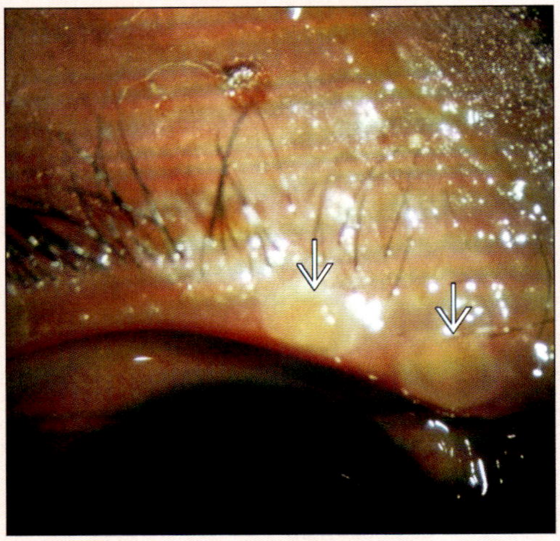

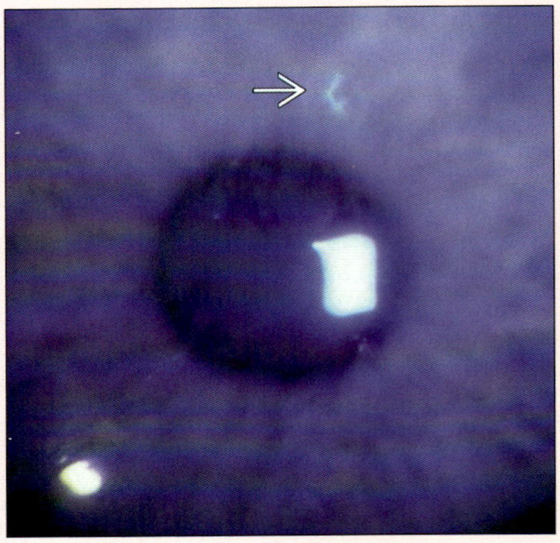

__(Left)__ External photo depicts small, grouped vesicles, which are often found in HSV infections. This patient also has noticeable edema of the upper and lower eyelids. __(Right)__ Slit-lamp photo demonstrates a corneal dendritic ulcer that has encroached upon the visual axis. Conjunctival hyperemia is also noted diffusely. Many patients with HSV conjunctivitis will also have a tender, palpable preauricular lymph node and conjunctival follicles.

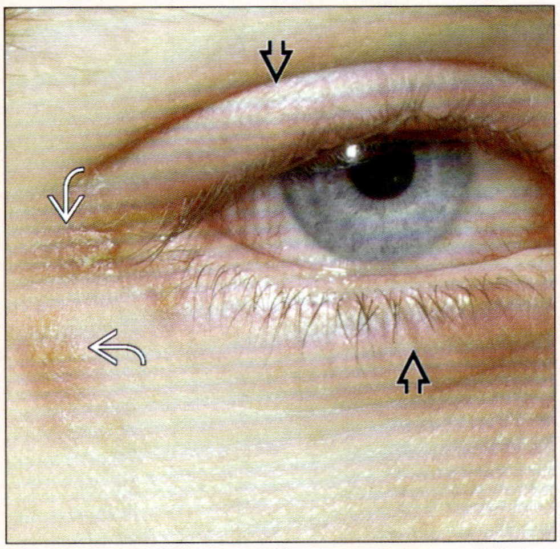

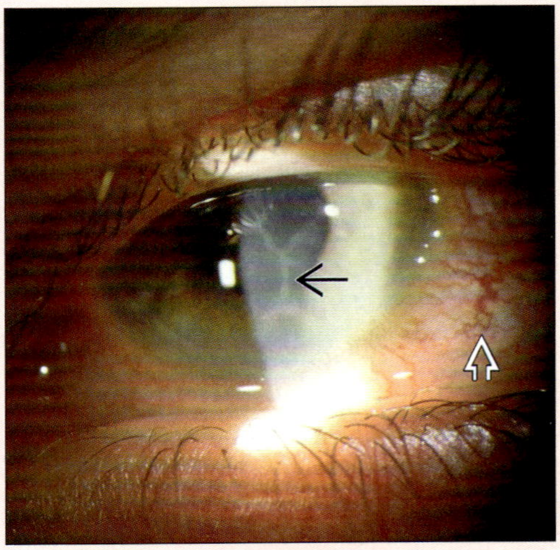

HERPES SIMPLEX VIRUS CONJUNCTIVITIS

INTRODUCTION

Abbreviations
- Herpes simplex virus (HSV)

Definitions
- Conjunctival inflammation caused by HSV

Subtypes
- HSV1 generally causes infection above waist
  - Mouth, face, eyes
- HSV2 generally causes infection below waist
  - Genital herpes
- Primary and recurrent infections

DEMOGRAPHICS

Etiology/Risk Factors
- Transmission of HSV occurs by contaminated secretions, direct contact with lesions, or exposure to asymptomatically shed viruses
  - Primary HSV infection is subclinical in most cases
    - Often causes mild fever, malaise, and upper respiratory tract infection

Epidemiology
- Ocular HSV incidence: 11.8 per 100,000 people in USA
- Nearly 100% of autopsy patients > 60 years of age have HSV in their trigeminal ganglia
- Most often contracted in adolescence and childhood

PRESENTATION

Symptoms
- Ocular irritation, lacrimation, watery discharge, foreign body sensation, and itching (usually unilateral)

Exam Findings
- Conjunctival hyperemia
- Conjunctival follicles, most often in fornices
- Tender, palpable preauricular lymph node
- Eyelid and conjunctival edema
- Single or grouped vesicles on skin or eyelid margin
  - Similar lesions may be found in mouth or nose
    - Stain lesions with rose bengal 1% or fluorescein
  - Nearly 25% of patients with HSV conjunctivitis have no cutaneous lesions
- Primary HSV typically presents as blepharoconjunctivitis, but patients can develop epithelial keratitis and dendritic ulcers
- Recurrent HSV can present with epithelial keratitis, blepharoconjunctivitis, stromal keratitis, disciform keratitis, &/or uveitis

DIFFERENTIAL DIAGNOSIS

Adenoviral Conjunctivitis
- More often bilateral and does not present with lid vesicles or dendritic ulcers
- May have conjunctival membranes/pseudomembranes

Herpes Zoster Virus Conjunctivitis
- Associated with painful vesicular rash that erupts in dermatomal distribution

EVALUATION/WORK-UP

Labs
- Laboratory investigation is needed only in atypical cases of HSV conjunctivitis
- Vesicular samples, conjunctival scrapings, and impression cytology specimens can be tested by
  - Cell culture (gold standard for HSV detection)
    - Results generally require > 48 hours
  - Enzyme Linked Viral Induced System (ELVIS)
    - Results obtained in 24 hours
    - Reliable alternative to normal cell culture
  - Polymerase chain reaction (PCR)
    - Detects viral DNA, can produce rapid results
  - Cytology and HSV antigen detection
- Serologic testing is generally helpful only when negative, as majority of adults are latently infected

Pathology
- Giemsa stain could show multinucleated giant cells and eosinophilic intranuclear inclusions

TREATMENT

Medical
- Treat with topical antiviral medications; commonly used regimens include
  - Trifluridine 1% drops 5-8x per day for 10 days
  - Vidarabine 3% (Vira-A; compounded) or ganciclovir (Zirgan) ophthalmic ointment 5x per day for 10 days
    - Topical antiviral treatment of HSV conjunctivitis with no corneal involvement is controversial as there is lack of evidence suggesting benefit
  - Surrounding skin lesions can be treated with acyclovir 5% dermatologic ointment 6x per day for 7 days
- Oral antiviral prophylaxis should be considered, especially for patients with recurrent corneal disease
- Steroids are contraindicated in HSV conjunctivitis
- Neonatal HSV conjunctivitis can be fatal
  - Treat with topical antivirals and IV acyclovir

Follow-Up
- Generally, in 2-3 days for all but very mild cases
  - Weekly thereafter until resolution of symptoms

Prognosis
- Uncomplicated HSV conjunctivitis typically resolves without treatment in 7-14 days

SELECTED REFERENCES

1. Young RC et al: Incidence, recurrence, and outcomes of herpes simplex virus eye disease in Olmsted County, Minnesota, 1976-2007: the effect of oral antiviral prophylaxis. Arch Ophthalmol. 128(9):1178-83, 2010
2. Kaye S et al: Herpes simplex keratitis. Prog Retin Eye Res. 25(4):355-80, 2006
3. Crist GA et al: Evaluation of the ELVIS plate method for the detection and typing of herpes simplex virus in clinical specimens. Diagn Microbiol Infect Dis. 49(3):173-7, 2004
4. Uchio E et al: Clinical and epidemiological features of acute follicular conjunctivitis with special reference to that caused by herpes simplex virus type 1. Br J Ophthalmol. 84(9):968-72, 2000
5. Jones B: The management of ocular herpes. Trans Ophthalmol Soc U K. 79:425-37, 1959

PARINAUD OCULOGLANDULAR CONJUNCTIVITIS

Key Facts

Introduction

- Granulomatous conjunctivitis with regional lymphadenopathy

Demographics

- Cat scratch disease (CSD) (most common)
  - Transmitted by cat scratch, bite, or lick
- Tularemia (common)
  - Infection comes through contact with rabbits, ticks, squirrels, and other animals
- Numerous other less common causes

Presentation

- CSD
  - Redness, irritation, foreign body sensation, and a watery, nonpurulent discharge
  - Conjunctival granulomatous lesions
  - Enlarged preauricular, submandibular, and cervical lymph nodes accompany the lesions or appear later
- Tularemia
  - Severe systemic symptoms are common, including fever, chills, headache, vomiting, and prostration
  - Conjunctival nodules with possible ulceration
  - Tender regional lymphadenopathy

Evaluation/Work-Up

- Elicit a thorough history, including animal exposure
- Serologic testing for typical CSD without complications to confirm diagnosis
- If unknown etiology, consider a variety of tests

Treatment

- Warm compresses for tender lymphadenopathy
- Antipyretics as needed
- Oral and topical antibiotics are used
  - Tailored to specific etiologic disease
- CSD generally has an excellent prognosis
  - Exam findings can take 1-2 months to resolve

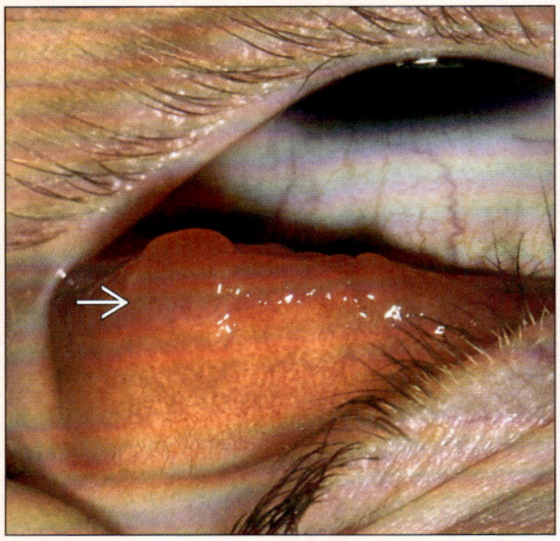

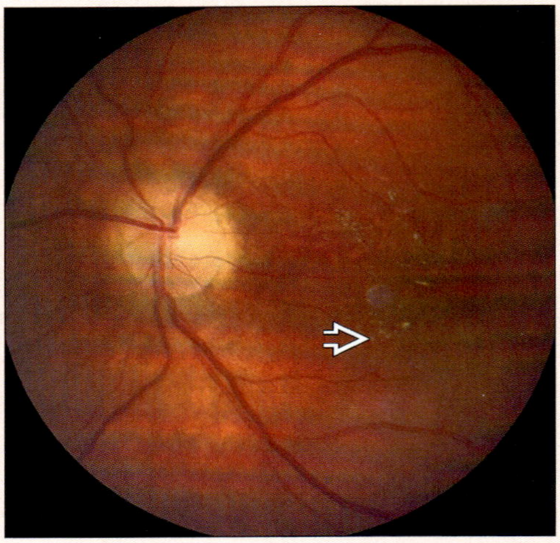

(Left) *This slit-lamp photo shows a patient with Parinaud oculoglandular conjunctivitis. This condition is characterized by granulomatous conjunctival lesions, which may be bulbar or palpebral →. (Courtesy C. Miller, MD.)* ***(Right)*** *This slit-lamp photo depicts neuroretinitis, which is also caused by Bartonella and is another manifestation of cat scratch disease in addition to Parinaud oculoglandular conjunctivitis. Numerous lipid exudates can be seen surrounding the macula →.*

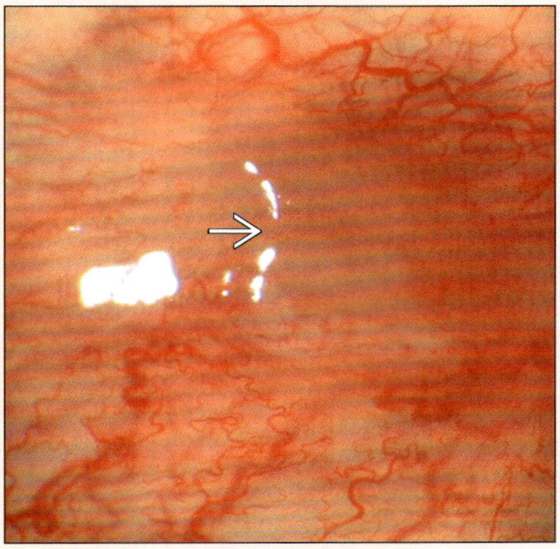

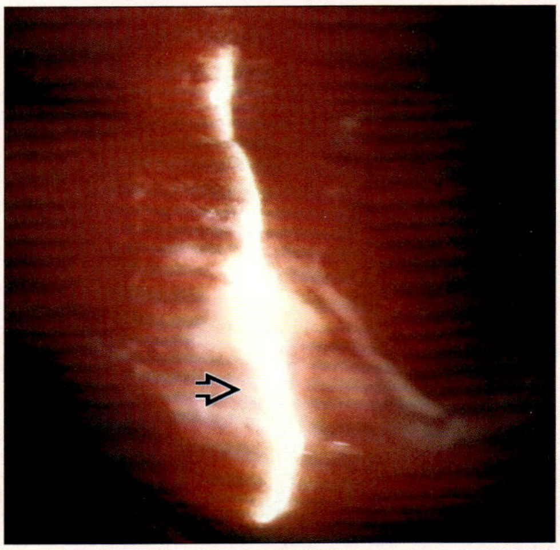

(Left) *This slit-lamp photo demonstrates a conjunctival granuloma →, which is typically seen in Parinaud oculoglandular conjunctivitis. Lesions are typically 3-4 mm in diameter and can be single or multiple, raised or flat, with variable coloration (red, white, yellow, or gray).* ***(Right)*** *This slit-lamp photo is of a patient with Parinaud oculoglandular conjunctivitis caused by tularemia. A granulomatous lesion is seen in the palpebral conjunctiva →. (Courtesy C. Miller, MD.)*

PARINAUD OCULOGLANDULAR CONJUNCTIVITIS

INTRODUCTION

Definitions

- Granulomatous conjunctivitis with lymphadenopathy

DEMOGRAPHICS

Etiology/Risk Factors

- Cat scratch disease (CSD) (most common)
  - Caused by *Bartonella henselae*
  - Transmitted by cat scratch, bite, or lick
- Tularemia (common)
  - Infection comes through contact with rabbits, ticks, squirrels, and other animals
- Sporotrichosis (common)
  - Caused by minor trauma and soil contamination
- Less common causes include TB and syphilis
- Numerous other rare causes

Epidemiology

- CDC estimates annual incidence of CSD in United States to be 1 in 10,000 people
  - Parinaud occurs in ~ 5-10% of CSD patients
    - 80% of cases are children and adolescents

PRESENTATION

Symptoms

- CSD symptoms typically develop 3-10 days after exposure and include
  - Irritation, foreign body sensation, and watery, nonpurulent discharge
  - Milder symptoms such as fever, headache, anorexia, and malaise in ~ 10-30% of patients
  - More severe symptoms such as encephalitis, hepatitis, and thrombocytopenic purpura in ~ 2% of patients
- Tularemia symptoms, which are commonly systemic and severe, include fever, chills, headache, vomiting, prostration, and occasionally death

Exam Findings

- CSD
  - Granulomatous lesions appear on the palpebral or bulbar conjunctiva 3-10 days after exposure
    - Lesions can be single or multiple, raised or flat, with variable coloration (red, white, yellow, or gray)
    - Lesions are 3-4 mm in diameter, typically surrounded by follicles
  - Enlarged preauricular, submandibular, and cervical lymph nodes accompany the lesions or appear later
    - Lymph nodes are firm and tender
    - ~ 10% become suppurative
- Tularemia findings include yellow conjunctival nodules with possible ulceration and necrosis, tender regional lymphadenopathy, and occasional corneal ulceration and endophthalmitis

DIFFERENTIAL DIAGNOSIS

Lymphoma

- Lymphadenopathy but without ocular symptoms
- Weight loss, night sweats, and fever are common

EVALUATION/WORK-UP

Labs

- Elicit a thorough history, including animal exposure
- Serologic testing for typical CSD without complications to confirm diagnosis
  - Indirect fluorescent antibody (IFA) or enzyme immunoassay (EIA) tests are available
  - Cat scratch skin test is no longer recommended
- If etiology is unknown (no history of cat contact), consider the following
  - Conjunctival cultures on blood, Löwenstein-Jensen, chocolate agar, Sabouraud, thioglycolate, and BHI media
  - Complete blood count, VDRL, FTA-ABS, ACE, PPD
  - Blood cultures if patient is febrile
  - Conjunctival biopsy with scrapings for acid-fast, Giemsa, and Gram stains
  - Serum IFA for other possible sources, including fungal

TREATMENT

Medical

- General treatment includes
  - Warm compresses for lymphadenopathy
  - Antipyretics as needed
- Treatment tailored to specific disease
  - CSD may resolve without treatment
    - Ideal treatment is undetermined, but the following antibiotics have shown success
      - Oral azithromycin, TMP-SMX, ciprofloxacin, doxycycline, or erythromycin
      - Oral rifampin can be used as adjuvant therapy
      - Topical antibiotics (e.g., gentamicin 4x per day)
  - Tularemia patients need medical supervision
    - IM streptomycin for 7 days is treatment of choice
    - Oral antibiotics (e.g., gentamicin, moxifloxacin, ciprofloxacin) are acceptable alternatives
    - Use gentamicin drops every 2 hours for 1 week, then 5x per day until resolved
  - Initiate typical antibiotic regimens for other causal diseases (e.g., penicillin for syphilis)

Follow-Up

- Repeat ophthalmic examination in 1-2 weeks

Prognosis

- CSD: Generally, excellent prognosis
  - Exam findings can take 1-2 months to resolve
- Tularemia: 2.5% mortality rate

SELECTED REFERENCES

1. Cunningham ET et al: Ocular bartonellosis. Am J Ophthalmol. 130(3):340-9, 2000
2. Ormerod LD et al: Ocular manifestations of cat-scratch disease. Curr Opin Ophthalmol. 10(3):209-16, 1999
3. Margileth AM: Cat scratch disease: no longer a diagnostic dilemma. Semin Vet Med Surg (Small Anim). 6(3):199-202, 1991
4. Rohrbach BW et al: Epidemiology and clinical characteristics of tularemia in Oklahoma, 1979 to 1985. South Med J. 84(9):1091-6, 1991

CHLAMYDIA TRACHOMATIS

Key Facts

Introduction

- Trachoma and adult chlamydial conjunctivitis are 2 important subtypes with ocular manifestations

Demographics

- **Trachoma**
  - Most cases result from direct eye-to-eye transmission
  - Global leading cause of preventable blindness
- **Adult inclusion (chlamydial) conjunctivitis (AIC)**
  - Autoinoculation of eye with genital secretions
  - Chlamydia is the most common STD, and AIC is seen in 0.2-3% of patients with urogenital chlamydia

Presentation

- **Trachoma**
  - Clinical diagnosis requires ≥ 2 of the following
  - Follicles on upper tarsal conjunctiva
  - Limbal follicles and their sequelae (Herbert pits)
  - Typical conjunctival scarring
  - Superior limbal vascular pannus
- AIC
  - Inferior tarsal conjunctival follicles
  - Palpable preauricular lymphadenopathy
  - Superficial punctate keratitis

Evaluation/Work-Up

- Diagnosis is usually made by history and clinical exam

Treatment

- **Trachoma**
  - Treatment was outlined in WHO "SAFE" strategy
  - Surgery for entropion/trichiasis
  - Antibiotics for infectious trachoma
  - Facial cleanliness to reduce transmission
  - Environmental improvements
  - May progress and cause blindness
- **Adult chlamydial conjunctivitis**
  - Patients need to be treated with systemic antibiotics

*(**Left**) This slit-lamp photo shows a superior palpebral follicular conjunctivitis ➔, which can be seen in trachoma. Follicles, most often found in the upper palpebral conjunctiva, can be elevated or flat; white, yellow, or gray in color; and can often become necrotic. (**Right**) This slit-lamp photo demonstrates Herbert pits ➔, which are circular depressions caused by limbal follicular regression and necrosis. This finding is virtually pathognomic of trachoma. (Courtesy C. Miller, MD.)*

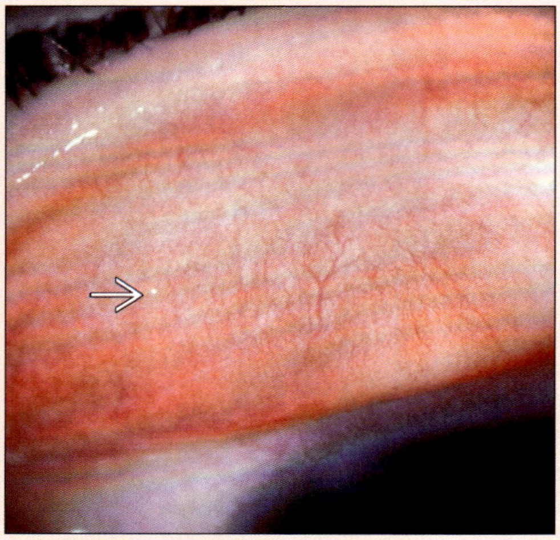

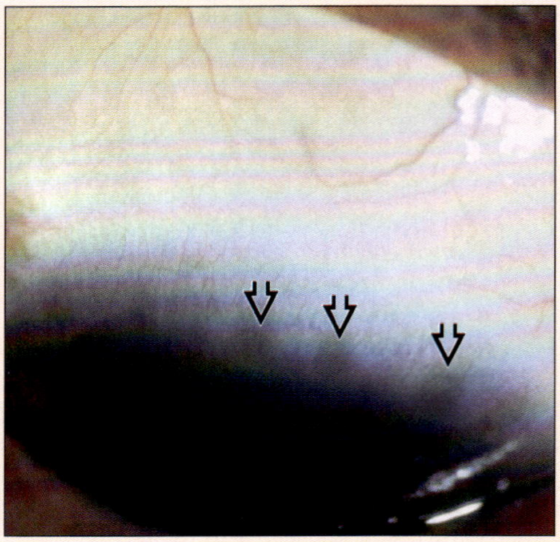

*(**Left**) This external photo shows a man who has trachoma of the left eye ➔. Patients often present with symptoms of mucopurulent discharge, tearing, foreign body sensation, hyperemia, photophobia, and eyelid edema. (Courtesy C. Miller, MD.) (**Right**) This Giemsa-stained pathology slide depicts the basophilic intracytoplasmic inclusion bodies ➔ seen in patients with Chlamydia trachomatis infection. Polymorphonuclear leukocytes and lymphocytes can also be seen in some cases. (Courtesy C. Miller, MD.)*

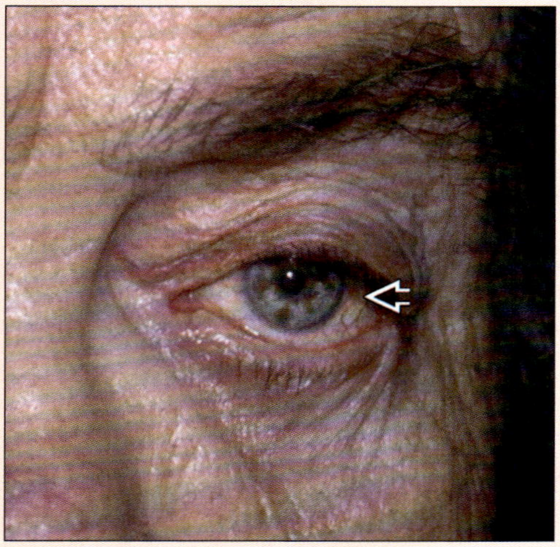

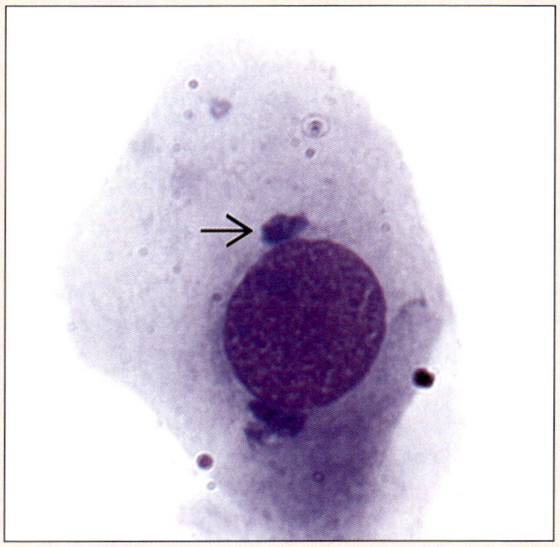

CHLAMYDIA TRACHOMATIS

INTRODUCTION

Definitions

- *Chlamydia trachomatis*, 1 of 3 bacterial species in the genus *Chlamydia*, is gram-negative obligate intracellular parasite

Subtypes

- Trachoma (serovars A-C)
- Adult inclusion (chlamydial) conjunctivitis (AIC) and neonatal inclusion (chlamydial) conjunctivitis (NIC) (serovars D-K)
  - Serovars D-K also cause
    - Pelvic inflammatory disease
    - Ectopic pregnancy
    - Urethritis
    - Neonatal pneumonia
- Lymphogranuloma venereum (LGV) (serovars L1-L3)
  - Ocular manifestations are very uncommon in LGV

DEMOGRAPHICS

Etiology/Risk Factors

- **Trachoma**
  - Most cases result from direct eye-to-eye transmission by intimate social or sexual contact
  - Can also occur by
    - Vector transmission
      - Flies
    - Household fomites
      - Towels
      - Bedding
      - Handkerchiefs
      - Washcloths
  - Bacterial and viral conjunctivitides create an environment that encourages the progression of nonblinding trachoma into blinding trachoma
  - Risk factors include
    - Poverty
    - Poor sanitation
    - Poor hygiene
    - Overcrowding
    - Lack of water
    - Contaminated eye makeup
- **AIC**
  - Infection arises from various sources, including
    - Autoinoculation of eye with genital secretions
    - Eye-to-eye transmission
    - Inadequately chlorinated swimming pool water

Epidemiology

- Trachoma affects ~ 84 million people globally
  - Leading infectious cause of blindness worldwide
    - 6 million people are estimated to be blind because of advanced trachoma
  - Active trachoma is most common in children < 5 years
  - More common in women than men
  - Endemic in over 50 countries, most prevalent in
    - Africa
      - Latin America
      - Middle East
      - Southwest Asia
      - Pacific Islands
      - Central Asia
      - Aboriginal communities in Australia
- Chlamydia infection is the most common sexually transmitted disease, with > 4 million cases annually
  - Most commonly seen in sexually active adolescents and young adults in developed countries
    - Adult chlamydial conjunctivitis is seen in 0.2-3% of patients with urogenital *Chlamydia* infection
      - AIC is the most common cause of chronic follicular conjunctivitis

PRESENTATION

Symptoms

- **Trachoma**
  - Mucopurulent discharge
  - Lacrimation
  - Foreign body sensation
  - Hyperemia
  - Photophobia
  - Eyelid edema
  - 5-10 day incubation period
  - Patients with active trachoma are often asymptomatic in initial stages
- **AIC**
  - Subacute onset of
    - Hyperemia
    - Lacrimation
    - Mattering of eyelids
    - Mild mucopurulent discharge
    - Papillary hypertrophy
  - Inquire about sexual symptoms and exposure
    - In females, the following can occur
      - Urethritis
      - Cervicitis
      - Dysuria
      - Discharge
      - Can progress to pelvic inflammatory disease
    - In males, the following can occur
      - Urethritis
      - Epididymitis
  - 5-14 day incubation period
    - Often becomes chronic and bilateral

Exam Findings

- **Trachoma**
  - Clinical diagnosis requires ≥ 2 of the following
    - Follicles on the upper tarsal conjunctiva
      - Can appear in multiple other locations
      - Often become necrotic
      - Typically white, gray, or yellow in color
      - 0.2-2 mm in diameter
      - Elevated or flat
      - Opaque or clear
    - Limbal follicles and their sequelae (Herbert pits)
      - Herbert pits are circular depressions caused by follicular regression and necrosis
    - Typical conjunctival scarring
      - Progresses from fine, linear, or stellate scarring of superior tarsus to broader, confluent deep scars (Arlt lines)
    - Vascular pannus most commonly found on superior limbus

CHLAMYDIA TRACHOMATIS

- Other findings include
  - Epithelial keratitis
  - Stromal infiltrates
  - Conjunctival papillae
  - Swelling of lymph nodes in front of ears
- Additional findings in more severe disease include
  - Corneal opacification
  - Trichiasis
  - Entropion
  - Corneal ulcers
  - Corneal vascularization
  - Dry eye
    - Caused by lacrimal gland duct scarring &/or goblet cell destruction
- World Health Organization (WHO) trachoma stages
  - TF (trachomatous inflammation: Follicular)
    - ≥ 5 superior tarsal follicles (≥ 0.5 mm in diameter)
  - TI (trachomatous inflammation: Intense)
    - Diffuse tarsal conjunctival inflammation with thickening obscuring > 50% of tarsal vessels
  - TS (trachomatous scarring)
    - Visible fibrous white tarsal bands or sheets
  - TT (trachomatous trichiasis)
    - Occurs if ≥ 1 eyelash is rubbing on eyeball
  - CO (corneal opacity)
    - Corneal opacity involving at least part of pupillary margin
- MacCallan system is an alternative staging system
  - Stage 1 (incipient trachoma)
    - Hyperemia of palpebral conjunctiva
    - Immature follicle
  - Stage 2 (established trachoma)
    - Appearance of mature follicle & papillae
    - Progressive corneal pannus
  - Stage 3 (cicatrizing trachoma)
    - Scarring of palpebral conjunctiva
    - Scars are easily visible as white bands
  - Stage 4 (healed trachoma)
    - Disease is cured or is not markable
    - Sequelae to cicatrization cause symptoms
- In general, there is an active inflammatory stage of trachoma (mainly seen in young children) and a chronic cicatricial stage (more often seen in adults)

- AIC
  - Inferior tarsal conjunctival follicles
  - Palpable preauricular lymphadenopathy
  - Superficial punctate keratitis
    - Yellow, peripheral subepithelial infiltrates may appear several weeks after initial symptom onset
  - Mild mucopurulent discharge
  - Superior corneal micropannus

DIFFERENTIAL DIAGNOSIS

Adenoviral Conjunctivitis

- Follicle location helps differentiate this from other causes
  - Upper tarsal conjunctiva
    - Most common in trachoma
  - Lower tarsal conjunctiva
    - Most common in adenoviral infections (epidemic keratoconjunctivitis) or AIC
- Adenoviral conjunctivitis is typically more acute
- Pannus and papillae are more often found in trachoma

Psittacosis

- Caused by *Chlamydia psittaci*
- History of bird exposure is common
- Also presents as chronic follicular conjunctivitis
  - Superior and inferior tarsal involvement

Acute Bacterial Conjunctivitis

- Trachoma should be suspected as the etiology of acute bacterial conjunctivitis if the following are present
  - Lymphoid follicles and diffuse conjunctival inflammation
  - Trichiasis
  - Incubation period is typically 5-12 days in trachoma and 24-72 hours in other causes of acute bacterial conjunctivitis (*Staphylococcus aureus*, *Haemophilus influenzae*, *Streptococcus pneumoniae*, *Moraxella catarrhalis*)

EVALUATION/WORK-UP

Labs

- Diagnosis is usually based on clinical exam findings
  - Obtain a detailed history for
    - Exposure to an endemic area (trachoma)
    - Sexually transmitted disease (AIC)
      - Vaginitis
      - Urethritis
      - Cervicitis
      - Rule out coinfection with other STDs before starting antibiotic therapy
- Laboratory investigations include
  - Cell culture isolation (McCoy)
  - Giemsa stain
    - Morphologic identification of chlamydial inclusions
  - Nucleic acid amplification tests (PCR, LCR)
    - PCR is current favored modality for detection
  - Direct fluorescein-conjugated monoclonal antibodies to species-specific (MOMP) or group-specific antigen (lipopolysaccharide [LPS])
  - Identification of chlamydial antigen by enzyme-labeled immunoassay
  - Multiple serologic tests
    - Antibody titers
    - Complement fixation tests
    - Indirect immunofluorescence
- Investigations are more useful for trachoma control programs than individual diagnoses

Pathology

- Giemsa stain shows
  - Basophilic intracytoplasmic inclusion bodies in epithelial cells, seen in clusters
  - Polymorphonuclear leukocytes
  - Lymphocytes

TREATMENT

Medical

- **Trachoma**
- Treatment and prevention was outlined in WHO "SAFE" strategy
  - Surgery for entropion/trichiasis
    - Bilamellar tarsal rotation (BTR) is preferred whether few or multiple lashes are involved
    - Following techniques are less effective than BTR but may be employed
      - Radiofrequency epilation
      - Hyfrecation
      - Cryotherapy
    - Rate of recurrence of trichiasis increases as disease progresses
    - Educating populations about importance of surgery remains an important challenge
    - Reasons patients do not present for surgery
      - Unaware of surgical options or availability
      - Lack of understanding of surgical benefit
      - Limited access to funds or transportation necessary for surgery
  - Antibiotics for infectious trachoma
    - Single dose of oral azithromycin 20 mg/kg is systemic treatment of choice
    - Acceptable systemic alternatives include a 2-week course of any of the following
      - Doxycycline 100 mg 2x a day
      - Tetracycline 250 mg 4x a day
      - Erythromycin 500 mg 4x a day
    - Topical erythromycin or 1% tetracycline ointment 2x a day for 6 weeks
      - Topical agents are reserved for situations in which oral azithromycin is not available
    - Do not use systemic tetracyclines in pregnant women, nursing mothers, and children < 8 years of age
      - Topical tetracycline is safe for use in pregnancy
    - Administer antibiotics to family members as well
  - Facial cleanliness to reduce transmission
    - Improving facial cleanliness is of paramount importance, as children with grossly visible nasal discharge, ocular discharge, or flies on their faces are at least 2x as likely to have active trachoma as children with clean faces
  - Environmental improvements
    - Hygiene
    - Sanitation
    - Access to free water
    - Control of disease-spreading flies
- Clinical stage helps shapes treatment plan
- WHO recommends community-based, mass antibiotic treatment when prevalence of active trachoma among 1- to 9-year-old children is > 10%
  - Annual treatment thereafter for 3 years, followed by a reassessment of disease prevalence
  - Annual treatment is continued until prevalence drops < 5%
- AIC
  - Patients need to be treated systemically with 1 of the following regimens
    - Doxycycline 100 mg 2x a day for 7 days
    - Tetracycline 250 mg 4x a day for 7 days
    - Erythromycin 500 mg 2x a day for 7 days
    - Azithromycin 1000 mg as a single dose
    - Topical antibiotics are not considered necessary but can provide relief for ocular symptoms
      - Erythromycin or tetracycline ointment 2-3x a day for 3 weeks
  - Treat sexual partners as well
  - Abstinence from sexual contact until 1 week after treatment termination
  - Refer to a genitourinary specialist to rule out other STDs such as syphilis or gonorrhea

Surgical

- Surgery for entropion/trichiasis

Follow-Up

- Typically every 2-3 weeks to start, then as needed

Prognosis

- **Trachoma**
  - Generally a good prognosis
    - Can be self-limiting, but treatment is curative and highly encouraged
    - Reinfection is common if sanitation, hygiene, and other risk factors are not adequately dealt with
  - May progress and cause severe conjunctival and corneal scarring, leading to blindness
- AIC
  - Generally, excellent prognosis
  - Often resolves without treatment in 6-18 months
  - With treatment, symptoms still may take weeks to resolve, and exam findings may persist for months

SELECTED REFERENCES

1. Evans JR et al: Antibiotics for trachoma. Cochrane Database Syst Rev. (3):CD001860, 2011
2. Taylor H: Trachoma: A Blinding Scourge from the Bronze Age to the Twenty-first Century. Melbourne: Centre for Eye Research Australia, 2008
3. Wright HR et al: Trachoma. Lancet. 371(9628):1945-54, 2008
4. Burton MJ: Trachoma: an overview. Br Med Bull. 84:99-116, 2007
5. Katusic D et al: Azithromycin vs doxycycline in the treatment of inclusion conjunctivitis. Am J Ophthalmol. 135(4):447-51, 2003
6. Dawson C: Flies and the elimination of blinding trachoma. Lancet. 353(9162):1376-7, 1999
7. Oliva MS et al: Evaluation of barriers to surgical compliance in the treatment of trichiasis. Int Ophthalmol. 21(4):235-41, 1997
8. Recommendations for the prevention and management of Chlamydia trachomatis infections et al: Centers for Disease Control and Prevention. MMWR Recomm Rep. 42(RR-12):1-39, 1993
9. Taylor HR et al: The natural history of endemic trachoma: a longitudinal study. Am J Trop Med Hyg. 46(5):552-9, 1992

MOLLUSCUM CONTAGIOSUM CONJUNCTIVITIS

Key Facts

Introduction

- Molluscum contagiosum (MC) conjunctivitis is conjunctival inflammation caused by MC virus

Demographics

- Follicular conjunctivitis is caused by toxic reaction or hypersensitivity response to viral protein particles shed into tear film from nearby lesions
- Spread by direct contact, normally hand to eye
- Can be transmitted sexually or during contact sports
- Peak incidence occurs during childhood
- More common in immunocompromised patients

Presentation

- Often asymptomatic, but may present with ocular irritation and redness
- Exam findings include small, elevated, dome-shaped umbilicated nodules with pearly borders and a waxy, curd-like core
- Lesions are typically small (2-6 mm in diameter) and found on eyelid or lid margin, often in clusters
- Conjunctival follicles, punctate epithelial keratopathy, and, less commonly, corneal pannus may develop

Evaluation/Work-Up

- Diagnosis usually made based on history and clinical exam
  - Typical lesions with follicular conjunctivitis
- HIV testing if patient has extensive lesions or is considered to be at high risk

Treatment

- Often resolves spontaneously without treatment
- Surgical options are preferred and include incision and curettage, complete excision, cryotherapy, and cautery
- Generally excellent prognosis
- Lesions typically resolve spontaneously over weeks to years, or quicker with surgery

__(Left)__ This slit-lamp photo is of a typical molluscum contagiosum (MC) lesion ➡ located on the medial upper eyelid margin of a 21-year-old patient. The lesion is an elevated, dome-shaped umbilicated nodule with a pearly border. __(Right)__ This slit-lamp photo shows a medial upper MC lesion ➡ with a view of hyperemic palpebral conjunctiva ⇨. MC follicular conjunctivitis is caused by a toxic reaction or hypersensitivity response to viral protein particles shed into the tear film from the lesion.

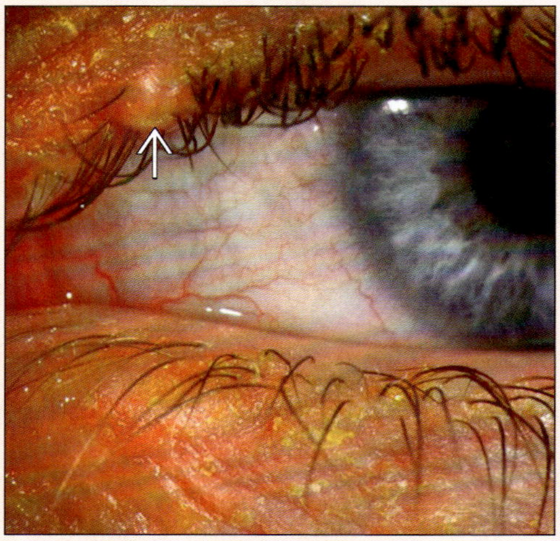

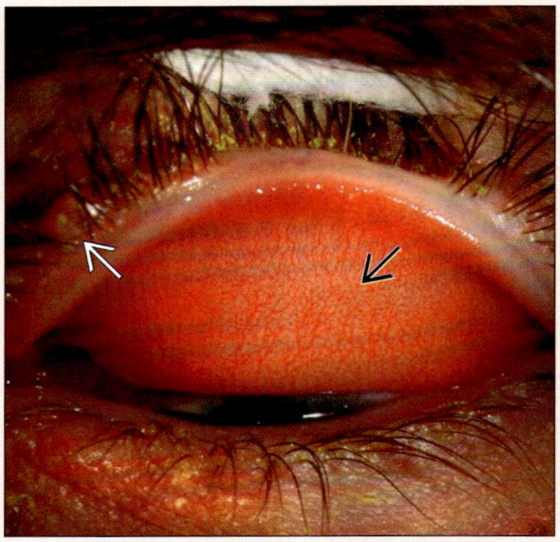

__(Left)__ This slit-lamp photo demonstrates an MC lesion ⇨ on the medial lower lid margin of a 16-year-old patient. Incision and curettage of the waxy, curd-like core (enough to cause bleeding) is an effective surgical treatment option. __(Right)__ This slit-lamp photo shows the same medial lower MC lesion ➡ and the secondary follicular conjunctivitis caused by its shed viral proteins and particles. The palpebral conjunctiva is hyperemic with several follicles dispersed throughout ⇨.

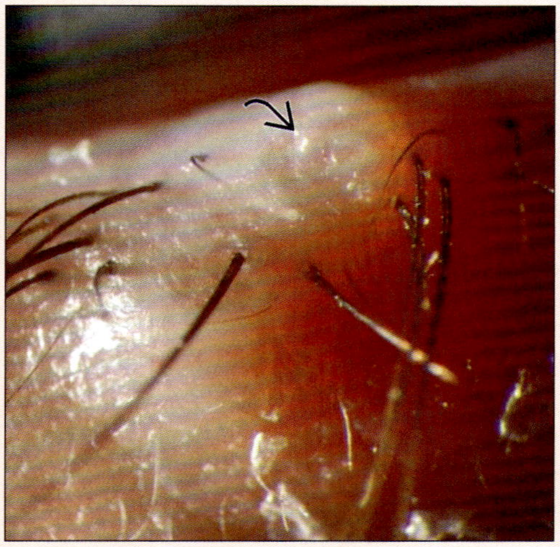

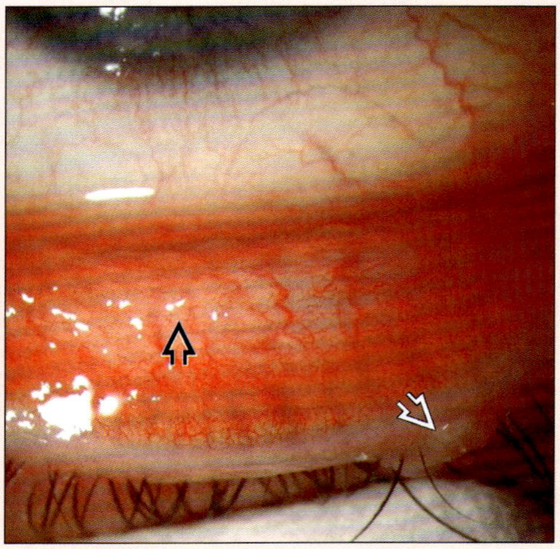

MOLLUSCUM CONTAGIOSUM CONJUNCTIVITIS

INTRODUCTION

Abbreviations
- Molluscum contagiosum (MC)

Definitions
- Conjunctival inflammation caused by DNA poxvirus

DEMOGRAPHICS

Etiology/Risk Factors
- Caused by infection with molluscum contagiosum virus, a DNA poxvirus
  - Follicular conjunctivitis is caused by a toxic reaction or hypersensitivity response to viral protein particles shed into tear film from nearby lesions
- Spread by direct contact, normally hand to eye
- Can be transmitted sexually or during contact sports
- More common in immunocompromised patients and in children with atopic dermatitis

Epidemiology
- Peak incidence occurs during childhood
  - 66% of cases occur < age of 40
- Estimated that < 5% of children have evidence of molluscum contagiosum virus

PRESENTATION

Symptoms
- Ocular irritation
- Redness
- Often asymptomatic

Exam Findings
- Small, elevated, dome-shaped umbilicated nodules with pearly borders and a waxy, curd-like core
- Lesions are typically small (2-6 mm in diameter) and found on eyelid or lid margin, often in clusters
  - Rarely found on conjunctiva
- Lesions are not always easily apparent
- Immunocompromised patients have lesions that appear with quicker onset and are more confluent, large, and numerous
- Conjunctival follicles, punctate epithelial keratopathy, and, less commonly, corneal pannus may develop
- Systemic lesions often found on fingers and around genital area
  - More common in immunocompromised patients

DIFFERENTIAL DIAGNOSIS

Basal Cell Carcinoma
- Lesions, usually solitary, may appear similar to MC
- No association with immunocompromised status
- Does not occur often in children
- Histology useful to differentiate from MC
- UV light is common risk factor, with lesions appearing mostly on face and head

Keratoacanthoma
- Lesions, usually solitary, may appear similar to MC
- No association with immunocompromised status
- Does not occur often in children
- More common in older adults with fair skin on sun-exposed, hair-bearing skin
- Histology useful to differentiate from MC

EVALUATION/WORK-UP

Labs
- Diagnosis usually made based on history and clinical exam
  - Typical lesions with follicular conjunctivitis
- HIV testing if patient has extensive lesions or is considered to be at high risk

Pathology
- Histology reveals central cavity of degenerated keratinocytes surrounded by keratinocytes that contain eosinophilic cytoplasmic inclusion bodies (Henderson-Patterson bodies)
- Biopsy if diagnosis is uncertain

TREATMENT

Medical
- Often resolves spontaneously without treatment; topical imiquimod 5% cream (Aldara) is becoming commonly used
- Nonocular lesions may be treated with cantharidin or podophyllotoxin
  - Do not use around eyes/eyelid

Surgical
- Incision and curettage
  - Core out center of lesion, enough to cause bleeding
    - Blades, jeweler's forceps commonly used
  - Treat with antibiotic ointment after curettage
- Complete excision
  - Can lead to scarring
- Cryotherapy
  - Can cause temporary or permanent pigment loss
- Cautery

Follow-Up
- Every 2-4 weeks until resolution of conjunctivitis

Prognosis
- Generally, excellent prognosis
  - Immunocompromised individuals have more extensive lesions
- Lesions typically resolve spontaneously over weeks to years or quicker with surgery
  - Conjunctivitis usually takes 1 month to resolve

SELECTED REFERENCES

1. Dohil MA et al: The epidemiology of molluscum contagiosum in children. J Am Acad Dermatol. 54(1):47-54, 2006
2. Schornack MM et al: Ocular manifestations of molluscum contagiosum. Clin Exp Optom. 89(6):390-3, 2006
3. Charles NC et al: Epibulbar molluscum contagiosum in acquired immune deficiency syndrome. Case report and review of the literature. Ophthalmology. 99(7):1123-6, 1992
4. Gonnering RS et al: Treatment of periorbital Molluscum contagiosum by incision and curettage. Ophthalmic Surg. 19(5):325-7, 1988

ALLERGIC CONJUNCTIVITIS

Key Facts

Introduction

- Seasonal allergic conjunctivitis (SAC)
- Perennial allergic conjunctivitis (PAC)

Demographics

- Mainly a type 1 (IgE mediated) hypersensitivity reaction that occurs after exposure to an allergen
- SAC allergens include pollens (tree, flower, grass) and ragweed, most often found in spring and summer
- PAC allergens include animal dander, house dust mites, mold spores, and fungi
- ~ 30% of people have allergic symptoms, with 40-80% of them having ocular involvement

Presentation

- Symptoms include itching, eyelid edema, conjunctival hyperemia, lacrimation, and photophobia
  - Occur rapidly after exposure to allergen and are bilateral, transient, and episodic
- Exam findings include erythematous and edematous eyelids, conjunctival hyperemia and papillae, mucoid or watery discharge, and chemosis

Evaluation/Work-Up

- Diagnosis is usually made by history and clinical exam

Treatment

- Depends upon severity of disease
- General treatment includes artificial tears, cool compresses, and avoiding known allergens
- Medications useful in allergic conjunctivitis include topical antihistamines ± vasoconstrictors, mast cell stabilizers, dual combinations of a mast cell stabilizer and an antihistamine, topical NSAIDs, topical corticosteroids, topical cyclosporine, and oral antihistamines
- Generally clears up with treatment but can often recur with repeat exposure to allergen

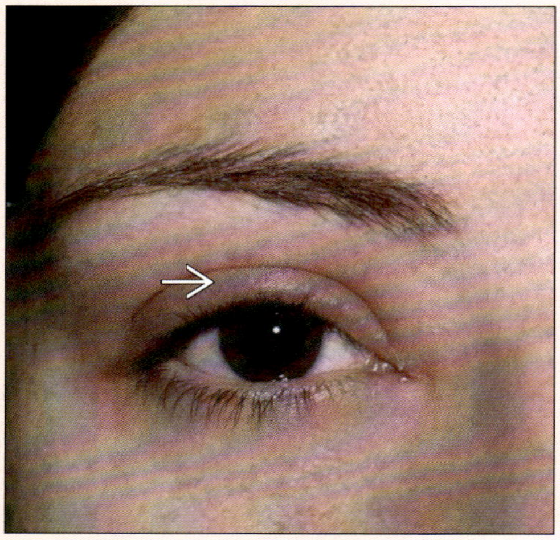

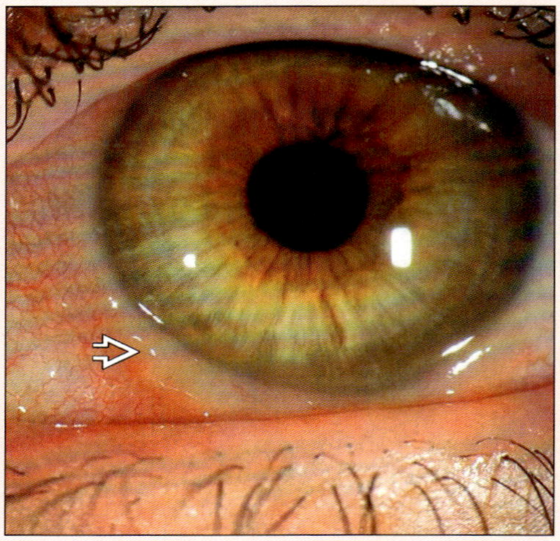

(Left) *This external photo depicts a female patient with allergic conjunctivitis. The most notable exam finding is the presence of edematous eyelids ➡. (Courtesy C. Miller, MD.)* ***(Right)*** *This slit-lamp photo shows a patient with allergic conjunctivitis ➡ with pronounced conjunctival hyperemia and chemosis. Allergic conjunctivitis is mainly a type I hypersensitivity reaction that occurs after exposure to an allergen, but it can also be a type IV hypersensitivity reaction to certain substances.*

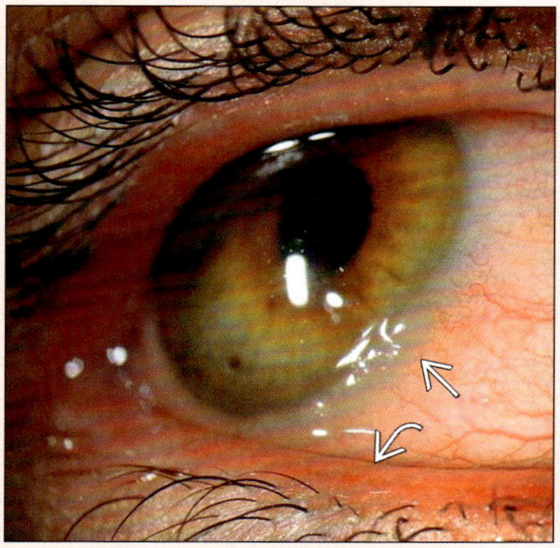

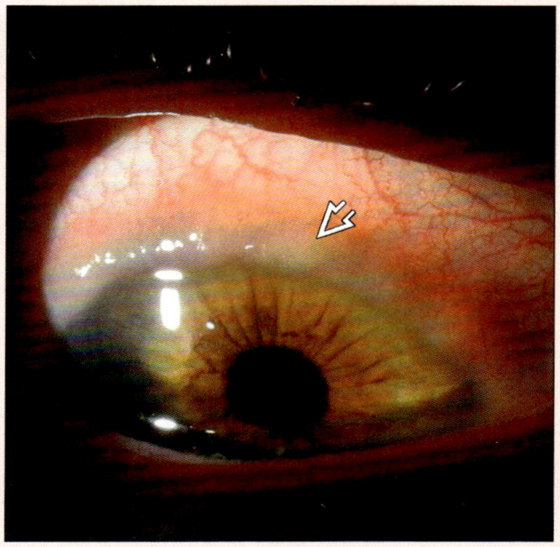

(Left) *This slit lamp photo demonstrates eyelid erythema ➡ and conjunctival hyperemia and chemosis ➡ that can be seen in patients with allergic conjunctivitis. This generally clears up with treatment but often recurs.* ***(Right)*** *This slit-lamp photo also shows a patient with allergic conjunctivitis ➡. Patients typically present with a chief complaint of ocular itching, normally bilateral in nature. Nonocular allergic symptoms such as rhinitis and asthma are also common.*

ALLERGIC CONJUNCTIVITIS

INTRODUCTION

Definitions
- Inflammation of the conjunctiva due to allergy

Subtypes
- Seasonal allergic conjunctivitis (SAC)
- Perennial allergic conjunctivitis (PAC)

DEMOGRAPHICS

Etiology/Risk Factors
- Mainly a type 1 (IgE mediated) hypersensitivity reaction that occurs after exposure to an allergen
  - SAC allergens include pollens (tree, flower, grass) and ragweed, most often found in spring and summer
  - PAC allergens include animal dander, house dust mites, mold spores, and fungi
- Can also be a type IV (cell mediated) hypersensitivity
  - Often from nickel or cosmetics
  - Less common cause of allergic conjunctivitis than type 1 hypersensitivity
- Family history of atopic disease increases risk

Epidemiology
- ~ 30% of people have allergic symptoms, with 40-80% of them having ocular involvement
- SAC is more common than PAC
- Incidence of PAC has recently been increasing

PRESENTATION

Symptoms
- Ocular itching is the main symptom
- Other common symptoms include eyelid edema, conjunctival hyperemia, lacrimation, and photophobia
  - Symptoms occur rapidly after exposure to allergen and are bilateral, transient, and episodic
- Nonocular allergic symptoms are common including rhinitis and asthma
- SAC occurs mainly in spring and summer
- PAC is milder than SAC
  - ~ 79% of PAC patients have seasonal exacerbations

Exam Findings
- Erythematous and edematous eyelids
- Conjunctival hyperemia and papillae
- Mucoid or watery discharge
- Chemosis

DIFFERENTIAL DIAGNOSIS

Infectious Conjunctivitis
- Does not present with itching

Dry Eye
- Typically involves the cornea, not the conjunctiva

EVALUATION/WORK-UP

Labs
- Diagnosis is usually made by history and clinical exam
- Conjunctival scrapings may demonstrate eosinophils
- Provocative challenge testing can be performed on the conjunctiva or skin but is rarely necessary for diagnosis
- Tear film can have elevated IgE and histamine levels

TREATMENT

Medical
- Treatment depends upon severity of disease
- General treatment includes artificial tears, cool compresses, and avoiding known allergens
  - Thorough cleaning of allergen-infested household items (e.g., linens) can be helpful
  - Mild cases can be resolved through general treatment
- Medications useful in allergic conjunctivitis include
  - Over-the-counter topical antihistamines ± vasoconstrictors (can help in mild cases)
    - Rebound hyperemia can be an issue
  - Prescription topical antihistamines reduce symptoms
    - Alcaftadine 0.25%, levocabastine 0.05%, and emedastine 0.05% 2x a day
  - Mast cell stabilizers are primarily for prophylaxis, as symptomatic relief is not found until several days after therapy initiation
    - Sodium cromoglycate 4%, pemirolast 0.1%, or lodoxamide 0.1% 4x a day
    - Nedocromil sodium 2% 2x a day
    - Best to use these 2 weeks before allergy season
  - Dual combinations of a mast cell stabilizer and an antihistamine are useful for prevention and treatment
    - Olopatadine 0.1%, azelastine 0.05%, ketotifen 0.025%, or epinastine 0.05% 2x a day
    - Olopatadine 0.2% 1x a day
  - Topical corticosteroids are effective but should be used sparingly in severe cases due to negative side effects
    - Common regimens include loteprednol 0.2% or dexamethasone 0.1% 4x a day for 7-14 days, followed by a taper
  - Topical NSAIDs may provide symptomatic relief but carry a small risk of corneal perforation
  - Topical cyclosporine 0.05% 2x a day is often helpful in patients refractory to other therapy
  - Oral antihistamines for systemic symptom relief

Follow-Up
- In 2 weeks, then as needed

Prognosis
- Generally clears up with treatment but can often reoccur with repeat exposure to allergen

SELECTED REFERENCES

1. Kari O et al: Updates in the treatment of ocular allergies. J Asthma Allergy. 3:149-58, 2010
2. Ono SJ et al: Allergic conjunctivitis: update on pathophysiology and prospects for future treatment. J Allergy Clin Immunol. 115(1):118-22, 2005
3. Brémond-Gignac D: The clinical spectrum of ocular allergy. Curr Allergy Asthma Rep. 2(4):321-4, 2002
4. Bielory L: Allergic and immunologic disorders of the eye. Part II: ocular allergy. J Allergy Clin Immunol. 106(6):1019-32, 2000
5. Friedlaender MH et al: Diagnosis of allergic conjunctivitis. Arch Ophthalmol. 102(8):1198-9, 1984

ATOPIC KERATOCONJUNCTIVITIS

Key Facts

Introduction

- Atopic keratoconjunctivitis (AKC)

Demographics

- Primarily, type IV hypersensitivity reaction with some involvement of type I hypersensitivity
- Atopic dermatitis is complicated by ocular involvement (AKC) in 25-42% of patients
- Asthma and eczema are both extremely common in patients with AKC
- Disease is chronic, with onset ranging from late teens through the 5th decade

Presentation

- Itching, photophobia, tearing, discharge, hyperemia, blurry vision, and pain
- Conjunctiva, lids, and cornea are usually involved
  - Retinal detachments, vitreous changes, and cataractous changes are also possible

Evaluation/Work-Up

- Diagnosis is usually made by history and clinical exam

Treatment

- Management of AKC is very similar to VKC
- Treatment more specific to AKC includes
  - Medications for atopic dermatitis and lid margin disease (e.g., topical steroid ophthalmic ointment, tacrolimus, and pimecrolimus)
  - Treat staphylococcal blepharitis if found
- Systemic treatment for AKC can include
  - Antihistamines
  - Immunosuppressives (e.g., steroids, tacrolimus) for ulcerative keratopathy, cases unresponsive to other therapy, or progressive cicatrization
- Follow-up every 1-3 days if a shield ulcer is present, otherwise, every few weeks
- Generally, good prognosis, with the disease typically becoming inactive during 5th decade of life

__(Left)__ Silt-lamp photo shows a patient with atopic keratoconjunctivitis (AKC) with prominent conjunctival hyperemia ⇒. Other common conjunctival findings in AKC include cicatricial changes, watery discharge, and a pale, milky-appearing edema. A gelatinous hyperplasia can also develop around the limbus. (Courtesy C. Miller, MD.) __(Right)__ This slit-lamp photo depicts a patient with superior palpebral conjunctival papillae ➡, often found in patients with AKC. Papillae are usually small to medium sized. (Courtesy C. Miller, MD.)

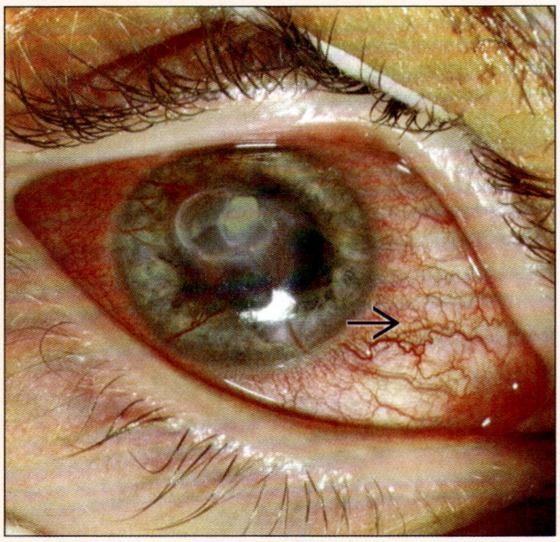

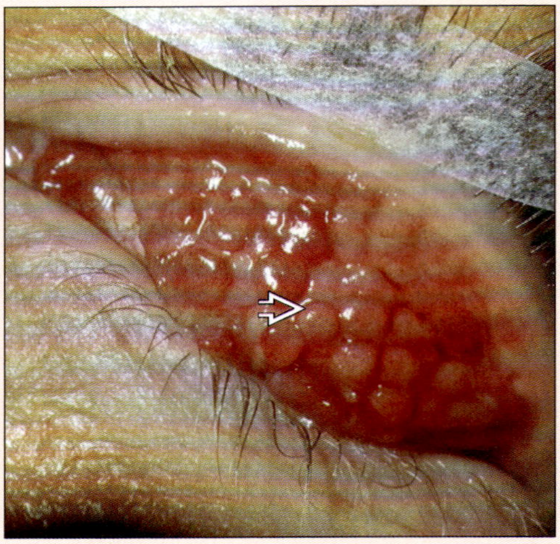

__(Left)__ This slit-lamp photo shows a patient with AKC and superior conjunctival papillae ⇨. Eyelids can also appear thick, erythematous, &/or edematous. (Courtesy C. Miller, MD.) __(Right)__ This slit-lamp photo demonstrates a patient with punctate epithelial erosions ➡, a finding that can be seen in patients with AKC. Other corneal findings include plaque formation, persistent epithelial defects, peripheral neovascularization, stromal scarring, corneal ulcers, or recurrent herpes simplex virus keratitis.

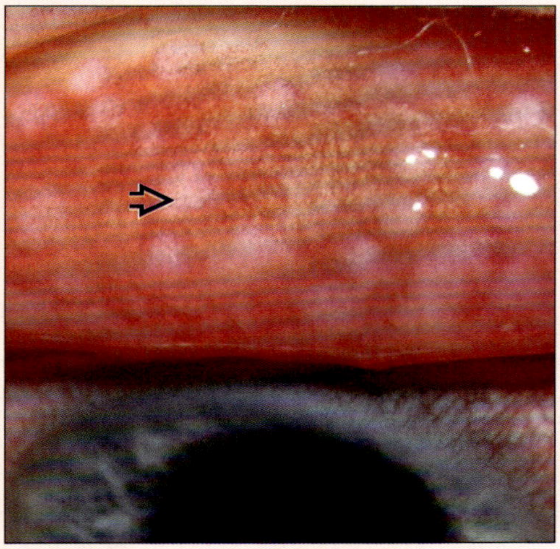

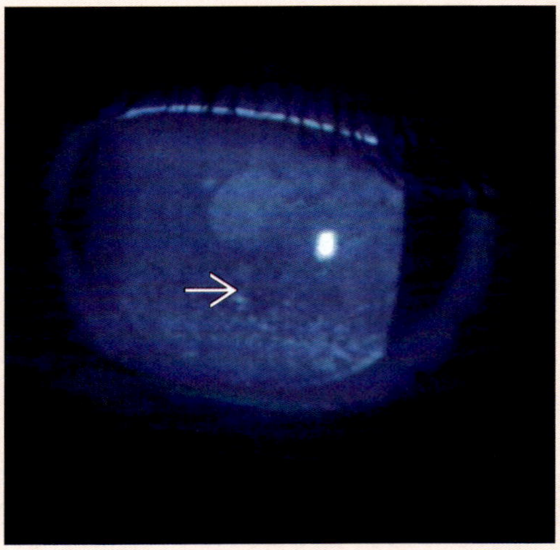

ATOPIC KERATOCONJUNCTIVITIS

INTRODUCTION

Abbreviations
- Atopic keratoconjunctivitis (AKC)

Definitions
- Chronic, bilateral inflammation of the conjunctiva and eyelids with potential corneal involvement

DEMOGRAPHICS

Etiology/Risk Factors
- Primarily, a type IV hypersensitivity reaction with some involvement of type I hypersensitivity
- Atopic dermatitis is complicated by ocular involvement (AKC) in 25-42% of patients
- Asthma and eczema are both extremely common in patients with AKC
- Most often perennial but can be seasonal
- ~ 5% of patients had vernal keratoconjunctivitis (VKC) in childhood
- T cell is primary effector cell in AKC and VKC

Epidemiology
- Disease is chronic, with onset being most common from late teens through the 5th decade
- No obvious racial, geographic, or gender predilection

PRESENTATION

Symptoms
- Itching, photophobia, tearing, discharge, hyperemia, blurry vision, pain
  - Similar to VKC but typically more chronic and severe

Exam Findings
- Conjunctival findings include
  - Mainly lower palpebral involvement
  - Small to medium papillae
  - Cicatricial changes with subepithelial fibrosis, symblepharon, and fornix foreshortening
  - Bulbar hyperemia and a pale, milky-appearing edema
  - Watery discharge
  - Gelatinous hyperplasia may occur around the limbus, with Horner-Trantas dots occasionally seen
- Skin and eyelid findings may include
  - Thick, erythematous, fissuring, and edematous lids
    - Severe edema leads to a single or double infraorbital lid crease (Dennie-Morgan line)
  - Chronic staphylococcal blepharitis (often associated with AKC)
  - Absent lateral eyebrow (Hertoghe sign)
  - Meibomianitis, madarosis, keratinization of the lid margin, trichiasis, punctal ectropion, and entropion
- Corneal findings include
  - Punctate epithelial erosions
  - Persistent epithelial defects
  - Plaque formation
  - Peripheral neovascularization and stromal scarring
  - Corneal ulcers, often with a microbial infection
  - Recurrent herpes simplex virus keratitis
- Lens changes include possible shield-shaped anterior or posterior subcapsular cataracts
- Retinal detachments and vitreous changes also possible

DIFFERENTIAL DIAGNOSIS

Vernal Keratoconjunctivitis
- Patients are typically young males in hot, dry climates who have seasonal symptoms, upper tarsal involvement, and little, if any, eyelid involvement

EVALUATION/WORK-UP

Labs
- Diagnosis is usually made by history and clinical exam
- Tears and serum may contain elevated IgE levels

Pathology
- Giemsa stain of a conjunctival scraping should demonstrate eosinophils and mast cells

TREATMENT

Medical
- Management of AKC is very similar to VKC, including
  - Tears, cool compresses, and allergen avoidance
  - Antihistamines ± vasoconstrictors
  - Mast cell stabilizers (can be used all year)
  - Topical corticosteroids, topical NSAIDs, and topical immunomodulators
  - AKC usually requires longer, more extensive treatment
- Treatment more unique to AKC includes
  - Medications for atopic dermatitis and lid margin disease; possible regimens include
    - Topical steroid ophthalmic ointment (e.g., fluorometholone 0.1% 4x per day)
    - Tacrolimus 0.03-0.1% ointment 2x per day (can also be used in the eye with a small cotton swab)
  - Staphylococcal blepharitis should be treated with appropriate lid hygiene and antibiotic therapy
  - Systemic treatment for AKC: Antihistamines or immunosuppressants (e.g., steroids, tacrolimus)

Surgical
- Shield ulcers may require debridement, superficial or phototherapeutic keratectomy, or keratectomy with amniotic graft to promote epithelial healing

Follow-Up
- If a shield ulcer is present, every 1-3 days, otherwise, every few weeks
- Taper medications where possible if symptoms improve

Prognosis
- Generally, good prognosis, with disease typically becoming inactive during 5th decade of life

SELECTED REFERENCES

1. Bielory B et al: Atopic dermatitis and keratoconjunctivitis. Immunol Allergy Clin North Am. 30(3):323-36, 2010
2. Zhan H et al: Clinical and immunological features of atopic keratoconjunctivitis. Int Ophthalmol Clin. 43(1):59-71, 2003
3. Tuft SJ et al: Clinical features of atopic keratoconjunctivitis. Ophthalmology. 98(2):150-8, 1991

CICATRICIAL PEMPHIGOID

Key Facts

Introduction

- Cicatricial pemphigoid (CP) is a chronic, autoimmune, and inflammatory subepithelial blistering disease that may involve skin and mucous membranes
- Ocular CP (OCP) is 1 of many CP subtypes

Demographics

- OCP is an autoimmune disease exhibiting a type II hypersensitivity reaction
- Average age of onset is 65 years

Presentation

- Nonspecific and includes insidious onset of ocular irritation, dry eye, tearing, and hyperemia
- Classic exam findings include chronic conjunctivitis and subepithelial fibrosis (stage 1), inferior forniceal shortening (stage 2), symblepharon formation (stage 3), and keratinization, ankyloblepharon, and obliteration of inferior fornix (stage 4)
- Subepidermal blisters, ulcers, scarring, and strictures may be found on other mucous membranes

Evaluation/Work-Up

- Detailed history and clinical exam, including exam of skin and mucous membranes, are crucial
- Biopsy should be sent of lesion (conjunctival or extraocular) for immunofluorescent and immunoperoxidase staining
- Early diagnosis is important to help prevent blindness

Treatment

- Multidisciplinary team approach is warranted
- Systemic immunomodulators and local therapy to reduce ocular complications (scarring, infection, dry eye) are mainstay of therapy
- Immunosuppress patients before any surgery
- OCP is generally a slow and progressive disease with an ultimately poor prognosis

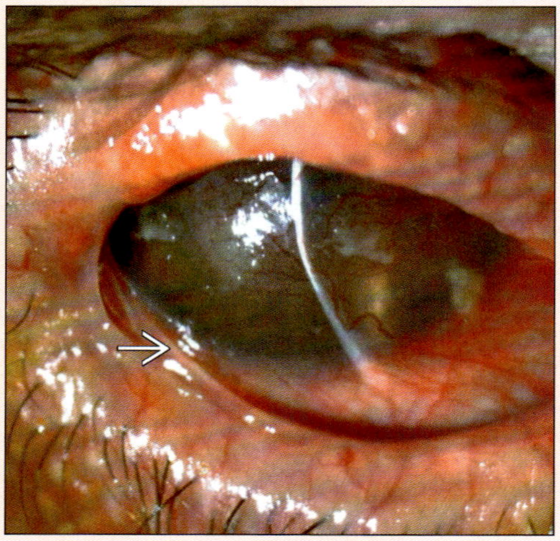
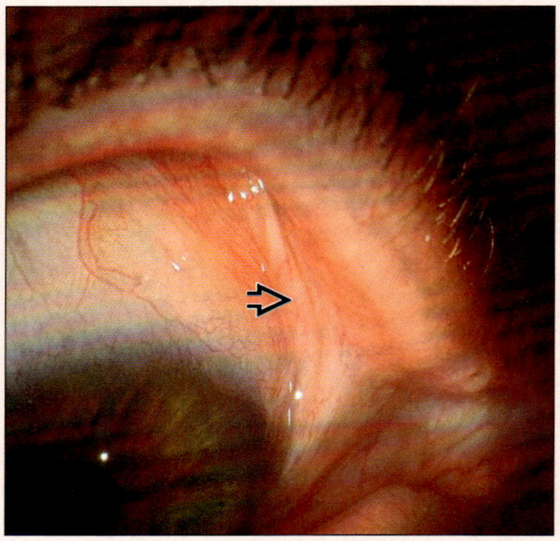

*(**Left**) This slit-lamp photo depicts symblepharon formation in the medial lower lid ➡. Symblepharon formation implies at least stage 3 disease. Stage 3 disease is further subdivided into 4 groups depending on the percentage of horizontal involvement by symblephera. (**Right**) This slit lamp photo demonstrates symblepharon formation in the lateral upper lid ⇨. Other ocular cicatricial pemphigoid (OCP) exam findings include trichiasis, entropion, and meibomian and lacrimal gland destruction. (Courtesy W. Nosé, MD.)*

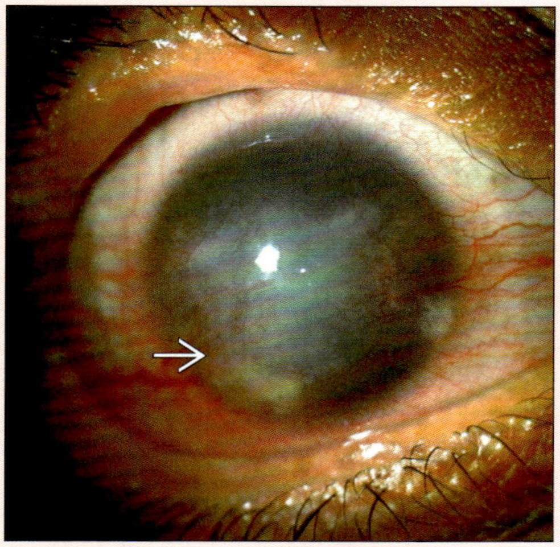
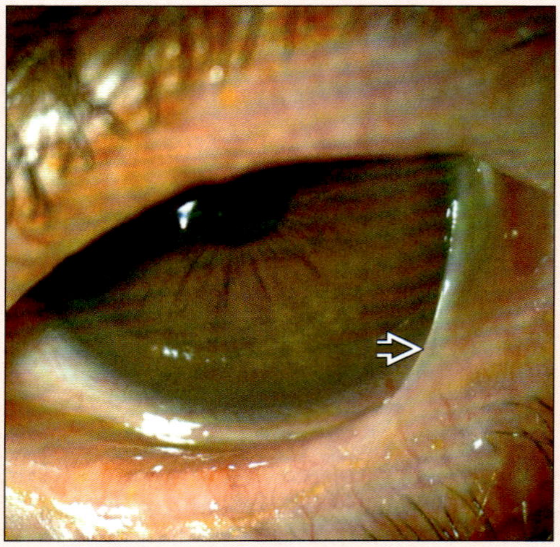

*(**Left**) This slit-lamp photo shows corneal keratinization that can occur in late stages of OCP ➡. Other corneal findings in OCP include ulceration, neovascularization, and scarring. (**Right**) This slit-lamp photo is of a patient with OCP and symblepharon formation in the lateral lower lid ⇨. Patients with this stage of disease typically have inferior forniceal shortening, which increases as the disease progresses until there is complete obliteration with end-stage disease. (Courtesy W. Nosé, MD.)*

CICATRICIAL PEMPHIGOID

INTRODUCTION

Abbreviations
- Cicatricial pemphigoid (CP)

Definitions
- Chronic, autoimmune, and inflammatory subepithelial blistering disease that may involve skin and mucous membranes
  - Also known as mucous membrane pemphigoid

Subtypes
- Ocular CP (OCP) is 1 of many CP subtypes

DEMOGRAPHICS

Etiology/Risk Factors
- OCP is an autoimmune disease exhibiting a type II hypersensitivity reaction
  - Autoantibodies bind to the conjunctival basement membrane (BM), leading to
    - Complement activation
      - Leads to destruction of conjunctival membrane
    - Inflammatory cell recruitment
      - IL1 and TNF-α
  - Production of these autoantibodies result from a combination of
    - Environmental triggers
      - Microbial organisms
      - Medications
    - Genetic susceptibility
      - Unknown gene in close linkage disequilibrium to HLA-DQβ1*0301 confers genetic susceptibility
  - α-6 β-4 integrin is an autoantibody that has been strongly linked to OCP

Epidemiology
- Reported incidence numbers range from 1 in 12,000 to 1 in 60,000 people
- Average age of onset is 65 years
  - Children are rarely affected
    - As of 2011, < 20 pediatric patients have been reported
- Affects females to males in 2-3:1 ratio
- No racial or geographical predilection has been discovered
- Discordant in monozygotic twins

PRESENTATION

Symptoms
- Nonspecific and include insidious onset of ocular
  - Irritation
  - Dry eye
  - Tearing
  - Hyperemia
- OCP is commonly misdiagnosed early on due to nonspecificity of these symptoms
- Findings are typically unilateral and progress to bilateral within 2 years
- Patients often have remissions and exacerbations

Exam Findings
- Ocular disease can be classified in 1 of 4 stages, depending on exam findings
  - Stage 1
    - Chronic conjunctivitis
      - Papillary
    - Subepithelial fibrosis
  - Stage 2
    - Inferior forniceal shortening
    - Further subdivided into 4 groups depending upon the % loss of inferior forniceal depth
      - A = 0-25%
      - B = 25-50%
      - C = 50-75%
      - D = 75-100%
  - Stage 3
    - Symblepharon formation
    - Increased forniceal shortening
    - Also subdivided into 4 groups, depending upon the % of horizontal involvement by symblephara
      - A = 0-25%
      - B = 25-50%
      - C = 50-75%
      - D = 75-100%
  - Stage 4 (end stage)
    - Keratinization
    - Ankyloblepharon (adhesions of the eyelid margins)
    - Obliteration of inferior fornix
  - Other OCP findings include
    - Trichiasis
    - Entropion
    - Lacrimal and meibomian gland duct obstruction
      - Resulting in dry eye
    - Secondary bacterial conjunctivitis
    - Corneal findings include
      - Ulceration
      - Neovascularization
      - Scarring
      - Opacification
- Systemic findings
  - Findings found on other mucous membranes include
    - Subepidermal blisters
    - Ulcers
    - Scarring
    - Strictures
  - Oral mucosa is most commonly affected and occurs in ~ 40% of OCP patients
    - Desquamative gingivitis is the most common oral manifestation
    - Erosions or vesicles may also appear on
      - Palate
      - Buccal mucosa
      - Tongue
      - Lip
      - Alveolar ridge
  - Laryngeal involvement can cause pain &/or hoarseness
  - Esophageal strictures can be life threatening
  - Nonmucosal skin vesicles or bullae, with possible erythematous plaques, may be present but are less common when compared to oral disease
    - Erythematous plaques lead to scarring

CICATRICIAL PEMPHIGOID

DIFFERENTIAL DIAGNOSIS

Allergic Causes of Cicatricial Conjunctivitis

- Stevens-Johnson syndrome
  - Similar symptoms, but more acute in onset than OCP
  - More likely to be caused by
    - Infections
      - Mycoplasma
      - Herpes
    - Drugs
      - Penicillins
      - Sulfas
      - Phenytoin
      - Other antibiotics
- Atopic keratoconjunctivitis
  - Primarily, a chronic type IV hypersensitivity reaction that presents with
    - Itching
    - Photophobia
    - Tearing
    - Discharge
    - Hyperemia
    - Blurry vision
    - Pain

Infectious Causes of Cicatricial Conjunctivitis

- Adenoviral infection
  - Presents with
    - Bilateral itching
    - Irritation
    - Foreign body sensation
    - Watery discharge
    - Tender preauricular lymphadenopathy
    - Conjunctival follicles
    - Eyelid edema
    - Eyelid erythema
- Trachoma
  - Presents in an endemic area with
    - Follicles on upper tarsal conjunctiva
    - Limbal follicles and their sequelae (Herbert pits)
    - Typical conjunctival scarring
    - Superior limbal vascular pannus
- Diphtheria conjunctivitis
  - Can present as a mild conjunctivitis or membranous conjunctivitis
  - May develop neurotoxicity due to diphtheria exotoxin
  - Often present with a respiratory infection

Traumatic Causes of Cicatricial Conjunctivitis

- Chemical or thermal burn
- Radiation exposure
- Other traumas
  - Detailed history should aid in diagnosis

Autoimmune Causes of Cicatricial Conjunctivitis

- Systemic lupus erythematosus
- Sarcoidosis
- Scleroderma
- Sjögren syndrome
- Epidermolysis bullosa acquisita
- Pemphigus vulgaris
- Linear IgA bullous disease
- Lichen planus
- Dermatitis herpetiformis
  - Systemic symptoms, laboratory tests, &/or direct and indirect immunofluorescence can aid in differentiating these diagnoses

Miscellaneous Causes of Cicatricial Conjunctivitis

- Porphyria cutanea tarda
  - Presents with
    - Fragile skin
    - Blistering of hands, arms, and face
  - Often induced by exposure to environmental factors
- Ocular rosacea
  - Presents as an inflammatory eruption of nose, cheeks, and forehead
    - Eruption is characterized by
      - Erythema
      - Pustules
      - Papules
      - Telangiectasias
- Drug induced (pseudopemphigoid)
  - Common causative drugs include
    - Echothiophate
    - Pilocarpine
    - Timolol
    - Epinephrine
    - Idoxuridine
    - Demecarium bromide
  - Disease progression halts once offending drug is discontinued
- Paraneoplastic pemphigus
  - Most commonly associated with B-cell lymphoma
  - Similar findings to pemphigus vulgaris
    - Use indirect immunofluorescence to distinguish
  - Xerophthalmia
    - Often caused by vitamin A deficiency
    - Presents with history of dry eye

EVALUATION/WORK-UP

Labs

- Detailed history and clinical exam, including exam of skin and mucous membranes, are crucial
- Early diagnosis is important to help prevent blindness
- Gram stain and culture of conjunctiva or cornea can be considered for suspected secondary bacterial infection

Pathology

- Biopsy of lesion should be sent (conjunctival or extraocular) for immunofluorescent and immunoperoxidase staining
  - Gold standard
  - Linear deposition of C3, IgM, IgG, and IgA along basement membrane are diagnostic of OCP
  - False-negative results can occur
  - Biopsy of perilesional tissue of an extraocular site is preferred, if possible
- An immunoblot analysis of patient serum can provide additional diagnostic evidence
- Conjunctival histology would show
  - Subepithelial inflammation
  - Submucosal scarring
  - Possible squamous metaplasia
  - Decreased goblet cells

- Perivasculitis
- Possible separation of epidermis from dermis

TREATMENT

Medical

- Multidisciplinary team approach is warranted, especially with use of immunomodulators; consider consulting oculoplastics, cornea, dermatology, ENT, gastroenterology, rheumatology, &/or oral surgeons
- Main goal of treatment is to prevent vision loss from scarring
- Local treatment
  - Aggressive lubrication with
    - Preservative-free ointments and tears
    - Possible punctal occlusion
      - Cautery typically more effective in OCP patients who have a higher rate of spontaneous extrusion of punctal plugs
    - Topical agents like tacrolimus, cyclosporine, or mitomycin C do not play a major role in treatment due to inability to suppress underlying immunologic problem
  - Treat chronic blepharitis with
    - Warm compresses
    - Antibiotic ointment
    - Good lid hygiene
    - Consider low-dose oral antibiotic like tetracycline
  - Retinoic acid may reduce keratinization
  - Topical steroids for adjuvant treatment
- Systemic treatment
  - Mild to moderate, slowly progressive disease can be treated with
    - Oral dapsone (starting dose 1 mg/kg per day and taper up to 100 mg per day)
      - Contraindicated in patients with G6PD deficiency or sulfa allergy
      - May be the best initial therapy
    - Mycophenolate mofetil (1 g 2x a day)
    - Methotrexate (15-25 mg weekly)
    - Azathioprine (2 mg/kg per day as initial dose)
  - Acute or rapidly progressive cases should be treated with
    - Oral prednisone 1 mg/kg per day
      - Gradually taper and discontinue it after 4-6 months
    - IV cyclophosphamide 2 mg/kg per day
      - Use IV cyclophosphamide for 6 months, then switch to an oral immunomodulator for a total treatment time of at least 2 years
      - Can be combined with prednisone in severe cases
- Combination of IVIG and rituximab has recently been shown to arrest OCP progression (comanage with a rheumatologist)
- Subconjunctival mitomycin C or steroid injection are not as effective but can be an alternative if systemic therapy is not feasible

Surgical

- Patients must be immunosuppressed before any surgical therapy can be performed
- Surgical therapy may be warranted for
  - Trichiasis
    - Cryotherapy
    - Laser ablation
  - Entropion
  - Dry eye
  - Persistent epithelial defects
- Mucous membrane autografting or amniotic membrane transplantation can reconstruct fornices and treat conjunctival keratinization
  - Buccal mucosa and hard palate can be used for grafting
- Limbal stem cell transfer may help ocular surface reconstruction, but is often unsuccessful
- Penetrating keratoplasty and Boston Keratoprosthesis (KPro) have a high failure rate

Follow-Up

- Every 1-2 weeks during acute exacerbations
- Every 1-3 months during remissions

Prognosis

- OCP is generally a slow and progressive disease with an ultimately poor prognosis
- Advancement to blindness from initial onset of OCP to end-stage disease can take from 10 to > 30 years
- Some patients may experience long-term remissions

SELECTED REFERENCES

1. Kirzhner M et al: Ocular cicatricial pemphigoid: a review of clinical features, immunopathology, differential diagnosis, and current management. Semin Ophthalmol. 26(4-5):270-7, 2011
2. Foster CS et al: Combination of rituximab and intravenous immunoglobulin for recalcitrant ocular cicatricial pemphigoid: a preliminary report. Ophthalmology. 117(5):861-9, 2010
3. Kharfi M et al: Early onset childhood cicatricial pemphigoid: a case report and review of the literature. Pediatr Dermatol. 27(2):119-24, 2010
4. Hingorani M et al: Ocular cicatricial pemphigoid. Curr Opin Allergy Clin Immunol. 6(5):373-8, 2006
5. Zerbe BL et al: Results from the multicenter Boston type 1 Keratoprosthesis study. Ophthalmology. 113(10):1779, 2006
6. Chang JH et al: Ocular cicatricial pemphigoid: manifestations and management. Curr Allergy Asthma Rep. 5(4):333-8, 2005
7. Holsclaw DS: Ocular cicatricial pemphigoid. Int Ophthalmol Clin. 38(4):89-106, 1998
8. Fiore PM et al: Drug-induced pemphigoid. A spectrum of diseases. Arch Ophthalmol. 105(12):1660-3, 1987
9. Foster CS: Cicatricial pemphigoid. Trans Am Ophthalmol Soc. 84:527-663, 1986

STEVENS-JOHNSON SYNDROME

Key Facts

Introduction
- Inflammatory disorder affecting skin and mucous membranes; toxic epidermal necrolysis (TEN) is a severe Stevens-Johnson syndrome (SJS) variant

Demographics
- Drugs and infections are most common causes
- Tends to affect younger adults but can arise at any age

Presentation
- Acute onset of rash, fever, malaise, arthralgia, headache, red eyes, and respiratory tract symptoms followed days later by skin and mucosal lesions
- Acute ocular findings include conjunctivitis, iritis, hyperemia, episcleritis, and hemorrhagic lid crusting
- Chronic ocular findings include symblepharon, cicatricial conjunctivitis, trichiasis, keratinization, entropion, tear deficiency or epiphora, and corneal scarring, ulcer, or neovascularization
- Systemic findings include "targetoid" skin lesions

Treatment
- Acute treatment includes lubrication, topical antibiotics, and amniotic membrane transplantation and prevention of symblepharon formation (using glass rods or rings to lyse symblephara early)
- Use of topical/systemic steroids is controversial (likely useful acutely, but be careful of causing or worsening corneal melt)
- Chronic treatment includes aggressive lubrication to treat dry eye, interventions for trichiasis, bandage soft contact lenses, topical retinoids, and mucous membrane or amniotic membrane grafts
- Penetrating keratoplasty is generally not effective
- Daily in-patient follow-up; weekly after discharge
- Mortality is ~ 1-5% for SJS and 25-35% for TEN patients

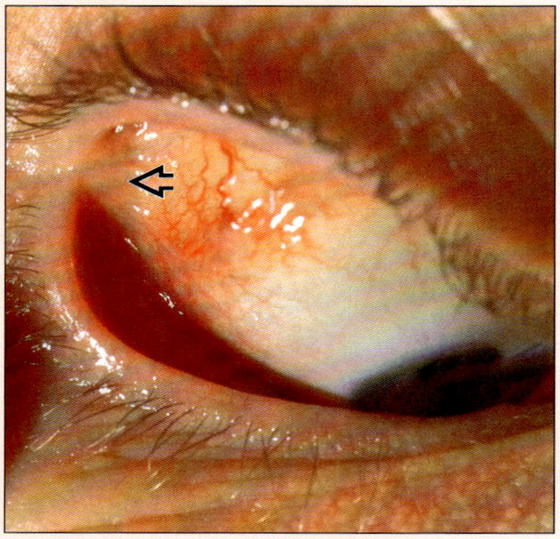
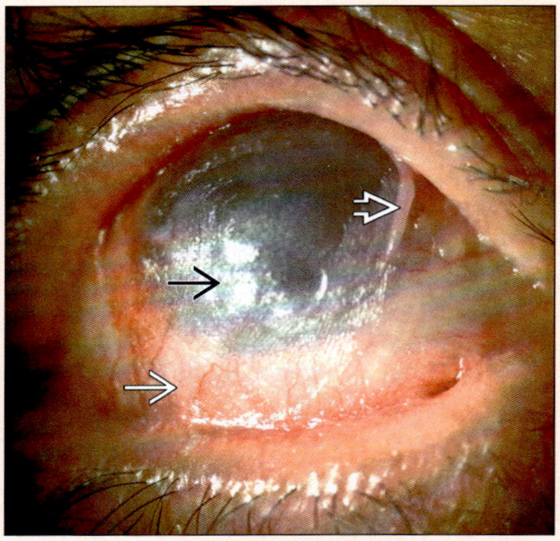

(Left) *This slit-lamp photo demonstrates lateral symblepharon formation in a patient with Stevens-Johnson syndrome (SJS) ⇨. SJS is thought to be a type IV hypersensitivity reaction with acute ocular complications in > 50% of patients. Systemic findings include "target" skin lesions.* ***(Right)*** *This slit-lamp photo is of a patient with SJS. Keratinization →, symblepharon ➡, and conjunctival hyperemia ➡ are observed. Drugs and infection are the most common causes of SJS. (Courtesy W. Nosé, MD.)*

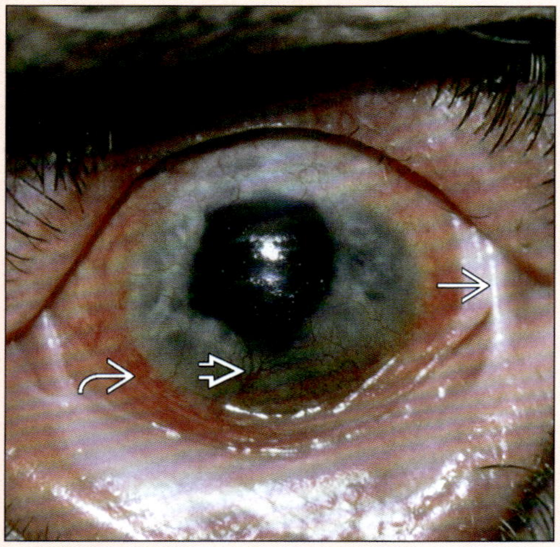
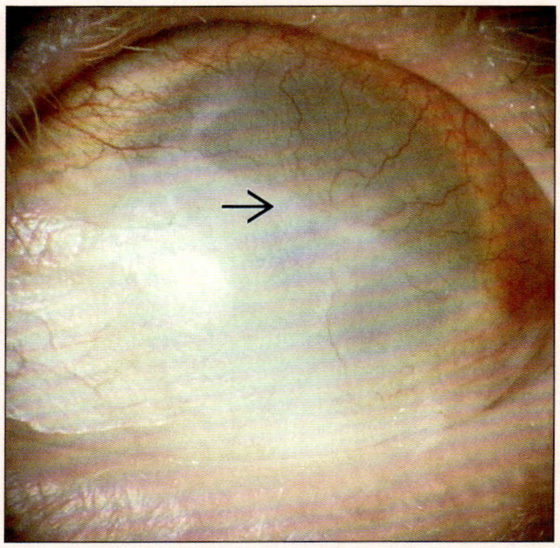

(Left) *This slit-lamp photo of a patient with SJS depicts symblepharon ➡, corneal neovascularization ➡, and marked conjunctival hyperemia ➡. (Courtesy C. Miller, MD.)* ***(Right)*** *This slit-lamp photo shows corneal keratinization that can occur in patients with chronic SJS →. Other chronic findings include symblepharon, cicatricial conjunctivitis, trichiasis, entropion, tear deficiency, posterior lid margin disease, and corneal scarring, ulcer, or neovascularization. (Courtesy C. Miller, MD.)*

STEVENS-JOHNSON SYNDROME

INTRODUCTION

Abbreviations
- Stevens-Johnson syndrome (SJS)

Definitions
- Inflammatory disorder affecting skin and mucous membranes
  - Very similar to erythema multiforme (EM) major but differs slightly in clinical features and etiology
    - EM major has mucosal erosions and acrally distributed typical target lesions; EM minor only affects skin
    - SJS also has mucosal erosions but differs in that it has atypical, flat target lesions &/or macular purpuric lesions; it has worse prognosis than EM

Subtypes
- Toxic epidermal necrolysis (TEN) is a severe SJS variant

DEMOGRAPHICS

Etiology/Risk Factors
- Thought to be a type IV hypersensitivity reaction
- Drugs (75% of cases) and infections are most common causes
  - Common causative drugs include
    - Antibiotics
      - Sulfonamides, tetracycline, trimethoprim, penicillins cephalosporins
    - Anticonvulsants
      - Carbamazepine, barbiturates, phenytoin
    - NSAIDs
    - Cardiovascular drugs
    - Other drugs
      - Allopurinol, cocaine, chlorpropamide, isoniazid, thiazide diuretics, aspirin
  - Common infections include herpes simplex virus, adenovirus, *Mycoplasma*, streptococci, measles, Epstein-Barr virus, enterovirus, *Yersinia*
- Less common causes include cancer, allergies, autoimmune disease

Epidemiology
- Tends to affect younger adults but can arise at any age
  - TEN patients are generally older than SJS patients
- Incidence of SJS/TEN is ~ 5 cases/million/year
  - Incidence varies depending on the trial
  - Women are at a 2:1 risk over men to contract TEN, while males are at a 2:1 risk over women for SJS
- More than 1/2 of SJS/TEN patients develop acute ocular complications
  - ~ 35% develop chronic ocular complications
  - ~ 25% develop severe ocular complications
- AIDS patients are at a higher risk for SJS/TEN
- HLA-Bw44 and HLA-B12 association with SJS

PRESENTATION

Symptoms
- Acute onset of
  - Rash
  - Fever
  - Malaise
  - Arthralgia
  - Pain
  - Headache
  - Red eyes
  - Respiratory tract symptoms
- These symptoms are followed days later by skin and mucosal lesions
- Symptoms make take 1-3 weeks to develop after exposure

Exam Findings
- Acute ocular findings (within 2 weeks of onset) include
  - Conjunctivitis, which can include any of the following characteristics
    - Mucopurulent
    - Papillary
    - Membranous
    - Pseudomembranous
  - Hyperemia
  - Episcleritis
  - Hemorrhagic lid crusting
  - Bullous rash of eyelid skin
  - Eyelid edema
  - Infection
  - Epithelial defects
  - Corneal ulcers
  - Anterior uveitis
- Chronic ocular findings can include
  - Symblepharon
  - Cicatricial conjunctivitis
  - Trichiasis
  - Keratinization
  - Entropion
  - Tear deficiency
  - Epiphora
  - Posterior lid margin disease
  - Corneal scarring
  - Corneal ulcer
  - Corneal neovascularization
  - Corneal perforation
- Systemic findings can include
  - Symmetric crops of skin lesions that develop every 2 weeks for about 6 weeks
  - Round, dusky red lesions that evolve into "target" lesions typically within 2 days
    - "Targetoid" maculopapular lesions have a red center surrounded by a pale zone and then a red ring
      - Usually found on hands, feet, and extremities but can also be on face and trunk
      - Heal after several weeks, leaving a pigmented scar
      - Lesions in SJS patients are atypical and flat while lesions in EM major patients are raised
    - Bullae, vesicles, and necrosis often develop
  - Blistering &/or hemorrhagic crusting of other mucosal surfaces like lips, tongue, and nose
- SJS involves < 10% of body surface area (BSA)
- TEN involves > 30% of BSA
- SJS/TEN overlap involves 10-30% of BSA
- Positive Nikolsky sign may be present
  - More common in TEN patients
- Mucous membranes are involved in > 90% of cases

STEVENS-JOHNSON SYNDROME

DIFFERENTIAL DIAGNOSIS

Systemic Differential Diagnosis

- Skin biopsies can help differentiate EM major, SJS, and TEN from the following disorders
  - Epidermolysis bullosa acquisita (EBA)
    - Acquired autoimmune disorder that presents either as a noninflammatory blistering disease or a generalized, inflammatory bullous disease
    - EBA antigen is part of type VII collagen
    - Ocular involvement is common and similar to ocular cicatricial pemphigoid, including
      - Symblepharon formation
      - Subepithelial vesicles
      - Corneal ulcers
      - Corneal opacification
    - Epidermolysis bullosa is different from EBA, being an inherited disease with recurrent skin blistering or erosions after minor trauma
  - Staphylococcal scalded skin syndrome
    - More common in infancy or childhood
    - Necrosis and inflammation usually absent
    - Blood and wound cultures can help differentiate
  - Pemphigus vulgaris
    - Flaccid intraepithelial bullae and erosions
      - Facial
      - Truncal
      - Mucosal
      - Oral mucosa generally involved before skin
  - Bullous pemphigoid
    - Characterized by
      - Tense subepithelial bullae
      - Erosions
      - Urticarial lesions
    - Rare mucosal involvement
    - Usually occurs in 7th and 8th decades
  - Paraneoplastic pemphigus
    - Most commonly associated with B-cell lymphoma
    - Similar findings to pemphigus vulgaris
      - Indirect immunofluorescence can differentiate
  - Toxic shock syndrome
    - Present with a sunburn-like rash and signs of sepsis
    - Usually caused by *Staphylococcus* or *Streptococcus*
    - Blood and wound cultures can help differentiate
  - Drug hypersensitivity syndrome
    - Characterized by
      - Fever
      - Widespread maculopapular erythematous rash
      - Internal organ involvement
      - Eosinophilia
      - Atypical lymphocytosis
  - Other
    - Bullous systemic lupus erythematosus
    - Burns
    - IgA
    - Bullous dermatosis
    - Viral exanthem
    - Exfoliative dermatitis
    - Graft-vs.-host disease
  - History, systemic symptoms, laboratory values, and other tests can help differentiate

Ocular Differential Diagnosis

- Ocular cicatricial pemphigoid
  - Presents with
    - Conjunctivitis
    - Subepithelial fibrosis
    - Inferior forniceal shortening
    - Symblepharon formation
    - Keratinization
    - Ankyloblepharon
    - Obliteration of inferior fornix
- Trachoma
  - Presents in an endemic area with
    - Follicles on upper tarsal conjunctiva
    - Limbal follicles and their sequelae (Herbert pits)
    - Typical conjunctival scarring
    - Superior limbal vascular pannus
- Severe chronic keratoconjunctivitis
  - Patient would have a history of chronic bacterial or viral conjunctivitis
- Adenoviral infection
  - Presents with
    - Tender preauricular lymphadenopathy
    - Watery discharge
    - Conjunctival follicles
    - Eyelid edema
    - Eyelid erythema
    - Foreign body sensation
    - Irritation
    - Itching
- Allergic conjunctivitis
  - Presents with
    - Itching
    - Eyelid edema
    - Hyperemia
    - Conjunctival papillae
    - Lacrimation
    - Mucoid or watery discharge
    - Chemosis

EVALUATION/WORK-UP

Labs

- Eyelid eversion is crucial to uncover all lesions
- Complete blood count

Pathology

- Diagnosis is usually made by history and clinical exam
- Skin biopsy in uncertain cases would reveal
  - Necrotic keratinocytes
  - Lymphocytic infiltrate at dermal-epidermal junction with vacuolar alterations
- Conjunctival biopsies in patients with active ocular disease would reveal
  - Subepithelial lymphocytic infiltration
    - Helper T cell most common
    - Present around vessel walls
  - Subepithelial plasma cells
- Total loss of palisades of Vogt (POV) should be observed in chronic cases
  - Absence of POV at limbal area implies an absence of corneal epithelial stem cells

STEVENS-JOHNSON SYNDROME

TREATMENT

Medical

- Patient should be admitted to hospital, preferably in an intensive burn care unit
  - Hospital team should manage systemic symptoms
  - Treatment includes
    - Immediately discontinuing or treating inciting factor
    - Monitoring fluid and electrolyte balance
    - Nutritional support
    - Wound care
    - Pain control
    - Respiratory therapy
  - Use of systemic steroids is controversial
    - High-dose, short-term systemic glucocorticoids seem to be beneficial in adults (but not children) with recent-onset SJS
      - However, steroid therapy does increase risk of GI hemorrhage, electrolyte imbalance, infection, and other complications
    - TEN patients have an increased risk of sepsis and should probably not receive glucocorticoids
    - IVIG seems to be useful in severe SJS/TEN adult and pediatric cases
- Acute ocular treatment includes
  - Aggressive lubrication
    - Preservative-free tears, gels, or ointments
  - Topical antibiotics for prophylaxis or infection
  - Amniotic membrane transplantation over entire ocular surface has shown long-term benefit
  - Efficacy of topical steroids is controversial
    - Can reduce inflammation but can make corneal melts worse
    - Immunosuppressants (cyclosporine 2% drops; tacrolimus ointment or tablets) can be considered in acute phase
    - Topical steroids and cycloplegic drops should be used in cases of anterior uveitis
  - Pseudomembrane/membrane peeling, lysis of symblepharon (using glass rods early), and symblepharon rings may help
- Chronic ocular treatment includes
  - Aggressive lubrication with possible punctal occlusion &/or tarsorrhaphy to treat dry eye
  - Established interventions for trichiasis
  - Soft contact lenses are often used to protect cornea from dry eye and aberrant lashes
  - Topical retinoids can minimize reverse corneal keratinization (vitamin A ointment)

Surgical

- Mucous membrane grafts or amniotic membrane grafts can be used to reconstruct fornices in chronic cases
- Amniotic membrane transplantation onto ocular surface can reduce destructive inflammation and ulcer formation in acute cases and prevent cicatricial change
- Penetrating keratoplasty is generally not effective due to ocular surface alterations and corneal neovascularization
- Permanent keratoprostheses may be required (high risk of corneal melt with type 1; would need type 2 Boston KPro with prophylactic tube)
- Other possible interventions include
  - Lamellar corneal grafting
  - Stem cell transplantation
    - Living-related or cadaveric conjunctival and limbal allografts

Follow-Up

- Daily while hospitalized and weekly after discharge
  - Important to watch for and treat complications, including infection and increased IOP

Prognosis

- Mortality rate is ~ 1-5% for SJS and 25-35% for TEN patients
  - Scorten Scale, a severity-of-illness scale that uses 7 independent risk factors for high mortality, can be used to predict the expected mortality rate for a particular patient
    - 7 independent risk factors are
      - Age > 40 years
      - Associated malignancy
      - Heart rate > 120 beats per minute
      - Serum BUN > 28 mg/dL
      - Detached or compromised body surface >10%
      - Serum bicarbonate < 20 mEq/L
      - Serum glucose > 252 mg/dL
    - Patients with 0-1 risk factors had an expected mortality rate of 3.2%; 2 risk factors: 12.1%; 3 risk factors: 35.3%; 4 risk factors: 58.3%; and ≥ 5 risk factors: 90%
  - Death typically secondary to sepsis
- Can last up to 6 weeks

SELECTED REFERENCES

1. Gerull R et al: Toxic epidermal necrolysis and Stevens-Johnson syndrome: a review. Crit Care Med. 39(6):1521-32, 2011
2. Mockenhaupt M: The current understanding of Stevens-Johnson syndrome and toxic epidermal necrolysis. Expert Rev Clin Immunol. 7(6):803-13; quiz 814-5, 2011
3. Shay E et al: Amniotic membrane transplantation as a new therapy for the acute ocular manifestations of Stevens-Johnson syndrome and toxic epidermal necrolysis. Surv Ophthalmol. 54(6):686-96, 2009
4. Sotozono C et al: Diagnosis and treatment of Stevens-Johnson syndrome and toxic epidermal necrolysis with ocular complications. Ophthalmology. 116(4):685-90, 2009
5. Gregory DG: The ophthalmologic management of acute Stevens-Johnson syndrome. Ocul Surf. 6(2):87-95, 2008
6. De Rojas MV et al: The natural history of Stevens Johnson syndrome: patterns of chronic ocular disease and the role of systemic immunosuppressive therapy. Br J Ophthalmol. 91(8):1048-53, 2007
7. Tsubota K et al: Clinical application of living-related conjunctival-limbal allograft. Am J Ophthalmol. 133(1):134-5, 2002
8. Bastuji-Garin S et al: SCORTEN: a severity-of-illness score for toxic epidermal necrolysis. J Invest Dermatol. 115(2):149-53, 2000

GIANT PAPILLARY CONJUNCTIVITIS

Key Facts

Introduction

- Giant papillary conjunctivitis (GPC) is a conjunctival inflammatory disorder associated with contact lens (CL) use or other mechanical trauma

Demographics

- GPC is caused by mechanical irritation &/or antigenic stimulation
  - CLs are most common cause
  - Variety of other causes (e.g., exposed suture)
  - Risk of GPC increases with soft CL, poorly fitted CL, and increased CL wearing time, age, and deposits
- Prevalence is estimated to be 1-5% of soft CL wearers and 1% of hard CL wearers

Presentation

- Symptoms include itching, CL discomfort &/or intolerance, blurry vision, mucoid discharge, foreign body sensation, and tearing
- Exam findings include superior tarsal conjunctival papillae > 0.3 mm in diameter, conjunctival hyperemia and thickening, and CL protein deposits

Treatment

- Removal of offending agents
  - Stop CL use for at least 2-4 weeks
  - Refit with new CL, improve lens hygiene, reduce CL wearing time, &/or switch from soft to hard CL
- Pharmacologic management includes topical mast cell stabilizers (MCSs), antihistamines, NSAIDs, &/or combination antihistamine/MCS drops
- Use short-term corticosteroids in severe cases
- Most cases resolve in < 1 week with treatment
- Most compliant patients will be able to resume CL use but should limit wear to < 6-8 hour/day and never sleep in them; if patient not able to do this, may need to permanently discontinue CL wear

__(Left)__ This slit-lamp photo shows giant papillary conjunctivitis (GPC) ➔. GPC involves the superior tarsal conjunctiva with papillae > 0.3 mm in diameter but can reach 1-2 mm. Papillae have a dilated vascular core surrounded by edema and inflammation that produces elevations. __(Right)__ This slit-lamp photo depicts GPC ⇨, which is caused by mechanical stimulation (contact lenses most common) or antigenic stimulation (environmental factors or other substances). (Courtesy C. Miller, MD.)

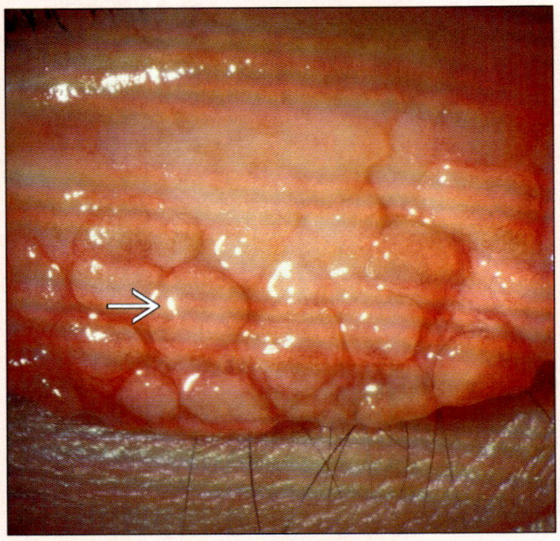

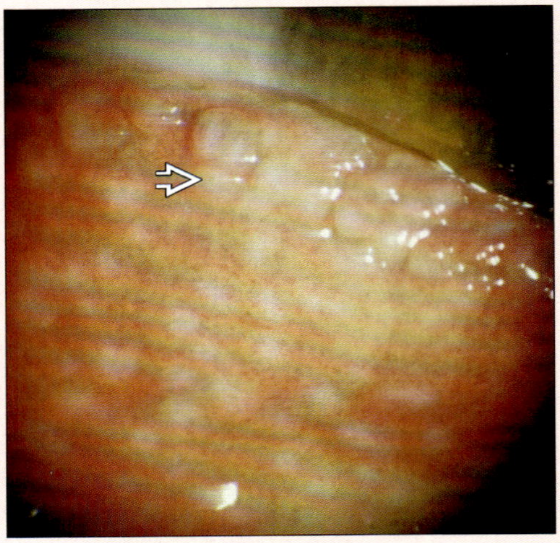

__(Left)__ This slit-lamp photo demonstrates follicular conjunctivitis ➔. In contrast to papillae, follicles are discrete, slightly elevated lesions of the conjunctiva with avascular cores. __(Right)__ This slit-lamp photo is of a patient with allergic conjunctivitis ⇨ with erythematous eyelids and conjunctival hyperemia. In GPC, an allergic immune response is mounted to antigens that come from environmental factors or substances (denatured proteins, debris) that have built up on a CL or other surface.

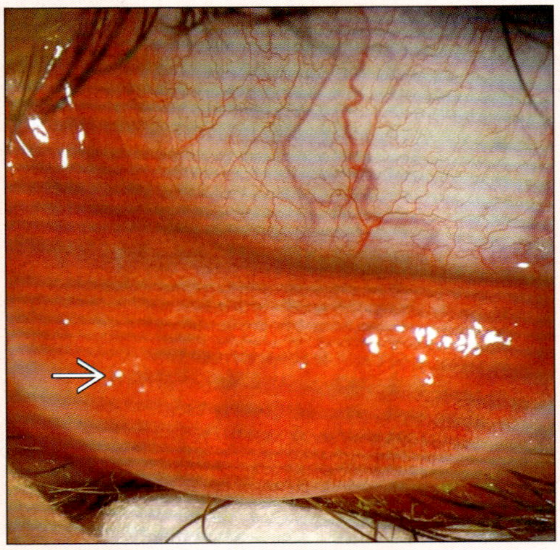

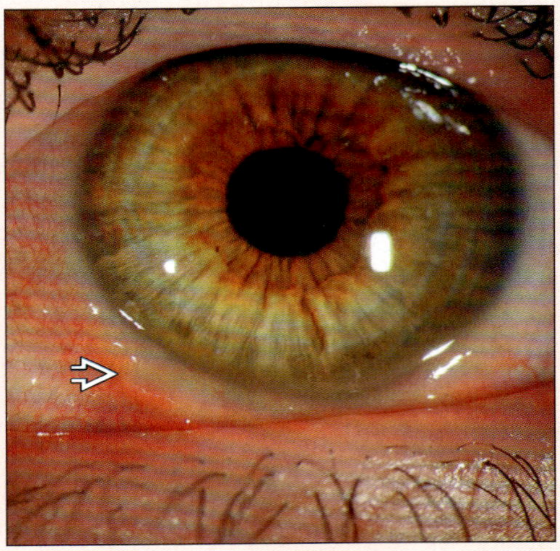

GIANT PAPILLARY CONJUNCTIVITIS

INTRODUCTION

Abbreviations

- Giant papillary conjunctivitis (GPC)

Definitions

- Inflammatory disorder involving superior tarsal conjunctiva, associated with contact lens (CL) or prosthesis use or other mechanical trauma

DEMOGRAPHICS

Etiology/Risk Factors

- GPC is caused by mechanical irritation &/or antigenic stimulation
  - Mechanical irritation can be caused by
    - CLs (most common cause)
      - Soft CL wearers are affected ~ 5x more frequently than hard CL wearers
      - Risk increases with increased CL wearing time, increased CL age, increased CL deposits, and poorly fitted CLs
    - Exposed sutures, ocular prosthesis, scleral buckle elements, band keratopathy, and filtering blebs
  - Antigenic stimulation
    - Allergic immune response is mounted to antigens that come from environmental factors or substances (denatured proteins, debris) that have built up on a CL or other surface
- Combination of type I and type IV hypersensitivity

Epidemiology

- Prevalence is estimated to be 1-5% of soft CL wearers and 1% of hard CL wearers

PRESENTATION

Symptoms

- On average, patients develop symptoms 8 months after beginning soft CL use and 8 years after beginning hard CL use
  - Itching (often continues after CL removal)
  - CL discomfort &/or intolerance, blurry vision
    - Leading to decreased CL use
  - Mucoid discharge, foreign body sensation, tearing

Exam Findings

- Conjunctival hyperemia and thickening
- Superior tarsal conjunctival papillae (need to flip upper lid to inspect tarsal surface)
  - > 0.3 mm in diameter
    - Often reach 1-2 mm in advanced disease
  - Involuted papillae can resemble follicles
- CL protein deposits
- Conjunctival opacification from cellular infiltration
- Degree of superior tarsal involvement varies

DIFFERENTIAL DIAGNOSIS

Vernal Keratoconjunctivitis (VKC)

- Typically affects young males in hot, dry climates
- Often associated with asthma and atopic dermatitis
- Not associated with CL or other mechanical trauma
- Histologic findings similar to GPC

EVALUATION/WORK-UP

Labs

- Diagnosis is usually made by history and clinical exam

Pathology

- Irregular conjunctival epithelial thickening over papillae with invaginations into the stroma
- Eosinophils, basophils, mast cells, lymphocytes, plasma cells, and fibroblast proliferation may be seen in biopsies of stroma and epithelium

TREATMENT

Medical

- Removal of offending agents
  - Stopping CL use for at least 2-4 weeks is preferable
  - Remove exposed sutures or scleral buckles, modify filtering bleb, &/or clean and polish prosthesis
- CL modifications
  - Refit the patient with new CLs
  - Reduce daily wearing time and improve lens hygiene
    - Use a preservative-free CL solution and saline and a hydrogen peroxide-based disinfectant
    - Use CL enzymatic cleaners at least 3x/week
  - Switch from extended-wear to daily-wear soft CLs
    - Daily disposable soft CLs are preferred
  - Switch to hard CLs if not improving
- Removal of offending agent and CL modifications are enough to resolve most mild to moderate GPC cases
- Pharmacologic management
  - Topical mast cell stabilizers (MCSs) (e.g., olopatadine, cromolyn)
    - Use at least until signs of GPC are gone
    - Most useful in early, mild cases
    - Can be used long term
  - Topical antihistamines, NSAIDs, or combination antihistamine/MCS drops are also beneficial
  - Topical corticosteroids can be used short term in severe cases not responding to other therapies
  - Topical tacrolimus ointment, 0.03% for severe, refractory GPC appears to be effective alternative

Follow-Up

- In 2-4 weeks, no CL use until symptoms have resolved
- Papillae may persist for months after symptoms resolve

Prognosis

- Most GPC cases resolve in < 1 week with treatment
- Most compliant patients will be able to resume CL use
  - Recurrences can be prevented with long-term MCS use
  - Long-term CL use is limited in a minority of patients

SELECTED REFERENCES

1. Donshik PC et al: Giant papillary conjunctivitis. Immunol Allergy Clin North Am. 28(1):83-103, vi, 2008
2. Elhers WH et al: Giant papillary conjunctivitis. Curr Opin Allergy Clin Immunol. 8(5):445-9, 2008
3. Kymionis GD et al: Tacrolimus ointment 0.03% in the eye for treatment of giant papillary conjunctivitis. Cornea. 27(2):228-9, 2008

LIGNEOUS CONJUNCTIVITIS

Key Facts

Introduction
- Chronic, pseudomembranous conjunctivitis typically associated with type I plasminogen deficiency

Demographics
- Absence of plasminogen leads to impaired fibrinolysis and buildup of fibrin-rich membranes
- Also caused by improper inflammatory response to tissue damage in genetically susceptible patients
  - Mostly seen with infection, local injury, and burns
- Very rare and occurs more often in young individuals

Presentation
- Symptoms include ocular irritation, tearing, foreign body sensation, photophobia, and pain
- Early-stage lesions are friable, elevated, and highly vascularized
- Lesions progress to become white, yellow, or red fibrin-rich pseudomembranes
  - Most commonly found on palpebral surfaces
  - Can develop wood-like (thick, firm) consistency with yellowish mucoid discharge over the lesion
- Generally, a systemic disease with possible extraocular involvement

Treatment
- Topical and systemic plasminogen or FFP with or without a plasminogen activator (tPA or uPA)
- Complete excision of lesions is necessary
- Post-excision therapy helps prevent recurrence
  - Continued topical and systemic plasminogen or FFP
  - Use a corticosteroid in combination with heparin &/ or 2% topical cyclosporin A
- Follow-up daily until no evidence of recurrence
- Treatment is improving with new therapies but still often leads to unsatisfactory results and recurrences

*(**Left**) This slit-lamp photo demonstrates a case of ligneous conjunctivitis (LC) →. Early-stage LC lesions are friable, elevated, and highly vascularized and later progress to become fibrin-rich pseudomembranes. They can develop a wood-like consistency. (Courtesy C. Miller, MD.) (**Right**) This slit-lamp photo depicts a patient with LC →, a condition usually associated with type I plasminogen deficiency and impaired fibrinolysis. Systemic symptoms are common. (Courtesy C. Miller, MD.)*

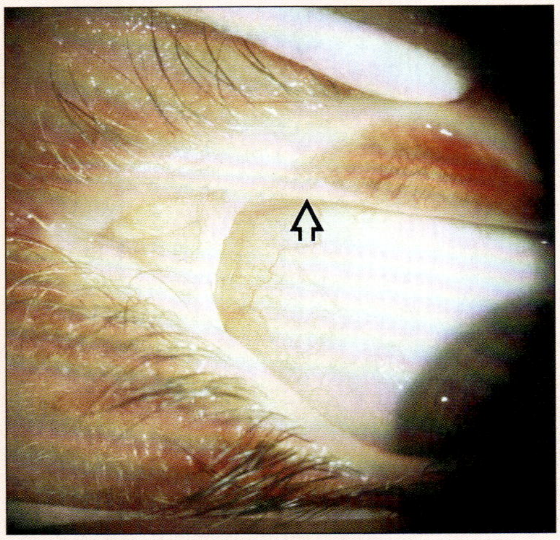

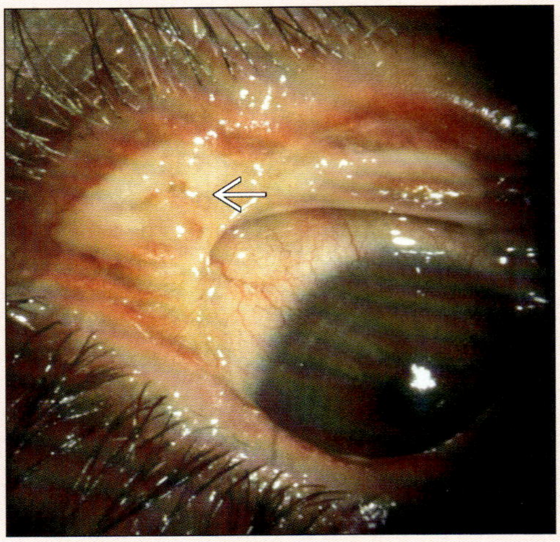

*(**Left**) Slit-lamp photo shows a pseudomembrane in a case of epidemic keratoconjunctivitis (EKC) →. LC can be differentiated from several types of pseudomembranous/ membranous conjunctivitis by history, clinical exam, conjunctival culture, and, if needed, a conjunctival biopsy. (Courtesy C. Miller, MD.) (**Right**) This slit-lamp photo shows EKC and a pseudomembrane →. Pseudomembranous/ membranous conjunctivitis causes include bacterial, viral, and chemical. (Courtesy C. Miller, MD.)*

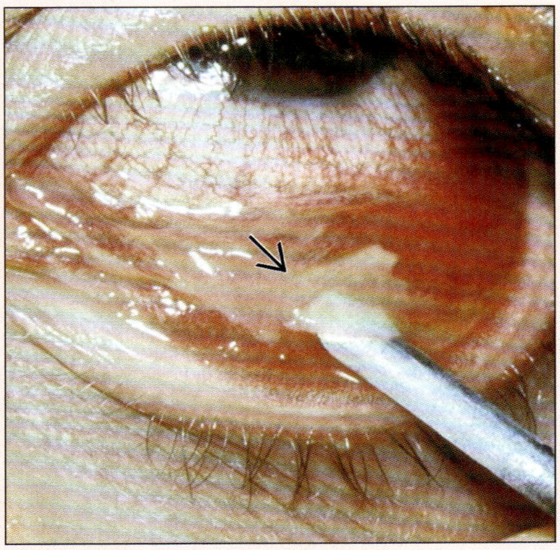

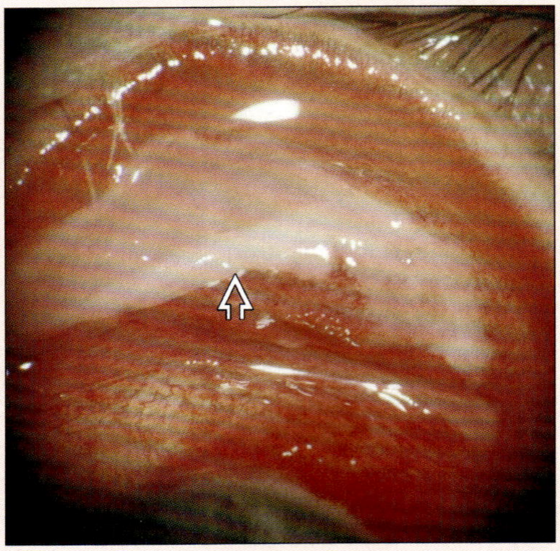

LIGNEOUS CONJUNCTIVITIS

INTRODUCTION

Abbreviations

- Ligneous conjunctivitis (LC)

Definitions

- Chronic, pseudomembranous conjunctivitis typically associated with plasminogen deficiency

DEMOGRAPHICS

Etiology/Risk Factors

- Most commonly due to a type I plasminogen deficiency
  - Autosomal recessive mode of inheritance
  - Absence of plasminogen leads to impaired fibrinolysis and buildup of fibrin-rich membranes
- Also caused by improper inflammatory response to tissue damage in genetically susceptible patients
  - Mostly seen with local injury (e.g., surgery or trauma), infection, and burns

Epidemiology

- Very rare
- Mean age of onset ranges from 13 to 16 years
  - Can occur at any age
- Median age of onset ranges from 3.5 to 5.5 years
- Slight female predominance (1.27:1)

PRESENTATION

Symptoms

- Early-stage symptoms include ocular irritation, tearing, and foreign body sensation
- Late-stage complaints include early-stage symptoms plus photophobia, pain, and cosmetic deformity

Exam Findings

- Early-stage lesions are friable, elevated, and highly vascularized
- Lesions progress to become white, yellow, or red fibrin-rich pseudomembranes
  - Most commonly found on palpebral surfaces but can also occur on bulbar conjunctiva
  - Can develop wood-like (thick, firm) consistency with yellowish mucoid discharge covering the lesion
- Severe cases may have corneal scarring and neovascularization
- Bilateral involvement is typical
- Generally, a systemic disease that often has extraocular involvement, including
  - Periodontal tissue, middle ear, lower and upper respiratory tract, kidney, and female genital tract
    - Life-threatening airway obstruction can occur with pulmonary involvement

DIFFERENTIAL DIAGNOSIS

Pseudomembranous/Membranous Conjunctivitis

- Other causes besides LC include bacteria, viruses, and chemicals
- Distinguish from LC by history, clinical exam, conjunctival culture, and, if needed, biopsy

EVALUATION/WORK-UP

Labs

- Conjunctival cultures to rule out bacterial pseudomembranous/membranous conjunctivitis
- Serum type 1 plasminogen

Pathology

- Large subepithelial or superficial deposits of fibrin and other plasma proteins under thinning epithelium
  - Granulation tissue, T lymphocytes, eosinophilic hyaline material, and IgG are commonly found

TREATMENT

Medical

- Topical and systemic plasminogen or FFP
  - Consider combining treatment with a plasminogen activator (tPA or uPA)
    - Softens pseudomembranes for easier excision

Surgical

- Before surgical intervention, obtain pulmonology consult to evaluate for possible respiratory complications
- Complete excision of lesions is necessary
  - With or without adjunctive cryotherapy or diathermy
  - Expect significant bleeding during surgery
  - Recurrences are common, especially if lesions are not completely removed
- Post-excision therapy helps prevent recurrence
  - Optimal treatment is not certain but can include
    - Topical and systemic plasminogen or FFP
    - Intensive therapy with a corticosteroid in combination with heparin &/or 2% topical cyclosporin A
      - Taper medications over the course of weeks
      - Treat until wound healing is complete with no sign of regrowth
      - Topical antibiotic is also recommended
    - Amniotic membrane transplantation has been effective
    - Other medications with some success include mitomycin C, azathioprine, hyaluronidase, and α-chymotrypsin

Follow-Up

- Daily after excision until no evidence of recurrence
- Daily debridement for recurrent lesions

Prognosis

- Resolution without treatment is uncommon
- Treatment is improving with new therapies but still often leads to unsatisfactory results and recurrences

SELECTED REFERENCES

1. Gürlü VP et al: Systemic and topical fresh-frozen plasma treatment in a newborn with ligneous conjunctivitis. Cornea. 27(4):501-3, 2008
2. Schuster V et al: Plasminogen deficiency. J Thromb Haemost. 5(12):2315-22, 2007
3. Heidemann DG et al: Treatment of ligneous conjunctivitis with topical plasmin and topical plasminogen. Cornea. 22(8):760-2, 2003

SUPERIOR LIMBIC KERATOCONJUNCTIVITIS

Key Facts

Introduction
- Recurrent inflammatory disorder involving superior cornea and conjunctiva

Demographics
- Exact etiology is unknown; thought to be due to mechanical trauma of superior palpebral and bulbar conjunctiva rubbing against each other

Presentation
- Ocular irritation, redness, foreign body sensation, burning, tearing, photophobia, mucoid discharge
- Chronic with frequent exacerbations and remissions
- Superior palpebral conjunctiva papillary reaction
- Thickened superior bulbar conjunctiva
- Superior limbal hypertrophy, corneal micropannus
- Fine punctate fluorescein and rose bengal staining of superior cornea, conjunctiva, and limbus
- Superior bulbar conjunctival and corneal filaments

Evaluation/Work-Up
- Diagnosis is usually made by history of ocular irritation and unique patterns of corneal and conjunctival staining and inflammation
- Thyroid function tests to evaluate for thyroid disease
  - Often associated with thyroid eye disease

Treatment
- Multiple options but no clear treatment of choice
- Conservative treatment for mild cases includes lubrication, punctal occlusion, topical cyclosporine
- Consider 0.5-1% silver nitrate, superior conjunctival resection, recession, thermocauterization or cryotherapy, supratarsal triamcinolone injection, soft CL, or pressure patch
- Prognosis generally excellent
- Follow-up every 2 weeks while symptomatic
- Usually lasts 1-10 years and resolves spontaneously

*(**Left**) This slit-lamp photo is of superior limbic keratoconjunctivitis (SLK). Hyperemic superior bulbar conjunctiva, superior limbal hypertrophy ➡, and corneal pannus can be observed. (Courtesy C. Miller, MD.) (**Right**) This slit-lamp photo demonstrates SLK ➡. The bulbar conjunctiva is thick and mildly hyperemic with extension onto the cornea. Redundancy of the superior bulbar conjunctiva can often be seen. The disease is often chronic and can have frequent exacerbations and remissions.*

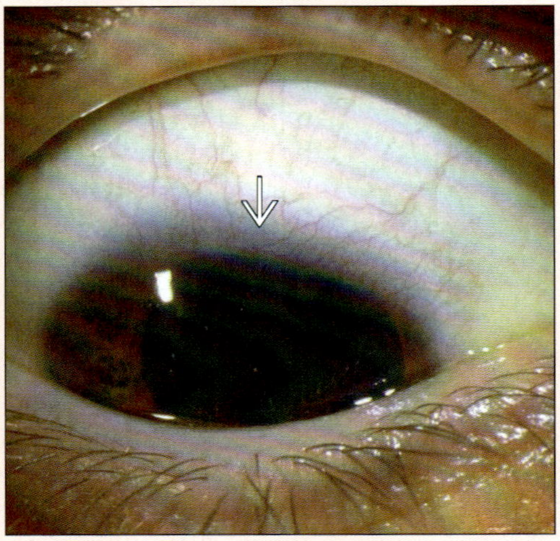

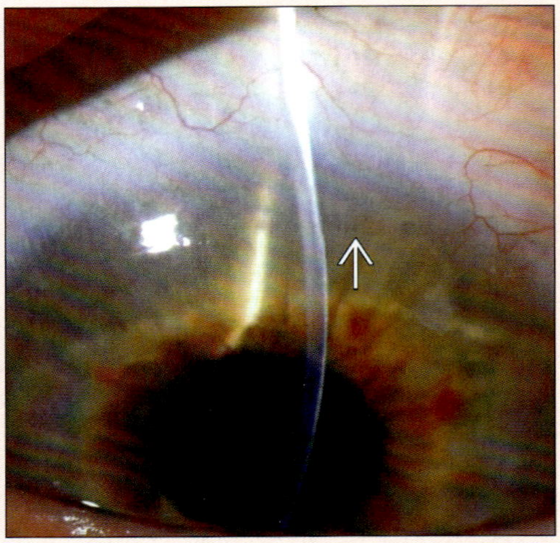

*(**Left**) This slit-lamp photo again shows SLK. Note the hyperemic superior bulbar conjunctiva ➡ and corneal pannus. SLK is thought to be secondary to mechanical trauma of the superior palpebral conjunctiva rubbing against the superior bulbar conjunctiva. (Courtesy C. Miller, MD.) (**Right**) This slit-lamp photo depicts SLK, which is often bilateral but can present asymmetrically. At times, superior conjunctival and corneal filaments may be seen.*

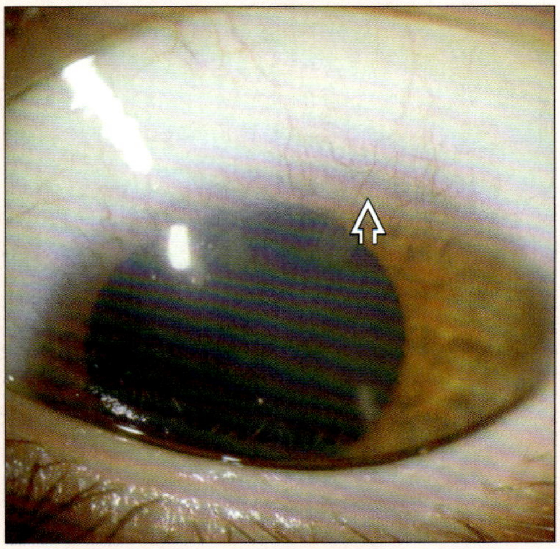

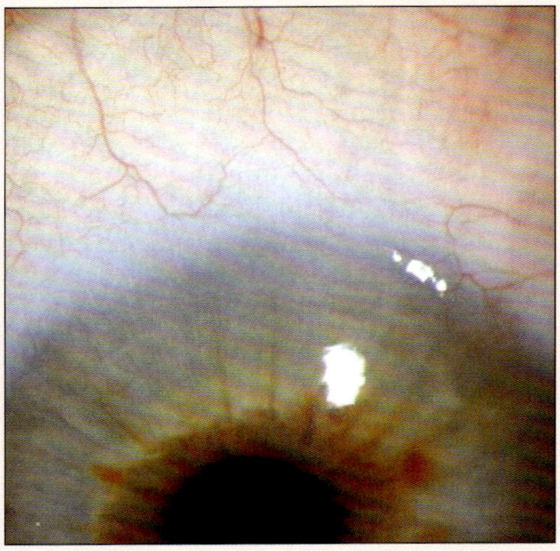

SUPERIOR LIMBIC KERATOCONJUNCTIVITIS

INTRODUCTION

Abbreviations
- Superior limbic keratoconjunctivitis (SLK)

Definitions
- Recurrent inflammatory disorder involving superior conjunctiva (bulbar and tarsal), superior limbus, and cornea

DEMOGRAPHICS

Etiology/Risk Factors
- Exact etiology is unknown
- Thought to be due to mechanical trauma of superior palpebral conjunctiva rubbing against superior bulbar conjunctiva
  - Causes of mechanical trauma in SLK include tight upper lids &/or loose, redundant conjunctival tissue
- Frequently associated with thyroid eye disease
  - Particularly hyperthyroidism
  - Present in ≥ 30% of SLK cases
- Other associations include keratoconjunctivitis sicca, blepharospasm, and hyperparathyroidism

Epidemiology
- Average age of onset ranges from 30-55 years
- Female:male = 3:1

PRESENTATION

Symptoms
- Ocular irritation, redness, foreign body sensation, burning, tearing, photophobia, mucoid discharge
- Chronic with frequent exacerbations and remissions

Exam Findings
- Typically a bilateral disease, but often asymmetric
- Fine papillary reaction of superior palpebral conjunctiva with a velvety appearance
- Thick, hyperemic superior bulbar conjunctiva
- Superior limbal hypertrophy, corneal micropannus
- Fine punctate fluorescein and rose bengal staining of superior cornea, conjunctiva, and limbus
- Superior conjunctival and corneal filaments
- Redundancy of superior bulbar conjunctiva
  - Seen with light downward pressure on upper lid

DIFFERENTIAL DIAGNOSIS

Contact Lens SLK (CL-SLK)
- Similar presentation as SLK but differs in the following
  - Keratinization is milder, no nuclear degradation
  - Minimal tarsal conjunctival involvement, no filaments, no association with thyroid disease, no female predilection
  - Signs and symptoms worsen with CL use
  - Can present with decreased visual acuity
  - Clinical changes thought to be due to thimerosal
- More correctly termed CL-induced keratoconjunctivitis

Dry Eye Syndrome
- Filaments occur in lower 1/2 of cornea, not in superior 1/2 as in SLK

EVALUATION/WORK-UP

Labs
- Diagnosis is usually made by history of ocular irritation and unique patterns of corneal and conjunctival staining and inflammation
  - Use fluorescein and rose bengal staining
- Thyroid function tests to evaluate for thyroid disease
- Schirmer test is decreased in some patients

Pathology
- Histologic examination of superior bulbar conjunctiva shows epithelial thickening and keratinization with loss of goblet cells
  - Epithelial cells and stroma can be edematous
  - Electron microscopy can demonstrate abnormal nuclear chromatin aggregation and distribution
- Superior tarsal conjunctiva histology depicts an infiltrate of neutrophils, lymphocytes, and plasma cells

TREATMENT

Medical
- Multiple options but no clear treatment of choice
- Conservative treatment for mild cases includes lubrication with preservative-free tears during day and ointment at night; punctal occlusion and cyclosporine 0.05% 2x daily may also be considered
- If the above measures do not alleviate symptoms, consider the following options
  - Apply 0.5-1% silver nitrate solution to anesthetized superior palpebral and bulbar conjunctiva
    - Use for ~ 15 seconds, and irrigate ocular surface with saline (do not use silver nitrate sticks)
    - Provides relief for 4-6 weeks; can be repeated
      - Can be reapplied 1 week after initial visit and repeated every 4-6 weeks thereafter
  - Soft contact lens or pressure patch
  - 10% N-acetylcysteine for mucous or filaments
  - Topical cromolyn and lodoxamide for symptom relief
  - Topical autologous serum, supratarsal triamcinolone injection, and retinoic acid can be beneficial
  - Steroids are not effective long term

Surgical
- Superior conjunctival resection (best combined with tenon layer excision in patients with a normal Schirmer test), thermocauterization, cryotherapy, or recession

Follow-Up
- Every 2 weeks while symptomatic

Prognosis
- Generally, excellent
- Usually lasts 1-10 years and resolves spontaneously

SELECTED REFERENCES

1. Sahin A et al: Topical cyclosporine a in the treatment of superior limbic keratoconjunctivitis: a long-term follow-up. Cornea. 27(2):193-5, 2008
2. Nelson JD: Superior limbic keratoconjunctivitis (SLK). Eye (Lond). 3 (Pt 2):180-9, 1989
3. Theodore FH et al: Superior limbic keratoconjunctivitis. Clinical and pathological correlations. Arch Ophthalmol. 84(4):481-4, 1970

TOXIC FOLLICULAR CONJUNCTIVITIS

Key Facts

Introduction
- Ocular toxicity induced by medication or other agent

Demographics
- Due to direct exposure of agent to ocular surface
  - Can be due to drug itself, its vehicle, or a preservative
- Probably result of mitogenic effect of some drugs
- Toxic keratoconjunctivitis (TKC) is most often caused by aminoglycosides, topical anesthetics, antineoplastic agents, antivirals, and preservatives
- Toxic follicular conjunctivitis (TFC) is most often caused by antiviral agents, cycloplegic agents, antiglaucoma agents, and epinephrine

Presentation
- Pain, foreign body sensation, photophobia, redness
- TKC findings include inferior punctate epithelial erosions, coarse keratopathy, vortex keratopathy, persistent epithelial defects, pseudodendrites, band keratopathy, neovascularization, and peripheral corneal infiltrates
- TFC findings include follicular reaction, usually palpebral but can include bulbar conjunctiva
  - Inferior tarsal conjunctiva and fornix most common

Evaluation/Work-Up
- Diagnosis is made by history and clinical exam
- Look for frequent drug instillation, multiple drug usage, and worsening symptoms upon instillation

Treatment
- Discontinue causative agent and use alternative medication, preferably preservative free
- Preservative-free artificial tears 4-8x per day
- Resolution of signs and symptoms varies from days to months after drug cessation
- Generally, excellent prognosis, but continued use of offending agent can lead to permanent changes

*(**Left**) Slit-lamp photo demonstrates superficial punctate keratopathy → in a patient with dry eye syndrome. Toxic follicular conjunctivitis (TFC) can be confused with dry eye syndrome, but dry eye syndrome does not improve with drug cessation. (**Right**) Slit-lamp photo shows lower palpebral follicular conjunctivitis → with hyperemia and follicles present. The most common locations for follicular reactions in TFC are the lower fornix and inferior palpebral conjunctiva.*

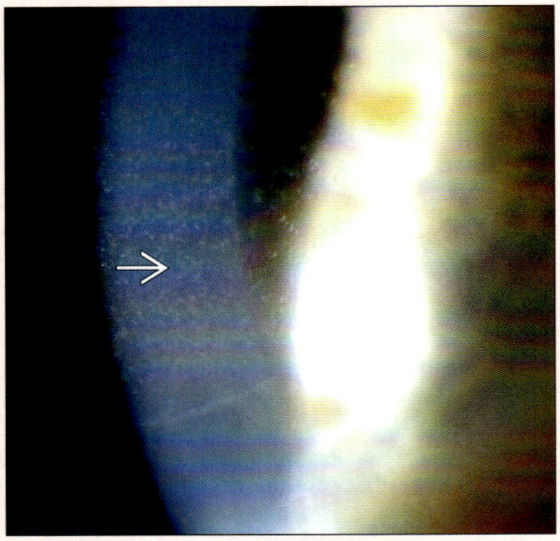

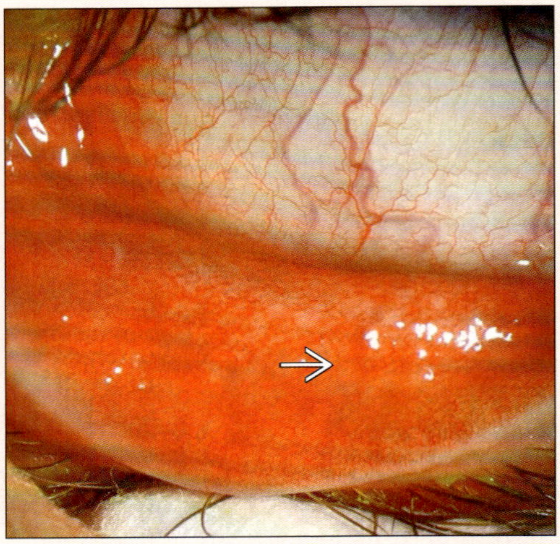

*(**Left**) This slit-lamp photo shows a patient with adenoviral conjunctivitis, which can be confused with TFC. Adenoviral conjunctivitis exam findings include conjunctival follicles →, hyperemia →, tender preauricular lymphadenopathy, and eyelid edema and erythema. (**Right**) Slit-lamp photo shows allergic conjunctivitis. Eyelid erythema → and conjunctival hyperemia and chemosis → are noted. Itching is much more common in these patients than in patients with TFC.*

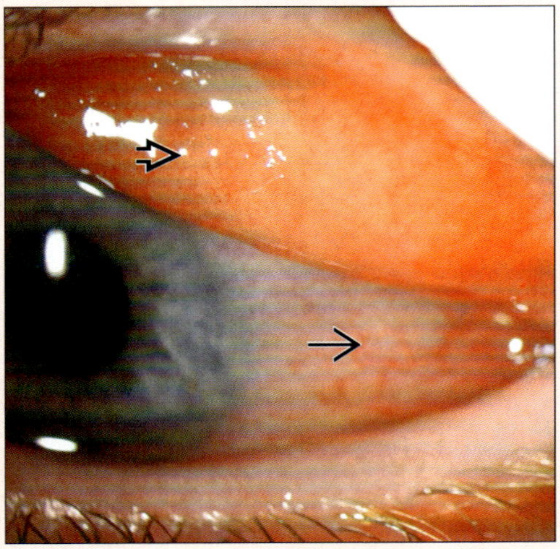

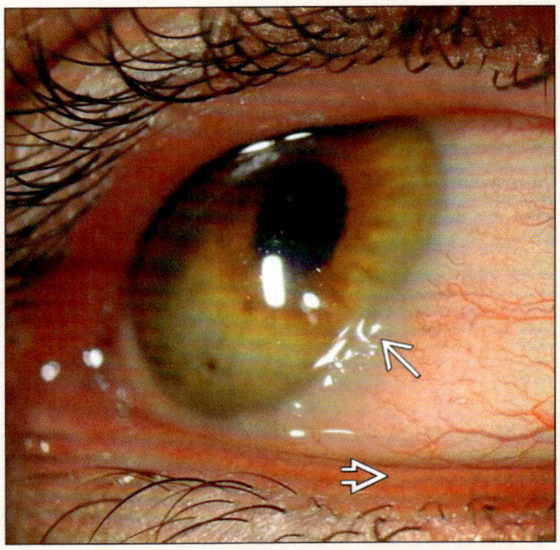

TOXIC FOLLICULAR CONJUNCTIVITIS

INTRODUCTION

Definitions
- Ocular toxicity induced by medication or other agent

Subtypes
- Toxic keratoconjunctivitis (TKC)
- Toxic follicular conjunctivitis (TFC)

DEMOGRAPHICS

Etiology/Risk Factors
- Result of direct exposure of an agent to ocular surface
  - Can be due to drug itself, its vehicle, or a preservative
  - Eye makeup, chlorine, and other environmental irritants can also be causative
- Corneal and conjunctival epithelium can retain agents for days after initial medication instillation
  - Tear deficiency or outflow obstruction increases risk
- Probably result of mitogenic effect of some drugs
- Most often occurs only after long-term drug use
- TKC is most often caused by aminoglycosides (neomycin, gentamicin), topical anesthetics (proparacaine), antineoplastic agents (mitomycin C), antivirals (idoxuridine, trifluorothymidine), and preservatives (benzalkonium chloride, thimerosal)
- TFC is most often caused by antiviral agents, antiglaucoma agents (brimonidine, pilocarpine, and many others), epinephrine, and cycloplegic agents

Epidemiology
- Somewhat common, difficult to estimate incidence or prevalence due to wide variety of offending agents
- TFC occurred in 9.6% of patients treated with brimonidine in 1 study

PRESENTATION

Symptoms
- Pain
- Foreign body sensation
- Photophobia
- Redness
- Tearing

Exam Findings
- TKC
  - Corneal findings include punctate epithelial erosions (usually inferior), coarse keratopathy, vortex keratopathy (whorl-like epithelial deposits), persistent epithelial defects, pseudodendrites, band keratopathy, neovascularization, and peripheral corneal infiltrates
- TFC
  - Follicular reaction, usually of palpebral conjunctiva but sometimes can include bulbar conjunctiva
    - Most common locations are lower fornix and inferior palpebral conjunctiva
  - Hyperemia and mild, if any, inferior punctate staining
- Reaction can also be papillary and lead to cicatrization
- Some patients may develop drug-induced pemphigoid, manifested by conjunctival scarring that leads to forniceal shortening and symblepharon formation

DIFFERENTIAL DIAGNOSIS

Dry Eye Syndrome
- Typically presents with abnormal tear film, scant tear meniscus, and decreased Schirmer test
- Generally, would not improve with drug cessation

Adenoviral Conjunctivitis
- Exam findings include tender preauricular adenopathy, conjunctival follicles and hyperemia, and eyelid edema and erythema
- Itching and watery discharge are common
- History of exposure often present

Atopic Keratoconjunctivitis
- Patients typically have history of asthma or eczema
- Itching much more common
- Disease is chronic

EVALUATION/WORK-UP

Labs
- Diagnosis is made by history and clinical exam
  - Look for frequent drug instillation, multiple drug usage, and worsening symptoms upon instillation
  - Rose bengal stain can aid in detecting early signs of corneal or conjunctival toxicity

Pathology
- Histology would reveal macrophages, lymphocytes, subepithelial fibrosis, epithelial cell death, plasma cell-membrane disruption, and microvilli loss
- Consider conjunctival biopsy if diagnosis is uncertain

TREATMENT

Medical
- Discontinue use of causative substance
  - Use alternative medication if needed, preferably preservative free
- Preservative-free artificial tears 4-8x per day
- Cold compresses 4x/day

Follow-Up
- 1-2 weeks
- Resolution of signs and symptoms varies from days to months after drug cessation

Prognosis
- Generally, excellent prognosis, but continued use of offending agent can lead to permanent changes

SELECTED REFERENCES

1. Adkins JC et al: Brimonidine. A review of its pharmacological properties and clinical potential in the management of open-angle glaucoma and ocular hypertension. Drugs Aging. 12(3):225-41, 1998
2. Liesegang TJ: Conjunctival changes associated with glaucoma therapy: implications for the external disease consultant and the treatment of glaucoma. Cornea. 17(6):574-83, 1998
3. Fiore PM et al: Drug-induced pemphigoid. A spectrum of diseases. Arch Ophthalmol. 105(12):1660-3, 1987

VERNAL CONJUNCTIVITIS

Key Facts

Introduction
- Bilateral, recurrent, self-limiting allergic inflammation of the conjunctiva
- Palpebral, limbal, and mixed subtypes

Demographics
- Most common during spring and summer but can be present year round, especially as disease progresses
- History of asthma, rhinitis, or eczema in most patients
- Typically occurs in young males living in hot climates

Presentation
- Itching, photophobia, tearing, foreign body sensation, hyperemia, burning, blepharospasm, discharge
- Palpebral vernal keratoconjunctivitis (VKC)
  - Involves upper palpebral conjunctiva
  - Flat-topped, polygonal, giant tarsal papillae are found
- Limbal VKC
  - Limbal papillae are gelatinous and confluent
- Corneal changes may include punctate epithelial erosions and keratitis, shield ulcers, subepithelial scars, and pseudogerontoxons

Evaluation/Work-Up
- Diagnosis is usually made by history and clinical exam

Treatment
- General treatment includes cool compresses, tears, climatotherapy, and allergen avoidance when possible
- Topical treatment includes
  - Antihistamines ± vasoconstrictors
  - Mast cell stabilizers (alone or in combo preparations)
  - Topical corticosteroids in short-term, high-dose regimens followed by a taper for severe cases
- Shield ulcers may require debridement or keratectomy to promote epithelial healing
- Generally good prognosis, with spontaneous resolution of disease after puberty

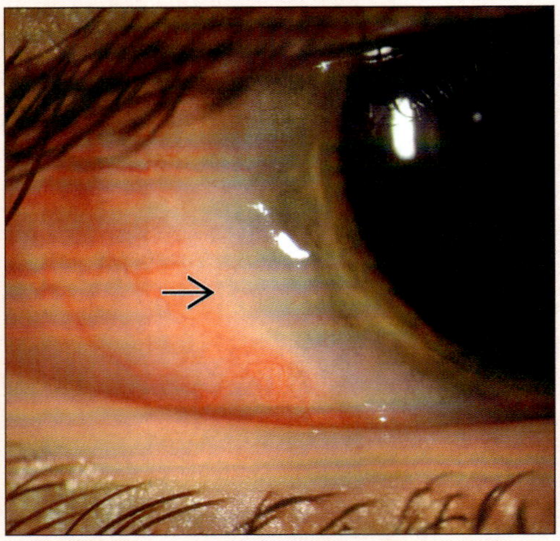
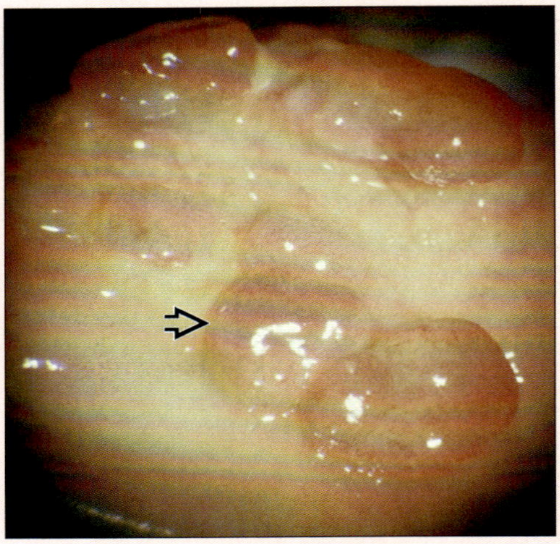

(Left) *This slit-lamp photo demonstrates vernal keratoconjunctivitis (VKC), with bulbar hyperemia and chemosis → evident. VKC involves type I and type IV hypersensitivity reactions and is most common during the spring and summer.* ***(Right)*** *This slit-lamp photo shows cobblestone papillae →, often seen with VKC. Papillary hypertrophy of the superior palpebral conjunctiva typically progresses to flat-topped, polygonal, giant tarsal papillae nicknamed cobblestone papillae. (Courtesy C. Miller, MD.)*

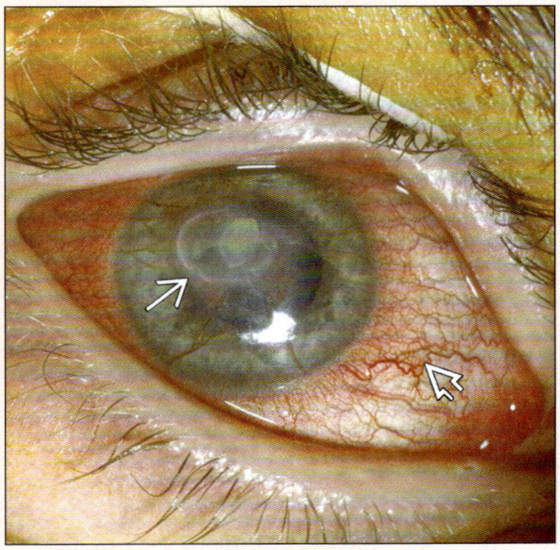
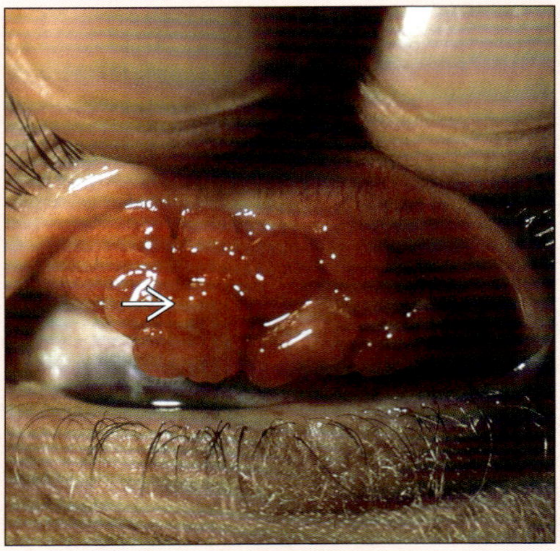

(Left) *External photo shows VKC with prominent, diffuse conjunctival hyperemia → and a shield ulcer →. VKC is often associated with other atopic manifestations, including asthma, rhinitis, or eczema, and is seen more often in hot, dry climates. (Courtesy C. Miller, MD.)* ***(Right)*** *This slit-lamp photo demonstrates cobblestone papillae of the superior palpebral conjunctiva →. A thick white discharge with sticky mucous filaments, termed ropy discharge, can often be seen. (Courtesy C. Miller, MD.)*

VERNAL CONJUNCTIVITIS

INTRODUCTION

Abbreviations

- Vernal keratoconjunctivitis (VKC)

Definitions

- Bilateral, recurrent, self-limiting allergic conjunctivitis

DEMOGRAPHICS

Etiology/Risk Factors

- Involves type I and type IV hypersensitivity reactions
- Most common during spring and summer but can be present year round, especially as disease progresses
- Often associated with other atopic manifestations
  - History of asthma, rhinitis, or eczema in most patients
  - Family history of atopic diseases in about 50% of cases

Epidemiology

- Onset is usually before 10 years of age
  - Generally resolves after puberty, 4-10 years after onset
- Before age 20, male to female ratio > 2:1
  - Gender difference almost neutral after age 20
- More common in hot, dry climates
  - West Africa, Mediterranean, and Middle East

PRESENTATION

Symptoms

- Itching, photophobia, tearing, foreign body sensation, hyperemia, burning, blepharospasm, discharge

Exam Findings

- Palpebral, limbal, and mixed subtypes
- Palpebral VKC
  - Involves upper palpebral conjunctiva
  - Thick, white discharge with sticky mucous filaments, termed ropy discharge
  - Bulbar hyperemia and chemosis
  - Diffuse superior palpebral papillae
    - Typically progresses to flat-topped, polygonal, giant tarsal papillae nicknamed cobblestone papillae
- Limbal VKC
  - Limbal papillae are gelatinous and confluent
  - Horner-Trantas dots (whitish raised limbal dots made up of epithelial cells and eosinophils) can be found
- Corneal changes may include
  - Punctate epithelial erosions and keratitis
  - Shield ulcers, which can impair epithelial healing
  - Subepithelial scar may appear with ulcer resolution
  - Pseudogerontoxon
    - Gray-white lipid deposition that may wax and wane in peripheral corneal stroma
      - Resembles arcus senilis

DIFFERENTIAL DIAGNOSIS

Atopic Keratoconjunctivitis (AKC)

- Generally has perennial symptoms, older patients, no gender predilection, lower tarsal involvement, and occasional corneal neovascularization and scarring

EVALUATION/WORK-UP

Labs

- Diagnosis is usually made by history and clinical exam

Pathology

- Conjunctival scraping would contain mast cells, eosinophils, and multiple other inflammatory cells

TREATMENT

Medical

- General treatment includes cool compresses, tears, climatotherapy, and allergen avoidance when possible
- Topical treatment
  - Antihistamines ± vasoconstrictors
    - Over the counter, suitable for mild VKC
  - Mast cell stabilizers
    - First-line of defense at onset of allergy season
    - Combo preparations of antihistamines and mast cell stabilizers are effective
    - Treatment should be started 2 weeks prior to allergy season and used throughout season
  - Topical corticosteroids
    - For severe cases or significant corneal involvement
      - Unfavorable long-term side effects limit use
    - Should be used in short-term, high-dose regimens followed by a taper
    - Supratarsal corticosteroid injection can be used to treat cases refractory to typical treatment
  - Topical NSAIDs can diminish itching
  - Immunomodulators
    - Cyclosporine 0.05% b.i.d. if not responding to steroids or if steroids are contraindicated
    - Maximum effect not seen for several weeks
- Shield ulcer merits treatment with a mast cell stabilizer, a topical corticosteroid, a topical antibiotic ointment, cycloplegic agent, and vitamin C/doxycycline to reduce melting
- Systemic anti-inflammatory therapy may be useful in severe cases not responsive to more traditional therapy

Surgical

- Shield ulcers may require debridement, superficial or phototherapeutic keratectomy, or keratectomy with amniotic graft to promote epithelial healing

Follow-Up

- Every 1 to 3 days if a shield ulcer is present, otherwise every few weeks
- Taper topical medications as symptoms improve

Prognosis

- Generally good, with spontaneous resolution of disease after puberty

SELECTED REFERENCES

1. Kumar S et al: Modern approach to managing vernal keratoconjunctivitis. Curr Allergy Asthma Rep. 10(3):155-62, 2010
2. Kumar S: Vernal keratoconjunctivitis: a major review. Acta Ophthalmol. 87(2):133-47, 2009
3. Buckley RJ: Vernal keratoconjunctivitis. Int Ophthalmol Clin. 28(4):303-8, 1988

CONJUNCTIVAL AND CORNEAL LACERATIONS

Key Facts

Introduction

- Conjunctival laceration: Superficial ocular injury that may or may not require surgical repair
- Partial-thickness corneal laceration: Descemet membrane not involved; thus, anterior chamber not violated
- Full-thickness corneal laceration or penetration: Constitutes open globe, ocular emergency

Demographics

- Corneal and conjunctival lacerations most commonly caused by blunt or penetrating trauma
- More common in young men

Treatment

- Conjunctival lacerations: Most heal without surgical intervention; treat with topical antibiotic ointment, pressure patch may be used for comfort
- Partial-thickness corneal laceration: Treat with antibiotic drops, cycloplegic agent, tetanus prophylaxis (for contaminated wounds), and bandage contact lens or pressure patch for comfort
- Full-thickness corneal laceration: Seidel (+), may have shallow anterior chamber, low IOP, peaked pupil, hyphema
    - Small slow-leaking and self-sealing lacerations may sometimes be managed with aqueous suppressants, bandage contact lens, and topical antibiotics or alternatively with pressure patch
    - Large or nonsealing wounds: Keep patient n.p.o. and admit to hospital, place eye shield, tetanus prophylaxis, start systemic antibiotics, and arrange emergent surgical repair
    - Cyanoacrylate glue may be used for cases with tissue loss or poorly sealing stellate wounds
- Intraocular foreign bodies and lens-corneal touch increase need for emergency intervention

*(**Left**) External photo shows a traumatic corneal laceration ➡ with iris prolapse ⇨. Some full-thickness lacerations are obvious on exam; however, most are not and require careful examination. (Courtesy R. Nosé, MD.) (**Right**) Slit-lamp photo shows a healing full-thickness corneal laceration following repair, with sutures still in place ➡. Further exploration should always be considered to exclude occult scleral lacerations extending posteriorly, especially when the corneal laceration extends to the limbus ⇨.*

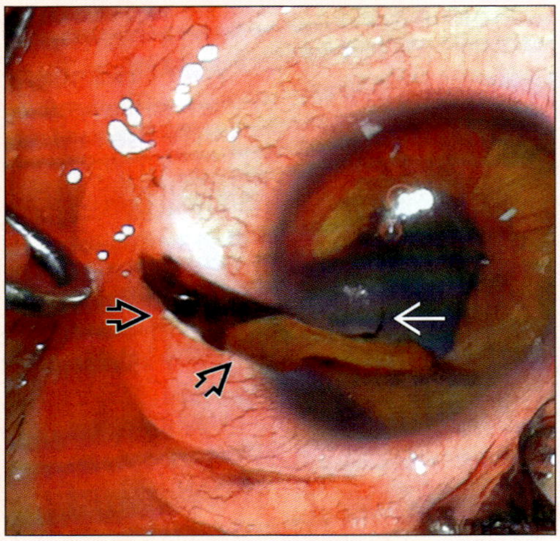

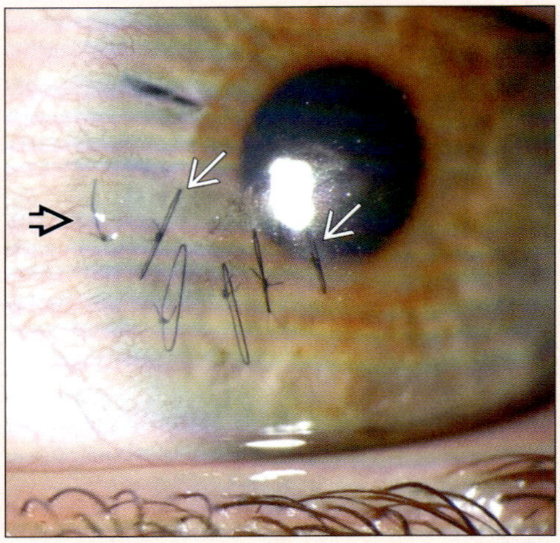

*(**Left**) Slit-lamp photo shows a stellate corneal laceration ➡. Stellate lacerations are typically the most difficult to make watertight. Careful thought should be given to suture placement prior to repair. Purse-string sutures may be helpful. (**Right**) Slit-lamp photo with cobalt blue light depicts a conjunctival laceration ➡ accentuated by fluorescein dye. Interrupted 6-O to 8-O absorbable sutures are traditionally used to repair larger conjunctival defects. Thorough evaluation should be performed to rule out deeper injury.*

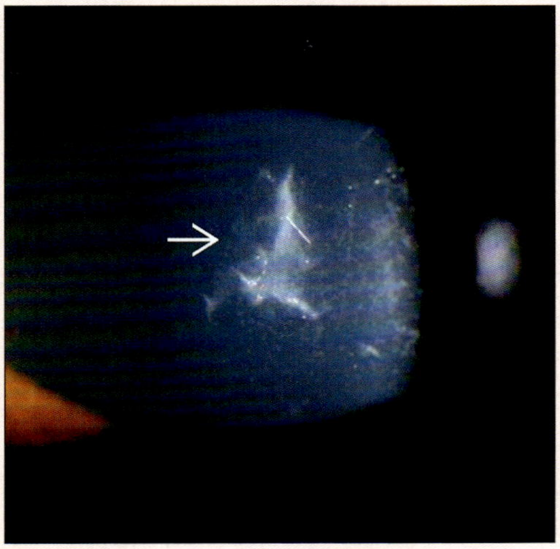

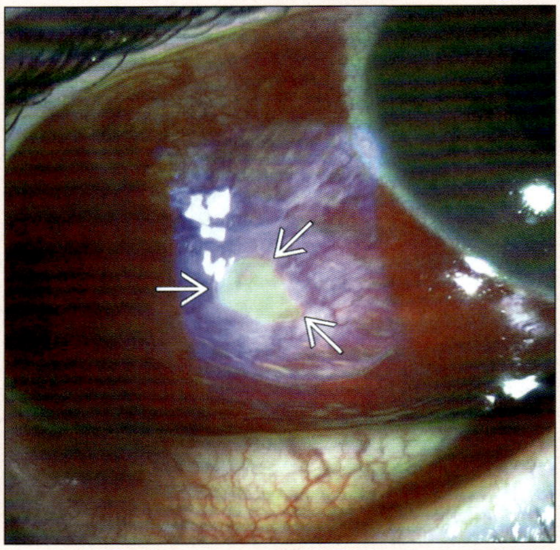

CONJUNCTIVAL AND CORNEAL LACERATIONS

INTRODUCTION

Definitions

- Lacerations of cornea or conjunctiva normally secondary to trauma

Subtypes

- Partial-thickness corneal laceration: Penetrates < 100% of cornea thickness, anterior chamber not violated
- Full-thickness corneal laceration: Open globe, ocular emergency

DEMOGRAPHICS

Etiology/Risk Factors

- Most commonly caused by blunt or penetrating ocular trauma
- High-risk activities ↑ ocular injury chance: Alcohol or narcotics use and high-risk sports and occupations without appropriate eye protection

Epidemiology

- Most commonly affects young males
- Average age of all ocular injuries: 29 years

PRESENTATION

Symptoms

- Mild to severe ocular pain, foreign body sensation, photophobia, epiphora, decreased vision, red eyes

Exam Findings

- Partial-thickness corneal laceration on exam
  - Seidel (-): Must rule out open globe, perform careful slit-lamp and funduscopic exam
- Full-thickness corneal laceration on slit-lamp exam
  - Seidel (+): Visualization of fluorescein stain over wound with cobalt blue light highlights aqueous leakage from wound
  - Low IOP: Avoid applanation tonometry if it will cause undue pressure on globe or if open globe suspected
  - Shallow anterior chamber, may have peaked iris if incarcerated in wound
- Conjunctival laceration: Conjunctival defect exposing underlying Tenon capsule and sclera on exam
  - Better visualized with fluorescein dye; may have associated conjunctival and subconjunctival hemorrhage
  - Must rule out open globe and occult injury on exam

EVALUATION/WORK-UP

Imaging

- CT scan of orbit with axial and coronal views for suspected open globe
- Seidel test to evaluate for leakage/rupture

TREATMENT

Medical

- Conjunctival lacerations: Most heal without need for surgical intervention; topical antibiotic ointment, pressure patch may be used for comfort
- Partial-thickness corneal laceration: Antibiotic drops, cycloplegic agent, tetanus prophylaxis for contaminated wounds, bandage contact lens or pressure patch for comfort
- Full-thickness corneal laceration (open globe): Once open-globe detected, defer further evaluation until in operating room to minimize further injury
  - Keep patient NPO and admit, place eye shield to protect eye, tetanus prophylaxis, start systemic antibiotics such as cefazolin and moxifloxacin, arrange emergent surgical repair
  - Small, slow-leaking, self-sealing lacerations may sometimes be managed with aqueous suppressants, bandage contact lens, and topical antibiotics; alternatively managed with pressure patch

Surgical

- Conjunctival laceration: Repair large lacerations > 1 cm with absorbable suture (typically 6-O to 8-O Vicryl)
- Partial-thickness corneal laceration: Deep lacerations with wound gape should be repaired to prevent corneal surface irregularities (typically 10-O nylon suture)
- Full-thickness corneal laceration: Explore adjacent sclera with appropriate conjunctival dissection to rule out injury of limbus and sclera, especially if laceration ends by limbus
  - Repair corneal lacerations with 10-O nylon sutures passed at 90% depth, use smaller passes for more central defects; needle bites should be vertical
  - Stellate lacerations may prove hard to repair and may require a purse-string suture or alternatively cyanoacrylate glue repair with placement of bandage contact lens
  - Cyanoacrylate glue may also be helpful in cases of tissue loss
  - Extensive corneal scarring resulting from laceration may eventually require lamellar or penetrating keratoplasty

Follow-Up

- Daily for corneal lacerations until there is no evidence of leakage or infection
- Weekly for uncomplicated conjunctival lacerations

Prognosis

- Depends on extent and concomitant ocular injury
- Prognostic indicators for open globes include
  - Type of injury
  - Location (anterior or posterior to rectus insertions) and extent of injury (> 1 cm)
  - Initial visual acuity
  - Presence of afferent pupillary defect
  - Lenticular involvement
  - Vitreous hemorrhage
  - Presence and type of intraocular foreign body

SELECTED REFERENCES

1. Ahmed Y et al: Endophthalmitis following open-globe injuries. Eye (Lond). 26(2):212-7, 2012
2. Castellarin AA et al: Open globe management. Compr Ophthalmol Update. 8(3):111-24, 2007
3. May DR et al: The epidemiology of serious eye injuries from the United States Eye Injury Registry. Graefes Arch Clin Exp Ophthalmol. 238(2):153-7, 2000

SUBCONJUNCTIVAL HEMORRHAGE

Key Facts

Introduction
- Blood located between conjunctiva and sclera

Demographics
- Caused by rupture or leakage of a small blood vessel
- Most cases are spontaneous, with no obvious cause
- May be caused by Valsalva maneuvers, vascular diseases (hypertension), trauma, acute conjunctivitis, anticoagulant and antiplatelet medications, high altitude, or underlying bleeding disorder
- Occurs frequently, incidence increases with age

Presentation
- Unilateral red eye, otherwise typically asymptomatic
- Collection of extravasated subconjunctival blood
  - Flat, red, demarcated, often focal but can be diffuse

Evaluation/Work-Up
- Ask about recent Valsalva maneuvers, medications, clotting disorders, contact lens use, trauma, vascular or systemic diseases, infection, and prior subconjunctival hemorrhages
- Check blood pressure
- Check IOP, extraocular motility (EOM), and resistance to retropulsion; look for signs of proptosis
  - If present, get CT scan in atraumatic cases to rule out orbital mass
- Rule out ruptured globe, orbital blowout fracture, and retrobulbar hemorrhage in traumatic cases
- For recurrent cases, obtain a complete blood count, prothrombin time, partial thromboplastin time, bleeding time, and protein C and protein S values

Treatment
- No medical treatment is typically necessary
- Artificial tears, cool/warm compresses for relief
- Follow-up for recurrence or if blood persists > 2 weeks
- Typically resolves spontaneously in 1-2 weeks
- Possible referral to internist depending on etiology

*(**Left**) This slit-lamp photo demonstrates a large subconjunctival hemorrhage that involves 360° of the conjunctiva. These events are typically unilateral and are most often spontaneous, with no obvious cause. (**Right**) This slit-lamp photo shows a temporal subconjunctival hemorrhage. Although most cases have no obvious cause, they may be caused by Valsalva maneuvers, vascular disease, trauma, an underlying bleeding disorder, or the use of anticoagulant or antiplatelet medications.*

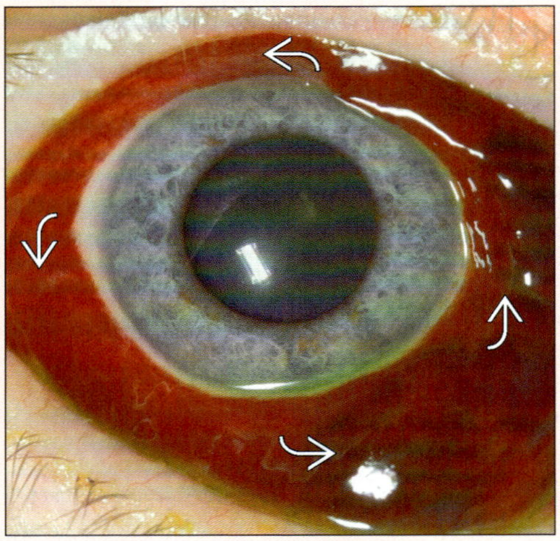

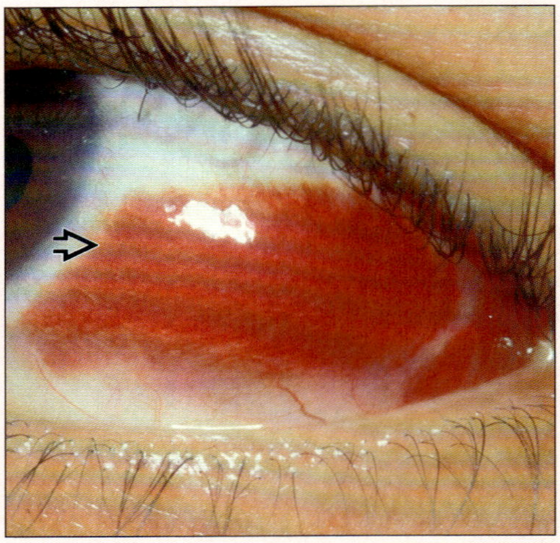

*(**Left**) This slit-lamp photo depicts another subconjunctival hemorrhage. Patients are typically asymptomatic except for cosmetic complaints. No blood should be found on the ocular surface. (Courtesy C. Miller, MD.) (**Right**) This slit-lamp photo shows a subconjunctival hemorrhage, which are typically flat, red, and demarcated. Though usually red, hemorrhages can vary from red to orange to yellow depending on the stage of blood resorption. They are caused by rupture or leakage of small blood vessels.*

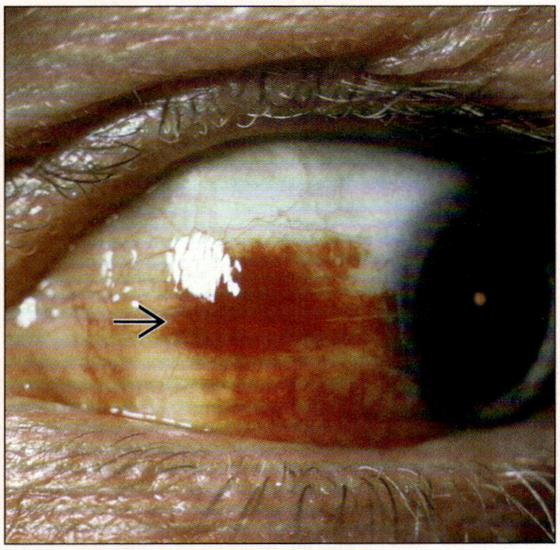

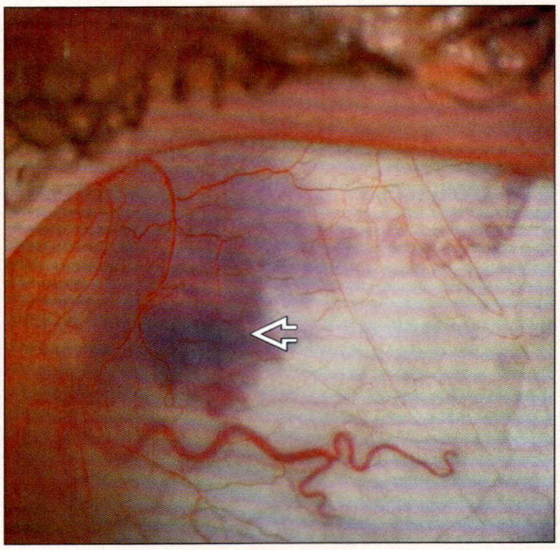

SUBCONJUNCTIVAL HEMORRHAGE

INTRODUCTION

Definitions
- Collection of blood located between conjunctiva and sclera

DEMOGRAPHICS

Etiology/Risk Factors
- Caused by rupture or leakage of small blood vessels
- Most cases are spontaneous, with no obvious cause
- May be caused by the following
  - Valsalva maneuvers
    - Coughing, sneezing, straining, vomiting, lifting
  - Vascular diseases
    - Hypertension: Major risk factor
    - Arteriolosclerosis and diabetes: Compromise vasculature integrity
  - Trauma
    - Isolated conjunctival injury
      - Surgery or subconjunctival injection
    - Eye rubbing
    - Contact-lens induced
      - Risk increases with conjunctivochalasis and pinguecula
    - Can be associated with retrobulbar hemorrhage, ruptured globe, and orbital blowout fracture
  - Acute conjunctivitis
  - Underlying bleeding disorder
    - Hemophilia, vitamin C deficiency
  - Anticoagulants or antiplatelet medications
    - Warfarin, aspirin, clopidogrel, vitamin E, garlic
  - Local vasculature anomalies
  - High altitude (mountaineering)

Epidemiology
- Occurs frequently
- More common in patients > 50 years of age

PRESENTATION

Symptoms
- Red eye (almost always unilateral)
  - Often quite dramatic and can frighten patients
- Otherwise, typically asymptomatic
  - Foreign body sensation may be present
- Often noticed when patient wakes up in the morning and looks in the mirror

Exam Findings
- Collection of extravasated subconjunctival blood
  - Flat, red, demarcated, often focal but can be diffuse
  - No blood should be on ocular surface
  - Usually red in color but can vary from red to orange to yellow depending on stage of blood resorption

DIFFERENTIAL DIAGNOSIS

Kaposi Sarcoma
- Violaceous vascular lesion of palpebral or bulbar conjunctiva that develops more gradually and occurs in immunocompromised patients

Acute Hemorrhagic Conjunctivitis
- Dramatic, sudden onset of painful follicular conjunctivitis with subconjunctival hemorrhages
  - Hemorrhages progress from petechial to confluent
  - Normally a highly contagious tropical disease that occurs in epidemics and resolves after 1-2 weeks
    - Normally caused by enterovirus type 70 and coxsackievirus A24 variant

EVALUATION/WORK-UP

Labs
- Diagnosis is usually made by history and clinical exam
  - Ask about recent Valsalva maneuvers, medications, clotting disorders, contact lens use, trauma, vascular or systemic diseases, infection, and prior subconjunctival hemorrhages
  - Check blood pressure
  - Check for orbital signs: ↑ IOP, extraocular motility (EOM), and resistance to retropulsion; look for signs of proptosis
    - If present in atraumatic cases, obtain CT scan to rule out orbital mass
  - Rule out ruptured globe, orbital blowout fracture, and retrobulbar hemorrhage in traumatic cases
- For recurrent cases, obtain complete blood count, prothrombin time, partial thromboplastin time, bleeding time, protein C and protein S testing
- Check for conjunctival laceration upon resolution

Imaging
- CT scan with and without contrast to rule out orbital mass for cases with increased IOP, decreased EOM, proptosis, &/or resistance to retropulsion

TREATMENT

Medical
- No medical treatment is typically necessary
- Artificial tears if ocular irritation is present
- Cool compresses followed by warm compresses for ~ 24 hours may provide relief and help blood resorb

Follow-Up
- None required unless blood continues to persist after 14 days or condition recurs
- Possible referral to an internist depending on etiology

Prognosis
- Typically resolves spontaneously in 1-2 weeks
  - Hemorrhage will appear larger on 2nd day because of blood redistribution but will soon decrease due to blood resorption

SELECTED REFERENCES

1. Mimura T et al: Contact lens-induced subconjunctival hemorrhage. Am J Ophthalmol. 150(5):656-665, 2010
2. Mimura T et al: Recent causes of subconjunctival hemorrhage. Ophthalmologica. 224(3):133-7, 2010
3. Curl A: Seeing red. A review of subconjunctival hemorrhage. Adv Nurse Pract. 7(3):77-8, 1999
4. Fukuyama J et al: Causes of subconjunctival hemorrhage. Ophthalmologica. 200(2):63-7, 1990

CONJUNCTIVOCHALASIS

Key Facts

Introduction
- Loose redundant conjunctiva, most commonly in inferior bulbar conjunctiva

Demographics
- Typically found in patients of advanced age or with history of chronic inflammation
- Matrix metalloproteinase overexpression and decreased lymphatic drainage have both been implicated in its development
- May be associated with dry eyes, blepharitis, or contact lens wear

Presentation
- Symptoms have wide range of severity, from asymptomatic to epiphora to severe ocular irritation and ocular surface disease
  - Commonly attributed to uneven tear film secondary to conjunctival folds
  - Conjunctival draping over inferior puncta may lead to epiphora
  - May develop inferior keratopathy secondary to dryness adjacent to conjunctival folds

Treatment
- Aggressive lubrication is mainstay of therapy
- Topical steroids and antihistamines may be added
- Surgery is considered for symptomatic cases refractory to conservative treatment
- Common surgical approaches include
  - Surgical excision of excess conjunctiva in crescent shape with suturing
  - Conjunctival excision with amniotic membrane grafting using either fibrin glue or sutures
  - Conjunctival suture fixation to underlying sclera
- Excellent prognosis

*(**Left**) Slit-lamp photo demonstrates multiple inferior conjunctival folds ➔ typically associated with moderate to severe conjunctivochalasis (**Right**) Fluorescein staining shows irregular tear distribution ➔ caused by excessive inferior conjunctival tissue and folds. This irregular pooling may cause or exacerbate ocular surface disease and contribute to many of the symptoms attributed to conjunctivochalasis, including tearing, foreign body sensation, and ocular irritation.*

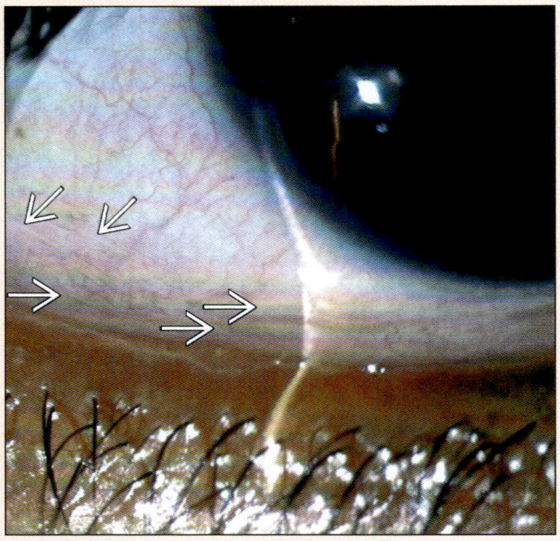

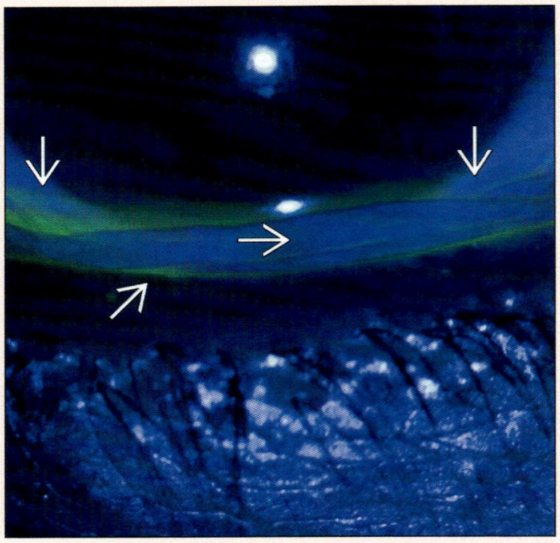

*(**Left**) External photo reveals mild draping of the redundant conjunctival tissue over the eyelid margin ↪. Irregular tear film pooling ➔ may contribute to frequent tearing, and, in severe cases, occlusion of the inferior puncta may lead to severe epiphora. (**Right**) This slit-lamp photo demonstrates exacerbation of conjunctivochalasis with downgaze. Patients may report increased symptoms in activities that involve downgaze, such as reading.*

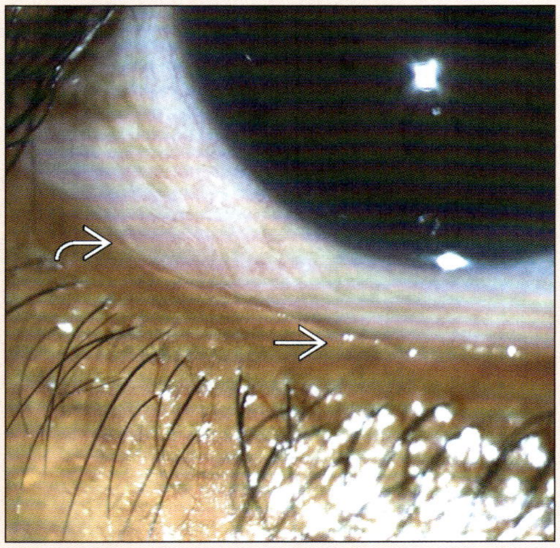

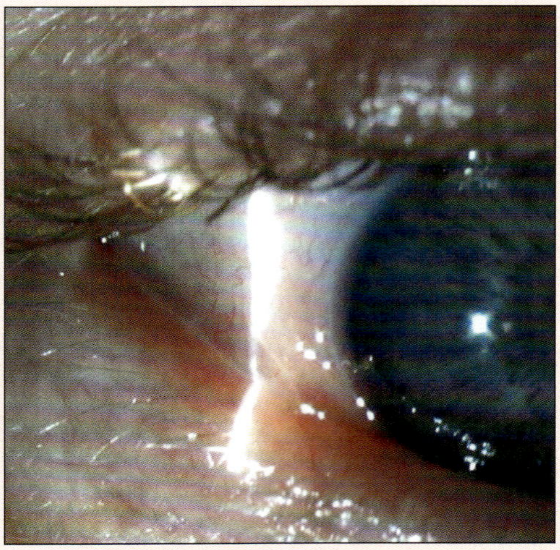

CONJUNCTIVOCHALASIS

INTRODUCTION

Abbreviations
- Conjunctivochalasis (CCh)

Definitions
- Redundant and loose conjunctiva, typically located between globe and inferior eyelid

DEMOGRAPHICS

Etiology/Risk Factors
- Typically found in patients of advanced age or with history of chronic inflammation
- Increased matrix metalloproteinase expression has been implicated as possible cause
- Another theory involves decreased lymphatic drainage from conjunctiva due to eyelid pressure

Epidemiology
- Most common in patients of advanced age
  - May affect 44-98% of patients > 60
- May be associated with
  - Dry eyes
  - Blepharitis
  - Contact lens wear

PRESENTATION

Symptoms
- May be asymptomatic
- Epiphora
  - Blockage of lower puncta by overhanging conjunctiva may cause tearing
- Ocular irritation secondary to ocular surface disease
  - Conjunctival folds cause uneven tear film and exposure
- Symptoms may be worsened with downgaze, e.g., when reading

Exam Findings
- Redundant conjunctival tissue, most commonly inferiorly
- Punctal occlusion from conjunctiva draping over eyelid margin
- May develop inferior keratopathy secondary to dryness
- Exacerbation of CCh with downgaze or digital pressure

DIFFERENTIAL DIAGNOSIS

Chemosis
- Conjunctiva is markedly edematous in contrast to CCh, where there is no edema

Conjunctivitis
- Usually presents with diffuse conjunctival inflammation
  - Minimal inflammation in CCh
    - If present, inflammation is localized to exposed conjunctiva inferiorly

Entropion
- Eyelid margin is abnormal, with eyelashes directed toward globe

EVALUATION/WORK-UP

Labs
- None

Pathology
- Histology may be normal or may show hyperplasia of conjunctival epithelium, decrease of elastic fiber, and chronic inflammation

TREATMENT

Medical
- Aggressive lubrication is mainstay of therapy
- Treatment of underlying condition
  - May add topical steroids and antihistamines
- Avoid UV exposure
- Nocturnal patching

Surgical
- Considered for symptomatic cases refractory to conservative treatment
- Common surgical approaches include
  - Surgical excision of excess conjunctiva in crescent shape with suturing
  - Conjunctival excision with amniotic membrane grafting with fibrin glue or sutures
  - Conjunctival fixation to underlying sclera
- Excellent prognosis with surgical treatment

Follow-Up
- Yearly for asymptomatic patients, every 3-6 months for symptomatic patients

Prognosis
- Excellent

SELECTED REFERENCES

1. Gumus K et al: Increasing prevalence and severity of conjunctivochalasis with aging detected by anterior segment optical coherence tomography. Am J Ophthalmol. 155(2):238-242, 2013
2. Mimura T et al: Changes of conjunctivochalasis with age in a hospital-based study. Am J Ophthalmol. 147(1):171-177, 2009
3. Yokoi N et al: Clinical impact of conjunctivochalasis on the ocular surface. Cornea. 24(8 Suppl):S24-S31, 2005
4. Watanabe A et al: Clinicopathologic study of conjunctivochalasis. Cornea. 23(3):294-8, 2004
5. Li DQ et al: Overexpression of MMP-1 and MMP-3 by cultured conjunctivochalasis fibroblasts. Invest Ophthalmol Vis Sci. 41(2):404-10, 2000
6. Meller D et al: Conjunctivochalasis: literature review and possible pathophysiology. Surv Ophthalmol. 43(3):225-32, 1998

PYOGENIC GRANULOMA

Key Facts

Introduction

- Benign vascular tumor of skin or mucosa
- Misnomered, as it does not contain granulomatous inflammation and is not suppurative

Demographics

- Proliferative fibrovascular response (granulation tissue) to tissue injury; common causes include inflammation, surgery, and trauma
  - Commonly occurs in association with chalazion or after strabismus surgery
- Lesions do not generally spontaneously occur
- Most common acquired eyelid vascular lesion
- Typically occurs in younger patients, with peak incidence in 2nd or 3rd decade of life

Presentation

- Findings include rapidly growing, painless eyelid or conjunctival mass with the following characteristics
  - Bright red or fleshy/pink, elevated, smooth, freely mobile, well vascularized, with possible superficial ulcerations of overlying epithelium

Evaluation/Work-Up

- Diagnosis is usually made based on history of tissue insult combined with clinical exam finding of rapidly growing, elevated, bright red mass
- Histology reveals granulation tissue, multiple capillaries, and chronic inflammatory cells

Treatment

- Topical and intralesional steroids are often curative
- Simple excision with cauterization to base and primary closure of conjunctiva are also curative
- Benign tumor with excellent prognosis
- May spontaneously involute, stabilize, or increase slowly in size without treatment
- Rate of recurrence: 0-15%

__(Left)__ This slit-lamp photo depicts a large pyogenic granuloma ⇒ that originates from the upper medial palpebral conjunctiva and protrudes over the eyelid margin. This elevated red-orange lesion appears smooth and is freely mobile. __(Right)__ This slit-lamp photo shows the same upper-medial pyogenic granuloma ➡ with the eyelid everted to view the broad base. Such lesions commonly occur in association with chalazion or at the site of other tissue insults, such as surgery, inflammation, or trauma.

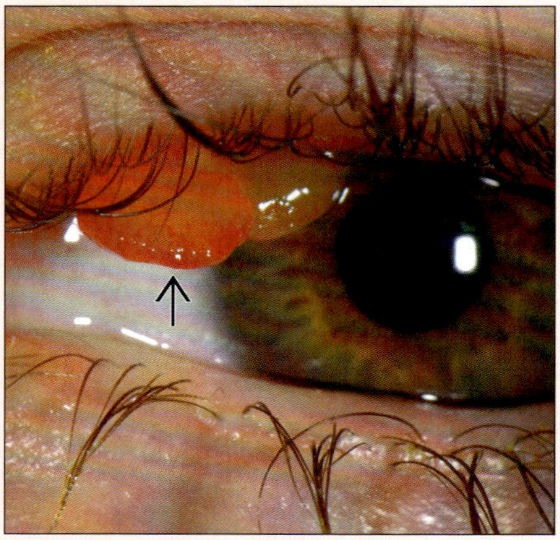

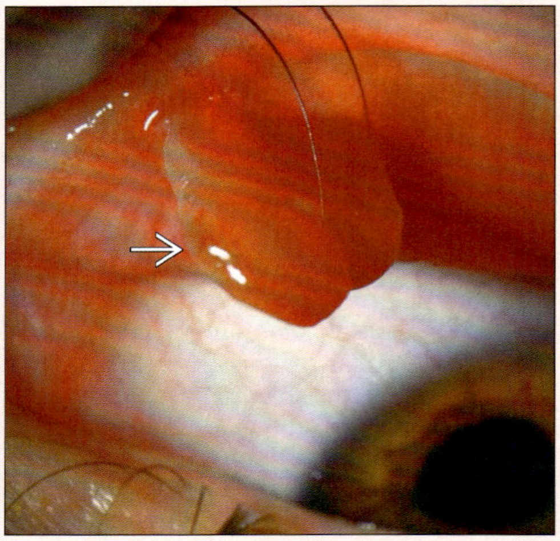

__(Left)__ This slit-lamp photo demonstrates a small pyogenic granuloma on the lower lateral palpebral conjunctiva ⇨. It appears well vascularized and would bleed easily if manipulated. __(Right)__ This slit-lamp photo is of a flesh-colored conjunctival pyogenic granule ⇒. Lesions that do not respond to steroid treatment will usually need simple excision with cautery at the base and primary closure of the surrounding conjunctiva. Recurrence rates are typically < 15%, depending on therapy choice.

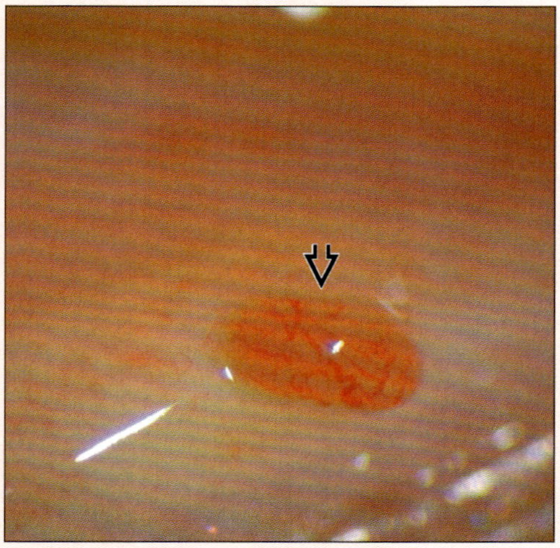

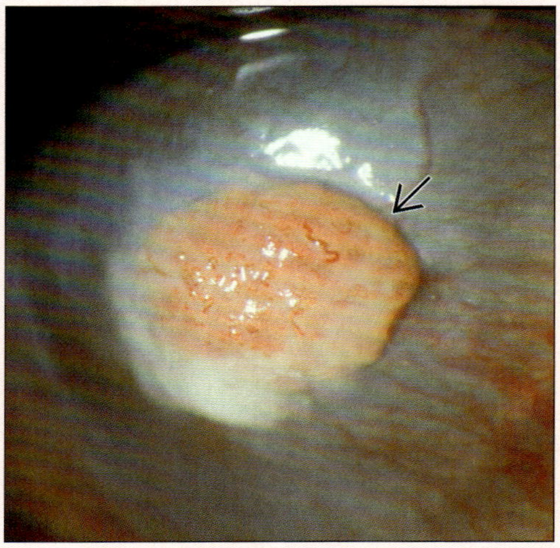

PYOGENIC GRANULOMA

INTRODUCTION

Definitions

- Benign vascular tumor of skin or mucosa
  - Misnomered, as it does not contain granulomatous inflammation and is not suppurative

DEMOGRAPHICS

Etiology/Risk Factors

- Proliferative fibrovascular response to tissue injury
- Common causes include
  - Inflammation
    - Often occurs at prior chalazion site or site of retained suture or foreign body
    - Infection
  - Surgery
    - Often seen after strabismus surgery
  - Trauma
- Generally, lesions do not occur spontaneously

Epidemiology

- Most common acquired eyelid vascular lesion
- Typically occurs in younger patients, with peak incidence in 2nd or 3rd decade of life

PRESENTATION

Symptoms

- Cosmetic complaint of rapidly growing, painless conjunctival or eyelid mass
- Ocular irritation secondary to mass
- Typically presents a few weeks after surgery for chalazion or strabismus

Exam Findings

- Rapidly growing mass, developing over days to weeks, with the following characteristics
  - Bright red or fleshy/pink
  - Elevated
  - Smooth
  - Freely mobile
  - Occurring at previous site of surgery
  - Well vascularized
    - Bleeds very easily
  - May adhere to surrounding surfaces
  - Superficial ulcerations of overlying epithelium
  - Stainable with fluorescein dye
- Can occur on skin or other mucosal surfaces

DIFFERENTIAL DIAGNOSIS

Kaposi Sarcoma

- Violaceous vascular lesion that develops more gradually and occurs in immunocompromised patients
- Does not usually occur over area of previous insult

Squamous Cell Carcinoma (SCC) Recurrence

- Pyogenic granuloma occurring at site of recently removed SCC can be misdiagnosed as recurrent SCC
  - SCCs are slow-growing, nonfriable lesions with hyperkeratotic surface
  - Use histologic examination to differentiate

Capillary Hemangioma

- Develop without history of previous ocular insult
- Bright red and protuberant
- Can be differentiated histologically, as it has more regular lobular architecture

EVALUATION/WORK-UP

Labs

- Diagnosis is usually made based on history of tissue insult combined with clinical exam finding of rapidly growing, elevated, bright red mass

Pathology

- Histology reveals loose stroma with
  - Granulation tissue
  - Multiple capillaries
    - Perpendicular to surface of lesion
  - Chronic inflammatory cells

TREATMENT

Medical

- Topical and intralesional steroids are often curative
  - Topical prednisolone 4x a day for 1-2 weeks
  - Add topical antibiotic if ocular infection is known to be present or suspected

Surgical

- Simple excision with cauterization to base is both diagnostic and curative
  - Used most commonly in lesions that persist after steroid treatment
  - Primary closure of surrounding conjunctiva is essential to prevent recurrence
    - Persistent granulation tissue can protrude through surface that has not reepithelialized
- Low-dose plaque radiotherapy has shown benefit in recurrent cases

Follow-Up

- None generally required

Prognosis

- Benign tumor, excellent prognosis
- May spontaneously involute, stabilize, or increase slowly in size without treatment
- 0-15% recurrence rate depending on choice of therapy

SELECTED REFERENCES

1. Ergün SS et al: Surgical treatment of giant pyogenic granuloma of the upper eyelid. Ann Ophthalmol (Skokie). 39(3):264-6, 2007
2. Giblin AV et al: Pyogenic granuloma - the quest for optimum treatment: audit of treatment of 408 cases. J Plast Reconstr Aesthet Surg. 60(9):1030-5, 2007
3. Gündüz K et al: Plaque radiation therapy for recurrent conjunctival pyogenic granuloma. Arch Ophthalmol. 116(4):538-9, 1998
4. Cameron JA et al: Pyogenic granulomas of the cornea. Ophthalmology. 102(11):1681-7, 1995
5. Ferry AP: Pyogenic granulomas of the eye and ocular adnexa: a study of 100 cases. Trans Am Ophthalmol Soc. 87:327-43; discussion 343-7, 1989

CONJUNCTIVAL PAPILLOMAS

Key Facts

Introduction

- Acquired benign tumor of the squamous epithelium of the conjunctiva

Demographics

- Associated with low-risk (most common) human papillomavirus (HPV) types 6 and 11 and high-risk HPV types 16, 18, and 33
- Acquired by children via vertical transmission
- Noninfectious papillomas are more common in adults
- Most common among people aged 20-39 years

Presentation

- Foreign body sensation, cosmetic complaint of a mass
- Typically unilateral but may be bilateral
- Appears as a pink, fibrovascular frond of tissue
- Lesion surface has red dots due to central vasculature
- Papillomas may have exophytic (pedunculated or sessile), mixed, or inverted (rare) growth pattern
- Can occur anywhere but most often located in inferior fornix, caruncle, and limbal areas
- Malignant transformation is suspected with inflammation, invasion, symblepharon formation, and increased keratinization

Evaluation/Work-Up

- Histology demonstrates a fibrovascular core covered by acanthotic, nonkeratinizing stratified epithelium

Treatment

- Observation for asymptomatic lesions
- Surgical excision with cryotherapy if lesion is symptomatic or concerning for malignancy
- Recurrences may be treated with topical mitomycin C, laser photocoagulation, topical or intralesional α-interferon, or oral cimetidine
- Often resolve spontaneously over months to years
- Generally benign; rarely undergo dysplastic change

*(**Left**) This slit-lamp photo demonstrates a conjunctival papilloma involving the right lower eyelid ➲. These lesions are typically unilateral and appear as pink, fibrovascular fronds of tissue. Patients most often present with cosmetic complaints or a foreign body sensation. (**Right**) This slit-lamp photo shows a pedunculated, exophytic conjunctival papilloma ➲. This particular lesion has a multilobulated appearance with smooth, clear epithelium and numerous visible underlying vessels.*

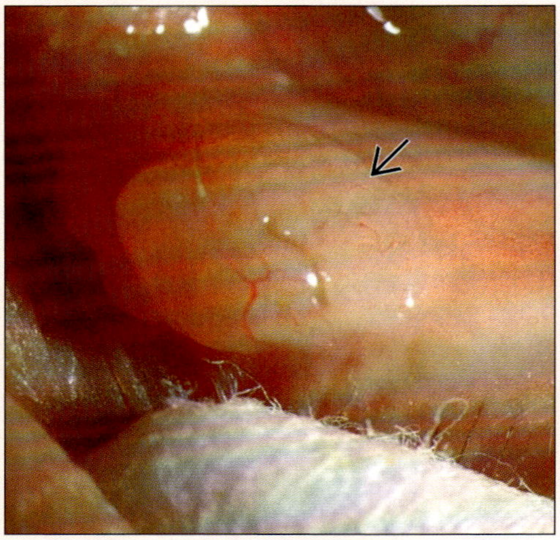

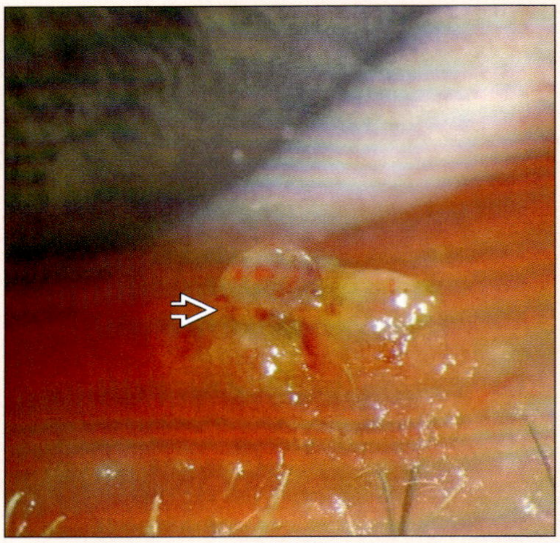

*(**Left**) This slit-lamp photo is of a bulbar conjunctival papilloma ➲. These lesions can occur anywhere but are most commonly found in the inferior fornix, caruncle, and limbal areas. Lesions can become confluent and involve the cornea or undergo malignant transformation. (**Right**) This slit-lamp photo depicts a sessile exophytic papilloma in the caruncle ➲ that is broad based, relatively flat, and has prominent vasculature. Inverted growth patterns are less common than exophytic growth patterns.*

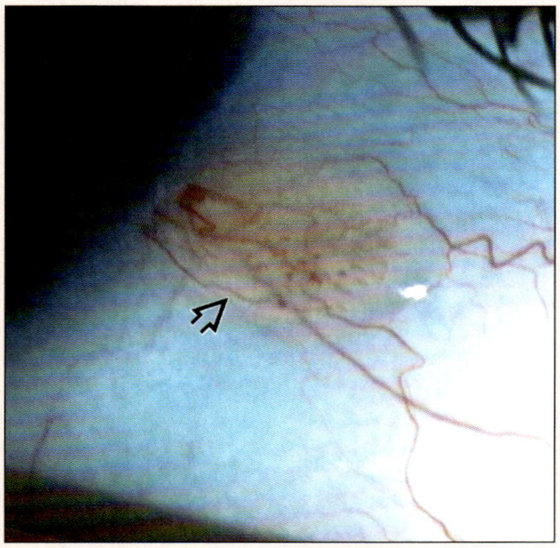

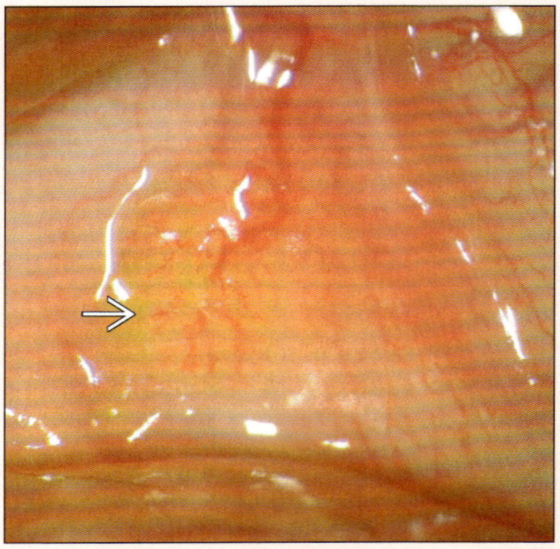

CONJUNCTIVAL PAPILLOMAS

INTRODUCTION

Definitions

- Acquired benign tumor of squamous epithelium of conjunctiva

DEMOGRAPHICS

Etiology/Risk Factors

- Associated with low-risk human papillomavirus (HPV) types 6 and 11 and high-risk HPV types 16, 18, and 33
  - ~ 81% of conjunctival papillomas have HPV
    - HPV types 6 and 11 are most commonly noted
  - Occurs in children by vertical transmission from a mother with an infected vagina
- Noninfectious papillomas are more common in adults

Epidemiology

- Relatively common occurrence
- Most common among people aged 20-39 years
- Slight male predominance (3:2)

PRESENTATION

Symptoms

- Foreign body sensation, cosmetic complaint of a mass
- Typically unilateral but may be bilateral

Exam Findings

- Appears as a pink, fibrovascular frond of tissue
- Lesion surface has red dots due to central vasculature
- Papillomas may have exophytic (pedunculated or sessile), mixed, or inverted (rare) growth pattern
  - Pedunculated exophytic lesions
    - Cauliflower-like lesions with fibrovascular core
    - Multilobulated appearance with smooth, clear epithelium and numerous visible underlying vessels
  - Sessile exophytic lesions
    - Broad-based, flat pink swellings with prominent vasculature
    - Glistening surface with numerous small red dots
    - Higher risk of malignant transformation
- Can occur anywhere but most often located in inferior fornix, caruncle, and limbal areas
- Lesions in children are generally small and multiple
- Lesions in adults are usually solitary but more extensive
- Lesions can become confluent and involve cornea
- Can appear pigmented in dark-skinned individuals
  - May be mistaken for malignant melanoma
- Malignant transformation is suspected with inflammation, invasion, symblepharon formation, and increased keratinization

DIFFERENTIAL DIAGNOSIS

Benign Hereditary Intraepithelial Dyskeratosis

- Rare autosomal dominant disorder that presents with bilateral hyperplastic, translucent juxtalimbal lesions
- Often with vessel dilation near lesion

Pseudoepitheliomatous Hyperplasia

- Benign, rapidly growing, white elevated nodule with a hyperkeratotic surface that develops due to irritation
- Lacks capillary fronds seen in conjunctival papillomas

Pyogenic Granuloma

- Proliferative fibrovascular response to injury
- Findings include a rapidly growing, painless eyelid or conjunctival mass that is bright red or pink, elevated, smooth, freely mobile, and well vascularized

Kaposi Sarcoma

- Violaceous vascular lesion that occurs in immunocompromised individuals

EVALUATION/WORK-UP

Labs

- Diagnosis is usually made by history and clinical exam

Pathology

- Histology demonstrates a fibrovascular core covered by acanthotic, nonkeratinizing stratified epithelium
- Goblet cells present in epithelium
- Papillomas caused by HPV may contain koilocytotic cells with irregular hyperchromatic nuclei surrounded by clear cytoplasm

TREATMENT

Medical

- Observation for asymptomatic lesions
- Recurrences may be treated with topical mitomycin C, laser photocoagulation, topical or intralesional α-interferon, or oral cimetidine

Surgical

- Surgical excision with 1 mm margin and cryotherapy to the base and surrounding areas
  - Incomplete excision often leads to recurrence and can stimulate further growth
  - Perform if symptomatic or concern for malignancy
  - Consider amniotic membrane transplantation for large papilloma excisions
- Minimized lesion manipulation during surgery to reduce risk of virus spreading to unaffected tissue

Follow-Up

- Periodic follow-up is recommended to monitor lesions &/or check for recurrence

Prognosis

- Often resolve spontaneously over months to years
- Generally benign; rarely undergo dysplastic change
  - Sessile lesions are more likely than pedunculated lesions to undergo malignant transformation

SELECTED REFERENCES

1. Sjö NC et al: Human papillomavirus in normal conjunctival tissue and in conjunctival papilloma: types and frequencies in a large series. Br J Ophthalmol. 91(8):1014-5, 2007
2. Chang SW et al: Oral cimetidine adjuvant therapy for recalcitrant, diffuse conjunctival papillomatosis. Cornea. 25(6):687-90, 2006
3. Shields CL et al: Tumors of the conjunctiva and cornea. Surv Ophthalmol. 49(1):3-24, 2004
4. Sjö NC et al: Human papillomavirus in conjunctival papilloma. Br J Ophthalmol. 85(7):785-7, 2001

CONJUNCTIVAL INTRAEPITHELIAL NEOPLASIA

Key Facts

Introduction

- CIN comprises dysplastic changes of conjunctiva ranging from dysplasia to carcinoma in situ and may be a precursor to SCC of conjunctiva
- Along with SCC, CIN is part of OSSN spectrum

Demographics

- Most common nonpigmented conjunctival tumor
- Most frequently seen in Caucasian males 65 and older by interpalpebral limbal conjunctiva
- Risk factors include UV exposure, HIV, HPV, and xeroderma pigmentosum

Presentation

- Patients are commonly asymptomatic but may have ocular pain, injection, and irritation
- Fleshy, sessile, usually located in the limbus and frequently appears gray-white and gelatinous, or may be papilliform in appearance

Treatment

- Medical treatment
  - Topical interferon-α-2b, mitomycin C, and 5-FU have all been used successfully
  - Interferon-α-2b is the most well-tolerated and least toxic topical treatment
- Surgical treatment
  - Gold standard is wide excision with 4 mm margins and cryotherapy to edges of resection
  - Alcohol epitheliectomy may be used for corneal involvement
  - Amniotic membrane grafting may be used to repair conjunctival defect
  - May recur with positive margins or residual microscopic disease
- Good prognosis with early detection and treatment

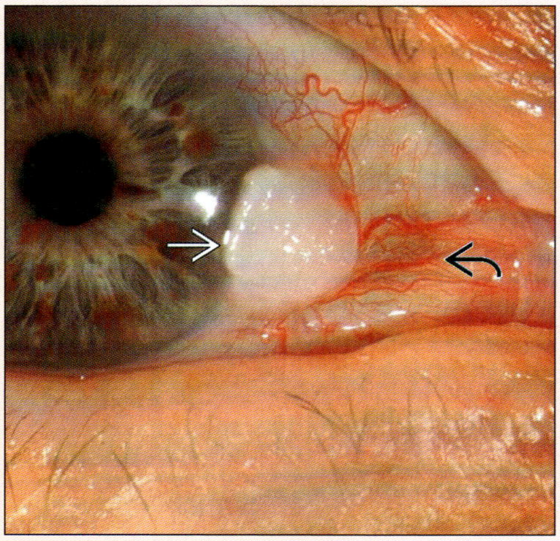

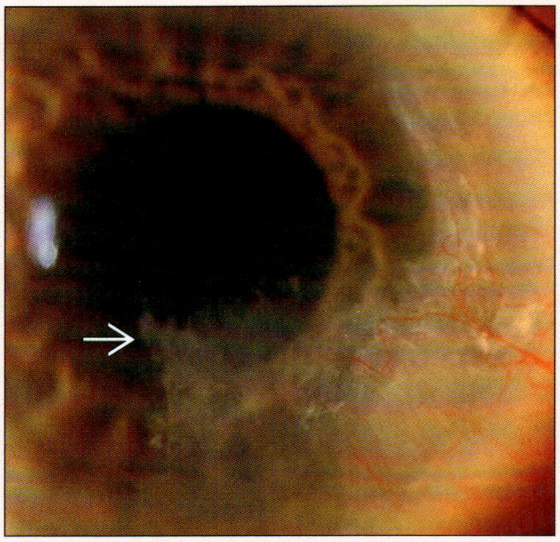

(Left) *This external photograph of a patient with conjunctival intraepithelial neoplasia (CIN) shows an elevated, opaque, gelatinous mass with substantial blood vessel recruitment, but without significant corneal involvement.* ***(Right)*** *This slit-lamp photograph of a patient with CIN depicts abnormal growth of fine translucent vascularized tissue extending from the conjunctiva to partially occlude the cornea. Ultra high-resolution OCT may help differentiate benign from neoplastic lesions.*

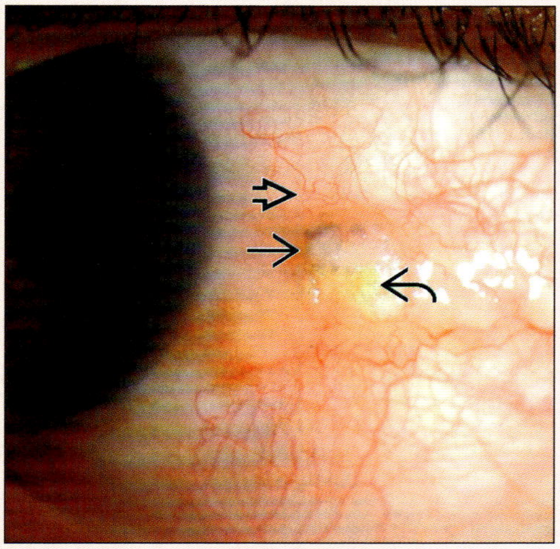

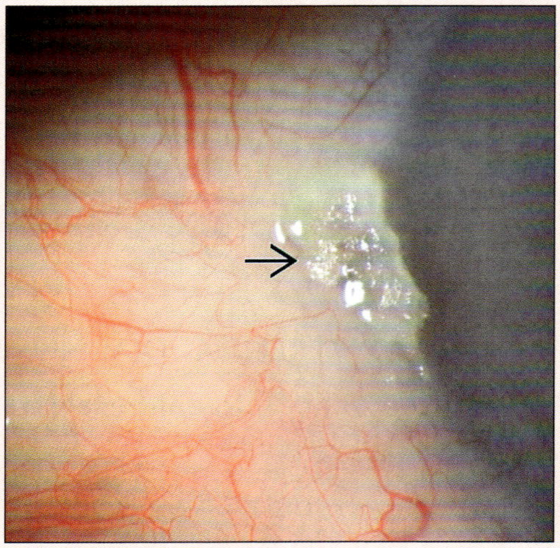

(Left) *This external photograph of a patient with CIN shows a nodular mass with increased vascularization surrounding the lesion. Additionally, the mass exhibits partial keratinization of the atypical epithelial cells, a finding occasionally present in CIN.* ***(Right)*** *This external photograph of a patient with CIN shows an opaque mass in the limbal conjunctiva with classic gelatinous appearance and mild leukoplakia. Surgical treatment includes wide resection with cryotherapy.*

CONJUNCTIVAL INTRAEPITHELIAL NEOPLASIA

INTRODUCTION

Abbreviations

- Conjunctival intraepithelial neoplasia (CIN)

Definitions

- Dysplastic changes of conjunctiva ranging from dysplasia to carcinoma in situ
- Precursor to squamous cell carcinoma (SCC)

Subtypes

- Ocular surface squamous neoplasia (OSSN) comprises both CIN and SCC

DEMOGRAPHICS

Etiology/Risk Factors

- Most frequently seen in older males with history of prolonged sun exposure
- More common in Caucasians
- Risk factors include UV exposure, HIV, HPV, xeroderma pigmentosum
- Tends to occur at earlier age in patients with xeroderma pigmentosum or HIV

Epidemiology

- Most common nonpigmented conjunctival tumor
- 0.02-1.9 cases per 100,000 people depending on location and risk factors

PRESENTATION

Symptoms

- May range from asymptomatic to ocular injection and pain

Exam Findings

- Sharply circumscribed limbus lesion, gray-white, gelatinous, opalescent, leukoplakic, or papilliform in appearance
- Usually unilateral and unifocal

DIFFERENTIAL DIAGNOSIS

Pterygium

- CIN usually possesses a gelatinous appearance with varying degrees of keratinization, in contrast to pterygia, which are more uniform and slow-growing fibrovascular tissues, though malignant cells may be present at the corneal edge of the pterygium

Squamous Cell Carcinoma

- Full-thickness conjunctival neoplasia with invasion of basement membrane into underlying stroma

EVALUATION/WORK-UP

Pathology

- Large or small squamous cells, may be spindled, with atypical mitotic figures at all levels of epithelium
- Dysplasia begins in basal layers and extends toward surface
- No invasion of epithelial basal membrane

Imaging

- Ultra high-resolution OCT
  - May help visualize subtle lesions that look benign clinically and monitor treatment response

TREATMENT

Medical

- Topical interferon-α-2b: 1 million IU/mL q.i.d. until resolution, and then treatment is continued for 1 additional month
  - Advantage: Treats microscopic disease and is less toxic to eye
  - Good nonsurgical alternative for compliant patients or patients with extensive involvement
  - Can also supplement with subconjunctival interferon-α-2b injection (10 million units)
- Mitomycin C 0.02% or 0.04%
  - q.i.d. for 1 week with 2-3 week breaks to allow for healing
  - Very painful and toxic to cornea, may cause punctal stenosis
- 5-FU 1%
  - q.i.d. for 1 week with 2-3 week breaks to allow for healing
  - Painful and toxic, less so than mitomycin C, however; may also cause punctal stenosis

Surgical

- Remains gold standard
- No-touch wide excision with alcohol epitheliectomy, superficial sclerectomy if necessary, 4 mm margins, and double-freeze, slow-thaw cryotherapy
- Amniotic membrane grafts may be used to cover conjunctival defect
- May have recurrence for unrecognized microscopic disease or positive margins
- May cause scarring, limbal stem cell deficiency, infection

Follow-Up

- Weekly to monthly while on topical therapy

Prognosis

- Good with early detection and treatment; low rate of metastasis

SELECTED REFERENCES

1. Galor A et al: Predictors of ocular surface squamous neoplasia recurrence after excisional surgery. Ophthalmology. 119(10):1974-81, 2012
2. Gupta N et al: Ocular surface squamous neoplasia in xeroderma pigmentosum: clinical spectrum and outcome. Graefes Arch Clin Exp Ophthalmol. 249(8):1217-21, 2011
3. Kiire CA et al: The aetiology and associations of conjunctival intraepithelial neoplasia. Br J Ophthalmol. 90(1):109-13, 2006
4. Scott IU et al: Human papillomavirus 16 and 18 expression in conjunctival intraepithelial neoplasia. Ophthalmology. 109(3):542-7, 2002

PRIMARY ACQUIRED MELANOSIS

Key Facts

Introduction
- Primary acquired melanosis (PAM)
- Acquired neoplastic proliferation of conjunctival melanocytes that can progress to melanoma

Demographics
- Most common in middle-aged light-skinned persons

Presentation
- Flat, irregular brown patch of noncystic pigmentation, most commonly on bulbar conjunctiva
- Cysts indicate benign melanoma
- Malignant transformation is suspected in lesions that are enlarging, thickening, well vascularized, nodular, multifocal, and nonbulbar

Evaluation/Work-Up
- Generally observe bulbar lesions with < 1 clock hour of conjunctival involvement
- Biopsy lesions with ≥ 3 clock hours of involvement
  - Biopsy all lesions suspicious for malignancy
- Histology will show 1 of the following
  - PAM without atypia, which carries no risk of malignant transformation
  - PAM with atypia, which has 46% chance of malignant transformation

Treatment
- Observe with photographs if not suspicious
- Small lesions should be completely excised
- Biopsy large or suspicious lesions from several sites
- If PAM without atypia, leave remainder untreated
- PAM with atypia needs to be either completely excised, if possible, or treated with mitomycin C, cryotherapy, or radiation therapy
  - May need amniotic membrane if large excision
- Lifelong follow-up due to malignant potential
- ~ 32% of all PAM lesions progress to malignant melanoma

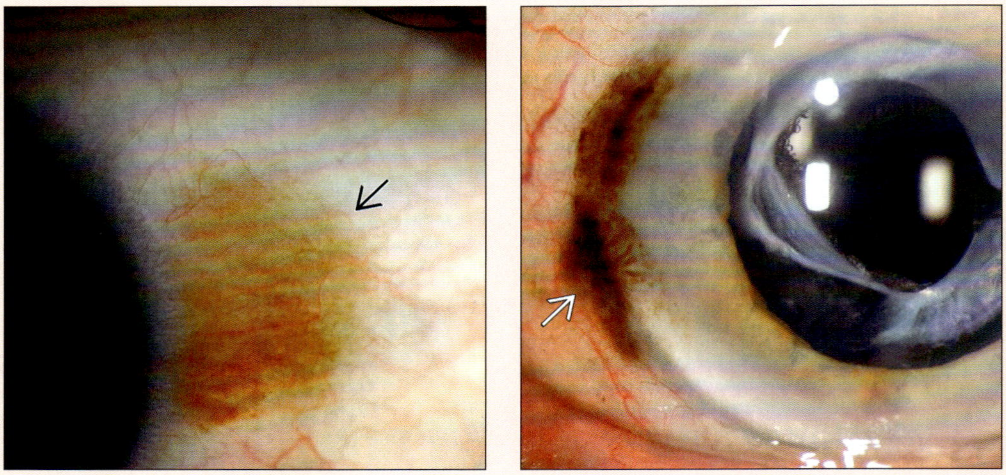

(Left) *Slit-lamp photo shows a flat, irregular brown patch of noncystic pigmentation typical of primary acquired melanosis (PAM) →. The bulbar conjunctiva is most commonly affected, especially the temporal and inferior quadrants.* ***(Right)*** *Slit-lamp photo depicts PAM of the temporal bulbar conjunctiva with corneal extension →. Transformation of PAM into malignant melanoma is suspected in lesions that are enlarging, thickening, well vascularized, nodular, multifocal, &/or nonbulbar.*

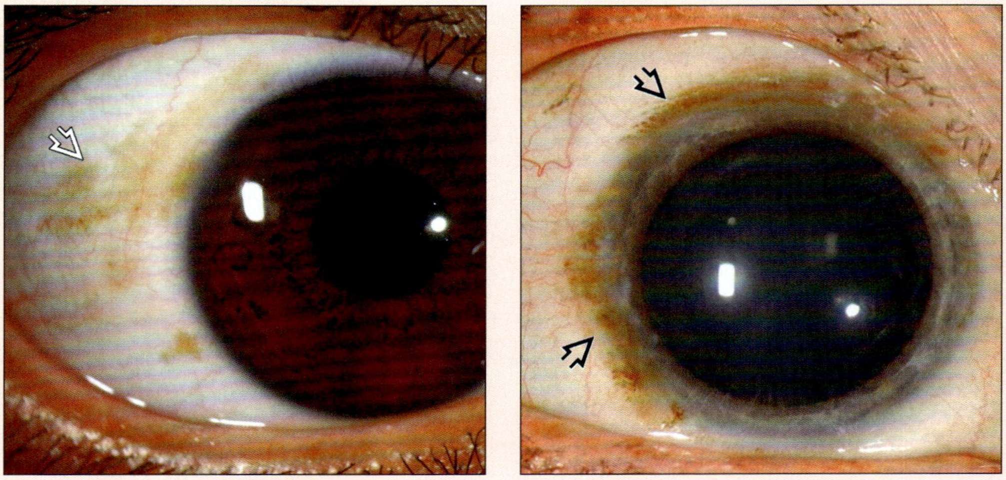

(Left) *Slit-lamp photo shows PAM of the temporal bulbar conjunctiva →.* ***(Right)*** *This slit-lamp photo is of PAM that involves > 6 clock hours of conjunctiva →. Lesions with ≥ 3 clock hours of involvement, or those that demonstrate increased thickness, pigmentation, vascularity, &/or spread, merit biopsy. Histology demonstrates either PAM without atypia (no risk of malignant transformation) or PAM with atypia (overall risk of malignant transformation is 46% but varies with degree of atypia).*

PRIMARY ACQUIRED MELANOSIS

INTRODUCTION

Abbreviations
- Primary acquired melanosis (PAM)

Definitions
- Acquired neoplastic proliferation of conjunctival melanocytes that can progress to melanoma

DEMOGRAPHICS

Etiology/Risk Factors
- Melanocyte dysplasia of unknown etiology
- Fair complexion is a risk factor

Epidemiology
- Most common in middle-aged light-skinned persons
  - Median age is 56 years

PRESENTATION

Symptoms
- Appearance of ocular pigmented lesion

Exam Findings
- Flat, irregular brown patch of noncystic pigmentation in conjunctiva
  - Most commonly on bulbar conjunctiva
    - Usually in temporal and inferior quadrants
    - Often adjacent to limbus
    - Microscopic view can show melanotic stippling beyond grossly visible margin of lesion
  - May occur in other locations
  - Amelanotic lesions are possible but uncommon
  - Can be moved over underlying sclera
- Lesions may remain stable, expand, shrink, &/or change color over time
  - Hormonal changes and inflammation may cause size fluctuation
  - Lesions often wax and wane
- Number of clock hours of involved conjunctiva can help predict malignant transformation risk
  - Lesions with < 1 hour of conjunctival involvement have low risk of malignant transformation
  - Lesions with ≥ 3 hours of conjunctival involvement have ≥ 20% chance of malignant transformation
- Presence of cysts indicate benign melanoma
- Malignant transformation is suspected in lesions that are enlarging, thickening, well vascularized, nodular, multifocal, and nonbulbar

DIFFERENTIAL DIAGNOSIS

Malignant Melanoma
- Presents as nodular, well-vascularized brown mass
- Usually fixed to underlying tissue

Conjunctival Nevus
- Appears during childhood with well-defined margin
- Small epithelial inclusion cysts are usually found

Benign Acquired Melanosis
- Bilateral, flat, irregular conjunctival brown patches
- Occur in people with dark skin pigmentation

EVALUATION/WORK-UP

Pathology
- Observe bulbar lesions with < 1 clock hour of conjunctival involvement
- Biopsy lesions with ≥ 3 clock hours of involvement
  - Lesions with increased thickness, pigmentation, vascularity, &/or spread also merit biopsy
- Histology will show 1 of the following
  - PAM without atypia
    - Benign proliferation of epithelial melanocytes confined to basal epithelial layer
    - No risk of malignant transformation
  - PAM with atypia
    - Atypical melanocytes (based on nuclear features) may be in epithelium or replace it with epithelioid (large hyperchromatic nuclei and prominent nucleoli) or spindle cells
    - Overall risk of malignant transformation for PAM with atypia is 46%
      - 20% risk if involvement is limited to basal epithelial layer
      - 75% risk if lesion is composed of epithelioid cells
      - 90% risk with intraepitheloid pagetoid spread
- Worrisome signs include increasing size, elevation, and change in color
  - Color change is not sign of malignancy if in context of puberty, pregnancy, or hormone/steroid use

TREATMENT

Medical
- Observe with photographs if not suspicious

Surgical
- Small lesions should be completely excised
- Biopsy large or suspicious lesions from several sites
  - If PAM without atypia, leave remainder untreated
  - PAM with atypia needs to be either completely excised, if possible, or treated with mitomycin C, cryotherapy, or radiation therapy
    - May need amniotic membrane if large excision

Follow-Up
- Every 6-12 months for PAM without atypia
- Lifelong follow-up due to malignant potential

Prognosis
- Varies depending on study
  - 35% of PAM lesions progressed and 12% underwent malignant transformation over 10-year interval
  - ~ 32% of all PAM lesions progress to malignancy
  - Overall risk for malignant transformation for PAM with atypia is 46%

SELECTED REFERENCES

1. Shields JA et al: Primary acquired melanosis of the conjunctiva: risks for progression to melanoma in 311 eyes. The 2006 Lorenz E. Zimmerman lecture. Ophthalmology. 115(3):511-519, 2008
2. Gloor P et al: Clinical characterization of primary acquired melanosis. Invest Ophthalmol Vis Sci. 36(8):1721-9, 1995
3. Folberg R et al: Primary acquired melanosis of the conjunctiva. Hum Pathol. 16(2):129-35, 1985

CONJUNCTIVAL LYMPHOID TUMORS

Key Facts

Introduction
- Spectrum of abnormal lymphocytic proliferations ranging from benign lymphoid hyperplasia to malignant lymphoma

Demographics
- Can be isolated or part of a systemic lymphoma
- Mean age ranges from 60-68 years
- Female predominance: 1.5-2:1
- Ocular adnexal lymphomas (OAL) represent ~ 6-8% of all extranodal lymphomas and 1% of all non-Hodgkin lymphomas (NHL)
  - ~ 28% of OAL are solely conjunctival

Presentation
- Present with ocular mass &/or irritation
- Usually unilateral, but bilateral in ~ 1/3 of cases
- Appear as mobile, pebbly, salmon-colored masses located in stroma or deep to Tenon fascia

Evaluation/Work-Up
- Refer to oncologist for systemic work-up
- Excisional or incisional biopsy is necessary to differentiate between benign lymphoid hyperplasia and malignant lymphoma (usually B-cell NHL)

Treatment
- Radiotherapy (external beam) is usually effective for all subtypes of conjunctival lymphoma
  - Systemic lymphoma requires systemic chemotherapy
- Alternatives include cryotherapy, local chemotherapy with topical mitomycin C, methotrexate, or interferon α-2b, and systemic rituximab
- Overall good prognosis; even those with systemic involvement generally respond favorably to treatment
- Systemic involvement is found in 17-31% of all patients with conjunctival lymphoid tumors
- Long-term follow-up is advised to monitor for recurrence or systemic involvement

__(Left)__ This slit lamp photo depicts a conjunctival lymphoma ⮕ in the right eye of a female patient who also has systemic lymphoma. Patients often present with cosmetic complaints, ocular irritation, &/or ptosis. (Courtesy C. Miller, MD.) __(Right)__ This slit lamp photo demonstrates lymphoid hyperplasia ⮕. Lymphoid tumors, like the one seen here, commonly appear as mobile, pebbly, salmon-colored masses located in the stroma or deep to Tenon fascia. (Courtesy C. Miller, MD.)

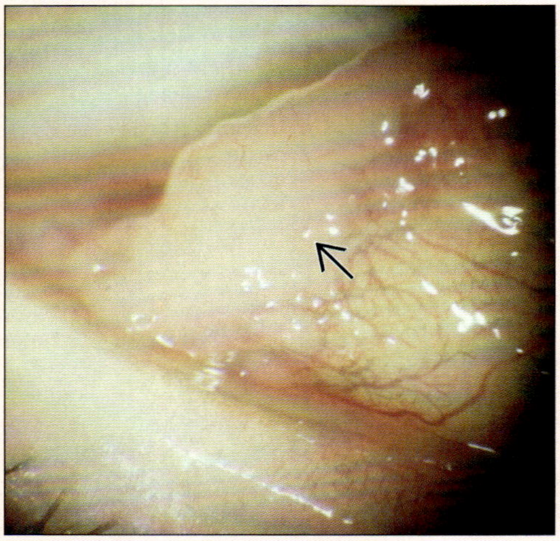

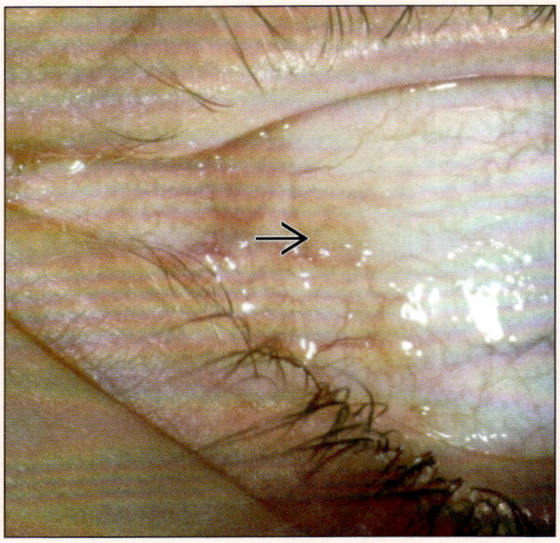

__(Left)__ This slit lamp photo depicts lymphoid hyperplasia ⮕. The most common location of lymphoid tumors is the inferior fornices. Tumors are often oval shaped when bulbar and parallel to the tarsal plate when forniceal in location. (Courtesy C. Miller, MD.) __(Right)__ This slit-lamp photo shows lymphoid hyperplasia in the left eye of a female patient ⮕. These tumors are often referred to as salmon patches due to their color, although the color can vary from pink to yellow to white. (Courtesy C. Miller, MD.)

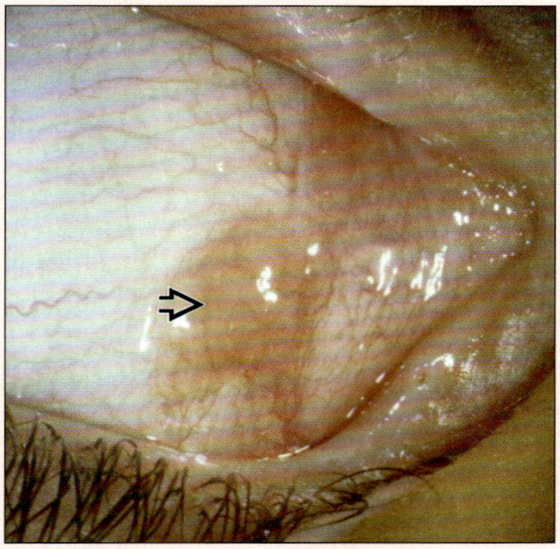

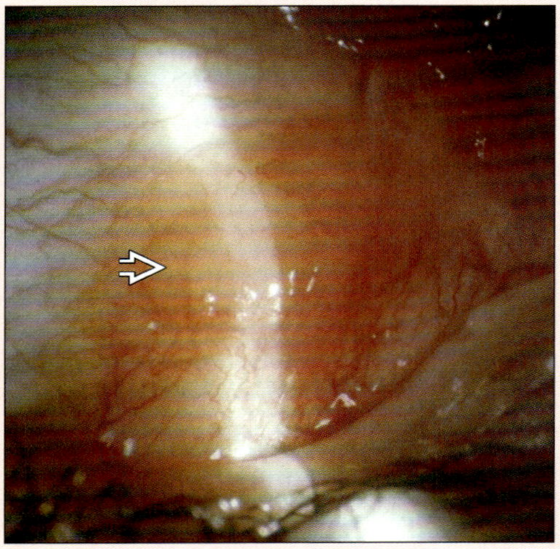

CONJUNCTIVAL LYMPHOID TUMORS

INTRODUCTION

Definitions

- Spectrum of abnormal lymphocytic proliferations ranging from benign, reactive lymphoid hyperplasia to malignant lymphoma

DEMOGRAPHICS

Etiology/Risk Factors

- Caused by abnormal lymphocytic proliferations
- Risk factors include older age, history of systemic lymphoma, and systemic immunosuppression
- Can be isolated or part of systemic lymphoma
- Risk of systemic involvement increases when lesions are bilateral, show malignant signs histopathologically, and have unfavorable lymphoma subtype

Epidemiology

- Mean age for conjunctival lymphoid disease ranges from 60-68 years
- Female predominance = 1.5-2:1
- Ocular adnexal lymphoma (OAL) represents ~ 6-8% of all extranodal lymphomas and 1% of all non-Hodgkin lymphomas
  - ~ 28% of OAL are solely conjunctival

PRESENTATION

Symptoms

- Cosmetic complaint of ocular mass
- Often present with ocular irritation or ptosis
- Usually unilateral, but bilateral in ~ 1/3 of cases

Exam Findings

- Appear as mobile, pebbly, salmon-colored masses located in stroma or deep to Tenon fascia
  - Color can vary from pink to yellow to white
  - Most often located in inferior fornices
  - Often oval shaped when bulbar and parallel to tarsal plate when forniceal in location
  - Often referred to as salmon patch due to color
- Can also masquerade as diffuse chronic conjunctivitis
- Can be mildly, moderately, or highly vascularized
- Painless proptosis &/or diplopia often found

DIFFERENTIAL DIAGNOSIS

Chronic Conjunctivitis

- Diffuse lymphoid tumor may present with chronic inflammation, follicles, and no elevated mass
- Biopsy suspected lymphoma in patients unresponsive to conjunctivitis treatment

Dermolipomas

- Round, well-circumscribed, elevated, smooth, soft, white-yellow nodules that are not freely mobile

EVALUATION/WORK-UP

Labs

- Work-up patients for presence of systemic disease
  - Refer to oncologist to help with systemic work-up

Pathology

- Excisional (if small) or incisional biopsy is necessary to differentiate between benign lymphoid hyperplasia and malignant lymphoma
  - Fresh, unfixed tissue required for pathologic studies
- Histologic examination reveals sheets of lymphocytes of varying shapes and sizes, depending on subtype
  - Cytomorphologic features are correlated to outcome
- Most OALs are extranodal B-cell non-Hodgkin type
  - Most common subtype is extranodal marginal-zone B-cell lymphoma (EMZL)
    - ~ 83% of patients have this subtype
    - Previously termed MALT lymphoma
    - Many other B-cell lymphoma subtypes can occur
  - T-cell lymphomas are rarely noted
- Most malignant lymphomas are monoclonal with no germinal centers whereas lymphoid hyperplasia is polyclonal with well-developed germinal centers

TREATMENT

Medical

- Topical steroids and excision for small lesions may be beneficial in symptomatic lymphoid hyperplasia
  - Can resolve spontaneously
- Radiotherapy (external beam) is effective for all subtypes of conjunctival lymphoma and is preferred treatment when possible
  - Systemic lymphoma requires systemic chemotherapy
- Alternatives include cryotherapy, local chemotherapy with topical mitomycin C, methotrexate, or interferon α-2b, and systemic rituximab
- Observation is possibility for low-grade lymphomas
  - Requires diligent follow-up

Follow-Up

- Long-term follow-up is advised to monitor for recurrence or systemic involvement
  - Every 6 months for 5 years, followed by yearly visits

Prognosis

- Overall good prognosis
  - Even those with systemic involvement generally respond favorably to treatment
- Systemic involvement is found in 17-31% of all patients with conjunctival lymphoid tumors
- Chances of developing systemic disease in patients with conjunctival lymphoid tumor but no systemic disease at evaluation were 7% after 1 year, 12% after 2 years, 15% after 5 years, and 28% after 10 years
- Conjunctival lymphomas have lower risk of systemic involvement and death when compared to other OAL

SELECTED REFERENCES

1. Ferry JA et al: Lymphoma of the ocular adnexa: A study of 353 cases. Am J Surg Pathol. 31(2):170-84, 2007
2. Bardenstein DS: Ocular adnexal lymphoma: classification, clinical disease, and molecular biology. Ophthalmol Clin North Am. 18(1):187-97, x, 2005
3. Tsai PS et al: Treatment of conjunctival lymphomas. Semin Ophthalmol. 20(4):239-46, 2005
4. Shields CL et al: Conjunctival lymphoid tumors: clinical analysis of 117 cases and relationship to systemic lymphoma. Ophthalmology. 108(5):979-84, 2001

MALIGNANT MELANOMA

Key Facts

Introduction
- Malignant melanocytic tumor of ocular surface

Demographics
- 70-75% of cases arise from PAM with atypia
- ~ 15-20% of cases arise from a preexisting nevus
- ~ 10% of cases arise de novo
- Increasing age, white race, and sun exposure (repeated, intense episodes) are common risk factors
- Incidence ranges from 0.2-0.8 per million in light-skinned populations

Presentation
- Elevated, nodular, well-vascularized, darkly pigmented lesion fixed to underlying tissue
- Can be multifocal with different areas of nodularity
- Generally on perilimbal bulbar conjunctiva
- Can spread to regional lymph nodes via lymphatics
- More distant metastasis can also occur

Evaluation/Work-Up
- Biopsy all lesions suspicious for melanoma
- Histology shows proliferation of atypical, pleomorphic melanocytes invading conjunctival substantia propria from epithelium

Treatment
- Diffuse melanoma is treated by excising localized nodules and using mitomycin C or cryotherapy
- Wide surgical resection for circumscribed lesions
  - Apply alcohol and supplement with cryotherapy
- Oncology consultation for systemic metastasis workup
- Exenteration has not shown mortality decrease
- Average 10-year mortality rate of 30%
- Unfavorable prognostic indicators include nonepibulbar location, lesions > 1.8 mm thick, multifocal tumors, lymphatic or orbital spread, recurrence, eyelid margin involvement, pagetoid spread, and melanomas arising de novo

__(Left)__ Slit-lamp photo shows inferior bulbar conjunctival melanoma. Melanomas can be multifocal with different areas of nodularity, as seen here ⇨. Large conjunctival feeding vessels can often be noted. (Courtesy C. Miller, MD.) __(Right)__ This slit-lamp photo demonstrates a temporal perilimbal conjunctival melanoma ➡. Conjunctival melanomas typically present as elevated, well-vascularized, nodular, darkly pigmented lesions. Intraocular and extraorbital extension may occur. (Courtesy W. Nosé, MD.)

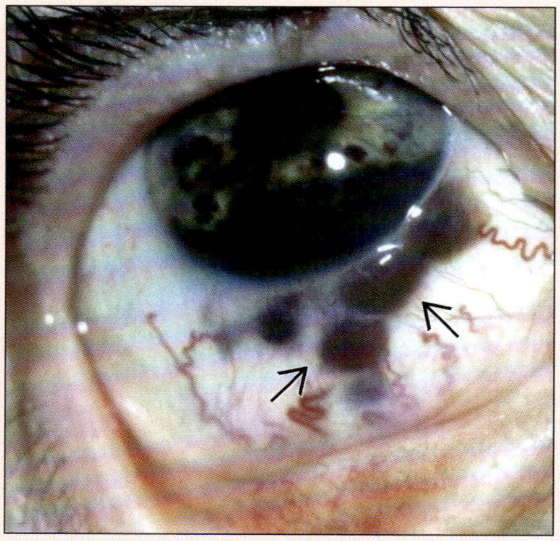

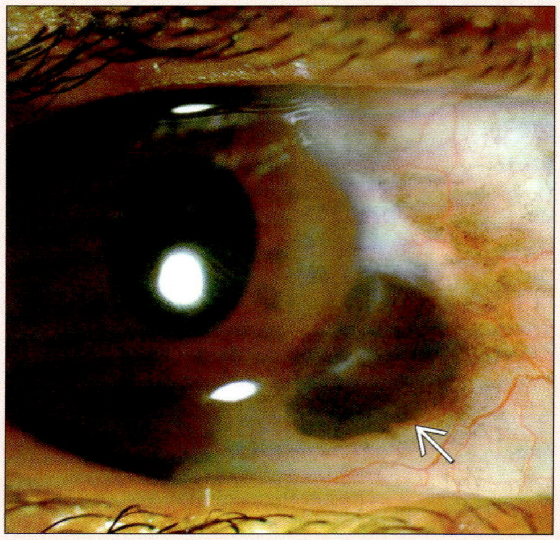

__(Left)__ This slit-lamp photo shows a superior bulbar conjunctival melanoma ⇨; 70-75% of melanomas arise from PAM with atypia, 15-20% from a preexisting nevus, and ~ 10% arise de novo. (Courtesy C. Miller, MD.) __(Right)__ This slit-lamp photo is of a temporal bulbar conjunctival melanoma ⇨. The perilimbal area is the most common location of conjunctival melanomas, but they can be found in other locations including nonbulbar, which carry a worse prognosis. (Courtesy C. Miller, MD.)

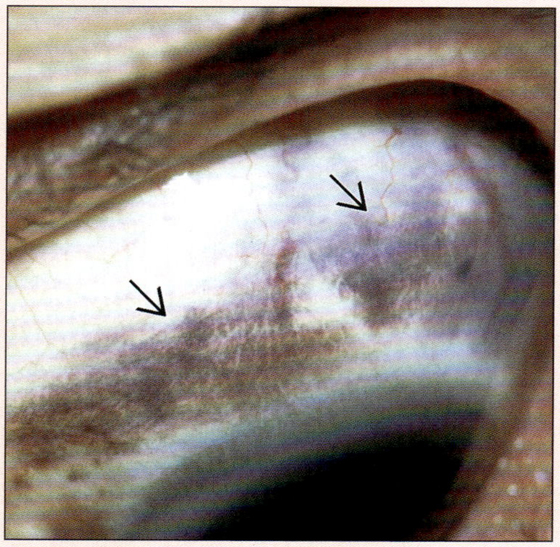

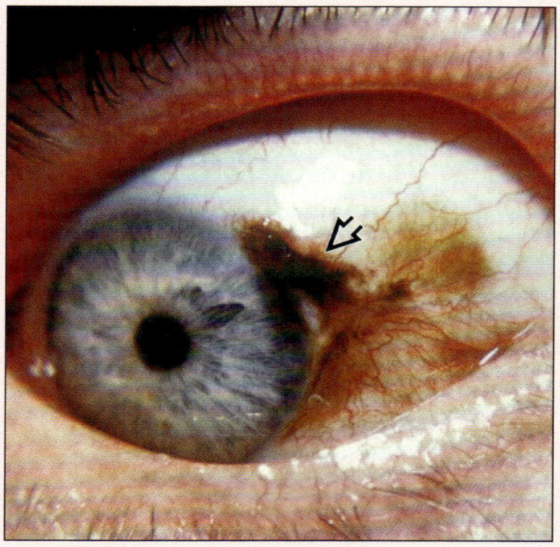

MALIGNANT MELANOMA

INTRODUCTION

Definitions

- Malignant melanocytic tumor of ocular surface

DEMOGRAPHICS

Etiology/Risk Factors

- Atypical melanocytes invade conjunctival substantia propria from epithelium
- 70-75% of cases arise from primary acquired melanosis (PAM) with atypia
- ~ 15-20% arise from preexisting nevus
- ~ 10% arise de novo
- Increasing age, white race, and sun exposure (repeated, intense episodes) are common risk factors

Epidemiology

- Incidence ranges from 0.2-0.8 per million in light-skinned populations
  - Incidence in dark-skinned persons is much smaller
  - Most common in 5th decade of life and beyond
  - Incidence has been increasing over recent years
  - 1/40th as common as choroidal melanoma

PRESENTATION

Symptoms

- Complaint of conjunctival mass, usually pigmented

Exam Findings

- Elevated, nodular, well-vascularized, darkly pigmented lesion (usually brown)
  - ~ 30% can be amelanotic and smooth
    - Recurrences are often amelanotic
  - Large conjunctival feeding vessel is often noted
  - Fixed to underlying tissues
  - Can be multifocal with different areas of nodularity
  - Size varies from 2 mm to > 10 mm in diameter
  - Generally on perilimbal bulbar conjunctiva
    - Can also be found on palpebral conjunctiva, fornices, caruncle, and plica semilunaris
      - Nonbulbar lesions usually have worse prognosis
- Intraocular and extraorbital extension may occur
- Can spread to regional lymph nodes via lymphatics
  - Preauricular lymph nodes are most commonly involved, followed by submandibular and cervical
- More distant metastasis can also occur in brain, lungs, liver, bone, and skin

DIFFERENTIAL DIAGNOSIS

Conjunctival Nevi

- Appear during childhood with well-defined margins
- Small epithelial inclusion cysts are usually found

Primary Acquired Melanosis

- Lesions are typically flat
  - Not as well vascularized; thinner, smaller, and can be moved over underlying sclera

Ocular Melanosis

- Congenital bulbar conjunctival pigmented lesions that normally occur 2 mm away from limbus

EVALUATION/WORK-UP

Labs

- Detailed ocular examination with dilated fundus exam, ultrasound biomicroscopy, and transillumination to check for underlying uveal melanoma
- Document lesion with photographs

Pathology

- Biopsy all lesions suspicious for melanoma
- Histology shows proliferation of atypical, pleomorphic melanocytes invading conjunctival substantia propria from epithelium
  - With atypical mitotic figures, prominent nucleoli, abundant cytoplasm, pagetoid spread, and spindle, epithelioid, balloon cells &/or polyhedral cells
- S100, Melan-A/MART-1, and HMB-45 stains identify melanocytes and can aid in diagnosis
  - Most useful in amelanotic lesions

TREATMENT

Medical

- Diffuse melanoma is treated by excising localized nodules and using mitomycin C or cryotherapy to diffusely involved areas
  - Short-term results suggest interferon α-2b can cause conjunctival melanoma regression
- Oncology consultation for systemic metastasis workup

Surgical

- Wide surgical resection with clear margins (4 mm) for circumscribed lesions
  - Apply alcohol and supplement with cryotherapy
  - Perform sentinal lymph node biopsy
  - Adjunctive radiotherapy if tumor extends to specimen's deep margin
  - Primary conjunctival closure is preferred, but larger resections may require amniotic or conjunctival grafts
- Treat recurrences with local resection and radiotherapy
- Exenteration has not been shown to decrease mortality and is only indicated for use in very advanced disease

Follow-Up

- Lifelong to monitor for signs of recurrence
  - Check liver function tests and head/neck lymph nodes periodically

Prognosis

- Average 10-year mortality rate of 30%
- Overall, ~ 25% risk of metastasis
- Unfavorable prognostic indicators include
  - Nonepibulbar location, lesions > 1.8 mm thick, multifocal tumors, lymphatic or orbital spread, recurrence, eyelid margin involvement, pagetoid spread, and melanomas arising de novo

SELECTED REFERENCES

1. Shields CL et al: Conjunctival melanoma: outcomes based on tumor origin in 382 consecutive cases. Ophthalmology. 118(2):389-95, 2011
2. Brownstein S: Malignant melanoma of the conjunctiva. Cancer Control. 11(5):310-6, 2004
3. Seregard S: Conjunctival melanoma. Surv Ophthalmol. 42(4):321-50, 1998

SQUAMOUS CELL CARCINOMA OF THE CONJUNCTIVA

Key Facts

Introduction

- Nonpigmented malignant tumor of ocular surface epithelium that may invade below basement membrane
- Also known as epithelioma

Demographics

- Occurs in elderly individuals with fair complexion and history of chronic sun exposure
- Most common conjunctival malignancy

Presentation

- Gelatinous thickening of limbal and bulbar conjunctiva in interpalpebral fissure zone
- Compared to BCC, SCC exhibits greater hyperkeratosis
- Lesion usually has broad base along limbus, sharp borders, and may exhibit leukoplakia
- Engorged and dilated conjunctival vessels feed tumor

Treatment

- If medical therapy (now primarily topical or subconjunctival interferon α-2b) fails, then surgery with wide excision followed by reconstruction
  - Histological exam on frozen section confirms tumor margins microscopically
- SCC of conjunctiva requires wide excision 4 mm beyond tumor margin, scleral flap beneath tumor, and cryotherapy to conjunctival margins; mitomycin C may be applied to scleral bed for 1-2 minutes
  - Amniotic membrane graft minimizes postoperative inflammation and allows for reepithelialization; may be utilized if area of surgical resection is large (> 4 contiguous clock hours)
- Corneal involvement requires surgical scraping of tumor cells with preservation of Bowman layer
- SCC extending into orbit requires exenteration of orbital contents

*(**Left**) Slit-lamp photo shows raised, gelatinous SCC with corkscrew vascular tufts and dilated vessels extending toward the lesion ➔. Leukoplakia may occur on the lesion's surface and represents hyperkeratosis, dyskeratosis, and parakeratosis of the conjunctival epithelium. (**Right**) This slit-lamp photo shows early-stage SCC with fimbriated conjunctival vessels ➔. Differential diagnosis includes squamous cell papilloma, a sessile or pedunculated mass that can be distinguished by biopsy and histopathology.*

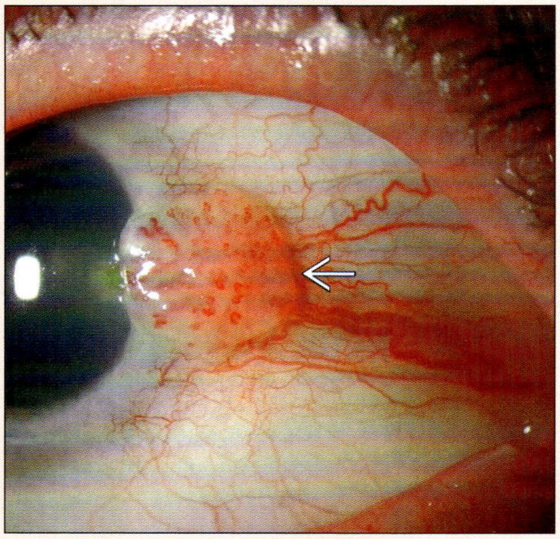

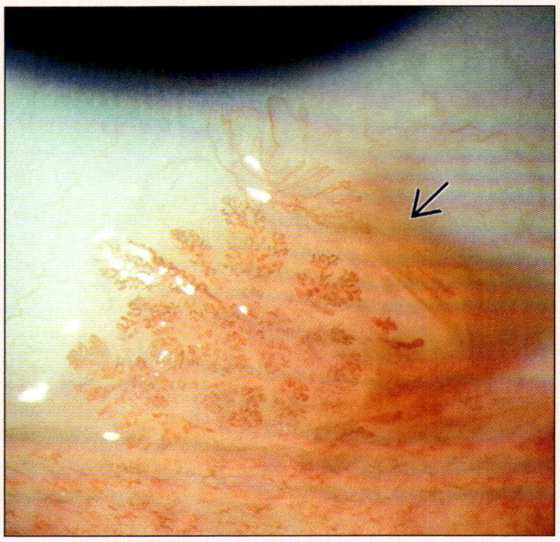

*(**Left**) Slit-lamp photo shows conjunctival SCC of the upper eyelid ➔. Histopathologic exam reveals partial- or full-thickness invasion. (Courtesy J. Dutton, MD, PhD.) (**Right**) Slit-lamp photo shows sessile conjunctival papilloma arising from superior fornix ➔. Lesion has fleshy, multilobulated appearance with smooth, clear epithelium and fibrovascular core of numerous corkscrew blood vessels. Multiple and extensive lesions may be found in immunocompromised patients. (Courtesy W. C. Fowler, MD).*

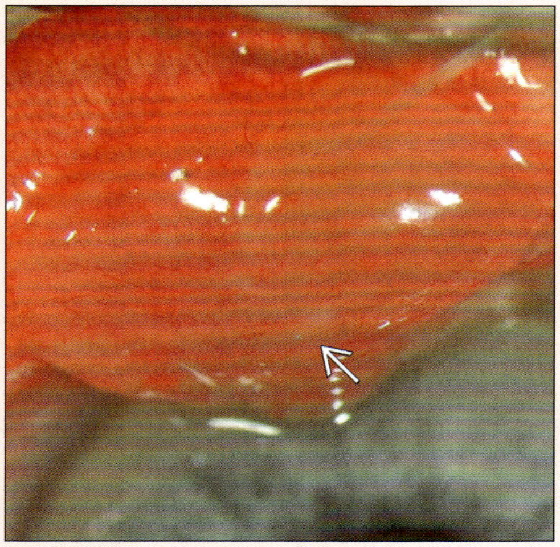

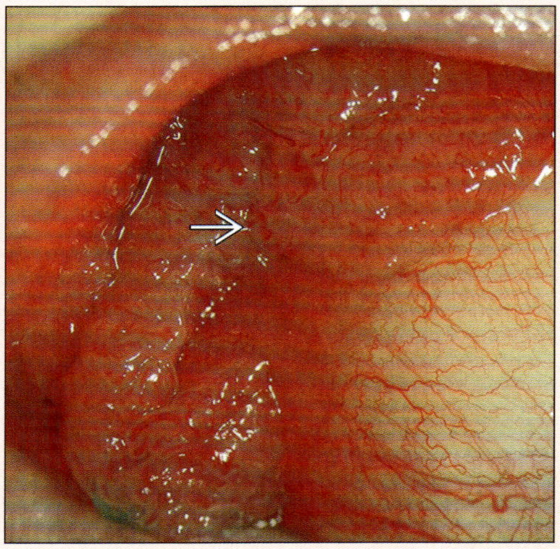

SQUAMOUS CELL CARCINOMA OF THE CONJUNCTIVA

INTRODUCTION

Abbreviations
- Squamous cell carcinoma (SCC)

Synonyms
- Epithelioma

Definitions
- Nonpigmented malignant tumor of ocular surface epithelium that may invade below basement membrane
- Conjunctival intraepithelial neoplasia (CIN), an SCC precursor, involves partial thickness of conjunctival epithelium and does not invade basement membrane
- Carcinoma in situ involves full thickness of conjunctival epithelium, invading basement membrane and underlying stroma or substantia propria
- 20% of SCC metastasizes to regional lymph nodes
- SCC more likely to cause distant metastases than BCC

DEMOGRAPHICS

Etiology/Risk Factors
- Occurs in elderly individuals with fair complexion and history of chronic sun exposure
- UVA/UVB radiation
- HPV: Types 6 and 8 cause benign neoplasm; types 16 and 18 cause malignant neoplasm
- Immunocompromised individuals (e.g., HIV patients)
- Younger individuals with albinism and genetic diseases such as xeroderma pigmentosum
- 2x more common in males than females

Epidemiology
- Most common conjunctival malignancy

PRESENTATION

Symptoms
- Irritation, foreign body sensation, redness, and visibly apparent growth(s) on ocular surface

Exam Findings
- Gelatinous thickening of limbal and bulbar conjunctiva in interpalpebral fissure zone
- Compared to BCC, SCC exhibits greater hyperkeratosis
- Lesion usually has broad base along limbus, sharp borders, and may exhibit leukoplakia
- Engorged and dilated, fimbriated conjunctival vessels feed tumor
- May exhibit perineural invasion
  - Trigeminal nerve involvement mimics tic douloureux
  - Orbital nerve involvement causes ophthalmoplegia
- May exhibit metastases to regional lymph nodes

DIFFERENTIAL DIAGNOSIS

Benign Lesions of Surface Epithelium
- Squamous papilloma, keratoacanthoma, actinic keratosis, pinguecula, pterygium

Malignant Lesions of Surface Epithelium
- Sebaceous gland carcinoma (SGC), malignant melanoma, MALT

EVALUATION/WORK-UP

Pathology
- Lesion is usually superficial with histologic invasion occurring beneath epithelial basement membrane but not penetrating Bowman layer or sclera

TREATMENT

Medical
- Chemotherapy
  - Topical mitomycin C, 5-fluorouracil, or interferon α-2b (which can be administered as eyedrops q.i.d. [1 million U/mL] or a subconjunctival/intratumoral injection [5-10 million U])
- Radiation therapy
  - May be used as adjunct to surgery, otherwise reserved for poor surgical candidates

Surgical
- If medical therapy (now primarily topical or subconjunctival interferon α-2b) fails, then surgery with wide excision followed by reconstruction
  - Histological exam on frozen section confirms tumor margins microscopically
- SCC of conjunctiva requires wide excision 4 mm beyond tumor margin, scleral flap beneath tumor, and cryotherapy to conjunctival margins; mitomycin C may be applied to scleral bed for 1-2 minutes
  - Amniotic membrane graft minimizes postoperative inflammation and allows for reepithelialization; may be utilized if area of surgical resection is large (> 4 contiguous clock hours)
- Corneal involvement requires surgical scraping of tumor cells with preservation of Bowman layer
  - Alcohol aids in delaminating epithelium
- SCC extending into orbit requires exenteration of orbital contents

Prognosis
- 5% recurrence rate despite tumor-free surgical margins
- Poor prognostic factors
  - Orbital extension, perineural invasion, immunosuppression, poorly differentiated tumor, metastasis

SELECTED REFERENCES

1. Shields CL et al: Tumors of the conjunctiva and cornea. Surv Ophthalmol. 49(1):3-24, 2004
2. Donaldson MJ et al: Squamous cell carcinoma of the eyelids. Br J Ophthalmol. 86(10):1161-5, 2002
3. McKelvie PA et al: Squamous cell carcinoma of the conjunctiva: a series of 26 cases. Br J Ophthalmol. 86(2):168-73, 2002
4. Shields CL et al: Topical mitomycin C for extensive, recurrent conjunctival-corneal squamous cell carcinoma. Am J Ophthalmol. 133(5):601-6, 2002
5. Midena E et al: Treatment of conjunctival squamous cell carcinoma with topical 5-fluorouracil. Br J Ophthalmol. 84(3):268-72, 2000
6. Lee GA et al: Ocular surface squamous neoplasia. Surv Ophthalmol. 39(6):429-50, 1995

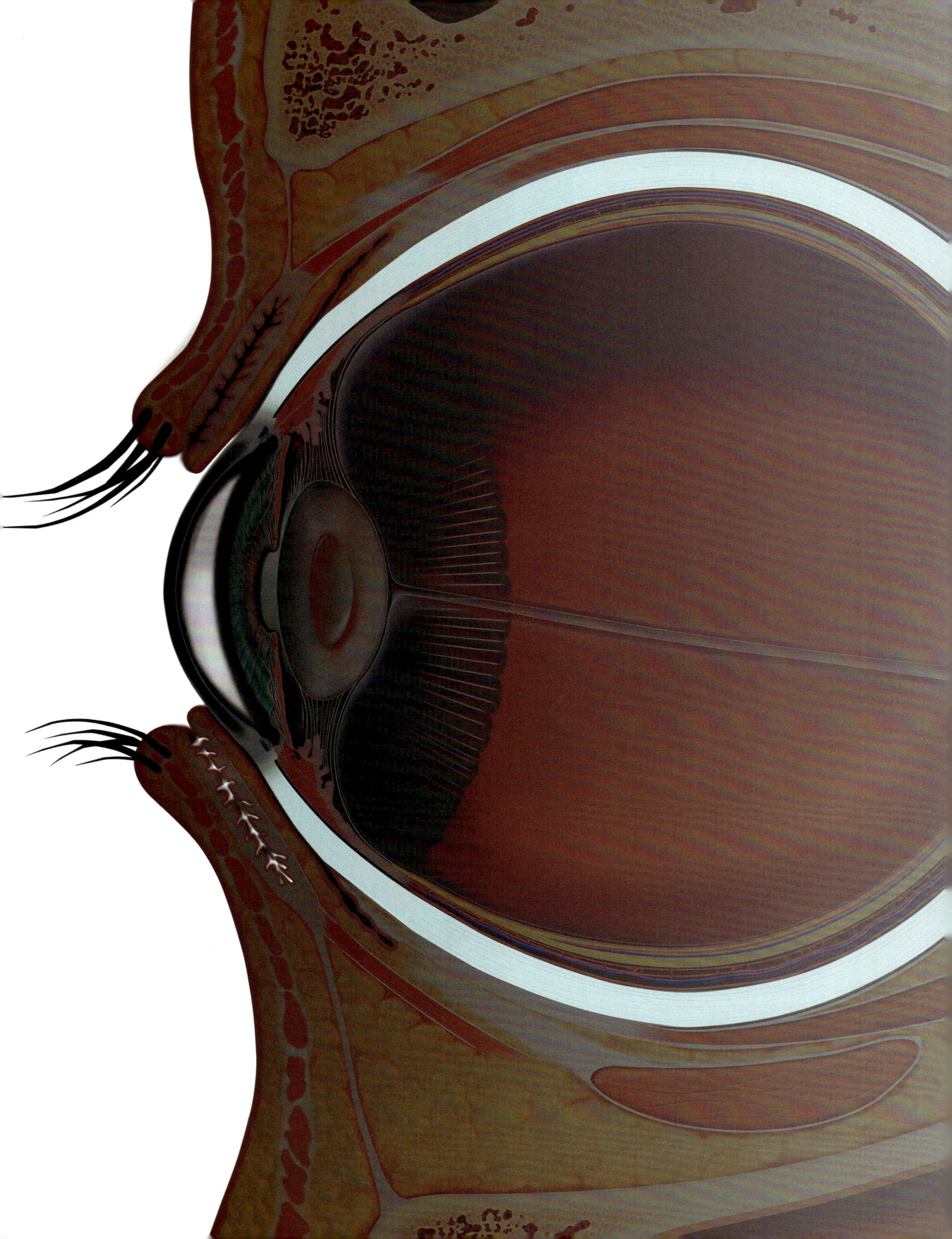

SECTION 2
Sclera

Introduction and Overview

Congenital Disorders

Infectious Disorders

Autoimmune and Inflammatory Disorders

Trauma

Vascular Disorders

SCLERA OVERVIEW

TERMINOLOGY

Definitions

- White outer layer of eye
- Continuous with cornea anteriorly (separated by limbus) and dura mater posteriorly

EMBRYOLOGY

Embryologic Events

- Most of the sclera is derived from neural crest
- Temporal portion of sclera derived from mesoderm
- Sclera is transparent early in gestation but becomes opaque prior to birth

SCLERAL ANATOMY, HISTOLOGY & FUNCTION

Anatomy

- Covers ~ 90% of eye outer coat
- Avascular structure
- At optic disc, outer 2/3 of sclera continues with dura mater
- Inner 1/3 joins with choroidal tissue to form lamina cribrosa
- Collagen of sclera is continuous with cornea anteriorly

4 Layers (Outer to Inner)

- Episclera
  - Composed of small bundles of collagen fibrils, fibrocytes, melanocytes, and elastin fibers
  - More vascular than scleral stroma
  - Connected to conjunctiva anteriorly
  - Anterior ciliary arteries provide anterior vascular supply
  - Posterior ciliary arteries provide posterior vascular supply
  - Tenon capsule: Thin membrane anterior of episclera separated by lymph space
- Stroma
  - 95% of total scleral thickness
  - Composed of dense collagen fibrils and some sclerocytes (similar to keratocytes of corneal stroma)
  - In contrast to corneal stroma, collagen fibrils (types 1, 3, 5) of scleral stroma are wider and more variable in diameter, spacing, size, and direction
    - Responsible for scleral opacity
- Lamina fusca
  - Brown, avascular, and very thin
  - Internal part of stroma where melanocytes reside
- Endothelium

Function

- Maintains shape of globe
- Protects intraocular components from trauma, light, and mechanical displacement
- Provides attachment for extraocular muscle insertions

DISEASES AFFECTING SCLERA

Congenital Diseases

- Epibulbar hamartomas and choristomas
  - Most common tumors of childhood
- Osteogenesis imperfecta, congenital glaucoma, or van der Hoeve syndrome
  - Blue-colored sclera (indicating thin sclera)
- Congenital scleral ectasia
- Anterior staphyloma
  - Protrusion of uveal tissue through cornea or sclera
  - Result of scleral weakening from inflammatory or degenerative processes

Scleral Inflammation

- Episcleritis
  - Benign and self-limiting
- Scleritis
  - Very serious and can cause blindness if not treated
  - One of few ocular emergencies
  - Associated with systemic inflammatory diseases

Infection

- Viral
  - Herpes simplex, herpes zoster
- Bacteria
  - *Pseudomonas aeruginosa*, *Streptococcus*, *Proteus*
- Fungi
  - *Aspergillus*
- *Acanthamoeba*

Metabolic Conditions

- Gout
  - Manifests as episcleritis or scleritis
- Cystinosis
  - Cystine crystals in episclera and superficial sclera
- Alkaptonuria
  - Melanin accumulation in light-exposed parts of sclera
- Porphyria
  - Can erode sclera
- Xanthomatosis
  - Yellow-white scleral deposits associated with abnormal lipid metabolism
- Hypercalcemia
  - White translucent plaques in all layers of sclera

Neoplasm

- Epithelial tumors associated with episclera
- Vascular tumors (e.g., hemangioma, angioma) involving episclera vessels
- Lymphoma infiltration of episclera
- Secondary cancer spread to episclera (e.g., dermolipoma, rhabdomyosarcoma)

Benign Scleral Degenerations

- Senile hyaline plaque
  - Circular depression of sclera between lateral or medial rectus muscles and limbus; no treatment required
- Spontaneous intercalary perforation
  - Hole in sclera without inflammation; no treatment required

RELATED REFERENCES

1. Watson PG et al: Scleral structure, organisation and disease. A review. Exp Eye Res. 78(3):609-23, 2004
2. Hogan MJ et al: Histology of the Human Eye: An Atlas and Textbook. Philadelphia: W. B. Saunders. 183, 1971

SCLERA ANATOMY AND HISTOLOGY

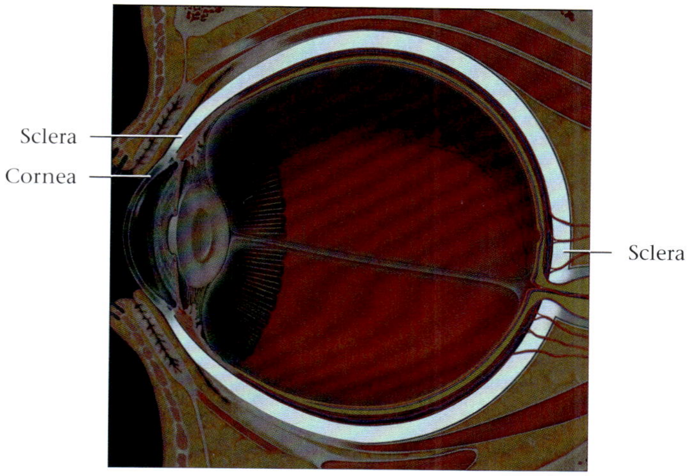

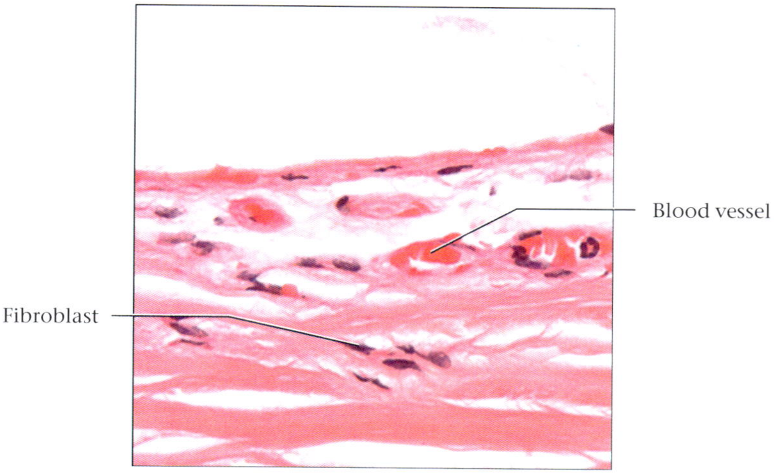

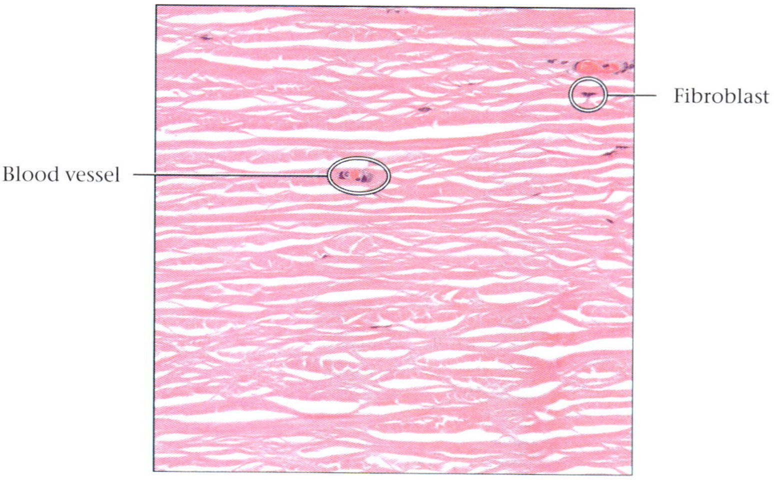

(Top) *The sclera is the white outer covering of the eye. It is continuous anteriorly with the cornea and is separated by the limbus. Posteriorly, it joins with the dura mater.* ***(Middle)*** *The episclera composes the outermost layer of the sclera and contains more numerous blood vessels admixed with collagen and fibroblasts. (Courtesy H. Brown, MD.)* ***(Bottom)*** *The middle portion, and the bulk of the sclera, is the scleral stroma. The stroma is composed of varying sizes of collagen fibers admixed with elastic fibers. Within the stroma, rare fibroblasts and blood vessels may be identified. (Courtesy H. Brown, MD.)*

EHLERS-DANLOS SYNDROME

Key Facts

Introduction

- Group of rare disorders affecting collagen formation
- Ocular involvement is common in type VI (ocular-scoliotic), rarely in type IV (arterial-ecchymotic)

Presentation

- Decreased distance visual acuity
- Monocular diplopia
- Red, painful eye
- Generalized soft tissue fragility, easy bruising
- Hyperextensible skin, hypermobile joints
- Poor wound healing
- Ophthalmic exam
  - Blue sclera
  - Ectopia lentis
  - Globe rupture with minimal trauma
  - Keratoconus, keratoglobus
  - Microcornea
  - Angioid streaks

Evaluation/Work-Up

- Molecular genetic testing
- Electron microscopy of skin → disturbed fibrillogenesis
- Biochemical testing of cultured dermal fibroblasts → abnormal migration of collagen chains
- Diagnosed with clinical exam and family history

Treatment

- Treat individual disease manifestations
- No specific treatment exists for Ehlers-Danlos syndrome
- Wound closure
  - Close dermal wounds in 2 layers, without tension
  - Close other wounds with generous, deep sutures
  - Sutures should be left in place 2x as long as usual
  - Tape skin at sutured wound edge to prevent scar
- Follow-up
  - Orthopedics, cardiology, physical therapy

*(**Left**) This external photograph demonstrates keratoconus. Note the angulated lower lid on downgaze due to corneal protrusion (Munson sign) ➔. This occurs because of defective collagen formation. Keratoconus is a frequent finding in Ehlers-Danlos syndrome. (**Right**) This external photograph demonstrates a subluxed crystalline lens ➔. This is a common finding in Ehlers-Danlos syndrome.*

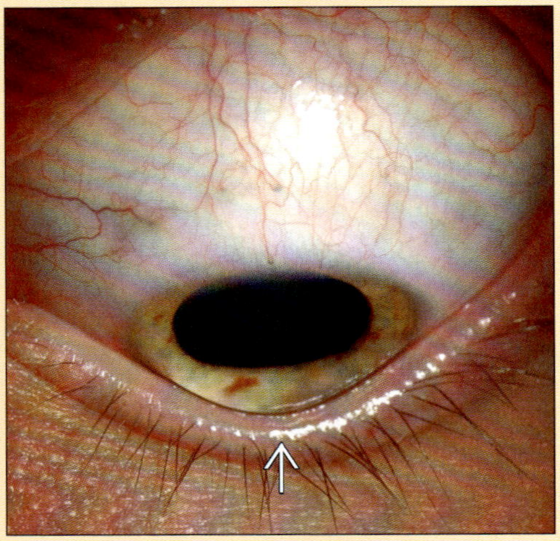

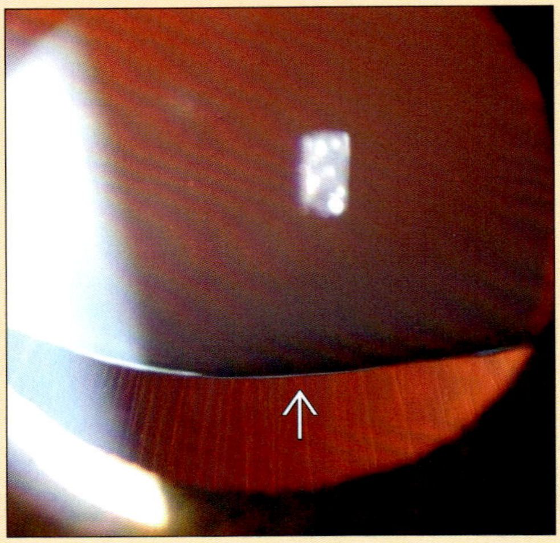

*(**Left**) This external photograph depicts blue sclera ➔. This is a typical finding in patients with Ehlers-Danlos syndrome and is indicative of thinning of the sclera that occurs due to problems with collagen formation. (**Right**) This fundus photograph depicts angioid streaks ➔. These streaks create a linear pattern beneath the retina and are a common finding in Ehlers-Danlos syndrome.*

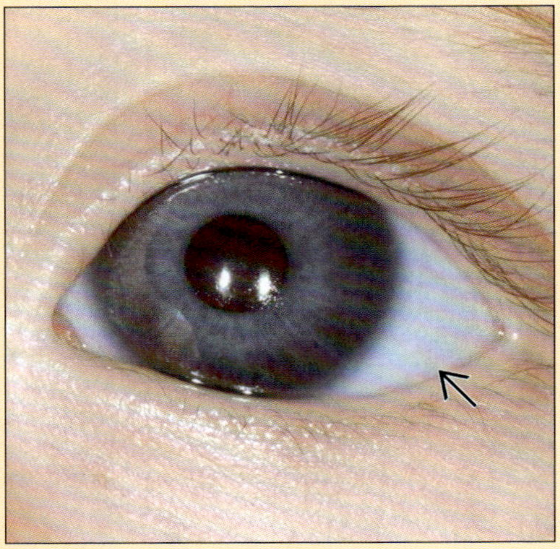

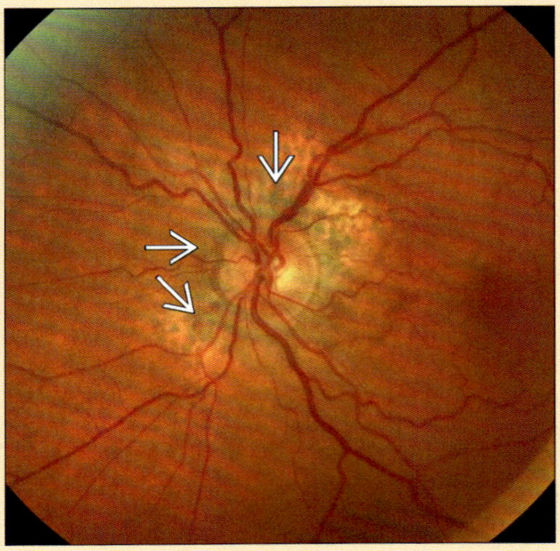

EHLERS-DANLOS SYNDROME

INTRODUCTION

Abbreviations
- Ehlers-Danlos syndrome (EDS)

Definitions
- Group of rare disorders affecting collagen formation

Subtypes
- > 10 types and subtypes
- Type VI (ocular-scoliotic)
  - Ocular involvement is common
- Type IV (arterial-ecchymotic)
  - Ocular involvement occurs, although rarely

DEMOGRAPHICS

Etiology/Risk Factors
- Autosomal dominant and recessive types
- Type VI (ocular-scoliotic) = deficient lysyl hydroxylase
  - *PLOD1* gene defect → abnormal collagen synthesis → weak connective tissues

Epidemiology
- 1/5,000 people, no racial predisposition

PRESENTATION

Symptoms
- Decreased distance visual acuity
- Monocular diplopia
- Red, painful eye
- Generalized soft tissue fragility, easy bruising
- Hyperextensible skin, hypermobile joints
- Poor wound healing

Exam Findings
- Ocular
  - Blue sclera
  - Ectopia lentis
  - Globe rupture with minimal trauma
  - Keratoconus, keratoglobus
  - Microcornea
  - Myopia
  - Retinal detachment
  - Angioid streaks, CNV
- Systemic findings
  - Generalized joint hypermobility/dislocation
  - Muscle hypotonia
  - Kyphoscoliosis
  - Cardiovascular abnormalities
  - Wide, atrophic, "cigarette paper" or papyraceous scars
  - Molluscoid pseudotumors over pressure points

DIFFERENTIAL DIAGNOSIS

Brittle Cornea Syndrome
- Similar ocular, systemic findings
- Skin hyperelasticity without fragility
- Normal lysyl hydroxylase activity

Osteogenesis Imperfecta
- Similar ocular and systemic findings
- Megalocornea
- Corneal arcus
- Bone fractures

EVALUATION/WORK-UP

Labs
- Molecular genetic testing
- Evaluation for disorders of hemostasis if bruising is present

Pathology
- Electron microscopy of skin → disturbed fibrillogenesis
- Biochemical testing of cultured dermal fibroblasts → abnormal migration of collagen chains

Imaging
- Electrocardiography and echocardiography

Diagnosis
- Established with clinical examination and history

TREATMENT

Medical
- Treat individual disease manifestations
- No specific treatment exists for EDS
- Physical therapy and non-weight-bearing exercise may reduce pain due to hypermobility
- Vitamin C (ascorbic acid) may reduce bruising

Surgical
- Wound closure
  - Close dermal wounds in 2 layers, without tension
  - Close other wounds with generous, deep sutures
  - Sutures should be left in place 2x as long as usual
  - Tape skin at sutured wound edge to prevent scar
- For dislocated lenses, need to fixate IOL to iris or to sclera or use Cionni ring to suture bag to sclera
- Treatment of CNV from angioid streaks

Follow-Up
- Routine ophthalmologic examinations
- Orthopedic surgery
- Physical therapy
- Cardiology
- Generalist

Prognosis
- Patients with EDS usually have normal life expectancy

SELECTED REFERENCES

1. Gharbiya M et al: Ocular features in joint hypermobility syndrome/ehlers-danlos syndrome hypermobility type: a clinical and in vivo confocal microscopy study. Am J Ophthalmol. 154(3):593-600, 2012
2. Malfait F et al. Ehlers-Danlos Syndrome, Classic Type. 1993-, 2007
3. Al-Hussain H et al: Brittle cornea syndrome and its delineation from the kyphoscoliotic type of Ehlers-Danlos syndrome (EDS VI): report on 23 patients and review of the literature. Am J Med Genet A. 124A(1):28-34, 2004
4. Beighton P et al: Ehlers-Danlos syndromes: revised nosology, Villefranche, 1997. Ehlers-Danlos National Foundation (USA) and Ehlers-Danlos Support Group (UK). Am J Med Genet. 77(1):31-7, 1998

OSTEOGENESIS IMPERFECTA

Key Facts

Introduction
- Osteogenesis imperfecta (OI) is an inherited disease resulting in defective connective tissue, most commonly caused by a deficiency in type I collagen
- Mutations in *COL1A1* and *COL1A2*, which encode type I collagen, account for 90% of cases
- Up to 12 different subtypes have been described
- Severity of OI (mild → severe)
  - Type I < IV < VI < VII < III < II

Demographics
- Estimated incidence is 1 per 20,000 births

Presentation
- Ocular findings
  - Blue sclera
  - Megalocornea
  - Corneal arcus
- Multiple fractures of different ages, pseudarthroses
- Dental hypoplasia
- Hearing loss
- Short stature, scoliosis
- Easy bruising, fragile skin

Evaluation/Work-Up
- Intrauterine biochemical/collagen analysis from chorionic villus sampling or amniocentesis
- Skeletal survey

Treatment
- Genetic counseling indicated in all cases
- No benefit from elective cesarean section
- Avoid instrument-assisted delivery
- Cyclic bisphosphonate therapy for severe OI
- Intramedullary rods to straighten and stabilize long bones

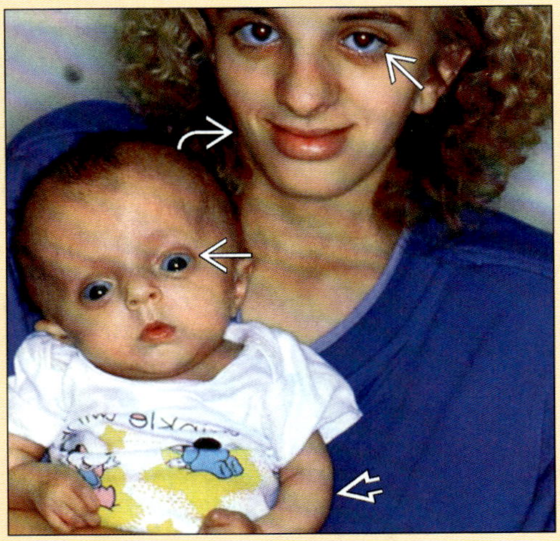
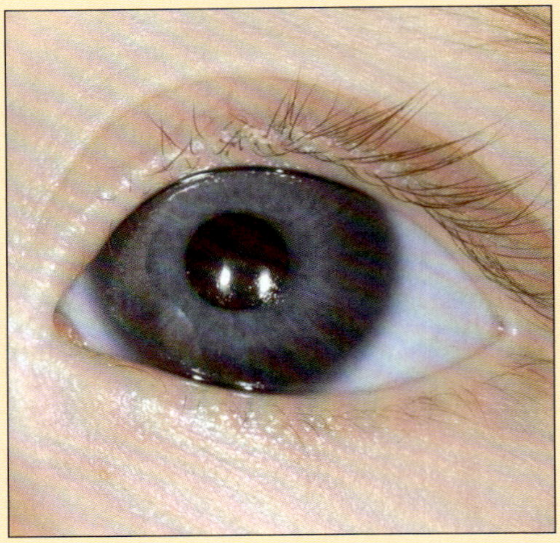

(Left) *Clinical photograph shows a mother and infant both affected with type IV osteogenesis imperfecta. Note the strikingly dark blue sclerae, triangular facies, and pseudoarthrosis.* ***(Right)*** *This clinical photograph demonstrates the faintly bluish sclera in a patient with osteogenesis imperfecta.*

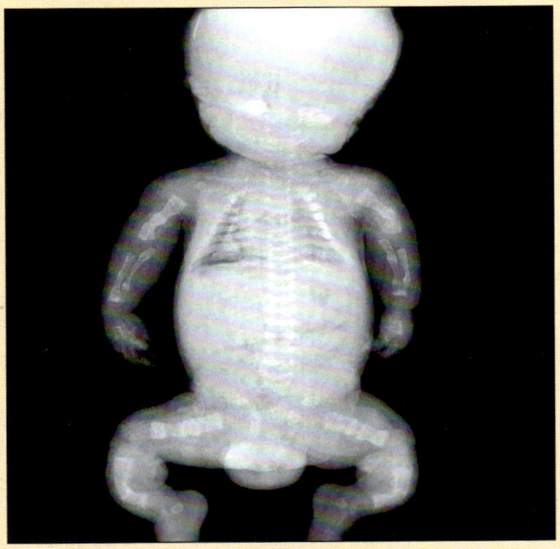
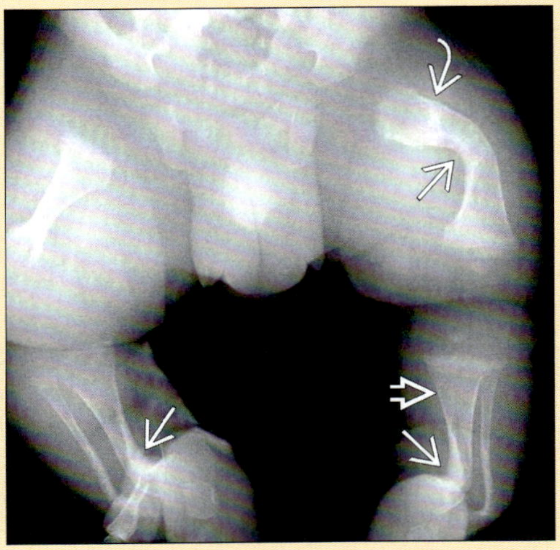

(Left) *Frontal radiograph of a fetus (suspected type II osteogenesis imperfecta) obtained during fetal-imaging autopsy demonstrates numerous fractures of all extremities and the ribs in varying states of repair as well as underossification of the calvarium.* ***(Right)*** *Anteroposterior radiograph of the lower extremities shows poorly ossified bones with thin cortices in a newborn with type IV osteogenesis imperfecta. Note the healed fracture and severe bowing.*

OSTEOGENESIS IMPERFECTA

INTRODUCTION

Abbreviations
- Osteogenesis imperfecta (OI)

Synonyms
- Brittle bone disease

Definitions
- Inherited disease resulting in defective connective tissue, most commonly caused by a deficiency in type I collagen

Pathology
- Mutation in *COL1A1* and *COL1A2*
  - Major components in type I collagen
  - Identified in 90% of cases
- Characteristic blue sclerae are caused by thinning or transparency of the scleral collagen

Subtypes
- Up to 12 different subtypes have been described
  - Type I
    - Fractures typically occur when child starts walking
    - Blue sclerae
  - Type II
    - Often lethal in utero or early infancy
    - Short, broad, deformed bones at birth
  - Type III
    - Multiple fractures at birth
    - Generalized osteopenia
    - Sclerae are white to grayish blue
    - Often nonambulatory
  - Type IV
    - Delayed presentation
    - Sclerae are white or grayish blue
  - Types V-XII
    - Non-type I collagen related, etiology unclear
- Severity of OI (mild → severe)
  - Type I < IV < VI < VII < III < II

DEMOGRAPHICS

Epidemiology
- Estimated incidence is 1 per 20,000 births

PRESENTATION

Exam Findings
- Ocular findings
  - Blue sclera, megalocornea, corneal arcus
- Multiple fractures of different ages, pseudarthroses
- Dental hypoplasia, hearing loss, short stature, scoliosis
- Easy bruising, fragile skin, joint laxity

DIFFERENTIAL DIAGNOSIS

Nonaccidental Trauma
- Bone fractures accompanied by retinal hemorrhages
- Normal bone mineral density
- Careful history and family evaluation required

Congenital Dwarfisms
- Common etiologies
  - Achondroplasia
  - Spondyloepiphyseal dysplasia
  - Thanatophoric dwarfism

Osteomalacia/Rickets
- Defective mineralization/calcification, "soft bones"
- Vitamin D deficiency

Hypophosphatasia
- Rare, autosomal disease resulting in generalized hypomineralization
- Fractures less common
- Low serum alkaline phosphatase in neonate

EVALUATION/WORK-UP

Labs
- While diagnosis is primarily clinical, DNA testing will often reveal mutations in *COL1A1* and *COL1A2*
  - Negative testing does not exclude the diagnosis due to non-type I collagen types (V-XII)
- Intrauterine biochemical/collagen analysis from chorionic villus sampling or amniocentesis

Imaging
- Skeletal survey
  - Multiple fractures of varying ages

TREATMENT

Perinatal
- Genetic counseling indicated in all cases
  - Types I-V are autosomal dominant
- No benefit from elective cesarean section
  - No increase in survival in lethal OI
  - No decrease in perinatal fractures in non-lethal OI
- Avoid instrument-assisted delivery

Medical
- Cyclic bisphosphonate therapy
  - Decreases bone turnover while increasing bone density
  - Decreases fracture rate

Surgical
- Intramedullary rods to straighten and stabilize long bones
- Spinal fusion for kyphoscoliosis
  - High risk of hardware mechanical failure

Prognosis
- Types I and IV
  - Normal to slightly shorter lifespan
- Type II
  - Perinatal lethal
- Type III
  - Significantly shortened lifespan

SELECTED REFERENCES

1. Hasegawa K et al: Growth of infants with osteogenesis imperfecta treated with bisphosphonate. Pediatr Int. 51(1):54-8, 2009
2. Marini JC: Osteogenesis imperfecta: comprehensive management. Adv Pediatr. 35:391-426, 1988

INFECTIOUS SCLERITIS

Key Facts

Introduction

- Infection of sclera from local or systemic source, leading to inflammation
- Primary
  - Disruption of scleral integrity, allowing entrance of pathogens
- Secondary
  - Extension or dissemination of extraocular infection into eye

Demographics

- Greater incidence in men than in women
- Not associated with systemic autoimmune disease
- Incidence of infectious scleritis is increasing

Presentation

- Intense pain in affected eye
- Conjunctival injection
- Decreased visual acuity
- Fever and other systemic manifestations of primary infection

Evaluation/Work-Up

- Orbital magnetic resonance (MR) imaging is useful in determining extent of infected tissue and posterior scleritis
- Ultrasonography
  - Demonstrates scleral thickness changes

Treatment

- Crucial to begin as soon as diagnosis of infectious scleritis has been made
- Antibiotic targeting identified pathogen
- Debridement surgery
- Anti-inflammatory drugs to alleviate pain
- Good prognosis if identified as infectious early and treated with debridement and antibiotics

__(Left)__ This external photo shows the characteristic appearance of HSV scleritis. Note the significant dilation of scleral blood vessels ⇒ and marked conjunctival injection over the primary site of infection. Also, note the violaceous hue in the area of scleritis ⇒. (Courtesy M. Moshirfar, MD.) __(Right)__ Ultrasound imaging illustrates scleral thickening. The normal human sclera averages 0.53 mm in the anterior portion of the eye. This sclera has a markedly increased thickness of 3.37 mm. (Courtesy A. Vitale, MD.)

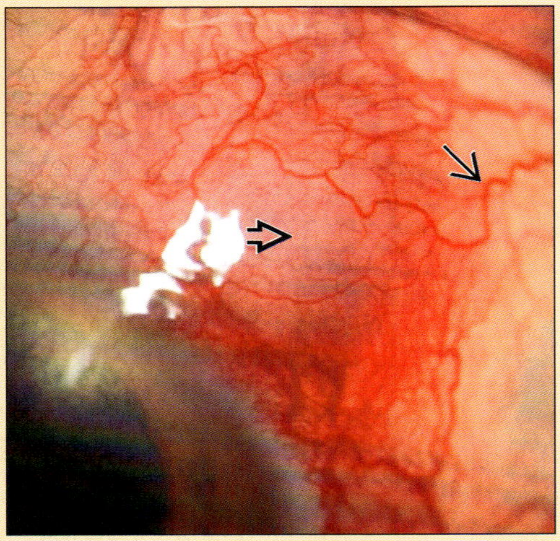

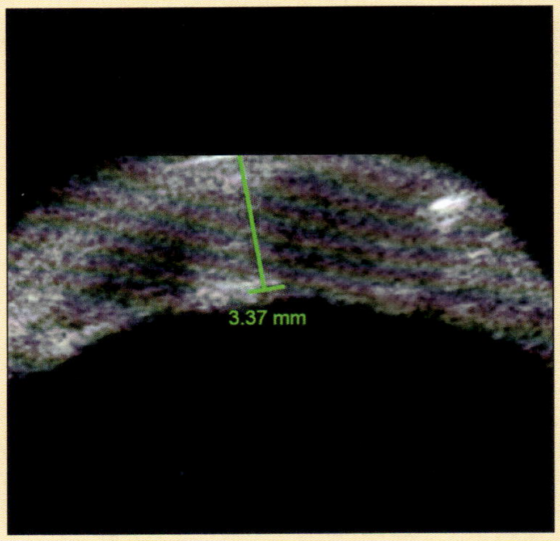

__(Left)__ One complication of infectious scleritis is scleral thinning that can lead to herniation of intraocular contents, known as a scleral staphyloma ⇒. Treatment involves a scleral patch graft. (Courtesy M. Mifflin, MD.) __(Right)__ Example shows intense temporal scleral injection that can be a feature of infectious scleritis. (Courtesy G. Jenkins, MD.)

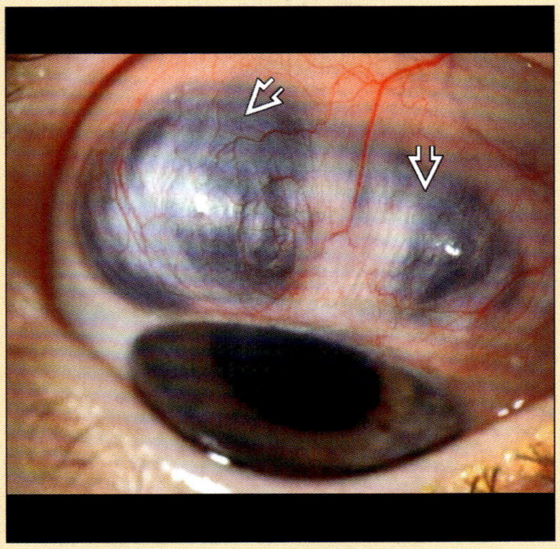

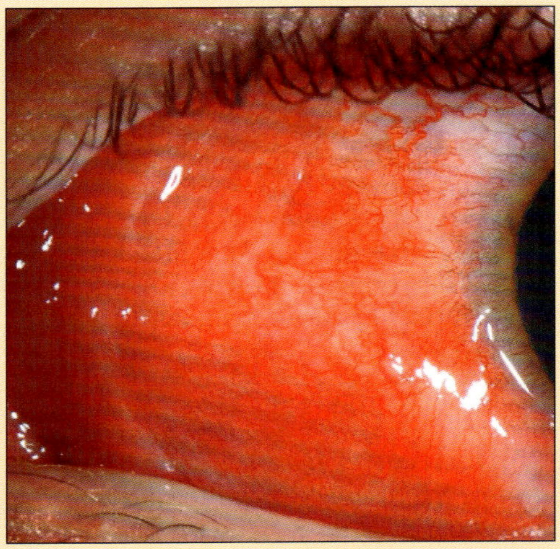

INFECTIOUS SCLERITIS

INTRODUCTION

Definitions

- Infection of sclera from local or systemic source, leading to inflammation, necrosis, or fistulization

Subtypes

- Primary
  - Disruption of scleral integrity, allowing entrance of pathogens
- Secondary
  - Extension or dissemination of extraocular infection into eye

DEMOGRAPHICS

Etiology/Risk Factors

- Common pathogens
  - *Pseudomonas, Mycobacterium tuberculosis, Mycobacterium leprae, Treponema pallidum, Borrelia Burgdorferi*, gram-positive cocci, gram-negative cocci, fungi, varicella zoster virus, and herpes simplex virus
- More common in eyes that have had
  - Spread of infection from adjacent sources
  - Radiation exposure (β radiation)
  - Surgery
    - Particularly pterygium or retinal surgery
  - Traumatic events that disrupt integrity of sclera

Epidemiology

- Incidence of infectious scleritis is increasing
- Immigrant populations: Undertreatment of many infections in 3rd world countries leads to incomplete elimination of underlying infection
- Greater incidence in men than women

PRESENTATION

Symptoms

- Intense pain in affected eye; responds poorly to analgesics
- Conjunctival injection
- Decreased visual acuity
- Pain that develops after initial healing of surgical site is highly indicative
- Lacrimation and photophobia
- Fever and chills

Exam Findings

- Significant dilation of scleral blood vessels
- Scleral nodules
- Scleral ectasia or melting
- Mycobacterial infections can cause fistulization

DIFFERENTIAL DIAGNOSIS

Necrotizing Scleritis

- Sclera may appear blue due to thinning of scleral tissue, revealing underlying choroid
- Slit-lamp exam will reveal avascular areas

Scleromalacia Perforans

- Nonpainful thinning and bluing of sclera
  - Lack of pain is due to necrosis of nociceptive nerve fibers
- Requires patch grafting

Episcleritis

- Pain and discomfort is generally mild
  - Eyes usually described as feeling "gritty"

EVALUATION/WORK-UP

Labs

- Specific microbiological tests for possible pathogens
- Culture with Gram stain of blood and scleral exudate

Pathology

- Biopsy can show different species (acid-fast stain for mycobacteria; Gomori methenamine silver for fungi)

Imaging

- Orbital magnetic resonance (MR) imaging is useful in determining extent of infected tissue and posterior scleritis
- Ultrasonography
  - Demonstrates scleral thickness changes

TREATMENT

Medical

- Crucial to begin treatment as soon as diagnosis of infectious scleritis has been made
- Antibiotic targeting identified pathogen, delivered
  - Systemically
  - Topically
  - Through subconjunctival injection

Surgical

- Debridement surgery with aggressive irrigation
  - Remove affected tissue and leave surgical defect open to ensure adequate exposure to topical antibiotics
- Enucleation
  - If infection does not respond to debridement with antibiotics and becomes necrotic

Follow-Up

- Within 1 week for
  - Medication dosage adjustment
  - Slit-lamp, funduscopic, and visual-acuity exam
- Look for complications of treatment, such as
  - Scleral staphyloma (scleral thinning requiring scleral patch graft)
  - Glaucoma
  - Phthisis bulbi

Prognosis

- Good prognosis if identified as infectious early and treated with debridement and antibiotics

SELECTED REFERENCES

1. Tittler EH et al: Early surgical debridement in the management of infectious scleritis after pterygium excision. J Ophthalmic Inflamm Infect. 2(2):81-7, 2012
2. Watson, P et al: The Sclera and Systemic Disorders. 3rd ed. London: JP Medical Ltd. 242-4, 2012
3. Reynolds MG et al: Treatment of infectious scleritis and keratoscleritis. Am J Ophthalmol. 112(5):543-7, 1991

EPISCLERITIS

Key Facts

Introduction

- Benign inflammatory condition of the episclera

Demographics

- No clear etiology in majority of cases
- Simple episcleritis ~ 75-85% of cases (F > M)
- Nodular episcleritis ~ 15-25% of cases

Presentation

- Simple episcleritis
  - Engorged episcleral vessels → eye redness
  - Acute onset (~ 30 min), diffuse or sectorial
  - Pain is mild or absent, rarely severe
  - Peaks at ~ 12 hours; resolves over several days
  - Diffuse edema in episcleral tissues
  - Gray deposits may be present
- Nodular episcleritis
  - Red areas increase in size, but their location does not change
  - Discomfort increases with redness
  - Nodules may be single or multiple and are tender, mobile, and nonnecrotic
  - Slit-lamp deep beam reflection is not displaced above scleral surface
  - Subacute onset over several days
- 2.5% epinephrine drops allow visualization of sclera

Evaluation/Work-Up

- Simple and nodular subtypes have similar pathology
- Normal anterior segment fluorescein angiography

Treatment

- None required in many cases
- Chilled artificial tears
- Weak topical steroid or oral NSAIDs, if needed
- Symptoms usually resolve in 7-10 days
- Recurrence is common

*(**Left**) This slit-lamp photograph shows very injected inferior conjunctiva in a patient with episcleritis. Vessel engorgement is most prominent in the superficial episcleral network ⇨ with the deep episcleral and conjunctival vessels less affected →. (**Right**) This slit-lamp photograph shows mildly injected conjunctiva associated with episcleritis. The eye redness of episcleritis can vary from a mild flush ⇨ to brick red and can be either diffuse or sectorial.*

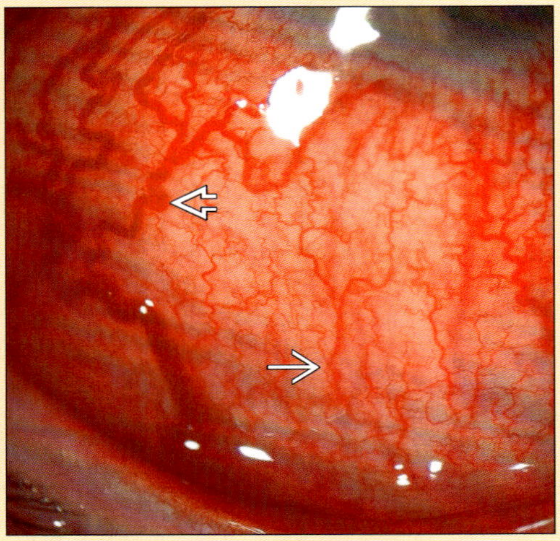

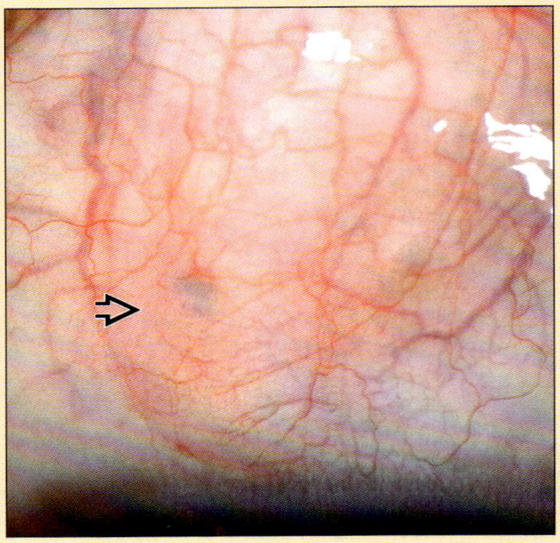

*(**Left**) This slit-lamp photograph shows severely injected conjunctiva with diffuse edema of the episcleral tissues ⇨, a common characteristic of episcleritis. (**Right**) This slit-lamp photograph shows moderately injected conjunctiva in a patient with episcleritis. Note the normal vessel architecture and radial position of the episcleral vessels ⇨.*

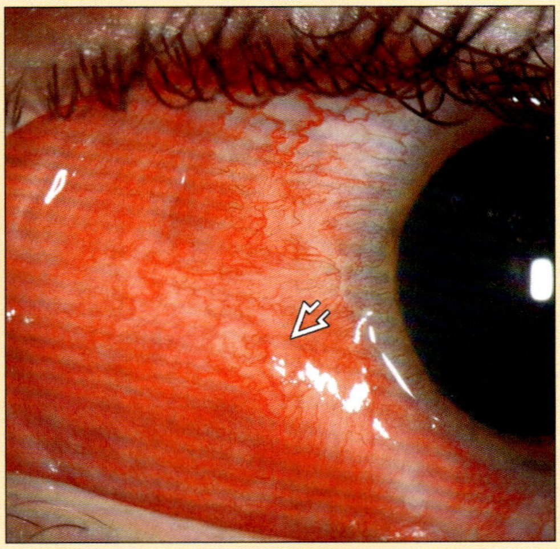

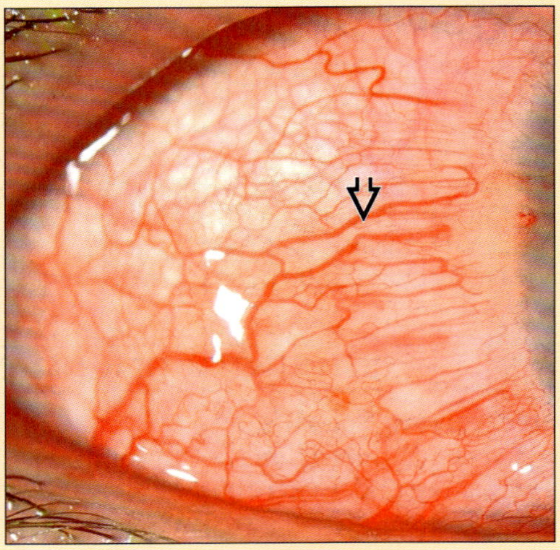

EPISCLERITIS

INTRODUCTION

Definitions

- Benign inflammatory condition of the episclera

Subtypes

- Simple episcleritis
- Nodular episcleritis

DEMOGRAPHICS

Etiology/Risk Factors

- No clear etiology in majority of cases
- Associated with
  - Rheumatoid arthritis (main association)
  - Immune-mediated conditions
    - Family history of atopy, penicillin sensitivity, Henoch-Schönlein purpura, erythema nodosum

Epidemiology

- Uncommon
- Simple episcleritis
  - ~ 75-85% of cases
  - Female predominance
- Nodular episcleritis
  - ~ 15-25% of cases

PRESENTATION

Symptoms

- Simple episcleritis
  - Eye redness (chief complaint)
    - Acute onset (~ 30 min), diffuse or sectorial
  - Discomfort
    - Pain is mild or absent, rarely severe
    - Sensations of heat, pricking
    - Localized to eye, may radiate to forehead
  - Lid edema is rare
  - Peaks at ~ 12 hours and resolves over several days
  - Recurrence is common
    - Attacks may be bilateral or jump from eye to eye
- Nodular episcleritis
  - Eye redness that slowly spreads
  - Discomfort increases as redness worsens
  - Subacute onset
    - Progressively worsens over several days
    - Usually, first noticed upon waking

Exam Findings

- Simple episcleritis
  - Engorged episcleral vessels
    - Affects superficial episcleral network > deep episcleral and conjunctival vessels
    - Normal vessel architecture and radial position
    - Generally blanch with phenylephrine drops
  - Edema: Diffuse in episcleral tissues
  - Gray deposits appear yellow under red-free light if present
  - Redness: Mild flush to brick red, diffuse or sectoral
- Nodular episcleritis
  - Localized edema with vascular congestion
  - Single or multiple, tender, mobile, nonnecrotic nodules
  - Almost always in interpalpebral fissure
  - Slit-lamp exam of nodules
    - Deep beam reflection is not displaced above sclera
  - Repeated attacks result in permanent alteration
    - Transparent sclera, dilation of vessels
- 2.5% epinephrine drops allow visualization of sclera
  - Conjunctival and episcleral vessels decongest
- Visual acuity, intraocular structures, and sclera are all unaffected

DIFFERENTIAL DIAGNOSIS

Scleritis

- More severe and destructive process
  - Severe boring pain, bluish tinge on exam
- Ocular morbidities, treatment modalities differ
- Associated with life-threatening diseases

EVALUATION/WORK-UP

Pathology

- Simple and nodular subtypes have similar pathology
  - Lymphocyte predominance with no mast cells, plasma cells, or eosinophils

Imaging

- Anterior segment fluorescein angiography
  - Normal vascular pattern with high flow rate

TREATMENT

Medical

- Treatment is similar for simple and nodular episcleritis
- Chilled artificial tears
- Weak topical steroid or oral NSAIDs, if needed
- No treatment is required in many cases

Follow-Up

- Suspicion of underlying condition if prolonged or very recurrent disease

Prognosis

- Symptoms usually resolve in 7-10 days
  - Nodular episcleritis takes longer to resolve
- Recurrence is common
  - Involvement often jumps from eye to eye
- Episcleritis does not progress to scleritis except when associated with vesicular stage of herpes zoster infection
  - Scleritis may develop 2-3 months later

SELECTED REFERENCES

1. Pavesio CE et al: Systemic disorders associated with episcleritis and scleritis. Curr Opin Ophthalmol. 12(6):471-8, 2001
2. Sainz de la Maza M et al: Severity of scleritis and episcleritis. Ophthalmology. 101(2):389-96, 1994
3. McGavin DD et al: Episcleritis and scleritis. A study of their clinical manifestations and association with rheumatoid arthritis. Br J Ophthalmol. 60(3):192-226, 1976
4. Watson PG et al: Scleritis and episcleritis. Br J Ophthalmol. 60(3):163-91, 1976

NECROTIZING SCLERITIS

Key Facts

Introduction
- Inflammation of the sclera leading to severe vasculitis, infarction, and ultimately, necrosis of involved sclera
- Subtypes
  - Necrotizing anterior scleritis
  - Necrotizing posterior scleritis

Demographics
- Least common form of scleritis, yet the most dangerous
- ~ 1/2 of scleritis cases are associated with systemic disease
  - Most commonly rheumatoid arthritis
- Greater incidence in women than in men
- Average age at onset is 68 years

Presentation
- Extreme tenderness with palpation of sclera
- Vasodilation of superficial scleral vessels
- Bluish discoloration of sclera on slit-lamp exam

Differential Diagnosis
- Episcleritis
- Paralimbic scleromalacia
- Infectious scleritis

Evaluation/Work-Up
- ESR
- Rheumatic factor, ANA, ANCA, PPD, RPR, FTA-ABS, CRP
- B-scan ultrasonography
- Anterior segment angiography

Treatment
- Corticosteroids
- Scleral patch graft
- Immunosuppression

*(**Left**) Note the area of avascular, necrotic sclera surrounded by edematous tissue. (Courtesy A. Vitale, MD.) (**Right**) External photo shows uveitis, which in necrotizing scleritis (NS) is caused when inflammation extends into the intraocular space. Presence of inflammatory cells in the vitreous and tissue damage are characteristic of uveitis. This is a sign of a worsening prognosis in NS. (Courtesy A. Vitale, MD.)*

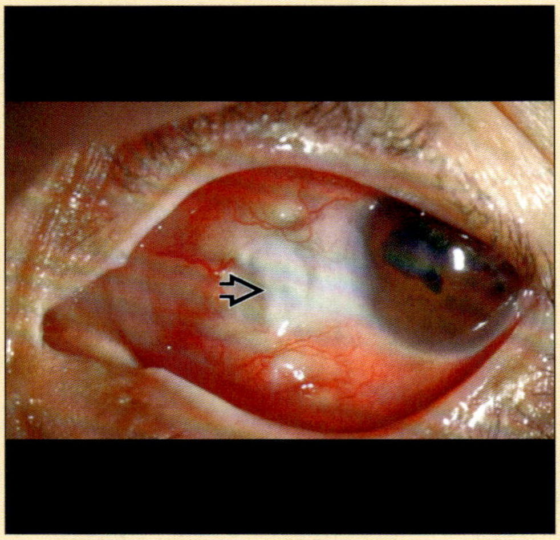

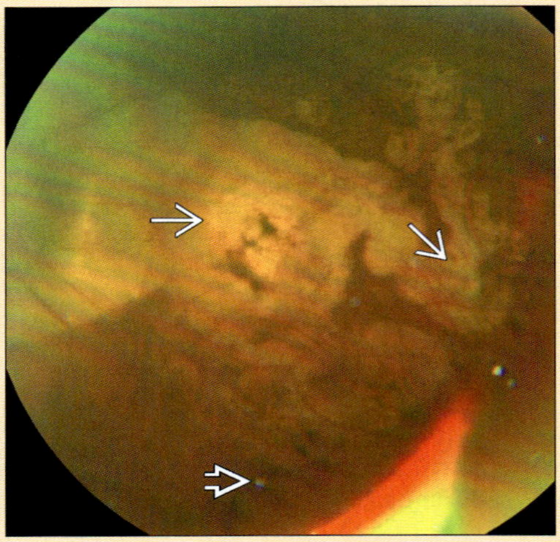

*(**Left**) Slit-lamp photo illustrates an example of the bluish scleral discoloration caused by the process of scleral thinning revealing the underlying choroid. (Courtesy A. Vitale, MD.) (**Right**) External photo shows an example of a staphyloma caused by weakening of the scleral tissue (due to necrotic thinning), leading to a bulging of the sclera. This serious complication of NS can rupture if left untreated. (Courtesy M. Mifflin, MD.)*

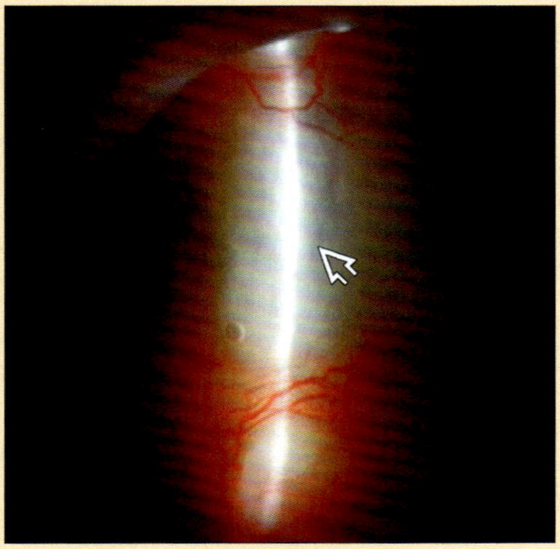

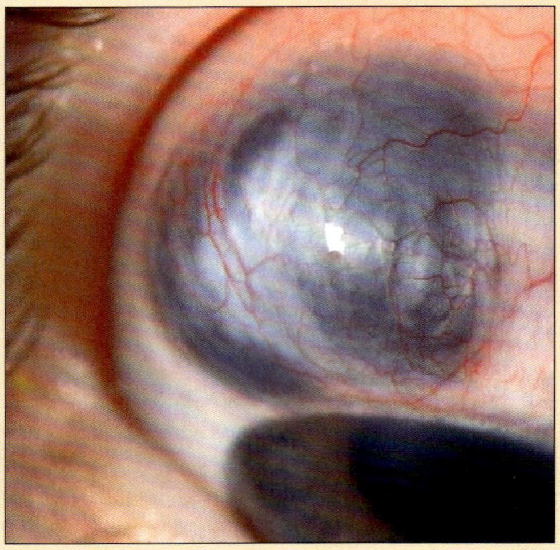

NECROTIZING SCLERITIS

INTRODUCTION

Abbreviations
- Necrotizing scleritis (NS)

Definitions
- Inflammation of the sclera, leading to severe vasculitis, infarction, and ultimately, necrosis of involved sclera

Subtypes
- Necrotizing anterior scleritis
  - Necrotizing anterior scleritis with inflammation
  - Necrotizing anterior scleritis without inflammation
  - Scleromalacia perforans
- Necrotizing posterior scleritis

DEMOGRAPHICS

Etiology/Risk Factors
- Least common form of scleritis, yet it is more dangerous than all other subtypes of scleral inflammation, with greatest potential for vision loss
- ~ 1/2 of scleritis cases are associated with systemic disease
  - Most common association: Rheumatoid arthritis
- Patients with systemic disease are more prone to having bilateral eye involvement

Epidemiology
- Greater incidence in women than in men
- Average age at onset is 68 years

PRESENTATION

Symptoms
- Generally presents unilaterally, but will likely involve the contralateral eye within 5-6 years
- Photophobia, lacrimation, and severe ocular and periorbital pain that gradually increases to an excruciating "boring" pain within weeks
  - During this time, there is extreme scleral tenderness
  - Severity of pain can interfere with sleep
- This constellation of symptoms should raise suspicion of NS in patients with rheumatoid arthritis, vasculitis, inflammatory bowel disease, and systemic lupus erythematous

Exam Findings
- Extreme tenderness with palpation of sclera
- Cells in anterior chamber
- Scleral edema
- Vasodilation of superficial scleral vessels (deep to conjunctival vessels)
- Inflammation and ulceration of cornea
- Slit-lamp findings
  - Deep episcleral vascular plexus dilation
  - Bluish discoloration of sclera caused by process of scleral thinning revealing the choroid
  - Blood vessel closure
  - Forward displacement of slit-lamp light beam due to scleral edema

DIFFERENTIAL DIAGNOSIS

Episcleritis
- Lacks eye pain and blue sclera of NS
- Ocular injection disappears with application of 10% phenylephrine in episcleritis

Paralimbic Scleromalacia
- Painless, noninflammatory thinning of sclera
  - Generally occurs at corneoscleral limbus

Infectious Scleritis
- Can be ruled out with tissue cultures
- Lacks boring eye pain of NS

EVALUATION/WORK-UP

Labs
- ESR
  - Will generally be elevated due to inflammatory component of NS
- Titers for: Rheumatoid factor, Lyme disease, antinuclear antibody, anti-neutrophil cytoplasmic antibodies
- Screen for tuberculosis and syphilis

Pathology
- Biopsy of scleral tissue
  - Inflammatory microangiopathy is indicative of NS

Imaging
- B-scan ultrasonography
  - Detects changes in thickness of sclera
    - Particularly useful in suspected posterior NS
- Anterior segment angiography
  - Detects necrotizing type arteriolar beading and for avascular areas

TREATMENT

Medical
- Corticosteroids
  - Systemic
  - Topical
- Immunosuppression: Anti-TNF-α agents (e.g., infliximab), cyclophosphamide, mycophenolate, tacrolimus
- Anti-collagenase: Vitamin C/doxycycline

Surgical
- Scleral patch graft (avoid unless absolutely necessary)

Prognosis
- If underlying systemic inflammatory disease can be identified and treated, ocular outcomes are greatly improved
- Scleral patch graphs help to improve integrity of sclera and prevent future complications

SELECTED REFERENCES

1. Okhravi N et al: Scleritis. Surv Ophthalmol. 50(4):351-63, 2005

SCLERITIS

Key Facts

Introduction

- Painful inflammation of sclera
- Anterior (more common) and posterior scleritis (more difficult to diagnose)
  - Necrotizing anterior scleritis is most severe but also rarest form
- May be 1st manifestation of a systemic disease (rheumatoid arthritis [RA], Wegener granulomatosis)

Demographics

- ~ 50% have no identifiable cause

Presentation

- Redness and severe eye pain
  - Eye pain that wakes patient in middle of night
  - Pain that radiates to forehead and temporal region
- Eye tender to palpation by applying pressure through eyelids

Evaluation/Work-Up

- Work-up for autoimmune/infectious disease including RA, lupus, polyarteritis nodosa, TB, Lyme disease, antiphospholipid syndrome, and Wegener granulomatosis
- Rule out episcleritis by phenylephrine test (will blanch vessels in episcleritis but not in scleritis)
- Presence of cells in the anterior chamber, bluish sclera, scleral thinning, or deep scleral vascular engorgement also indicate scleritis

Treatment

- NSAIDs for mild disease; steroids or cyclophosphamide for more severe
- Treat underlying cause

*(**Left**) This external photograph depicts a case of scleritis. Note the dilated vessels and the deep erythema of the of the sclera. (**Right**) This external photograph shows diffuse scleritis with associated diffuse erythema and swelling. The swelling is demonstrated by the elevation of the conjunctiva.*

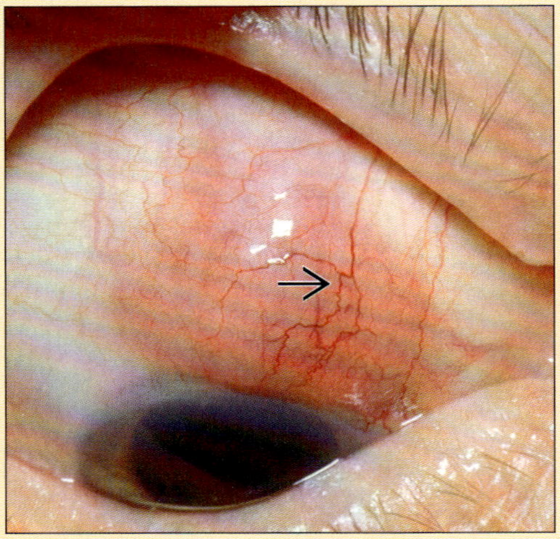

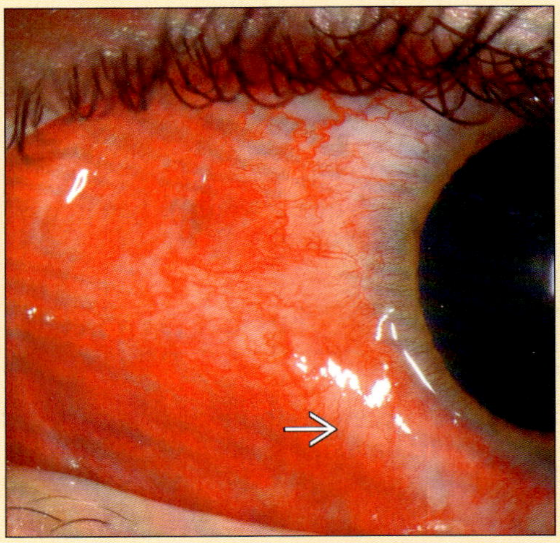

*(**Left**) This external photograph demonstrates diffuse anterior scleritis in a left eye. This eye is at risk of scleromalacia perforans due to thinning of the sclera. (**Right**) This external photograph illustrates a mild presentation of nodular anterior scleritis in the lateral aspect of the left eye.*

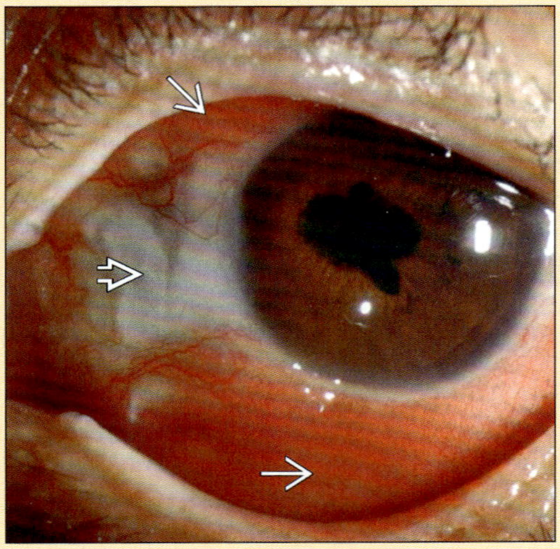

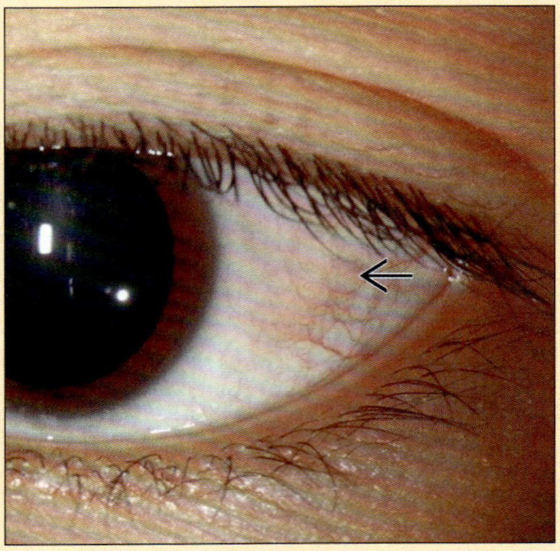

SCLERITIS

INTRODUCTION

Definitions
- Chronic inflammatory response centered on sclera
- Usually involves adjacent episclera, cornea, and uvea

Subtypes
- Anatomic: Anterior or posterior scleritis (or both)
  - Anterior scleritis: Diffuse (most common), nodular, and necrotizing (rare and most severe)
  - Posterior scleritis: Diffuse or nodular
  - Scleromalacia perforans: Scleritis variant; necrotic thinning of sclera without inflammation
- Diagnostic: Infectious (local or systemic) and noninfectious (immune disease)

DEMOGRAPHICS

Etiology/Risk Factors
- Up to 50% of cases are associated with systemic autoimmune disease or vasculitis
- Rheumatoid arthritis (RA) is most common associated systemic disease

Epidemiology
- Mean age of onset is 50 years
- Women account for 2/3 of cases
- Bilateral involvement in 30-50% of patients
- Can be self-limited with complete resolution after treatment
- Can be chronic with need for continuing immunosuppression

PRESENTATION

Symptoms
- Ocular redness and pain
  - Severe, boring pain
  - Retrobulbar pain
  - Radiates to forehead and temporal region
  - Worse at night
  - Severe pain that wakes patient early in the morning

Exam Findings
- Eye tender to palpation by applying pressure through eyelids
- Diffuse redness
- Presence of nodules
- Scleral necrosis
- Anterior chamber cells
- Raised intraocular pressure
- Presence of vitreous cells

DIFFERENTIAL DIAGNOSIS

Noninfectious
- Episcleritis
  - Blanching of superficial episcleral vessels by 10% phenylephrine in episcleritis but not in scleritis
  - Patients complain of redness and eye discomfort (not severe pain)
  - Not vision threatening
- Conjunctivitis: Sticky discharge with itch
- Uveitis: Does not cause a painful/tender eye

Infectious
- Viruses (e.g., syphilis, herpes simplex virus, varicella zoster virus), bacteria (tuberculosis), and fungi

EVALUATION/WORK-UP

Labs
- Urinalysis (UA), ANCA antibodies
- Rheumatoid factor (RF) and anti-citrullinated peptide/protein antibodies (ACPA) for RA
- Antinuclear antibodies (ANA), extractable nuclear antigens (ENA) and DNA for systemic lupus erythematosus (SLE)

Pathology
- Chronic granulomatous disorder (fibrinoid necrosis, polymorphonuclear cells, lymphocytes, plasma cells, macrophages)

Imaging
- Chest x-ray
  - Exclude pulmonary complications of granulomatosis with polyangiitis, RA, and Wegener
  - Help diagnose TB or sarcoidosis
- Ultrasonography
  - For diagnosing posterior scleritis, which shows a thickened eye wall

TREATMENT

Medical
- Oral NSAIDs for mild forms of scleritis (diffuse and nodular anterior scleritis)
- Oral prednisone (1 mg/kg/day)
- Steroid + cyclophosphamide for severe scleritis or refractive disease

Surgical
- Scleral or corneal perforation: Emergency graft procedure (scleral or corneal graft) is necessary

Follow-Up
- Periodic review of systems for those diagnosed with scleritis without systemic disease (increased 50x compared to general population for RA)

Prognosis
- Involvement of peripheral cornea in anterior scleritis indicates severe disease
- Necrotizing scleritis also sign of vision-threatening disease
- Poor visual outcome for eyes with scleral or corneal perforation

SELECTED REFERENCES

1. Wakefield D et al: Scleritis: Immunopathogenesis and molecular basis for therapy. Prog Retin Eye Res. 35:44-62, 2013
2. Sims J: Scleritis: presentations, disease associations and management. Postgrad Med J. 88(1046):713-8, 2012
3. Watson PG et al: Scleral structure, organisation and disease. A review. Exp Eye Res. 78(3):609-23, 2004

RUPTURED GLOBE

Key Facts

Introduction

- Full-thickness injury to cornea or sclera resulting from blunt, penetrating, or perforating trauma

Presentation

- Careful examination is required so as to not place pressure on eye and risk extruding intraocular contents
- Once diagnosis of ruptured globe is made by slit-lamp or penlight examination, further examination should wait until time of surgical repair in OR
- Prolapse of iris, lens, ciliary body, or vitreous may be present
- Very little evidence of trauma may be visible anteriorly
- Suspect posterior rupture when asymmetry of anterior chamber exists
- Measurement is contraindicated to avoid pressure on globe

Evaluation/Work-Up

- B-scan ultrasonography (generally not advisable as it can put pressure on globe)
- CT superior to plain radiography for detection of intraocular FB; MRI is more sensitive for soft tissue but should be avoided if there is any risk of metallic IOFB

Treatment

- Patient should be immediately placed on bed rest; cover eye with shield or Styrofoam cup
- Document tetanus status and update as indicated
- Systemic antibiotics should be administered within 6 hours
- Primary closure of globe should be priority with later vitreoretinal evaluation
- Most globes can be closed within 24 hours; if there is IOFB or lens-corneal touch, close as soon as possible, preferably within 6 hours

__(Left)__ Axial NECT of a child who was accidentally shot with a BB gun shows that the left globe is ruptured and there is a radiodense foreign body ➔ (a BB) within the vitreous chamber. __(Right)__ Axial NECT in a patient who sustained a shotgun injury to the face shows shrapnel ➔ in the sclera posteriorly. The globe was ruptured, and there is intraocular hemorrhage ➔. An additional foreign body artifact is noted on the left ➔.

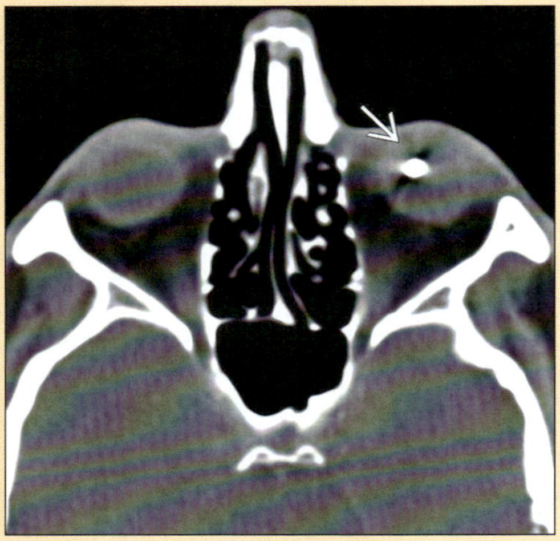

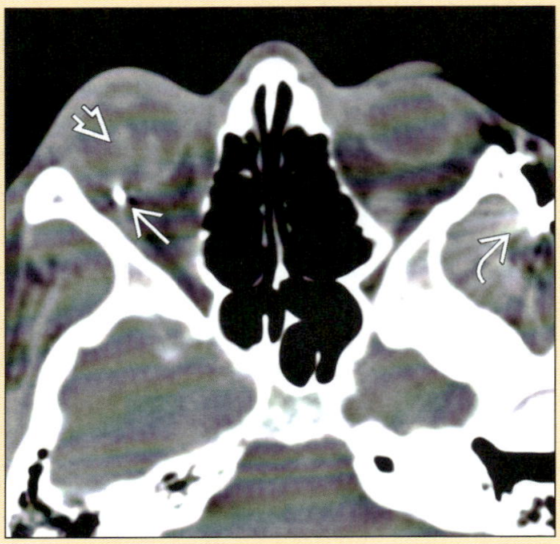

__(Left)__ This slit-lamp photo shows a patient with an anterior penetrating injury, which required suturing of the cornea and eventual cataract surgery. __(Right)__ This fundus photo shows a penetrating injury with a retinal detachment and large inferonasal retinal break.

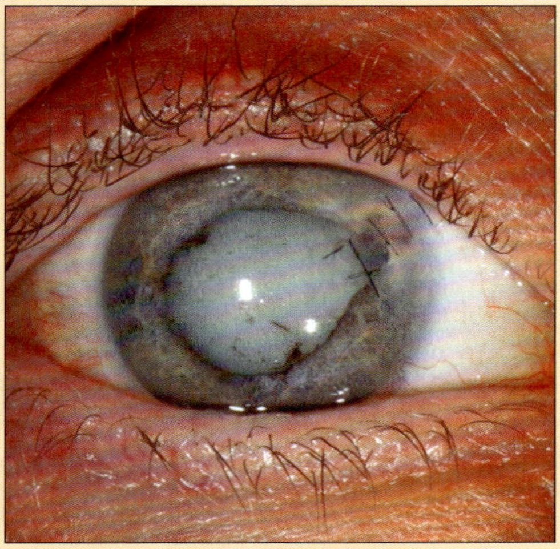

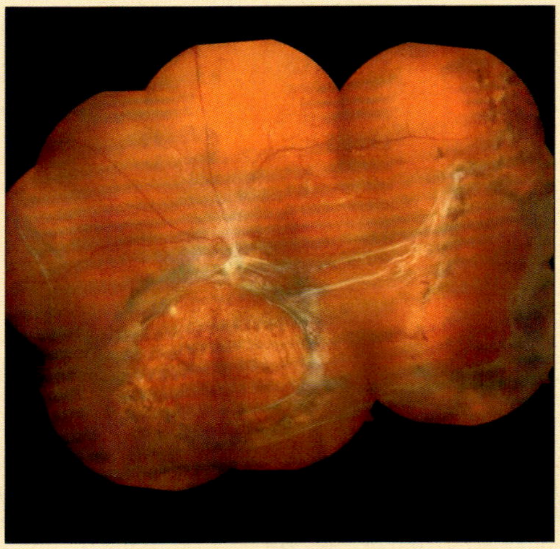

RUPTURED GLOBE

INTRODUCTION

Synonyms
- Open globe

Definitions
- Full-thickness injury to cornea or sclera resulting from blunt, penetrating, or perforating trauma
- Intraocular contents may be extruded

Subtypes
- Anterior
- Posterior
  - Difficult to visualize by examination, often requires imaging for diagnosis
- Blunt injury
  - Causes IOP to increase to point of rupture
- Penetrating injury
  - Entrance wound only
- Perforating injury
  - Both entrance and exit wounds are present

DEMOGRAPHICS

Etiology/Risk Factors
- Majority of ruptured globes occur in males (3:1)
  - Men more frequently present with penetrating trauma
  - Women more commonly rupture a globe secondary to blunt trauma
- Globe ruptures typically occur in younger individuals
  - Most common causes: Motor vehicle accidents, assault, sporting activities, and workplace accidents
- Substance abuse

Epidemiology
- 2 million eye injuries in USA annually
- 20-40% of open globe cases have associated intraocular foreign body (FB)

Primary Prevention
- Ruptured globe often results in catastrophic visual loss
- Eye protection should be worn during high-risk activities

PRESENTATION

Symptoms
- History of blunt or penetrating trauma
  - Pain
  - Poor visual acuity
  - Double vision

Exam Findings
- Careful examination is required so as to not place pressure on eye and risk extruding intraocular contents
- Once diagnosis of ruptured globe is made by slit-lamp or penlight examination, further examination should wait until time of surgical repair in OR
- Ruptured globes most commonly occur anteriorly in vicinity of canal of Schlemm
  - Evaluate for prolapse of iris, lens, ciliary body, and vitreous
- Occult posterior rupture
  - Very little evidence of trauma may be visible anteriorly
  - Suspect posterior rupture when asymmetry of anterior chamber exists
- Cornea and sclera
  - Full-thickness laceration to cornea or sclera will be present
    - Fluorescein may be helpful to identify entry wound
    - Evaluate for leakage of aqueous humor using fluorescein dye (positive Seidel sign)
  - IOP likely to be low
    - Measurement is contraindicated to avoid pressure on globe
- Iris
  - Transillumination defects
  - Iridodialysis
- Pupil
  - Irregularities common
    - Peaked pupil
    - Teardrop shape
- Anterior chamber (AC)
  - Asymmetry in AC depth between traumatic and normal eye
  - Hyphema
  - Lens dislocation or subluxation
  - Traumatic cataract may result
- Posterior segment
  - Vitreous hemorrhage
    - Often obscures posterior examination
  - Retinal detachment
  - Traumatic optic neuropathy
- Orbits
  - Periorbital ecchymosis
  - Orbital rim fracture
  - Enophthalmos (recession of globe within orbit)
  - Exophthalmos may be present if there is an associated retrobulbar hemorrhage
- Eyelid and conjunctiva
  - Conjunctival hemorrhage is often present
    - Subconjunctival edema and hemorrhage may mask ruptured globe
  - Lacerations
- Evaluate for intraocular FB

DIFFERENTIAL DIAGNOSIS

Corneal Laceration
- Partial-thickness laceration
- No entry to anterior chamber
  - Seidel test may be performed by applying fluorescein to cornea
    - Negative test (no dilution or change in color under a cobalt blue filter) will result if globe is not ruptured
- Anterior chamber depth should be symmetrical

Scleral Laceration
- Partial-thickness laceration
- No entry to intraocular space

Retinal Detachment
- Elevation of retina
- Flashes of light
- Floaters
- Patient complains of a "curtain" or "shadow" moving over visual field

RUPTURED GLOBE

- May occur in combination with ruptured globe

Vitreous Hemorrhage

- Loss of vision or hazy vision
- Obscured view of retina
- Mild relative afferent pupillary defect (RAPD)
- Common in open globe injuries

EVALUATION/WORK-UP

Imaging

- B-scan ultrasonography
  - Helpful in identifying ruptured globe, intraocular FB (IOFB), hemorrhage, and retinal detachment
  - Avoid placing pressure on globe during imaging study
- Plain radiographs
  - Indicated if radiopaque FB is suspected
- CT scan
  - Superior to plain radiography for detection of IOFB
  - Demonstrates anatomy of intracranial, orbital, facial, and intraocular structures
- MRI
  - Superior to CT at detecting globe injuries, including posterior rupture
    - **Do not** perform MRI if there is risk of a metallic intraocular FB
  - Inferior to CT for detection of bony injury

TREATMENT

Medical

- Patient should be immediately placed on bed rest
- Document tetanus status and update as indicated
- Systemic antibiotics should be administered within 6 hours
  - Adults
    - Vancomycin 1 g IV q. 12 hours + ceftazidime 1 g IV q. 8 hours for 2 days &/or moxifloxacin 400 mg p.o. q. daily x 7 days
  - Children < 12 years
    - Give cefazolin 25-50 mg/kg/day IV divided into 3 doses
    - Also give gentamicin 2 mg/kg IV q. 8 hours
- Consider topical antibiotic, steroid, and cycloplegia
- Administer antiemetic (prochlorperazine or ondansetron) for nausea and vomiting to prevent Valsalva

Surgical

- Once diagnosis of ruptured globe is made, further evaluation should be reserved until time of surgical repair in OR
- Retrieval of any retained FB
  - Culture of any FB material
- Viable uveal tissue should be reposited if possible
- Primary closure of globe should be priority with later vitreoretinal evaluation
- Enucleation
  - Primary enucleation reserved only for severe injuries with no chance of restoring vision
  - Secondary enucleation may be considered after primary repair if eye is severely damaged or uncomfortable
    - Should occur within 10 days of original injury to avoid remote possibility of sympathetic ophthalmitis
- Most globes can be closed within 24 hours; if there is IOFB or lens-corneal touch, close as soon as possible, preferably within 6 hours

Complications

- Bacterial endophthalmitis occurs in ~ 7% of ocular penetrating trauma cases
  - *Staphylococcus*, *Streptococcus*, and *Bacillus* species are most often isolated
  - *Bacillus* more commonly encountered with injuries contaminated by soil
  - *Eikenella* for dog bites
  - *Pasteurella multocida* for cat bites

Follow-Up

- Urgent surgical attention required upon diagnosis

Prognosis

- Globe rupture associated with high risk of vision loss
  - Predictors of poor visual potential
    - Light perception vision or worse at presentation
    - Wounds that extend posterior to rectus muscle plane
    - Wounds > 1 cm
- Study in pediatric population suffering from ruptured globes showed that > 50% of patients achieved best corrected visual acuity of 20/40 or better at 2 year follow-up

SELECTED REFERENCES

1. Bunting H et al: Prediction of visual outcomes after open globe injury in children: a 17-year Canadian experience. J AAPOS. 17(1):43-8, 2013
2. Burstein ES et al: Traumatic ruptured globe eye injuries in a large urban center. Clin Ophthalmol. 7:485-8, 2013
3. Castellarin AA et al: Open globe management. Compr Ophthalmol Update. 8(3):111-24, 2007
4. Mittra RA et al: Controversies in the management of open-globe injuries involving the posterior segment. Surv Ophthalmol. 44(3):215-25, 1999

RUPTURED GLOBE

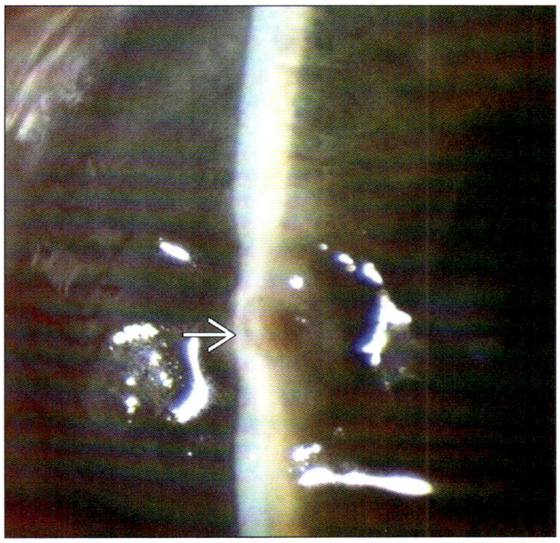

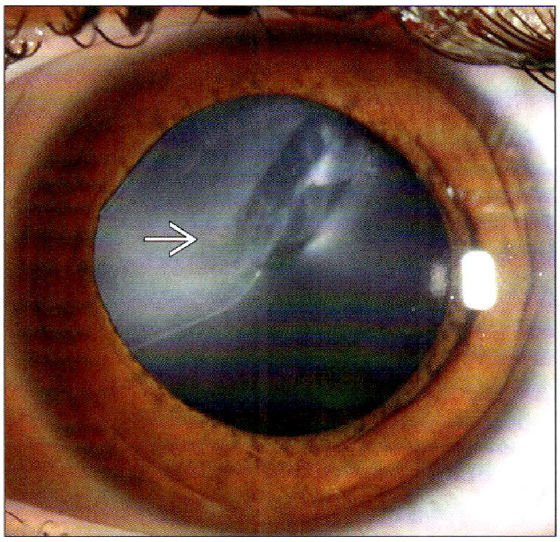

(Left) *This slit-lamp photograph shows a ruptured globe that occurred secondary to penetrating cornea trauma* ➔*. Recognizing that this is an open globe may be difficult, making evaluation for leakage of aqueous humor using fluorescein dye important.* ***(Right)*** *This external photograph shows an eye that suffered a corneal rupture and subsequently developed a traumatic cataract* ➔*.*

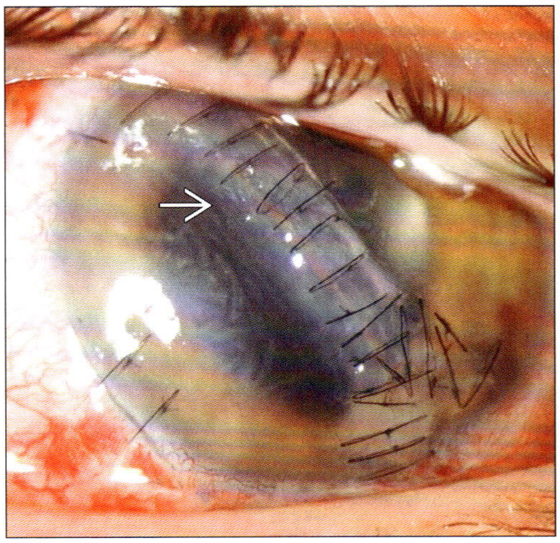

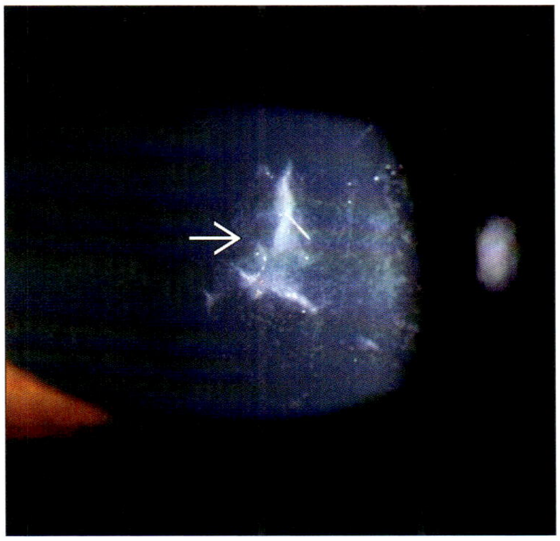

(Left) *This external photograph shows an eye with an open globe secondary to a corneal laceration after repair* ➔*. This eye has a poor visual prognosis due to the involvement of the central cornea in addition to the ruptured globe.* ***(Right)*** *This slit-lamp photograph shows corneal trauma with a possible full-thickness corneal injury* ➔*. Stellate corneal lacerations can be difficult to repair and make water-tight. Purse-string sutures are advisable for stellate lacerations.*

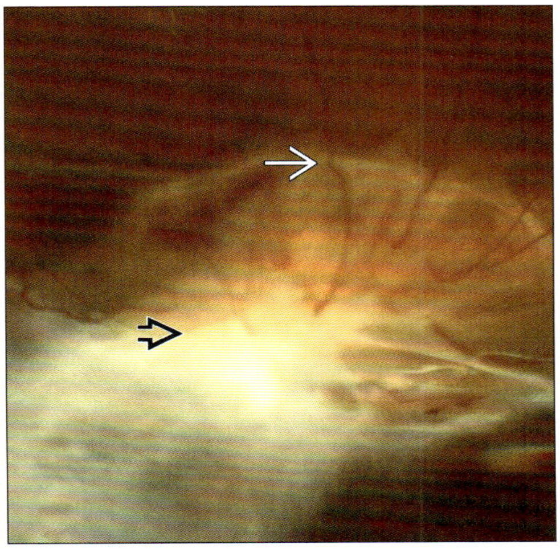

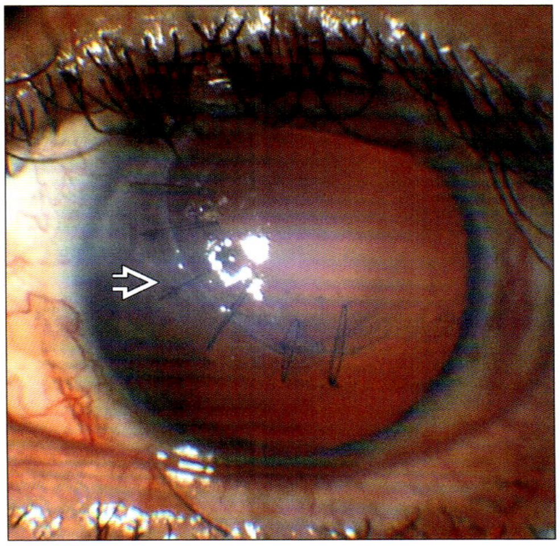

(Left) *This fundus photograph shows retinal detachment* ⇨ *and fibrosis that developed as the result of a ruptured globe. Note the course of the vessels* ➔ *as they run with the elevated and detached retina.* ***(Right)*** *This external photograph shows a ruptured globe after repair* ⇨*. Prompt repair of ruptured globes is necessary to reduce the risk of endophthalmitis.*

SCLEROMALACIA PERFORANS

Key Facts

Introduction
- Type of necrotizing anterior scleritis
  - Minimal or no adjacent inflammation

Demographics
- Case reports in various autoimmune diseases
  - Rheumatoid arthritis (RA) most frequently
- High rheumatoid factor (RF) titer
  - Associated with severe disease
- Longstanding RA
- Very rare
- Female predominant

Presentation
- Most cases are asymptomatic
- Painless, perilimbal scleral plaques
  - Little or no surrounding inflammation
  - Yellow-white or grey-black in color
  - Often necrotic
- Slowly progressive scleral thinning may result in exposure of underlying uvea

Treatment
- Prevention
  - Early anti-inflammatory therapy
  - Disease-modifying antirheumatoid drugs (DMARDs)
- Active disease
  - DMARDs (should be started if not previously prescribed)
- Repair of scleral perforation or extensive thinning
  - Difficult but necessary to avoid phthisis bulbi
  - Various materials used for repair
  - Fresh or preserved donor sclera
  - Periosteum
  - Fascia lata
- No effective treatment for scleral thinning
- Spontaneous perforation is rare
- Case reports of good response

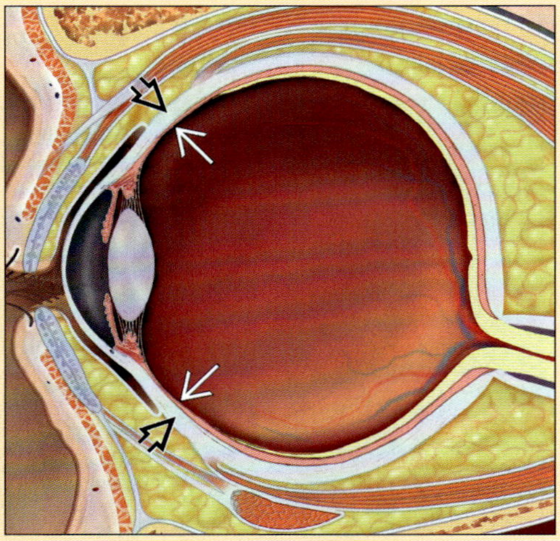
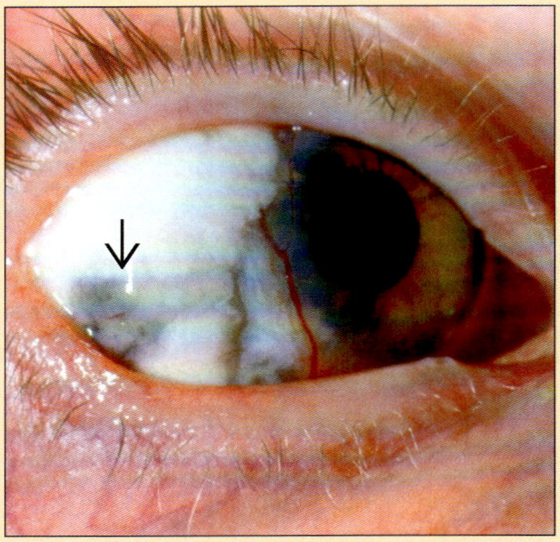

(Left) *This illustration demonstrates the normal anatomy of the eye. Scleromalacia perforans affects the perilimbal sclera ⇨, which necroses and sloughs, often exposing the underlying uveal tissue ➔.* ***(Right)*** *This external photograph shows scleromalacia perforans →. Note the perilimbal location of the plaque with no evidence of surrounding inflammation. Plaques often appear yellow-white or gray-black in color, with darker black areas denoting exposure of underlying uvea.*

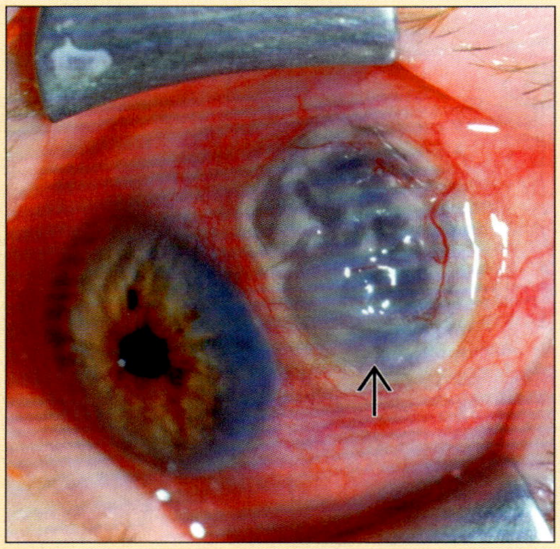
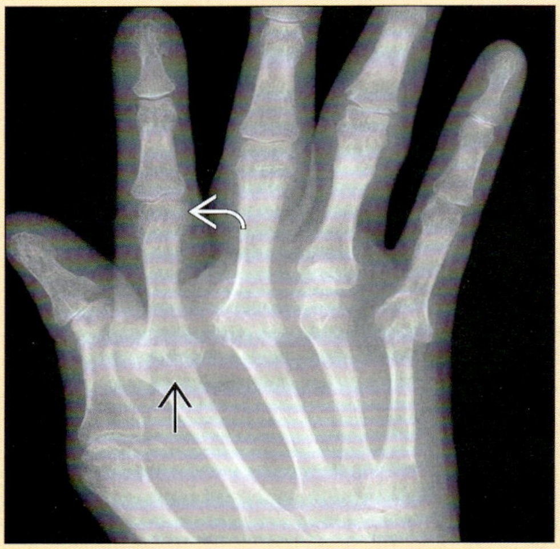

(Left) *This external photograph shows significant scleral thinning → as a result of scleromalacia perforans. Histopathologic examination of these plaques is similar to that of rheumatoid nodules.* ***(Right)*** *This radiograph shows the right hand of a patient with RA, the most common cause of scleromalacia perforans. Note the articular manifestations of RA including ulnar deviation at the metacarpophalangeal joints → and bony erosions ➔ involving multiple joints.*

SCLEROMALACIA PERFORANS

INTRODUCTION

Definitions
- Rare form of necrotizing anterior scleritis
  - Minimal or no adjacent inflammation

DEMOGRAPHICS

Etiology/Risk Factors
- Cases reported in various autoimmune diseases
  - Rheumatoid arthritis (RA)
    - Most common
  - Crohn disease
  - Systemic lupus erythematosus
  - Periarteritis nodosa
  - Granulomatosis with polyangiitis (Wegener)
  - Ulcerative colitis
- High rheumatoid factor (RF) titer associated with
  - Severe disease
  - Unremitting disease
  - Nodules
  - Other extraarticular lesions
- Pathogenesis
  - Likely related to immune complex deposition

Epidemiology
- Very rare
- Female predominant

PRESENTATION

Symptoms
- Most cases are asymptomatic
  - Advanced disease at presentation is possible

Exam Findings
- Painless, perilimbal scleral plaques
  - Little or no surrounding inflammation
  - Yellow-white or grey-black in color
  - Often necrotic
    - Necrotic plaques may slough, resulting in scleral defects
    - Necrotic areas may enlarge and coalesce
- Slowly progressive scleral thinning may result in exposure of underlying uvea

DIFFERENTIAL DIAGNOSIS

Necrotizing Anterior Scleritis With Inflammation
- Severe, persistent pain and edema
- Aggressive disease with poor prognosis

Scleral Hyaline Plaque
- Oval, dark-gray lesion
- Located near insertion of lateral rectus muscles

Nodular, Nonnecrotizing Anterior Scleritis
- Pain, redness
- Tender globe

EVALUATION/WORK-UP

Labs
- RF titer
  - Helpful for risk assessment

Pathology
- Scleral nodules
  - Histopathologically similar to rheumatoid nodules

TREATMENT

Medical
- Prevention
  - Early anti-inflammatory therapy in RA patients
  - Disease-modifying antirheumatoid drugs (DMARDs)
- Active disease
  - DMARDs
    - Should be started if not previously prescribed
    - Case reports of good response
- Use IOP-lowering agents to reduce scleral stress
- Oral vitamin C + doxycycline to reduce scleral thinning

Surgical
- Repair of scleral perforation or extensive thinning
  - Difficult but necessary to avoid phthisis bulbi
  - Various materials used for repair
    - Fresh or preserved donor sclera
    - Periosteum
    - Fascia lata
- No effective treatment for scleral thinning

Follow-Up
- RA patients with high RF titers
  - Regular, careful examinations
  - Aggressive treatment with DMARDs
- Other at-risk patients
  - Regular, careful examinations

Prognosis
- Spontaneous perforation is rare
  - Exception: High-pressure glaucoma

SELECTED REFERENCES

1. Ranjan A et al: Ahmed glaucoma valve surgery for necrotizing scleritis with secondary glaucoma. Int Ophthalmol. Epub ahead of print, 2013
2. Reddy SC et al: Bilateral scleromalacia perforans and peripheral corneal thinning in Wegener's granulomatosis. Int J Ophthalmol. 4(4):439-42, 2011
3. Herrera-Esparza R et al: Infliximab treatment in a case of rheumatoid scleromalacia perforans. Reumatismo. 61(3):212-5, 2009
4. Wu CC et al: Rare extra-articular manifestation of rheumatoid arthritis: scleromalacia perforans. Kaohsiung J Med Sci. 21(5):233-5, 2005
5. Riono WP et al: Scleritis: a clinicopathologic study of 55 cases. Ophthalmology. 106(7):1328-33, 1999
6. Sainz de la Maza M et al: Scleritis associated with systemic vasculitic diseases. Ophthalmology. 102(4):687-92, 1995
7. Sainz de la Maza M et al: Severity of scleritis and episcleritis. Ophthalmology. 101(2):389-96, 1994

SECTION 3
Cornea

Introduction and Overview

Congenital Disorders

Infectious Disorders

Autoimmune and Inflammatory Disorders

Trauma

Vascular Disorders

Degenerations

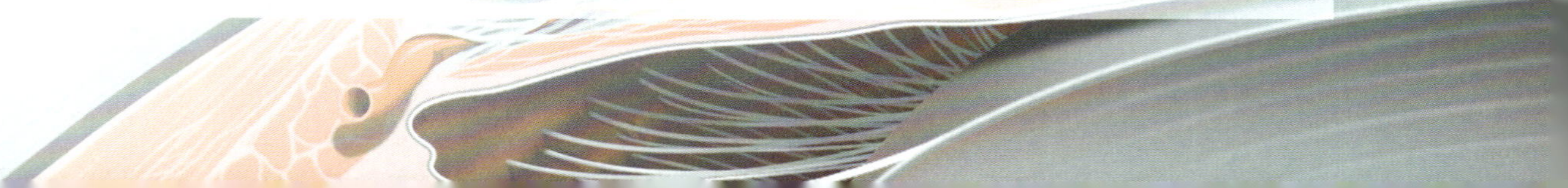

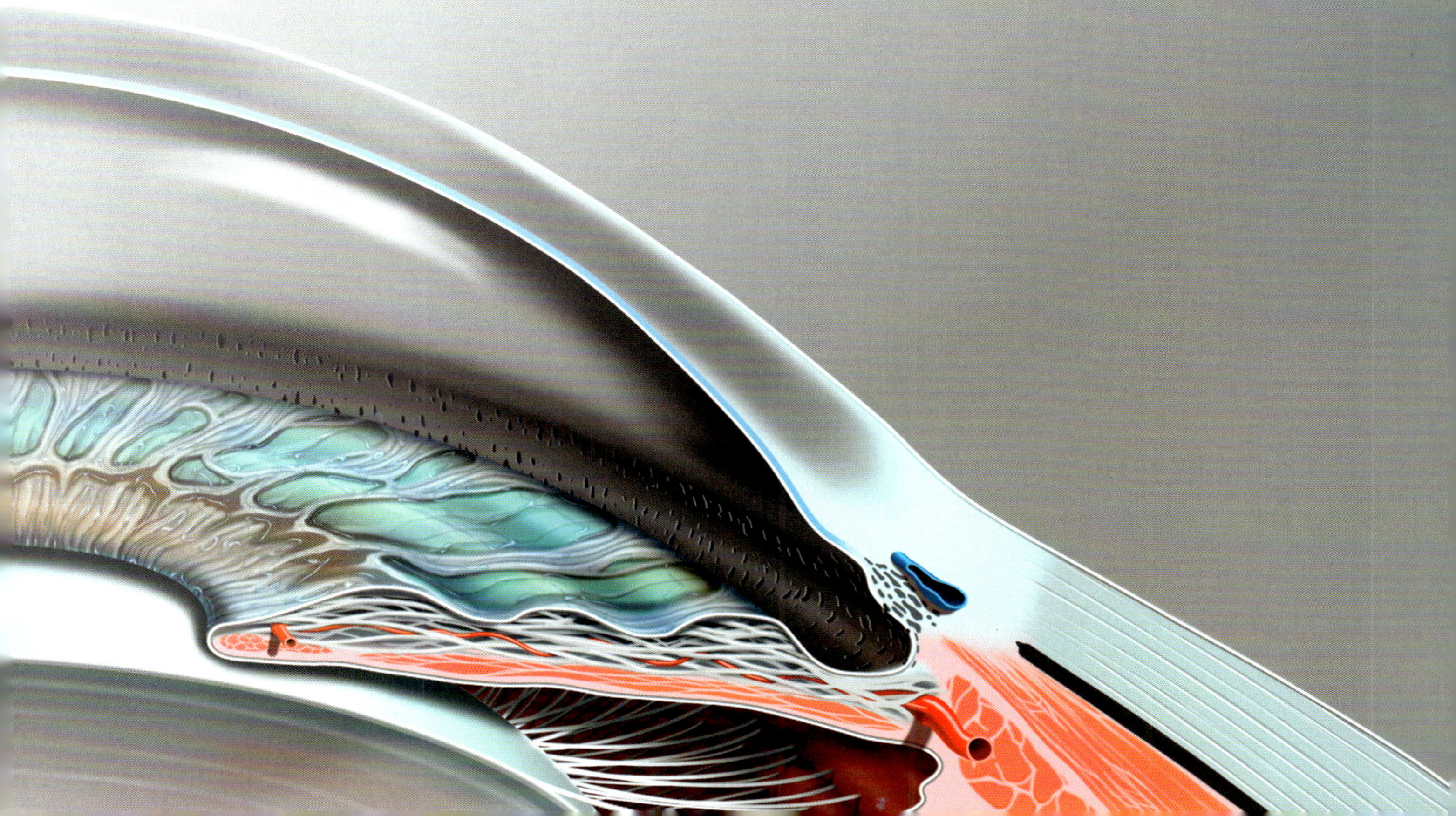

MAJOR CLINICAL STUDIES: CORNEA

TERMINOLOGY

Abbreviations

- Herpetic eye disease (HED), corneal refractive surgery (CRS), corneal cross-linking (CXL), riboflavin collagen cross-linking (RCXL), corneal ectasia (CE)

COLLABORATIVE CORNEAL TRANSPLANTATION STUDIES

Objective and Principal Conclusions

- Assess effectiveness of histocompatibility matching in high-risk keratoplasty patients
- Determine risk factors for graft failure
- Crossmatching & HLA matching do not affect graft survival, but ABO blood group matching reduces graft failure by 50%

Inclusion Criteria

- Age ≥ 10 years
- 2-4 quadrants of corneal stroma vascularization or a history of allograft rejection in transplant eye
- No xerophthalmia, severe exposure keratopathy or other condition that ↑ risk of nonrejection graft failure
- No systemic diseases or medications that alter immune system

Randomization Method

- Crossmatch study: Randomized study to assess effectiveness of crossmatching in preventing graft rejection among high-risk patients with lymphocytotoxic antibodies
- Antigen-matching study: Prospective, double-masked, observational study of effectiveness of HLA-A, HLA-B, & HLA-DR donor-recipient matching in high-risk patients who had no lymphocytotoxic antibodies

Results

- Risk factors for graft failure: Young age, number of previous grafts, prior anterior segment surgery, preoperative glaucoma, quadrants of anterior synechiae, quadrants of stromal vessel, primary diagnosis of chemical burn
- Anti-class 1 lymphocytotoxic antibodies in sera are associated with immune graft rejection
- HLA matching did not affect graft survival or graft rejection, nor did a positive donor-recipient crossmatch
- ABO blood group matching reduced risk of graft failure from rejection by ~ 50% in high-risk patients (2 or more risk factors)
- Development of rejection was associated with increasing corneal thickness (> 0.59 mm was risk factor)

HED STUDY 2 (HEDS-2)

Objective

- Determine role of acyclovir in management of HED
- HSV epithelial keratitis trial (HEDS-EKT)
  - Determine ability of oral acyclovir given during treatment of acute HSV keratitis in preventing future stromal keratitis or iridocyclitis
- Acyclovir prevention trial (HEDS-APT)
  - Evaluate efficacy of long-term acyclovir in patients with history of HSV eye disease (but no current active disease) in preventing recurrent HSV eye disease
- Addition of oral acyclovir to topical trifluridine does not prevent stromal keratitis or iritis but does ↓ recurrences & severity

Inclusion Criteria

- Age ≥ 18 years
- HEDS-EKT: Active acute HSV keratitis, onset ≤ 7 days
  - Dendritic or geographic keratitis
- HEDS-APT: Ocular HSV infection within 1 year
  - Blepharitis, conjunctivitis, keratitis, or iridocyclitis
  - Infection active & untreated for prior 30 days

Randomization Method

- 2 randomized, placebo-controlled trials
- HEDS-EKT
  - All patients treated with topical antiviral
  - Randomized to additional oral acyclovir or placebo
    - Acyclovir 400 mg 5x per day for 21 days
- HEDS-APT
  - Randomized to oral acyclovir or placebo for 1 year
    - Acyclovir 400 mg 2x per day
  - Patients who developed HSV eye disease treated with topical corticosteroids & antivirals as indicated; continued to receive oral acyclovir or placebo

Results

- HEDS-EKT
  - No benefit from addition of oral acyclovir to treatment with topical trifluridine in preventing development of stromal keratitis or iritis
  - Risk of stromal keratitis or iridocyclitis was quite low in year following an episode of epithelial keratitis treated with topical trifluridine alone
- HEDS-APT
  - Oral acyclovir reduced probability of developing recurrent HED by 41%
  - 50% reduction in rate of severe HED, stromal keratitis
  - Oral acyclovir reduced incidence of epithelial keratitis from 11% to 9% & stromal keratitis from 13% to 8%
  - 4% in acyclovir group & 9% in placebo group had multiple occurrences of HED

ECTASIA RISK ASSESSMENT POST CRS

Objective and Principal Conclusion

- Increase understanding of epidemiologic risk factors for corneal ectasia (CE) following excimer laser cornea refractive surgery (ELCRS)
- Risk factors for CE: Abnormal topography, thin residual stromal bed, younger age, corneal thickness, & degree of myopia

Inclusion Criteria

- Cases of CE following ELCRS from 1997 to December 2005 found in a literature search: CE, keratectasia, keratoectasia, iatrogenic ectasia, keratoconus, & LASIK
- Unpublished cases of CE following ELCRS at authors' institution from 1998 to 2005
- Control group was patients undergoing uneventful LASIK with uncomplicated postoperative course

Randomization Method

- No randomization due to observational study

Results

- Risk factors for developing CE in order of decreasing correlation

- Abnormal preoperative topography
- Residual stromal bed (RSB) thickness < 300 μm ($P < .001$)
- Younger age ($P < .0001$ for age < 30 years)
- Thinner preoperative corneal thickness ($P = .01$)
- Degree of myopia preoperatively ($P = .3$ for myopia worse than -8.00 D)

LONG-TERM RESULTS OF RIBOFLAVIN ULTRAVIOLET A CXL FOR KERATOCONUS IN ITALY: SIENA EYE CROSS STUDY

Objective

- Determine long-term results of CXL
- CXL provides long-term stability of keratoconus without relevant side effects

Inclusion Criteria

- Age: 10-40 years
- Minimum corneal thickness: ≥ 400 μm
- Topographic mean: K ≤ 55 diopters
- Clear cornea without Vogt striae or scars
- No current eye infections, history of herpetic illness, autoimmune disease, or current pregnancy

Randomization

- No randomization as all participants were treated with combined riboflavin ultraviolet A collagen cross-linking

Results

- At 4 years, mean hyperopic shift of 1.87 ± 0.98 diopters
- UDVA improved by 2.85 ± 0.81 Snellen lines at 4 years
- Mean K value decreased by 2.26 ± 0.68 at 4 years
- ↓ in coma aberration with corneal symmetry improvement was seen in > 85%
- No significant changes in IOP, central retinal thickness on OCT, endothelial density loss

PROSPECTIVE RANDOMIZED BILATERAL EYE COMPARISON TRIAL OF HIGHER FLUENCE, SHORTER DURATION ULTRAVIOLET A RADIATION, & RCXL FOR PROGRESSIVE KERATOCONUS

Objective and Principal Conclusion

- Evaluate safety & efficacy of higher fluence CXL
- CXL with higher fluence UV light & shorter exposure time is safe & effective with
  - Results in stabilizing CE without adverse effects
  - Offers more comfort than standard CXL routine

Inclusion Criteria

- Age ≥ 18 years
- Diagnosis of bilateral keratoconus
- Minimum corneal thickness ≥ 450 μm

Randomization Method

- High-fluence CXL: 1 eye received CXL with 7 mW/cm² for 15 minutes
- Low-fluence CXL: Fellow eye received CXL with 3 mW/cm² for 30 minutes

Results

- High-fluence CXL is faster procedure with 1/2 the radiation exposure time
- All participants returned to preoperative visual function with no epithelial defects by week 1
- Uncorrected distance visual acuity (UDVA) change from pre- to postoperative was comparable in both groups
  - High fluence: Change from 20/60 to 20/38; low fluence: Change from 20/62 to 20/40
- Corrected distance visual acuity (CDVA) change from preoperative to postoperative was 20/30 to 20/25 in both groups
- Change in refractive cylinder was -2.9 diopters in high-fluence group & -2.8 diopters in low-fluence group
- Endothelial cell count decreased by 100 in high-fluence group & decreased by 250 in low-fluence group

PATIENT SUBJECTIVE VISUAL FUNCTION AFTER CXL FOR KERATOCONUS & CE

Objective and Principal Conclusions

- Assess changes in subjective visual function after CXL

Inclusion Criteria

- Age ≥ 14 years
- Diagnosis of keratoconus or LASIK-induced CE
- Inferior:superior ratio > 1.5 on topography mapping
- CDVA worse than 20/20
- Exclusion criteria: History of corneal surgery (other than LASIK), corneal pachymetry < 300 μm, chemical injury to cornea or delayed epithelial healing, pregnancy or lactation during study

Randomization Method

- All participants were treated with CXL & completed questionnaire rating visual symptoms from 1 to 5

Results

- Patients noted subjective improvement in visual symptoms 1 year following CXL, including night driving, reading, diplopia, glare, halo, starbursts, & foreign body sensation
- No associations between change in any symptom & changes in CDVA

RELATED REFERENCES

1. National Institutes of Health, National Eye Institute: Collaborative Corneal Transplantation Studies (CCTS). http://www.nei.nih.gov/neitrials/static/study36.asp. Updated October 21, 1999. Accessed September 6, 2013
2. National Institutes of Health, National Eye Institute: Herpetic Eye Disease Study (HEDS) II. http://www.nei.nih.gov/neitrials/static/study38.asp. Updated October 22, 1999. Accessed September 6, 2013
3. Brooks NO et al: Patient subjective visual function after corneal collagen crosslinking for keratoconus and corneal ectasia. J Cataract Refract Surg. 38(4):615-9, 2012
4. Kanellopoulos AJ: Long term results of a prospective randomized bilateral eye comparison trial of higher fluence, shorter duration ultraviolet A radiation, and riboflavin collagen cross linking for progressive keratoconus. Clin Ophthalmol. 6:97-101, 2012
5. Caporossi A et al: Long-term results of riboflavin ultraviolet a corneal collagen cross-linking for keratoconus in Italy: the Siena eye cross study. Am J Ophthalmol. 149(4):585-93, 2010
6. Randleman JB et al: Risk assessment for ectasia after corneal refractive surgery. Ophthalmology. 115(1):37-50, 2008

CORNEA OVERVIEW

TERMINOLOGY

Definitions

- Transparent, avascular connective tissue at anterior, external surface of eye encircled by highly vascular limbus
  - Connective tissue of the cornea transitions to opaque sclera and translucent conjunctiva at limbus

CORNEAL FUNCTION

Clinical Importance and Optical Properties

- Cornea comprises 1 of 3 main components of the external surface of the eye, along with the sclera and conjunctiva
  - Fibrous collagen gives cornea and sclera mechanical strength, maintains shape of eye, and helps create a protective sheath around ocular contents
- Cornea protects eye by acting as a structural and immunologic barrier for deeper ocular segments
- Cornea also occupies 1/3 of outer sheath of eye and creates anterior refractive surface
  - Accounts for 2/3 of total refractive power of eye
    - Corneal contour, surface smoothness, thickness, transparency, integrity of corneal layers, and refractive index are crucial for clear vision and good optical functioning
  - Shape of cornea is prolate, with a steeper central portion and flatter periphery; creates aspherical, convex anterior surface
    - Appears somewhat elliptical because vertical meridian is shorter than horizontal meridian
    - Scleral tissue extends slightly further along superior and inferior aspects of anterior corneal margin than temporal and nasal aspects
  - Corneal measurements
    - Horizontal diameter: 11-12 mm
    - Vertical diameter: 9-11 mm
    - Central thickness: 0.55 mm
    - Peripheral thickness: 0.7-0.8 mm
    - Refractive power: 40-44 diopters

CORNEAL ANATOMY AND PHYSIOLOGY

Histological Layers

- Anterior surface of cornea is covered by tear film; posterior surface is in direct contact with aqueous humor
- Cornea itself is composed of 5 layers
  - 3 cellular layers: Epithelium, stroma, endothelium
  - 2 interface layers: Bowman membrane, Descemet membrane
- Tear film
  - Covers anterior surface of cornea to create a smooth optical interface with air and to keep epithelial surface hydrated
  - Acts as lubricant, nutrient source, and immunologic barrier for corneal epithelium
  - Tear film is composed of 3 layers
    - Lipid layer: Outermost layer; secreted by meibomian glands
    - Aqueous layer: Middle layer; secreted by main and accessory lacrimal glands
    - Mucous layer: Innermost layer; secreted by conjunctival goblet cells
- Epithelium
  - Composed of 4-6 cell layers of stratified, nonkeratinized squamous epithelium that are 40-50 μm thick
  - Develops from surface ectoderm at 5-6 weeks gestation
  - Mucous layer of tear film (produced by conjunctival goblet cells) is in direct contact with glycocalyx (formed by corneal epithelial cells)
    - Hydrophilic nature of this interaction decreases surface tension so tear film can spread smoothly and evenly over corneal surface to create a smooth optical surface during blinking
  - Superficial epithelial cells
    - Flat, polygonal, terminally differentiated epithelial cells that are 2-4 cell layers deep
    - Microvilli and microplicae increase surface area of each epithelial cell for better oxygen and nutrient uptake from tear film; also allow better adherence of tear film mucous layer to corneal surface
    - Tight junctions and desmosomes keep tear film, microbes, and other substances from penetrating intercellular space and deeper corneal layers
  - Suprabasal epithelial cells (wing cells)
    - Wing cells lie below superficial epithelial cell layer and are 2-3 cell layers deep
    - Exhibit an intermediate state of differentiation between superficial and basal epithelial cells
    - Connected by desmosomes and gap junctions
  - Basal epithelial cells
    - Basal cell layer is deepest layer of corneal epithelium; attached to basement membrane and in contact with Bowman membrane
    - Composed of a single layer of columnar epithelium
    - Cells proliferate via mitosis and differentiate into wing cells and then superficial epithelial cells as they move to surface of corneal epithelium
    - Corneal epithelial cells turnover and desquamate into tear film every 1-2 weeks
    - Neighboring cells interdigitate via desmosomes, gap junctions, and hemidesmosomes
    - Basal cells adhere to basement membrane via hemidesmosomes and secrete type VII collagen, which creates fibrils that anchor hemidesmosomes with type I collagen in stroma
    - Limbal palisades of Vogt are nests of stem cells, which regenerate corneal epithelium and stroma
- Bowman membrane
  - 12-15 μm thick zone of acellular, membrane-like tissue composed of type I and type III collagen secreted by stromal keratocytes
  - Situated anterior to stroma and functions in giving cornea its shape
- Stroma
  - 90% of corneal thickness attributed to stroma, which consists mostly of extracellular matrix (ECM) + keratocytes (i.e., corneal fibroblasts) & nerve fibers
    - Type I fibers are arranged in parallel bundles called fibrils, which form 200-300 uniform stromal lamellae; also contain smaller amounts of type III, V, and VI collagen

- Fibrils are surrounded by ECM that hydrates cornea and gives it structure; glycosaminoglycans between collagen fibers absorb and retain water
- Stromal keratocytes are scattered between stromal lamellae and maintain stromal ECM
- Uniform arrangement of collagen fibers allows for mechanical strength, shaping, and corneal transparency
- Mean diameter of collagen fibers and mean distance between them are < 1/2 wavelength of visible light; allows for clear passage of light through cornea
- Stromal layer is thicker peripherally than in central cornea

- Descemet membrane
  - 8-10 μm layer of type IV collagen and laminin that lies posterior to stroma and anterior to endothelium
  - Acts as basement membrane of endothelium and is secreted by endothelial cells
- Endothelium
  - 5 μm thick, single layer of hexagon-shaped cells at posterior surface of Descemet membrane
  - Endothelial cells are derived from neuroectoderm
  - Endothelial cells interdigitate with junctional complexes such as zonula occludens, macula occludens, and macula adherens
  - Cell surface facing aqueous humor has microvilli and folds that allow for increased surface area of contact with aqueous humor
  - Physiologic function of endothelium is to regulate water content of corneal stroma
    - Solutes and nutrients from aqueous humor leak into superficial corneal layers
    - Ion transport systems in endothelial cells actively pump water from stroma into aqueous humor via Na+/K+ ATPase pumps and carbonic anhydrase

CORNEAL INNERVATION

Nerve Supply

- Corneal tissue is one of the most sensitive in the body due to its dense innervation
- Sensory nerves are derived from nasociliary branch of ophthalmic division of trigeminal nerve, primarily entering at 3- and 9-o'clock
- Nerves enter stroma in a radial pattern, with thick trunks that form a plexiform network
  - Trunks pass through Bowman membrane and create a rich neural plexus beneath basal epithelium

CORNEAL VASCULATURE

Oxygen and Nutrient Supply

- Cornea is an avascular tissue and must obtain nutrients and other blood components from blood circulating through limbal vessels
  - Limbal vessels are derived from anterior ciliary artery, which branches from ophthalmic artery
    - Anastomoses with vessels from facial branch of external carotid artery to create limbal arcade around cornea
- Oxygen is mostly obtained via diffusion from tear film and its direct interface with air; a small portion of oxygen is derived from limbal circulation and aqueous humor
- Glucose is obtained via diffusion from aqueous humor

CORNEAL INFLAMMATION

Superficial Lesions

- Punctate epithelial erosions (PEE)
  - Pinpoint epithelial defects that stain with fluorescein or rose bengal
- Punctate epithelial keratopathy (PEK)
  - Tiny, focal, granular lesions of corneal epithelium caused by swelling of epithelial cells; stain better with rose bengal than fluorescein
- Filamentary keratitis
  - Mucous filaments lined with epithelial cells that have a "head" attached to corneal surface and a "tail" that floats freely in tear film
- Edema
  - Swelling within cornea
    - Severe cases may be associated with vesicles and bullae
- Neovascularization
  - Ingrowth of blood vessels from limbal vascular plexus into avascular cornea
    - Occurs secondary to chronic hypoxia and inflammation
    - May occur superficially or deeper within stroma

Deep Lesions

- Infiltrates
  - Local or diffuse areas of granular, gray-white opacities in stroma
    - Composed of leukocytes and cellular debris secondary to stromal inflammation
- Ulcers
  - Disruption of corneal epithelium with possible stromal involvement
    - Occur secondary to inflammation or infection
- Lipid deposition
  - Occurs as a result of chronic inflammation and leakage from neovessels secondary to corneal neovascularization
- Folds and breaks in Descemet membrane
  - May occur secondary to inflammation, trauma, pathologic conditions, or aqueous in corneal stroma

RELATED REFERENCES

1. Dua HS et al: Human corneal anatomy redefined: a novel pre-Descemet's layer (Dua's layer). Ophthalmology. 120(9):1778-85, 2013
2. Smolek MK et al: Cornea. In Tasman W: Duane's Foundations of Clinical Ophthalmology. Philadelphia: Lippincott Williams & Wilkins, 2006. http://www.oculist.net/downaton502/prof/ebook/duanes/pages/v7/v7c008.html. Accessed June 13, 2013
3. DelMonte DW et al: Anatomy and physiology of the cornea. J Cataract Refract Surg. 37(3):588-98, 2011
4. Kanski J: Cornea. In Clinical Ophthalmology: A Systematic Approach. 6th ed. Oxford: Butterworth-Heinemann. 250-54, 2007
5. Tuft S: The normal cornea. In Spalton D et al: Atlas of Clinical Ophthalmology. 3rd ed. Oxford: Mosby Elsevier. 147-185, 2006
6. Krachmer J et al: Cornea. In Krachmer et al: Cornea: Fundamentals, Diagnosis, and Management. Vol. 1. 2nd ed. Philadelphia: Elsevier Mosby. 3-26, 2005

NORMAL CORNEA

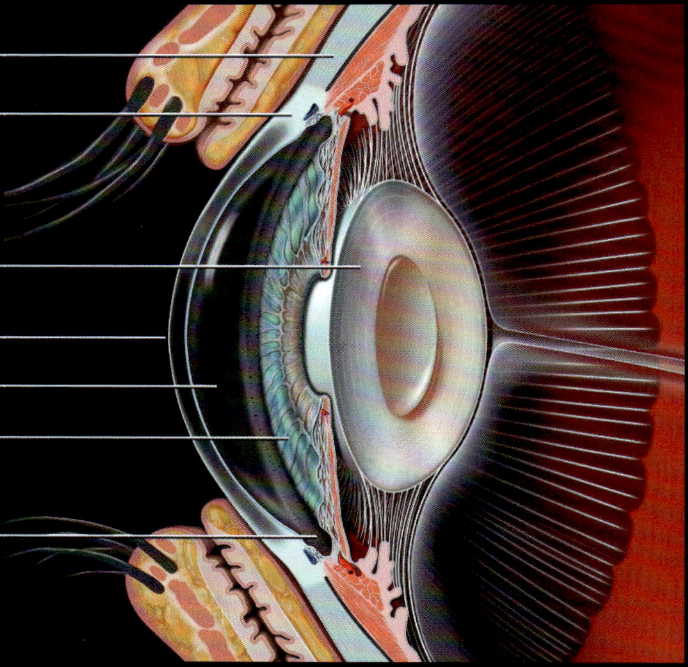

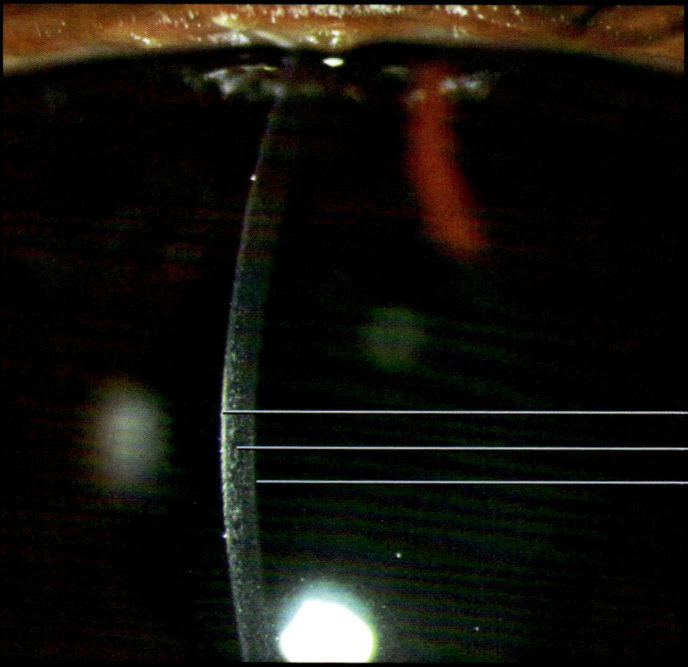

(Top) *The transparent, avascular cornea occupies 1/3 of the outer ocular sheath and protects the inner ocular structures. Corneal connective tissue transitions to the opaque sclera and translucent conjunctiva at the limbus. As the anterior external refractive surface, the cornea accounts for 2/3 of the total refractive power of the eye.* ***(Bottom)*** *Thin-block slit-lamp illumination distinguishes the corneal epithelial, stromal, and endothelial layers. The epithelium appears as a bright, reflective anterior curve, the stroma appears clear and compact, and the contour of the endothelium is smooth and slightly less bright than the epithelium. Each of these layers can be disrupted in various ways by different ocular disorders.*

MICROSCOPIC FEATURES

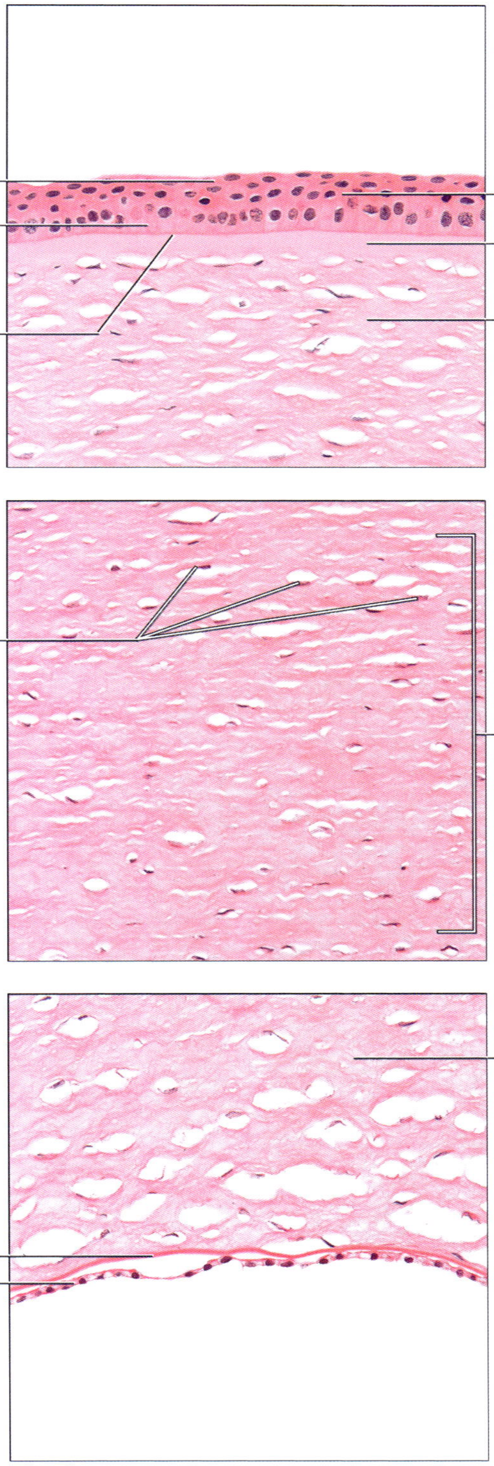

(Top) *The stratified nonkeratinized squamous corneal epithelium is composed of columnar basal cells that sit on the Bowman membrane and proliferate via mitosis. Basal cells differentiate into wing cells, and wing cells then flatten as they rise to the corneal surface to become superficial epithelial cells. The superficial cells turn over and desquamate into the tear film every 1-2 weeks. (Courtesy H. Brown, MD.)* ***(Middle)*** *The corneal stroma comprises 90% of corneal thickness and is composed of regularly spaced collagen fibers embedded in an extracellular matrix. This arrangement allows mechanical strength, shaping, and transparency. No blood vessels or lymphatics are present in the stroma. Note that cleft-like spaces are secondary to tissue fixation/processing. (Courtesy H. Brown, MD.)* ***(Bottom)*** *The posterior cornea is lined by a single layer of hexagonally shaped endothelial cells that sit on the Descemet membrane. The endothelium is responsible for regulating the water content of the stroma. (Courtesy H. Brown, MD.)*

ANTERIOR SEGMENT OCT

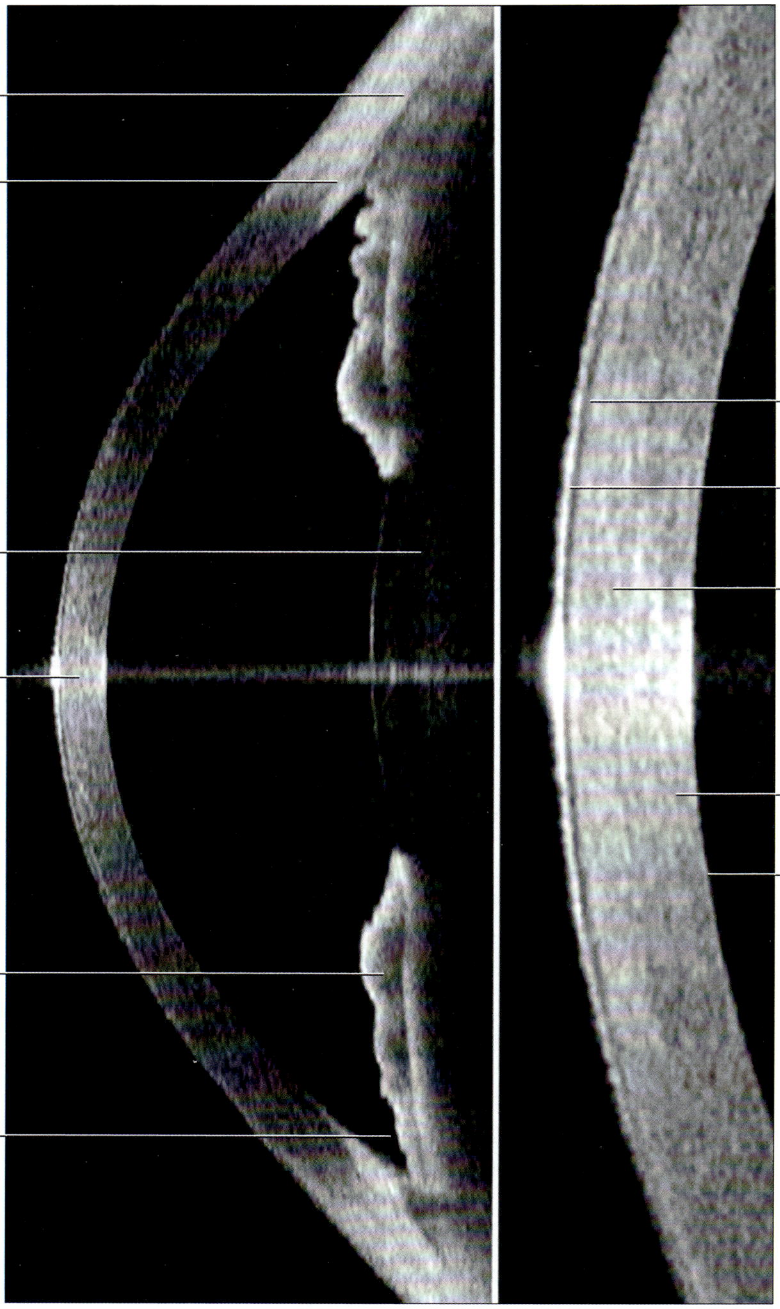

Anterior segment OCT is a high-resolution, cross-sectional imaging modality that shows the normal contours of the cornea, iris, and lens. This test is particularly useful as an adjunct to gonioscopy in visualizing the iridocorneal angle for glaucoma evaluation. Under high magnification, anterior segment OCT also reveals all 5 layers of the cornea.

CORNEAL MAPPING

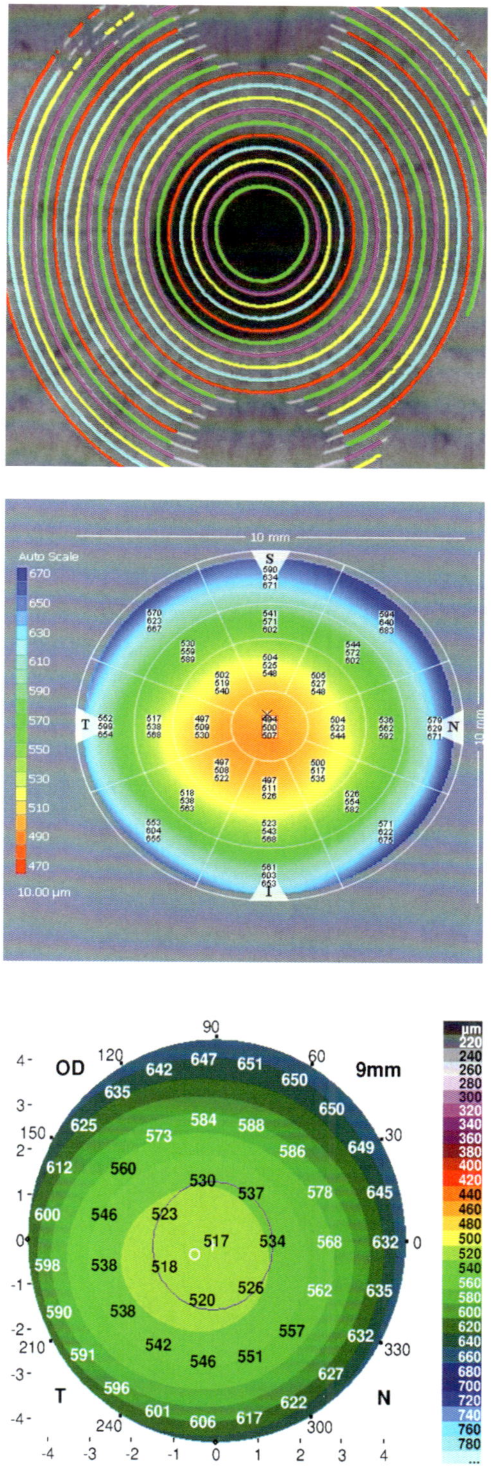

(Top) *Videokeratography is a noninvasive diagnostic imaging technique that uses a pattern of concentric rings to qualitatively visualize the steepness of curvature of the cornea. This imaging modality is useful in contact lens fitting and for diagnosis of conditions that manifest with high or irregular astigmatism.* ***(Middle)*** *A corneal topography elevation map demonstrates how a subject's corneal curvature differs from a baseline computer-generated reference image. The warmer colors on the color map (red, orange, and yellow) represent areas that are higher or steeper than the reference surface, whereas cooler colors (green and blue) represent lower or flatter regions.* ***(Bottom)*** *Pachymetry mapping outlines corneal thickness and detects irregularities by providing high, low, and average corneal thickness measurements for multiple points along the cornea. The central portion of a pachymetry map represents the geometric or anatomic center, which is the thinnest part of the cornea.*

GRANULAR/LATTICE/MACULAR DYSTROPHY

Key Facts

Introduction
- Progressive, bilateral, noninflammatory opacification of corneal stroma caused by deposition of abnormal metabolic byproducts

Granular Dystrophy
- Discrete opacities in central anterior stroma with clear corneal zones between lesions
- Amorphous hyaline deposits in stroma, which stain bright red with Masson trichrome

Lattice Dystrophy
- Refractile, fine lattice lines in anterior stroma
- Amyloid deposits stain with Congo red and have green birefringence with polarization

Macular Dystrophy
- Diffuse opacities in corneal stroma that extend limbus to limbus; no clear zones between lesions
- Mucopolysaccharide aggregation in stroma, which stains with Alcian blue

Treatment
- Medical: Treat recurrent erosions with bandage contacts and artificial tears; reduce photophobia with tinted contacts
- Surgical: Granular dystrophy
  - Penetrating keratoplasty (PK), penetrating corneolimbal keratoplasty (PCLK), or deep anterior lamellar keratoplasty (DALK) if vision markedly reduced
  - Manage superficial opacities with lamellar keratoplasty or phototherapeutic keratectomy (PTK)
- Surgical: Lattice and macular dystrophy
  - PK, PLCK, or DALK

*(**Left**) Granular dystrophy exhibits various discrete, centrally located stromal opacities ↗ with peripheral limbal sparing ↗. (Courtesy W. Nosé, MD.) (**Right**) Gray-white, crumb-like lesions with sharp borders occur in the anterior to mid-stroma ↗. The intervening cornea between lesions is clear → but becomes hazy as the disease advances. Vision may be unaffected in early disease, but with progression, patients complain of photophobia due to light scattering by these lesions.*

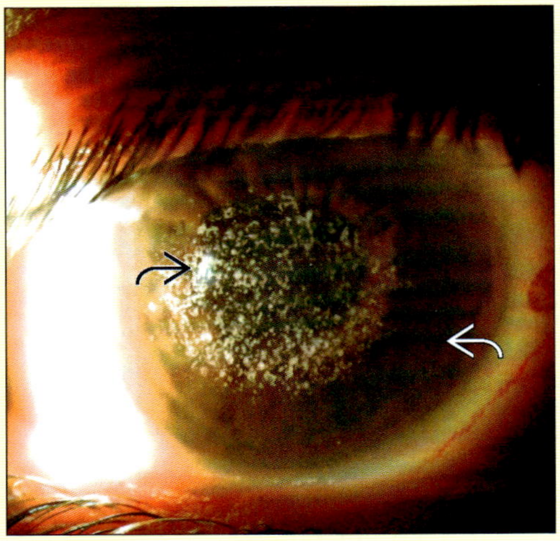

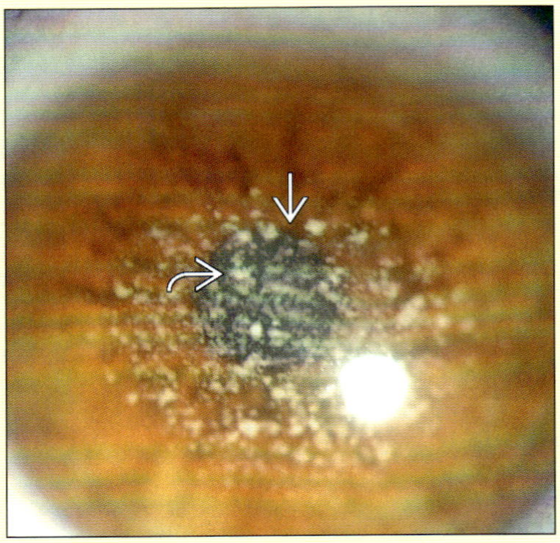

*(**Left**) High magnification shows superficial granular irregularities and a diffuse, ground-glass appearance →. Direct illumination makes lesions look opaque ↗; retroillumination reveals they are translucent →. (**Right**) Red-reflex illumination shows lattice dystrophy with radially oriented, overlapping, linear lines that create branching refractile opacities in the anterior stroma →. Central corneal haze occurs in advanced disease. (Courtesy W. Nosé, MD.)*

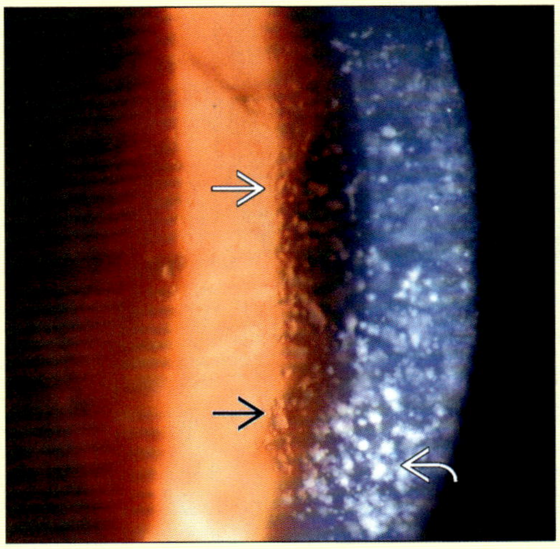

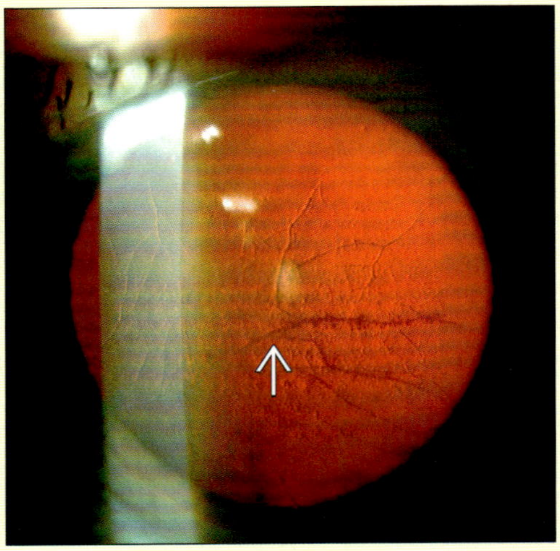

GRANULAR/LATTICE/MACULAR DYSTROPHY

INTRODUCTION

Definitions

- Progressive, bilateral, noninflammatory opacification of corneal stroma caused by deposition of abnormal metabolic byproducts secondary to genetic defects
  - Granular dystrophy: *GCD1*, Groenouw type 1
  - Lattice dystrophy: Type 1 (Biber-Haab-Dimmer), type 2 (Meretoja syndrome), type 3 and 3A
  - Macular dystrophy: Groenouw type 2

DEMOGRAPHICS

Etiology/Risk Factors

- **Granular dystrophy type 1**
  - Autosomal dominant (AD) inheritance pattern; affected gene loci at 5q31
- **Lattice dystrophy**
  - Type 1: AD inheritance; affected gene loci at 5q31
  - Type 2: AD inheritance; affected gene loci at 9q34
  - Type 3: Autosomal recessive (AR) inheritance (type 3); AD inheritance (type 3A); affected gene loci at 5q31
- **Macular dystrophy**
  - AR inheritance pattern; affected gene loci at 16q22

Epidemiology

- *BIGH3* gene mutations in 5q31 region for granular, lattice, and Avellino dystrophies (Avellino = granular + lattice)
- **Granular dystrophy**
  - Onset in 1st or 2nd decade of life; similar exam findings within families
- **Lattice dystrophy**
  - Type 1 onset in 1st decade, type 2 in 3rd decade, type 3 and 3A in 4th and 6th decades
- **Macular dystrophy**
  - Least common, but most severe stromal dystrophy; onset in 1st decade

PRESENTATION

Symptoms

- **Granular dystrophy**
  - Vision unaffected in early stages, but patient may complain of mild photophobia from light scattering by corneal lesions
  - Advanced disease impairs vision and corneal sensation
- **Lattice dystrophy**
  - Stromal haze gradually impairs vision; recurrent erosions common
- **Macular dystrophy**
  - Progressive vision loss, irritation, photophobia

Exam Findings

- **Granular dystrophy**
  - Bilateral deposition of small, white, well-demarcated opacities in central anterior stroma
  - Opacities are shaped like drops, crumbs, rings, or snowflakes; deposition pattern is ray- or disc-shaped or may resemble Christmas tree pattern
  - Stroma between opacities initially clear, but individual lesions then grow in size and number and may coalesce; deposits extend deeper and more peripherally, sparing of 2-3 mm of limbal area; further confluence causes diffuse haze in intervening stroma
- **Lattice dystrophy**
  - Type 1
    - Refractile, anterior stromal dots coalesce into fine lattice lines
    - Lesions progress to thread-like or thick, radially branching lines; lines can extend into deep stroma and epithelium
    - Stroma between dots and lines initially clear, but opacities can coalesce and cause central haze in anterior and middle stroma over time
  - Type 2
    - Systemic amyloidosis associated with corneal dystrophy, occurs later in onset
    - Glaucoma and pseudoexfoliation common
    - Fewer radial lattice lines, mostly in peripheral cornea
  - Type 3
    - Thick lines that extend limbus to limbus
- **Macular dystrophy**
  - Anterior and central stromal haze
    - Eventually extends peripherally up to limbus
    - Causes increasing opacification of entire cornea thickness by 2nd decade of life
  - Corneal thinning over time
  - Multiple dense, white nodules with indistinct borders in anterior stroma centrally and posterior stroma peripherally; cause irregularity of corneal surface
  - Limbus-limbus with no clear zones in between lesions (both unlike granular or lattice dystrophy)

DIFFERENTIAL DIAGNOSIS

Granular Dystrophy Type 2 (Avellino Dystrophy = Granular + Lattice)

- AD inheritance; variant of granular dystrophy type 1, causing both granular and lattice corneal deposits
- Symptoms: Glare, decreased vision, foreign body sensation, recurrent painful epithelial erosions
- Signs
  - Bilateral, asymmetric, discrete, gray-white granular deposits in anterior stroma
  - Lattice lesions in middle to posterior stroma
  - Anterior stromal haze between deposits
- Treatment: Superficial debridement, lamellar keratoplasty, or excimer laser phototherapeutic keratectomy (PTK); penetrating keratoplasty (PK) for deeper involvement

Meesmann Corneal Dystrophy (Juvenile Epithelial Dystrophy)

- Rare autosomal recessive dystrophy of anterior corneal epithelium (with deposits of peculiar substance) manifesting in 1st few years of life
- Signs
  - Clusters of multiple small, clear intraepithelial microcysts or vesicles containing degenerated epithelium; lesions are roughly equal in size
  - Corneal surface appears smooth since microcysts are small and limited to epithelium
  - Cysts are mostly located in visual axis and midperiphery, but visual impairment is none or mild

- Cornea rarely clouds and recurrent erosions are uncommon
- Treatment: Surgical intervention rarely necessary; soft contact lenses may decrease size of microcysts

Reis-Buckler Corneal Dystrophy

- Also known as Thiel-Behnke dystrophy or corneal dystrophy of Bowman layer type 1
- Symptoms: Irritation, photophobia, decreased vision
- Signs
  - Reticular corneal opacities
  - Honeycomb or ring-like pattern of opacification in central cornea by 2nd-3rd decades of life
  - Opacification spares peripheral cornea
  - Diffuse superficial stromal haze occurs with progressive scarring of Bowman layer, corneal thickening, irregular astigmatism, and decreased corneal sensation
  - Recurrent painful corneal epithelial erosions
  - Corneal nerves appear prominently
- Treatment: Superficial keratectomy; lamellar or PK in severe cases

Fuchs Endothelial Dystrophy

- Posterior corneal dystrophy of endothelium that develops during middle age
- Signs
  - Thickening of Descemet membrane
  - Corneal endothelial cells become attenuated and reduced in number, causing stromal edema and distorted vision
  - More severe visual impairment occurs with progressive epithelial edema
  - Painful, focal epithelial bullae
- Treatment
  - Medical management: Topical hypertonic saline, therapeutic soft contact lenses
  - Surgical management: Descemet membrane stripping with endothelial keratoplasty (DSEK) or PK

Congenital Hereditary Endothelial Dystrophy

- Rare posterior membrane dystrophy with corneal clouding apparent in 1st 6 months of life
- Signs
  - Bilateral, symmetric, noninflammatory corneal opacification without clear zones; extends to limbus
  - Significant corneal thickening with edema; haziness in all corneal layers
  - Patients with significant visual impairment exhibit fine nystagmus
- Type 1: AD inheritance
  - Signs: Corneal edema and pain; cornea is clear at birth but clouds in early infancy
- Type 2: AR inheritance; more common
  - Signs: Corneal edema and cloudiness at birth; nystagmus

EVALUATION/WORK-UP

Pathology

- **Granular dystrophy**
  - Amorphous hyaline deposits in stroma stain bright red with Masson trichrome
- **Lattice dystrophy**
  - Amyloid deposits stain with Congo red, crystal violet, and have green birefringence with polarized filter
- **Macular dystrophy**
  - Aggregation of glycosaminoglycans and mucopolysaccharides between stromal lamellae stain with Alcian blue or colloidal iron

Mnemonic for Corneal Dystrophies and Stains

- **M**arilyn: **M**acular dystrophy
- **M**onroe: **M**ucopolysaccharide
- **A**lways: **A**lcian blue stain
- **G**ets: **G**ranular dystrophy
- **H**er: **H**yaline
- **M**an in: **M**asson trichrome stain
- **L**os: **L**attice dystrophy
- **A**ngeles: **A**myloid
- **C**alifornia: **C**ongo red

TREATMENT

Medical

- Treat recurrent epithelial erosions with bandage contacts and artificial tears; reduce photophobia with tinted contacts

Surgical

- **Granular dystrophy**
  - PK if vision markedly reduced
  - Manage superficial opacities with epithelial scraping, superficial keratectomy, or lamellar keratoplasty
  - PTK with argon-fluoride excimer laser for superficial recurrences
- **Lattice and macular dystrophy**
  - PK is surgical procedure of choice, but PTK and lamellar keratoplasty may also be successful
- PK is standard approach
  - Penetrating corneolimbal keratoplasty (PCLK) provides anatomic gene therapy with donor limbal stem cells
  - Deep anterior lamellar keratoplasty (DALK) can be considered to preserve host endothelium

Prognosis

- **Granular dystrophy**
  - Recurrence in grafts as early as 1 year after surgery
- **Lattice dystrophy**
  - Higher recurrence rate than granular and macular dystrophy
- **Macular dystrophy**
  - Recurrence has same pattern as primary dystrophy; involves superficial and deep peripheral donor stroma

SELECTED REFERENCES

1. Schmedt T et al: Molecular bases of corneal endothelial dystrophies. Exp Eye Res. 95(1):24-34, 2012
2. Klintworth GK: Corneal dystrophies. Orphanet J Rare Dis. 4:7, 2009

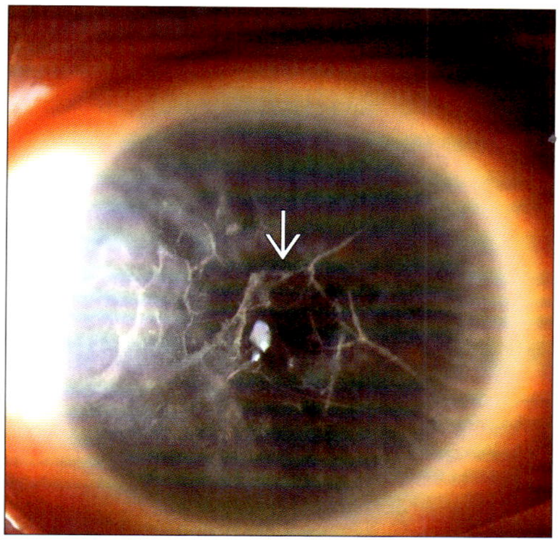

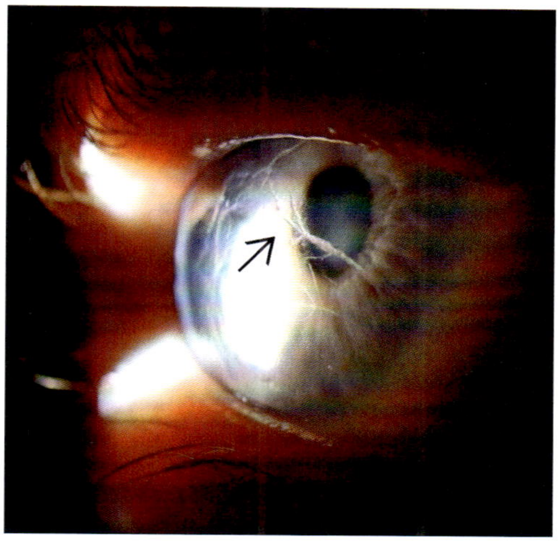

(Left) *Filamentous lattice lines occupy the central cornea* → *and typically do not extend to the peripheral cornea or limbus. Clear spaces between lesions in early disease progressively take on a ground-glass appearance as they become opacified over time.* ***(Right)*** *An oblique view of the eye reveals glass-like lattice lines with a double contour* →*. Over time, these anterior stromal lesions progress to more nodular, thread-like, and thicker linear lesions that extend deeper into the stroma.*

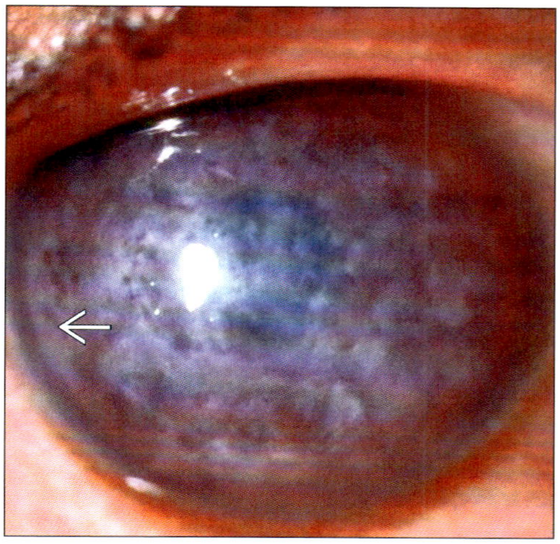

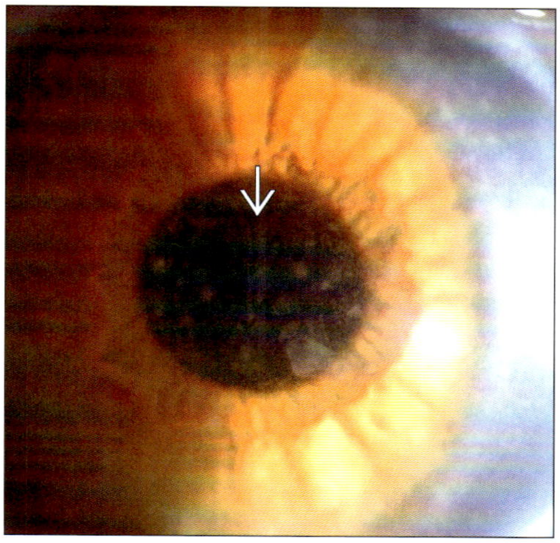

(Left) *Macular dystrophy is characterized by multiple diffuse, gray-white opacities in the corneal stroma that extend into the peripheral cornea* →*. Stromal opacities involve the full thickness of the cornea, without clear zones between lesions. Lesions in the central cornea are more superficial than those in the periphery. Central corneal thinning may occur, and significant corneal guttata may be present. (Courtesy W. Nosé, MD.)* ***(Right)*** *Even in early disease, macular dystrophy exhibits stromal haze between opacities* →*.*

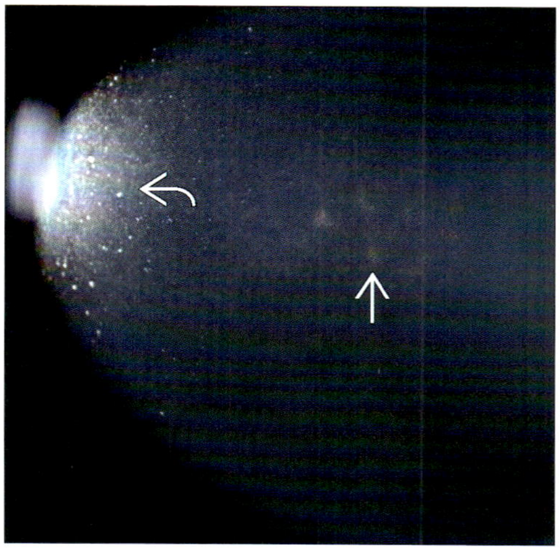

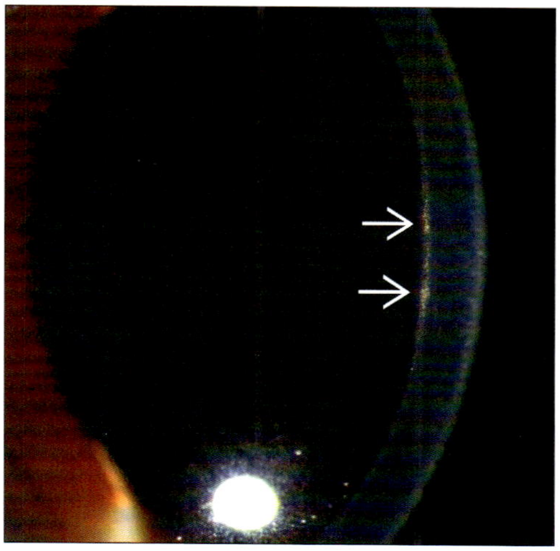

(Left) *In Fuchs dystrophy, multiple guttata form in the central portion of the Descemet membrane* →*. In the early stage of Fuchs dystrophy, these guttata can lead to pigment dusting on the endothelium* →*. As the condition progresses, the guttata increase in number and become confluent, giving the endothelium a characteristic "beaten metal" appearance.* ***(Right)*** *This slit-lamp photograph demonstrates pigment deposition on the corneal endothelium under a higher magnification slit-lamp beam* →*.*

PETERS ANOMALY

Key Facts

Introduction

- Congenital disorder involving dysgenesis of the anterior segment during development
  - Lens placode does not separate or separates late in embryology from the cornea
- Type I (without lens involvement)
  - Typically unilateral and consists of corneal opacity and iridocorneal adhesions
- Type II (with lens involvement)
  - Frequently bilateral and consists of corneal opacity and iridocorneal adhesions and lens abnormalities

Presentation

- Corneal opacity of varying degrees, usually centrally located and may be bilateral
- Glaucoma
- Often, iris strands extend from iris collarettes to peripheral margin of posterior corneal defect
- Systemic physical exam findings may include developmental delay, congenital heart disease, external ear abnormalities, central nervous system structural abnormalities, genitourinary abnormalities, hearing loss, cleft lip and palate, and spinal defects

Treatment

- Monitor for elevated IOP, signs of glaucoma, and amblyopia
- Cornea transplant and cataract extraction if necessary
  - Urgent procedure if unilateral
- Eye exams every 6-12 months, lifelong
  - May need contacts or glasses

*(**Left**) These light micrographs demonstrate the corneal histopathology associated with Peters anomaly (top image, H&E; bottom image, PAS). Note the disorganized epithelium and thickened Bowman layer. The PAS stain highlights the thin epithelial basement membrane, which emphasizes the unstained, enlarged Bowman layer. (**Right**) Slit-lamp photo depicts a leukoma, or white corneal opacity. Leukoma is one of the hallmark findings in Peters anomaly and leads to an abnormal red reflex.*

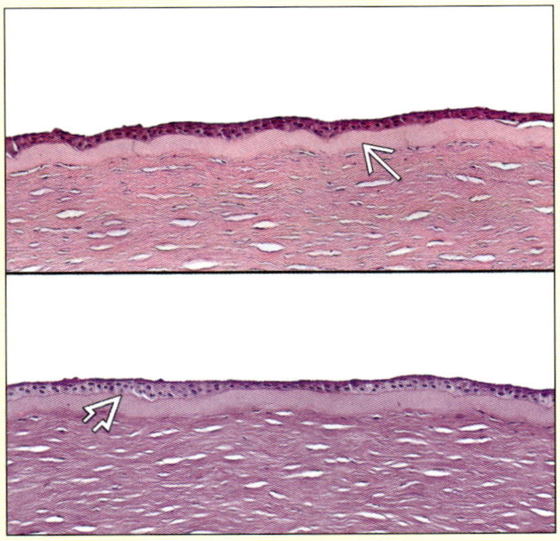

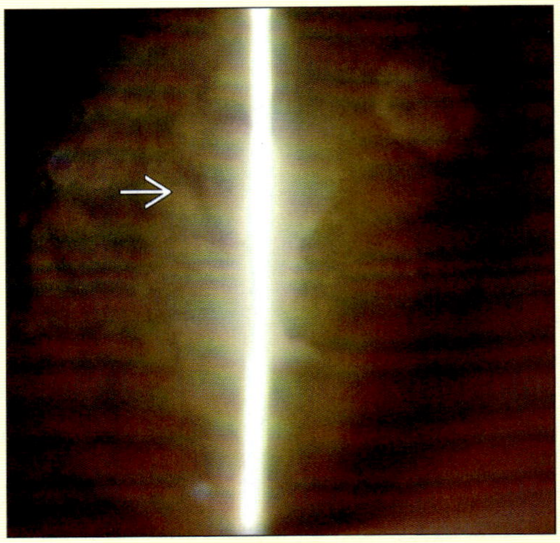

*(**Left**) Slit-lamp photograph shows an eye with a congenital cataract, which is found in type II Peters anomaly. (**Right**) Slit-lamp photograph shows the iris of a patient with Axenfeld-Reiger syndrome (ARS). ARS is an important differential diagnosis for Peters anomaly. Note the iridocorneal adhesions attached to the posterior embryotoxon. The posterior embryotoxon is a prominent Schwalbe line that is displaced anteriorly, a feature associated with ARS.*

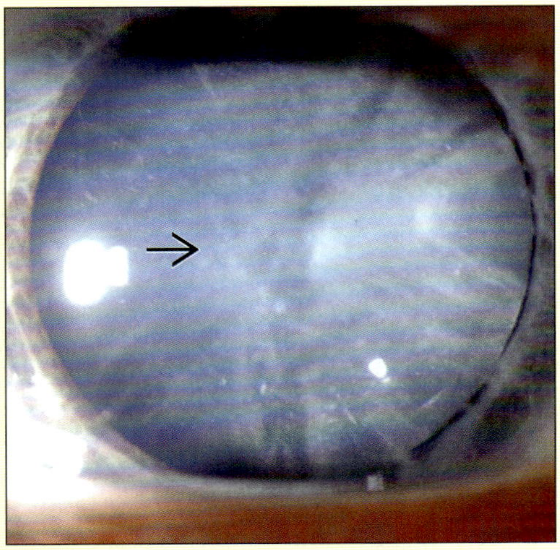

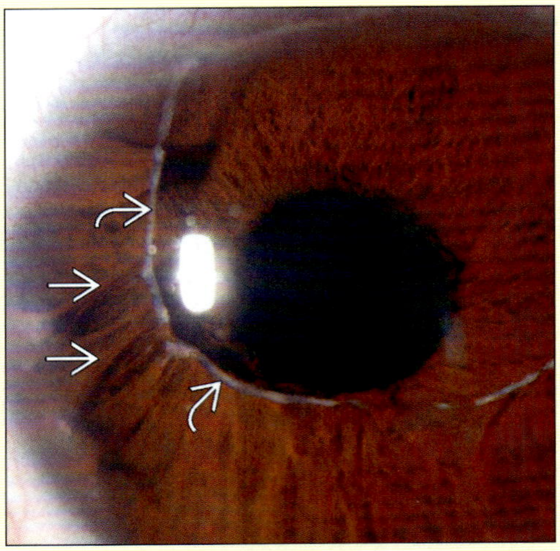

PETERS ANOMALY

INTRODUCTION

Definitions
- Congenital anterior segment dysgenesis, characterized by central corneal opacity with endothelial and Descemet membrane defects

Subtypes
- Type I (without lens involvement)
  - Typically unilateral and consists of corneal opacity and iridocorneal adhesions
  - Peripheral edema regresses over time as surrounding endothelium repairs endothelial and Descemet membrane defects
  - May be associated with sclerocornea, microcornea, and infantile glaucoma
- Type II (with lens involvement)
  - Frequently bilateral and consists of a corneal opacity and iridocorneal adhesions and lens abnormalities
  - Variable degrees of keratolenticular adherence and cataract formation
  - Often associated with additional ocular abnormalities including microphthalmos, colobomas, persistent hyperplastic primary vitreous, and optic nerve hypoplasia
  - Often associated with systemic abnormalities including congenital cardiac disease, external ear malformation, central nervous system defects, genitourinary abnormalities, hearing loss, and cleft lip/palate

DEMOGRAPHICS

Etiology/Risk Factors
- Premature infants; fetal alcohol syndrome

Epidemiology
- Most cases are sporadic
- *PAX6* gene associated with aniridia; *PITX2* and *FOXC1* genes associated with Axenfeld-Rieger syndrome; *CYP1B1* gene associated with primary congenital glaucoma

PRESENTATION

Symptoms
- Congenital, central, corneal opacification

Exam Findings
- Abnormal red reflex with a corneal leukoma from central corneal opacity
- May have cataracts
- Elevated intraocular pressure (IOP)
- Often, iris strands extend from iris collarettes to peripheral margin of posterior corneal defect
- Systemic findings may include developmental delay, congenital heart disease, external ear abnormalities, central nervous system structural abnormalities, genitourinary abnormalities, hearing loss, cleft lip and palate, and spinal defects

DIFFERENTIAL DIAGNOSIS

Primary Congenital Glaucoma
- Corneal opacity is diffuse
- Associated with Haab striae and buphthalmos

Mucopolysaccharidoses
- Corneal opacity is diffuse

Congenital Hereditary Endothelial Dystrophy
- Corneal opacity is diffuse

Birth Trauma
- Typically unilateral with breaks in Descemet membrane (typically vertical)

Axenfeld-Rieger Anomaly/Syndrome
- Bilateral and presents with posterior embryotoxon (a prominent, anteriorly displaced Schwalbe line)

Iridocorneal Endothelial Syndrome
- Iris atrophy, corneal endotheliopathy, corneal edema, and prominent iris nevi
- Corneal endothelium has a fine hammered metal appearance

EVALUATION/WORK-UP

Imaging
- B-scan ultrasound to evaluate anterior segment

TREATMENT

Medical
- Treat glaucoma with topical medications or oral carbonic anhydrase inhibitors

Surgical
- Penetrating keratoplasty and cataract extraction
- Glaucoma procedures such as trabeculectomy or tube-shunt procedures
- Iridoplasty for reformation of iris

Follow-Up
- Eye exams every 6-12 months, lifelong; monitor IOP and amblyopia
- Associated systemic findings are managed by a pediatric specialist

Prognosis
- Early keratoplasty, aggressive glaucoma and amblyopia management can obtain graft clarity
- Congenital glaucoma is independent predictor of graft failure

SELECTED REFERENCES

1. Zaidman GW et al: Long-term visual prognosis in children after corneal transplant surgery for Peters anomaly type I. Am J Ophthalmol. 144(1):104-108, 2007
2. Yang LL et al: Peters' anomaly. A synopsis of surgical management and visual outcome. Ophthalmol Clin North Am. 14(3):467-77, 2001

WILSON DISEASE

Key Facts

Demographics
- Mutations of *ATP7B* gene, which codes for copper-dependent P-type ATPase, a copper transport protein found on Golgi apparatus and canalicular membrane

Presentation
- Corneal Kayser-Fleischer ring
  - Descemet membrane copper deposits
  - Appears superiorly 1st, then joins deposits inferiorly
- Sunflower cataract
  - Cuprous oxide deposition in anterior lens capsule and subcapsular cortex
- Both ring and cataract are reversible with treatment

Evaluation/Work-Up
- Low serum ceruloplasmin
- Increased free copper in serum
- Increased urine copper
- Most reliable test is hepatic copper concentration
- Slit lamp: Look for Kayser-Fleischer ring or sunflower cataract
- Gonioscopy: Helpful to find Kayser-Fleischer when not seen with slit lamp

Treatment
- Copper chelators: Penicillamine, trientine, ammonium tetrathiomolybdate
- Zinc: Induces intestinal metallothionein

Follow-up/Prognosis
- Regression of Kayser-Fleischer ring indicates effective treatment
- With effective medical therapy &/or liver transplant, Kayser-Fleischer rings disappear, corneal changes may remain present

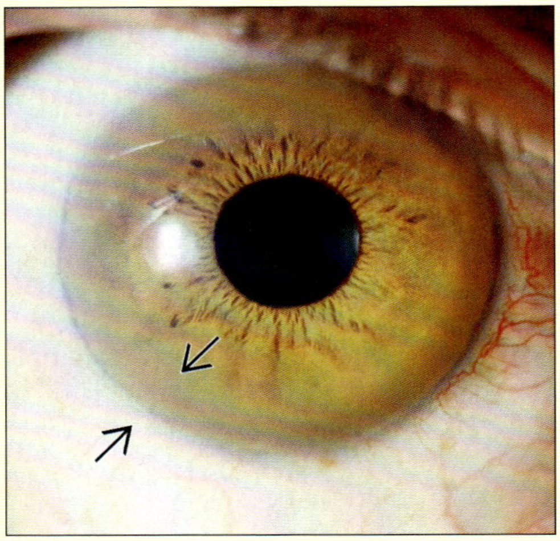
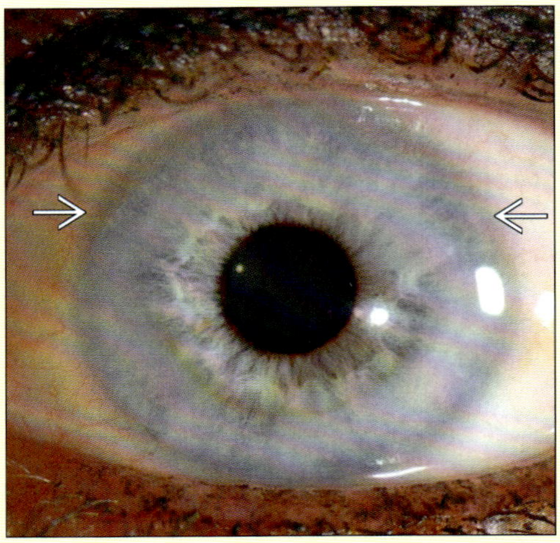

(Left) *Clinical photograph of Kayser-Fleischer ring shows brown deposits of copper at the periphery of the cornea →. (Courtesy S. Uwaydat, MD.)* ***(Right)*** *This external photograph depicts a Kayser-Fleischer ring → on the superior border of Descemet membrane. Deposits typically appear superiorly 1st before joining deposits inferiorly. (Courtesy M. Moshirfar, MD.)*

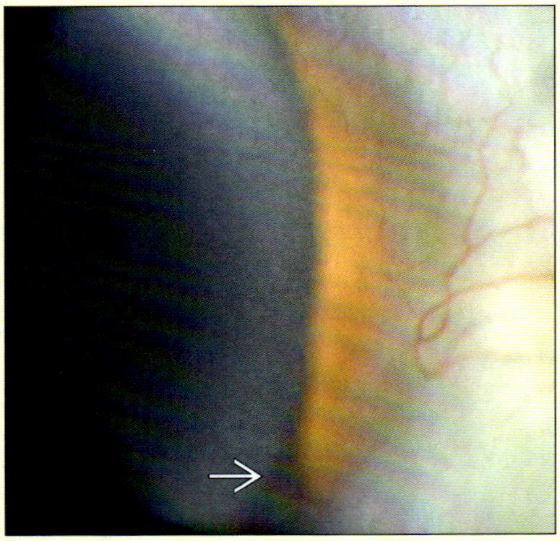
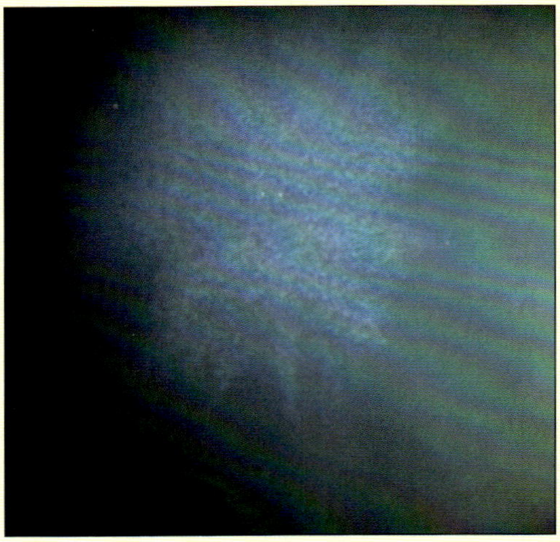

(Left) *This slit-lamp photograph shows a Kayser-Fleischer ring, which may appear in patients with Wilson disease. The ring is due to deposition of copper → on Descemet membrane on the periphery of the cornea. (Courtesy R. Cameron, MD.)* ***(Right)*** *This slit-lamp photograph depicts a sunflower cataract in a patient with Wilson disease. These cataracts result from anterior lens capsule and subcapsular cortex cuprous oxide deposits. (Courtesy R. Cameron, MD.)*

WILSON DISEASE

INTRODUCTION

Synonyms

- Hepatolenticular degeneration

Definitions

- Autosomal recessive inherited mutation of copper transport protein that leads to increased copper levels

DEMOGRAPHICS

Etiology/Risk Factors

- Mutations of *ATP7B* gene, which codes for copper-dependent P-type ATPase, a copper transport protein found on Golgi apparatus and on canalicular membrane
  - Inability to excrete copper in bile leads to its accumulation in liver and various tissues
  - Inability to transport copper into Golgi apparatus makes it unavailable for synthesis of ceruloplasmin, leading to release of apoceruloplasmin into serum and its rapid degradation
    - Ceruloplasmin functions as a plasma ferroxidase, oxidizing ferrous iron for subsequent transfer to plasma apotransferrin, making it available for hemoglobin biosynthesis

Epidemiology

- Incidence ~ 1 in 30,000 people

PRESENTATION

Symptoms

- Neurologic
  - Dorsal midbrain syndrome → light-near dissociation of the pupils, convergence-retraction nystagmus, upgaze paresis
- Symptoms of acute liver and renal failure, cirrhosis
- Rare: Night blindness, optic neuritis, exotropic strabismus, slowed saccades

Exam Findings

- Corneal Kayser-Fleischer ring
  - Descemet membrane copper deposits
  - Appears superiorly first, then joins deposits inferiorly
- Sunflower cataract
  - Anterior lens capsule and subcapsular cortex cuprous oxide deposits

DIFFERENTIAL DIAGNOSIS

Primary Biliary Cirrhosis

- Kayser-Fleischer ring present but without neurologic symptoms and normal serum ceruloplasm level

Chronic Active Hepatitis

- Kayser-Fleischer ring with normal ceruloplasm

Multiple Myeloma

- Kayser-Fleischer ring with normal ceruloplasm

Cholestasis

- Kayser-Fleischer ring with normal ceruloplasm

Chalcosis

- Due to copper-containing foreign body, leads to severe inflammation and retinal toxicity

EVALUATION/WORK-UP

Labs

- Low serum ceruloplasmin: Not sensitive or specific
- Increased free copper in serum
- Increased urine copper
- Most reliable test is hepatic copper concentration
- Genetic testing is definitive

Pathology

- Kayser-Fleischer ring: Copper deposits in Descemet membrane
- Sunflower cataract: Subcapsular cortex and anterior lens capsule cuprous oxide deposits
- Liver histology
  - Early disease → steatosis, Mallory hyaline, and glycogenated nuclei and mimics steatohepatitis
  - Intermediate disease → chronic hepatitis with fibrosis or cirrhosis
  - Fulminant → parenchymal necrosis and collapse
- Histochemical stains
  - Rhodanine and rubeanic acid stains show copper in periportal hepatocytes
  - Orcein or aldehyde fuchsin stains may show granules in periportal hepatocytes

Imaging

- Slit lamp: Look for Kayser-Fleischer ring or sunflower cataract
- Gonioscopy: Helpful to find Kayser-Fleischer when not seen with slit lamp

TREATMENT

Medical

- Copper chelators
  - Penicillamine: Binds copper and excretes in urine, also leads to sequestration of free intracellular copper
  - Trientine
  - Ammonium tetrathiomolybdate: Inhibits copper absorption and is excreted in bile
- Zinc: Induces intestinal metallothionein
  - Enterocyte copper binding, lost when enterocytes shed

Surgical

- Liver transplant for fulminant hepatic failure or failed medical therapy

Prognosis

- With effective medical therapy &/or liver transplant, Kayser-Fleischer rings and sunflower cataract can disappear, corneal changes may remain present
- Death if untreated

SELECTED REFERENCES

1. Huster D: Wilson disease. Best Pract Res Clin Gastroenterol. 24(5):531-9, 2010

ENDOTHELIAL DYSTROPHIES

Key Facts

Introduction

- Progressive, bilateral, noninflammatory, degenerative disease of corneal endothelium marked by endothelial cell dysfunction resulting in corneal edema and ultimately corneal decompensation

Presentation

- **Fuchs** visual symptoms may be worse in the morning secondary to recurrent erosions from ruptured bullae
  - Fuchs hallmark is central corneal guttata
- **CHED** presents with bilateral edematous and cloudy corneas with a diffuse gray-blue ground-glass coloring
- **PPMD** hallmark is a scalloped lesion on the posterior cornea; often, lesions are isolated or in lines, clusters, or confluent groups but by definition are polymorphous

Evaluation/Work-Up

- Specular and confocal microscopy can provide endothelial cell counts and may show pathological changes in corneal layers

Treatment

- Descemet stripping automated endothelial keratoplasty (DSAEK) is a good treatment option for Fuchs, CHED, and PPMD
- Fuchs
  - Use of hypertonic saline solutions or ointments (Muro, dextran, albumin), increase evaporative tear loss with blow dryer, and reduce IOP when necessary
  - When supportive medical management is no longer sufficient, DSAEK is performed
- Follow-up
  - Every 3-12 months to assess corneal edema and IOP

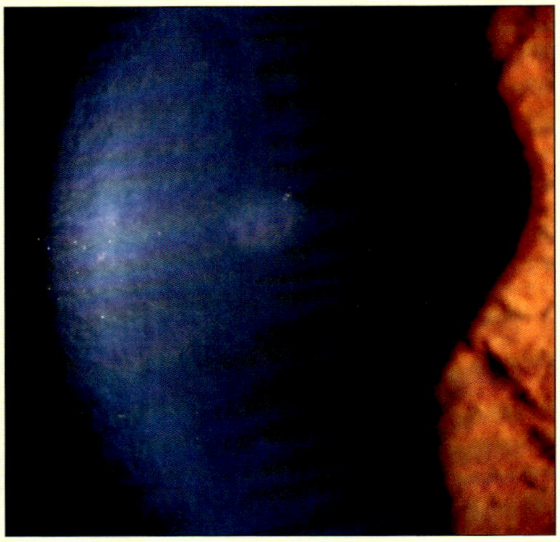

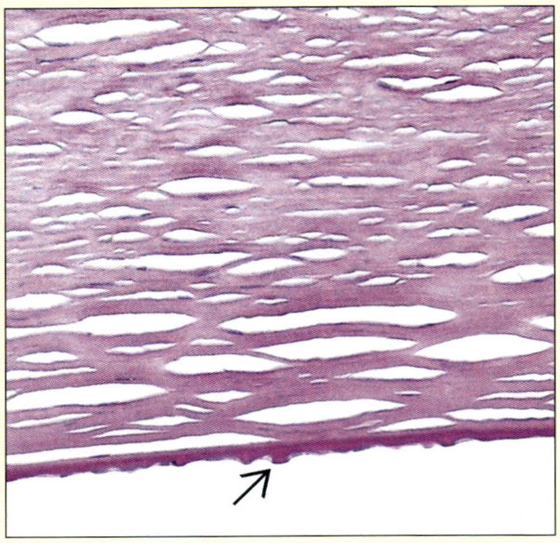

(Left) *This slit-lamp photo highlights the characteristic guttata present on the endothelium in a patient with Fuchs endothelial dystrophy. Some guttata have become confluent, giving the endothelium a hammered metal appearance. There is also mild corneal edema.* ***(Right)*** *Periodic acid-Schiff light micrograph shows the corneal stroma and Descemet membrane from a patient with Fuchs endothelial dystrophy. Note the thickened Descemet membrane, absent endothelial layer, and anvil-shaped guttata ⇒.*

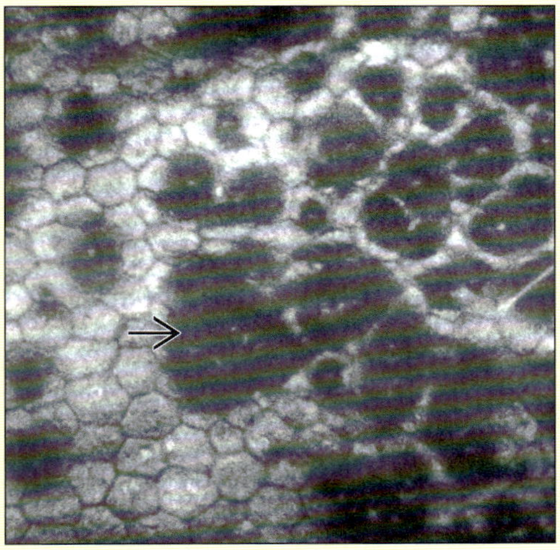

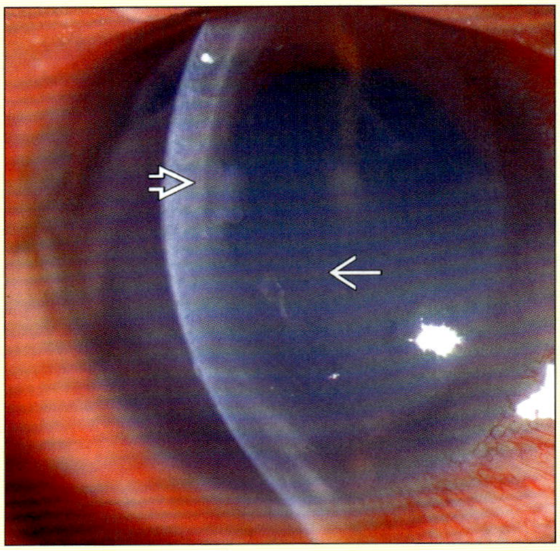

(Left) *Confocal microscopy of the corneal endothelial layer shows multiple areas of guttata (dark gray patches ⇒) in a patient with Fuchs endothelial dystrophy.* ***(Right)*** *This slit-lamp photo shows an eye with congenital hereditary endothelial dystrophy (CHED). Note the characteristic edematous and cloudy cornea with a diffuse gray-blue ground-glass coloring ➡. Also note the absence of corneal guttata ➡. This condition is typically bilateral.*

ENDOTHELIAL DYSTROPHIES

INTRODUCTION

Definitions
- Progressive, bilateral, noninflammatory, degenerative disease of corneal endothelium marked by endothelial cell dysfunction resulting in corneal edema and ultimately corneal decompensation

Subtypes
- Fuchs endothelial dystrophy (Fuchs)
- Congenital hereditary endothelial dystrophy (CHED)
- Posterior polymorphous dystrophy (PPMD)

DEMOGRAPHICS

Etiology/Risk Factors
- Endothelial dystrophies are most commonly inherited disorders

Epidemiology
- **Fuchs**
  - Rarely symptomatic before age 50
- **CHED**
  - Rare autosomal dominant and recessive condition
- **PPMD**
  - Rare inherited disease with an autosomal dominant pattern with variable penetrance, occasionally autosomal recessive

PRESENTATION

Symptoms
- Worsening vision with glare and blurring
- Severe pain may occur secondary to recurrent erosions due to ruptured bullae, often experienced upon eye opening in the morning

Exam Findings
- **Fuchs**
  - Hallmark is central corneal guttata
- **CHED**
  - Bilateral edematous and cloudy corneas with a diffuse gray-blue ground-glass coloring
  - Corneal thickness is 2-3x normal, normal corneal diameter, normal IOP
  - Epithelial surface is irregular, no corneal guttata
- **PPMD**
  - Hallmark is a vesicular lesion on posterior cornea; often lesions are isolated or in lines or clusters
  - Peripheral anterior synechiae are characteristic

DIFFERENTIAL DIAGNOSIS

Fuchs
- Bullous keratopathy, Hassall-Henle bodies

CHED
- Congenital glaucoma, macular dystrophy, mucopolysaccharidosis, intrauterine infection, birth trauma

PPMD
- Tears in Descemet membrane, iridocorneal endothelial (ICE) syndrome, interstitial keratitis

EVALUATION/WORK-UP

Labs
- Visante OCT or Pentacam

Pathology
- **Fuchs**
  - Thickened Descemet membrane with anvil-shaped guttae and attenuated endothelium (H&E and PAS)
- **CHED**
  - Descemet membrane is thickened with an attenuated endothelial layer, but no guttata are present
- **PPMD**
  - Light microscopy shows small pits in posterior cornea, multilayered endothelium, and attenuated Descemet membrane with complete discontinuities

Imaging
- Specular and confocal microscopy can provide endothelial cell counts and may show pathological changes in corneal layers

TREATMENT

Medical
- For corneal edema, hypertonic saline solutions/ointments (Muro, dextran, albumin) or blow dryer to increase evaporative tear loss
- Reduce IOP when necessary

Surgical
- **Fuchs**
  - When supportive medical management is no longer sufficient, Descemet stripping automated endothelial keratoplasty (DSAEK) is performed
- **CHED**
  - Penetrating keratoplasty (PK) or DSAEK (with accompanying peripheral iridotomy to prevent block if patient is phakic) is indicated with loss of fixation or development of nystagmus
- **PPMD**
  - PK or DSAEK may be offered for corneal opacification (depending on extent of opacification into stroma)

Follow-Up
- Every 3-12 months to assess corneal edema and IOP

Prognosis
- **Fuchs**
  - Ultimately, PK or DSAEK, or emerging procedure, Descemet membrane endothelial keratoplasty, (DMEK) will be required
- **CHED**
  - Visual potential may vary due to other visual rehabilitation and amblyogenic factors
- **PPMD**
  - Typically, a nonprogressive dystrophy without vision impairment

SELECTED REFERENCES

1. Özdemir B et al: Penetrating keratoplasty in congenital hereditary endothelial dystrophy. Cornea. 31(4):359-65, 2012
2. Waring GO 3rd et al: Corneal dystrophies. II. Endothelial dystrophies. Surv Ophthalmol. 23(3):147-68, 1978

EPITHELIAL AND SUBEPITHELIAL DYSTROPHIES

Key Facts

Introduction

- Anterior corneal dystrophies characterized by recurrent corneal erosions; small, intraepithelial dots; or subepithelial ridges and lines representing abnormal corneal epithelium

Demographics

- Most corneal dystrophies have autosomal dominant pattern

Presentation

- Symptoms vary and often fluctuate and range from asymptomatic to painful
- Corneal erosions can be visually significant and rarely proceed to scarring
- Features may be variable, absent, or only subtle in fellow eye
  - Hallmark intraepithelial microcysts ("dots")
  - Irregular, gray, geographical patches surrounding microcysts ("maps")
  - Subepithelial ridges or contoured concentric lines ("fingerprint")

Treatment

- Hypertonic drops (5% NaCl) t.i.d. and ointment q.h.s.
- Prophylactic supportive therapies
  - Artificial tears q.i.d. and p.r.n., ointments q.h.s. and t.i.d., punctal plugs, blindfolds, or moisture chamber goggles while sleeping
- Prognosis
  - EBMD/ABMD symptoms fluctuate but typically do not progress over time
  - Management of recurrent corneal erosions with conservative therapy will reduce frequency and severity of attacks

*(**Left**) This slit-lamp photograph depicts the irregular, gray, geographical patches seen in anterior basement membrane dystrophy (ABMD). These lesions are often referred to as the classic "maps" seen in this disease. (**Right**) This slit-lamp photograph shows the hallmark intraepithelial microcysts seen in ABMD. These lesions are referred to as "dots" and are 1 of the 3 classic findings in ABMD.*

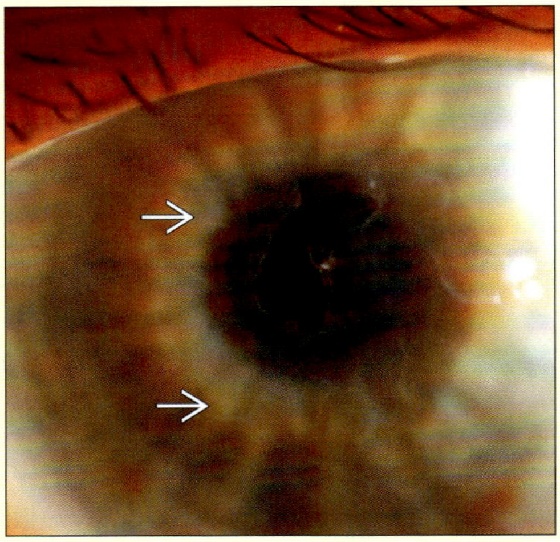

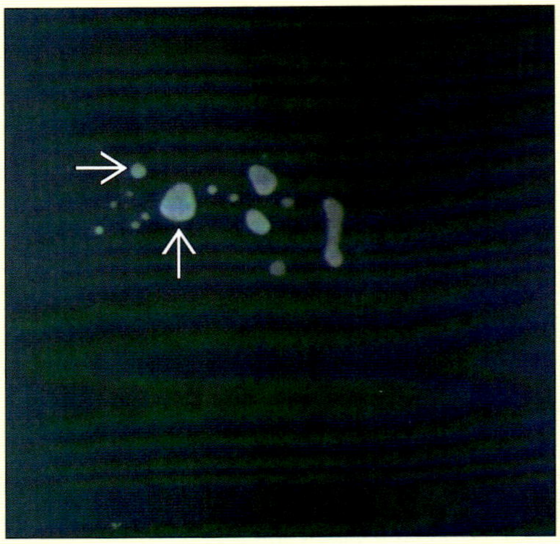

*(**Left**) This slit-lamp photograph demonstrates subepithelial ridges and contoured concentric lines that are often seen in ABMD. These whorls are often referred to as "fingerprints" and are considered 1 of the 3 classic findings in ABMD. (**Right**) This slit-lamp photograph shows an eye with ABMD. Note the irregular, gray geographic patch and associated contoured concentric line. Often, findings in ABMD are more subtle than depicted here.*

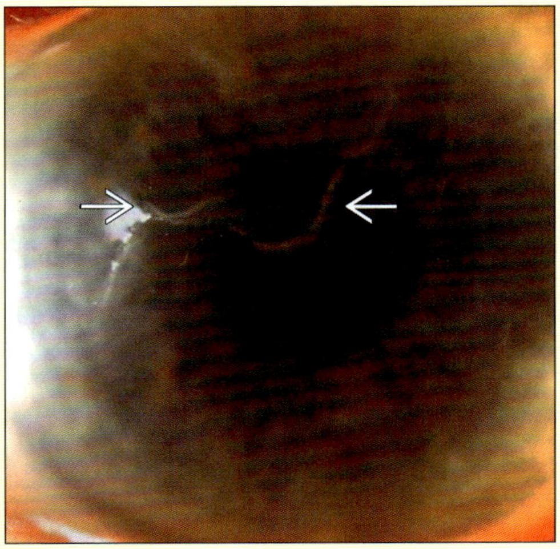

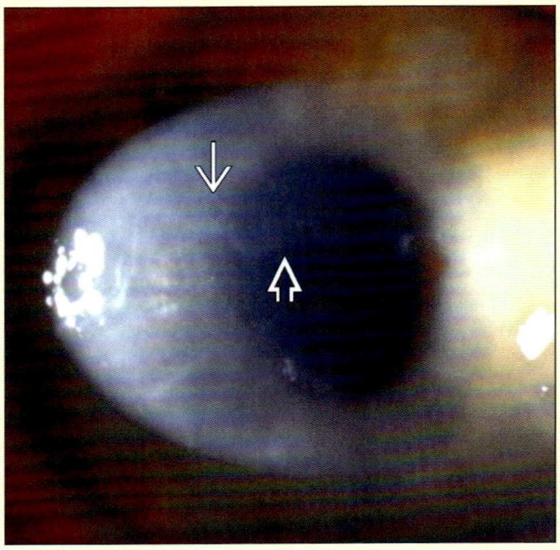

EPITHELIAL AND SUBEPITHELIAL DYSTROPHIES

INTRODUCTION

Definitions

- Noninfectious, noninflammatory, bilateral, and progressive corneal opacity or alteration involving corneal epithelium, epithelial basement membrane (BM), or Bowman membrane
- Anterior corneal dystrophies characterized by recurrent corneal erosions; small, intraepithelial dots; or subepithelial ridges and lines representing abnormal corneal epithelium

Subtypes

- **Recurrent corneal erosion**
  - Causes can be traumatic, dystrophic, or idiopathic
- **Epithelial basement membrane dystrophy (EBMD)/ anterior basement membrane dystrophy (ABMD)**
  - Involve epithelial layer and epithelial BM with subsequent epithelial changes
    - EBMD (most common)
    - Meesmann dystrophy
    - Lisch epithelial corneal dystrophy (LECD)
- **Bowman membrane dystrophies**
  - Typically involve abnormalities within the epithelium, BM, Bowman membrane, and extend into the superficial stroma
  - Corneal dystrophy of Bowman layer I (CDB I), a.k.a. Reis-Bucklers dystrophy
  - Corneal dystrophy of Bowman layer II (CDB II), a.k.a. Thiel-Behnke dystrophy

DEMOGRAPHICS

Etiology/Risk Factors

- Most commonly autosomal dominant

Epidemiology

- EBMD is estimated to affect 2-43% of population
  - 1/2 of patients with recurrent erosions have EBMD; female predominance
  - Symptoms often appear in 4th decade

PRESENTATION

Symptoms

- Variable and often fluctuating and ranging from asymptomatic to painful
  - Corneal erosions may progress to scarring
    - Transient symptoms, lasting minutes to days
    - Fluctuating visual acuity without discomfort
    - Pain or irritation
    - Blurred vision associated with minimal, irregular astigmatism from uneven corneal surface

Exam Findings

- Slit-lamp exam
  - **EBMD**
    - Features may be asymmetrical, variable, or absent
    - Lesions may be seen in isolation or combination and are best visualized by retroillumination with fluorescein staining
      - Hallmark intraepithelial microcysts ("dots") surrounded by irregular, gray, geographical patches ("maps")
      - Subepithelial ridges or contoured concentric lines ("fingerprint") that may have bleb-like changes (clear, round, bubble-like defects within epithelial and basal layers)

DIFFERENTIAL DIAGNOSIS

Recurrent Corneal Erosion/Abrasion

- Traumatic, mechanical

Infectious Keratitis

- Herpes simplex or herpes zoster

EVALUATION/WORK-UP

Pathology

- EBMD, light microscopy
  - Absence of hemidesmosomes of basal cells
  - Abnormal multilamellar areas of thickened BM extending into epithelium ("fingerprints")
  - Normally maturing epithelial cells get trapped beneath this extended BM, forming microcysts composed of cellular and nuclear debris ("dots")

TREATMENT

Medical

- EBMD/ABMD
  - Corneal erosions
    - 5% NaCl drops t.i.d. and ointment q.h.s.
    - Acute episodes: Consider patching, short-term collagen shields, or bandage contact lenses
    - Recalcitrant recurrent corneal erosions: Consider topical corticosteroids and doxycycline or matrix metalloproteinase (MMP) inhibitors
  - Prophylactic supportive therapies
    - Artificial tears q.i.d. and p.r.n., ointments q.h.s. and t.i.d., punctal plugs, blindfolds, or moisture chamber goggles while sleeping

Surgical

- Recurrent corneal erosions (RCE)
  - Corneal anterior stromal puncture for recalcitrant RCE
  - Excimer laser phototherapeutic keratectomy (PTK)
- EBMD/ABMD
  - Mechanical debridement and superficial keratectomy followed with a bandage contact lens, nonsteroidal drops, and topical antibiotics
  - Diamond burr superficial keratectomy
  - Excimer laser PTK

Prognosis

- EBMD/ABMD symptoms fluctuate but typically do not progress over time
- Management of recurrent corneal erosions with conservative therapy ↓ frequency, severity of attacks

SELECTED REFERENCES

1. Weiss JS et al: The IC3D classification of the corneal dystrophies. Cornea. 27 Suppl 2:S1-83, 2008
2. Waring GO 3rd et al: Corneal dystrophies. I. Dystrophies of the epithelium, Bowman's layer and stroma. Surv Ophthalmol. 23(2):71-122, 1978

ACANTHAMOEBA KERATITIS

Key Facts

Introduction
- Microbial keratitis caused by *Acanthamoeba* protozoa

Demographics
- Acanthamoebae are ubiquitous protozoa commonly found in soil and water
- Exist in trophozoite or dormant double-walled cyst form
- Vast majority of cases (85%) are related to contact lens use and improper care

Presentation
- Severe pain, usually described as out of proportion to exam findings
- Blurred vision, photophobia
- Dendritic epithelial lesion
- Diffuse punctate epitheliopathy
- Radial perineuritis with enlarged corneal nerves
- Scleritis or limbitis
- Ring-shaped infiltrate of cornea with stromal opacification, vascularization, and melt in severe cases

Differential Diagnosis
- Herpetic keratitis
  - Resembles early forms of AK, especially with dendritic presentation
  - Confusion is common cause of treatment delay
- Anesthetic abuse
  - May also produce ring-shaped corneal infiltrate

Treatment
- Controversial, commonly biguanides with diamidines
  - Polyhexamethylene biguanide (PHMB) 0.02% or chlorhexidine 0.02%
  - Propamidine isethionate 0.1% (Brolene) or hexamidine diisethionate 0.1% (Desomodine)
- May also incorporate aminoglycosides or imidazoles/triazoles

*(**Left**) Pathology smear shows classic double-walled Acanthamoeba cyst with outer → & inner ➔ walls clearly visible. This morphology contributes to protozoan's resiliency and high rate of treatment. Acanthamoeba is ubiquitous in soil & water but predominantly infects contact lens wearers. (**Right**) In vivo confocal microscopy shows Acanthamoeba cysts → in corneal stroma. This real-time diagnostic technique is useful in differentiating acanthamoeba keratitis (AK) from other causes of keratitis and is not invasive.*

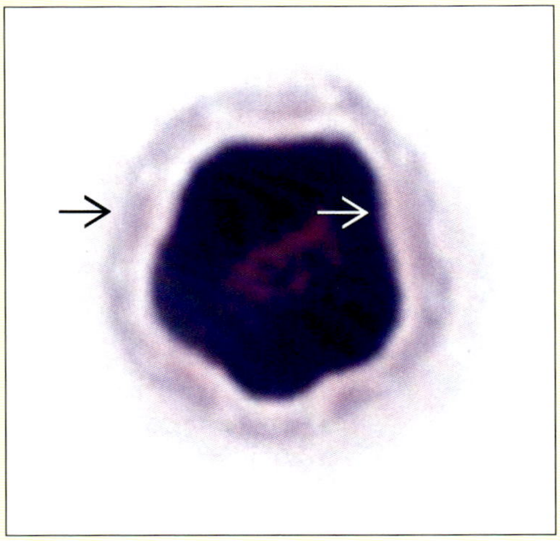

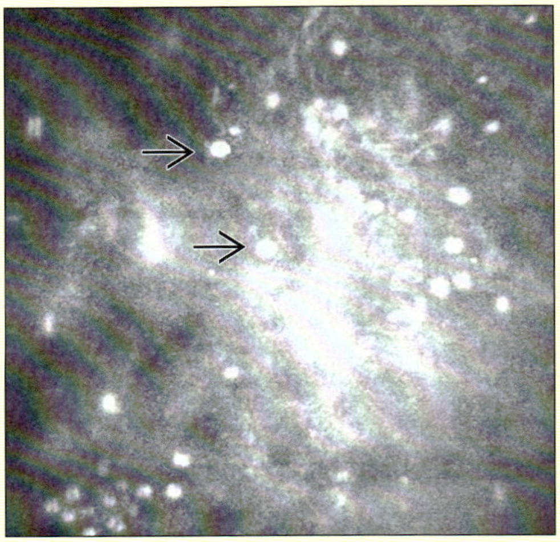

*(**Left**) Slit-lamp photo shows classic ring-shaped corneal infiltrate ➔ found in AK, which facilitates diagnosis in later stages of disease. AK is commonly confused with HSV keratitis in earlier stages & usually only suspected after treatment failure. (**Right**) Slit-lamp photo shows advanced AK with severe limbitis/scleritis ➔, a large hypopyon ↩, & diffuse corneal infiltrate & melt ⇨. This case was delayed diagnosis with poor prognosis & high likelihood of recurrence after corneal transplant. (Courtesy W. Nosé, MD.)*

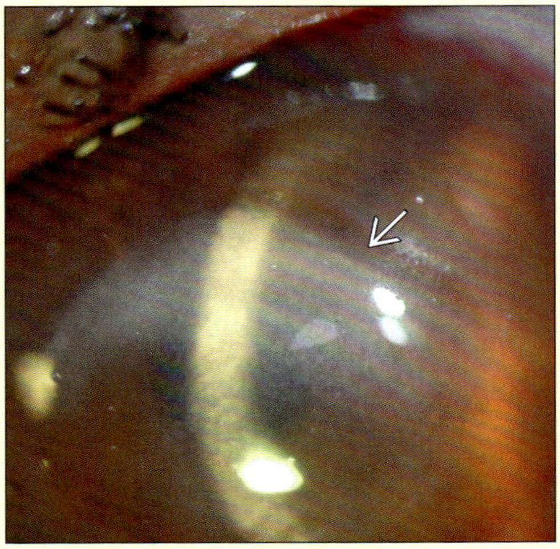

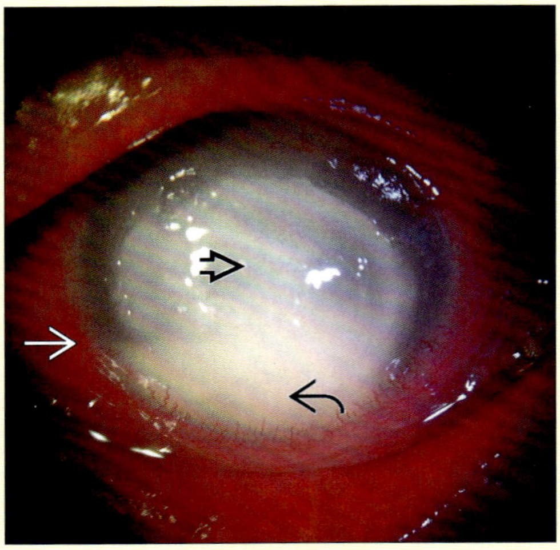

ACANTHAMOEBA KERATITIS

INTRODUCTION

Abbreviations
- Acanthamoeba keratitis (AK)

Definitions
- Microbial keratitis caused by *Acanthamoeba* protozoa

DEMOGRAPHICS

Etiology/Risk Factors
- Acanthamoebae are ubiquitous protozoa commonly found in soil and water
  - Exist in trophozoite or dormant double-walled cyst form
  - No human or animal vectors, with 0 person-to-person transmissibility
- Vast majority of cases related to contact lens use (85%)
  - Risk factors include
    - Swimming with contact lenses
    - Trauma to cornea
    - Improper storing and handling of contact lenses
      - Cleaning contact lenses with tap water
      - Using homemade saline solution

Epidemiology
- 1-2 cases per million contact lens wearers

PRESENTATION

Symptoms
- Severe pain, usually described as out of proportion to exam findings
- Blurred vision
- Photophobia

Exam Findings
- Early
  - Dendritic epithelial lesion
  - Diffuse punctate epitheliopathy
- Mid
  - Gray-white superficial stromal infiltrates, usually in central cornea
  - Radial perineuritis with enlarged corneal nerves
  - Scleritis or limbitis
- Late
  - Ring-shaped infiltrate of cornea with stromal opacification, vascularization, and melt in severe cases

DIFFERENTIAL DIAGNOSIS

Herpetic Keratitis
- Resembles early forms of AK, especially with dendritic presentation or ring infiltrate in stromal disease
  - HK responds to antivirals and corticosteroids unlike AK
  - Confusion is common cause of treatment delay for AK

Bacterial or Fungal Keratitis
- History, confocal microscopy, cultures, and biopsy results are helpful in differentiating these from AK

Anesthetic Abuse
- May also produce ring-shaped corneal infiltrate
  - Pain and inflammation usually greater in AK

EVALUATION/WORK-UP

Labs
- Organisms and cysts may be visualized in stained corneal scrapings
  - Calcofluor white, Giemsa, periodic acid-Schiff, and acridine orange are commonly used stains
- Cultured in nonnutrient agar with *Escherichia Coli* overlay
- Real-time PCR

Imaging
- Confocal microscopy allows visualization of cysts in vivo

TREATMENT

Medical
- No consensus; however, mainstay of therapy includes biguanides with diamidines
  - Biguanides
    - Chlorhexidine 0.02%
    - Polyhexamethylene biguanide (PHMB) 0.02%; derived from common pool cleaner
  - Diamidines
    - Propamidine isethionate 0.1% (Brolene) or hexamidine diisethionate 0.1% (Desomedine)
    - IV pentamidine is another alternative
  - Aminoglycosides
  - Imidazoles or triazoles (oral fluconazole and oral itraconazole) can be adjunctive therapies

Surgical
- Penetrating keratoplasty (PK)
  - Reserved for progressive disease with threatened corneal perforation or for corneal scarring
  - High risk of recurrence even in apparently quiet eyes
  - Recommend waiting 3-12 months after full-course amebicidal treatment ends prior to attempting PK to reduce recurrence rates

Follow-Up
- Every 1-2 days until there is demonstrated improvement

Prognosis
- Varies with disease stage at presentation; good prognosis with early treatment

SELECTED REFERENCES

1. Carvalho FR et al: Twenty years of acanthamoeba keratitis. Cornea. 28(5):516-9, 2009
2. Dart JK et al: Acanthamoeba keratitis: diagnosis and treatment update 2009. Am J Ophthalmol. 148(4):487-499, 2009
3. Ibrahim YW et al: Factors affecting the epidemiology of Acanthamoeba keratitis. Ophthalmic Epidemiol. 14(2):53-60, 2007
4. Seal DV et al: Acanthamoeba keratitis. Br J Ophthalmol. 87(4):516-7, 2003
5. Seal DV: Acanthamoeba keratitis update-incidence, molecular epidemiology and new drugs for treatment. Eye (Lond). 17(8):893-905, 2003

BACTERIAL KERATITIS

Key Facts

Introduction
- Bacterial infection of cornea

Etiology/Risk Factors
- Contact lenses (overnight use is biggest risk)
- Trauma, including surgeries
- Contaminated eyedrops
- Topical steroids

Presentation
- Severe pain
- Eye discharge
- Photophobia
- Decreased vision
- Cells, flare, or hypopyon
- Stromal inflammation and ulceration
- Focal infiltrate

Evaluation/Work-Up
- Gram stains and cultures if central, refractory, or large lesion, or if there is anterior chamber cell
- Slit-lamp photography

Treatment
- Topical broad-spectrum antibiotics (4th generation quinolone or fortifieds)
- Taper medications if clinical improvement
- Severe cases: Hospitalization with frequent administration of drops and systemic antibiotics

Microbiology: Most Common Agents
- *Staphylococcus aureus*, *Streptococcus pneumoniae*, *Pseudomonas aeruginosa*, Enterobacteriaceae

Prognosis
- Can lead to stromal scarring and decreased vision
- Severe cases → corneal perforation and loss of eye

*(**Left**) This slit-lamp photograph shows a fluorescein-stained eye with a severe bacterial ulcer ➔. The infection in this eye resulted in perforation of the cornea. Corneal perforation is one of the most serious potential complications of bacterial keratitis. (**Right**) This external photograph of bacterial keratitis demonstrates the irregular corneal surface caused by the ulcer ➔. This ulcer is in the visual axis and resulted in decreased vision.*

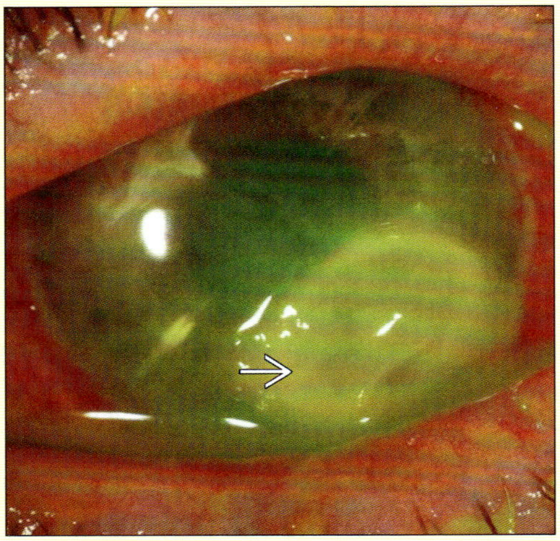

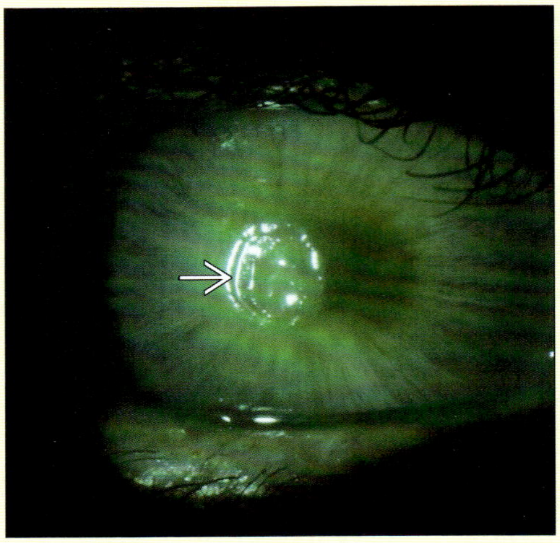

*(**Left**) This external photograph shows a large bacterial ulcer involving the visual axis ➔. Note the associated hypopyon ➔. (**Right**) This external photograph shows bacterial keratitis ➔. Note the associated haziness of the cornea caused by corneal edema from the local inflammatory reaction ➔. There is also marked hyperemia of the conjunctival and limbal vessels ➔.*

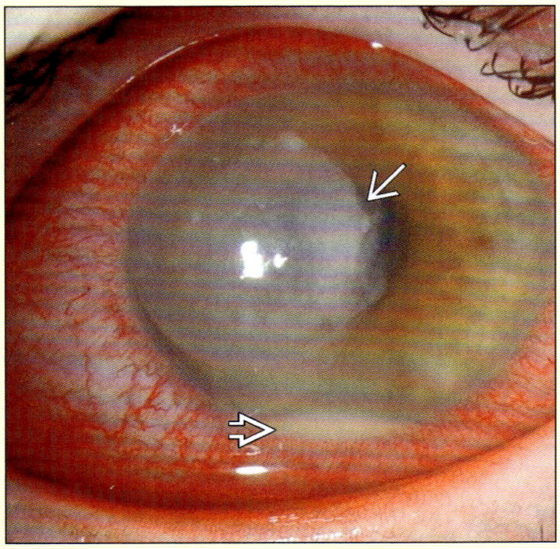

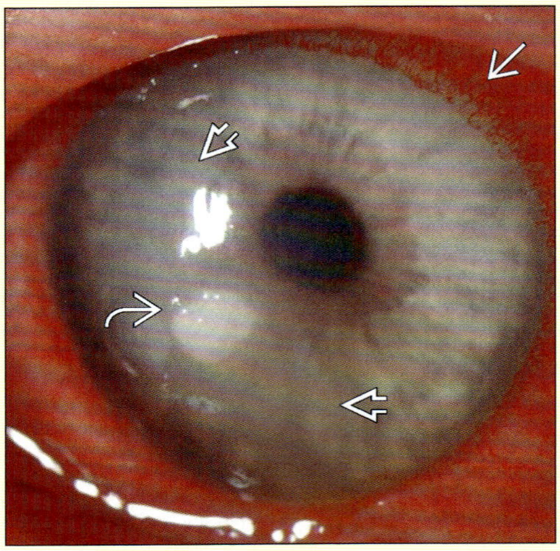

BACTERIAL KERATITIS

INTRODUCTION

Definitions

- Bacterial infection of cornea

DEMOGRAPHICS

Etiology/Risk Factors

- Contact lenses, trauma, surgeries, topical steroids, immunosuppression, dryness, diabetes, scars, surface irritation

Epidemiology

- 10-20x more likely with overnight contact lens use
- 0.02% per year with rigid contact lenses
- 0.02-0.04% per year with daily-wear soft contact lens
- 0.1-0.2% per year with extended-wear soft contact lenses

PRESENTATION

Symptoms

- Pain, discharge, photophobia, reduced vision

Exam Findings

- Stromal and upper lid edema
- Anterior chamber inflammation ± hypopyon
- Focal infiltrate
  - At least 1.0-1.5 mm
  - Usually yellow-white and opaque
  - Often irregular in shape
- Stromal inflammation and ulceration
- Conjunctival injection

DIFFERENTIAL DIAGNOSIS

Contact Lens-Induced Peripheral Ulcer

- Inflammatory reaction of the cornea characterized by focal excavation of epithelium and infiltration and necrosis of anterior stoma
  - Bowman layer remains intact

Fungal Keratitis

- Dingy white, dry infiltrate with feathery borders; satellite lesions often present
- Often follows trauma with organic/vegetable matter or in setting of steroid use
  - e.g., *Aspergillus*, *Fusarium*, *Candida albicans*

Viral Keratitis

- Herpes simplex virus
  - Dendritic ulcer, focal endotheliitis, eyelid vesicles
- Ebstein-Barr virus
- Varicella zoster virus

Parasitic Keratitis

- Photophobia, severe pain, and pseudodendrites
- Acanthamoeba

EVALUATION/WORK-UP

Labs

- Cultures
  - Corneal scraping and contact lens
  - Blood and chocolate agars and thioglycolate
- Gram stain: Corneal scraping

Pathology

- *Staphylococcus*
- *Streptococcus*
- *Pseudomonas aeruginosa*
- Enterobacteriaceae

Imaging

- Slit-lamp photography
  - Used to follow disease progression

TREATMENT

Medical

- Low-risk patient
  - Topical broad-spectrum antibiotics
    - Generally start with a broad-spectrum quinolone
      - Loading dose: 1 drop every 2 minutes for 5 applications
      - Followed by administration every 30 minutes for first 12-24 hours
      - Alternate drugs when multiple antibiotics used
- Severe risk patient
  - Fortified antibiotic choices: Cefazolin (50 mg/mL), vancomycin (25 mg/mL), or tobramycin (15 mg/mL)
  - Subconjunctival antibiotic injections
    - Every 12-24 hours at different sites for first 24-48 hours
  - Parenteral antibiotics
    - Severe keratitis with risk of perforation
    - Perforation with risk of intraocular spread
    - Contiguous scleral involvement
  - Hospitalization

Surgical

- Penetrating keratoplasty
  - With large perforation or necrotic cornea
- Corneal patch grafting

Follow-Up

- Taper medications if clinical improvement

Prognosis

- Stromal scarring with variable visual outcome
- Severe: Corneal perforation and loss of eye

SELECTED REFERENCES

1. Hindman HB et al: Rationale for adjunctive topical corticosteroids in bacterial keratitis. Arch Ophthalmol. 127(1):97-102, 2009
2. Aasuri MK et al: Differential diagnosis of microbial keratitis and contact lens-induced peripheral ulcer. Eye Contact Lens. 29(1 Suppl):S60-2; discussion S83-4, S192-4, 2003
3. O'Brien TP: Management of bacterial keratitis: beyond exorcism towards consideration of organism and host factors. Eye (Lond). 17(8):957-74, 2003
4. Liesegang TJ: Contact lens-related microbial keratitis: Part I: Epidemiology. Cornea. 16(2):125-31, 1997
5. Asbell P et al: Ulcerative keratitis. Survey of 30 years' laboratory experience. Arch Ophthalmol. 100(1):77-80, 1982

FUNGAL KERATITIS

Key Facts

Introduction
- Corneal disease caused by filamentous fungi or yeast

Demographics
- Fungi infiltrate corneal stroma through epithelial defect (causing stromal inflammation, tissue necrosis)
- More common in tropical and developing countries than in temperate countries
- Constitutes < 5-10% of reported corneal infections in USA; most cases occur in warm southern states

Presentation
- Filamentous fungal keratitis appears with dry or roughly textured, grayish-white, elevated infiltrates; branching ulcers; filamentous or feathery margins; &/ or satellite lesions
- Severe conjunctival injection, suppuration, stromal infiltration, anterior chamber inflammation, or hypopyon may occur with progression of infection
- Ring infiltrate and endothelial plaque are also indicative of fungal keratitis

Evaluation/Work-Up
- Lab work-up necessary since clinical diagnosis of fungal keratitis is difficult; requires direct microscopy, staining, culture, and possible corneal biopsy for histopathologic exam

Treatment
- Principal drugs for medical treatment: Polyenes, azoles, pyrimidines (e.g., amphotericin B, natamycin, voriconazole, flucytosine)
- Surgical treatment: Periodic debridement of necrotic tissue, penetrating keratoplasty (PK), deep anterior lamellar keratoplasty (DALK); collagen cross-linking is an emerging alternative

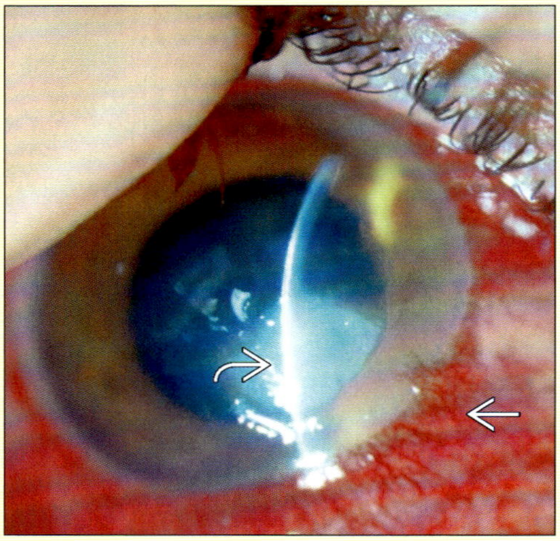
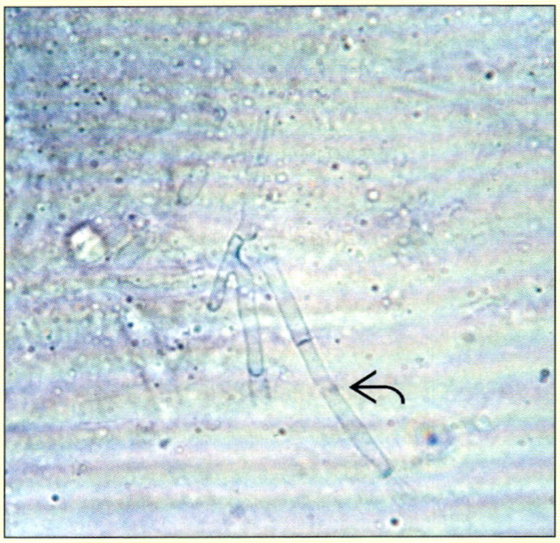

(Left) *Clinical photo shows infectious corneal ulcer ➡ with overlying epithelial defect and localized stromal infiltrate in paracentral nasal quadrant of right eye. Moderate surrounding edema and hyperemia are present ➡. Patient initially admitted to hospital and treated with scopolamine b.i.d. and fortified vancomycin and gentamicin q.30 minutes around the clock. (Courtesy K. Cohen, MD.)* ***(Right)*** *KOH preparation of corneal scrapings reveals Fusarium fungal hyphae ➡. (Courtesy K. Cohen, MD.)*

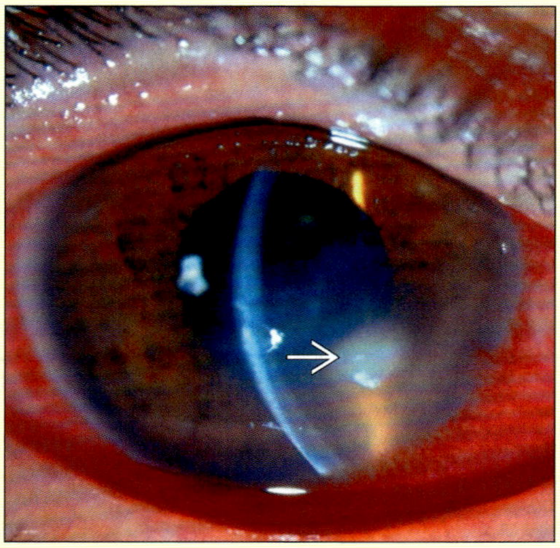
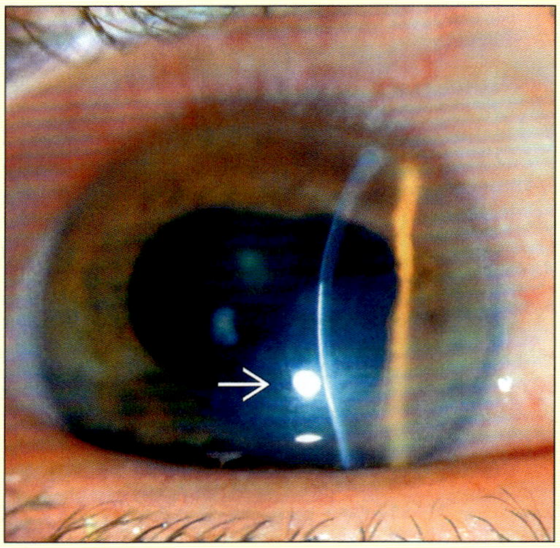

(Left) *Fusarium keratitis was subsequently treated with IV voriconazole and topical natamycin and moxifloxacin. Corneal infiltrate showed improvement 2 weeks after initiating antifungals ➡. (Courtesy K. Cohen, MD.)* ***(Right)*** *Four weeks after diagnosis and treatment, the cornea exhibits a large inferonasal anterior stromal scar with mild thinning ➡, minimal punctate fluorescein staining, and peripheral superficial vascularization. (Courtesy K. Cohen, MD.)*

FUNGAL KERATITIS

INTRODUCTION

Definitions

- Corneal disease caused by filamentous fungi or yeast

DEMOGRAPHICS

Etiology/Risk Factors

- Fungi infiltrate corneal stroma through epithelial defect, causing stromal inflammation and tissue necrosis
  - Can invade past Descemet membrane into anterior chamber, iris, and lens or outward to sclera
    - Invasion of these avascular tissues is difficult to treat since medications cannot effectively reach them
- Risk factors
  - Ocular trauma, especially from outdoor work (e.g., gardening) where agricultural tools can cause ocular injury from plant matter
  - Contact lens wear
  - Topical corticosteroids, which can increase fungal organism virulence and decrease corneal immunity to infection
  - Immunosuppression secondary to systemic disease or systemic corticosteroid use
  - Chronic vernal or allergic keratoconjunctivitis
  - Chronic neurotrophic ulcers secondary to VZV or HSV
  - Incisions from refractive surgery and keratoplasty

Epidemiology

- More common in tropical and developing countries than in temperate countries
- Constitutes < 5-10% of reported corneal infections in USA; most cases occur in warm southern states
- Septate filamentous fungi, especially *Fusarium* and *Aspergillus*, are most common organisms in tropical climates
- *Candida*, the most common cause of yeast keratitis, is most common in temperate climates
- Incidence of fungal keratitis is < bacterial keratitis

PRESENTATION

Symptoms

- Eye pain and redness
- Blurred vision
- Light sensitivity
- Excessive tearing or discharge

Exam Findings

- Insidious inflammatory signs during initial period
- Filamentous fungal keratitis appears with dry or roughly textured, grayish-white, elevated infiltrates; branching ulcers; filamentous or feathery margins; &/ or satellite lesions
- Severe conjunctival injection, suppuration, stromal infiltration, anterior chamber inflammation, or hypopyon may occur with progression of infection
- Endothelial plaque are also indicative of fungal keratitis (but can also occur in CMV)

DIFFERENTIAL DIAGNOSIS

Bacterial Keratitis

- Most common cause of infectious keratitis
- Occurs from bacterial invasion through defect in corneal epithelium
- Signs: Conjunctival injection, focal white infiltrates, corneal thinning, stromal edema, endothelial inflammatory plaque, Descemet folds, mucopurulent discharge, anterior chamber reaction, and hypopyon

Herpes Simplex Keratitis

- Caused by HSV1 and HSV2; reactivation of virus can lead to recurrent keratitis
- Signs: Multiple, small, branching dendritic lesions of corneal epithelium; vesicular lesions on eyelids or ocular adnexa; bulbar follicles; decreased corneal sensation

Acanthamoeba Keratitis

- Related to swimming with contact lenses and use of tap water for cleaning of contact lenses
- Signs: Severe eye pain and corneal ring ulcer

EVALUATION/WORK-UP

Labs

- Lab work-up necessary since clinical diagnosis of fungal keratitis is difficult
- Direct microscopy
  - Treat specimen with 10% KOH preparation to dissolve human tissue and reveal fungal structures
  - Negative results of direct microscopy do not rule out fungal infection; staining and culture are necessary for definitive diagnosis
- Stains
  - Gram stain: Demonstrates darkened fungal walls
  - Giemsa stain: Shows contrast between walls and highlighted cytoplasm
  - Ink-potassium hydroxide stain: Demonstrates dark outline of fungal walls
  - Gomori methenamine-silver stain: Best demonstrates fungal organisms but time-consuming and difficult to perform
- Culture media
  - Culturing allows for identification of fungi and determination of sensitivity to antifungal agents
  - Sheep blood agar, chocolate agar, Sabouraud dextrose agar, thioglycollate broth, or brain-heart infusion broth
  - Incubate cultures for 2-4 weeks; for fungal cultures, growth occurs optimally at 25-30°C and for yeasts at 35-37°C
- Corneal scraping for initial debridement of organisms and epithelium
- Corneal biopsy for histopathologic exam may be necessary if corneal scrapings are negative on smear or culture
- Anterior chamber tap for aspiration of hypopyon or endothelial plaque if fungus penetrates beyond Descemet membrane
- In contact lens wearers, obtain cultures or smears from lenses, storage containers, and cleaning solutions

FUNGAL KERATITIS

Pathology

- Fungal isolates are classified into following 3 groups
  - Moniliaceae: Nonpigmented filamentary fungi (e.g., *Fusarium* and *Aspergillus* species)
  - Dematiaceae: Pigmented filamentary fungi (e.g., *Curvularia* species)
  - Yeasts (including *Candida* species)

Imaging

- In vivo confocal microscopy (IVCM)
  - Noninvasive imaging technique used to examine all layers of live cornea for detection of microbial structures
  - High sensitivity and specificity in detecting fungal elements due to ↑ ability to differentiate hyperreflective elements of filamentous fungi and pseudohyphae of yeast from corneal epithelial and stromal nerves

TREATMENT

Medical

- Principle drugs for treatment
  - Polyenes
    - Amphotericin B (0.15-0.30%): Drug of choice for *Candida* and *Aspergillus*
    - Natamycin (5%): Initial topical antifungal of choice for filamentous fungal keratitis (e.g., *Fusarium*)
  - Azoles and pyrimidines
    - Alternative agents when fungal ulcer is very advanced or does not improve with polyenes
    - Imidazoles: Effective in treating superficial infections
      - Miconazole: Useful for poorly responsive *Aspergillus* infections
      - Ketoconazole: Effective against both yeast and filamentous organisms (e.g., *Aspergillus*, *Candida*, *Curvularia*, *Fusarium*)
    - Triazoles
      - Fluconazole: Effective against *Candida*; consider oral fluconazole for deep fungal keratitis that threatens anterior chamber involvement
      - Voriconazole: Effective for treatment of fungal keratitis that is unresponsive to traditional treatment
      - Itraconazole: Useful for *Aspergillus*, *Blastomyces*, and *Histoplasma* species
    - Pyrimidines
      - Flucytosine: Effective against *Candida*, but fungal organisms develop rapid resistance; thus, administer in combination with azole (for *Aspergillus*) or amphotericin B (for *Candida*)
  - Debridement of corneal epithelium is necessary for penetration of topical antifungals when fungi infiltrate deeply into stroma
  - Reserve subconjunctival injections and systemic antifungal treatment for severe keratitis, scleritis, and endophthalmitis
  - Topical steroids
    - Consider after epithelium has closed, when the infection is well controlled (or over) and excessive inflammation/fibrosis appears to be causing vision loss
    - Continue use of topical antifungal when initiating topical steroid and for 1 month after cessation of systemic antifungals to ensure there is no recurrence of fungi

Surgical

- Surgical disease in many parts of the world because of delays in initiating medical treatment or inability to obtain antifungal medications
  - 24-48 hour periodic debridement with spatula or blade performed with slit lamp under local anesthesia helps debride necrotic tissue and decreases fungal organism load, also enhances antifungal penetration
- Penetrating keratoplasty (PK)
  - Performed to prevent scleral or intraocular extension when medical treatment fails and keratitis progresses; try to avoid surgery in active infection unless tectonic keratoplasty is absolutely necessary
  - Less advanced cases may be treated with lamellar keratoplasty, but if depth of infection is questionable, full-thickness PK is preferred; may need to irrigate anterior chamber intraoperatively with antifungals
  - Complications include graft rejection, irregular astigmatism, and corneal opacification leading to visual impairment
- Deep anterior lamellar keratoplasty (DALK)
  - Corneal stroma is removed, but recipient's Descemet membrane and endothelium are preserved
  - Fewer risks compared to PK but carries potential for decreased visual acuity due to opacification of interface layers
- Riboflavin and UVA collagen cross-linking
  - Riboflavin eyedrop is instilled onto cornea; UVA radiation cross-links riboflavin with collagen
    - Cross-linking ↑ corneal integrity and ↓ susceptibility to collagen breakdown and melting
    - UV light eradicates fungal organisms through oxidation

Follow-Up

- Treat patient with topical antifungals postoperatively and follow for the course of several months, also consider systemic antifungal treatment
- Extend length of topical and systemic antifungal treatment if margins of corneal biopsy specimen reveal fungal organisms

Prognosis

- Depends on extent of corneal involvement at presentation, patient's health condition (e.g., healthy vs. immunocompromised), and length of time to culture-confirmed clinical diagnosis
- Good prognosis for mild infections and infections with early microbiologic diagnosis
- Very poor prognosis if disease progresses into sclera or globe due to difficulty in controlling and eradicating infection
- ~ 1/3 of fungal infections fail medical treatment or result in corneal perforation

SELECTED REFERENCES

1. Garg P: Fungal, mycobacterial, and nocardia infections and the eye: an update. Eye (Lond). 26(2):245-51, 2012

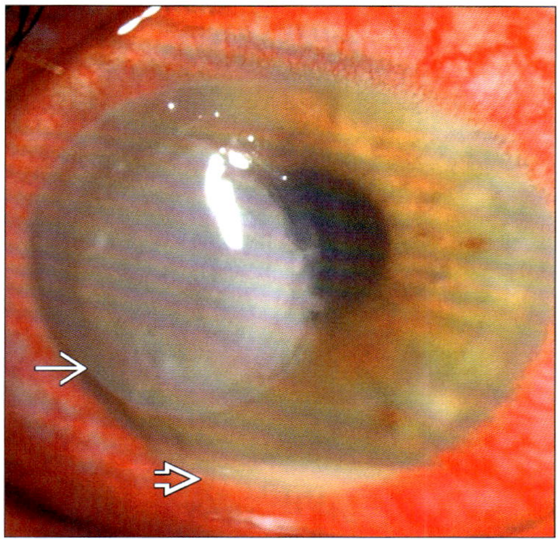
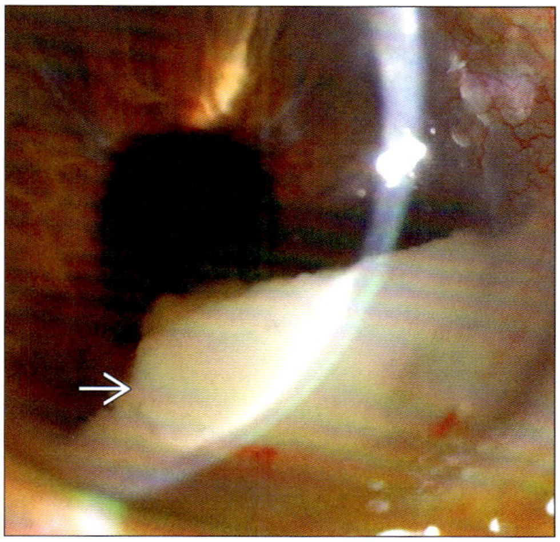

(Left) *This slit-lamp photograph demonstrates fungal keratitis ➔ and an associated hypopyon ➔. A hypopyon may develop in an eye with fungal keratitis, even in the absence of corneal perforation. Other findings in fungal keratitis include severe conjunctival injection and anterior chamber inflammation.* ***(Right)*** *This slit-lamp photograph shows a patient with fungal keratitis and a resulting endothelial plaque ➔. Inflammatory endothelial plaques are a typical finding in fungal keratitis.*

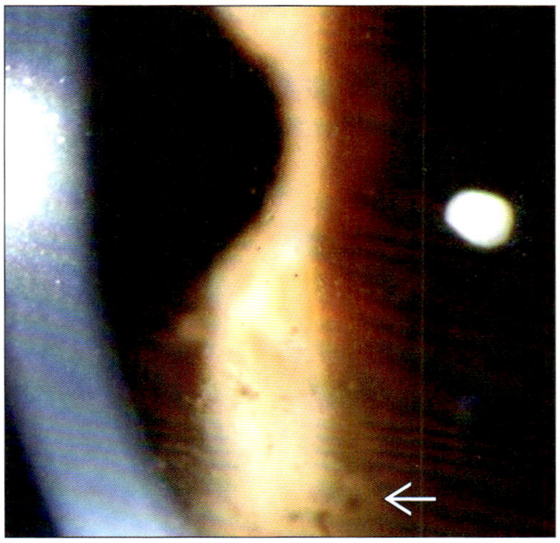
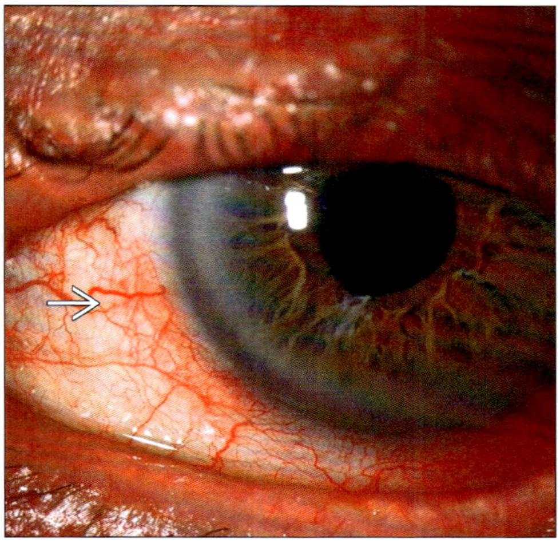

(Left) *This slit-lamp photograph shows endothelial debris ➔ in a patient with fungal keratitis. Fungal keratitis can invade past the Descemet membrane into the anterior chamber, iris, and lens or outward to the sclera.* ***(Right)*** *This external photograph demonstrates conjunctival injection ➔ in a patient with a fungal eye infection. Conjunctival injection with surface pain warrants a careful corneal examination. The patient was subsequently diagnosed with fungal endophthalmitis.*

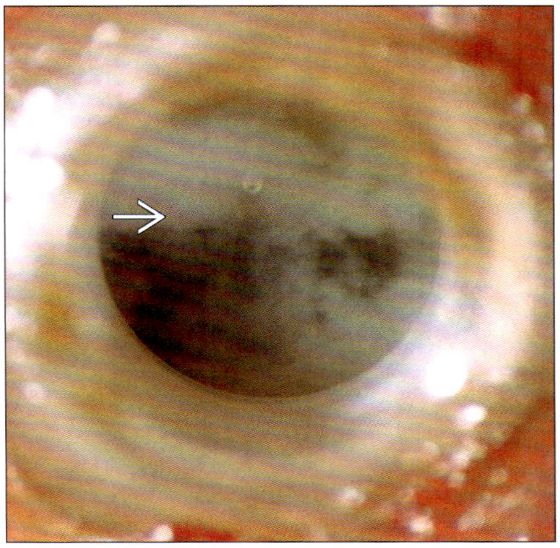
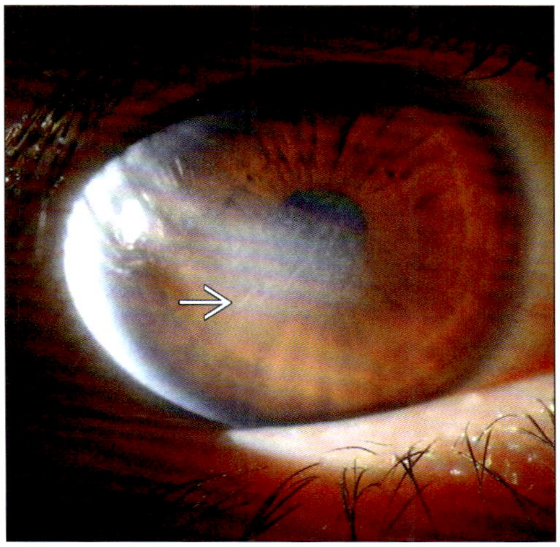

(Left) *This external photograph shows an eye that has undergone the placement of a keratoprosthesis with subsequent development of fungal keratitis and endophthalmitis ➔. Keratoprosthesis implantation is a risk factor for fungal keratitis.* ***(Right)*** *This slit-lamp photograph depicts an eye infected with Acanthamoeba keratitis, which is an important differential diagnosis for fungal keratitis. Note the subepithelial infiltrates ➔ that are typical of Acanthamoeba infections.*

HERPES ZOSTER VIRUS KERATITIS

Key Facts

Introduction
- Herpes zoster ophthalmicus (HZO): Ocular manifestation of unilateral painful skin rash that results from reactivation of varicella zoster virus (VZV) involving ophthalmic division of trigeminal nerve (CNV1)

Demographics
- Elderly and immunocompromised patients are most commonly affected

Presentation
- Prodromal period of influenza-like illness including fever, malaise, headache, ipsilateral lymphadenopathy, and eye pain prior to development of skin rash
- Acute, painful, vesicular rash erupts along distribution of dermatome associated with ophthalmic branch of trigeminal nerve
- Cornea is involved in ~ 65% of HZO cases

Evaluation/Work-Up
- Diagnosis of HZO is based primarily on clinical history and physical findings

Treatment
- Acyclovir (800 mg, 5x daily) for 7-10 days, or valacyclovir (1,000 mg, 3x daily) for 7-14 days, or famciclovir (500 mg, 3x daily) for 7 days
- Monitor every 1-7 days acutely and every 3-12 months after resolution
- Prognosis is greatly variable depending on acute manifestations and long-term sequelae
- Most common complication is post-herpetic neuralgia
- Zoster vaccine boosts cell-mediated immunity response to VZV and may be effective in preventing both HZO and post-herpetic neuralgia

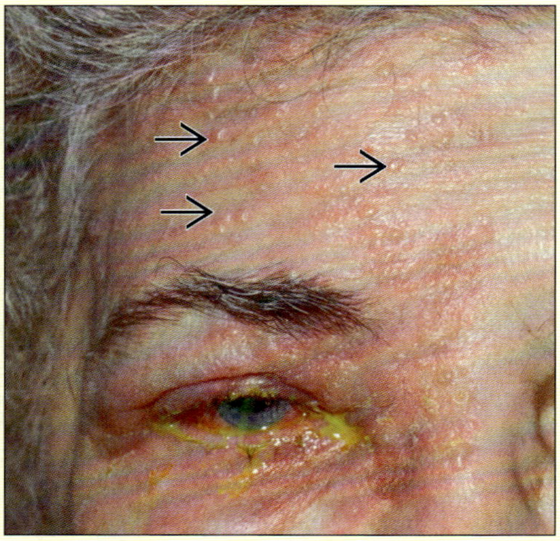
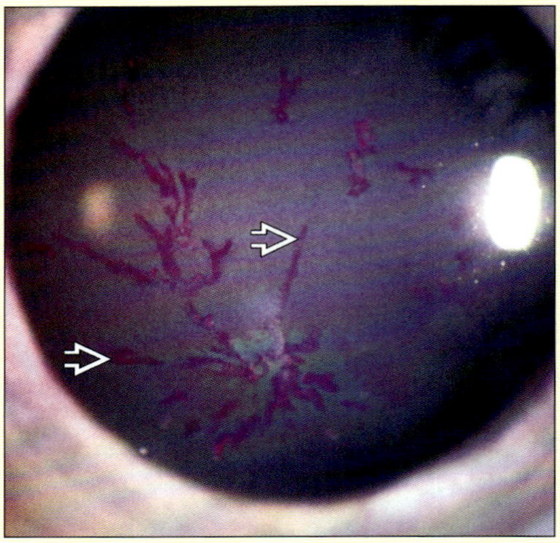

(Left) *External photo shows multiple raised skin lesions associated with shingles* ⇨*. The rash is classically described as "dew on rose petal." Note that the rash is distributed in the typical dermatomal pattern.* ***(Right)*** *Varicella zoster virus (VZV), a common cause of neurotrophic keratopathy, exhibits characteristic pseudodendritic staining. Note the absence of terminal bulbs at the tips of the dendrites* ⇨*, making VZV more likely than herpes simplex virus (HSV).*

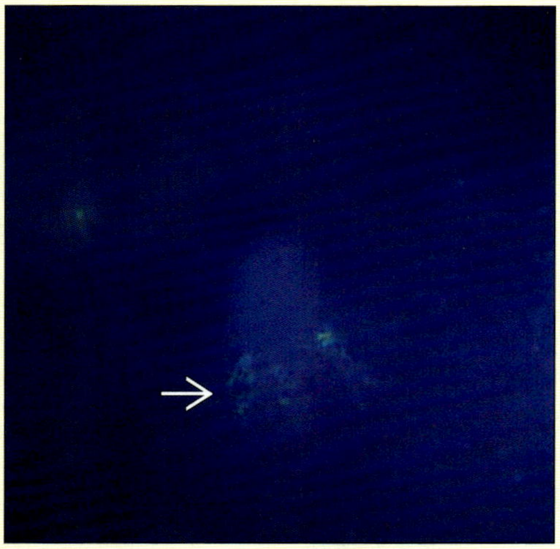
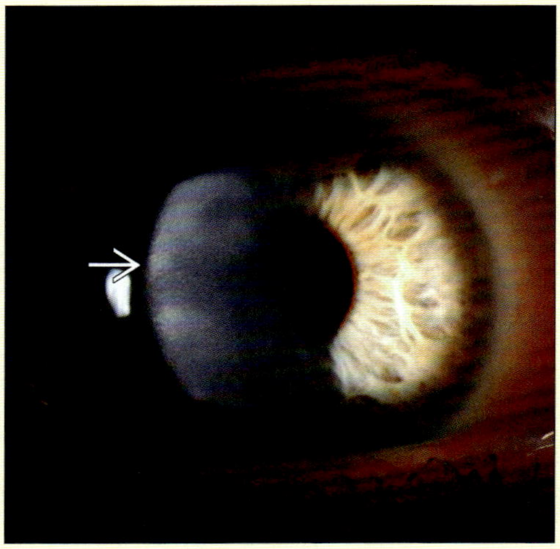

(Left) *Slit-lamp photo shows epithelial punctate staining* ➡ *seen in a patient with herpes zoster virus keratitis. Epithelial punctate keratitis is a common finding in herpes zoster virus keratitis.* ***(Right)*** *Slit-lamp photo depicts epithelial punctate keratitis* ➡ *in a patient with an herpes zoster virus infection. This image is shown without fluorescein dye and is viewed as mild haziness.*

HERPES ZOSTER VIRUS KERATITIS

INTRODUCTION

Definitions

- Herpes zoster ophthalmicus (HZO): Ocular manifestation of unilateral painful skin rash that results from reactivation of varicella zoster virus (VZV) involving ophthalmic division of trigeminal nerve (CN5)

Subtypes

- Zoster sine herpete
  - Presents with clinical symptoms of HZO but without rash

DEMOGRAPHICS

Etiology/Risk Factors

- Initial exposure to VZV (chickenpox) is prerequisite
- VZV-specific immunity and cell-mediated immunity (CMI) declines with age
- Immunosuppression (HIV, AIDS, immunosuppressive therapy)
- Acute or chronic diseases (malignancies and infections)

Epidemiology

- 20-30% of population will be affected by herpes zoster (HZ)
  - 10-20% of those affected by HZ will have HZO
    - 50% of patients with HZO will have ocular involvement
- Elderly and immunocompromised patients are most commonly affected
- Incidence is less among blacks

PRESENTATION

Symptoms

- Prodromal period of influenza-like illness including fever, malaise, headache, ipsilateral lymphadenopathy, and eye pain prior to development of skin rash
- Acute, painful, vesicular rash erupts along distribution of dermatome associated with ophthalmic branch of trigeminal nerve
- Rash evolves through stages including erythematous lesions, macules, papules, vesicles, pustules, and crusts
- Pain, decreased vision, ocular irritation, photophobia, and epiphora are common

Exam Findings

- Ocular manifestations of HZO
  - Potential ocular manifestations of HZO are numerous and generally result of either direct viral invasion, secondary inflammation, vasculitis, neuritis, &/or fibrosis
  - **HZ keratopathy/keratitis**
    - Cornea is involved in ~ 65% of HZO cases
    - **Punctate epithelial keratitis (acute or chronic)**
      - Pseudodendrites are typically smaller and snake-like without terminal end-bulb formations (distinguishing feature from HSV)
      - Lesions stain mildly with fluorescein and variably with rose bengal dye
      - Debridement of these lesions causes less damage to epithelium
      - Chronic form is characterized by epithelial mucous plaques or delayed pseudodendrites that occur several months or years after cutaneous eruption
    - **Nummular (coin-shaped) anterior stromal infiltrates**
      - Superficial, granular anterior stromal opacities are at areas of prior acute epithelial keratitis
    - **Disciform keratitis**
      - Central, well-defined, disc-shaped area of diffuse stromal edema without vascularization
      - May develop weeks to months after original cutaneous eruption and often recurs
    - **Limbal vascular (fascicular) keratitis**
      - Vessels grow from limbus toward lipid infiltrates associated with episcleral or scleral inflammation
      - Immune-complex vasculitis leading to corneal edema, intense vascularization, and possible lipid deposition with subsequent scarring
    - **Serpiginous ulceration**
      - Large geographic ulcers cause entire epithelium to slough
      - Can mimic HSV infection with ulceration leading to corneal melting without secondary pannus or vascularization
    - **Neurotrophic keratitis**
      - HZO causes nerve damage, which leads to profoundly diminished corneal sensation and subsequent loss of corneal epithelial integrity and tear dysfunction
      - Characterized by inferior, horizontally oval, epithelial defect with rolled-under edges
      - Ulcers do not readily epithelialize and lead to corneal melting, descemetocele formation, and ultimately, corneal perforation
    - **Exposure keratopathy**
      - Similar to neurotrophic keratitis, except caused from HZO-induced cicatricial eyelid changes
      - Corneal desiccation
- Extraocular manifestations
  - Vesicular and erythematous involvement of CNV1 dermatome, ipsilateral forehead, and upper eyelid
  - Hutchinson sign (skin lesions of nose and a strong predictor of ocular inflammation and corneal denervation)
  - Retrobulbar neuritis, exophthalmos, lid retraction, ptosis, and extraocular muscle palsies
  - Orbital apex syndrome may occur related to vasculitis of orbital apex with involvement of CN3, CN4, or CN6

DIFFERENTIAL DIAGNOSIS

Exanthems

- Contact dermatitis
- Vaccinia dermatitis
- Eczema herpeticum
- Eczema vaccinatum
- Impetigo contagiosum
- Enterovirus-associated exanthema
- Drug eruptions/adverse reactions

Keratitis

- Mooren ulcer

HERPES ZOSTER VIRUS KERATITIS

- Corneal abrasion
- Vernal keratoconjunctivitis
- Keratoconjunctivitis sicca (dry eye syndrome)
- Sterile corneal foreign body
- Staphylococcal hypersensitivity
- Hypoxic or toxic corneal irritation

EVALUATION/WORK-UP

Labs
- Can be helpful with unusual presentations among HIV and immunocompromised patients
- Tzanck smear
- Direct fluorescent antibody (DFA) testing or PCR
  - Can differentiate between HSV and VZV infections
  - Must transport specimen to lab quickly and on ice (4°C)

Pathology
- Histopathology
  - Intraepidermal vesicle shows ballooning degeneration and acantholysis or keratinocytes
  - Multinucleated giant cells
  - Lymphocytic infiltrate throughout tissue
  - Underlying leukoclastic vasculitis may be prominent finding and differentiate zoster from other herpetic infections

TREATMENT

Medical
- Cutaneous manifestations of HZ is self-limiting and treatment with analgesics, cool compresses, and physical cleansing of skin is adequate
- Aggressive treatment and follow-up monitoring are required for HZO
- Topical anesthetics should never be prescribed because of corneal toxicity
- Antiviral medication
  - Acyclovir (800 mg, 5x daily) for 7-10 days or valacyclovir (1,000 mg, 3x daily) for 7-14 days or famciclovir (500 mg, 3x daily) for 7 days
    - May accelerate resolution of skin lesions, shorten duration of pain, reduce viral shedding, and decrease post-herpetic neuralgia (PHN) if administered within 72 hours of onset
    - May decrease incidence of dendritic and stromal keratitis and anterior uveitis
    - Intravenous acyclovir is recommended in immunocompromised patients
- Topical steroids for sclerokeratitis, keratouveitis, interstitial keratitis, anterior stromal infiltrates, and disciform keratitis
  - 1% prednisolone acetate eye drops every 3 hours for severe disease or q.i.d. for less severe cases and tapered slowly
- Neurotrophic keratitis is treated with preservative-free artificial tears, eye lubricants, punctal occlusion, pressure patching, or soft contact lenses
  - Steroids should be avoided because of risk of keratolysis (if there is corneal thinning, use medroxyprogesterone drops, and oral vitamin C + doxycycline)
- Topical cycloplegics to prevent ciliary spasm associated with HZO

Follow-Up
- Monitor every 1-7 days during acute episode
- Follow-up every 3-12 months after remission to monitor for delayed sequelae
- Viral prophylaxis may be considered if recurrence is suspected
  - Acyclovir (400 mg, 2x daily)

Prognosis
- Greatly variable depending on acute manifestations and long-term sequelae
- Uncomplicated rash typically resolves within 10-15 days
  - Complications include secondary bacterial infection, residual ptosis, lid scarring, deep scalp pitting, entropion, ectropion, loss of normal pigmentation, or lid necrosis
- Most common complication is post-herpetic neuralgia (PHN)
  - Neuropathic pain syndrome that persists after dermatomal rash has healed
  - PHN has variable course and can develop up to 1 year after acute episode has resolved
  - Many manifestations of neuropathic pain including allodynia, deep aching pain, sharp intermittent pain, or piercing pain
  - PHN requires diligent pain management with topical analgesics, opioids, tricyclic antidepressants, anti-seizure drugs, or combinations
- Common neurological complications of HZO include acute neuralgia and PHN

Prevention
- Zoster vaccine boosts CMI response to VZV and may be effective in preventing both HZ and PHN

SELECTED REFERENCES

1. Kaufman SC: Anterior segment complications of herpes zoster ophthalmicus. Ophthalmology. 115(2 Suppl):S24-32, 2008
2. Liesegang TJ: Herpes zoster ophthalmicus natural history, risk factors, clinical presentation, and morbidity. Ophthalmology. 115(2 Suppl):S3-12, 2008
3. Opstelten W et al: Treatment of herpes zoster. Can Fam Physician. 54(3):373-7, 2008
4. Weinberg JM: Herpes zoster: epidemiology, natural history, and common complications. J Am Acad Dermatol. 57(6 Suppl):S130-5, 2007

HERPES ZOSTER VIRUS KERATITIS

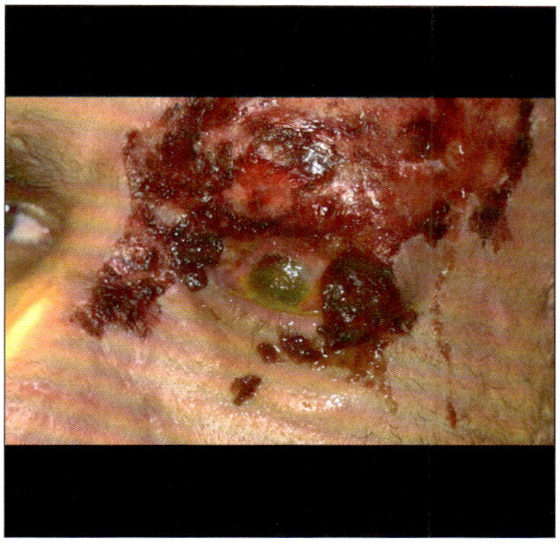

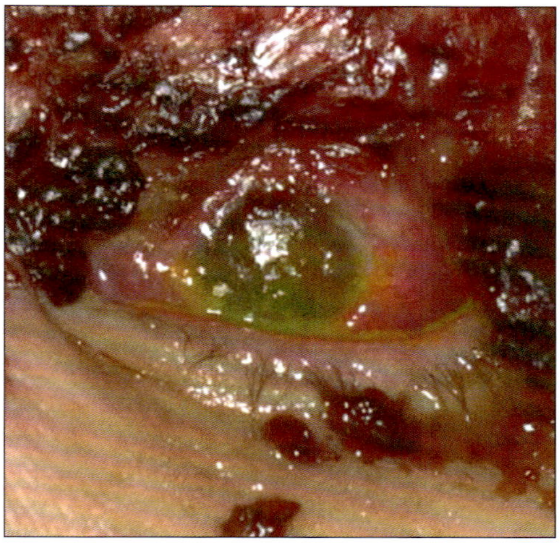

(Left) *This external photo of a patient with severe, ulcerative herpes zoster virus shows the rash in the typical dermatomal pattern. This patient presents with the rash in the CNV1 distribution. While the rash is typically more mild in nature, it can occasionally become ulcerative, as depicted here.* ***(Right)*** *This external photo shows a closer view of the eye of the same patient. Notice the damage and irregularity of the cornea and conjunctiva.*

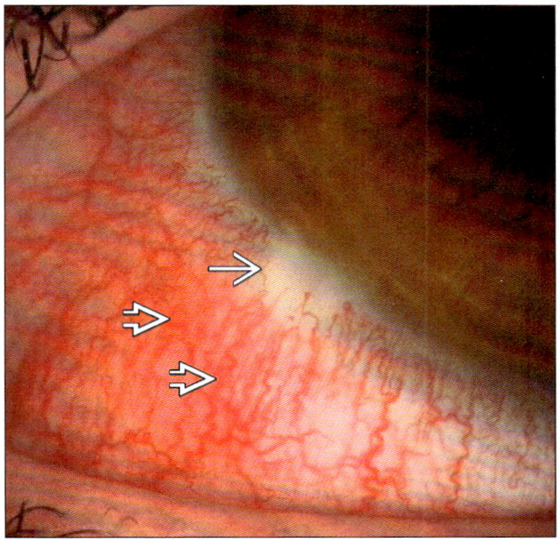

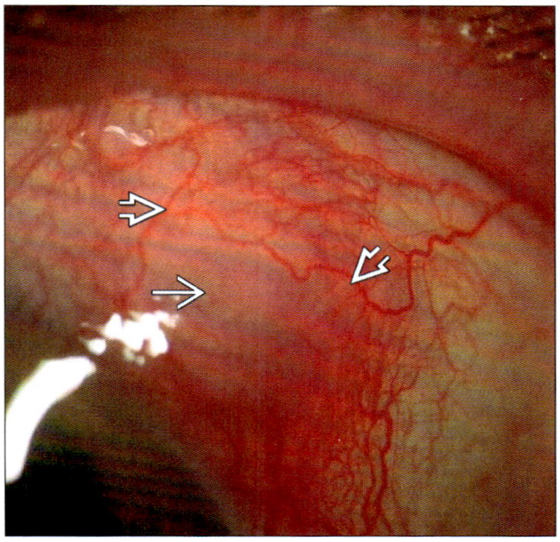

(Left) *This slit-lamp photo shows the eye of a patient with herpes zoster virus infection. Note the engorged, inflamed vessels* ➔ *and the inflammatory infiltrate present at the limbal margin* ➔. ***(Right)*** *This slit-lamp photo shows the eye of a patient with scleritis secondary to an herpes zoster virus infection. Note the inflamed vessels* ➔ *and deep purplish hue of the sclera* ➔.

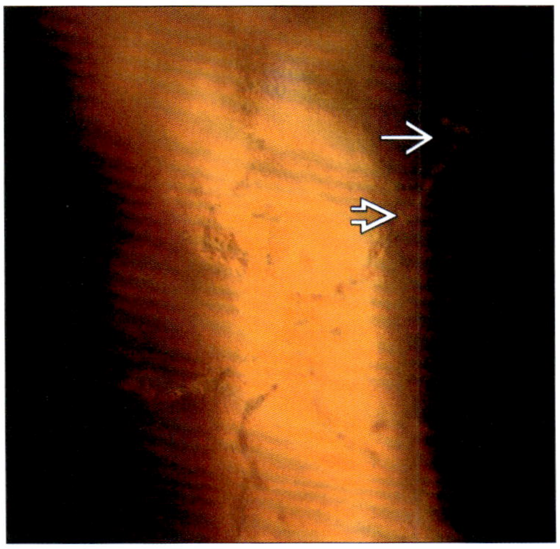

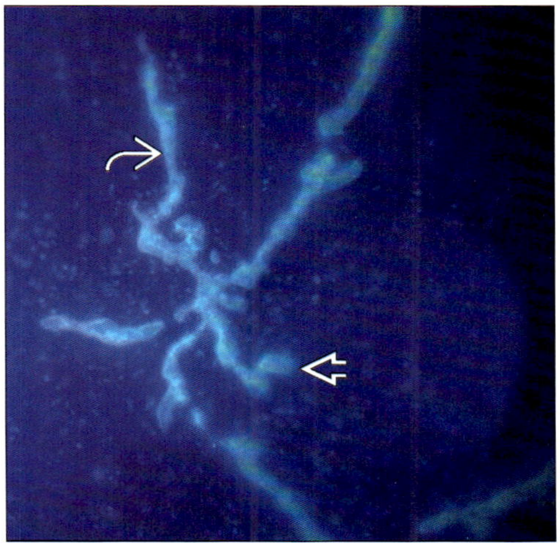

(Left) *This slit-lamp photo shows a lesion in a patient with herpes simplex virus keratitis. This lesion has the typical "dendrite" pattern with long branches* ➔ *and terminal bulbs* ➔. ***(Right)*** *This slit-lamp photo with fluorescein staining shows long branches* ➔ *and terminal bulbs* ➔ *in the dendrites of herpes simplex virus keratitis.*

HERPES SIMPLEX VIRUS KERATITIS

Key Facts

Introduction

- Corneal infection and inflammation caused by herpes simplex virus (HSV)

Presentation

- HSV epithelial keratitis
  - Characterized by corneal vesicles, dendritic lesions, and geographic ulcers
- Immune stromal keratitis (nonnecrotizing)
  - Focal or diffuse stromal inflammation; ghost-like superficial stromal opacities at sites of previous dendrites and ghost vessels in areas of previous stromal neovascularization
- Interstitial stromal keratitis (necrotizing)
  - Dense stromal cellular infiltrates with overlying stromal ulceration and necrosis; also keratic precipitates and anterior chamber inflammation
- Disciform endotheliitis
  - Circular areas of stromal edema with underlying endothelial keratic precipitates secondary to endothelial inflammation
- Neurotrophic keratopathy
  - Punctate epithelial erosions, ulcers, and impaired corneal sensation from nerve damage

Treatment

- HSV epithelial keratitis
  - Typical antivirals: Topical trifluorothymidine or ganciclovir; oral acyclovir, valacyclovir, or famciclovir
- Immune/interstitial stromal keratitis & disciform endotheliitis
  - Combination of topical corticosteroids and antivirals; long-term treatment with both to prevent recurrence
- Neurotrophic keratopathy
  - Manage with preservative-free lubricants, ointments, collagenase inhibitors, amniotic membrane graft, and bandage contact lenses

*(**Left**) HSV keratitis begins with granular punctate epithelial lesions that coalesce into single or multiple linear dendritic lesions with branching terminal bulbs ➡. Lesions typically follow the nerve pattern of the cornea. Formation of central epithelial defects leads to ulceration through the basement membrane. (Courtesy I. Porter, MD.) (**Right**) The ulcer bed stains with fluorescein ➡, but the corneal epithelium at the edges typically stains better with rose bengal. (Courtesy I. Porter, MD.)*

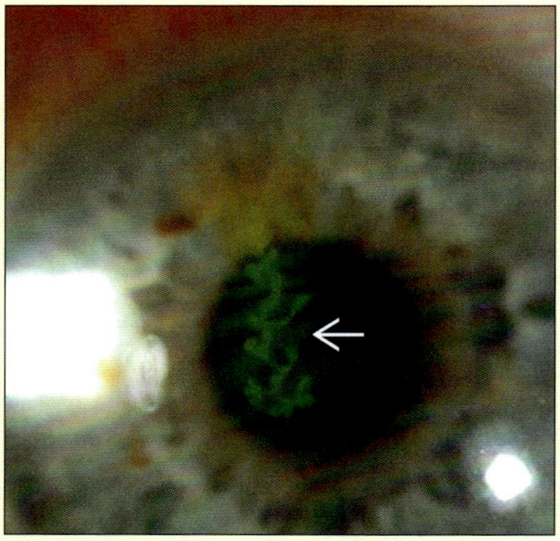

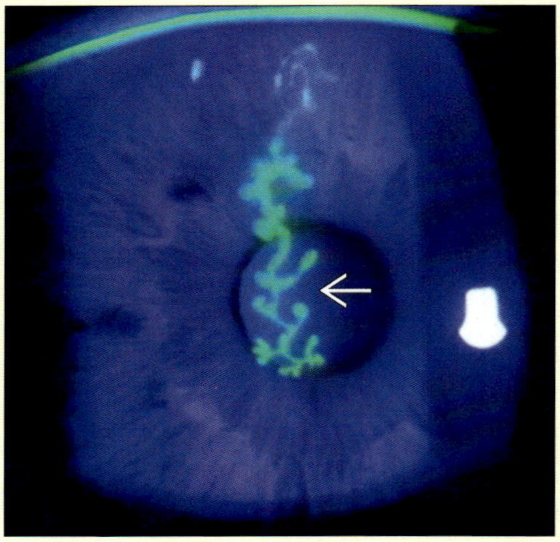

*(**Left**) If several dendrites coalesce, they form a wider, irregular geographic epithelial ulcer ➡ with scalloped edges. These ulcers are slow to heal and are more likely to lead to scarring. In contrast, neurotrophic ulcers tend to be roughly oval in shape and have smoother borders. (**Right**) Fluorescein staining under cobalt-blue filtered light allows for better visualization of the geographic ulcer bed ➡.*

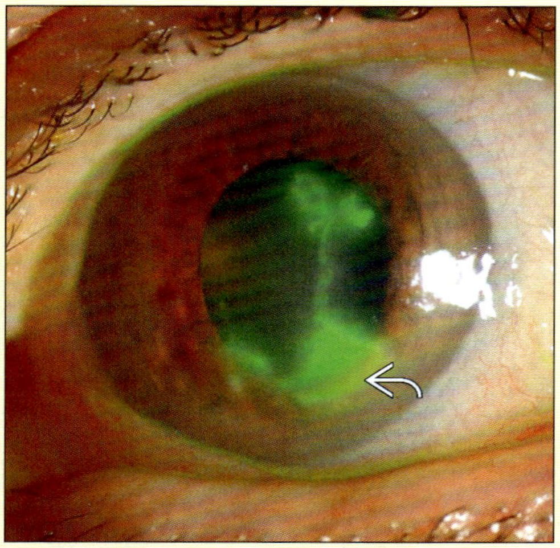

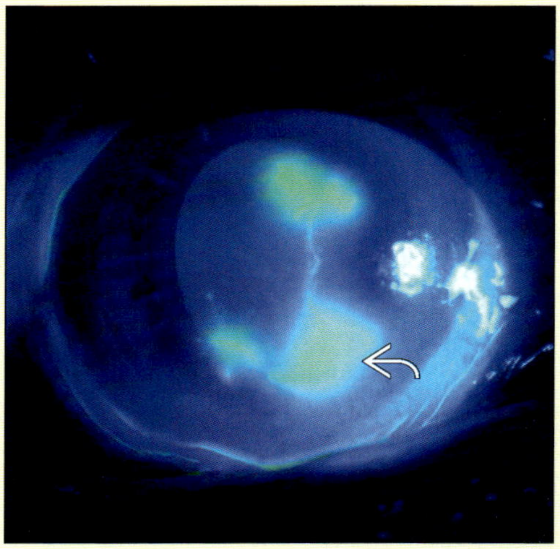

HERPES SIMPLEX VIRUS KERATITIS

INTRODUCTION

Definitions

- Corneal infection and inflammation caused by herpes simplex virus (HSV)

DEMOGRAPHICS

Etiology/Risk Factors

- HSV1: Causes ocular and oropharynx infections
- HSV2: Causes genital infections
- Primary HSV infection occurs from direct contact of skin or mucosal surfaces; ocular disease usually occurs from HSV recurrence after a latent phase rather than primary infection
  - HSV enters sensory neurons and remains latent in sensory ganglia; in ocular disease, HSV is latent in trigeminal ganglion
  - Virus does not replicate during latent phase
  - Latency is interrupted by triggers such as UV laser treatment, topical medications (e.g., epinephrine, β-blockers, prostaglandins), immunosuppression
  - Reactivated infectious viral particles travel to neuron endings and spread within corneal basal epithelial cells

Epidemiology

- HSV1 is endemic in human populations, with 90% having circulating antibodies against the virus
- Ocular involvement in < 5% of primary infections; most infections are from recurrent disease
- Ocular HSV tends to occur unilaterally, with most recurrences in same eye
- Prevalence in USA is ~ 150 per 100,000, with estimated 20,000 new cases, and 48,000 episodes annually
- Major cause of blindness from corneal scarring and opacity worldwide

PRESENTATION

Symptoms

- Acute onset pain, blurry vision, photophobia, redness, tearing

Exam Findings

- HSV epithelial keratitis
  - Most frequent type of ocular HSV infection
  - Characterized by dendritic lesions and geographic ulcers
    - Active viral infection begins with granular punctate epithelial lesions forming small, raised, clear vesicles
    - Single or multiple linear branching dendritic lesions are < 1 mm to several mm in length with branching terminal bulbs
    - Epithelial borders contain actively proliferating virus, and central epithelial defects ulcerate through basement membrane
    - Geographic ulcers are characterized by an irregular, nonlinear shape and scalloped borders; slow to heal and more likely to cause scarring
    - Active epithelial HSV lesions at limbus can lead to marginal keratitis with limbal dendrites and neovascularization of underlying stroma
- Immune stromal keratitis (nonnecrotizing)
  - 20-60% of chronic recurrent corneal HSV infections
  - Stromal disease may result from active viral infection or immune and inflammatory reaction to infection
    - Ghost-like superficial stromal opacities at sites of previous dendrites
    - Focal or diffuse stromal inflammation; may create ring- or coin-shaped infiltrates composed of viral antigens complexed with antibodies and complement
    - Stromal neovascularization may occur in long-term disease; blood vessels regress with treatment, leaving stromal scarring and nonperfused vascular channels called ghost vessels
    - Stromal thinning, fibrosis, pannus, and lipid deposits from stromal vessels
- Interstitial stromal keratitis (necrotizing)
  - Less common than immune stromal keratitis
    - Dense stromal cellular infiltrates with overlying stromal ulceration and necrosis
    - Corneal endothelial white cell deposits, keratic precipitates, and anterior chamber inflammation with possible hypopyon or hyphema
    - Viral replication in stromal keratocytes with severe inflammation can lead to corneal thinning and perforation
- Disciform endotheliitis
  - May be caused by immune reaction to viral antigens in corneal endothelial cells
    - Circular areas of stromal edema with underlying endothelial keratic precipitates secondary to endothelial inflammation; usually in central or paracentral cornea
    - Stromal edema overlying focal keratic precipitates is usually herpetic in origin
- Neurotrophic keratopathy
  - Occurs in patients with prior HSV epithelial infection
  - Caused by impaired corneal innervation and decreased tear formation
    - Punctate epithelial erosions create irregular corneal surface in early disease
    - Erosions can become persistent epithelial defects, leading to stromal ulceration, scarring, neovascularization, necrosis, corneal perforation, &/or secondary bacterial infection
    - Ulcers are oval in shape with smooth borders; often located in central or inferior paracentral cornea
    - Corneal hypesthesia or anesthesia occurs from corneal nerve damage

DIFFERENTIAL DIAGNOSIS

Corneal Abrasion

- Defect in epithelial surface of cornea secondary to mechanical trauma, foreign body, contact lens wear, or chemical or flash burns
- Signs: Epithelial defect with possible stromal involvement; roughened corneal light reflex in area of denuded epithelium; loose epithelium, stromal infiltrate; and anterior chamber reaction, if exam is done 12-24 hours after injury

HERPES SIMPLEX VIRUS KERATITIS

Recurrent Corneal Erosions
- Patients with history of previous corneal abrasions may experience spontaneous sloughing of new epithelium secondary to abnormal basement membrane attachments after healing; erosions occur without ocular trauma as inciting event

Herpes Zoster Ophthalmicus
- Caused by varicella zoster virus (VZV) reactivation in ophthalmic division of trigeminal nerve
- Signs: Painful, unilateral, facial skin rash with macules, papules, vesicles, pustules, and crusting lesions in ophthalmic dermatomal distribution of trigeminal nerve (i.e., involving eye and ocular adnexa)

Bacterial Keratitis
- Most common cause of infectious keratitis; occurs when bacteria invade a corneal epithelial defect
- Signs: Conjunctival injection, focal white infiltrates, corneal thinning, stromal edema, endothelial plaque, Descemet folds, mucopurulent discharge, anterior chamber reaction, and hypopyon

Fungal Keratitis
- Corneal disease caused by filamentous fungi or yeast infiltrating corneal stroma through epithelial defect
- Filamentous fungal keratitis shows dry or roughly textured, gray-white, elevated infiltrates; branching ulcers; feathery margins; &/or satellite lesions
- Signs: Severe conjunctival injection, suppuration, stromal infiltration, anterior chamber reaction, or hypopyon as infection progresses; ring infiltrate and endothelial plaque are indicative

Syphilitic Interstitial Keratitis
- Nonulcerative inflammation of corneal stroma secondary to syphilis infection
- Signs: Corneal neovascularization, stromal inflammation, anterior uveitis, dense stromal necrosis, scarring, ghost vessel formation

EVALUATION/WORK-UP

Labs
- Viral cultures: 70% sensitive when obtained within several days of disease onset; ELISA and PCR are alternatives
  - PCR: Detection of viral DNA in tear samples, corneal epithelium, or anterior chamber tap; does not distinguish between active or latent HSV infection since PCR is also positive with inactive virus

Pathology
- HSV keratitis is most often diagnosed based on characteristic clinical findings, but lab testing may be necessary in severe cases with atypical findings and high suspicion for HSV infection
  - Epithelial scrapings with Giemsa stain; may show multinucleated giant cells; negative cytology does not exclude HSV

TREATMENT

Medical
- HSV epithelial keratitis
  - Treatment based on whether disease is caused by active viral infection or as response to past infection
  - Topical glucocorticoids discouraged in active HSV infection since they worsen epithelial lesions
  - Topical &/or oral antiviral therapy is standard treatment for dendritic and geographic keratitis; most patients improve within 1-2 weeks using
    - Trifluorothymidine 1% eyedrops q.2 hours (9x/day) until epithelium closes; begin taper after 1st week
    - Topical ganciclovir 0.15% gel 5x daily until epithelial healing occurs, then t.i.d. for 1 week
    - Oral acyclovir 800 mg 5x daily; similar effectiveness to topical eyedrops and avoids corneal epithelial toxicity
    - Valacyclovir 1 g p.o. b.i.d. and famciclovir 500 mg p.o. t.i.d. are also effective
- Immune and interstitial stromal keratitis
  - Combination of topical corticosteroids and antivirals; long-term treatment with both to prevent recurrence
- Disciform endotheliitis
  - Combined topical glucocorticoids and prophylactic antivirals; long-term treatment with both to prevent recurrence
- Neurotrophic keratopathy
  - Manage with preservative-free lubricants, bandage contact lenses, and eyelid patching
  - Use vitamin C 1 g p.o. q.i.d.; medroxyprogesterone 1% drops q.i.d.; doxycycline 100 mg p.o. b.i.d. to prevent corneal melting

Surgical
- Nonhealing ulcers may require tarsorrhaphy
- Corneal transplantation if scarring significantly decreases vision or in cases of perforation
  - Transplants have high rejection rate due to corneal neovascularization and HSV keratitis recurrence; graft survival is improved with acyclovir prophylaxis

Prognosis
- Generally good but varies depending on disease severity and number of infection recurrences
- In patients with recurrent HSV keratitis, ongoing oral antivirals for at least 1 year are suggested for disease suppression
  - Valacyclovir 500 mg daily
  - Acyclovir 400 mg daily

SELECTED REFERENCES

1. Sugar A: Herpes simplex keratitis. In Trobe J et al: UpToDate. Waltham, 2013
2. Farooq AV et al: Herpes simplex epithelial and stromal keratitis: an epidemiologic update. Surv Ophthalmol. 57(5):448-62, 2012
3. Wilhelmus KR: Antiviral treatment and other therapeutic interventions for herpes simplex virus epithelial keratitis. Cochrane Database Syst Rev. (12):CD002898, 2010
4. Knickelbein JE et al: Management of herpes simplex virus stromal keratitis: an evidence-based review. Surv Ophthalmol. 54(2):226-34, 2009
5. Suzuki T et al: Corneal endotheliitis. Semin Ophthalmol. 23(4):235-40, 2008
6. Toma HS et al: Ocular HSV-1 latency, reactivation and recurrent disease. Semin Ophthalmol. 23(4):249-73, 2008
7. Bonini S et al: Neurotrophic keratitis. Eye (Lond). 17(8):989-95, 2003

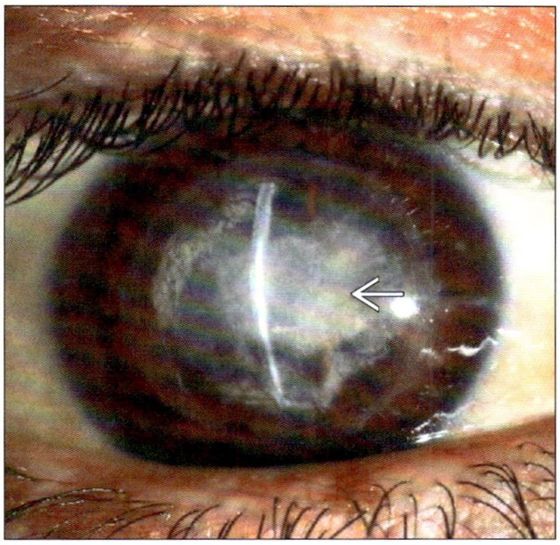

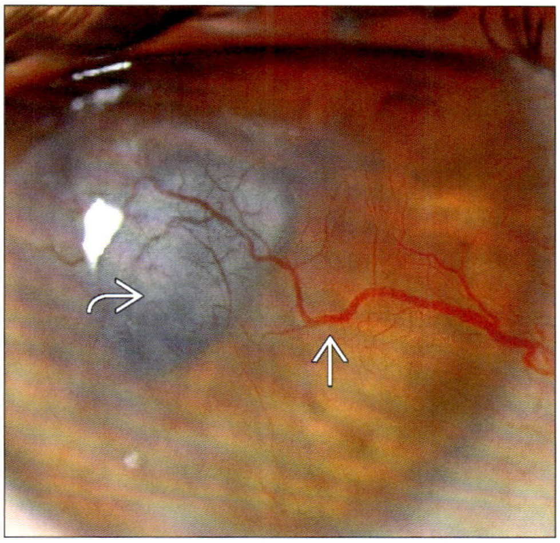

(Left) *Interstitial stromal keratitis leads to dense stromal cellular infiltrates with overlying stromal ulceration and necrosis ➡. Severe inflammation can lead to corneal thinning and perforation.* ***(Right)*** *Immune stromal keratitis leads to focal or diffuse stromal inflammation, neovascularization ➡, and fibrosis ➡. Blood vessels regress with treatment, leaving behind stromal scarring and nonperfused vascular channels called ghost vessels.*

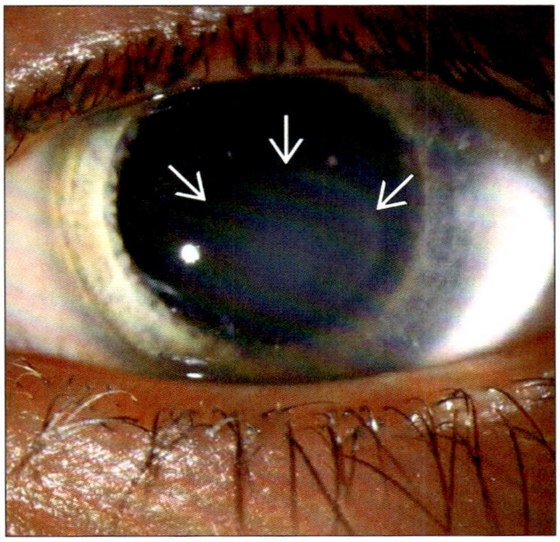

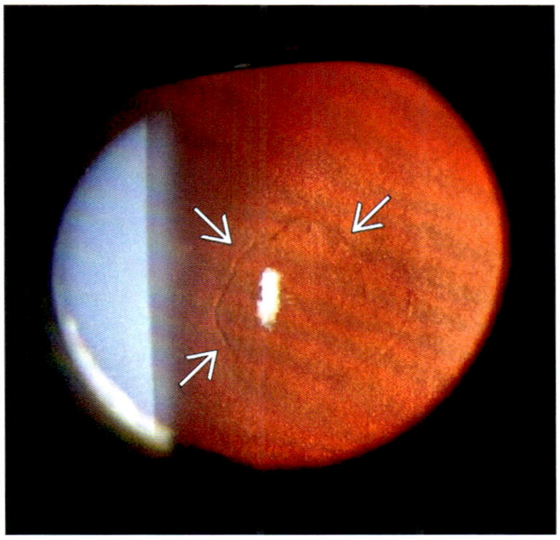

(Left) *Disciform endotheliitis presents with a well-demarcated, circular area of stromal edema ➡ in the central or paracentral cornea. In contrast, diffuse endotheliitis exhibits scattered keratic precipitates in a previous disciform area. Linear endotheliitis exhibits a line of keratic precipitates that progress from the limbus to the central cornea, with peripheral corneal edema behind the line of precipitates.* ***(Right)*** *Retroillumination allows for better visualization of stromal edema ➡.*

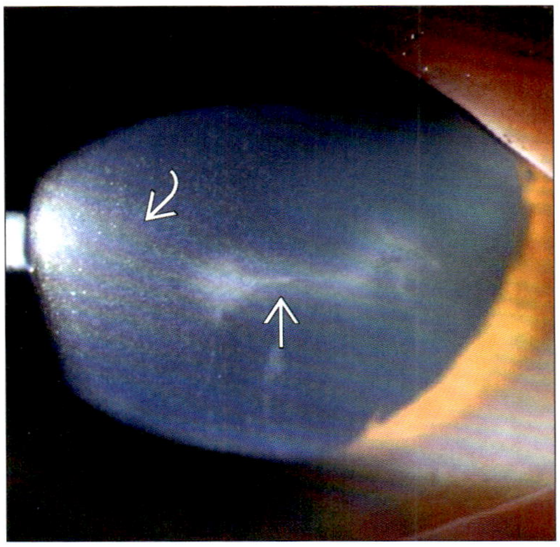

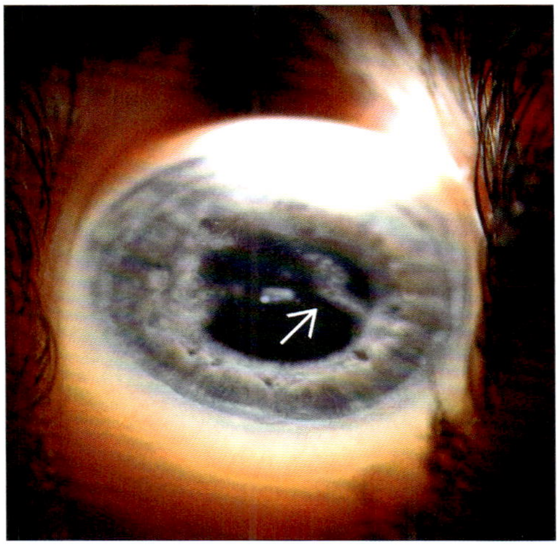

(Left) *Punctate epithelial erosions ➡ create an irregular corneal surface in early neurotrophic keratopathy. These erosions can become persistent epithelial defects ➡, leading to stromal ulceration and scarring. Neurotrophic ulcers typically occur in the central or inferior paracentral interpalpebral fissure zone.* ***(Right)*** *Following resolution of primary HSV infection, a ghost dendrite ➡ may be visualized beneath the area where epithelial ulceration occurred previously.*

Key Facts

Introduction
- Nonulcerative inflammatory reaction within corneal stroma that appears as white opacities in absence of endothelial or epithelial disease

Demographics
- Most cases in USA related to herpes simplex virus or syphilis, although interstitial keratitis (IK) has a wide range of etiologies
- Syphilitic IK: Generally caused by congenital syphilis
  - Manifests in childhood or teen years
- Acquired IK: Commonly between 3rd and 5th decades

Presentation
- Symptoms: Photophobia, pain, blepharospasm, ↓ visual acuity
- Signs: Corneal edema and neovascularization (salmon patch of Hutchinson), ghost vessels, stromal white cell infiltrate

Differential Diagnosis
- Infection: Viral, bacterial, parasitic
- Autoimmune
- Cogan syndrome

Evaluation/Work-Up
- Detailed history includes exposure history to insects/animals, travel history, risk of STDs, contact lens wear, and constitutional symptoms including hearing loss and shortness of breath

Treatment
- Inflammation: Treat with corticosteroids to prevent scarring
- Treat underlying etiology
- Wait until disease is quiescent to perform penetrating keratoplasty if transplant is necessary

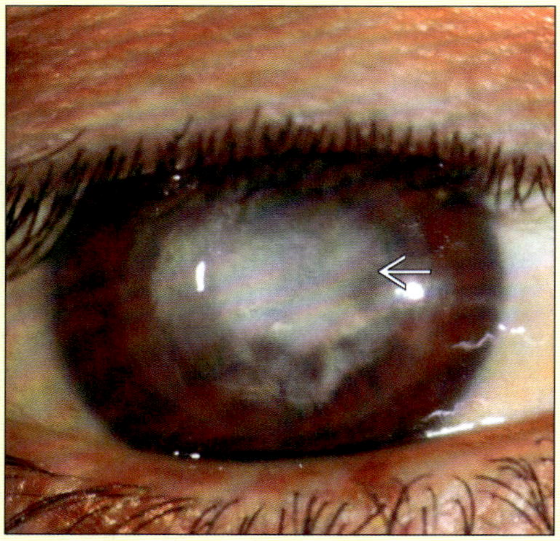
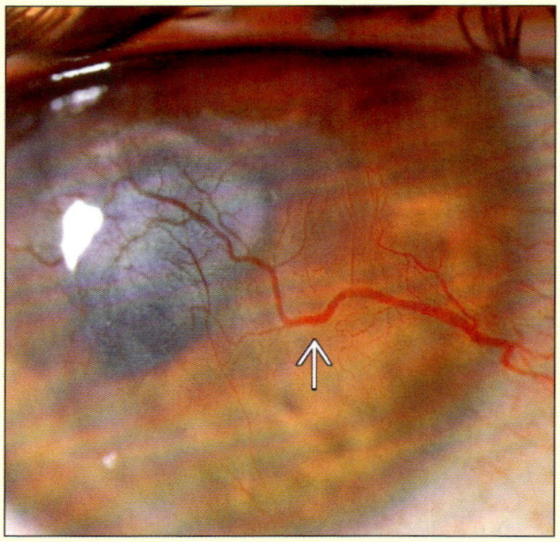

(Left) *Note the salmon patch ➔ in this external photograph. In interstitial keratitis secondary to syphilis, the salmon-patch appearance of the cornea is often one of the first findings.* ***(Right)*** *Corneal neovascularization ➔ is a common sign in patients presenting with interstitial keratitis secondary to Cogan syndrome.*

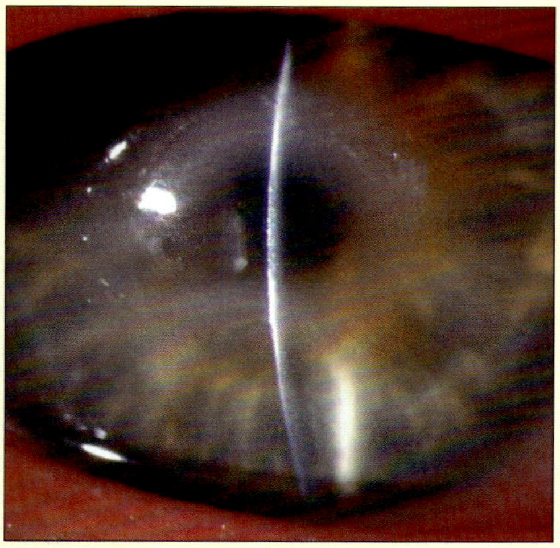
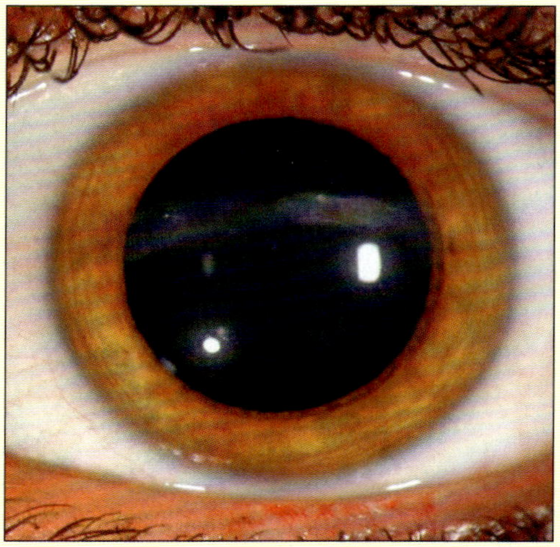

(Left) *This slit-lamp photograph demonstrates haziness from interstitial keratitis that has progressed centrally.* ***(Right)*** *This slit-lamp photograph demonstrates linear interstitial keratitis, which is often idiopathic and occurs in a horizontal linear pattern.*

INTERSTITIAL KERATITIS

INTRODUCTION

Abbreviations
- Interstitial keratitis (IK)

Definitions
- Nonulcerative inflammatory reaction of corneal stroma that appears as small, white, stromal opacities or as dense, white cellular infiltrate in absence of epithelial or endothelial disease

DEMOGRAPHICS

Etiology/Risk Factors
- Viral: HSV, HZV, EBV, human T-lymphotropic virus 1 (HLTV1), mumps, measles, vaccinia, variola
- Bacterial: Syphilis, Lyme disease, tuberculosis, leprosy, brucellosis, leptospirosis
- Parasitic: Acanthamoeba, onchocerciasis, leishmaniasis, trypanosomiasis, microsporidiosis
- Immune: Cogan syndrome, sarcoidosis, rheumatoid arthritis (RA), Wegener granulomatosis, polyarteritis nodosa
- Mycosis fungoides
- Risk factors vary according to etiology

Epidemiology
- Most common causes in USA: HSV and syphilis

PRESENTATION

Symptoms
- Photophobia, pain, blepharospasm, and sometimes visual acuity deficits

Exam Findings
- Corneal edema and white cell infiltrates without significant necrosis or suppuration
- Stromal neovascularization: Salmon patch of Hutchinson when cornea exhibits a pinkish color
- Ghost vessels: Regressed corneal vessels when disease is quiescent
- Lipid keratopathy
- May see associated anterior uveitis, scleritis, &/or retinal vasculitis
- Bilateral in 80-90% of cases

DIFFERENTIAL DIAGNOSIS

Infection
- Viral, bacterial, and parasitic etiologies

Autoimmune Disease
- RA, sarcoidosis, Wegener granulomatosis, polyarteritis nodosa

Cogan Syndrome
- Triad of nonsyphilitic IK, vestibuloauditory disease (e.g., tinnitus, vertigo, vomiting), and autoimmune disease

Episcleritis/Scleritis/Uveitis
- Inflammation within episcleral, scleral, and uveal tissues, respectively

EVALUATION/WORK-UP

Labs
- Syphilis serologies: RPR/VDRL and FTA-ABS, PPD, Lyme titers, HIV testing (if syphilis positive), CBC, ACE test
- Leukocytosis and ↑ ESR/CRP if Cogan syndrome suspect

Imaging
- CXR: Tuberculosis/sarcoidosis
- Consider MRI/audiology testing if patient is a Cogan syndrome suspect

Diagnostic Procedures
- Slit-lamp exam
- Dilated exam
- Corneal pachymetry and IOP
- Confocal microscopy may be helpful to distinguish fungal and acanthamoebal keratitis

TREATMENT

Medical
- Anterior ocular inflammation: Topical corticosteroids, mydriatics for comfort, topical or oral NSAIDs for evidence of episcleritis/scleritis
- Posterior ocular inflammation: Systemic corticosteroids
- Treatment regimen based on etiology
  - Syphilitic IK is same as that for neurosyphilis: Aqueous penicillin G followed by benzathine penicillin
  - Herpetic IK: Topical steroids combined with topical antiviral agents (trifluridine)

Surgical
- Can perform a penetrating keratoplasty (PKP) for corneal opacity once ocular inflammation has become quiescent

Follow-Up
- Reduce corticosteroids to lowest effective dosage based on resolving inflammation and regression of corneal neovascularization
- Monitor for side effects of corticosteroid therapy and systemic antibiotic therapy
- Routine follow-up for patients undergoing PKP to assess for graft rejection, neovascularization, wound healing, IOP, cataract formation, and secondary infection
- Consider infectious disease consultation for infectious IK and ENT for suspected cases of Cogan syndrome

Prognosis
- Visual acuity generally preserved with appropriate treatment in case of permanent corneal scarring
- Surgical treatment often successful if underlying cause of IK is controlled

SELECTED REFERENCES

1. Murphy G et al: Cogan's syndrome: present and future directions. Rheumatol Int. 29(10):1117-21, 2009
2. Knox CM et al: Interstitial keratitis. Int Ophthalmol Clin. 38(4):183-95, 1998
3. Schwartz GS et al: Etiology of immune stromal (interstitial) keratitis. Cornea. 17(3):278-81, 1998

PHLYCTENULOSIS

Key Facts

Introduction
- Phlyctenular keratoconjunctivitis (PKC)
- Nonspecific inflammatory type of microbiallergic conjunctivitis affecting the cornea and conjunctiva in pediatric populations

Demographics
- Most commonly associated with chronic staphylococcal blepharoconjunctivitis and tuberculosis

Presentation
- Small, slightly elevated, pale pink or yellow nodules surrounded by a hyperemic response in the peripheral cornea or conjunctiva near the limbus
- Lid disease such as chalazia or blepharitis

Differential Diagnosis
- Staphylococcal infection
- Mycobacterial infection (tuberculosis, avium complex, or leprosy)
- Treponemal infection (syphilis)
- Pingueculitis
- Sarcoid nodule
- Bacterial keratitis
- Herpes simplex viral infection

Evaluation/Work-Up
- Tuberculosis purified protein derivative (PPD) skin test and possible chest x-ray

Treatment
- Lid hygiene
- Successful treatment and resolution with oral antibiotics and topical steroids

*(**Left**) This is a slit-lamp photo of the eye of a patient with phlyctenulosis. Note the wedge-shaped superficial corneal neovascularization ➔. (**Right**) This slit-lamp photo is of the eye of a patient with phlyctenulosis. Note the corneal thickening at the site of corneal neovascularization ➔.*

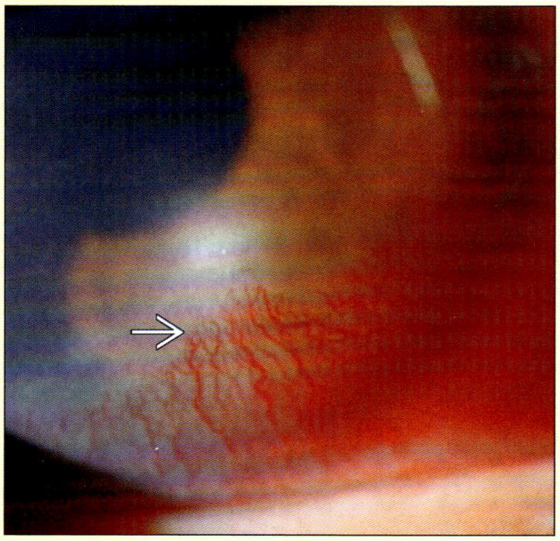

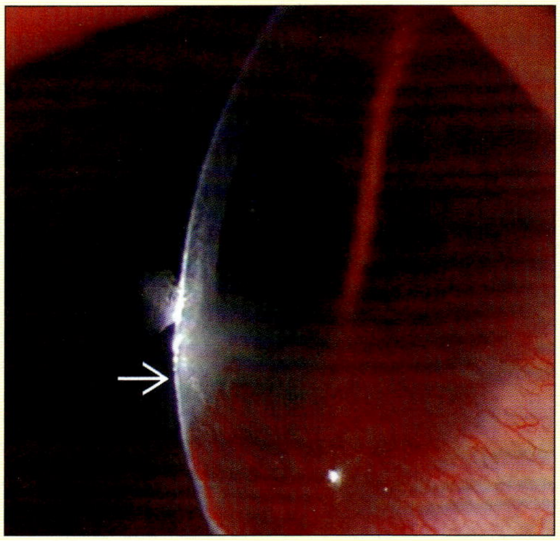

*(**Left**) This slit-lamp photo of a patient with phlyctenulosis demonstrates conjunctival injection associated with this condition. (**Right**) This slit-lamp photo is of the eye of a patient with a pinguecula ➔. An inflamed pinguecula is an important consideration in the differential diagnosis of phlyctenulosis. A pinguecula does not involve the cornea.*

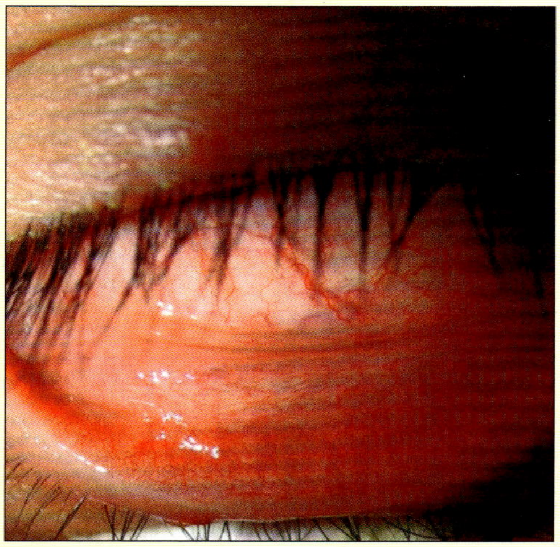

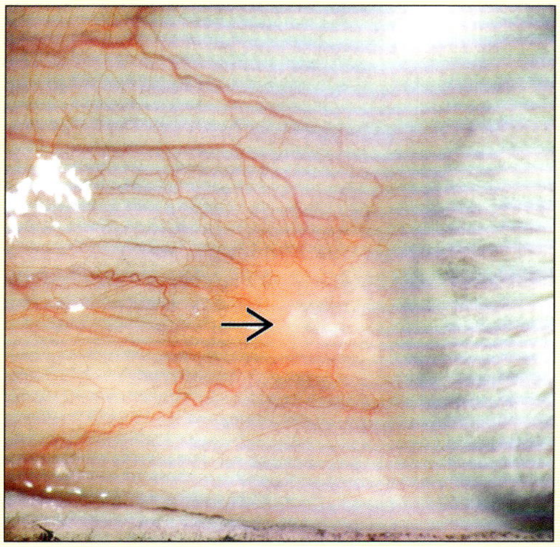

PHLYCTENULOSIS

INTRODUCTION

Synonyms
- Phlyctenular keratoconjunctivitis (PKC)
- Scrofulous ophthalmia

Definitions
- Nonspecific inflammatory type of microbiallergic conjunctivitis affecting the cornea and conjunctiva in pediatric populations
- Type IV delayed hypersensitivity response to bacterial, fungal, or parasitic antigens

DEMOGRAPHICS

Etiology/Risk Factors
- Most commonly associated with chronic staphylococcal blepharoconjunctivitis and tuberculosis

Epidemiology
- Most frequently occurs in children and young adults

PRESENTATION

Symptoms
- Ocular irritation, red eye, tearing
- Blepharospasm
- Mild to severe photophobia
- Often a history of similar episodes

Exam Findings
- Small, slightly elevated, pale pink or yellow nodules surrounded by a hyperemic response in the peripheral cornea or conjunctiva near the limbus
  - Focal injection of conjunctiva
- Corneal infiltrates, possibly corneal scarring
  - Progression of the ulcer from the periphery toward the center of the cornea
  - Absence of keratic precipitates or anterior chamber reaction
- Lid disease such as chalazia or blepharitis
- If related to staphylococcal infection, may be rope-like mucopurulent discharge
- Demarcating margin

DIFFERENTIAL DIAGNOSIS

Infectious Disease Etiologies
- Staphylococcal infection
- Mycobacterial infection (tuberculosis, avium complex, or leprosy)
- Treponemal infection (syphilis)

Pingueculitis
- Pinguecula may become acutely irritated, hyperemic, and vascularized
- No corneal involvement

Sarcoid Nodule
- Histopathology shows noncaseating epithelioid granulomas with giant cells

Bacterial Keratitis
- Often teenagers with contact lens wear

Trachomatous Pannus
- More often seen superiorly
- Herbert pits (small gaps in a pannus from resolved limbal follicles)

Microbial Ulcer
- Lack of demarcating margin
- More central corneal position
- Typically greater degree of pain
- May be associated with iritis &/or hypopyon
- Conjunctiva has a generalized pattern of injection

Herpes Simplex Virus
- Shows dendrites or geographic epithelial ulcer
- Foreign body sensation

Keratoconus
- Teenager with irregular astigmatism

Nodular Episcleritis
- No ulceration
- Time course is typically longer (2-3 weeks)

EVALUATION/WORK-UP

Labs
- Tuberculosis purified protein derivative (PPD) skin test and possible chest x-ray
- Consider conjunctival culture for bacteria, virus, or fungus

Pathology
- Exact mechanism is unknown
- Histology shows lymphocytes, histocytes, and plasma cells

TREATMENT

Medical
- Lid hygiene
- Systemic antibiotics for nontuberculous phlyctenulosis
  - Oral tetracycline (250 mg, 2-3x daily until the resolution of symptoms for 3 weeks)
- Short course of topical antibiotic-corticosteroid combination ointment or drops

Follow-Up
- Weekly until signs and symptoms resolve

Prognosis
- Successful treatment and resolution with oral antibiotics and topical steroids
- May recur, requiring more prolonged prophylactic oral antibiotic therapy for any associated blepharitis

SELECTED REFERENCES

1. Zaidman GW: The pediatric corneal infiltrate. Curr Opin Ophthalmol. 22(4):261-6, 2011
2. Farpour B et al: Diagnosis and management of chronic blepharokeratoconjunctivitis in children. J Pediatr Ophthalmol Strabismus. 38(4):207-12, 2001
3. Rohatgi J et al: Phlyctenular eye disease: a reappraisal. Jpn J Ophthalmol. 44(2):146-50, 2000

STAPHYLOCOCCAL HYPERSENSITIVITY

Key Facts

Introduction
- Type 2 hypersensitivity reaction to host's antibodies to staphylococcal antigens
- Also called staph marginal ulcer and staphylococcal keratitis
- Associated with anterior blepharitis and ocular rosacea

Presentation
- Red eye
- Photophobia
- Foreign body sensation
- Conjunctival injection
- Subepithelial corneal infiltrates
- Infiltrates may progress and develop shallow ulceration
- Rarely develop anterior chamber inflammation
- Anterior blepharitis

Evaluation/Work-Up
- If there is concern for bacterial keratitis, consider ulcer scraping and sending for cultures
- Slit-lamp exam with fluorescein stain

Treatment
- Treat blepharitis
  - Lid hygiene
  - Warm compresses
  - Lid scrubs
  - Lid massage
  - Erythromycin ointment
- Treat inflammation if hypersensitivity reaction does not improve with treatment of blepharitis
  - Low-dose topical steroid such as loteprednol 0.2-0.5% or prednisolone 0.25%

*(**Left**) This external photograph shows an eye with staphylococcal hypersensitivity. Typical findings for staphylococcal hypersensitivity reactions include conjunctival injection, worse in a defined sector →, and mild corneal haziness →. (**Right**) This slit-lamp photograph shows an eye with a staphylococcal hypersensitivity reaction. Note the presence of inferior punctate epithelial defects → and a mild area of corneal haziness →.*

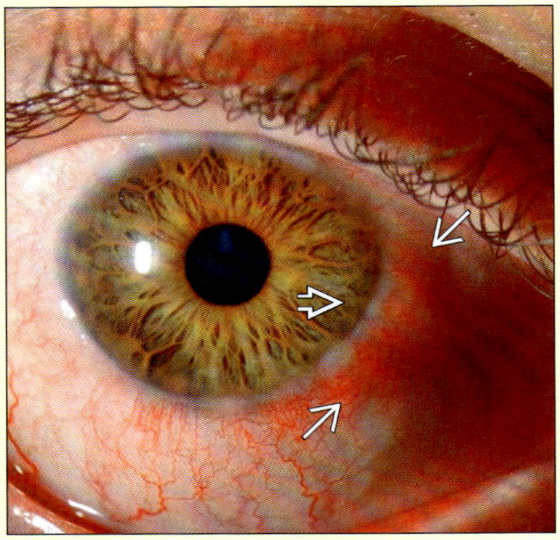

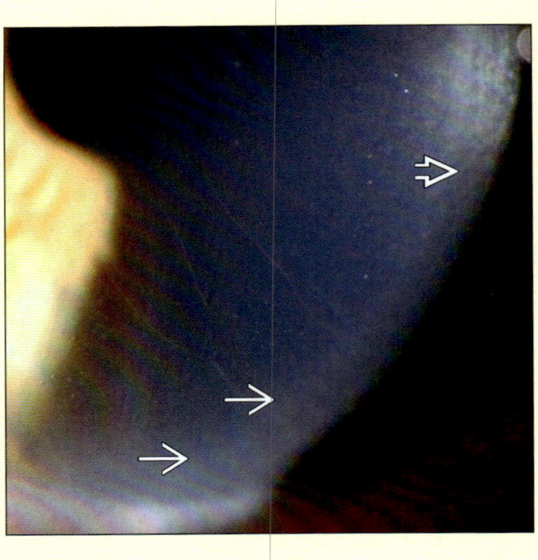

*(**Left**) This external photograph shows anterior blepharitis →, likely caused by Staphylococcus. This condition can lead to staphylococcal hypersensitivity. The infiltrates seen in staphylococcal hypersensitivity are an autoimmune reaction that occurs secondary to the blepharitis. (**Right**) This external photograph shows an eye with a bacterial corneal ulcer →. Bacterial keratitis is an important differential for a staphylococcal hypersensitivity and is associated with a more obvious ulcer and staining.*

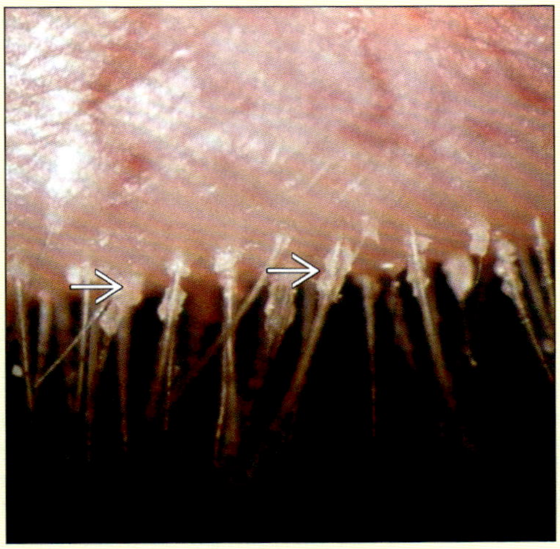

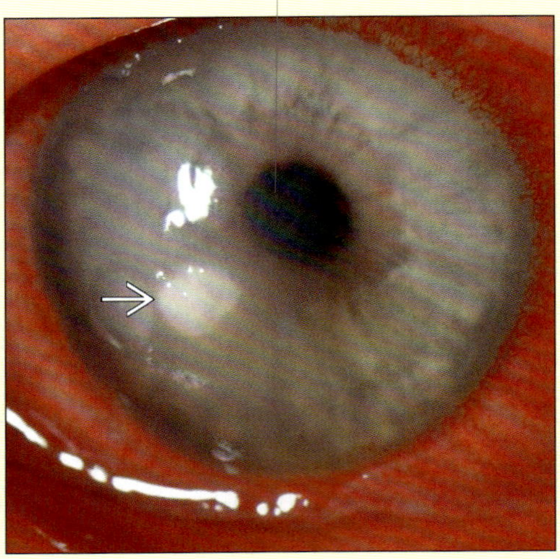

STAPHYLOCOCCAL HYPERSENSITIVITY

INTRODUCTION

Synonyms
- Staph marginal ulcer
- Staphylococcal hypersensitivity keratitis

Definitions
- Inflammation and infiltration of cornea caused by a type 2 hypersensitivity reaction
- Type 2 hypersensitivity reactions are antibody-mediated formation of membrane attack complexes
  - These cause cell lysis and destruction, leading to local inflammation

DEMOGRAPHICS

Etiology/Risk Factors
- Type II hypersensitivity reaction to host's antibodies to staphylococcal antigens
- Associated with anterior blepharitis
  - Anterior blepharitis specifically refers to inflammation of epidermis surrounding eyelashes and their follicles
  - Most anterior blepharitis is caused by *Staphylococcus*
- Associated with ocular rosacea

PRESENTATION

Symptoms
- Red eye
- Photophobia
- Dry eye
- Foreign body sensation
- Corneal hazing
- Patients also report symptoms of blepharitis, which include the above symptoms and
  - Burning
  - Tearing/Watering
  - Crusting
  - Pain
  - Decreased Vision

Exam Findings
- Conjunctival injection
  - Typically localized to the sites of hypersensitivity and corneal involvement
- Subepithelial corneal infiltrates
  - Classically have clear area between infiltrate and limbus
- Infiltrates may progress and develop shallow ulceration
  - This is termed staph marginal ulceration
  - These shallow ulcerations can also present as punctate epithelial defects
- Rarely develop anterior chamber inflammation
  - Typically very mild if present
- Anterior blepharitis
  - Lash crusting
- Phlyctenules can be present and may be from *Staphylococcus* but should prompt consideration of TB or other granulomatous conditions as well

DIFFERENTIAL DIAGNOSIS

Bacterial Keratitis
- Typically more painful
- Ulcer is typically more defined and deeper
- Often associated with more significant conjunctival and anterior chamber inflammation

Terrien Marginal Degeneration
- Slowly progressive, idiopathic disorder
- Causes peripheral corneal thinning
- Associated with lipid deposition and vascularization
- Typically starts at superonasal quadrant as fine, yellow-white punctate stromal opacities that can spread circumferentially around cornea

EVALUATION/WORK-UP

Labs
- If there is concern for bacterial keratitis, consider ulcer scraping and sending for cultures

Work-Up
- Intraocular pressure check
- Slit-lamp examination with fluorescein stain to detect ulcerations or punctate epithelial defects if present

TREATMENT

Medical
- Treat blepharitis
  - Lid hygiene
    - Warm compresses multiple times throughout the day
    - Lid scrubs to help with blepharitis and crusting
    - Lid massage
  - Antibiotics
    - Erythromycin ointment
    - Consider addition of fluoroquinolone antibiotic if not responsive
    - Consider addition of oral antibiotic such as doxycycline or minocycline
- Treat inflammation if hypersensitivity reaction does not improve with treatment of blepharitis
  - Low-dose topical steroid such as loteprednol 0.2-0.5%, prednisolone 0.25%
    - Slow taper prior to cessation

Follow-Up
- Within 1 week, at which time the addition of other antibiotics/steroids are considered

Prognosis
- Reaction responds well to medical treatment and with treatment prognosis is full resolution
- In rare cases, without treatment, corneal scarring can occur, which can lead to decreased vision

SELECTED REFERENCES

1. Mondino BJ: Inflammatory diseases of the peripheral cornea. Ophthalmology. 95(4):463-72, 1988
2. Chignell AH et al: Marginal ulceration of the cornea. Br J Ophthalmol. 54(7):433-40, 1970

CONTACT LENS-RELATED INFLAMMATION

Key Facts

Introduction

- Ocular inflammation, hypoxia, &/or neovascularization secondary to contact lens wear

Demographics

- Giant papillary conjunctivitis (GPC): Inflammatory hypertrophy of upper eyelid conjunctiva
  - Secondary to chronic mechanical trauma from foreign body
  - Secondary to delayed hypersensitivity reaction against debris and mucus on contact lens surface
- Corneal hypoxia: Decreased corneal oxygen diffusion secondary to contact lens acting as barrier; chronic limbal trauma causes neovascularization into peripheral cornea (micropannus)

Presentation

- GPC: Hypertrophic papillae surrounded by thickened superior tarsal conjunctiva and prominent vessels
- Corneal hypoxia: Conjunctival hyperemia, micropannus, fine punctate epitheliopathy over corneal surface

Treatment

- GPC: Total discontinuation of contact lens wear for a few weeks should eliminate symptoms and then limited wear can be reintroduced
  - If patient wishes to continue lens wear, management should focus on decreasing length of time lenses are worn, type of lenses, and lens care regimen
- Corneal hypoxia: Resolves with discontinuation of lens wear; reducing contact lens wear time and using soft lenses with higher oxygen permeability decreases progression of neovascularization and microcysts
  - < 2 mm of vessel growth into cornea is tolerable; > 2 mm of growth merits discontinuation of contact lens wear

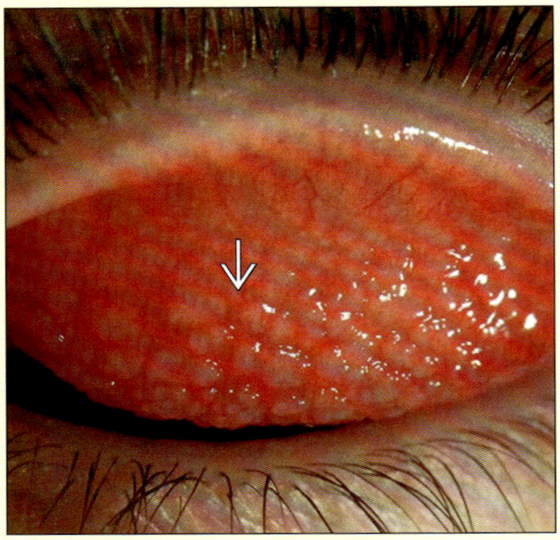
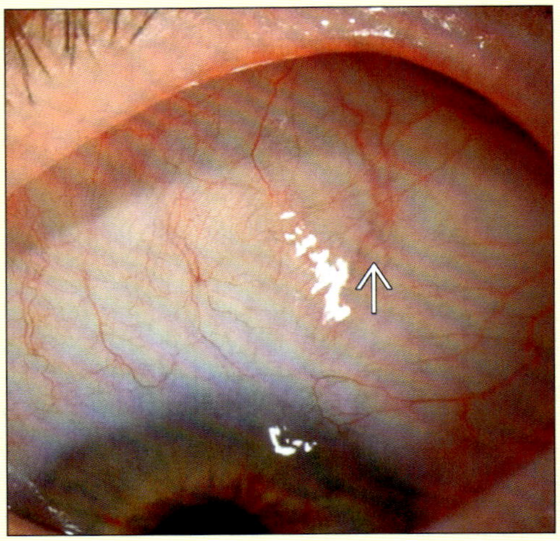

(Left) *GPC occurs from mechanical irritation of the tarsal conjunctiva by contact lens wear and inflammatory reaction to antigens on the lens surface. Hypertrophic papillae ⮕ develop in response to debris coating the lens, leading to a cycle of inflammation and further formation of lens deposits. (Courtesy J. B. Baldwin, OD, PhD.)* ***(Right)*** *CL-SLK occurs from inflammation of superior bulbar conjunctiva and limbus ⮕, epithelial keratitis, and papillary hypertrophy of the upper tarsal conjunctiva.*

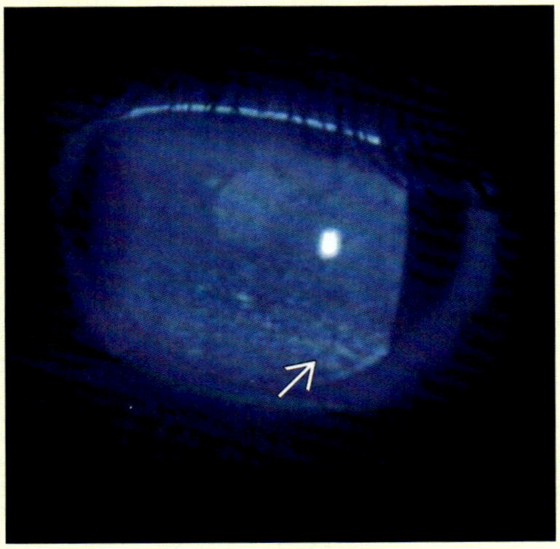
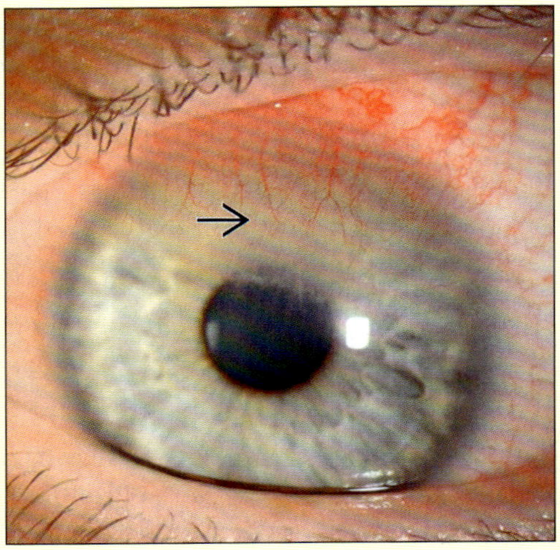

(Left) *Punctate epitheliopathy is visualized with fluorescein dye ⮕ and occurs when contact lens overwear damages the corneal surface. Central staining occurs when a lens is flat compared to the cornea. Peripheral staining occurs when a lens is too steep for the cornea. Staining in the interpalpebral fissure zone occurs from dryness due to lid elevation by the lens.* ***(Right)*** *Prolonged contact lens-associated inflammation can lead to hypoxia and the formation of fibrovascular corneal pannus ⮕.*

CONTACT LENS-RELATED INFLAMMATION

INTRODUCTION

Definitions

- Ocular inflammation, hypoxia, &/or neovascularization secondary to contact lens wear

DEMOGRAPHICS

Etiology/Risk Factors

- Giant papillary conjunctivitis (GPC): Inflammatory hypertrophy of upper eyelid conjunctiva
  - Secondary to chronic mechanical trauma from foreign body (e.g., soft contact lenses, gas-permeable contact lenses, ocular prosthesis, sutures, filtering blebs)
  - Secondary to delayed hypersensitivity reaction against cellular and protein debris and mucus on the contact lens surface
  - Risk factors: Large amount of lens deposits, large-sized lenses, prolonged or overnight contact lens wear
- Corneal hypoxia: Decreased corneal oxygen diffusion secondary to contact lens acting as barrier
  - Can cause epithelial cell death
  - Chronic limbal trauma causes angiogenic molecule release (e.g., VEGF), which causes neovascularization into peripheral cornea (micropannus)
  - Risk factors: Prolonged or overnight contact lens wear

Epidemiology

- GPC and corneal hypoxia with micropannus are more common in soft contact lens wearers; less frequent in hard or rigid gas-permeable lens wearers

PRESENTATION

Symptoms

- GPC: Redness, itching, foreign body sensation, mucous discharge
- Corneal hypoxia: Mild discomfort and inflammation can progress to blurry vision, pain, conjunctival injection, photophobia

Exam Findings

- GPC
  - Hypertrophic papillae surrounded by thickened superior tarsal conjunctiva and prominent vessels
  - Increased mucus production and mucus coating on contact lens surface
  - Excessive contact lens movement with blinking
- Corneal hypoxia
  - Conjunctival hyperemia, micropannus, and fine punctate epitheliopathy over corneal surface
  - Soft lenses frequently produce superficial corneal neovascularization near superior limbus due to chronic hypoxia
    - Chronic hypoxia also decreases corneal sensation
  - Patients sleeping in extended wear soft lenses may develop transparent epithelial inclusions (microcysts) and subepithelial infiltrates
  - Due to altered corneal physiology, contact lens wearers have thinner epithelial layer with larger superficial epithelial cells

DIFFERENTIAL DIAGNOSIS

Allergic Conjunctivitis

- Bulbar &/or palpebral conjunctival inflammation due to reaction against pollen, dander, mold, or other allergy-causing substances

Bacterial Conjunctivitis

- Bulbar &/or palpebral conjunctival inflammation caused by *Staphylococci*, *Streptococci*, *Chlamydia*, and *Gonococci*

Viral Conjunctivitis

- Bulbar &/or palpebral conjunctival inflammation caused by adenoviruses, picornaviruses, HSV, VZV, etc.

Superior Limbic Keratoconjunctivitis (SLK)

- Immunologic reaction in peripheral conjunctiva caused by contact lens wear (CL-SLK); similar to Theodore superior limbic keratoconjunctivitis

TREATMENT

Medical

- GPC: Focus treatment on reducing contact between conjunctiva and protein deposits on contact lens surface
  - Papillae remain long after symptoms disappear and can take many months to resolve
  - Total discontinuation of contact lens wear for few weeks should eliminate symptoms and then limited wear can be reintroduced
  - If patient wishes to continue lens wear, management should focus on decreasing length of time lenses are worn, type of lenses, and lens care regimen
    - Rigid gas-permeable lenses have surface that resists protein deposit formation; smaller size also decreases contact with conjunctiva
    - Disposable soft contact lenses avoid build-up of protein deposits since they are replaced frequently
    - Disinfection with hydrogen peroxide, preservative-free solution, and frequent enzymatic cleaning (1-2 times weekly) effectively removes protein
  - Short course of topical corticosteroids will initially reduce symptoms, but long-term use is discouraged due to complication risks
  - Overnight contact lens wear strongly discouraged to relieve GPC symptoms and reduce bacterial keratitis risk
  - Topical olopatadine drops can be useful
- Corneal hypoxia: Resolves with discontinuation of lens wear; reducing contact lens wear time and using soft lenses with higher oxygen permeability decreases progression of neovascularization and microcysts
  - < 2 mm of vessel growth into cornea is tolerable; > 2 mm of growth merits discontinuation of contact lens wear

SELECTED REFERENCES

1. Donshik PC et al: Giant papillary conjunctivitis. Immunol Allergy Clin North Am. 28(1):83-103, vi, 2008
2. Dillehay SM: Does the level of available oxygen impact comfort in contact lens wear?: A review of the literature. Eye Contact Lens. 33(3):148-55, 2007

PERIPHERAL ULCERATIVE KERATITIS

Key Facts

Introduction
- Crescent-shaped peripheral corneal ulcer within 2 mm of limbus
- Peripheral cornea adjacent to vasculature, giving access to inflammatory cell infiltration
- Cornea stromal thinning can lead to perforation and permanent loss of vision

Demographics
- Associated with systemic inflammatory (autoimmune) conditions
- Rheumatoid arthritis present in 34-42% of peripheral ulcerative keratitis

Presentation
- Eye pain
- Redness
- Tearing
- Photophobia
- Decreased vision

Evaluation/Work-Up
- History and labs for systemic inflammatory disease
- Cultures for bacteria, viruses, and fungi

Treatment
- Minimize inflammation with glucocorticoids + cyclophosphamide
- Infliximab for cases refractory to conventional immunomodulatory treatment
- Prophylaxis for infection
- Alternative immunosuppressants: Tacrolimus, mycophenolate, azathioprine
- Vitamin C, doxycycline, medroxyprogesterone acetate help thwart collagenase and used to slow corneal melting
- Surgery to prevent corneal perforation by corneal or scleral graft

(Left) *This slit-lamp photograph shows an eye with bilateral peripheral ulcerative keratitis (PUK). Note the crescent-shaped ulceration present in the periphery of the cornea →. PUK is often associated with systemic autoimmune disease.* ***(Right)*** *This slit-lamp photograph depicts an eye with PUK. The area of thinning is most obvious when illuminated by the slit-lamp beam ⇨. Also note the associated vessel engorgement →, a finding seen in PUK.*

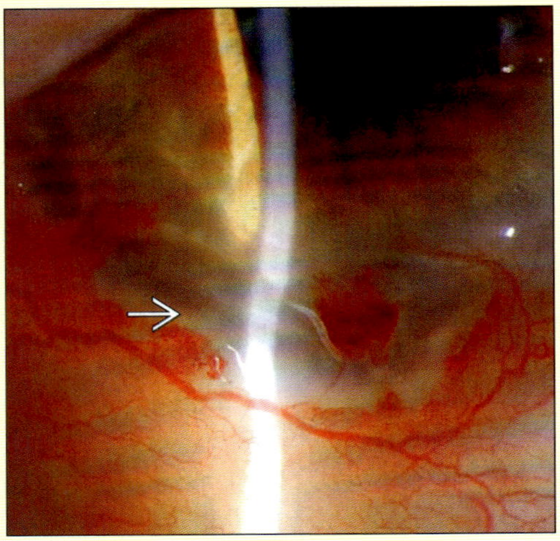

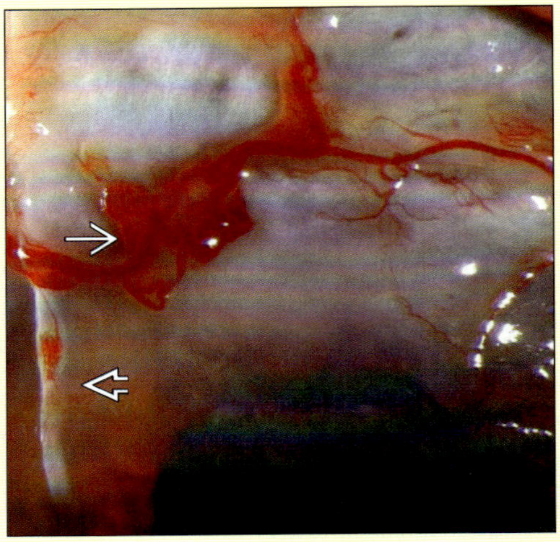

(Left) *This slit-lamp photograph of a patient with PUK shows findings of intraocular inflammation, including anterior chamber pigment → and pigment adhered to the corneal endothelium ⇨. PUK may be associated with intraocular inflammation.* ***(Right)*** *This external photo provides an example of Terrien marginal degeneration with circumferential peripheral corneal thinning ⇨. Terrien marginal degeneration is a slowly progressive, idiopathic disorder that causes peripheral corneal thinning.*

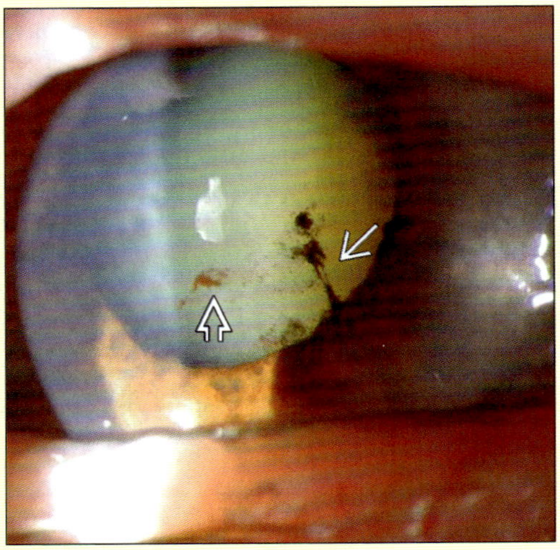

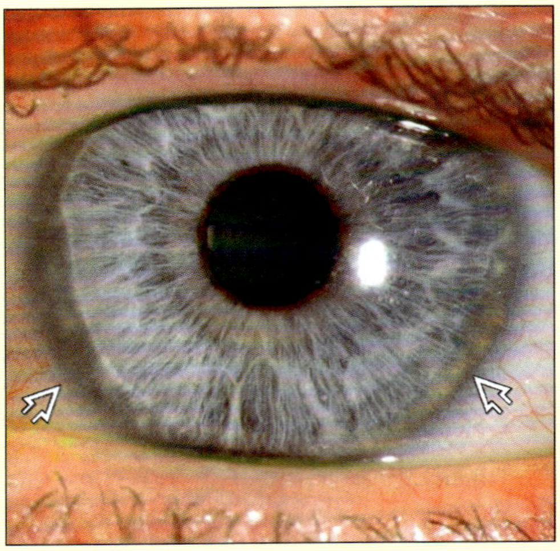

PERIPHERAL ULCERATIVE KERATITIS

INTRODUCTION

Abbreviations
- Peripheral ulcerative keratitis (PUK)

Definitions
- Ocular inflammatory disease resulting in peripheral corneal thinning
- Most severe disease sequelae is corneal melt syndrome (corneal perforation), leading to abrupt and permanent vision loss

Subtypes
- Mooren ulcer
  - Extreme eye pain, no associated scleral involvement or systemic findings

DEMOGRAPHICS

Etiology/Risk Factors
- Associated with systemic inflammatory conditions (RA most common followed by Wegener granulomatosis)
- Ocular and systemic infections
  - Bacteria (*Staphylococcus* and *Streptococcus*), spirochetes (*Treponema pallidum*), mycobacteria (TB), viruses (hepatitis C, herpes simplex, varicella zoster), acanthamoeba, fungi

Epidemiology
- 3:1,000,000/year with no gender predilection
- Bilateral in 40% of cases

PRESENTATION

Symptoms
- Eye pain, redness, tearing, photophobia, decreased vision

Exam Findings
- Crescent-shaped peripheral corneal ulcer with stromal thinning
- Presence of inflammatory cells within the stroma, conjunctiva, and sclera (unlike Terrien marginal degeneration)

DIFFERENTIAL DIAGNOSIS

Systemic Disease
- Autoimmune vasculitic disease
  - RA, Wegener granulomatosis, relapsing polychondritis, SLE, polyarteritis nodosa, Sjögren syndrome
- Dermatologic
  - Acne rosacea, cicatricial pemphigoid, Stevens-Johnson syndrome
- Inflammatory bowel disease

Ocular
- Infection, trauma, abnormalities of eyelids/lashes, local/autoimmune (Mooren ulcer, allograft reaction)

EVALUATION/WORK-UP

Labs
- CBC, CMP, UA and micro, antineutrophil cytoplasmic antibody assay (ANCA), antinuclear antibody (ANA), rheumatoid factor (RF), anti-cyclic citrullinated peptide antibodies (anti-CCP), rapid plasma reagin (RPR), corneal cultures for bacteria, virus, and fungi
- Hepatitis B and hepatitis C common in Mooren ulcer

Pathology
- Peripheral predilection of disease from vascular juxtaposition of peripheral cornea
- Abnormal T-cell response resulting in antibody production and deposition of immune complexes
- Neutrophils and macrophages are recruited, releasing collagenases and proteases, leading to destruction of stroma

Imaging
- Chest x-ray, sacroiliac joint x-ray, CT scan of sinuses

TREATMENT

Medical
- Systemic immunosuppression with prednisone (1 mg/kg/day with max of 60 mg/day) or methylprednisolone (1 g/day x 3 days) followed by tapering schedule
- Steroid sparing agents used for impending perforation, ineffective steroid treatment, or patients with RA
  - Alkylating agents: Cyclophosphamide
  - Antimetabolites: Methotrexate, azathioprine, mycophenolate mofetil, tacrolimus
  - Biologics: Infliximab, rituximab
- Prophylaxis for *Pneumocystis jiroveci (carinii)* with trimethoprim-sulfamethoxazole (1 single-strength tablet daily)
- Vitamin C 1 gm p.o. q.i.d., doxycycline 100 mg p.o. b.i.d., Provera 1% drops q.i.d. all help reduce corneal melting

Surgical
- Resection of conjunctival tissue adjacent to PUK to decrease spread of inflammatory cells is controversial
- Surgery is indicated for corneal perforation or to decrease risk of perforation from severe corneal thinning
  - Tissue adhesive bandage contact lens, lamellar graft, or tectonic corneal grafting

Follow-Up
- Close follow-up and regular laboratory surveillance from medication side effects

Prognosis
- Visual prognosis correlated with ocular disease severity

SELECTED REFERENCES

1. Yagci A: Update on peripheral ulcerative keratitis. Clin Ophthalmol. 6:747-54, 2012
2. Galor A et al: Scleritis and peripheral ulcerative keratitis. Rheum Dis Clin North Am. 33(4):835-54, vii, 2007

RHEUMATOID ARTHRITIS

Key Facts

Introduction

- Chronic, systemic, inflammatory autoimmune disease involving joints and other extraarticular manifestations, including ocular involvement

Presentation

- Ocular conditions associated with rheumatoid arthritis (RA): Keratoconjunctivitis sicca (KCS), episcleritis, diffuse anterior scleritis, nodular scleritis, necrotizing scleritis with inflammation, scleromalacia perforans, RA-associated keratitis (corneal inflammation and melt)

Treatment

- KCS: Early, aggressive treatment necessary to prevent corneal ulcers and scarring; treatment usually progresses in stepwise fashion according to severity of dry eye disease (topical cyclosporine or steroids necessary before punctal plugs)
- Episcleritis: Preservative-free topical lubricants as needed, topical or oral NSAIDs, topical glucocorticoids (e.g., fluorometholone)
- Nonnecrotizing scleritis (diffuse or nodular scleritis): Treat mild cases with NSAIDs; treat moderate to severe cases with prednisone
- Necrotizing scleritis or scleritis unresponsive to NSAIDs and prednisone only: Treat with prednisone plus methotrexate, oral cyclophosphamide, cyclosporine, or azathioprine
  - Eye protection and treatment of systemic RA are of utmost importance
- RA-associated keratitis: Oral corticosteroids and topical cyclosporin A; use topical corticosteroids with caution since they can accelerate thinning and perforation
- Collagenase inhibitors to prevent melting; consider TNF-α inhibitors for long-term control in consultation with rheumatologist

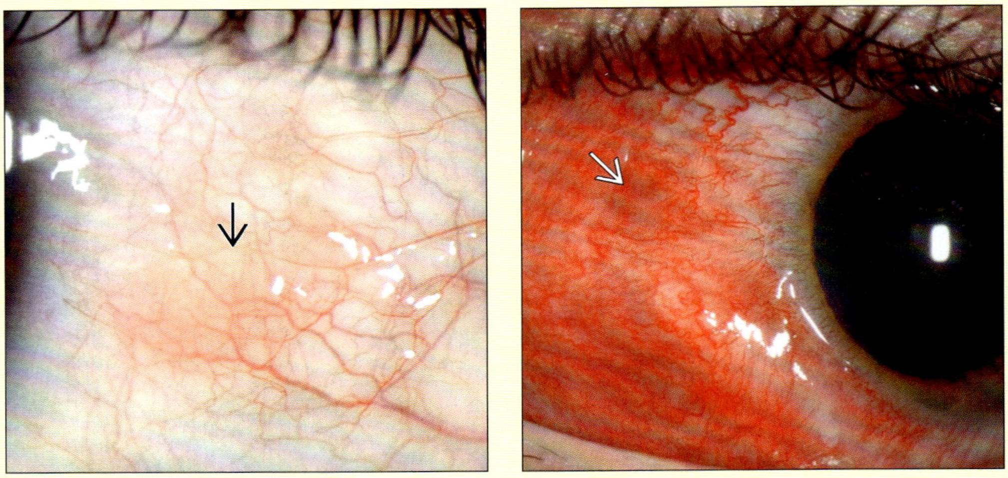

(Left) *Nodular episcleritis demonstrates edema in the area of the nodule with surrounding congestion ⇨. Episcleritis typically presents with localized superficial episcleral vessel congestion, slight congestion of conjunctival vessels, and edema. The sclera is not involved.* ***(Right)*** *Diffuse anterior scleritis is characterized by widespread inflammation ➡. Unlike episcleritis, engorged vessels do not blanch with application of topical phenylephrine 2.5%.*

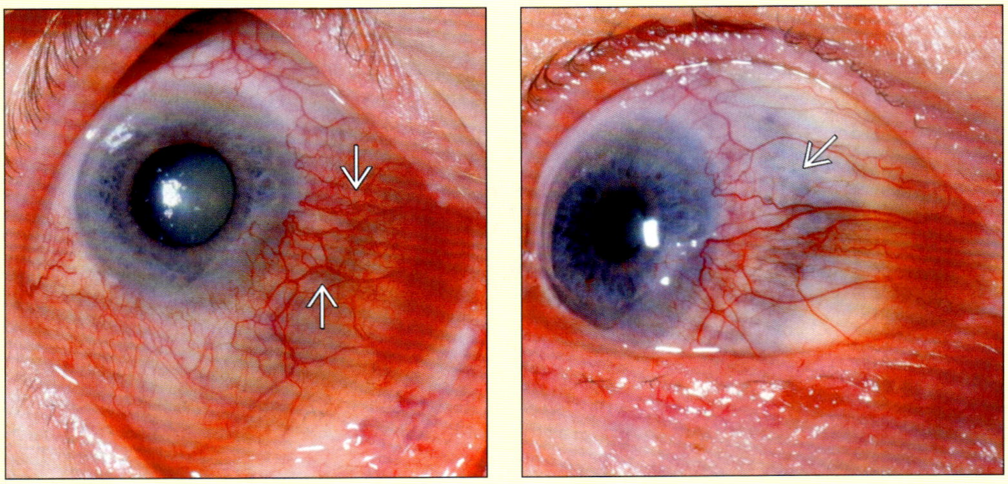

(Left) *Scleritis causes severe penetrating ocular pain that radiates to other areas of the head and face and awakens patients from sleep. Scleral vessels are significantly dilated along with overlying vessels of the episclera and bulbar conjunctiva ➡. (Courtesy K. Cohen, MD.)* ***(Right)*** *In severe cases of necrotizing scleritis with inflammation, the sclera may become transparent due to chronic inflammation, revealing the underlying dark blue color of the choroid ➡. (Courtesy K. Cohen, MD.)*

RHEUMATOID ARTHRITIS

INTRODUCTION

Abbreviations

- Rheumatoid arthritis (RA)

Definitions

- Chronic, systemic, inflammatory autoimmune disease involving joints and other extraarticular manifestations, including ocular involvement

DEMOGRAPHICS

Etiology/Risk Factors

- Exact causes unknown, but it may be triggered by a combination of factors: Abnormal autoimmune response, genetic susceptibility, and some environmental or biologic triggers (e.g., viral infection or hormonal changes)
- Risk factors: Female sex (2-3x higher incidence compared to males), positive family history, smoking

Epidemiology

- Prevalence ranges from 0.5-1.0% in general population
- 1.5 million adults in USA have RA
  - Keratoconjunctivitis sicca (KCS): 15-25% of RA patients
  - Episcleritis: Up to 11% of RA patients
  - Scleritis: Up to 20% of RA patients
- Commonly begins between 40-60 years of age

PRESENTATION

Symptoms

- KCS: Dryness, foreign body sensation, burning, irritation, photophobia, mucus discharge
- Episcleritis: Redness, discomfort without pain
- Scleritis: Redness, photophobia, severe pain (especially in necrotizing scleritis with inflammation), deep red or purple discoloration of sclera

Exam Findings

- KCS
  - Most common ophthalmic manifestation of RA
  - Commonly occurs from Sjögren syndrome secondary to RA (i.e., secondary Sjögren syndrome)
    - Sjögren triad: Mucosal dryness (dry eyes = KCS, dry mouth = xerostomia), positive minor salivary gland biopsy, positive anti-SSA or anti-SSB antibodies
  - Slit-lamp exam reveals conjunctival injection, superficial punctate keratopathy
  - Schirmer test shows decreased tear production and low tear meniscus
  - Lissamine green, rose bengal, or fluorescein staining reveals devitalized epithelium and poor mucin coverage on conjunctiva and cornea
    - KCS starts with nasal and temporal interpalpebral conjunctiva staining and eventually becomes diffuse over entire corneal surface
  - Filamentary keratitis may occur when epithelial debris and mucus strands adhere to corneal surface
  - Severe KCS may lead to corneal melting
- Episcleritis
  - Focal or diffuse acute onset of episcleral inflammation with intense episcleral injection and edema; no scleral edema or thinning
  - Presents with painless, bright red superficial episcleral vessels that move with the episclera; scleritis exhibits intense pain and deep-red or purplish scleral vessels adherent to sclera
  - Episcleritis is benign and self-limited
    - To distinguish episcleritis from scleritis, instill 1-2 drops of topical phenylephrine 2.5% to affected eye; dilated vessels caused by episcleritis will blanch whereas those caused by scleritis remain dilated
- Scleritis
  - Diffuse anterior scleritis
    - Most common and least severe type of scleritis
    - Ocular surface inflammation with scleral and episcleral chemosis
    - Engorged scleral vessels do not blanch with topical phenylephrine eyedrops
  - Nodular scleritis
    - Single or multiple firm and tender scleral nodules
  - Necrotizing scleritis with inflammation
    - Severe scleral inflammation, edema, and necrosis
    - Acute episodes have worse epithelial defects, scleral thinning, stromal loss, and necrosis
    - Higher incidence of concurrent bacterial and fungal infections during acute episodes
  - Necrotizing scleritis without inflammation (scleromalacia perforans)
    - Severe scleral thinning with yellow-white necrotic scleral lesions
    - No ocular inflammation or pain
    - Severe scleral thinning creates areas of blue, gray, or brown discoloration where uvea is covered by only conjunctiva and episclera
    - Patients with longstanding RA require thorough eye exam since they may have scleral thinning without discomfort or other symptoms
- RA-associated keratitis (corneal inflammation and melt)
  - Corneal collagen breakdown secondary to inflammation in corneal extracellular matrix
  - Associated with concurrent scleritis
  - Types of inflammation
    - Peripheral ulcerative keratitis (PUK)
      - Most common form of corneal melt
      - Proinflammatory cytokines and proteases worsen stromal breakdown
      - Can lead to globe rupture
    - Sclerosing keratitis: Occurs adjacent to active region of scleritis; thickening, vascularization, and opacification of peripheral cornea
    - Acute stromal keratitis: Stromal edema and infiltrates; corneal neovascularization and thinning
    - Keratolysis: Loss of corneal stroma (typically central, inferocentral, or at limbus in a gutter pattern) without infiltrate

RHEUMATOID ARTHRITIS

DIFFERENTIAL DIAGNOSIS

Primary Sjögren Syndrome

- Inflammatory autoimmune disease affecting lacrimal and salivary glands but with no other associated rheumatologic disease
- Signs: KCS, dysphagia, swelling of glands around face and neck, and dryness in nasal passages, mouth, throat, vagina, and skin

Juvenile Idiopathic Arthritis

- Group of autoimmune diseases leading to chronic joint inflammation in children
- Signs: Decreased visual acuity, band keratopathy, synechiae, cataracts, or increased intraocular pressure

Systemic Lupus Erythematosus

- Systemic autoimmune connective tissue disease that affects the joints, skin, kidneys, lungs, nervous system, serous membranes, &/or other bodily organs
- Signs: KCS, uveitis, episcleritis, scleritis, keratitis, discoid lupus rash over eyelids, optic neuritis, ischemic optic neuropathy

Seronegative Spondyloarthropathies

- Types: Ankylosing spondylitis, Reiter syndrome, psoriatic arthritis
- Signs: Unilateral or bilateral uveitis and anterior chamber inflammation

TREATMENT

Medical

- KCS: Early and aggressive treatment necessary to prevent corneal ulcers and scarring; treatment usually progresses in stepwise fashion according to severity of dry eye disease
  - Ocular surface lubrication with preservative-free artificial tears, gels, &/or ointments is mainstay treatment for mild to moderate dry eye symptoms due to aqueous-deficient tear film
  - Long-term eyelid hygiene with lid scrubs thickens lipid layer of tear film
  - Topical cyclosporin A used b.i.d. for a few months decreases dry eye symptoms and inflammation by increasing aqueous layer of tear film and goblet cell density
  - Topical or oral tetracyclines (e.g., doxycycline) are effective in treating eyelid margin disease (e.g., meibomian gland dysfunction or meibomitis)
  - Oral omega-3 fatty acids provide anti-inflammatory effect for treatment of dry eye and eyelid margin disease
  - Wearing moisture chamber goggles and using a room humidifier while sleeping may also be beneficial
  - Slow-release artificial ophthalmic inserts can provide continuous lubrication
  - Severe KCS may require temporary occlusion of lacrimal puncta with dissolvable collagen plugs or permanent silicone plugs to increase tear meniscus by decreasing tear drainage (use after inflammation control with cyclosporine or steroids)
- Episcleritis
  - Preservative-free topical lubricants as needed
  - Topical NSAID such as diclofenac q.i.d.
  - Topical glucocorticoids such as fluorometholone acetate 0.1% q.i.d. or prednisolone acetate 1% q.i.d.
  - Oral NSAID such as indomethacin 25 mg t.i.d.
- Scleritis
  - Nonnecrotizing scleritis (diffuse or nodular scleritis)
    - Mild cases: Begin with NSAIDs (e.g., indomethacin 75 mg b.i.d. or naproxen 375-500 mg b.i.d.)
    - Moderate to severe cases: Begin with prednisone 1 mg/kg per day and alter dosage based on response
  - Necrotizing scleritis or scleritis unresponsive to NSAIDs and prednisone only
    - Add methotrexate 10-20 mg per week or oral cyclophosphamide 1-2.5 mg/kg per day to prednisone; taper prednisone after about 3 weeks, once scleritis improves
    - If necessary, cyclosporine 2-5 mg/kg per day or azathioprine 1-2 mg/kg per day are also useful in combination with prednisone
    - Eye protection and treatment of systemic RA are of utmost importance
    - Consider TNF-α inhibitors for long-term control in consultation with rheumatologist
- RA-associated keratitis
  - Oral corticosteroids and topical cyclosporin A
  - Use topical corticosteroids with caution, as they can accelerate thinning and perforation
  - Melts: Vitamin C 1 g p.o. q.i.d., doxycycline 100 mg p.o. b.i.d., medroxyprogesterone 1% eyedrops q.i.d.

Surgical

- KCS
  - If punctal occlusion with plugs is ineffective, thermal punctal cautery may be performed to permanently close puncta; begin with lower puncta and proceed to upper puncta, if necessary
  - Lateral tarsorrhaphy and use of a bandage contact lens may be necessary in patients with nonhealing epithelial defects or corneal ulcers secondary to KCS or keratolysis or exposure keratitis
- Scleritis
  - Necrotizing scleritis with severe scleral thinning or threatened globe perforation may require urgent tectonic grafts with corneal and scleral tissue
- Use amniotic membrane for corneal or scleral melts as adjunct to immunosuppressants and tectonic tissue

Prognosis

- RA patients with scleritis have worse ocular prognosis than those with episcleritis
- RA patients with scleritis may have more advanced joint disease and extraarticular manifestations than those without scleritis
- Necrotizing scleritis ± inflammation: Severe scleral thinning puts patients at high risk of globe rupture and loss of eye secondary to even minor trauma

SELECTED REFERENCES

1. Akpek EK et al: Treatment of Sjögren's syndrome-associated dry eye an evidence-based review. Ophthalmology. 118(7):1242-52, 2011
2. Galor A et al: Scleritis and peripheral ulcerative keratitis. Rheum Dis Clin North Am. 33(4):835-54, vii, 2007
3. Smith JR et al: Therapy insight: scleritis and its relationship to systemic autoimmune disease. Nat Clin Pract Rheumatol. 3(4):219-26, 2007

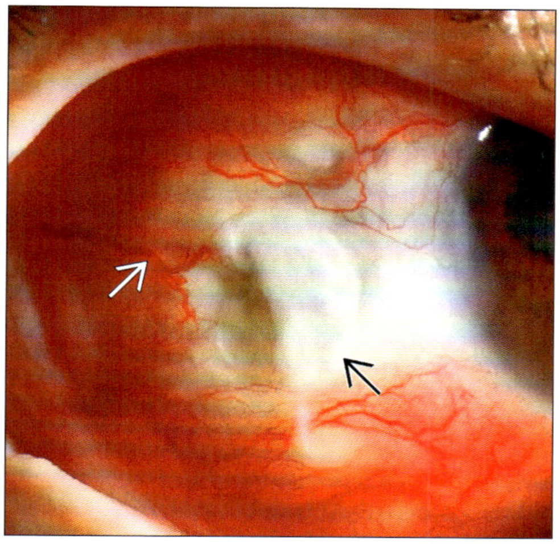

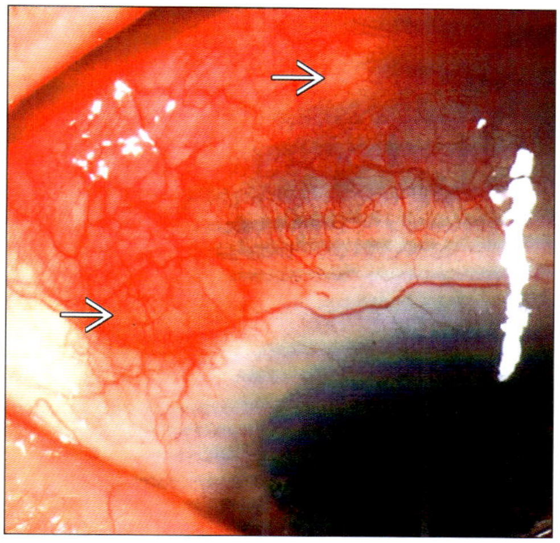

(Left) *Diffuse anterior scleritis is characterized by widespread inflammation, conjunctival vessel dilation and distortion ➔, edema, and conjunctival chemosis ➔.* ***(Right)*** *Nodular scleritis presents with small, tender, thickened scleral nodules ➔ that are clearly visible on the surface of the eye or by lifting the upper or lower eyelids. The formation of these nodules represents generalized ocular inflammation, with the areas surrounding the nodules exhibiting deep, intense inflammation.*

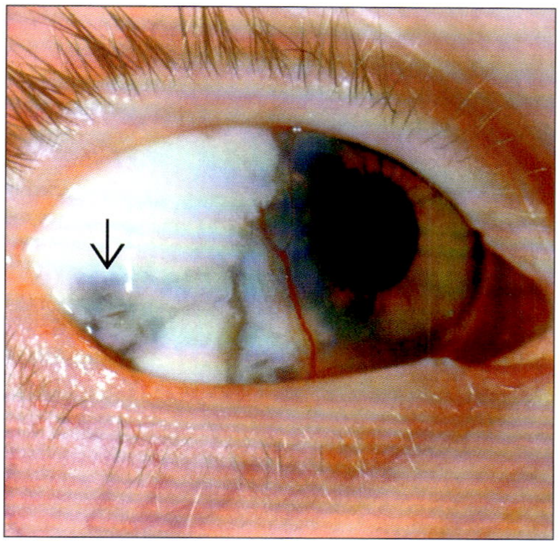

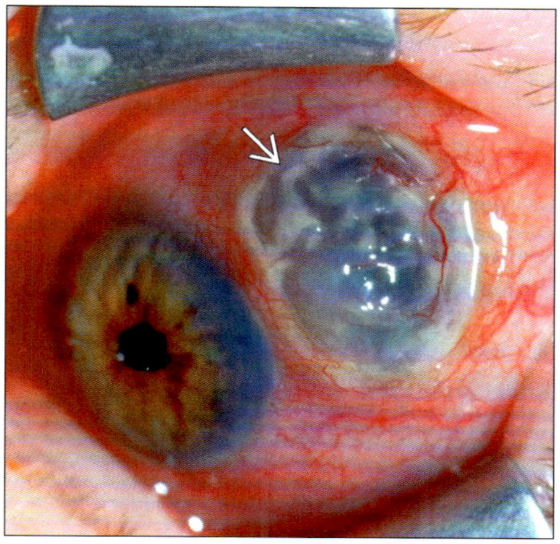

(Left) *Longstanding polyarticular RA leads to the development of scleromalacia perforans ➔, especially in female patients. (Courtesy K. Cohen, MD.)* ***(Right)*** *Scleromalacia perforans exhibits significant scleral thinning in discrete areas, causing necrotic outpouchings of underlying choroid ➔. The anterior sclera loses its episcleral covering, necrotic slough eventually separates or is absorbed, and the choroid is left covered only by conjunctiva or is completely exposed. (Courtesy K. Cohen, MD.)*

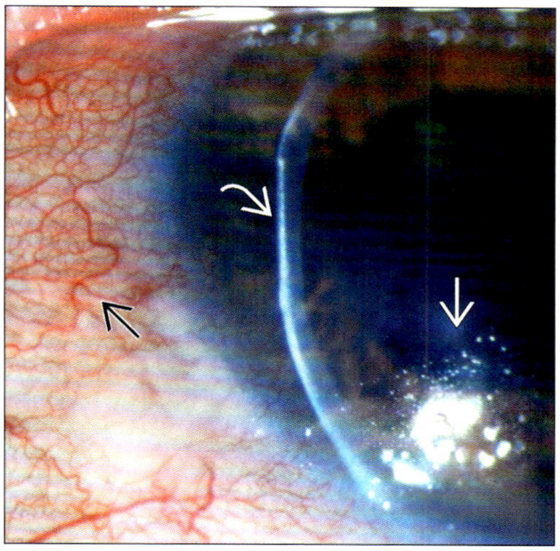

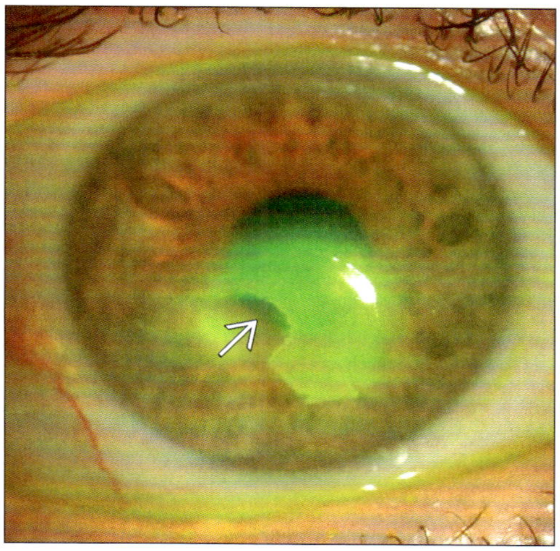

(Left) *Severe KCS leads to superficial punctate keratopathy ➔, conjunctival injection ➔, inflammatory infiltrate, and eventual corneal thinning ➔. (Courtesy K. Cohen, MD.)* ***(Right)*** *Corneal melt from PUK reveals a noninfiltrating corneal ulcer ➔ with surrounding inflammatory infiltrate and conjunctival injection. This condition is a harbinger of systemic vasculitis in RA patients, requiring aggressive immunosuppression to avoid the associated morbidity and mortality of this stage of RA.*

CHEMICAL BURN

Key Facts

Introduction
- Severity of chemical burn injury depends on inciting agent, surface area of burn, length of exposure, and depth of penetration
- Alkaline injuries more severe due to saponification of phospholipid membranes, resulting in continuous cell destruction
- Most serious alkali injuries are associated with exposures to ammonia and lye
- Acidic injury is usually localized and less severe
- Sulfuric acid is most common "acid burn," while hydrofluoric acid (HF) is one of the most caustic

Demographics
- Common in males in industrial accidents

Presentation
- Eye pain, photophobia, blurry or decreased vision, blepharospasm, conjunctival redness
- Fluorescein exam with slit-lamp examination: Chemosis, corneal opacification, epithelial defects, limbal ischemia

Treatment
- Irrigate until pH normalization
- Topical proparacaine (0.5%) and IV analgesic for comfort and prevention of blepharospasm
- Elevated intraocular pressure: Carbonic anhydrase inhibitors
- Prevention of synechiae: Cycloplegic eye drops (cyclopentolate 0.5%) or atropine drops
- Epithelial defects: Tetracycline ointment &/or systemic antibiotics
- Severe epithelial defects: Amnionic membrane grafting
- Ocular surface reconstruction with limbal stem cell transplantation and systemic immunosuppression; keratoprosthesis is alternative

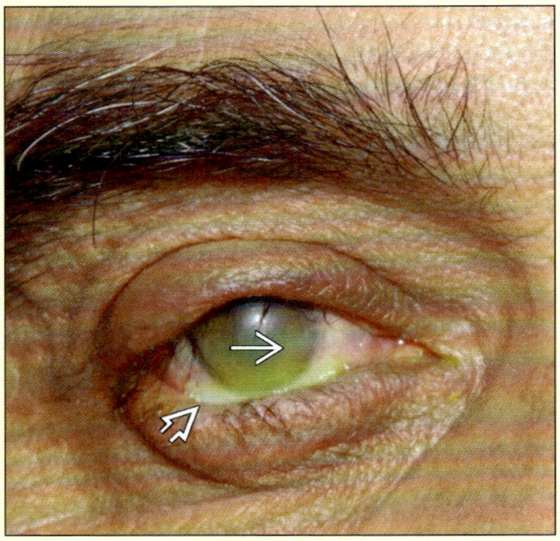

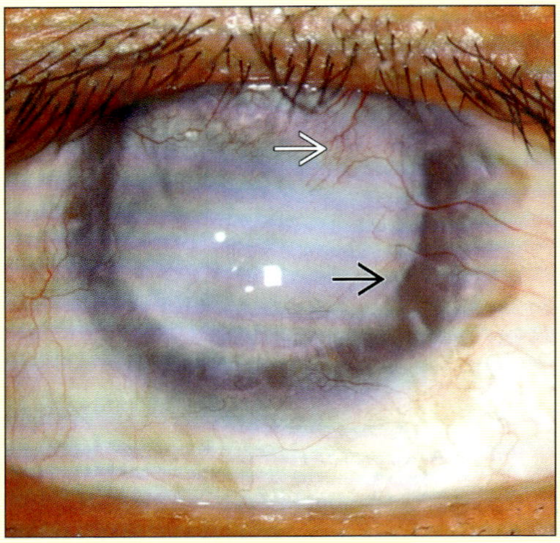

(Left) *External photograph shows corneal opacification and discoloration, which occurs in penetrating chemical injuries such as alkaline chemical exposure ➔. The blanched area absent of vasculature, near the inferior corneal-conjunctival border, suggests limbal ischemia ➔.* ***(Right)*** *External photograph shows corneal opacification after a penetrating keratoplasty (corneal transplant) ➔ as a result of a chemical burn. Vascularization of the cornea has occurred post transplant ➔.*

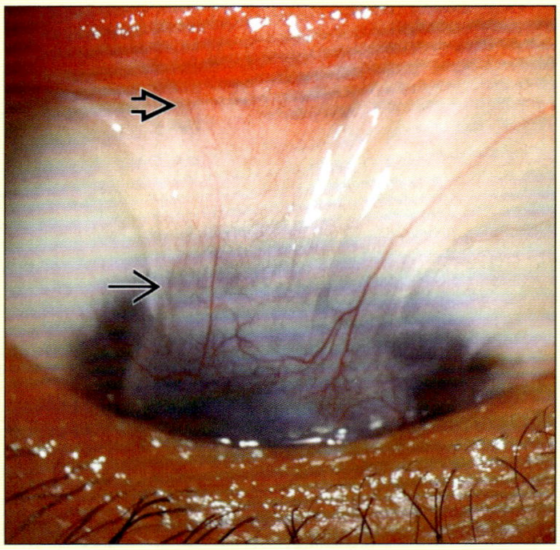

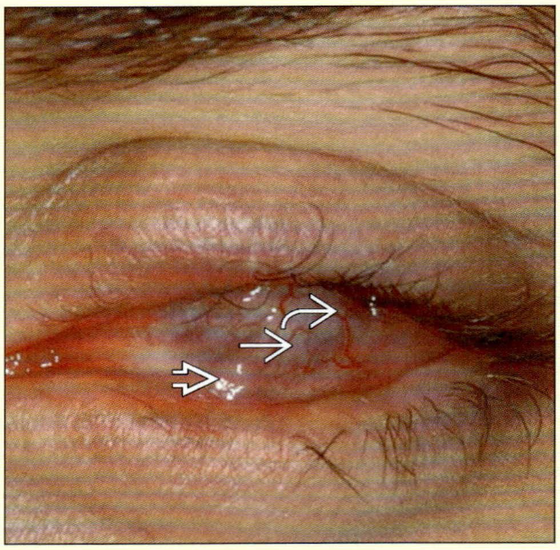

(Left) *This external photograph shows marked conjunctivalization and vascularization of the cornea due to a chemical burn ➔. A symblepharon has also formed, which is a common finding in severe chemical injuries ➔.* ***(Right)*** *This external photograph shows vascularization of the cornea due to thermal injury, which needs to be differentiated from chemical injury ➔. Symblepharon formation ➔ and conjunctivalization of the cornea ➔ are evident.*

CHEMICAL BURN

INTRODUCTION

Definitions

- Chemical exposure resulting in damage to conjunctiva, cornea, and anterior segment of the eye
- Severity of chemical burn injury depends on inciting agent, surface area of burn, and length of exposure

Subtypes

- Alkaline injuries
  - Result in liquefactive necrosis
  - Typically more severe than acidic injuries due to saponification and penetration through cornea, resulting in continuous cell destruction
  - Strong alkaline agents penetrate the anterior chamber causing inflammation of the iris, lens, and ciliary body
  - Most serious alkali injuries are associated with exposures to ammonia and lye
  - Common agents
    - Ammonia (cleansers, fertilizer, hair dyes)
    - Magnesium hydroxide (fireworks)
    - Calcium carbonate (lime)
    - Sodium hydroxide (lye)
    - Potassium hydroxide (oven or drain cleaners)
    - Sodium or potassium hydroxide (swimming pool cleaner, air bag aerosol)
- Acidic injuries
  - Result in coagulative necrosis due to denatured proteins that help limit ocular penetration
  - Acidic injury is usually localized and less severe; however, exposure to acids with pH of 2.5 or less can have similar destructive power to alkaline chemicals
  - Common agents
    - Acetic acid (hair relaxer, vinegar)
    - Hydrochloric acid (toilet bowl cleaner, grout cleaner, rust stain remover, swimming pool cleaner)
    - Hydrofluoric acid (glass etching, silicone production, rust removal, leather tanning fluid, high octane gasoline)
    - Phosphoric acid (rust remover, toilet bowl cleaner)

DEMOGRAPHICS

Etiology/Risk Factors

- Common in males in industrial accidents

Epidemiology

- Chemical burns are a leading cause of work-related eye injury treated in United States

PRESENTATION

Symptoms

- Eye pain, photophobia, blurry vision, blepharospasm, conjunctival redness

Exam Findings

- Fluorescein exam with slit-lamp examination: Chemosis, corneal opacification, epithelial defects, limbal ischemia
- Sweep fornices and evert eyelids: Foreign bodies embedded in any part of the ocular structures
- Tonometry: High intraocular pressure as a result of periorbital edema or inflammation of trabecular meshwork

DIFFERENTIAL DIAGNOSIS

Thermal Burn

- Injury is usually limited to superficial epithelium
- Eyelid involvement is common

TREATMENT

Medical

- Immediate irrigation on site with tap water
- Repeat irrigation with saline at hospital, then check pH at 30 minutes and then every 15 minutes until neutralization to pH of 7.4
- IV analgesic for comfort
- Topical and systemic ascorbic acid (1 g p.o. q.i.d.) to promote collagen growth and wound healing
- Carbonic anhydrase inhibitors for high IOP
- Cycloplegic eye drops (cyclopentolate 0.5%) for prevention of synechiae
- Consider moisture chamber goggles, bandage contact lenses, large-diameter gas-permeable scleral contact lens for epithelial defects
- Doxycycline and Provera 1% drops to prevent melting

Surgical

- Amnionic membrane grafting for severe epithelial defects
- Ocular surface reconstruction with corneal stem cell transplantation (limbal stem cell transplants) from healthy fellow eye or cadaver tissue
  - Systemic immunosuppression may be necessary in cadaveric transplants
- If cornea transplant fails or is at high risk for failure, consider keratoprosthesis

Follow-Up

- During early repair stages (< 3 weeks)
  - Monitor closely for epithelial healing: If no reepithelialization of the cornea, this would confirm the total lack of limbal stem cell activity

Prognosis

- Damage may be irreversible
- Intact vasculature has better prognosis
- Loss of perilimbal epithelium has poor prognosis

SELECTED REFERENCES

1. Lin A et al: Management of ocular conditions in the burn unit: thermal and chemical burns and Stevens-Johnson syndrome/toxic epidermal necrolysis. J Burn Care Res. 32(5):547-60, 2011
2. Fish R et al: Management of ocular thermal and chemical injuries, including amniotic membrane therapy. Curr Opin Ophthalmol. 21(4):317-21, 2010
3. Spector J et al: Chemical, thermal, and biological ocular exposures. Emerg Med Clin North Am. 26(1):125-36, vii, 2008
4. Xiang H et al: Work-related eye injuries treated in hospital emergency departments in the US. Am J Ind Med. 48(1):57-62, 2005

CORNEAL ABRASION

Key Facts

Introduction

- Defect in epithelial surface of cornea secondary to mechanical trauma, foreign body, contact lens wear, or chemical or flash burns

Presentation

- Symptoms
  - Pain, photophobia, foreign body sensation, tearing, blurry vision
- Work-up
  - Slit-lamp exam with both direct illumination and fluorescein dye to delineate edges of epithelial defect
  - If exam is done soon after injury, corneal stroma will appear clear
  - If exam is done within 12-24 hours after injury, stromal infiltrate and anterior chamber cell and flare reaction may be present

Treatment

- Topical anesthetic, such as proparacaine 0.5%, provides rapid pain relief, but frequent use retards epithelial healing; use only to facilitate the eye exam (do **not** give to patient)
- Short-acting cycloplegic drops relieve pain from reflex ciliary spasm; use for small to moderately sized abrasions that are expected to heal within 12-24 hours
- Long-acting cycloplegic drops should be used for larger epithelial defects, which may take longer to heal
- Although patching has been mainstay in corneal abrasion treatment for many years, recent evidence suggests using only for treatment of large abrasions (> 10 mm) or in patients who may rub their eyes (e.g., children, patients with cognitive disabilities)
- Soft bandage contact lenses: Alternative to patching
- Antibiotics (erythromycin or bacitracin ointment)

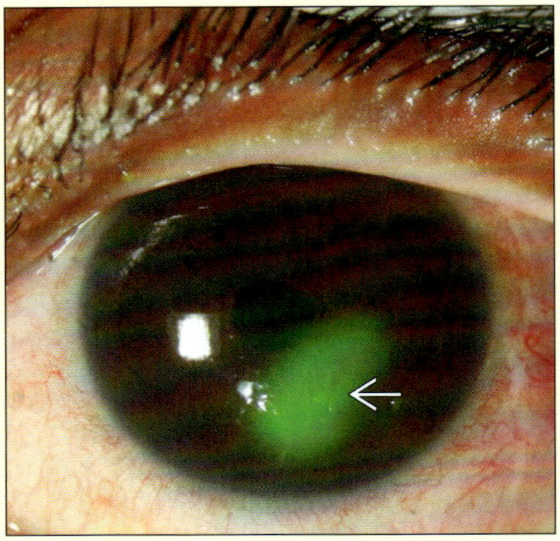

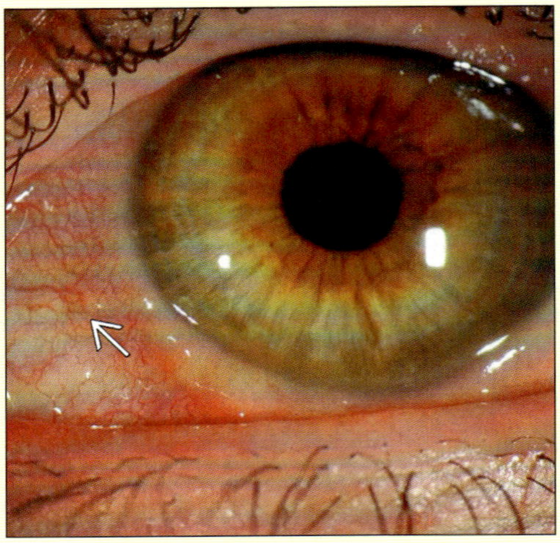

(Left) *Slit-lamp examination with both direct illumination and fluorescein dye helps confirm the diagnosis of corneal abrasion by delineating the edges of the epithelial defect ➔. (Courtesy J. Wrzosek, MD.)* ***(Right)*** *Diffuse conjunctival injection ➔ and ciliary flush are common findings in patients with corneal abrasion. In addition to the extreme pain of the corneal injury itself, patients usually complain of pain secondary to the inflammation associated with a corneal abrasion.*

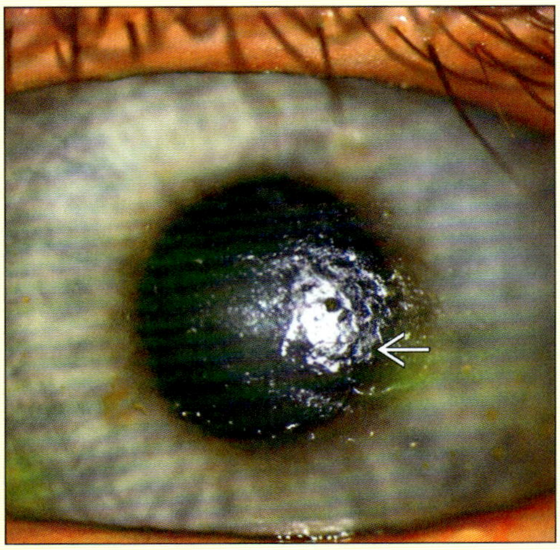

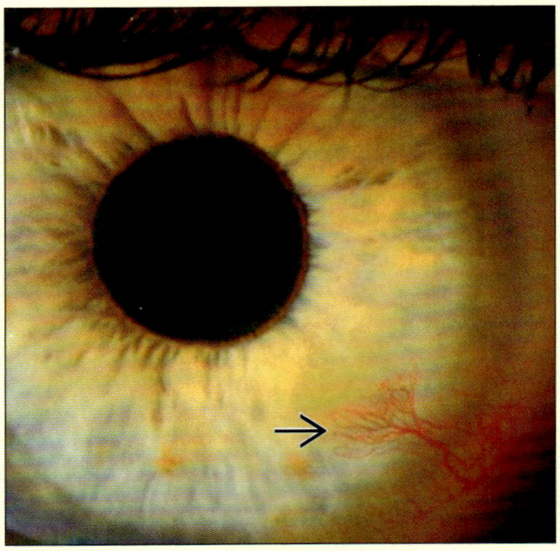

(Left) *The corneal light reflex can appear rough in the area where corneal epithelium has been denuded ➔. In cases of injury with a sharp object, a partial-thickness corneal flap or complete avulsion of corneal epithelium and exposure of bare stroma may also be present.* ***(Right)*** *Corneal neovascularization ➔, an in-growth of blood vessels into the avascular corneal tissue, may occur as a long-term sequelae of a corneal abrasion and can lead to scarring and subsequent visual impairment.*

CORNEAL ABRASION

INTRODUCTION

Definitions

- Defect in epithelial surface of cornea

DEMOGRAPHICS

Etiology/Risk Factors

- Mechanical trauma
- Foreign body
- Contact lens wear
- Chemical or flash burns

Epidemiology

- Higher risk in manufacturing, service, and construction industries

PRESENTATION

Symptoms

- Pain; often out of proportion to degree of injury
- Photophobia
- Foreign body sensation
- Tearing
- Blurry vision

Exam Findings

- Slit-lamp exam with both direct illumination and fluorescein dye to delineate edges of epithelial defect
  - Determine extent of abrasion and underlying stromal involvement and presence of any other associated injuries (e.g., globe perforation)
  - Corneal light reflex appears rough in area of denuded epithelium; flap of loose epithelium may be seen
  - If exam is done soon after injury, corneal stroma will appear clear
  - If exam is done within 12-24 hours after injury, stromal infiltrate and anterior chamber cell and flare reaction may be present

DIFFERENTIAL DIAGNOSIS

Occult Injury/Globe Perforation

- Maintain high index of suspicion since high-velocity injury with sharp foreign body is not uncommon in metal and machine workers
- Thorough slit-lamp exam is required since object may pass completely through cornea with only small epithelial injury

Microbial Keratitis

- Risk of microbial infection increases when break in corneal epithelium allows microbes in tear film to access underlying ocular structures and tissues
- Examine abraded cornea for signs of corneal infiltrate that may indicate developing infection

Recurrent Corneal Erosions

- Patients with history of previous corneal abrasions may experience spontaneous sloughing of new epithelium secondary to abnormal basement membrane attachments after healing
  - Occur without ocular trauma as inciting event

Stromal Abrasion

- Injury from tangential blow to eye with abrasive or sharp object; seen in sports (e.g., basketball) where individual receives fingernail injury to eye
- Results in partial-thickness corneal flap or complete avulsion of corneal epithelium and exposure of bare stroma

TREATMENT

Medical

- Topical anesthetic, such as proparacaine 0.5%, provides rapid pain relief, but frequent use retards epithelial healing; use only to facilitate the eye exam (do **not** give to patient)
- Cycloplegic eyedrops
  - Short-acting cycloplegic drops (cyclopentolate 0.5-1%) relieve pain from reflex ciliary spasm; use for small to moderately sized abrasions that are expected to heal within 12 to 24 hours
  - Long-acting cycloplegic drops (homatropine hydrobromide 5% or scopolamine hydrobromide 0.25%) should be used for larger epithelial defects, which may take longer to heal
- Tight patching
  - Although patching has been a mainstay in corneal abrasion treatment for many years, recent evidence suggests using it only for treatment of large abrasions (> 10 mm) or in patients who may rub their eyes (e.g., children, patients with cognitive disabilities)
    - Pros of patching: Reduces ocular pain and discomfort; facilitates epithelial healing process by eliminating blinking
    - Cons of patching: Patient cannot use both eyes for seeing; may retard reepithelialization by decreasing oxygenation of cornea; may increase risk of developing microbial keratitis by allowing microorganisms to replicate in tear film
- Soft bandage contact lenses: Alternative to patching
  - Decrease ocular pain and discomfort, protect corneal epithelium, facilitate healing, allow patient to continue activities of daily living
- Antibiotics: For prophylaxis against microbial keratitis
  - For uncomplicated abrasions, use erythromycin 0.5% ointment, polymyxin B/trimethoprim solution, or sulfacetamide 10% ointment or solution q.i.d. until patient is asymptomatic for 24 hours
  - Avoid preparations containing topical steroids, because steroids may delay healing and increase susceptibility to infection

Prognosis

- Most abrasions heal spontaneously in 24-48 hours
- Abrasions with stromal involvement often lead to scarring
- Wearing protective eyewear is of utmost importance in prevention of abrading and foreign body injuries

SELECTED REFERENCES

1. Wipperman JL et al: Evaluation and management of corneal abrasions. Am Fam Physician. 87(2):114-20, 2013
2. Turner A et al: Patching for corneal abrasion. Cochrane Database Syst Rev. (2):CD004764, 2006

SURFACE FOREIGN BODIES

Key Facts

Introduction

- Foreign material that is embedded superficially or deeply on corneal or conjunctival surface; material is usually of metal, glass, plastic, or organic origin

Demographics

- Most common form of ocular trauma
- Ocular injury frequently occurs during occupational activities such as grinding, welding, hammering, &/or drilling without wearing protective eyewear

Presentation

- Corneal foreign bodies
  - Multiple foreign bodies occur commonly and may be lodged superficially or embedded deep within cornea
  - As metallic and iron foreign bodies come in contact with tear film, oxidation often leaves rust rings in surrounding corneal tissue
- Conjunctival foreign bodies
  - Careful eversion and examination of upper and lower eyelid conjunctiva is necessary as foreign bodies can become embedded in superior tarsal plate or eyelid margin

Treatment

- Corneal foreign bodies
  - Superficial foreign bodies may be removed at slit-lamp exam with a moist cotton swab after instilling a topical anesthetic eyedrop
  - If material is more deeply embedded, attempt removal with topical anesthesia and forceps or a tuberculin syringe with 30-g needle
- Conjunctival foreign bodies
  - Irrigate fornices with saline solution
  - Remove embedded foreign material with moist cotton swab, forceps, or hypodermic needle

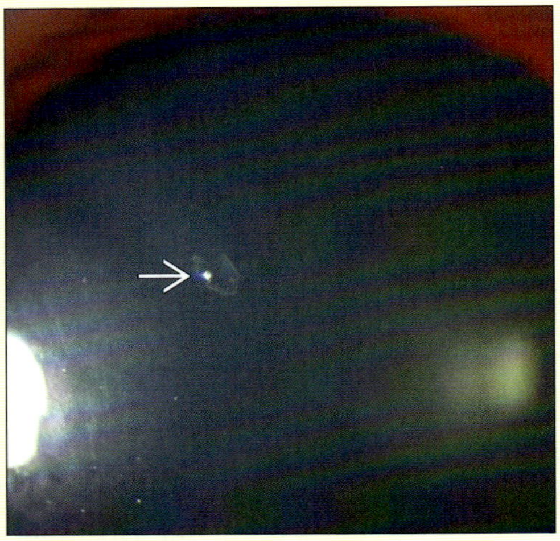
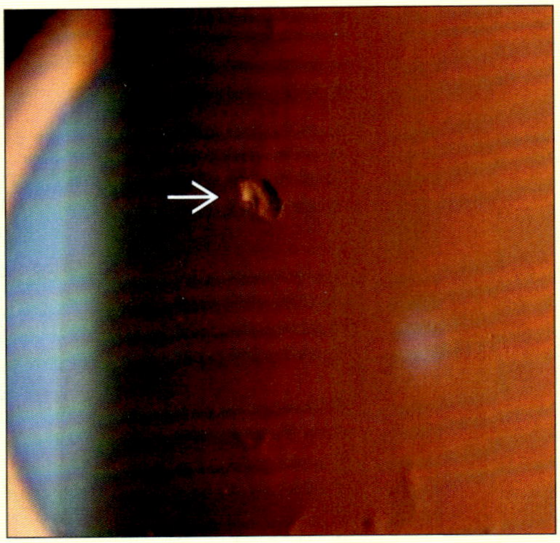

***(Left)** This slit-lamp photograph shows a faintly visible superficial foreign body on the surface of the cornea ➡. Discomfort caused by even a small corneal body can be quite severe. Any patient complaining of a foreign body sensation therefore merits a careful corneal surface examination. **(Right)** This slit-lamp photograph depicts the same foreign body viewed using the technique of retroillumination ➡. Retroillumination often facilitates visualization of small foreign bodies.*

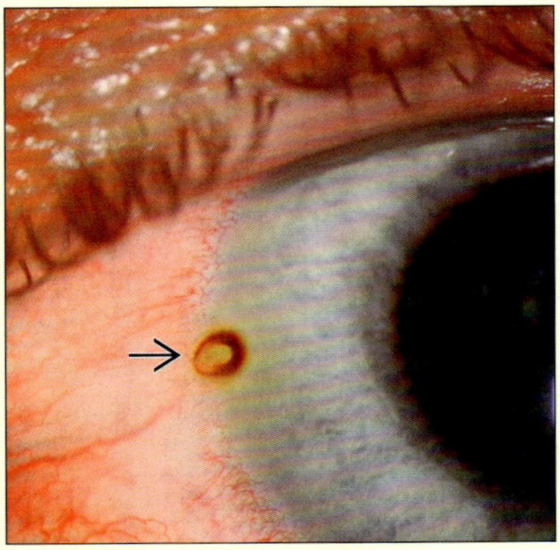
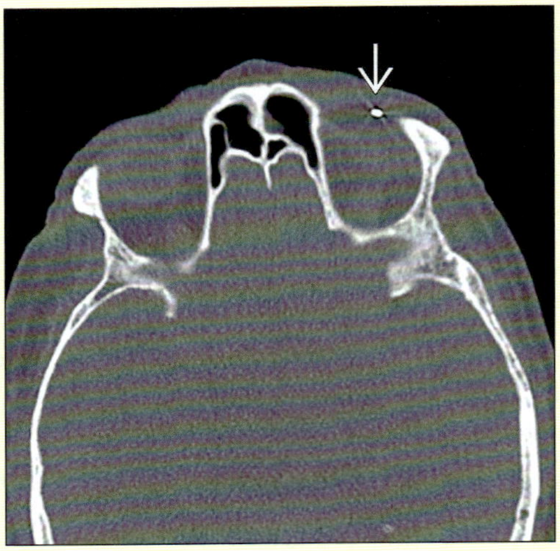

***(Left)** Metallic foreign bodies often leave rust rings in surrounding corneal tissue ➡. A rust ring can be pro-inflammatory and may be removed by scraping with a small needle or by applying an automated burr to the affected cornea. **(Right)** This CT scan shows a metallic foreign body on the surface of the eye ➡. CT and MRI are useful if external exam alone does not reveal whether a foreign body has penetrated the globe. However, an MRI is contraindicated when a metallic foreign body is suspected.*

SURFACE FOREIGN BODIES

INTRODUCTION

Definitions

- Foreign material that is embedded superficially or deeply on corneal or conjunctival surface; material is usually of metal, glass, plastic, or organic origin

DEMOGRAPHICS

Etiology/Risk Factors

- Ocular injury frequently occurs during occupational activities such as grinding, welding, hammering, &/or drilling without wearing protective eyewear
- Higher risk in manufacturing, service, and construction industries

Epidemiology

- Most common form of ocular trauma
- Higher incidence in men

PRESENTATION

Symptoms

- Foreign body sensation, irritation and tearing, eye pain, eye redness, photophobia

Exam Findings

- Thorough slit-lamp exam of entire eye to rule out intraocular foreign bodies
- Corneal foreign bodies
  - High magnification and narrow slit beam reveal stromal depth of foreign material in cornea
  - Multiple foreign bodies occur commonly and may be lodged superficially or embedded deep within cornea
  - Fluorescein staining reveals pooling in and around epithelial defects and irregularities
  - Seidel test helps to rule out corneal perforation if foreign body is deeply embedded
  - As metallic and iron foreign bodies come in contact with tear film, oxidation often leaves rust rings in surrounding corneal tissue
- Conjunctival foreign bodies
  - Careful eversion and examination of upper and lower eyelid conjunctiva is necessary as foreign bodies can become embedded in superior tarsal plate or eyelid margin
  - In cases of embedded foreign bodies in upper eyelid, fluorescein staining often reveals vertical corneal abrasions

DIFFERENTIAL DIAGNOSIS

Corneal Abrasion

- Mechanical trauma to eye resulting from dry eye syndrome, superficial foreign body injuries, &/or contact lens wear
- Results in corneal epithelial defect from scraping or denudation
- Foreign bodies are not retained

Intraocular Foreign Bodies

- Penetrating ocular injury in which foreign material is retained in globe or orbit
- CT scan is imaging study of choice for diagnosis
- If risk of endophthalmitis and scarring is high, emergent surgery is necessary

EVALUATION/WORK-UP

Imaging

- To rule out intraocular or intraorbital foreign body, consider B-scan ultrasound or orbital CT scan
- If possible history of metallic foreign body, avoid MRI and consider orbital x-ray films as initial test

TREATMENT

Medical

- Corneal foreign bodies
  - Superficial foreign bodies may be removed at slit lamp with a moist cotton swab after instilling a topical anesthetic eyedrop
  - If material is more deeply embedded, attempt removal with topical anesthesia and forceps or a tuberculin syringe with a 30-g needle
    - Avoid aggressive attempts at removal under slit lamp as this may result in aqueous humor leakage and collapse of anterior chamber
  - Remove rust rings by scraping with a small needle or by applying an automated burr to affected cornea
- Conjunctival foreign bodies
  - Retract upper and lower eyelids with Desmarres retractor
  - Irrigate fornices with saline solution
  - Remove embedded foreign material with moist cotton swab, forceps, or hypodermic needle
- Following removal of foreign body, patient should receive topical broad-spectrum antibiotic (e.g., moxifloxacin)
- Give topical NSAID (e.g., ketorolac 0.5%) and short-acting cycloplegic eyedrop for severe ocular discomfort or inflammation
- Higher incidence of inflammation and microbial contamination if foreign body is of plant, insect, or other organic origin
  - If infection develops, appropriate work-up with lab studies, cultures, biopsies, etc., is indicated

Surgical

- If perforation and anterior chamber involvement is suspected or present, foreign body should be removed under sterile conditions

Prognosis

- Irregular astigmatism, glare, and decreased vision can occur if a foreign body penetrates beyond Bowman layer and leaves a scar in the visual axis
- Most foreign body injuries are not severe and do not have significant morbidity
- Wearing protective eyewear is of utmost importance in preventing foreign body injuries

SELECTED REFERENCES

1. Gumus K et al: Corneal injury from a metallic foreign body: an occupational hazard. Eye Contact Lens. 33(5):259-60, 2007

NEUROTROPHIC KERATOPATHY

Key Facts

Introduction

- Keratitis that develops due to abnormal corneal sensation and interrupted trophic stimulation due to a lesion of the trigeminal nerve (CN5), which innervates the cornea

Demographics

- Most common causes are varicella zoster and herpes simplex keratitis

Presentation

- 3 stages of neurotrophic keratitis
- Decreased corneal sensation
- Decreased aqueous tear production

Evaluation/Work-Up

- Culture stromal infiltrate for bacteria prior to instituting antibiotic treatment
- Culture or immunofluorescence staining for herpes simplex or herpes zoster when suspected
- If associated neurologic deficit, consider MRI of brain and orbits

Treatment

- Pharmacologic treatment varies according to stage of keratopathy
- Copious lubrication with preservative-free artificial tears, gels, and ointments
- Avoid topical corticosteroids or NSAIDs, which can decrease corneal sensitivity or increase collagenase activity
- Surgical intervention may be considered for stage 2 or 3 neurotrophic keratopathy
- Monitor stage 1 disease every 3-7 days until resolution
- Monitor stage 2 disease every 1-2 days
- Hospitalization is necessary for stage 3 neurotrophic keratopathy

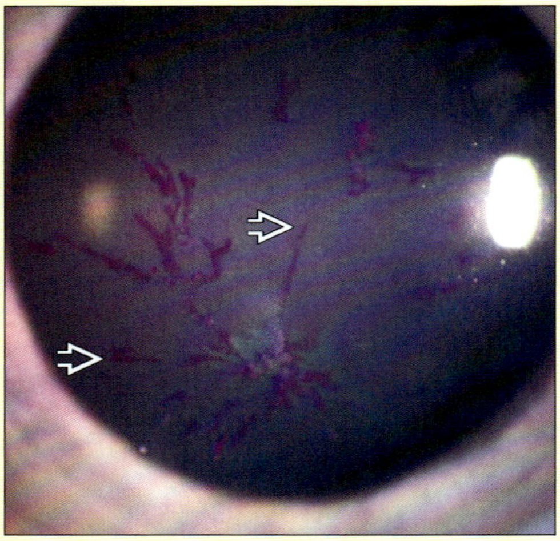
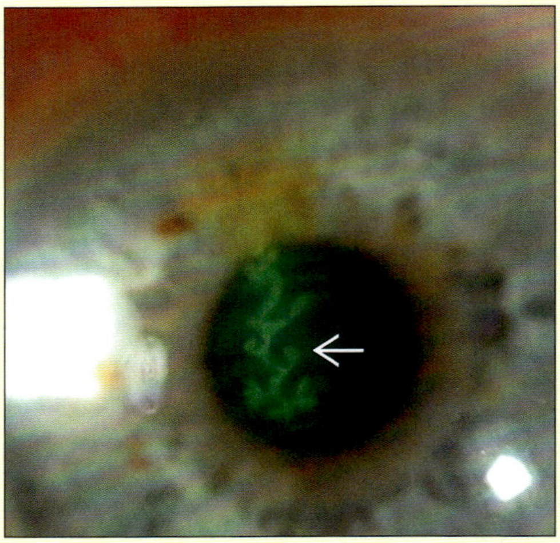

(Left) *Varicella zoster virus (VZV), a common cause of neurotrophic keratopathy, exhibits characteristic pseudodendritic staining. Note the absence of terminal bulbs at the tips of the dendrites ➯, making VZV more likely than herpes simplex virus (HSV).* ***(Right)*** *HSV, another common etiology of neurotrophic keratopathy, presents with characteristic dendritic lesions with branching terminal bulbs ➯.*

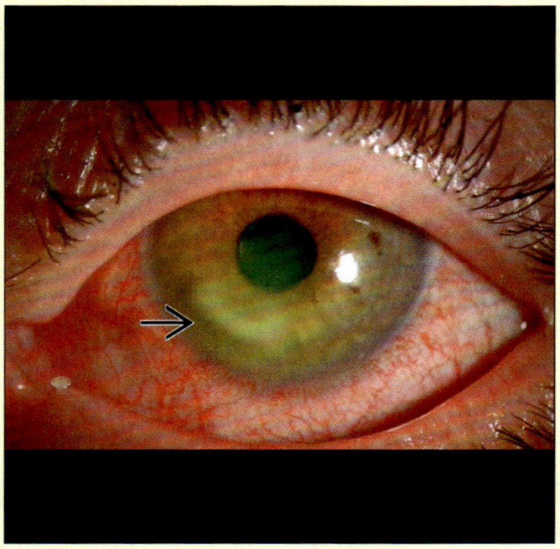
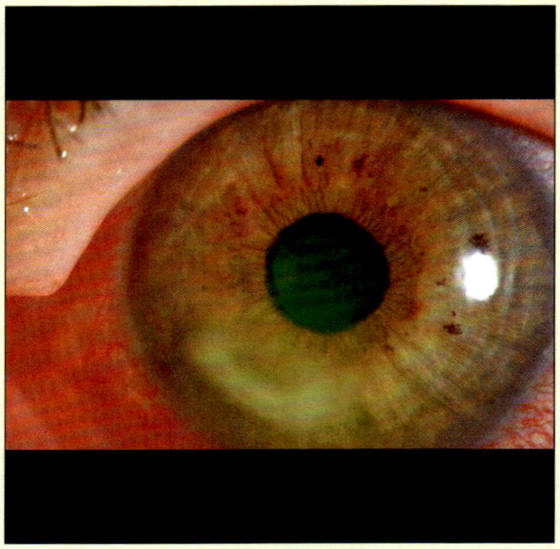

(Left) *Slit-lamp photo demonstrates a paracentral oval-shaped ulcer in the lower cornea ➔, typical of neurotrophic keratopathy. This stage 2 lesion should be monitored closely given concern for development of stromal melting and potential perforation.* ***(Right)*** *A magnified image shows the same patient. Prior to instituting antibiotic treatment, it is important to culture the stromal infiltrate for bacteria. If HSV or VZV is suspected, viral culture and immunofluorescence staining is critical as well.*

NEUROTROPHIC KERATOPATHY

INTRODUCTION

Definitions

- Keratitis that develops due to abnormal corneal sensation and interrupted trophic stimulation due to a lesion of the trigeminal nerve (CN5), which innervates the cornea

DEMOGRAPHICS

Etiology/Risk Factors

- Most common causes are varicella zoster and herpes simplex keratitis
- Trigeminal dysfunction with corneal ulceration
  - Traumatic damage to CN5 (ophthalmic branch)
  - Stroke, aneurysm, or brainstem hemorrhages
  - Irradiation exposure to the eye or orbit
  - Multiple sclerosis
  - Toxic chemical reactions
- Diabetes mellitus
- Contact lens use
- Abuse of topical anesthetics or nonsteroidal anti-inflammatory drugs (NSAIDs)

PRESENTATION

Symptoms

- Can vary depending on degree of keratitis
- Red eye
- Foreign body sensation
- Blurred vision
- Lid edema

Exam Findings

- 3 stages of neurotrophic keratitis
  - **Stage 1**: Subtle irregular corneal surface and developing punctate keratitis; decreased tear break-up time
  - **Stage 2**: Obvious epithelial defect associated with mild anterior stromal inflammation; epithelium surrounding defect is often swollen and gray and partially elevated; may develop folds in Descemet membrane; typically a paracentral oval-shaped ulcer develops in lower, exposed cornea
  - **Stage 3**: Corneal stromal melting with potential perforation

Physical Exam

- Decreased corneal sensation
  - Cranial nerve exam to evaluate hypesthesia
- May have decreased conjunctival sensation
- Excess mucous production resulting from increased conjunctival epithelial turnover
- Decreased aqueous tear production

DIFFERENTIAL DIAGNOSIS

Decreased Corneal Sensation

- Lesions to the ophthalmic division of CN5
  - Surgery, acoustic neuroma, trauma
- Infectious disease
  - Herpes simplex or zoster
- Contact lens wear
- Diabetes
- Topical pharmaceutical agents
  - Anesthetics, β-blockers, NSAIDs

EVALUATION/WORK-UP

Labs

- Culture stromal infiltrate for bacteria prior to instituting antibiotic treatment
- Culture or immunofluorescence staining for herpes simplex or herpes zoster when suspected
- Impression cytology may be performed to evaluate for limbal deficiency

Imaging

- If associated neurologic deficit, consider MRI of brain and orbits

TREATMENT

Medical

- Pharmacologic treatment varies according to stage of keratopathy
  - Vitamin C, doxycycline, topical Provera 1% drops help prevent corneal melting
  - Albumin drops and bandage contact lens can promote reepithelialization
- Copious lubrication with preservative-free artificial tears, gels, and ointments
- Avoid topical corticosteroids or NSAIDs, which decrease corneal sensitivity or increase collagenase
- Reevaluate topical ocular treatments and systemic medications that may contribute to decreased corneal sensation or ocular surface disease
- Treat any underlying causes of trigeminal nerve injury

Surgical

- Surgical intervention may be considered for stage 2 or 3 neurotrophic keratopathy
  - Lid closure procedures including lateral tarsorrhaphy, palpebral spring, or botulinum A toxin injection into levator muscle
- Procedures to repair persistent epithelial defect
  - Conjunctival flap or amniotic membrane transplant
- Procedures to repair ulceration
  - Penetrating or lamellar keratoplasty
  - Multilayer amniotic membrane transplantation for large defects
  - Cyanoacrylate glue with bandage contact lens for small defects (< 2 mm)

Follow-Up

- Monitor stage 1 disease every 3-7 days until resolution
- Monitor stage 2 disease every 1-2 days
- Stage 3 needs surgery &/or inpatient follow-up
- Consult neurologist for associated neurologic deficits

Prognosis

- Depends on severity, duration, and comorbidities

SELECTED REFERENCES

1. Goins KM: New insights into the diagnosis and treatment of neurotrophic keratopathy. Ocul Surf. 3(2):96-110, 2005

RECURRENT CORNEAL EROSION

Key Facts

Introduction

- Condition caused by defective epithelial adhesion to underlying basement membrane (BM)
- Can cause corneal scarring, infection, and permanent vision loss if not treated properly

Demographics

- Risk factors: Ocular trauma &/or various genetically mediated corneal dystrophies
- Epidemiology: More common in the developing world where corneal health is compromised due to malnutrition and among middle-aged and elderly patients

Presentation

- Symptoms include pain, photophobia, visual acuity deficits, and sometimes foreign body sensation

Differential Diagnosis

- Must consider HSV infection, abrasion, foreign body, complications secondary to contact lens use, corneal dystrophies, and various eyelid pathologies

Evaluation/Work-Up

- Slit-lamp exam is mainstay of evaluation

Treatment

- Goals: Relieve pain and promote corneal reepithelialization and reestablishment of competent BM
- Conservative medical therapy generally produces excellent results but should not be prolonged (> 1 month) if unsuccessful
- For medically refractory cases, surgical modalities should be considered given their relatively high success rate and low risk of complication

(Left) *This external photograph shows epithelial erosion on the surface of the cornea. Note how the epithelium is incorrectly adhering to the corneal surface ➡, resulting in corneal epithelial sloughing.* ***(Right)*** *This external photograph shows epithelial aggregates caused by corneal erosion. Note how the corneal epithelium begins to separate from the underlying corneal surface ➡.*

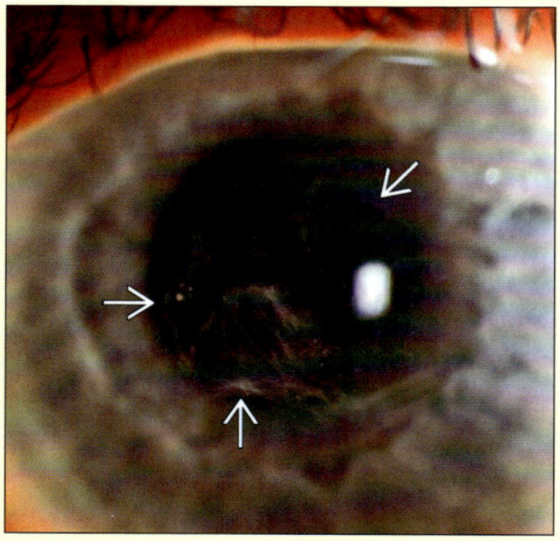

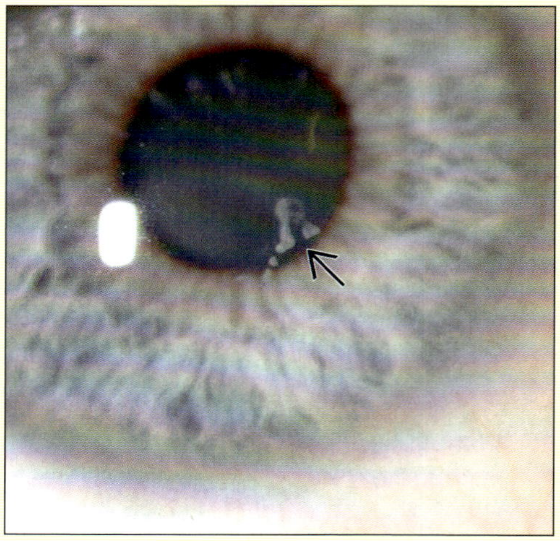

(Left) *This slit-lamp photograph depicts corneal erosion with an associated infiltrate ➡. Note the change in clarity between the normal and the eroded cornea. This is due to degradation of the corneal epithelium.* ***(Right)*** *This external photograph shows erosion of the cornea. Note the subtle circumferential corneal haze surrounding the pupil. This photograph also shows healing epithelium ➡, characterized by its ridged surface.*

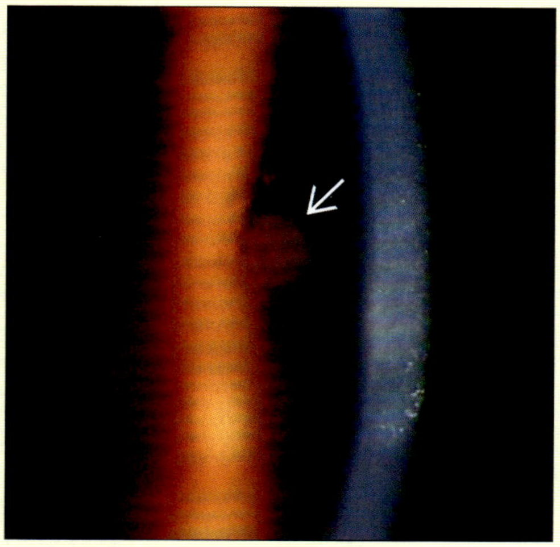

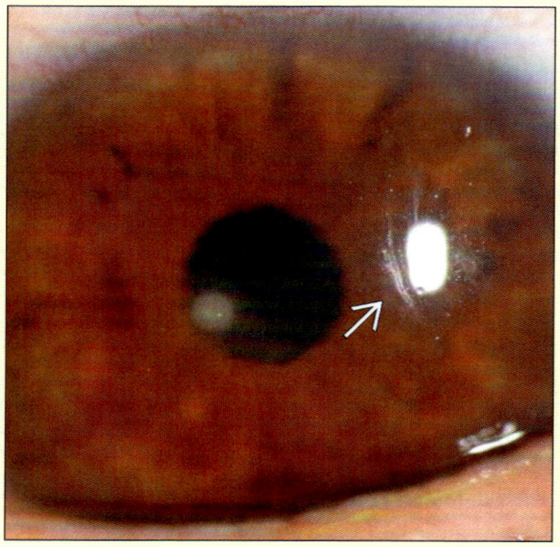

RECURRENT CORNEAL EROSION

INTRODUCTION

Abbreviations

- Recurrent corneal erosion (RCE)

Definitions

- Characterized by corneal epithelial breakdown due to defective epithelial adhesion to underlying basement membrane (BM) (a.k.a. Bowman layer)

DEMOGRAPHICS

Etiology/Risk Factors

- Primary (or genetically mediated) causes
  - Anterior BM dystrophies: Map-dot-fingerprint dystrophy, Cogan dystrophy
  - BM dystrophies: Reis-Buckler dystrophy (type 1 and type 2)
  - Stromal dystrophies: Lattice dystrophy, macular dystrophy, granular dystrophy
- Secondary (or acquired) causes
  - Traumatic epithelial abrasions, LASIK, or bacterial ulcers
  - Herpetic infection, meibomian gland dysfunction, keratoconjunctivitis sicca, Salzmann nodular degeneration, band keratopathy, epidermolysis bullosa, diabetes mellitus

Epidemiology

- RCE most likely to develop in those who have had a previous corneal abrasion that was sharp, clean, and linear (e.g., fingernail or paper cut)
- Incidence of recurrence after traumatic abrasion: 1 in 150
- Generally occurs after 4th decade of life
- More frequent in females than males
- More common in developing countries where malnutrition plays a significant role in health of cornea

PRESENTATION

Symptoms

- Pain, redness, photophobia, tearing, blurry vision, and foreign body sensation, and patients sometimes complain of pain in the morning upon wakening

Exam Findings

- Epithelial loss, bullae, epithelial filament formation; may also see a brownish granular edema that occupies anterior stroma &/or pseudodendrites
- Macroform erosions: Large area of epithelial separation from cornea, persists for several days, traumatic in origin
- Microform erosions: Intraepithelial microcysts with a minor break in epithelium, last for hours and occur at night or in the morning, associated with epithelial BM dystrophy

DIFFERENTIAL DIAGNOSIS

Corneal Lesion Secondary to

- HSV keratitis
- Abrasion
- Foreign body
- Contact lens complications
- Keratoconjunctivitis sicca
- Genetic dystrophies
- Floppy eyelid syndrome
- Roughening of tarsal plate
- Neurotrophic keratitis

EVALUATION/WORK-UP

Imaging

- Corneal topographic analysis: May see corneal microdepressions, which is important because epithelial abnormalities may not be evident on slit-lamp exam in some patients presenting with frank symptoms

Other Tests

- Slit-lamp exam: Must rule out corneal perforation first; use fluorescein to stain corneal erosions &/or 1% rose bengal to stain intact, but devitalized, epithelium

TREATMENT

Medical

- Conservative management: Patching for 1-2 days; cycloplegia and topical lubrication; temporary soft bandage contact lens; NSAIDs to relieve pain; instruct patients to move eyes slowly upon waking
- Refractory cases: Long-term soft bandage contact lens, oral tetracycline/doxycycline, care of associated lid pathology

Surgical

- Epithelial debridement: Debridement of loose epithelium to promote healing from healthy epithelial edge
- Anterior stromal puncture: Enhances epithelial adhesion to BM by scar formation; not advisable if erosions lie on visual axis
- Phototherapeutic keratectomy: Partial ablation of the BM to give a smooth bed for epithelium (risks inducing presbyopia or hyperopia)
- Diamond burr Bowman polishing: Involves debriding loose sheets of epithelium and polishing entire corneal surface with fine diamond burr (can be combined with others)

Follow-Up

- Regular follow-up care for months to years based on clinical picture

Prognosis

- Most patients heal completely and will not have any more episodes if treated properly and do not have underlying corneal dystrophy

SELECTED REFERENCES

1. Ewald M et al: Review of diagnosis and management of recurrent erosion syndrome. Curr Opin Ophthalmol. 20(4):287-91, 2009
2. Ramamurthi S et al: Pathogenesis, clinical features and management of recurrent corneal erosions. Eye (Lond). 20(6):635-44, 2006

THERMAL/ULTRAVIOLET KERATOPATHY

Key Facts

Introduction
- Ultraviolet (UV) keratopathy: Injury to cornea due to UV radiation
- Thermal keratopathy: Thermal burn injury to cornea

Demographics
- UV keratopathy
  - High-energy photons in short UV light wavelengths cause cellular photochemical damage
- Thermal keratopathy
  - Flame burns: Injury caused by fire, radiant heat, or flash burns
  - Contact burns: More common; caused by contact with hot objects or liquids

Presentation
- Irritation, pain, photophobia, foreign body sensation, decreased corneal sensation
- UV keratopathy
  - Lid edema, conjunctival hyperemia, superficial punctate keratitis
- Thermal keratopathy
  - Mild burns damage epithelium; severe burns damage deep tissue layers

Treatment
- Short-acting cycloplegic eyedrop relieves pain from ciliary spasm or iridocyclitis
- UV keratopathy
  - Topical anesthetic for rapid pain relief and to facilitate eye exam only
  - NSAIDs and bland ointment for pain management; patching for < 24 hours
- Thermal keratopathy
  - Short corticosteroid course may be necessary for treating iridocyclitis
  - Topical antibiotics to prevent infection and decrease risk of corneal ulcers from infection

__(Left)__ Slit-lamp photo shows an absent corneal light reflex and diffuse uptake of fluorescein over the entire surface of the cornea exposed to UV light ➡. Conjunctival hyperemia is present ➡. Higher magnification will reveal diffuse superficial punctate keratitis. __(Right)__ Thermal burn secondary to firework injury exhibits severe corneal edema, opacity, and deepithelialization ⇨. Conjunctival hyperemia, hemorrhagic exudate, and external eyelid burns are also evident ➡. (Courtesy K. Cohen, MD.)

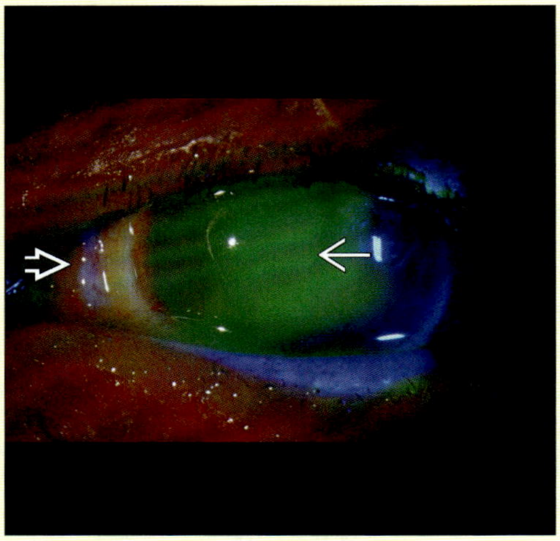

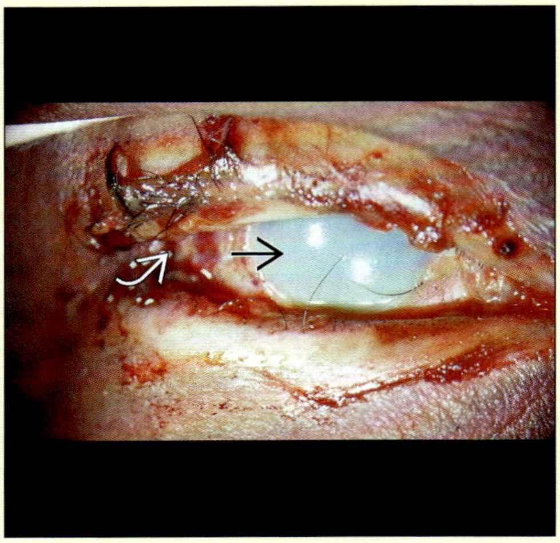

__(Left)__ Photo shows thermal injury 1 day after amniotic membrane graft/ conjunctivoplasty ➡. Interrupted nylon sutures around the limbus and running sutures join the peripheral membrane with Tenon capsule and remaining conjunctiva. (Courtesy K. Cohen, MD.) __(Right)__ One week after surgery, the graft is in place and the eye has healing burns, mild exposure, superior/ inferior symblepharon, and improved edema ⇨. Descemet membrane is swollen. (Courtesy K. Cohen, MD.)

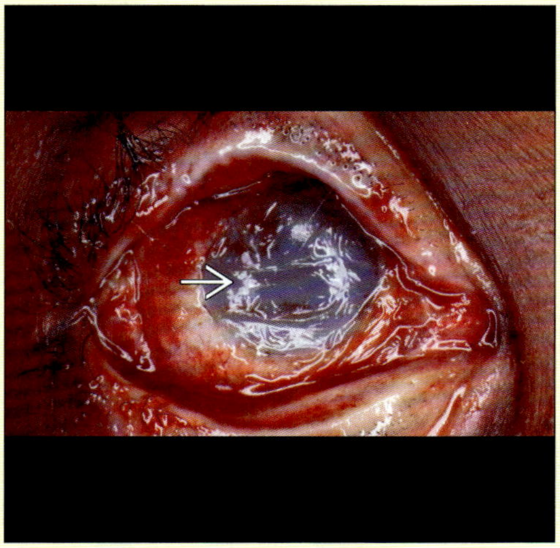

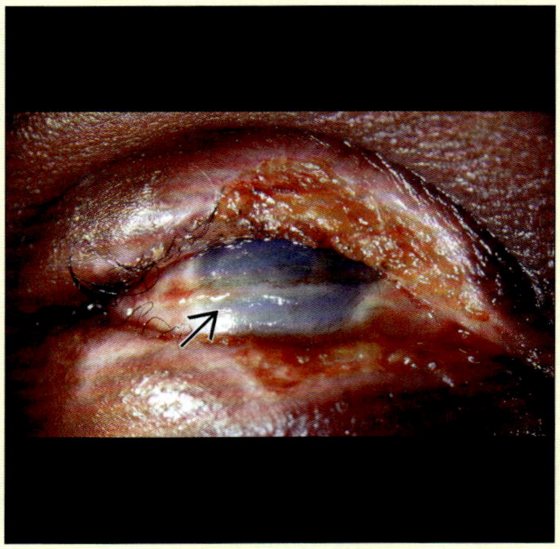

THERMAL/ULTRAVIOLET KERATOPATHY

INTRODUCTION

Definitions

- Injuries secondary to radiant energy
  - Ultraviolet (UV) keratopathy: Injury to cornea due to UV radiation
  - Thermal keratopathy: Thermal burn injury to cornea

DEMOGRAPHICS

Etiology/Risk Factors

- UV keratopathy
  - Most common cause of ocular radiation injury
  - Most visible light is transmitted through cornea, but as light wavelengths decrease, greater amounts of UV light are absorbed
    - High-energy photons in short UV light wavelengths inhibit mitosis, damage cells via photochemical reactions in nucleic acids and proteins, and loosen the epithelial layer
    - Cornea is most sensitive to damage at 260-280 nm wavelengths
    - Epithelial damage is cumulative
  - Mechanism of injury
    - Unprotected sun exposure, either directly or from highly reflective snow (snow blindness); arc welding; electrical sparks; and suntanning beds
    - Injury prevention: Eye protection with welding goggles and helmet, sunglasses, snow goggles that block UV light
- Thermal keratopathy
  - Flame burns: Corneal injury caused by fire, radiant heat, or flash burns
    - Commonly involve face and eyelids; corneal damage less common due to rapid-reflex eyelid closure, Bell phenomenon, and thermal insulation by eyelids
  - Contact burns: More common corneal injury caused by contact with hot objects or liquids
  - Clinical presentation depends on temperature of causative agent, duration of exposure to heat source, and area of cornea affected

Epidemiology

- 20% of significant facial burns involve eyes
- 31% of eye burn injuries involve cornea, and 7% of these result in permanent scarring
- Curling irons are frequent cause of corneal contact burns in United States

PRESENTATION

Symptoms

- Irritation, pain, photophobia, foreign body sensation, decreased corneal sensation
- UV keratopathy: Symptoms usually delayed 6-12 hours after exposure because of brief loss of corneal sensation; may be caused by photochemical injury

Exam Findings

- UV keratopathy
  - Loss of corneal light reflex
  - Lid edema and conjunctival hyperemia
  - Fluorescein staining shows rough epithelial surface with superficial punctate keratitis (SPK) erosions and defects covering area of cornea exposed to UV light
  - Lens involvement rare; only with intense exposure
- Thermal keratopathy
  - Mild burns
    - Stromal shrinkage, coagulation, and abrasion as epithelium sloughs
  - Severe burns (e.g., from molten metal or glass) involve deep corneal tissue layers
    - Cause tissue opacity with ground-glass appearance
    - Eschar formation with sloughing and tissue thinning
    - Corneal curvature change secondary to tissue remodeling

DIFFERENTIAL DIAGNOSIS

Conjunctivitis

- Inflammation of conjunctiva due to viruses, bacteria, or other irritants

Corneal Ulceration and Ulcerative Keratitis

- Mostly due to infectious causes, such as bacterial invasion of traumatic break in corneal epithelium; may be due to abrasion, foreign body, tear insufficiency, malnutrition, or contact lens overwear

Iritis and Uveitis

- Inflammation of iris, ciliary body, and choroid; caused by autoimmune disorders, infection, toxin exposure

TREATMENT

Medical

- Short-acting cycloplegic drop (cyclopentolate 0.5-1%) relieves pain from reflex ciliary spasm or iridocyclitis
- UV keratopathy
  - Topical anesthetic such as proparacaine 0.5% provides rapid pain relief, but frequent use retards epithelial healing; use only to facilitate eye exam
  - NSAIDs and bland ointment for pain management
  - Patch < 24 hours so reepithelialization is not delayed
- Thermal keratopathy
  - Short corticosteroid course may be necessary for treating iridocyclitis
  - Topical antibiotics to prevent infection and decrease risk of corneal ulcers

Surgical

- Thermal burns may require debridement of damaged and granulated tissue; full-thickness skin graft and tarsorrhaphy minimize eyelid scarring and ectropion

Prognosis

- UV keratopathy: Reepithelialization usually occurs within 36-72 hours; long-term sequelae rare
- Thermal keratopathy: Severe burns can cause permanent scarring

SELECTED REFERENCES

1. Roberts JE: Ocular phototoxicity. J Photochem Photobiol B. 64(2-3):136-43, 2001

CORNEAL NEOVASCULARIZATION

Key Facts

Introduction

- In-growth of blood vessels from the limbal vascular plexus into avascular cornea; occurs secondary to chronic hypoxia and inflammation

Demographics

- Cornea is naturally avascular and has an "angiogenic privilege" that is maintained by balance between antiangiogenic and angiogenic molecules
  - Chemical, mechanical, traumatic, degenerative, or infectious insults to eye trigger inflammatory and immune-mediated pathways that upregulate vascular endothelial growth factor (VEGF) expression, leading to growth of new vessels (neovessels) from the limbus into the corneal stroma

Presentation

- Superficial neovascularization
  - Single or multiple tortuous vessels seen in anterior stroma under low magnification
  - In-growth of vessels up to 4 mm into cornea
- Deep neovascularization
  - Caused by stromal vessels with branching pattern; may be accompanied by nerve fibers
  - In-growth of vessels > 4 mm into cornea

Treatment

- Topical corticosteroids are mainstay of neovascularization treatment; suppress actively proliferating corneal vessels with their anti-inflammatory properties and also inhibit proinflammatory cytokines
- Topical or subconjunctival anti-VEGF agents, such as bevacizumab, are useful adjunct to steroid treatment
- Surgical: Photodynamic therapy or superficial keratectomy ± amniotic membrane or limbal stem cell transplantation

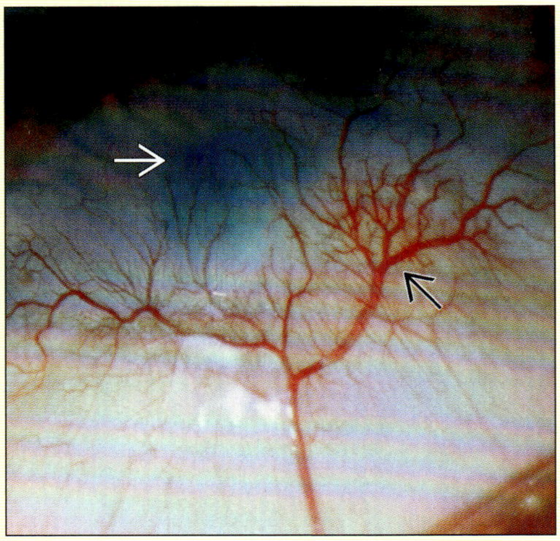

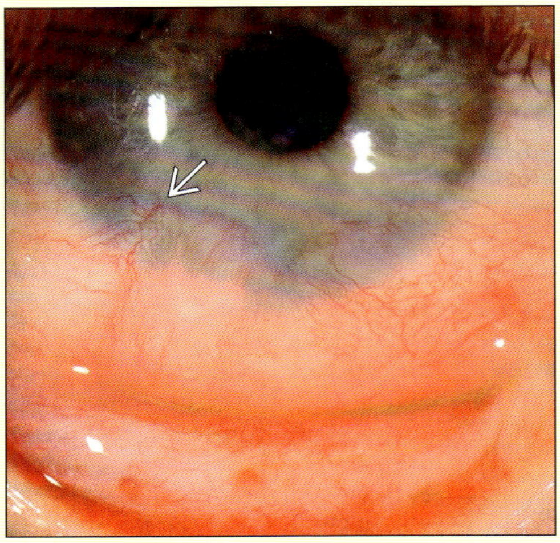

(Left) *Slit-lamp photo shows corneal scarring with conjunctival overgrowth and scarring ⇒ secondary to an alkali burn. Vascularization extends from the conjunctiva into the corneal stroma ⇒. An amniotic membrane graft is necessary to remove the conjunctival overgrowth from the cornea so that the surface of the eye can heal. (Courtesy K. Cohen, MD).* ***(Right)*** *Resolved epithelial HSV lesions at the limbus can cause marginal keratitis with limbal dendrites and neovascularization of underlying stroma ⇒.*

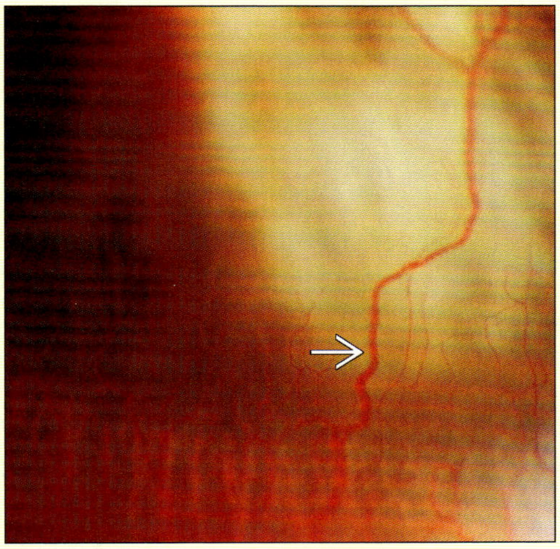

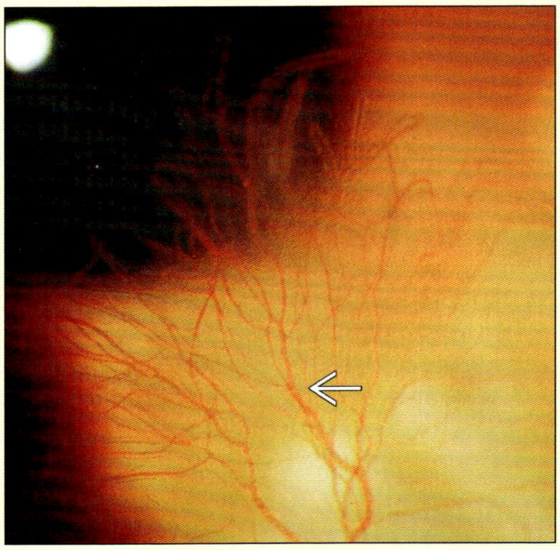

(Left) *Corneal NV begins with angiogenesis, in which new vessels form from the preexisting vascular network of the corneal limbus ⇒. This condition occurs when the balance between angiogenic and antiangiogenic factors tips toward upregulation of angiogenic factors.* ***(Right)*** *Deep stromal neovascularization occurs secondary to chronic hypoxia and can lead to active inflammation and a fibrovascular response, causing neovessels ⇒ to grow > 4 mm beyond the limbus and into the cornea.*

CORNEAL NEOVASCULARIZATION

INTRODUCTION

Abbreviations

- Neovascularization (NV)

Definitions

- In-growth of blood vessels from limbal vascular plexus into avascular cornea; occurs secondary to chronic hypoxia and inflammation

DEMOGRAPHICS

Etiology/Risk Factors

- Cornea is naturally avascular and has "angiogenic privilege," which is maintained by balance between antiangiogenic and angiogenic molecules
  - Ocular insults trigger inflammatory and immune-mediated pathways that upregulate vascular endothelial growth factor (VEGF) expression, leading to new vessel growth (neovessels) from limbus into corneal stroma
  - NV begins with vasodilation of limbal vessels and leukocytosis → upregulation of VEGF and other angiogenic molecules → vascular bud formation around the cornea → bud growth into neovessels, anastomosis into a network, and growth toward a site of corneal injury
- Risk factors
  - Contact lens overwear, infection, trauma, chemical burns, graft rejection, immunologic diseases, corneal degeneration
  - Anterior segment pathologies such as blepharitis, conjunctivitis, and keratitis
  - Intraocular conditions such as uveitis and glaucoma

Epidemiology

- 1.4 million patients in USA are at risk of developing NV
- 4% of USA population has corneal NV

PRESENTATION

Symptoms

- Redness, irritation, pain, tearing, photophobia, contact lens intolerance, blurry vision

Exam Findings

- Slit-lamp examination with direct illumination &/or retroillumination reveals vessels growing into cornea from the limbus
  - Superficial NV: Single or multiple tortuous vessels seen in anterior stroma under low magnification
    - In-growth of vessels up to 4 mm into cornea
    - Most common with contact lens wear; also occurs in blepharitis, superior limbic keratoconjunctivitis, and vernal conjunctivitis
  - Deep NV: Caused by stromal vessels with branching pattern; may be accompanied by nerve fibers
    - In-growth of vessels > 4 mm into cornea
    - Occur secondary to chronic inflammation (e.g., contact lens overwear, blepharoconjunctivitis, keratitis, chemical injuries, graft rejection)
  - Lipid deposition may appear as yellow-white opacities around or in front of stromal vessels
- Gonioscopy to examine iris angle for NV
- Test corneal sensation if there is concern for HSV keratitis; contact lens-related NV does not reduce corneal sensation whereas HSV keratitis does

DIFFERENTIAL DIAGNOSIS

Infectious

- Diseases: HSV keratitis, HZV keratitis, syphilis, candidiasis, aspergillosis, onchocerciasis

Inflammatory

- Graft rejection, papulopustular rosacea, Stevens-Johnson syndrome, graft-vs.-host disease, pemphigoid, atopic conjunctivitis

Traumatic

- Alkali burns, contact lenses, ulceration

Degenerative

- Terrien marginal degeneration, pterygium, aniridia

TREATMENT

Medical

- Topical corticosteroids are mainstay of NV treatment; suppress actively proliferating corneal vessels with their anti-inflammatory properties and also inhibit proinflammatory cytokines
  - Long-term side effects include glaucoma and cataracts
  - Examples: Hydrocortisone, cortisone, dexamethasone, prednisone, and triamcinolone acetonide
- Topical or subconjunctival anti-VEGF agents, such as bevacizumab, are useful adjunct to steroid treatment
  - Bevacizumab is most effective on acutely developing neovessels that are still dependent on VEGF for growth

Surgical

- Photodynamic therapy (PDT)
  - Photosensitizing agent is injected into systemic circulation or applied topically to eye; a laser beam activates agent and allows for selective occlusion of vessels in which photosensitizing agent has accumulated
- Superficial keratectomy
  - Corneal epithelium and superficial vessels are scraped with a blade, leaving Bowman layer intact; subconjunctival bevacizumab is injected next to neovessel
  - Amniotic membrane or limbal stem cell transplantation also helps restore the ocular surface by decreasing angiogenic stimuli and increasing antiangiogenic factors

SELECTED REFERENCES

1. Gupta D et al: Treatments for corneal neovascularization: a review. Cornea. 30(8):927-38, 2011
2. Maddula S et al: Horizons in therapy for corneal angiogenesis. Ophthalmology. 118(3):591-9, 2011
3. Qazi Y et al: Mediators of ocular angiogenesis. J Genet. 88(4):495-515, 2009
4. Chang JH et al: Corneal neovascularization. Curr Opin Ophthalmol. 12(4):242-9, 2001

BULLOUS KERATOPATHY

Key Facts

Introduction

- Persistent and irreversible corneal edema with epithelial or subepithelial bullae due to endothelial dysfunction

Demographics

- Estimates show an incidence of 0.1% of patients undergoing cataract will develop pseudophakic bullous keratopathy (PBK)

Presentation

- Poor vision &/or halos
- Bullae rupture results in pain, photophobia, and epiphora

Evaluation/Work-Up

- Cell density < 300-500 cells/mm² typically results in corneal edema
- Permanent corneal edema is observed when central pachymetry is > 590 microns in a pseudophakic eye

Treatment

- Topical hypertonic saline solutions (5% NaCl ointment/drops) improve vision; albumin and dextran are alternatives
- Extended-wear hydrophilic contact lenses alleviate pain associated with epithelial bullae and improve vision by smoothing the corneal surface
- Reduce IOP if needed
- Monitor acute ruptured bullae every 24-48 hours until epithelium heals; if no acute signs, follow-up every 1-6 months
- Descemet stripping automated endothelial keratoplasty (DSAEK) or penetrating keratoplasty (PKP)
- Intraocular lens (IOL) explantation/exchange (especially if there is an anterior chamber IOL)
- Prognosis is determined by the patient's visual acuity and functional capacity

*(**Left**) Slit-lamp photograph shows pseudophakic bullous keratopathy. Note the presence of the anterior chamber IOL. There is diffuse corneal edema with a large epithelial defect, likely from a ruptured bullae. (**Right**) This light micrograph of a corneal button shows a separation ➡ between the epithelium and the Bowman layer indicative of a corneal bullae (H&E, original magnification 200x). Note the folds in the Descemet membrane ➡ along with a markedly attenuated endothelium ⇨.*

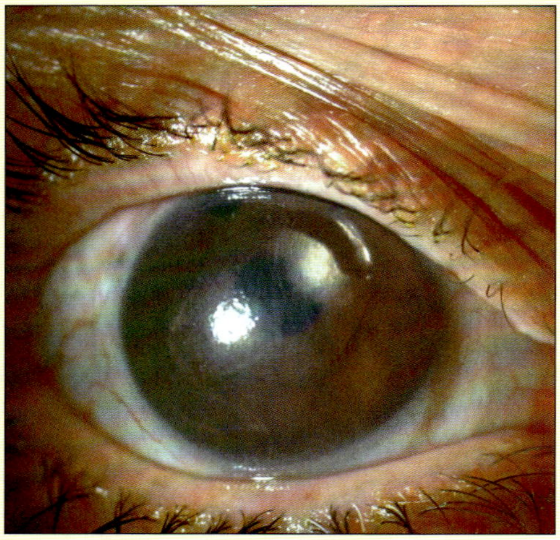

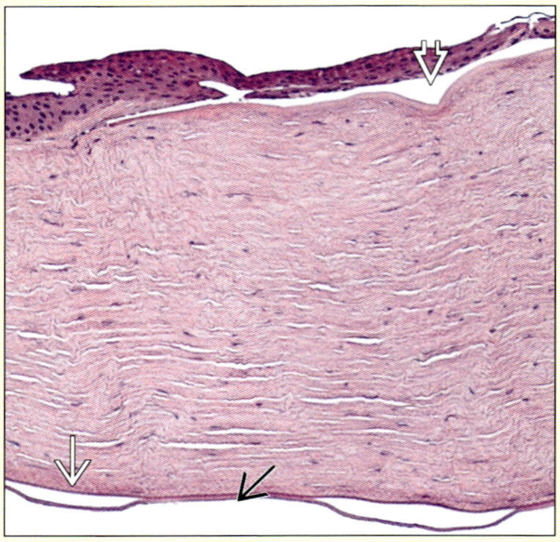

*(**Left**) Slit-lamp photo demonstrates pseudophakic bullous keratopathy induced by an anterior chamber IOL. Note the diffuse corneal edema and multiple folds in the Descemet membrane. (**Right**) Slit-lamp photo demonstrates the increased corneal thickness highlighted by the slit-beam. Note the diffuse corneal edema, folds in the Descemet membrane, and roughened corneal surface, likely due to bullae or epithelial defects.*

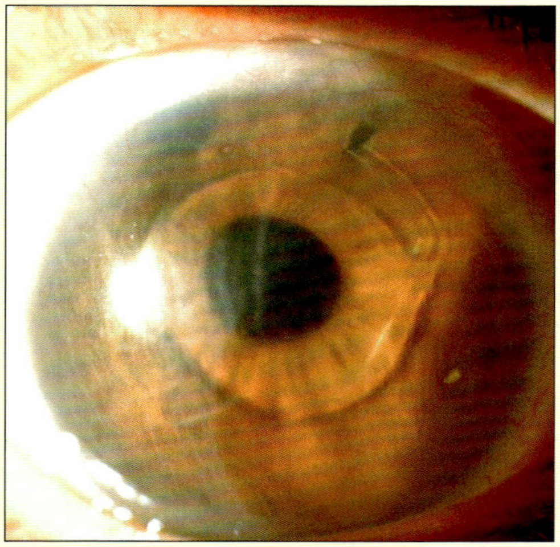

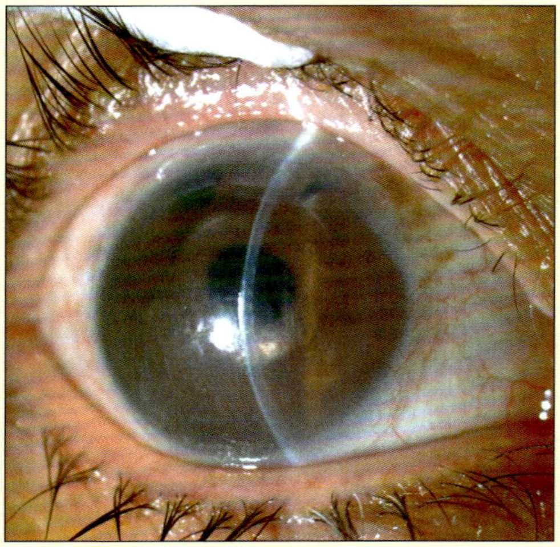

BULLOUS KERATOPATHY

INTRODUCTION

Abbreviations

- Bullous keratopathy (BK)

Definitions

- Irreversible corneal edema with epithelial/subepithelial bullae due to endothelial dysfunction

Subtypes

- Pseudophakic BK (PBK)
  - Corneal edema due to endothelial damage caused by cataract surgery or malposition of the IOL
- Aphakic BK (ABK)
  - Corneal edema resulting from endothelial dysfunction caused by surgical trauma during lens extraction

DEMOGRAPHICS

Etiology/Risk Factors

- Endothelial cells normally maintain the cornea in a relatively dehydrated state; dysfunctional endothelial cells result in corneal swelling of all layers
- Endothelial disease/dystrophy or cell loss
- Intraoperative endothelial cell trauma
- Specific IOLs have a higher risk of PBK
  - Iris-sutured IOLs
  - Anterior chamber lenses with closed-loop haptics
- Excessive inflammation or prolonged increased intraocular pressure (IOP), postoperatively
- Pseudoexfoliation syndrome

Epidemiology

- Estimated 0.1% of patients undergoing cataract will develop PBK

PRESENTATION

Symptoms

- Poor vision &/or halos
- Discomfort, pain, &/or foreign body sensation

Exam Findings

- Slit-lamp exam
  - Folds in Descemet membrane
  - Diffuse corneal thickening
  - Edematous epithelial layer
  - Vesicles and bullae on the corneal surface

DIFFERENTIAL DIAGNOSIS

Postoperative Corneal Edema

- Surgical trauma: Instruments, IOL, irrigating solutions, ultrasonic vibrations, nuclear fragments, prior surgery

Endothelial Disease

- Fuchs endothelial dystrophy, posterior polymorphous dystrophy, congenital hereditary endothelial syndrome

Toxic Anterior Segment Syndrome

- Preservatives, residual detergents on instruments, incorrect solutions/concentrations

EVALUATION/WORK-UP

Pathology

- Bullae may rupture with subsequent corneal nerve ending exposure that manifests as pain
- Histopathology
  - Markedly attenuated endothelium
  - Bullous detachments between the epithelium and Bowman layer
  - Desquamating epithelial cells with hydropic changes

Imaging

- Pachymetry measures corneal thickness
  - Permanent corneal edema is observed when central pachymetry is > 590 microns in a pseudophakic eye
- Endothelial specular microscopy can determine endothelial cell counts and cell morphology
  - Cell density < 300-500 cells/mm² typically results in corneal edema

TREATMENT

Medical

- Topical hypertonic saline solutions help dehydrate the cornea and improve vision
  - 5% NaCl ointment/drops
  - Albumin 5%; dextran 10% or 20% are alternatives
- Extended-wear hydrophilic contact lenses can alleviate pain associated with epithelial bullae and improve vision by smoothing the corneal surface
  - Careful monitoring is necessary as there is an increased risk of corneal infection with these extended-wear hydrophilic contact lenses
- Reduce IOP if needed

Surgical

- Pain management
  - Conjunctival flap or amniotic membrane
  - Cauterization of Bowman layer
  - Anterior stromal micropuncture and phototherapeutic keratectomy
- Descemet stripping automated endothelial keratoplasty (DSAEK) or penetrating keratoplasty (PKP)
- IOL explantation/exchange (especially if there is anterior chamber IOL)

Follow-Up

- Acute ruptured bullae should be monitored every 24-48 hours until the epithelial defect heals
- If no acute signs, follow-up every 1-6 months, depending on symptoms

Prognosis

- Determined by patient's visual acuity and functional capacity

SELECTED REFERENCES

1. Sheldon CA et al: Correlation of clinical and pathologic diagnoses of corneal disease in penetrating keratoplasties in Vancouver: a 10-year review. Can J Ophthalmol. 47(1):5-10, 2012
2. Mamalis N: Explantation of intraocular lenses. Curr Opin Ophthalmol. 11(4):289-95, 2000

DELLEN

Key Facts

Introduction
- Small, localized excavation at peripheral cornea margin

Demographics
- Associated with paralimbal elevations or abnormal blinking
- Most often occurs as postoperative complication with excessive or elevated limbal tissue
- Causes include
  - Pterygia
  - Pingueculae
  - Dermoids
  - Filtering blebs
  - Chemosis
  - Pyogenic granulomas

Presentation
- Enhanced fluorescein pooling at corneal depression
- Epithelium is intact
- Usually there is a small elevation in juxtalimbal conjunctiva impairing tear film coverage

Treatment
- Corneal lubrication with artificial tears and ointment
- Patching and contact lenses can reduce elevation and irritation
- Typically resolves rapidly with appropriate lubrication and patching
- Can consider
  - Vitamin C orally
  - Oral doxycycline
  - Topical medroxyprogesterone
- Remove or treat primary cause of dellen

*(**Left**) This external photograph depicts a large conjunctival nevus ➡ with a resulting dellen ⇨. The elevation from nevi is a common cause of dellen. (**Right**) This slit-lamp photograph shows a closer view of the nevus with associated dellen from the previous image. Note the pooling of Rose Bengal stain in the dellen ➡. Pooling of stain such as this is a characteristic feature of dellen.*

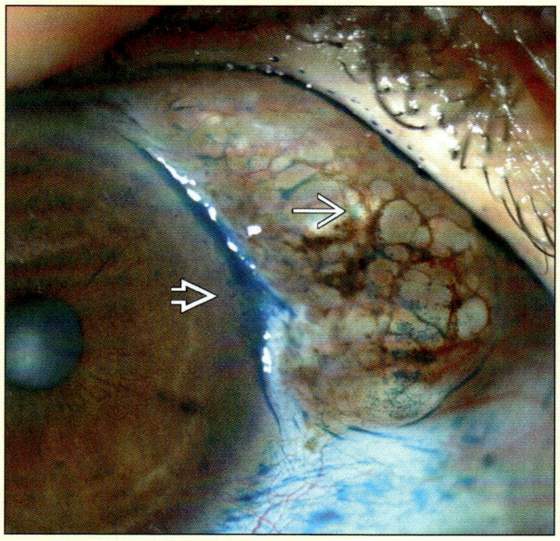

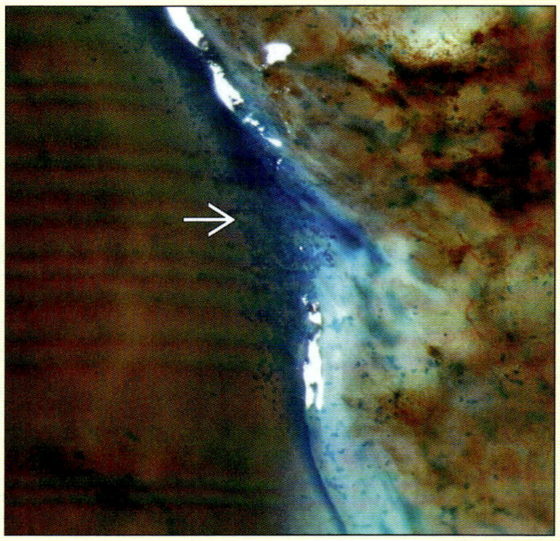

*(**Left**) This external photograph depicts a dermoid cyst that encroaches on the cornea →. Dermoids are a common cause of dellen. (**Right**) H&E light micrograph of a dellen shows the shallow excavation and dehydration of the cornea at a site with previous trauma (likely an incision or suture site) with focally thinned stroma. Epithelial break is artifactual change from processing the tissue.*

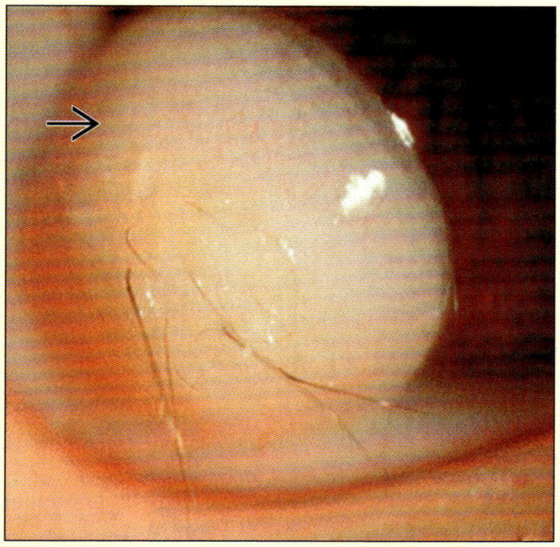

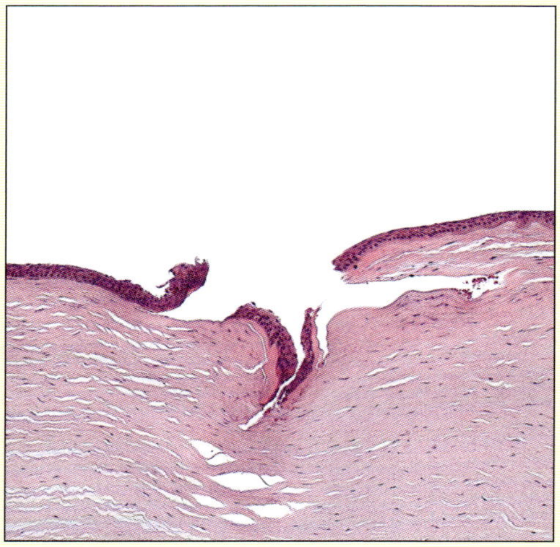

DELLEN

INTRODUCTION

Definitions

- Small, localized excavation at peripheral cornea margin

DEMOGRAPHICS

Etiology/Risk Factors

- Associated with paralimbal elevations or abnormal blinking with impaired tear film coverage
  - Associated raised limbal lesions include
    - Pterygia
    - Pingueculae
    - Dermoids
    - Filtering blebs
    - Chemosis
    - Pyogenic granulomas

Epidemiology

- Most often occurs as postoperative complication with excessive or elevated limbal tissue

PRESENTATION

Symptoms

- Pain or foreign body sensation

Exam Findings

- Slit lamp
  - Appears as a divot with abrupt elevation and hazy base
  - Region of opaque or clear, thin, epithelialized cornea
  - Typically observed in peripheral cornea
  - Enhanced fluorescein pooling at corneal depression

DIFFERENTIAL DIAGNOSIS

Corneal Arcus

- Opaque circumferential deposition of lipid in corneal stroma at limbus

Terrien Marginal Degeneration

- Progressive, bilateral, asymmetrical corneal thinning disorder
- Progresses from fine stromal lipid deposition to circumferential thinning with mild vascularization

Mooren Ulcer

- Idiopathic, noninfectious, progressive ulceration of peripheral cornea

Pellucid Marginal Degeneration

- Progressive, bilateral, noninflammatory, peripheral corneal thinning disorder
- Inferior cornea shows a peripheral band of thinning with surrounding corneal ectasia

Rheumatoid Arthritis

- Typically causes limbal guttering
  - ± neovascularization
- Systemic diagnosis is usually already present
- There is usually an epithelial defect

EVALUATION/WORK-UP

Pathology

- Inadequate tear coverage
  - Causes tissue dehydration and thinning
- Occurs most often following procedures involving a paralimbal elevation
  - Paralimbal elevation induces break in precorneal oily tear layer
    - Results in focal dehydration and subsequent corneal thinning
- Epithelium is intact
  - Fluorescein will confirm pooling, not punctate staining, because epithelial layer is not degenerating

TREATMENT

Medical

- Corneal lubrication
  - Artificial tears and ointment
- Patching and contact lenses
  - Can help to reduce elevation and irritation
- Additional treatments to consider
  - Vitamin C
    - 1,000 mg p.o. q.i.d.
  - Doxycycline
    - 100 mg p.o. b.i.d.
  - Medroxyprogesterone can be helpful
    - 1% drops q.i.d.

Surgical

- Remove or treat primary cause of dellen

Prognosis

- Typically resolves rapidly with appropriate lubrication and patching

SELECTED REFERENCES

1. Ono T et al: Ocular surface complications after trabeculectomy: incidence, risk factors, time course and prognosis. Ophthalmologica. 230(2):93-9, 2013
2. Kymionis GD et al: Treatment of corneal dellen with a large diameter soft contact lens. Cont Lens Anterior Eye. 34(6):290-2, 2011
3. Moshirfar M et al: Salzmann's-like nodular degeneration following laser in situ keratomileusis. J Cataract Refract Surg. 31(10):2021-5, 2005
4. Lee DH et al: Scleral dellen after bilateral adjustable suture medial rectus muscle resection. J AAPOS. 7(3):221-2, 2003
5. Baum JL et al: On the nature of dellen. Arch Ophthalmol. 79(6):657-62, 1968

KERATOCONUS

Key Facts

Introduction

- Bilateral noninflammatory corneal ectasia due to central or paracentral corneal thinning

Demographics

- Unknown etiology, with multifactorial genetic and environmental contributors
  - Eye rubbing and contact lens wear implicated

Presentation

- Irregular astigmatism: Best corrected visual acuity worse than 20/20 in moderate to advanced disease
- Central or paracentral corneal thinning: Leads to conical corneal protrusion

Differential Diagnosis

- Pellucid marginal degeneration: Corneal thinning occurs inferiorly, close to the limbus, with corneal protrusion above area of thinning
- Terrien marginal degeneration: May have superior or inferior corneal thinning adjacent to limbus

Evaluation/Work-Up

- Computerized corneal topography/tomography

Treatment

- Rigid gas-permeable contact lenses improve visual acuity caused by irregular astigmatism and ectasia
- Intracorneal ring segments may improve visual acuity in rigid gas-permeable-intolerant patients and delay need for corneal transplant
- Corneal cross-linking with riboflavin and UVA light may delay progression
- Penetrating keratoplasty is definitive treatment for advanced disease or corneal scarring; DALK is emerging as alternative with less long-term rejection
  - 93-96% success rate with very low recurrence rate

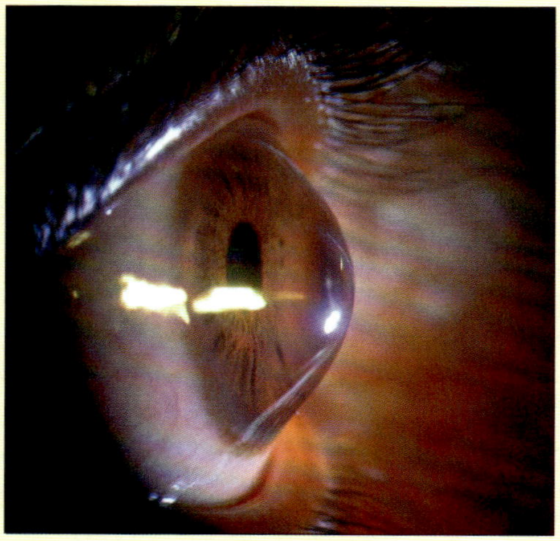

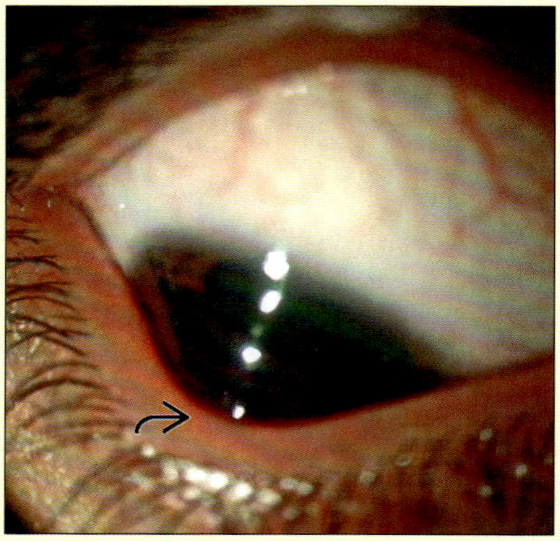

(Left) *In keratoconus, as the name implies, corneal thinning causes a central conical corneal protrusion that severely limits vision secondary to irregular astigmatism. (Courtesy W. Nosé, MD.)* ***(Right)*** *The conical cornea causes a pronounced V-shaped indentation of the lower eyelid on downgaze →, called Munson sign. Other diagnostic findings include central or paracentral stromal thinning, Rizzuti sign, Fleischer ring, Vogt striae, and anterior stromal scars. (Courtesy W. Nosé, MD.)*

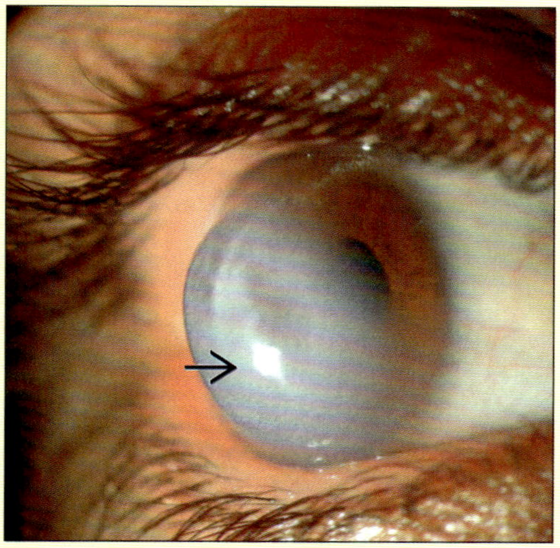

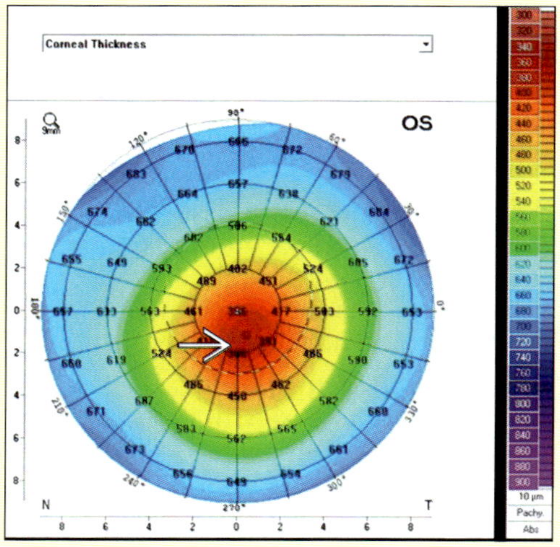

(Left) *Acute corneal hydrops → in a patient with keratoconus. Hydrops is an acute decompensation of the cornea secondary to tears in Descemet allowing imbibition of aqueous into corneal stroma. Hydrops may last for weeks to months and may result in corneal scarring. Hypertonic saline drops may be used to speed resolution. (Courtesy W. Nosé, MD.)* ***(Right)*** *Pentacam pachymetric map shows inferior central corneal thinning, which corresponds to area of greatest steepening →.*

KERATOCONUS

INTRODUCTION

Abbreviations

- Keratoconus (KC or KCN)

Definitions

- Bilateral noninflammatory corneal ectasia due to central or paracentral corneal thinning

Subtypes

- Forme fruste keratoconus: Preclinical keratoconus with early topographic changes

DEMOGRAPHICS

Etiology/Risk Factors

- Unknown etiology, with multifactorial genetic and environmental contributors
  - Positive family history in 6-10% of patients
  - Associated with Down syndrome, Marfan syndrome, mitral valve prolapse, atopy, Leber congenital amaurosis, sleep apnea, floppy eyelid syndrome
  - Eye rubbing and contact lens wear implicated
- Onset in early adolescence, stabilizes by age 30-40

Epidemiology

- ~ 1 per 2,000

PRESENTATION

Symptoms

- Decreased vision, progressive increase in myopia and astigmatism, sudden onset of pain accompanied by vision loss in acute hydrops

Exam Findings

- Irregular astigmatism: Best corrected visual acuity worse than 20/20 in moderate to advanced disease; can lead to scissoring on retinoscopic evaluation of red reflex
- Central or paracentral corneal thinning: Leads to conical corneal protrusion
- Munson sign: V-shaped eyelid contour on downgaze
- Rizzuti sign: Sharply focused beam of light in nasal limbus produced by lateral illumination of cornea
- Fleischer ring: Basal epithelial iron line around cone, most common inferiorly
- Vogt striae: Vertical lines in Descemet that disappear with digital pressure
- Oil droplet sign: Found on retroillumination
- Hydrops: Corneal edema secondary to breaks in Descemet membrane

DIFFERENTIAL DIAGNOSIS

Pellucid Marginal Degeneration (PMD)

- Corneal thinning occurs inferiorly, close to limbus, with corneal protrusion above area of thinning

Terrien Marginal Degeneration

- May have superior or inferior corneal thinning adjacent to limbus; usually accompanies pannus formation and lipid deposition, differentiating it from PMD

EVALUATION/WORK-UP

Pathology

- Histopathologic examination may show stromal thinning and breaks in Bowman layer, breaks in Descemet with endothelial scrolling, new endothelium, stromal scarring

Imaging

- Keratometry: Increased central corneal Ks above 47.2 and inter-eye asymmetry of > 2 D are suggestive of KC
- Computerized corneal topography/tomography
  - Shows central or paracentral thinning
  - I:S ratio (inferior vs. superior corneal asymmetry) > 1.4
  - Advanced software algorithms for early detection available; allows for enhanced screening; especially useful for refractive surgery patients

TREATMENT

Medical

- Discourage eye rubbing or treat underlying atopic/allergic condition
- Rigid gas-permeable (RGP) contact lenses: Used for vision that can no longer be spectacle corrected
  - Piggyback lenses (hard on top of soft) or soft permeable lenses (soft skirt, hard center) are good alternatives as well if RGP lenses do not stay in
- Corneal cross-linking with riboflavin and UVA light shows promise in delaying progression
- Hypertonic saline drops, injection of SF6 gas into anterior chamber, and bandage contact lens: Decrease edema and improve comfort for acute hydrops
  - SF6 usually treats hydrops within 1-2 weeks whereas it might take ≥ 8 weeks to recover on its own

Surgical

- Intracorneal ring segments (Intacs) may improve visual acuity in RGP-intolerant patients and delay need for corneal transplant
- Penetrating keratoplasty (PK): Definitive treatment for advanced disease or corneal scarring; need to remove all diseased tissue (so typically decenter trephine inferiorly)
  - 10-20% of KC patients eventually require PK
  - 93-96% success rate with very low recurrence rate
  - Deep anterior lamellar keratoplasty (sparing of Descemet and endothelium) decreases rejection

Follow-Up

- Depends on severity; every 6-12 months for mild disease, every 1-2 weeks for patients with hydrops

Prognosis

- Excellent prognosis
- Very low recurrence rate in graft after PK

SELECTED REFERENCES

1. Sugar J et al: What causes keratoconus? Cornea. 31(6):716-9, 2012
2. Rabinowitz YS: Keratoconus. Surv Ophthalmol. 42(4):297-319, 1998
3. Krachmer JH et al: Keratoconus and related noninflammatory corneal thinning disorders. Surv Ophthalmol. 28(4):293-322, 1984

PELLUCID MARGINAL DEGENERATION

Key Facts

Introduction

- Bilateral corneal ectatic disorder that causes inferior peripheral corneal thinning in crescent fashion from 4-o'clock to 8-o'clock positions

Presentation

- Inferior corneal thinning 1-2 mm wide and separated from limbus by 1-2 mm of clear, normal cornea
- Corneal bulge superior to area of thinning occurs from normal thickness cornea above and below area of PMD
  - Classic "beer belly" contour in side profile
- High, progressive, irregular astigmatism against the rule

Evaluation/Work-Up

- Corneal topography shows "butterfly" pattern with vertical flattening of cornea, inferior annular corneal steepening, and central astigmatism against the rule
- Pachymetry mapping reveals thinning

Treatment

- Mild cases corrected with glasses or contact lenses
- High irregular astigmatism may be treated with large-diameter, rigid, gas-permeable contact lenses, but stable, long-term fit is difficult to achieve due to contour abnormality
- Scleral lenses or hybrid lenses with rigid gas-permeable center and soft hydrophilic "skirt" may be successful
- Severe cases require surgical management: Large-diameter or eccentric penetrating keratoplasty close to the limbus is necessary to encompass area of peripheral thinning
  - This type of surgery is technically difficult, and graft is prone to rejection; collagen cross-linking is emerging therapy
- Patients with PMD are poor candidates for refractive surgery because of potential for poor outcome and risk of surgical procedure stimulating progressive ectasia

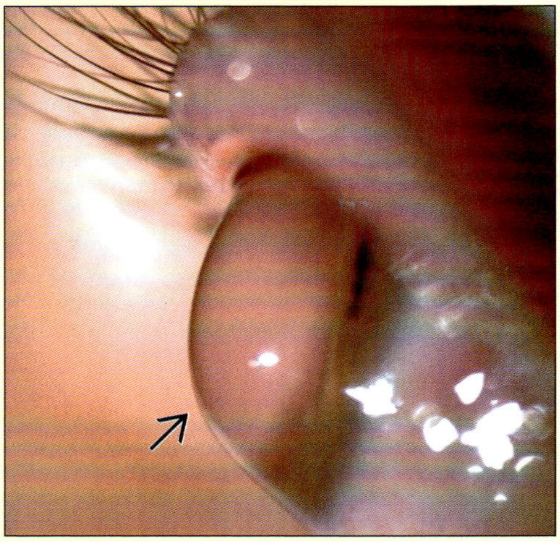
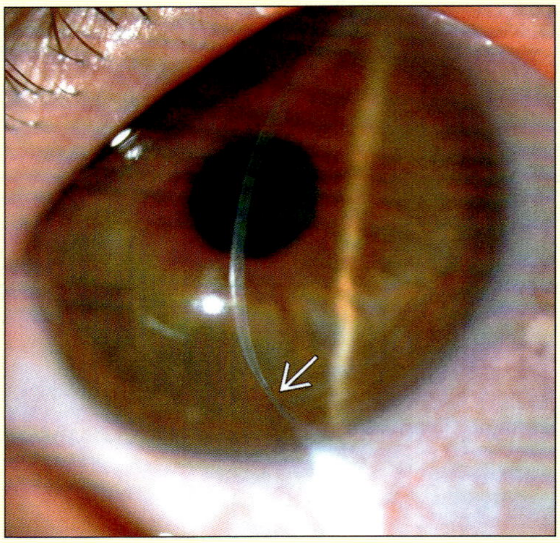

*(**Left**) The classic "beer belly" contour of pellucid marginal degeneration (PMD) can be seen in side profile ⇒. Normal-thickness cornea above and below the area of PMD creates a corneal bulge superior to the area of thinning. (Courtesy W. Nosé, MD.) (**Right**) PMD typically shows a peripheral band of thinning in inferior cornea from 4- to 8-o'clock positions. The narrowing of the slit-beam in the inferior cornea is 1-2 mm wide ➡ and is separated from the limbus by 1-2 mm of clear, normal cornea. (Courtesy W. Nosé, MD.)*

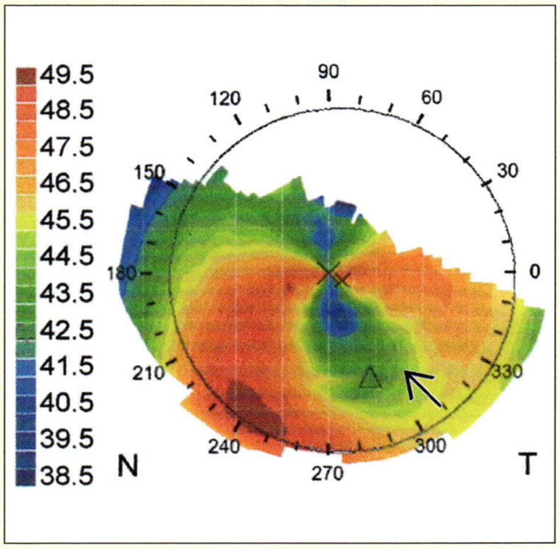

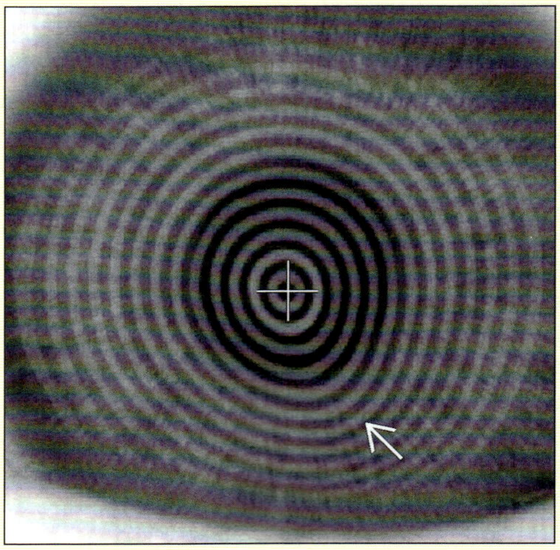

*(**Left**) Corneal topography usually shows the classic "crab claw" pattern ⇒ with flattening of the central cornea along a vertical axis, steepening of the inferior corneal periphery, and mid peripheral cornea gradually decreasing in power above the inferior oblique meridians. Pachymetry reveals thinning. (**Right**) Videokeratoscopy of PMD shows a typical pear-shaped pattern of light rings with compression of the inferior rings ➡. (Courtesy J. B. Baldwin, OD, PhD.)*

PELLUCID MARGINAL DEGENERATION

INTRODUCTION

Abbreviations

- Pellucid marginal degeneration (PMD)

Definitions

- Bilateral corneal ectatic disorder that causes inferior peripheral corneal thinning in crescent fashion from 4-o'clock to 8-o'clock positions

DEMOGRAPHICS

Etiology/Risk Factors

- Idiopathic; may be phenotypic variation of keratoconus &/or keratoglobus

Epidemiology

- Rare condition
- Onset between 2nd and 5th decades of life
- Higher incidence in males compared to females
- High astigmatism or ectasia on corneal topography have been described in asymptomatic family members of PMD patients
- Atypical cases: Unilateral or superior thinning; thinning beyond inferior 4-o'clock position

PRESENTATION

Symptoms

- Blurry and decreased vision from irregular astigmatism

Exam Findings

- Most commonly occurs bilaterally
- Inferior corneal thinning is 1-2 mm wide and separated from limbus by 1-2 mm of clear, normal cornea
- Corneal bulge superior to area of thinning occurs from normal thickness cornea above and below area of PMD
  - Classic "beer belly" contour in side profile
- No cone shape, inflammation, vascularization, scarring, iron ring, Fleischer ring, lipid deposition, or infiltrate present
- Descemet folds concentric with inferior limbus disappear with application of pressure to cornea
- Breaks in Descemet membrane above the area of progressive thinning can lead to acute hydrops
- High, progressive, irregular, against-the-rule astigmatism

DIFFERENTIAL DIAGNOSIS

Keratoconus

- Thinning and steepening of cornea; creates conical protrusion at area of maximal thinning
- Vogt striae, Fleischer ring, Munson sign, Rizutti phenomenon
- Differentiate from PMD by corneal topography and pachymetry

Keratoglobus

- Diffuse thinning of cornea, greatest in periphery
- No Vogt striae, scarring, Fleischer ring, lipid deposition, or corneal vascularization

Terrien Marginal Degeneration

- Marginal thinning begins superiorly and progresses circumferentially, extending to inferior cornea; creates furrow near limbus with lipid deposition
- High astigmatism from thinning of superior and inferior peripheral cornea and steepening of interpalpebral peripheral cornea

Mooren Ulcer

- Painful inflammatory thinning of peripheral cornea with epithelial defect and ulceration
- Scarring and vascularization with stromal thinning

Furrow Degeneration

- Bilateral, noninflammatory, occurs in elderly in arcus

EVALUATION/WORK-UP

Pathology

- Epithelium, Descemet membrane, and endothelium are typically normal
- Increased stromal mucopolysaccharides, breaks in Bowman layer, irregular arrangement of stroma
- Weakening of collagen in corneal stroma could underlie PMD-associated thinning

Imaging

- Corneal topography shows "butterfly" or "crab claw" pattern with vertical flattening of cornea, inferior annular corneal steepening, and central astigmatism against the rule
- Pachymetry mapping reveals thinning much inferior to the apex (unlike keratoconus where apex is the thinnest point)

TREATMENT

Medical

- Mild cases corrected with glasses or contact lenses
- High irregular astigmatism may be treated with large-diameter, rigid, gas-permeable contact lenses, but a stable, long-term fit is difficult to achieve
- Scleral lenses or hybrid lenses with rigid gas-permeable center and soft hydrophilic "skirt" may be successful

Surgical

- Severe cases require surgical management: Large-diameter or eccentric penetrating keratoplasty close to limbus is necessary to encompass peripheral thinning
  - Difficult, and graft is prone to rejection
- Patients with PMD are poor candidates for refractive surgery because of potential for poor outcome and risk that surgical procedure may worsen ectasia
- Alternative surgical procedures: Thermokeratoplasty, crescentic lamellar keratoplasty, epikeratoplasty, and crescentic or wedge excision
- Collagen cross-linking is emerging alternative

SELECTED REFERENCES

1. Jinabhai A et al: Pellucid corneal marginal degeneration: A review. Cont Lens Anterior Eye. 34(2):56-63, 2011
2. Tzelikis PF et al: Management of pellucid marginal corneal degeneration. Cornea. 24(5):555-60, 2005

TERRIEN MARGINAL DEGENERATION

Key Facts

Introduction
- Slowly progressive, idiopathic disorder that causes peripheral corneal thinning

Demographics
- Unknown etiology; most cases are noninflammatory
- Most commonly affects males 20-40 years of age

Presentation
- Asymptomatic peripheral corneal lesions
  - Typically bilateral, often asymmetric
- Starts at superonasal quadrant as fine, yellow-white punctate stromal opacities that can spread circumferentially around cornea
  - Lucid area between leading edge and limbus
- Followed by development of vascular pannus with lipid deposition and scarring at leading edge
- Thinning begins between lipid deposition and limbus
- Against-the-rule astigmatism typically develops

Evaluation/Work-Up
- Diagnosis usually made based on history and clinical exam
- Histologic examination demonstrates
  - Subepithelial fibrillar collagen degeneration
  - Histiocytes with phagocytized collagen material
- Corneal topography can aid in diagnosis

Treatment
- Vitamin C/doxycycline/topical medroxyprogesterone acetate to reduce melting risk
- Glasses or rigid contact lenses to treat astigmatism
- Surgery may be indicated for perforation, impending perforation, &/or severe astigmatism
  - Perforation occurs in ~ 15% of patients
- Glue + amniotic membrane may be alternatives to grafting
- Monitor regularly due to lifelong perforation risk
- Disease progression is typically slow

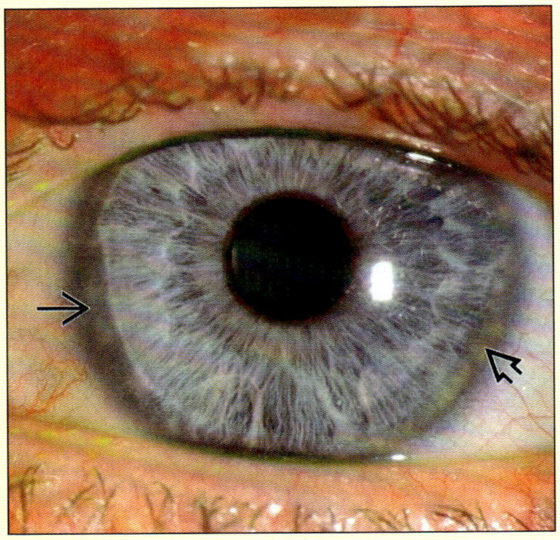
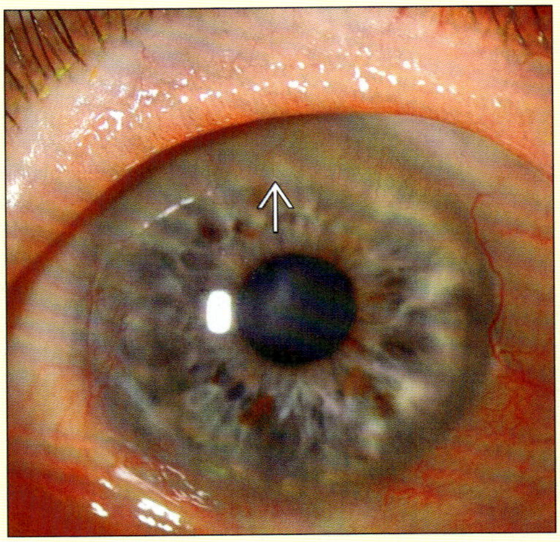

(Left) *This slit-lamp photo is of a patient with Terrien marginal degeneration with circumferential peripheral corneal thinning ⇨. The disease typically begins in the superonasal quadrant as a fine, yellow-white punctate stromal opacity that spreads circumferentially. A lucid area between the leading edge and limbus is seen →.* ***(Right)*** *This slit-lamp photo depicts an inflamed eye with circumferential peripheral thinning and vascular pannus formation, most severe in the superior cornea ➡.*

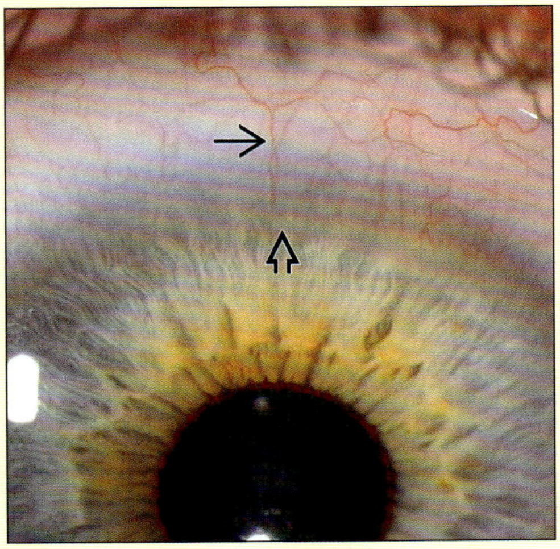
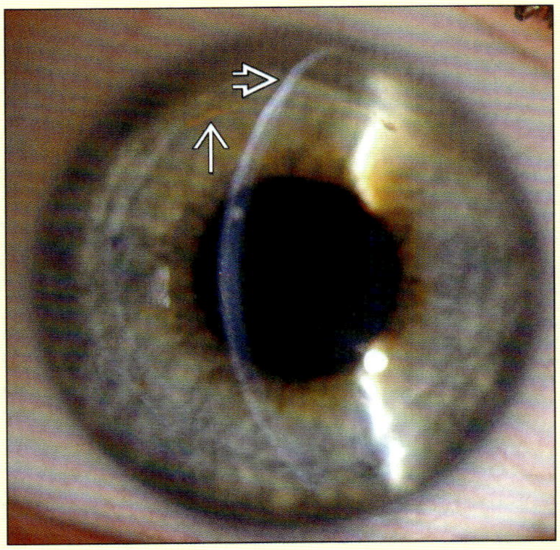

(Left) *This slit-lamp photo shows a vascular pannus, commonly associated with this disease ⇨. Superficial vascularization is seen from the limbal arcades extending to the lesion →.* ***(Right)*** *This slit-lamp photo demonstrates the peripheral corneal thinning that occurs in Terrien marginal degeneration. The slit-lamp beam ➡ clearly shows corneal thinning extending from the leading edge of the vascular pannus to the limbus. A lipid deposition ➡ can be seen at the leading edge.*

TERRIEN MARGINAL DEGENERATION

INTRODUCTION

Definitions

- Slowly progressive, idiopathic disorder that causes peripheral corneal thinning with associated lipid deposition and vascularization

DEMOGRAPHICS

Etiology/Risk Factors

- Unknown etiology
- Majority of cases are noninflammatory
  - Some inflammatory cases have been reported
    - Mainly in younger age groups
- Has been associated with posterior polymorphic dystrophy, erythema elevatum diutinum, and anterior basement membrane dystrophy

Epidemiology

- Can occur at any age, but most commonly affects those 10-40 years of age
- M:F = 3:1
- Up to 1/3 of cases are inflammatory

PRESENTATION

Symptoms

- Asymptomatic peripheral corneal lesions
  - Typically bilateral but often asymmetric
- Inflammatory cases can present with painful, recurrent episodes of scleritis or episcleritis
- Decreased visual acuity in advanced cases

Exam Findings

- Starts at superonasal quadrant as fine, yellow-white punctate stromal opacities that can spread circumferentially around cornea
  - Lucid area between leading edge and limbus
- Followed by development of vascular pannus with lipid deposition and scarring at leading edge
  - Superficial vascularization is found from limbal arcades extending to lesion
- Epithelium remains intact
- Thinning begins between lipid deposition and limbus
- Against-the-rule astigmatism typically develops
- Progressive thinning leads to peripheral gutter with steep central edge and gently sloped peripheral edge
- Other possible findings include corneal ectasia, corneal hydrops, pseudopterygia, and perforation
  - Perforation rarely occurs spontaneously but can occur with minor trauma

DIFFERENTIAL DIAGNOSIS

Mooren Ulcer

- Rapidly progressive, nonpurulent, inflammatory, painful peripheral corneal ulcer
- Findings include epithelial cell loss and an overhanging ledge of tissue extending from central margin

Pellucid Marginal Degeneration

- Painless, inferior peripheral corneal thinning

Marginal Furrow Degeneration

- Painless avascular degeneration with mild, or absent, corneal thinning peripheral to arcus senilis

EVALUATION/WORK-UP

Labs

- Diagnosis usually made based on history and clinical exam

Pathology

- Histologic examination demonstrates
  - Subepithelial fibrillar collagen degeneration
  - Histiocytes with phagocytized collagen material
  - Evidence of increased lysosomal activity
  - Thick, thin, or normal epithelium
  - Fragmented or absent Bowman layer
  - Possible break in Descemet membrane

Imaging

- Corneal topography can aid in diagnosis

TREATMENT

Medical

- Vitamin C 1 g q.i.d. and doxycycline 100 mg p.o. b.i.d. may slow down thinning; topical medroxyprogesterone acetate may be of benefit
- Use glasses or rigid contact lenses to treat astigmatism
  - Soft bandage lens with rigid gas-permeable lens piggyback may be necessary due to astigmatism
  - Safety glasses should be worn if thinning is severe
- Inflammatory cases should be treated with topical lubricants and mild steroids
  - Steroids should be used with caution because of increased risk of corneal thinning

Surgical

- Surgery may be indicated for perforation, impending perforation, &/or severe astigmatism
  - Crescent-shaped lamellar or full-thickness patch grafts are often utilized
    - Large eccentric full-thickness grafts may also be used but carry increased risk of rejection
- Corneal glue + amniotic membrane may be alternatives to large corneal surgeries

Follow-Up

- Monitor regularly due to lifelong perforation risk

Prognosis

- Disease progression is typically slow
- Usually can be managed with glasses/contact lenses
- Perforation occurs in ~ 15% of patients

SELECTED REFERENCES

1. Wagoner MD et al: Terrien's marginal degeneration associated with posterior polymorphous dystrophy. Cornea. 18(5):612-5, 1999
2. Beauchamp GR: Terrien's marginal corneal degeneration. J Pediatr Ophthalmol Strabismus. 19(2):97-9, 1982
3. Austin P et al: Inflammatory Terrien's marginal corneal disease. Am J Ophthalmol. 92(2):189-92, 1981

PTERYGIUM/PINGUECULA

Key Facts

Introduction
- Pterygium: Wing-shaped mass of fibrovascular, degenerative bulbar conjunctival tissue extending across limbus onto cornea
- Pinguecula: Benign, whitish-yellow, elevated bulbar conjunctival mass composed of degenerating subepithelial stromal collagen fibers

Demographics
- Caused by actinic UV radiation exposure and microtrauma from wind, sand, dust, surface dryness

Presentation
- Usually asymptomatic, but inflammation can cause dryness, redness, irritation, foreign body sensation
- Located in interpalpebral zone; more frequently found at nasal rather than temporal limbus; pinguecula does not cross limbus whereas pterygium does

Evaluation/Work-Up
- Histopathology demonstrates excessive elastin production by damaged fibroblasts and abnormal maturation and degeneration of collagen fibers

Treatment
- Medical
  - Acute inflammation can be treated with lubricant eyedrops, topical corticosteroids, or topical NSAIDs
- Surgical
  - Pterygium: Surgery necessary when medical management fails, pterygium interferes with visual axis, or for cosmetic purposes; various surgical techniques available
  - Pinguecula: Excised if chronic inflammation present, lesion interferes with contact lens wear, or for cosmetic reasons

__(Left)__ Slit-lamp photo shows yellow, fleshy, raised pinguecula in interpalpebral zone of conjunctiva at 8-o'clock position →. Lesion does not cross the limbus of the cornea and does not affect vision but may cause irritation and foreign body sensation if it becomes elevated. __(Right)__ Slit-lamp photo at higher magnification shows elevation of pinguecula →. Significant elevation close to the limbus can interfere with contact lens wear due to edge lift.

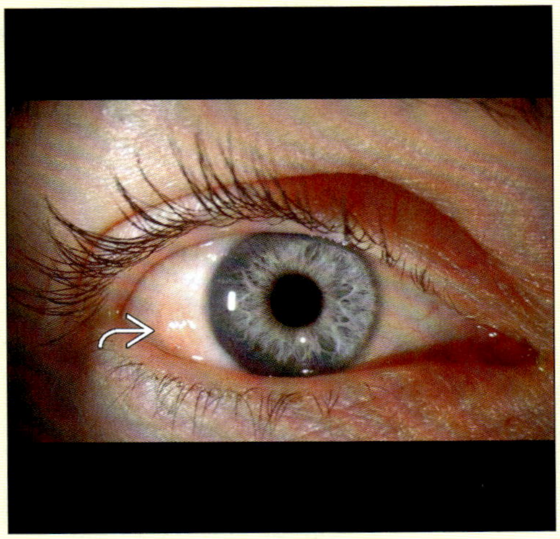

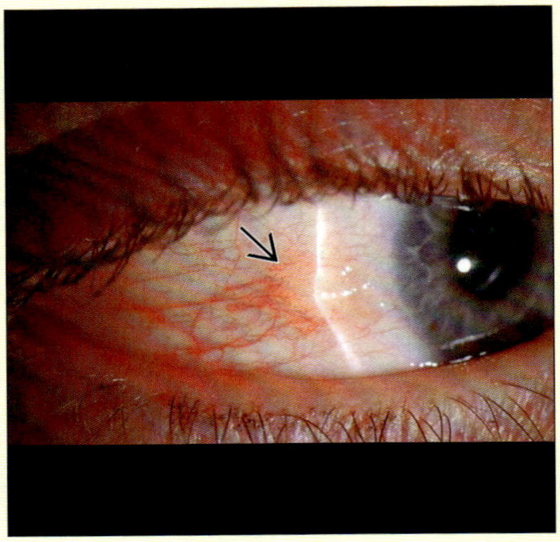

__(Left)__ Slit-lamp photo shows fibrovascular pterygium with triangular shape →. The head extends past the limbus and onto the cornea. At higher magnification, a chronic lesion would have a pigmented epithelial iron line anterior to the cap. __(Right)__ Slit-lamp photo shows a large, vascular pterygium extending from the nasal interpalpebral conjunctiva, crossing the limbus, and encroaching on the visual axis →. A pterygium this large can affect the shape of the corneal surface, leading to astigmatism.

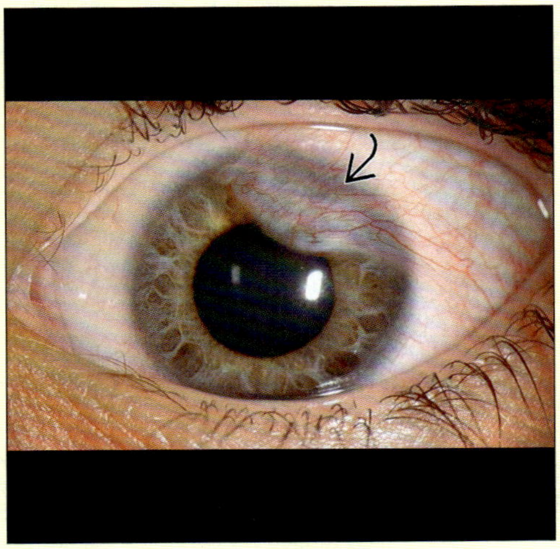

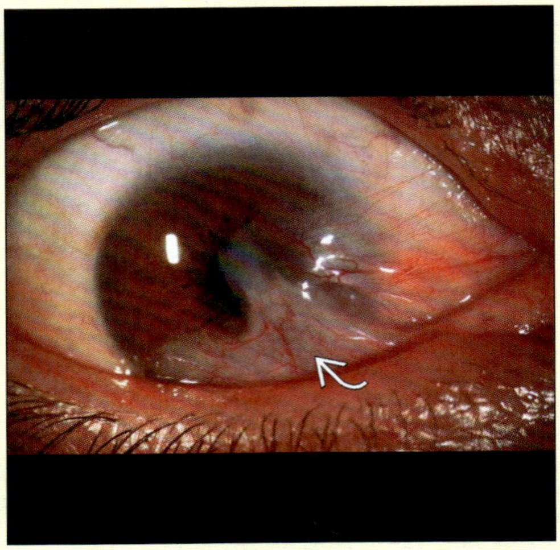

PTERYGIUM/PINGUECULA

INTRODUCTION

Definitions

- Pterygium: Wing-shaped mass of fibrovascular, degenerative bulbar conjunctival tissue extending across limbus onto cornea
- Pinguecula: Benign, whitish-yellow, elevated bulbar conjunctival mass composed of degenerating subepithelial stromal collagen fibers

DEMOGRAPHICS

Etiology/Risk Factors

- Primary risk factor is actinic UV radiation exposure
- Microtrauma: Wind, sand, dust, surface dryness

Epidemiology

- Prevalence increases with age
- Pterygium prevalence increases in populations closer to equator
- More common in men than in women (likely due to occupational differences with men more likely to work in construction, landscaping, etc.)

PRESENTATION

Symptoms

- Both lesions are mostly asymptomatic
- Inflammation can cause dryness, redness, irritation, foreign body sensation
- May cause visual changes from increased astigmatism
- Dellen can occur at head of pterygium that is especially elevated, interfering with uniformity of tear film and causing irritation and grittiness

Exam Findings

- Pinguecula
  - Usually in both eyes
  - Located paralimbally in interpalpebral zone, with nasal location more common than temporal
  - May exhibit calcification
  - If it crosses limbus, then it is termed pterygium
- Pterygium
  - Located in interpalpebral zone, with nasal location more common than temporal
  - Tissue grows across limbus and onto cornea, destroying Bowman layer
  - 3 distinct parts
    - Cap: Flat, leading edge that destroys Bowman layer; may see dellen, areas of drying, or iron line (Stocker line) anteriorly due to impaired tear film coverage
    - Head: Thick, fibrovascular segment located behind cap and attached to cornea
    - Body or tail: Mobile segment of bulbar conjunctiva with distinct edges

DIFFERENTIAL DIAGNOSIS

Pseudopterygium

- Conjunctival adherence to peripheral cornea due to inflammation from corneal ulcer, trauma, or chemical or thermal injury; occurs at any point around limbus; lacks firm adhesion throughout underlying structures

SCC and Conjunctival Carcinoma In Situ

- Rare; does not exhibit typical pterygium shape; may occur at any position around cornea

Corneal Micropannus

- History of trachoma or hypoxia secondary to excessive contact lens wear

EVALUATION/WORK-UP

Pathology

- Both pinguecula and pterygium have similar histopathology
  - Conjunctival epithelium may be normal, hyperkeratotic, or atrophic
  - UV radiation causes excessive elastin production by increased numbers of damaged fibroblasts
  - Abnormal collagen fiber maturation and degeneration
  - Subepithelial fibrovascular tissue and hyalinization of substantia propria
  - Collections of eosinophilic granular material

TREATMENT

Medical

- Treat acute inflammation with lubricant eyedrops, topical corticosteroids, or topical NSAIDs

Surgical

- Pinguecula
  - Excision necessary if chronic inflammation present, lesion interferes with contact lens wear, or for cosmetic reasons
- Pterygium
  - Surgical correction necessary when pterygium interferes with visual axis, medical management fails, or for cosmetic purposes
    - Simple excision (bare scleral technique): All remnants of pterygium are excised, leaving underlying sclera exposed; associated with high recurrence rate, which may be more aggressive than initial lesion
    - Conjunctival flap
    - Conjunctival autograft: Most popular current approach; donor tissue harvested from superior paralimbal area
    - Amniotic membrane transplantation
    - Lamellar keratoplasty may be required if corneal thinning is significant
    - Adjunctive treatments: Chemotherapy (mitomycin C [fairly common], thiotepa), β-irradiation (rarely used)
    - Fibrin glue can be used to reduce or eliminate need for sutures

SELECTED REFERENCES

1. Todani A et al: Pterygium: current concepts in pathogenesis and treatment. Int Ophthalmol Clin. 49(1):21-30, 2009
2. Hirst LW: The treatment of pterygium. Surv Ophthalmol. 48(2):145-80, 2003
3. Austin P et al: Elastodysplasia and elastodystrophy as the pathologic bases of ocular pterygia and pinguecula. Ophthalmology. 90(1):96-109, 1983

CORNEAL GRAFT REJECTION

Key Facts

Introduction

- Immune-mediated inflammation and edema in a primary graft that has been clear for at least 2 weeks or in a regraft that has been clear for 1 week

Presentation

- Conjunctival vessel dilation, ciliary flush, tissue edema, anterior chamber cell/flare
- Small, scattered, hazy subepithelial infiltrates in central donor cornea are early sign of rejection
- Epithelial rejection: 10% of patients experiencing graft rejection; occurs 1-13 months postoperatively
- Stromal/subepithelial: Infiltrates on donor cornea and anterior chamber reaction; necrosis if rejection is severe
- Endothelial: Most common and severe type (8-37% of cases); endothelial keratic precipitates on donor tissue create Khodadoust line

Treatment

- Prompt, aggressive therapy necessary in all corneal transplant recipients experiencing graft rejection regardless of clinical type
- Treat epithelial and stromal rejection aggressively with topical corticosteroids since both can precede endothelial rejection
- Aggressive treatment for endothelial rejection with hourly topical corticosteroids for 2-3 days, then q. 2 hours while awake; steroid ointment at bedtime
- Severe endothelial rejections, recurrent rejections, or high-risk patient
  - Subconjunctival corticosteroid injection, collagen shield soaked in corticosteroid and applied to cornea combined with frequent corticosteroid eyedrops, systemic corticosteroids, pulsed IV steroids
  - Bevacizumab, tacrolimus, and cyclosporine can be useful adjuncts in acute or maintenance therapy

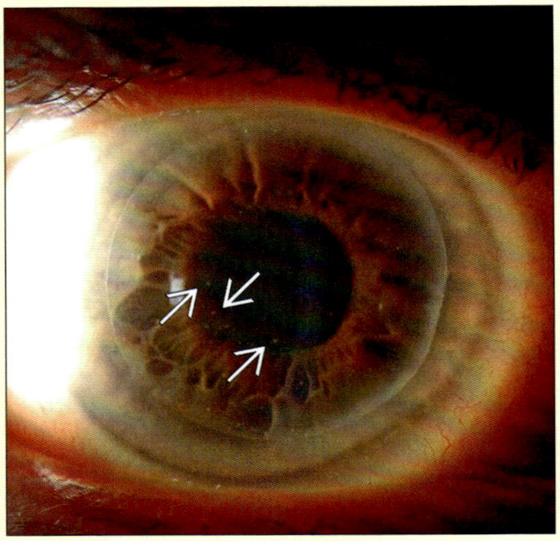

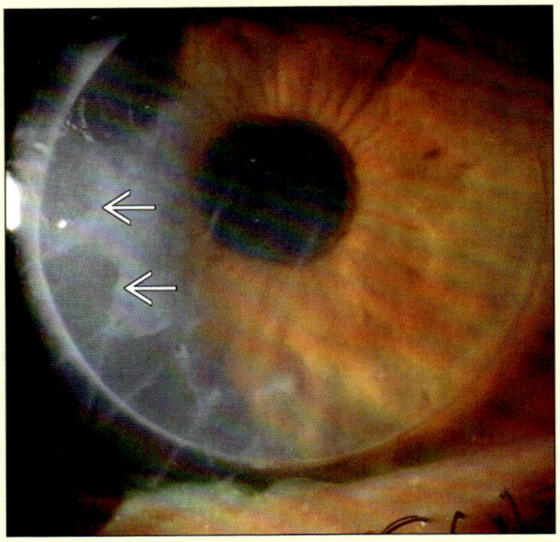

(Left) *Diffuse endothelial keratic precipitates ➔ scattered across the donor graft endothelium are an indication of allograft rejection.* ***(Right)*** *Another sign of corneal allograft rejection is an advancing rejection line (Khodadoust line) ➔ that generally originates in a vascularized area and extends across the donor cornea. As the line advances, endothelial cells are destroyed, and keratic precipitates are deposited. Graft edema and Descemet folds can also be seen within the affected area.*

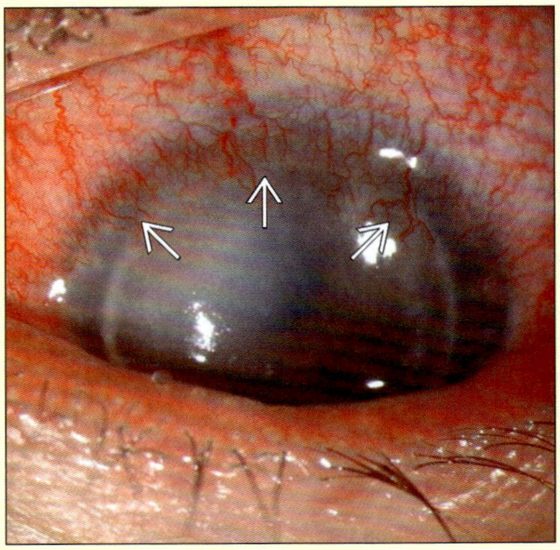

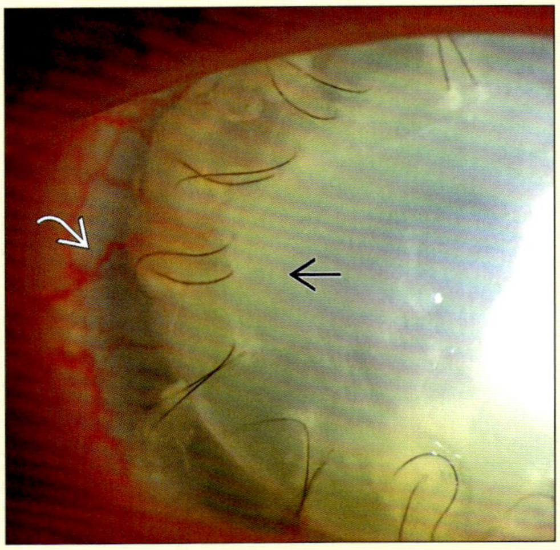

(Left) *Avascularity of the normal cornea grants immunologic privilege to corneal tissue. Corneal neovascularization ➔ induces an immune response by creating a route for immune mediators to enter a graft. The donor cornea thus becomes infiltrated with immune cells that lead to graft rejection.* ***(Right)*** *Severe rejection of all corneal layers results in stromal necrosis ➔ with stromal edema and neovascularization ➔.*

CORNEAL GRAFT REJECTION

INTRODUCTION

Definitions

- Immune-mediated inflammation and edema in a primary graft that has been clear for at least 2 weeks or in a regraft that has been clear for 1 week

DEMOGRAPHICS

Etiology/Risk Factors

- Age of graft recipient is < 40 years old
- Host corneal stromal vascularization pre- or postoperatively
- Grafts > 8 mm in diameter or eccentric grafts
- Loose sutures; can induce neovascularization or inflammation
- Active infection or inflammation at time of surgery
- Prior graft failure or rejection

PRESENTATION

Symptoms

- Redness, decreased &/or blurry vision, photophobia, discomfort lasting more than a few hours

Exam Findings

- Conjunctival vessel dilation, ciliary flush, tissue edema, anterior chamber reaction
- Small, scattered, hazy subepithelial infiltrates in central donor cornea are early sign of rejection
- 3 clinical forms of rejection
  - Epithelial rejection
    - Occurs in 10% of patients experiencing graft rejection; occurs 1-13 months postoperatively
    - Lymphocytes create elevated ridge of epithelial tissue that moves centrally
    - Rejection of epithelium occurs if host cells begin to replace donor epithelium
    - Responds well to topical steroid treatment
  - Stromal/subepithelial rejection
    - Stromal/subepithelial infiltrates on donor cornea and anterior chamber reaction
    - Neovascularization and stromal necrosis occur if rejection is severe or prolonged
    - Responds well to topical steroid treatment
  - Endothelial rejection
    - Most common and severe type (8-37% of cases)
    - Causes severe endothelial cell loss and decompensation
    - Endothelial keratic precipitates on donor tissue form a linear rejection line of leukocytes migrating from peripheral to central cornea (Khodadoust line)
    - Stromal edema and anterior chamber reaction
    - Donor cornea endothelial cells destroyed by host immune response can only be replaced by regraft

DIFFERENTIAL DIAGNOSIS

Herpes Simplex Keratouveitis

- Signs: Dendritic epithelial lesions, anterior chamber reaction, keratic precipitates in peripheral host endothelium

Herpes Zoster Ophthalmicus

- Signs: Anterior chamber reaction, diffuse keratic precipitates

Epithelial Downgrowth

- Migration of corneal or conjunctival epithelial tissue from peripheral cornea at site of previous penetration or perforation and across posterior graft surface
- Composed of single layer of epithelial cells; advancing edge is multilayered, thickened, and scalloped
- Differentiate from rejection with steroid therapy since epithelial downgrowth will not respond to steroids

TREATMENT

Medical

- Prompt, aggressive therapy necessary in all corneal transplant recipients experiencing graft rejection regardless of clinical type
- Treat epithelial and stromal rejection aggressively since both can precede more severe endothelial rejection
  - Topical corticosteroids (e.g., dexamethasone 0.1%, prednisolone acetate 1%) administered 4-6x/day until rejection signs resolve
  - Monitor closely for improvement and to ensure that endothelial rejection is not developing
- Aggressive treatment for endothelial rejection
  - Hourly topical corticosteroids for 2-3 days, then q. 2 hours while awake; steroid ointment at bedtime; difluprednate 0.05% can be given q. 3 hours
  - Continue therapy until signs of rejection resolve, then taper eyedrops over several weeks to a few months
  - If no response, continue therapy for at least 3 weeks before judging graft has failed
- Severe endothelial rejections, recurrent rejections, or high-risk patient
  - Subconjunctival corticosteroid injection (e.g., triamcinolone 8 mg, dexamethasone phosphate 2 mg, betamethasone 3 mg in 0.5 mL)
  - Collagen shield soaked in corticosteroid and applied to cornea combined with frequent steroid eyedrops
  - Systemic corticosteroids (e.g., oral prednisone 60-80 mg q.d. x 1-2 weeks before tapering)
  - Pulsed IV steroids (e.g., single 500 mg IV dose of methylprednisolone) may be more effective than oral prednisone
  - Subconjunctival bevacizumab fights corneal neovessels inciting rejection (2.5 mg in 0.1 mL injected contiguous to vessels)
- Frequent corticosteroid use can increase IOP; monitor closely and, if necessary, control with eyedrops to prevent glaucoma and improve graft survival

Follow-Up

- In high-risk patients, ↑ topical steroid frequency &/or adjuvants like topical cyclosporine 2% (not Restasis) or tacrolimus 0.03% ointment can ↓ recurrence; oral tacrolimus (1-3 mg p.o. b.i.d.) is alternative

SELECTED REFERENCES

1. Tan DT et al: Corneal transplantation. Lancet. 379(9827):1749-61, 2012

REFRACTIVE SURGERY COMPLICATIONS

Key Facts

Introduction
- Refractive surgery is a broad category of procedures to improve refraction
- Most common reason to have refractive surgery: Patient free from prescription glasses or contact lenses
- Most common procedure: Laser assisted in situ keratomileusis (LASIK)

LASIK
- Most common corneal refractive procedure
- Used for correction of myopia (up to 15 D), hyperopia (up to 6 D), and astigmatism (up to 6 D)
- General procedure
  - Create a cornea flap with a laser (excimer or femtosecond) or microkeratome
  - Lift flap towards hinge to expose corneal stroma
  - Corneal stroma remodeling then ensues with a laser

Demographics
- Patient screening is important to detect presence of possible risk factors for development of surgical complications of LASIK
- Contraindications for LASIK
  - Unstable refraction
  - Thin corneas
  - Severe dry eyes
  - Keratoconus and other corneal abnormalities

Complications of LASIK
- Diffuse lamellar keratitis (DLK)
- Epithelial ingrowth
- Dry eye disease
- LASIK-induced keratectasia
- Intraoperative flap complications
- Infection
- Flap striae or dislocation

*(**Left**) This external photograph shows post-LASIK epithelial ingrowth. Note both the small as well as large "bubbling" structures beneath the circular flap ➡, denoting growth of epithelial cells into the corneal stroma. (**Right**) This external photograph shows a corneal laceration due to a LASIK complication. Note the laceration ➡ penetrating towards the center of the LASIK flap.*

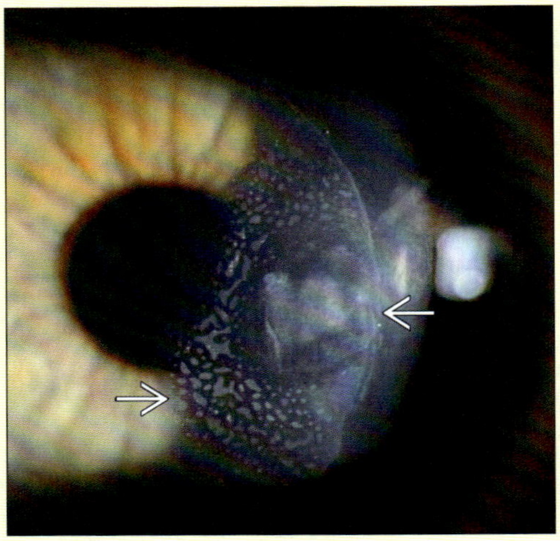

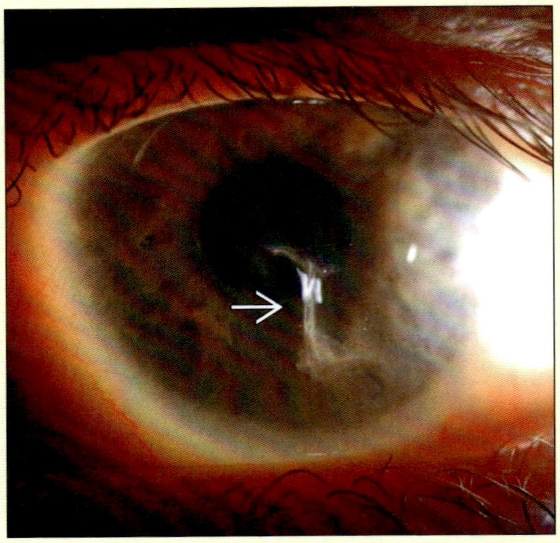

*(**Left**) This slit-lamp photo shows corneal dryness, a common finding after LASIK surgery. Note the spotted abrasions across the cornea that have the appearance of rock chips in a car windshield →. Post-LASIK eye drops can help mitigate corneal dryness. (**Right**) This external photograph shows melting of the corneal flap. Note the bubbling appearance of the cornea ➡. This finding is often a progression of epithelial ingrowth and results from ischemia or necrosis of the ingrown epithelium.*

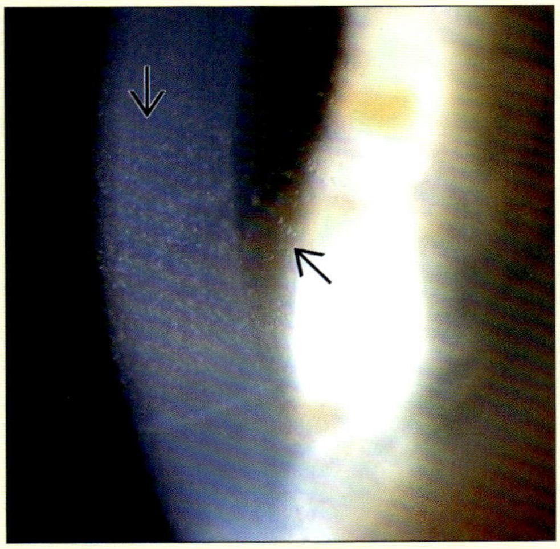

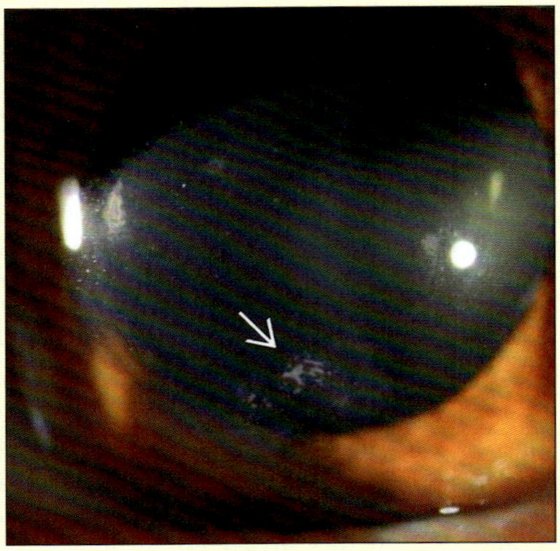

REFRACTIVE SURGERY COMPLICATIONS

INTRODUCTION

Definitions

- Refractive surgery: General term for different procedures that reduce or cure common eye problems such as myopia (nearsightedness), hyperopia (farsightedness), and astigmatism

Subtypes

- Laser-assisted in situ keratomileusis (LASIK)
  - Most common corneal refractive procedure
  - Used for correction of myopia (up to 15 D), hyperopia (up to 6 D), and astigmatism (up to 6 D)
- Photorefractive keratectomy (PRK)

DEMOGRAPHICS

Epidemiology

- > 1.5 million refractive surgeries done in USA each year
- Most common procedure done on myopic eyes ± astigmatism

Contraindications to LASIK and PRK

- Absolute contraindications
  - Unstable refraction
  - Cataract
  - Very thin central cornea (< 500 microns)
    - Postoperative stromal bed thickness < 270-300 μm
    - Risk for development of corneal ectasia
  - Ocular or systemic diseases
    - Glaucoma
    - External eye disease
    - Connective tissue disease
    - Immunodeficiency
    - Severe dry eye
    - Ectasias (e.g., keratoconus)
    - Corneal vascularization
    - Uveitis
    - Retinal disease (e.g., diabetic retinopathy)
  - Irregular corneal topography
  - Significant corneal scarring
- History of ocular herpes simplex or herpes zoster infection
  - Risk for corneal perforation from HSV reactivation
- Pregnancy
- Medications (e.g., isotretinoin, amiodarone)

Patient Screening

- Detailed ophthalmic history and exam
  - History of refractive surgery
  - History of amblyopia or strabismus
  - Family history of corneal ecstatic disorders
  - History of retinal disease and glaucoma
  - Ocular dominance, visual acuity, refraction, slit-lamp exam, pupillometry
- Corneal pachymetry
- Corneal topography
- IOP measurement
- Dilated funduscopy

COMPLICATIONS OF LASIK OR PRK

Flap Complications

- Intraoperative complications
  - Incomplete/buttonholed/irregular/free caps
  - Epithelial abrasion
    - Prevent with corneal lubrication
    - Increases diffuse lamellar keratitis (DLK), epithelial ingrowth, and keratolysis
  - Corneoscleral perforation
- Postoperative complications
  - Flap striae
  - Flap displacement/slippage
  - Interface debris, infections, heme, and fluid (can increase risk of DLK)

Ablation Complications

- Central islands
- Decentration

Others

- DLK, a.k.a. sands of Sahara syndrome
  - Presents 1-6 days after LASIK (peak incidence is day 3)
  - Stromal inflammation with decreased vision and pain
  - Must exclude infection
  - Treat with aggressive topical and systemic steroids
- Epithelial ingrowth
  - Most is self-limiting
  - 1-2% may require surgery because of visual loss, increased refractive error, flap melt, or keratolysis; suture or glue to prevent recurrence
  - More likely with flap relift (especially after 3 years) than primary LASIK
  - More likely with mechanical microkeratomes
- Dry eye disease
  - May affect up to 50% of patients
  - Risk factors include: Dry eye, Asian, female, need for higher correction/greater stromal ablation, thick corneal flap, superior flap hinge, narrow flap hinge
  - Treatment includes topical cyclosporine
- Infectious keratitis
  - Rare but very serious complication (1:1000-5000)
- LASIK-induced keratectasia
  - Progressive inferior corneal steepening, loss of uncorrected visual acuity (UCVA) and best-corrected visual acuity (BCVA), increasing myopia and astigmatism
  - Risk factors include young age, abnormal corneal topography, thin cornea/stroma

PRK Complications

- Haze: Treat with aggressive steroids
- Persistent epithelial defect: Treat with ointment, albumin, bandage contact lens, vitamin C

Posterior Segment Complications

- Retinal detachment

SELECTED REFERENCES

1. Sutton GL et al: Laser in situ keratomileusis in 2010 - a review. Clin Experiment Ophthalmol. 38(2):192-210, 2010
2. Varley GA et al: LASIK for hyperopia, hyperopic astigmatism, and mixed astigmatism: a report by the American Academy of Ophthalmology. Ophthalmology. 111(8):1604-17, 2004

BAND KERATOPATHY

Key Facts

Introduction

- Chronic degenerative condition characterized by dystrophic calcification of the cornea; typically, in a distinctive band-like pattern

Demographics

- Possible etiologies
  - Chronic ocular disease
  - Hypercalcemia
  - Gout
  - Chemical irritant exposure

Presentation

- Often asymptomatic but can present with a foreign body sensation, decreased visual acuity, tearing, photophobia, or cosmetic complaint
- Exam shows a grayish-white interpalpebral corneal opacification
  - Typically starts at corneal periphery at 3- and 9-o'clock positions
  - Central spread occurs as disease progresses
  - Holes can be present in plaque and give a Swiss cheese-like appearance

Evaluation/Work-Up

- Work-up for possible systemic causes may be prudent in cases of unknown etiology

Treatment

- Mild cases may be treated with artificial tear drops
- Moderate to severe cases typically require chelation with disodium ethylenediaminetetraacetate (EDTA)
- Excimer laser phototherapeutic keratectomy has been effectively performed to treat more severe cases
- Generally, a progressive condition
- Recurrences are common, especially if underlying cause cannot be corrected

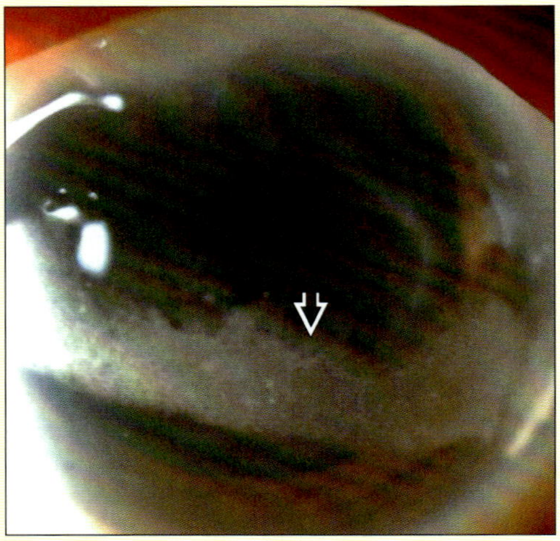

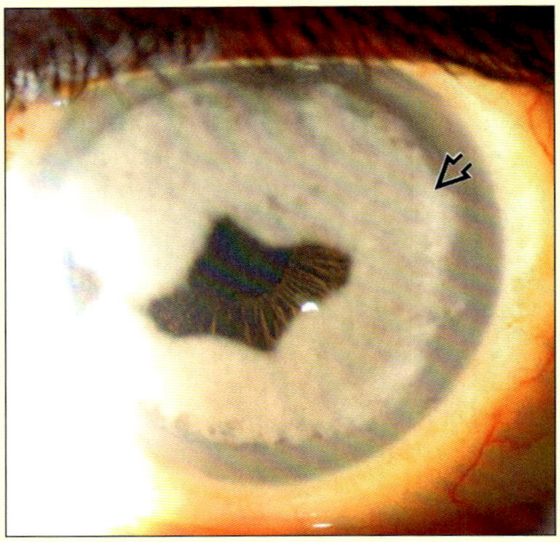

(Left) *This slit-lamp photo demonstrates band keratopathy ➡. The typical pattern starts at the peripheral cornea at the 3- and 9-o'clock positions but can spread more centrally as the disease progresses.* ***(Right)*** *Extensive band keratopathy ➡ is seen here with a sharply demarcated peripheral edge (typical) separated from the limbus by a clear corneal zone. This lucent zone is thought to be secondary to buffering from limbal vessels or lack of Bowman layer at the periphery.*

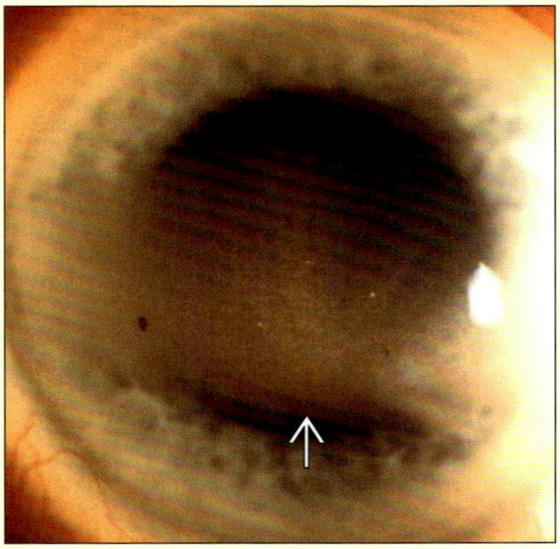

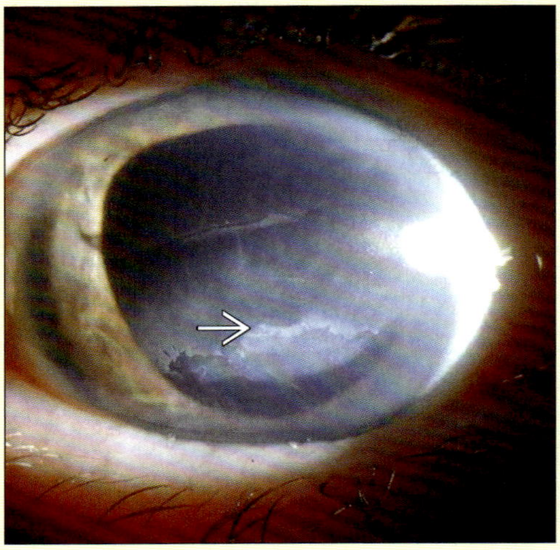

(Left) *This slit-lamp photo shows band keratopathy that started in the 3- and 9-o'clock positions and spread centrally ➡. Patients can be asymptomatic but may present with a foreign body sensation, cosmetic complaint, or vision loss.* ***(Right)*** *This slit-lamp photo shows a patient who has band keratopathy ➡. There are a variety of etiologies for this degenerative condition including chronic ocular disease, hypercalcemia, gout, chemical irritant exposure, or silicone oil in the anterior chamber.*

BAND KERATOPATHY

INTRODUCTION

Definitions

- Chronic degenerative condition characterized by dystrophic calcification of the cornea
  - Typically, in a distinctive band-like pattern in middle part of cornea (interpalpebral zone)

DEMOGRAPHICS

Etiology/Risk Factors

- Chronic ocular disease
  - Chronic uveitis (juvenile rheumatoid arthritis), interstitial keratitis, corneal edema, glaucoma, phthisis bulbi
- Hypercalcemia
  - Hyperparathyroidism, sarcoidosis, vitamin D toxicity, milk-alkali syndrome, renal failure, hypophosphatemia, Paget disease, multiple myeloma, metastatic neoplasm to bone
- Gout
- Chemical irritant exposure
  - Mercury fumes or preservatives
    - Can be found in ophthalmic medications
- Silicone oil in anterior chamber

Epidemiology

- No age predilection

PRESENTATION

Symptoms

- Often asymptomatic but can present with foreign body sensation, decreased vision, tearing, photophobia, or a cosmetic complaint of a white spot on cornea

Exam Findings

- Grayish-white interpalpebral corneal opacification from calcification
  - Typically starts at the corneal periphery at 3- and 9-o'clock positions
    - Sharply demarcated peripheral edge separated from the limbus by a clear corneal zone
      - Lucent areas may be due to buffering from limbal vessels or lack of peripheral Bowman layer
    - Chronic uveitic cases may begin centrally
  - Calcium deposit at level of Bowman membrane
  - Central spread occurs as disease progresses
  - Holes can be present in plaque and give a Swiss cheese-like appearance
    - Appear where nerve endings perforate Bowman membrane

DIFFERENTIAL DIAGNOSIS

Lipid Keratopathy

- White-yellow infiltrate with feathery edges and neovascularization (NV) going to center
- Can be primary (spontaneous, rare) or secondary (from HSV, old scar, or old NV)

EVALUATION/WORK-UP

Labs

- Diagnosis is usually made by history and clinical exam
- Work-up for possible systemic causes may be prudent in cases of unknown etiology
  - Serum calcium, phosphorus, albumin, magnesium, renal function, and uric acid levels
  - PTH or calcitonin may be dysregulated

Pathology

- Histopathology shows calcium deposition involving Bowman layer and superficial corneal stroma
- Fine basophilic granules, which can later coalesce, can be noted at Bowman layer
- Fibrous pannus can separate epithelium and Bowman layer

TREATMENT

Medical

- Mild cases may be treated with artificial tears/gels
- Moderate to severe cases typically require chelation with disodium ethylenediaminetetraacetate (EDTA)
  - First, anesthetize eye with topical anesthetic
  - Debride corneal epithelium (EDTA will not penetrate epithelium)
  - Apply EDTA (0.05 molar concentration) to calcified areas with a saturated cellulose sponge
    - Continue application until calcium is removed (carefully scrape off with a blade)
    - Adequate chelation may take between 10 and 30 minutes
    - Can give maintenance 2% EDTA drops to prevent or slow recurrence
  - Irrigate with normal saline, apply antibiotic ointment, provide post-procedure analgesia, and instruct pressure patch application for 24 hours
- Treat cause if there is a systemic problem

Surgical

- Excimer laser phototherapeutic keratectomy has been effectively performed to treat more severe cases
- Amniotic membrane can help restore a stable ocular surface after surgical removal of band keratopathy

Follow-Up

- Every 1-2 days until epithelium has healed after removal
- Check every 6-12 months for evidence of recurrence

Prognosis

- Generally, progressive
  - Often at a slow rate but can be quite rapid (weeks) in patients with severely dry eyes
- Recurrences are common, especially if underlying cause cannot be corrected

SELECTED REFERENCES

1. Jhanji V et al: Corneal calcific band keratopathy. Curr Opin Ophthalmol. 22(4):283-9, 2011
2. Anderson DF et al: Amniotic membrane transplantation after the primary surgical management of band keratopathy. Cornea. 20(4):354-61, 2001

DRY EYE SYNDROME

Key Facts

Introduction
- Inadequacy in tear film or function that results in instability, causing visual disturbance and discomfort and potentially damaging the ocular surface
- Keratitis conjunctivitis sicca (KCS)/dry eye syndrome (DES) is a chronic condition marked by exacerbations and remissions with a variable prognosis depending on underlying cause and severity
- Categorized into 2 main subtypes: Tear deficient and evaporative

Demographics
- Dry eye classification/etiology

Presentation
- Symptom questionnaires assist with clinical diagnosis
  - Foreign body sensation or dryness
  - Ocular irritation
  - Hyperemia
  - Epiphora
- Slit-lamp exam
  - Tear meniscus abnormalities
  - Conjunctivochalasis
  - Fluorescein staining
  - Interpalpebral staining of nasal or inferior cornea
  - Punctate epithelial defects
- Tear break-up time (TBUT) measures tear stability; abnormal < 10 seconds
- Schirmer test measures tear volume; abnormal < 5 mm; DES screening criteria < 10 mm in 5 minutes

Treatment
- Treat underlying cause
- Artificial tears (preservative free if used > q. 3 h), lubricating gels and ointments
- Education and environmental modifications
- Reevaluation of systemic and topical medications

Tear Deficient	
Sjogren syndrome	**Autoimmune and connective tissue disease** Rheumatoid arthritis, systemic lupus erythematosus, systemic sclerosis, Wegener granulomatosis, ocular rosacea
Non-Sjogren syndrome	**Lacrimal disease or obstruction** Congenital or acquired, trachoma, cicatricial pemphigoid, erythema multiforme, burns (chemical, thermal), sarcoid, HIV, graft-vs.-host disease, xerophthalmia, lacrimal gland ablation, orbital surgery **Tear reflex abnormality** Neurotrophic keratitis, CN (7, 5) palsies, contact lens wear, corneal surgery **Medications** Antihistamines, β-blockers, decongestants, oral contraceptives, hormone replacement therapy

Evaporative	
Oil deficiency	Meibomian gland dysfunction, blepharitis
Eyelid abnormality	Blink abnormalities, palpebral fissure abnormalities, lagophthalmos, thyroid orbitopathy, floppy eyelid syndrome, lid-surface incongruities, blepharoplasty
Ocular surface disease	Xerophthalmia, xerosis, allergy, vitamin A deficiency
Contact lens wear	Overuse of contacts can induce or exacerbate ocular surface disease
Medications	Topical medications with preservatives, Accutane

This overview outlines dry eye syndrome, a multifactorial disease, by the most common etiologies. The major classifications, aqueous tear deficient and evaporative, are designated by the most prominent pathological features leading to dry eye disease. These categories are not mutually exclusive. Both subtypes may coexist and conditions may evolve over time or become exacerbated by environmental factors to develop features associated with another major mechanism.

DRY EYE SYNDROME

INTRODUCTION

Abbreviations
- Dry eye syndrome (DES)

Synonyms
- Keratoconjunctivitis sicca (KCS); keratitis sicca (KS)

Definitions
- Inadequacy in tear film or function that results in instability, causing visual disturbance and discomfort and potentially damaging ocular surface

Subtypes
- Tear deficient
  - DES with Sjögren syndrome (SS)
  - DES without SS
- Evaporative
  - Intrinsic or extrinsic pathological etiologies can result in dysregulation of tear film or ocular surface, which causes tears to evaporate at a faster rate

DEMOGRAPHICS

Dry Eye Classification/Etiology
- General classification scheme serves as a guide and best clinical judgment is necessary for accurate diagnosis
- Conditions may be primary or secondary causes
  - Autoimmune diseases
    - Sjögren syndrome
    - Rheumatoid arthritis
    - Systemic lupus erythematosus
    - Granulomatosis polyangiitis (formerly Wegener granulomatosis)
    - Systemic sclerosis
    - Ocular rosacea
  - Lacrimal disease/obstruction
    - Congenital or acquired lacrimal gland disease
    - Sarcoid
    - HIV
    - Graft vs. host disease
    - Trachoma
    - Cicatricial pemphigoid
    - Erythema multiforme
    - Burns (chemical, thermal)
  - Thyroid orbitopathy
  - Tear reflex abnormality
    - Neurotrophic keratopathy
    - Contact lens
    - CN5 or CN7 palsy
  - Oil deficiency
    - Meibomian gland disease
    - Blepharitis (anterior or posterior)
  - Eyelid abnormality
    - Blink abnormality
    - Palpebral fissure abnormality
    - Lid-corneal surface incongruity
    - Lagophthalmos
    - Floppy eyelid syndrome
  - Ocular surface changes
    - Xerophthalmia
    - Xerosis
  - Medication
    - OCPs
    - HRT
    - Antihistamines
    - β-blockers
  - Iatrogenic
    - Corneal surgery
    - Orbital surgery
    - Eyelid surgery, especially blepharoplasty
  - Nutritional deficiency
    - Vitamin A deficiency
  - Decrease in androgen production
    - Menopause
    - Pregnancy

Epidemiology
- ~ 15-35% of population
- Women > men
- More common among elderly

PRESENTATION

Symptoms
- Symptom questionnaires assist with clinical diagnosis
  - Ocular Surface Disease Index questionnaire is most widely used
- Foreign body sensation, dryness, irritation
- Conjunctival injection or hyperemia
- Epiphora
- Fluctuating or blurry visual acuity
- Photophobia
- Symptoms are exacerbated by environmental conditions (dry and arid, smoke, computer screens)

Exam Findings
- Slit-lamp exam
  - Tear meniscus abnormalities
    - Decreased meniscus height, depth, or flattened curvature
  - Conjunctivochalasis
  - Epitheliopathy: Staining
    - Fluorescein (stains devitalized cells and basement membrane)
      - Interpalpebral staining of nasal or inferior cornea
      - Punctate epithelial defects
    - Rose bengal (stains cells lacking mucin coating)
      - Linear staining of inferior conjunctiva and cornea is characteristic in meibomian gland dysfunction (MGD)
      - Scoring system: Intensity 0-3 in 3 regions: Nasal conjunctiva, temporal conjunctiva, and cornea; DES ≥ 3.5
    - Lissamine green (devitalized cells and cells lacking mucin coating)
  - Tear break-up time (TBUT) measures tear stability
    - Abnormal < 10 sec
  - Schirmer test measures tear volume
    - Abnormal < 5 mm
    - DES screening criteria < 10 mm in 5 minutes
  - Signs of MGD
    - Anterior/posterior blepharitis
      - Erythema and crusting at lid margin surrounding lashes
      - Collarettes, scurf, sleeves: Refers to epithelialized greasy material adherent to bases of lashes

DRY EYE SYNDROME

DIFFERENTIAL DIAGNOSIS

Conjunctivitis
- Allergic
- Bacterial
- Viral
- Atopic
- Superior limbic keratoconjunctivitis

Keratitis
- Filamentary
- Interstitial

Infectious
- Herpes simplex virus (HSV)
- Herpes zoster virus (HZV)
- Chlamydia

Keratopathy
- Neurotrophic
- Pseudophakic
- Thygeson superficial punctate keratopathy

Corneal Abnormalities
- Abrasion
- Erosion
- Foreign body
- Mucous plaques

EVALUATION/WORK-UP

Labs
- For SS DES
  - Autoantibodies to Ro (SSA) or La (SSB) antigens or a combination
- Quantification of tear components
  - Lipid
    - High pressure lipid chromatography (HPLC)
    - Gas chromatography with mass spectroscopy (GC-MS)
  - Aqueous proteins
    - ELISA to analyze tear lysozyme, tear lactoferrin, epidermal growth factor, aquaporin 5, lipocalin, and IgA
  - Tear-film osmolarity (elevated in DES)
  - Mucin
    - Evaluate mRNA expression using impression cytology, immunofluorescence, flow cytometry, ELISA, or immunoblotting
- Impression cytology to monitor ocular surface changes
- Additional tests
  - Tear stability analysis system (TSAS)
  - Tear function index (TFI)
  - Tear ferning test (TFT)

Pathology
- Light microscopy
  - Conjunctival epithelial cells show squamous metaplasia with fewer goblet cells, cellular enlargement, increased nuclear:cytoplasmic ratio, and possible keratinization
  - Lacrimal gland and conjunctiva may show lymphocytic infiltrate
  - In MGD, lacrimal glands show hyperkeratinization, loss of glandular architecture, and dilation and obstruction of ductules
  - In SS, lacrimal glands show a progressive lymphocytic infiltrate and disorganized glandular architecture

TREATMENT

Medical
- Treat underlying cause
  - Treatment of systemic disorders (SS, RA, thyroid)
    - Treat dry mouth with Salagen or Neutrasal in Sjögren syndrome
  - MGD (Lid hygiene, doxycycline 100 mg q.d. or b.i.d.)
- First-line treatment
  - Artificial tears (preservative free if used > q. 3 h), lubricating gels and ointments
  - Education and environmental modifications
  - Reevaluation of systemic and topical medications
- Second-line treatment
  - Anti-inflammatory agents (topical cyclosporine 0.05%), corticosteroids, or systemic omega-3 fatty acids)
  - Secretagogues
  - Punctal plugs
  - Tetracyclines (treat meibomitis or rosacea)
  - Moisture chamber goggles
- Third-line treatment
  - Autologous serum drops
  - Contact lenses (scleral lenses)
- Fourth-line treatment
  - Systemic anti-inflammatories or immunosuppressants

Surgical
- Eyelid reconstruction or temporary tarsorrhaphy may be indicated for patients with DES secondary to exposure keratopathy
- Surgical occlusion of puncta (electrocauterization)
- Conjunctival flap
- Amniotic membrane transplant

Follow-Up
- Dependent on symptoms

Prognosis
- Chronic condition with a variable prognosis depending on underlying cause and severity
- Mild to moderate DES is typically managed well with artificial tears, lubricating gels and ointments

SELECTED REFERENCES

1. Foulks GN et al: Improving awareness, identification, and management of meibomian gland dysfunction. Ophthalmology. 119(10 Suppl):S1-12, 2012
2. Tong L et al: Choice of artificial tear formulation for patients with dry eye: where do we start? Cornea. 31 Suppl 1:S32-6, 2012
3. Management and therapy of dry eye disease: report of the Management and Therapy Subcommittee of the International Dry Eye WorkShop (2007). Ocul Surf. 5(2):163-78, 2007

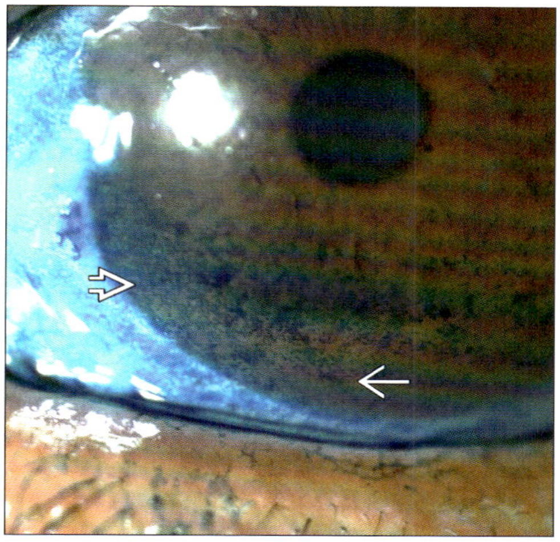

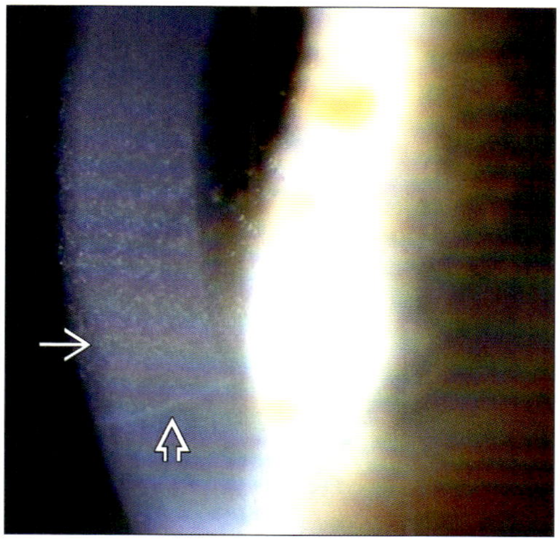

(Left) *This external photograph demonstrates an eye with severe dry eye. Note the multiple punctate areas of staining ➡, which in areas become confluent ➡.* ***(Right)*** *This slit-lamp photograph shows punctate corneal defects ➡ in a patient post LASIK treatment. Note the visible margin of the LASIK flap ➡. LASIK is a risk factor for developing dry eye syndrome (DES).*

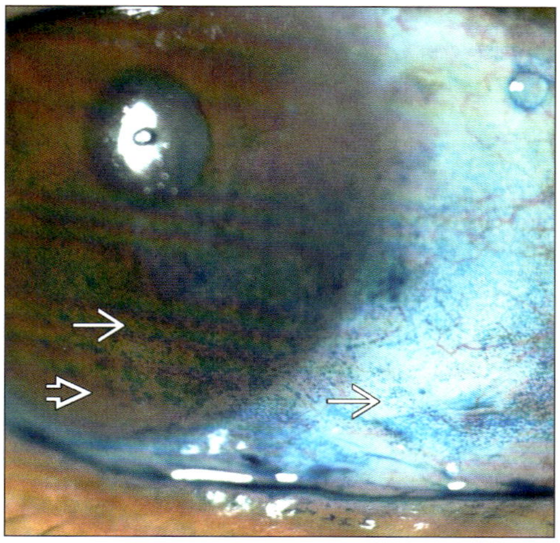

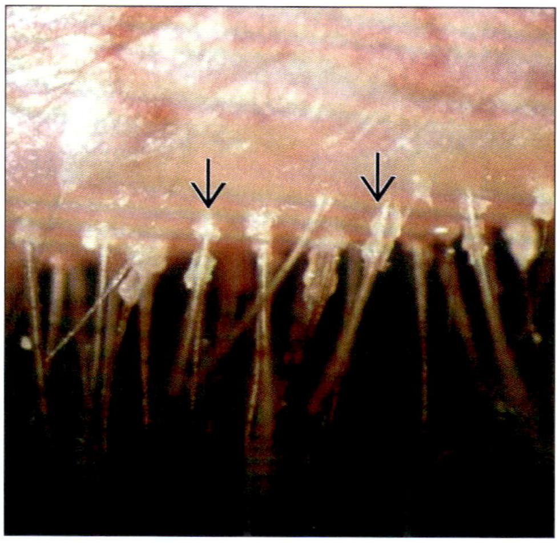

(Left) *This slit-lamp photograph demonstrates punctate staining of the cornea ➡, suggesting damage to the surface epithelium caused by dry eye. This damage is often limited to the exposed area of the eye in the intrapalpebral fissure. Manual retraction of the eyelid can reveal a demarcation between healthy and exposed cornea ➡.* ***(Right)*** *This external photograph shows crusting around the lashes →, suggestive of anterior blepharitis. Blepharitis is often associated with DES.*

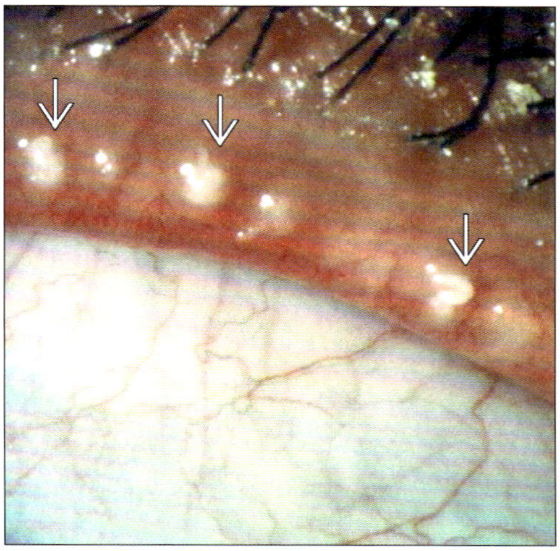

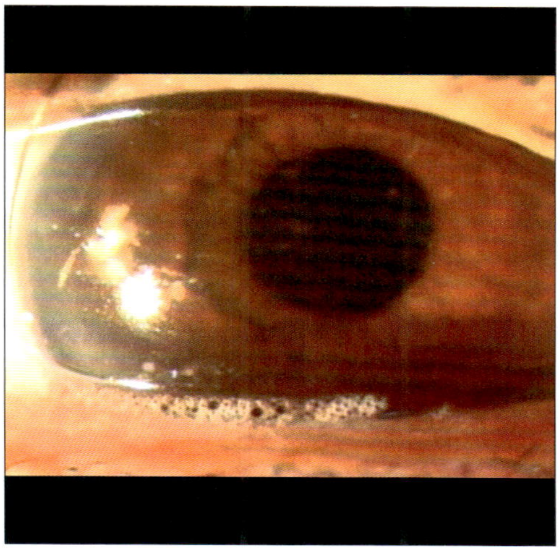

(Left) *This external photograph shows capping of the meibomian glands ➡, suggestive of meibomian gland dysfunction (MGD), which is also known as posterior blepharitis. MGD is associated with DES. In MGD, the meibomian glands are unable to produce adequate oil for the lubricating and superficial layers of the tear film. This can lead to increased evaporation of the aqueous layer of the tear film and dry eye.* ***(Right)*** *This external photograph shows foamy tears, which are suggestive of MGD.*

EXPOSURE KERATOPATHY

Key Facts

Introduction
- Excessive ocular surface exposure leading to increased evaporative tear loss and subsequent irritation of corneal surface

Demographics
- Common associations include any impairment of eyelid function or eyelid malposition
- Causes can include traumatic, neurological, mechanical, psychiatric, psychological, or a medication side effect
- Proptosis or lid retraction
- Impaired or reduced blinking

Presentation
- Ocular irritation, blurry vision, tearing, red eyes, dryness, or pain
- Foreign body sensation, grittiness
- Silt-lamp exam: Punctate epithelial defects in interpalpebral fissure

Evaluation/Work-Up
- Evaluate for history of previous surgery, thyroid disease, or Bell palsy
- Evaluate for secondary corneal infection

Treatment
- Obtunded or sedated patients in ICU/OR should be treated with lubricating ointment and eyelid taping
- Artificial, preservative-free tears and ointments; may tape lids closed with antibiotic ointment
- Tarsorrhaphy or surgical reconstruction of eyelid
- Orbital decompression (for proptosis)
- Reevaluate daily if corneal ulceration present; weekly to monthly if less corneal involvement

*(**Left**) This external photograph shows the eye of a patient with exposure keratopathy as a complication from blepharoplasty. Note the enlarged interpalpebral fissure and the excessive amount of scleral exposure inferiorly ⇨. (**Right**) This external photograph demonstrates punctate staining on the epithelial surface of a patient with exposure keratopathy →. Note the distribution of the staining on the inferior aspect of the cornea ➡.*

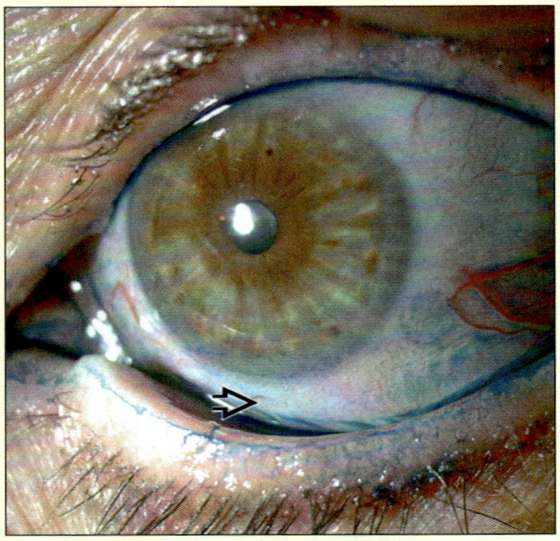

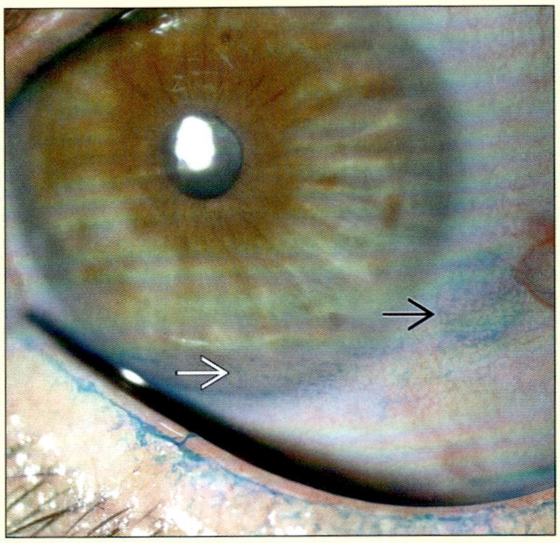

*(**Left**) This slit-lamp photograph shows multiple punctate lesions on the corneal surface ➡ that become confluent ➡ in places. In the setting of a patient with a clinical history concerning for corneal exposure, this finding is suggestive of exposure keratopathy. (**Right**) Axial T1WI C+ FS MRI shows classic findings of Bell palsy with the fundal "tuft" sign ➡ as well as labyrinthine ➡ and tympanic ➡ facial nerve segment enhancement. Bell palsy is a risk factor for exposure keratopathy.*

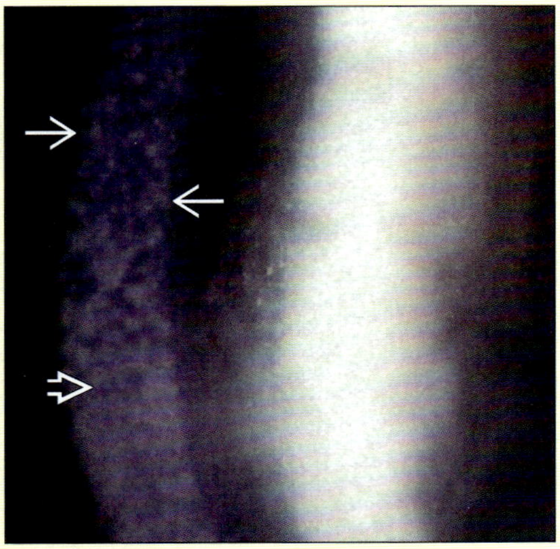

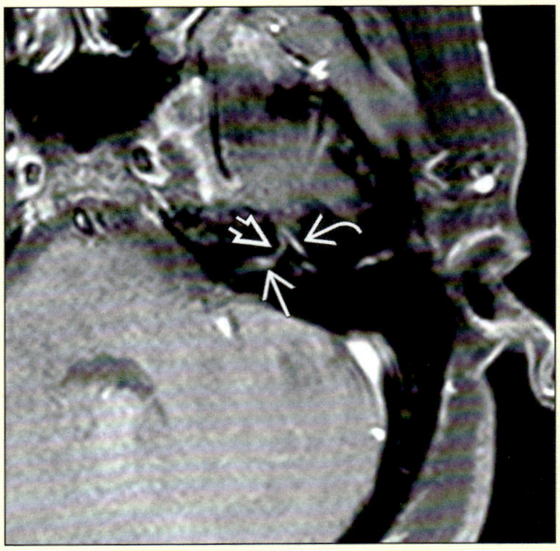

EXPOSURE KERATOPATHY

INTRODUCTION

Definitions

- Excessive ocular surface exposure leading to increased evaporative tear loss and subsequent irritation of corneal surface

DEMOGRAPHICS

Etiology/Risk Factors

- Common associations include any impairment of eyelid function or eyelid malposition
  - Causes can include traumatic, neurological, mechanical, psychiatric, psychological, or a medication side effect
    - Examples: Orbicularis oculi weakness, sedation or altered mental status (ICU care), eyelid deformity (e.g., ectropion, scarring from trauma, chemical burn, or herpes zoster ophthalmicus), after ptosis repair or blepharoplasty procedures, floppy eyelid syndrome
  - Lagophthalmos: Incomplete or defective eyelid closure
    - Nocturnal: Failure to close eyes during sleep
    - Paralytic : Facial nerve paralysis secondary to Bell palsy, trauma, infections, tumors
    - Cicatricial: After trauma or surgery
  - Proptosis or lid retraction
    - Thyroid or Graves orbitopathy
    - Orbital tumors
- Impaired or reduced blinking
  - Poor blink rate with Parkinson disease
  - Postoperative laser assisted in situ keratomileusis (LASIK)
  - Reduced blink rate associated with computer and reading tasks
  - Contact lens wear

PRESENTATION

Symptoms

- Ocular irritation, blurry vision, tearing, red eyes, dryness, or pain
- Foreign body sensation, grittiness
- Can be worse in morning

Exam Findings

- Slit-lamp exam
  - Incomplete or abnormal eyelid closure
    - Eyelid deformity
  - Punctate epithelial defects
    - Located in lower 1/3 of cornea or within palpebral fissure
    - Enhanced with fluorescein stain
  - May also have
    - Conjunctival injection
    - Chemosis
    - Corneal erosion
    - Corneal ulceration &/or infiltrate
    - Decreased tear break-up time

EVALUATION/WORK-UP

History

- Evaluate for history of previous surgery, thyroid disease, or Bell palsy
- Evaluate medications that enhance corneal dryness

Physical

- Evaluate eyelid laxity and closure with degree of corneal exposure (close lids gently)
- Assess Bell phenomenon (close lids tightly against resistance; eyes should roll upward under eyelids)
- Decreased corneal sensation increases risk for corneal complications (assess sensation prior to anesthetic drops)
- Evaluate for secondary corneal infection (e.g., anterior chamber reaction, severe conjunctival injection, corneal infiltrate)

Labs

- Thyroid evaluation if thyroid orbitopathy suspected

TREATMENT

Prevention

- Patients who are obtunded or sedated (ICU or critical care) should be treated with lubricating ointment
- Behavior modification to enhance blink efficiency (e.g., increasing blinking at computer)
- Avoid exacerbating environmental factors (e.g., smoke, arid environments)

Medical

- Treat underlying cause
- Artificial, preservative-free tears and ointments or gels
- May tape lids closed with antibiotic ointment
- Bandage contact lens, moisture chambers, humidifier, oral vitamin C or doxycycline, topical medroxyprogesterone, or albumin drops may be of use

Surgical

- Punctal occlusion plugs
- Partial tarsorrhaphy: May be temporary or permanent
- Surgical reconstruction of eyelid
- Eyelid weighted implant (for CN7 palsy)
- Orbital decompression (for proptosis)
- Conjunctival flap or amniotic membrane graft (for severe corneal decompensation)

Follow-Up

- Reevaluate daily if corneal ulceration present
- Follow-up in weeks to months for less severe corneal involvement

Prognosis

- Depends on location, extent, degree, and etiology of condition

SELECTED REFERENCES

1. Pereira MV et al: Lagophthalmos. Semin Ophthalmol. 25(3):72-8, 2010
2. McMonnies CW: Incomplete blinking: exposure keratopathy, lid wiper epitheliopathy, dry eye, refractive surgery, and dry contact lenses. Cont Lens Anterior Eye. 30(1):37-51, 2007

FILAMENTARY KERATOPATHY

Key Facts

Introduction
- Chronic, recurrent condition characterized by presence of filaments consisting of mucous strands on surface of corneal epithelium
- Common condition; typically a sign of severe ocular surface disease

Demographics
- Most commonly associated with keratoconjunctivitis sicca

Presentation
- Hallmark feature is filaments or strands of degenerated epithelial cells and mucous depositions
- These filaments stain with fluorescein and rose bengal dyes

Differential Diagnosis
- Superior limbic keratoconjunctivitis
- Bullous keratopathy
- Prolonged patching following ocular surgery
- HSV

Treatment
- Lubricate with a mucolytic agent to dissolve mucous filaments and deposits (acetylcysteine 10% drops)
- NSAIDs (diclofenac)
- Hypertonic solutions to enhance adhesion of loose epithelium (5% saline drops)
- Treat any underlying dry eye disease as symptoms will recur if underlying etiology is not properly addressed
- Prognosis depends on underlying cause and treatment approach
- May resolve within weeks to months, or may persist for several months

__(Left)__ This external photograph shows multiple filaments ➔ composed of degenerated epithelium surrounded by mucous. These filaments remain attached to the cornea at one end and are a critical finding for filamentary keratopathy. __(Right)__ Filaments ➔ can be stained and easily visualized with fluorescein.

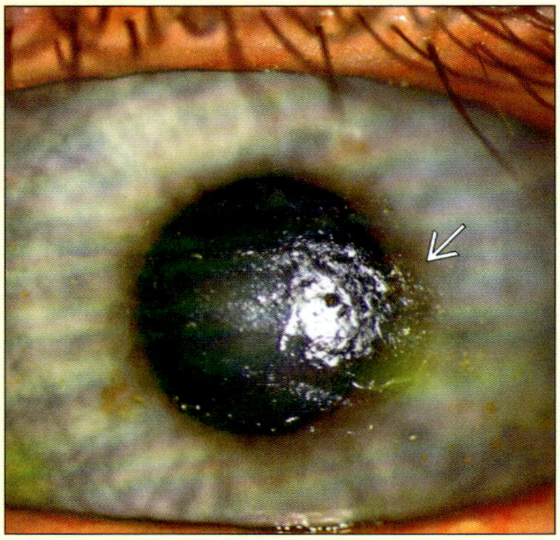

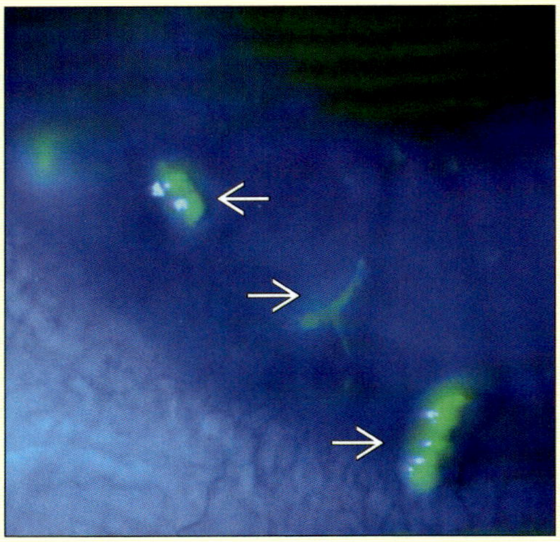

__(Left)__ Small defects are occasionally visualized at the base of filaments. In this external photo, the multiple defects are apparent. __(Right)__ Patients with filamentary keratopathy often have persistent foreign-body sensations. Prolonged irritation may lead to inflammation, as seen in this external photograph

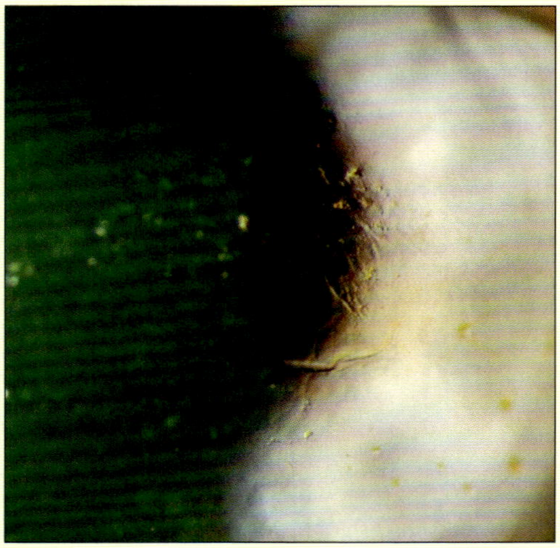

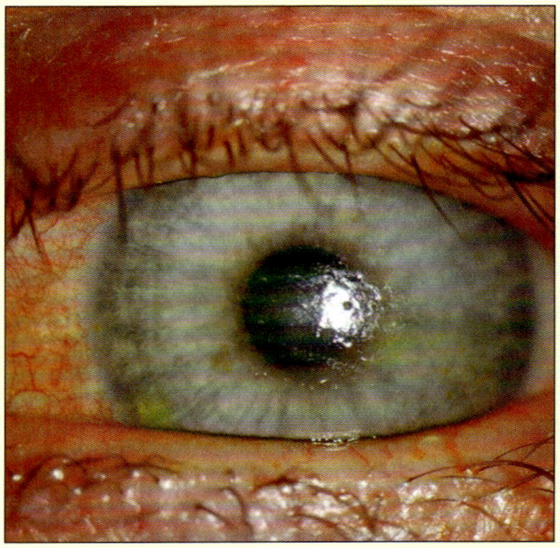

FILAMENTARY KERATOPATHY

INTRODUCTION

Abbreviations
- Filamentary keratopathy (FK)

Definitions
- Chronic, recurrent condition characterized by presence of filaments consisting of mucous strands on corneal epithelium surface
- Common condition; typically a sign of severe ocular surface disease

DEMOGRAPHICS

Etiology/Risk Factors
- Common associations
  - Keratoconjunctivitis sicca
  - Epithelial defects
  - Epitheliopathies (recurrent erosion syndrome, drug toxicity, aerosol keratitis, radiation keratitis)
  - Superior limbic keratoconjunctivitis
  - Bullous keratopathy
  - Neurotrophic keratopathy
  - Herpetic keratitis
  - Recent procedures (cataract surgery, refractive surgery, corneal graft)
  - Prolonged patching (postoperative)
  - Excessive contact lens wear
  - Systemic disorders (diabetes, psoriasis, connective tissue disorders)
  - Immune deficiencies

Epidemiology
- Women > men
- Elderly

PRESENTATION

Symptoms
- Discomfort
- Foreign body sensation
- Redness
- Photophobia

Exam Findings
- Filaments (hallmark feature)
  - Strands of degenerated epithelial cells and mucous
  - Move with blinking, attached at one end to corneal epithelium
  - Stain with rose bengal or fluorescein
- Small epithelial defect often present at base of filament
- Chronic filaments can form plaques
- Reduced tear break-up time
- Punctate epithelial keratopathy

DIFFERENTIAL DIAGNOSIS

Ocular Surface Disease
- Dry eye syndrome
- Bullous keratopathy
- Neurotrophic keratopathy
- Epitheliopathies
- Prolonged patching following ocular surgery

Keratitis
- Bacterial, viral, fungal
- Superior limbic keratoconjunctivitis

Trauma
- Corneal abrasion

EVALUATION/WORK-UP

Pathology
- Mucin, a soluble component of tear film, becomes compromised and precipitates out into strands
- Weak area of corneal epithelium acts as a focus for deposition of mucous and cellular debris
- Mucous strands lined with epithelium become anchored at one end to corneal surface

TREATMENT

Medical
- Lubrication with a mucolytic agent to dissolve mucous filaments and deposits
  - 5% or 10% acetylcysteine drops q.i.d.
- NSAIDs (diclofenac)
- Hypertonic solutions to enhance adhesion of loose epithelium
  - 5% saline drops q.i.d. or ointment at bedtime
- Soft bandage contact lens (BCTL) with high oxygen permeability to protect cornea from repetitive irritation secondary to blinking
  - Use prophylactic antibiotic drops b.i.d. to t.i.d. with BCTL
- Treat any underlying dry eye disease
  - Copious lubrication with preservative-free artificial tears and ointment
- Review any medications that may induce ocular surface toxicity

Surgical
- Debridement of filaments using jeweler's forceps under topical anesthesia

Follow-Up
- May manage this condition for prolonged periods
- Must treat underlying etiology once filaments dissipate

Prognosis
- Depends on underlying cause and treatment approach
- May resolve within weeks to months, or may persist for several months
- May recur if underlying etiology is not properly addressed

SELECTED REFERENCES

1. Diller R et al: A case report and review of filamentary keratitis. Optometry. 76(1):30-6, 2005
2. Albietz J et al: Management of filamentary keratitis associated with aqueous-deficient dry eye. Optom Vis Sci. 80(6):420-30, 2003

THYGESON SUPERFICIAL PUNCTATE KERATITIS

Key Facts

Introduction

- Transient, bilateral, recurrent superficial keratitis with minimal or no stromal or conjunctival involvement
- Unclear etiology and pathogenesis

Presentation

- Ocular irritation, photophobia, dry eyes, blurry vision, foreign body sensation
- May be unilateral but more commonly bilateral
- Multiple small, elevated, randomly distributed, white-gray intraepithelial lumps scattered in cornea; inverse staining with fluorescein due to elevation
- Differentiated from superficial punctate keratitis (SPK) from other causes (e.g., neurotrophic, dry eye, and toxic) by random distribution, elevation, and no staining with fluorescein
- Minimal or no conjunctival injection

Differential Diagnosis

- Adenoviral conjunctivitis: Subepithelial infiltrates may sometimes be found, which may be confused for TSPK; however, these are not elevated and easily distinguished from TSPK
- Dry eye syndrome: May have filaments, punctate epithelial erosions, or SPK; usually clustered in interpalpebral zone instead of randomly distributed, and stain with fluorescein
- HSV keratitis: May present with SPK and have similar symptoms; however, there is usually significant injection and pain, unlike TSPK

Treatment

- Aggressive lubrication with artificial tears and ointments
- Topical steroid eye drops
- Cyclosporin A may be considered as addition or alternative to steroid eye drops

*(**Left**) Slit-lamp photograph shows common findings in Thygeson superficial punctate keratitis (TSPK). Note the reflective white-gray bumps ➔ on the corneal surface. There is usually minimal ocular inflammation accompanying these findings. (**Right**) Slit-lamp photograph shows the elevated lesions in more detail. Note the circular white reflections (which do not stain) augmented by fluorescein dye. These intraepithelial lesions ➔ look as if they are puckering out from the corneal surface.*

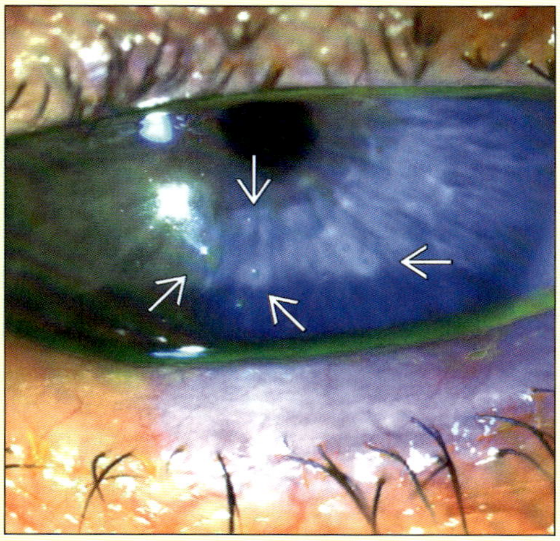

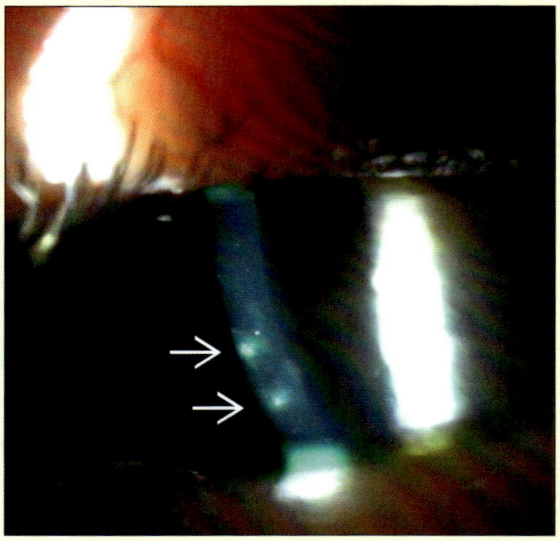

*(**Left**) Slit-lamp photograph shows a different form of superficial punctate keratopathy (SPK) diffusely distributed throughout the interpalpebral zone in a patient with severe dry eye ➔. Note the diffuse staining with fluorescein dye. (**Right**) Slit-lamp photo depicts SPK ➔ as seen in exposure keratopathy and dry eye. This form of SPK contrasts to the intraepithelial lesions in TSPK, which do not stain and appear elevated. TSPK lesions are also diffusely distributed throughout the cornea instead of clustered, as shown here.*

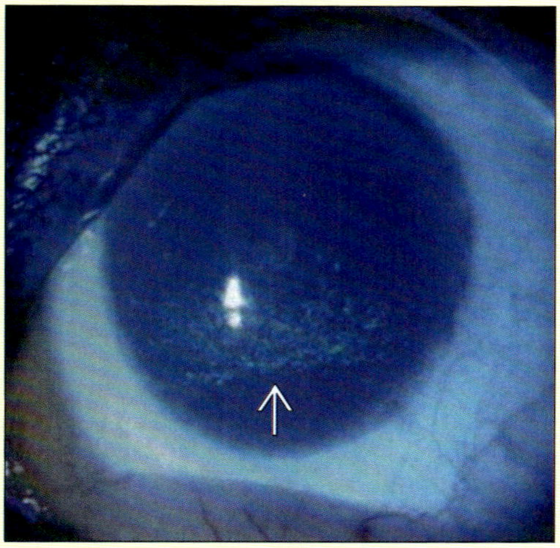

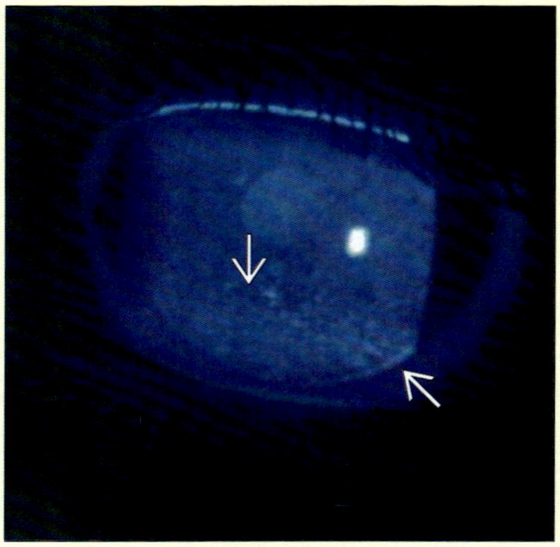

THYGESON SUPERFICIAL PUNCTATE KERATITIS

INTRODUCTION

Abbreviations
- Thygeson superficial punctate keratitis (TSPK)

Definitions
- Transient, bilateral, recurrent superficial keratitis consisting of multiple elevated intraepithelial white or gray epithelial lesions with minimal or no stromal or conjunctival involvement

DEMOGRAPHICS

Etiology/Risk Factors
- Unclear etiology and pathogenesis
- Associated with HLA-DR3
- Associations with viral infections have been suggested; no definitive evidence of a causal relationship
- Attacks may last months and may go into remission for years

Epidemiology
- Rare
- Affects all races, genders, and ages

PRESENTATION

Symptoms
- Foreign body sensation, ocular irritation, photophobia, dry eyes, blurry vision, epiphora
  - May be unilateral but more commonly bilateral

Exam Findings
- Multiple small, elevated, randomly distributed, white-gray intraepithelial lumps scattered in cornea
  - Inverse staining with fluorescein due to elevation
- Minimal or no conjunctival injection
- Corneal and conjunctival sensation normally intact
- May cause corneal scarring (rare)

DIFFERENTIAL DIAGNOSIS

Adenoviral Conjunctivitis
- Conjunctiva are usually injected and edematous and no corneal intraepithelial lumps are found
  - Subepithelial infiltrates may sometimes be found in severe cases
    - However, these are not elevated and easily distinguished from TSPK on slit-lamp exam

Dry Eye Syndrome
- Severe cases may have filaments, punctate epithelial erosions, or superficial punctate keratopathy (SPK), which might vaguely resemble TSPK
  - However, TSPK is not clustered in interpalpebral zone and instead is uniformly distributed throughout cornea

Herpes Simplex Virus (HSV) Keratitis
- May have similar symptoms and present with SPK
  - Differentiating features: Sensation may be decreased; lesions stain with fluorescein; HSV is commonly unilateral and is usually accompanied by conjunctival injection

EVALUATION/WORK-UP

Pathology
- Histological features of TSPK include intracellular and intercellular edema at epithelial level

Imaging
- None necessary
- Confocal imaging of TSPK demonstrates considerable abnormalities in subepithelial nerve plexus, Bowman membrane, and anterior stroma related to disease duration

TREATMENT

Medical
- Aggressive lubrication with artificial tears/ointments
- Topical steroid eye drops improve symptoms and clinical signs but are difficult to wean
- Steroids should be tapered to minimum amount necessary to achieve remission
  - Patients on steroids should have their intraocular pressures closely monitored
- Cyclosporin A (2%) may be considered as addition or alternative to steroid eye drops (useful in patients with contraindication to steroid treatment)

Surgical
- No definitive data is present on benefit of surgical treatment
- Case reports of photorefractive keratectomy (PRK) or phototherapeutic keratectomy (PTK) have showed some success

Follow-Up
- Weekly until symptoms improve
- May be prolonged according to symptoms and findings

Prognosis
- Excellent

SELECTED REFERENCES

1. Fintelmann RE et al: Thygeson superficial punctate keratitis and scarring. Cornea. 31(12):1446-8, 2012
2. Kobayashi A et al: In vivo laser confocal microscopy findings of Thygeson superficial punctate keratitis. Cornea. 30(6):675-80, 2011
3. Nagra PK et al: Thygeson's superficial punctate keratitis: ten years' experience. Ophthalmology. 111(1):34-7, 2004
4. Netto MV et al: Thygeson's superficial punctate keratitis recurrence after laser in situ keratomileusis. Am J Ophthalmol. 138(3):507-8, 2004
5. Watson SL et al: Confocal microscopy of Thygeson's superficial punctate keratopathy. Cornea. 22(4):294-9, 2003
6. Goldstein MH et al: PRK-pTK as a treatment for a patient with Thygeson's superficial punctate keratopathy. CLAO J. 28(4):172-3, 2002
7. Fite SW et al: Photorefractive keratectomy for myopia in the setting of Thygeson's superficial punctate keratitis. Cornea. 20(4):425-6, 2001
8. Goldberg DB et al: Management of Thygeson's superficial punctate keratitis. Am J Ophthalmol. 89(1):22-4, 1980
9. Thygeson P: Superficial punctate keratitis. J Am Med Assoc. 144(18):1544-9, 1950

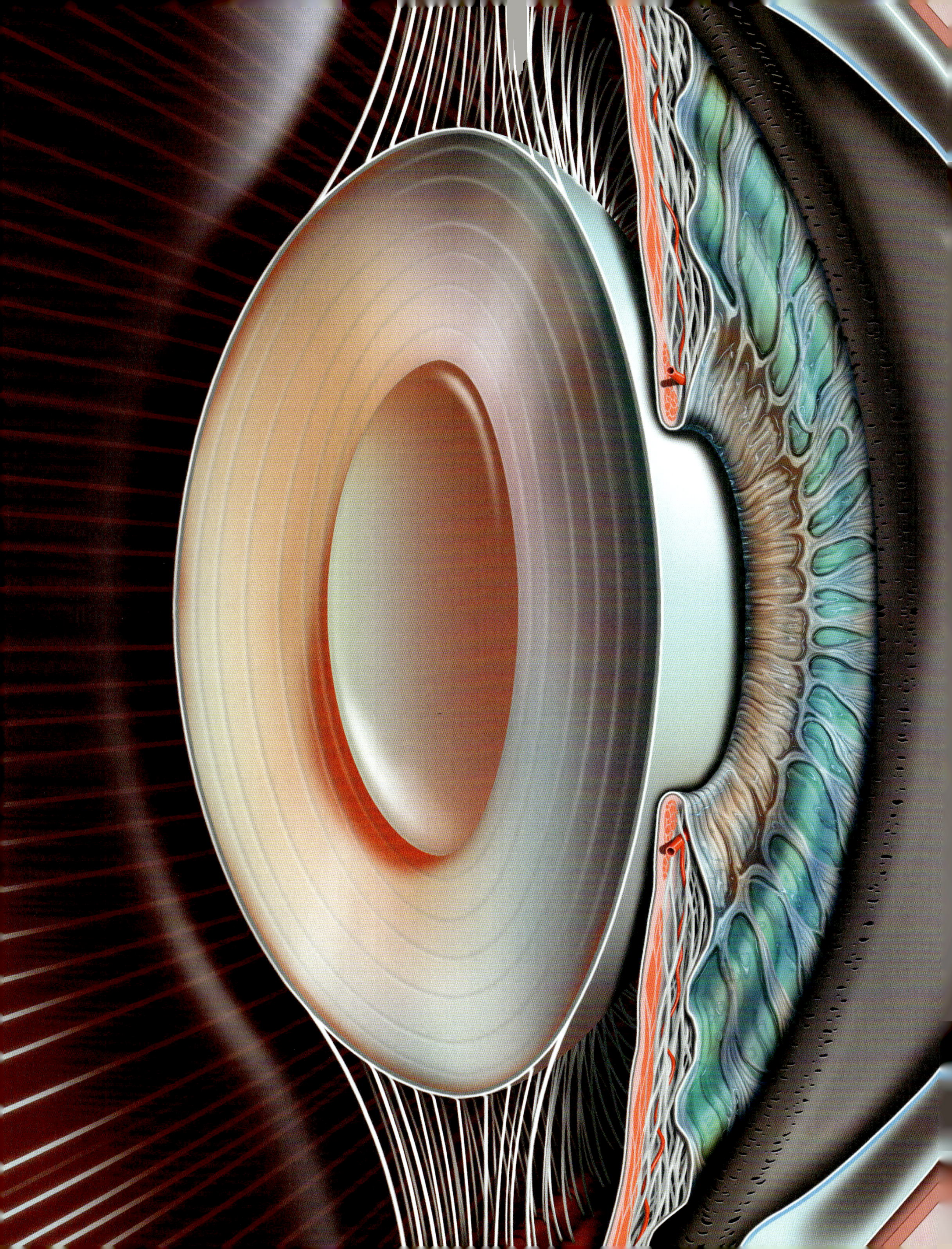

SECTION 1
Cataracts and Other Disorders of the Lens

Introduction and Overview

Congenital Disorders

Trauma

Degenerations

Treatment-Related Disorders

Miscellaneous

LENS AND CATARACT OVERVIEW

GROSS ANATOMY

Lens Anatomy

- Biconcave structure separating anterior and posterior chambers
- Capsule
  - Acellular layer rich in type IV collagen that encloses lens material
  - Thicker anteriorly (8-14 µm) than posteriorly (2-3 µm), and equator is thicker than center
- Epithelium
  - Lays deep to anterior capsule
  - Cuboidal cells in center that do not undergo mitosis
  - Columnar cells in periphery that undergo mitosis
    - Nearly 2 million lens fibers are produced per lifetime
- Fibers
  - Nucleus consists of lens fibers laid down prior to birth
    - Clinical "nucleus" seen on slit-lamp exam also contains deep cortical fibers laid down after birth
    - Nucleus contains nondividing older cells
    - Located in central lens
  - Cortex is composed of recently formed fibers from dividing cells
    - Located in peripheral lens and surrounds the nucleus
  - Lens sutures represent origination of fibers prior to migration and outward growth
    - Located centrally in lens nucleus
    - Anterior suture appears as an upright "Y"
    - Posterior suture appears as a "λ" (or Mercedes sign)
- Zonules
  - Sheets of fibrillin that attach lens capsule to ciliary body
  - From anterior to posterior, zonules attach to lens pre-equatorially, equatorially, and post-equatorially

Lens Physiology

- Composed of 65% water and 35% protein
- Relatively hypoxic structure, with mostly anaerobic energy production
- Peripheral lens fibers synthesize protein, mostly crystallin
  - Crystallin gives lens its high refractive index
  - Minimal lens fiber scatter secondary to thin lens fiber membranes, small interfiber spaces, tightly packed crystallin, absence of blood vessels, loss of organelles within cells

Lens Dimensions

- Thickness: 4 mm
- Radius of curvature
  - Anteriorly ~ 10 mm
  - Posteriorly ~ 6 mm
- Lens strength/power: 18-20 diopters
- Refractive index: 1.386

CATARACTS

Age of Onset

- Congenital (newborns or infants)
- Juvenile or presenile
- Age-related or senile

Morphology

- Fiber based: Cataract pattern follows anatomical structure of lens, either along a suture or within nucleus or cortex
- Non-fiber based: Random distribution of cataract

Grade

- Defines degree of lens opacification
- Lens Opacities Classification System III (LOCS III) is often used

Maturity

- Immature: Incomplete opacification
- Mature: Total opacification
- Hypermature: Lysis of cortex material → shrinkage of cortex and wrinkling of capsule
- Morgagnian: Liquefaction of cortex → hard nucleus drops inferiorly within capsule

Type

- Sutural: Along central "Y" suture
  - Congenital: Nonprogressive, appears at birth
  - Concussion: Lens fiber separation allows fluid to enter between fibers and creates a flower appearance
  - Storage disorder: Seen in Fabry disease or mannosidosis; often originates in posterior lens
  - Deposition disorder: Deposits of copper, gold, silver, iron, or chlorpromazine in anterior lens
- Nuclear: Within nucleus
  - Congenital: Nonprogressive, can be limited to embryonic nucleus or more involved
  - Age related: Causes light scattering and brunescence due to brown chromophores
- Lamellar: Within peripheral nucleus
  - Congenital/infantile: Localized to a particular layer of lens ± extensions (riders); can be inherited or secondary to rubella, diabetes, galactosemia, or hypocalcemia
- Coronary: Within deep cortex
  - Sporadic: Round opacities form a crown-like appearance; can be inherited but not always
- Cortical: Within peripheral cortex
  - Age related: Spoke-like opacities in superficial layers of cortex
- Subcapsular: Just within capsule in far cortex periphery
  - Age related or presenile: Granular material directly beneath capsule; posterior is more common than anterior location; associated with diabetes, corticosteroid use, uveitis, and radiation, prior vitrectomy
- Polar: Within central anterior or posterior pole of lens capsule ± lens involvement
  - Congenital anterior: Seen in persistent pupillary membrane, anterior lenticonus, Peters anomaly
  - Congenital posterior: Seen in persistent hyperplastic primary vitreous, Mittendorf dots, posterior lenticonus; associated with remnants of tunica vasculosa lentis; ↑ risk of capsule rupture and vitreous loss
- Diffuse: Within entire lens
  - Congenital: Focal blue dot opacities; seen in Lowe syndrome carriers
  - Age related: Christmas tree cataracts with highly reflective crystalline opacities

LENS ANATOMY AND HISTOLOGY

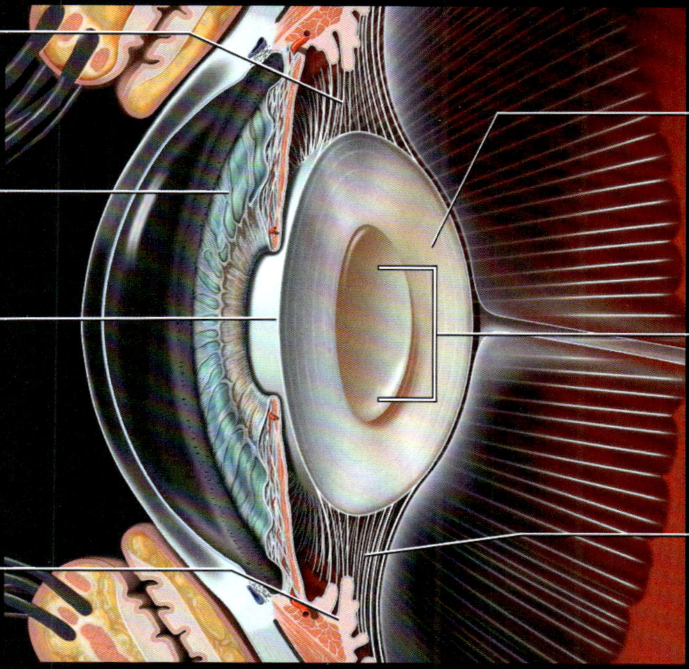

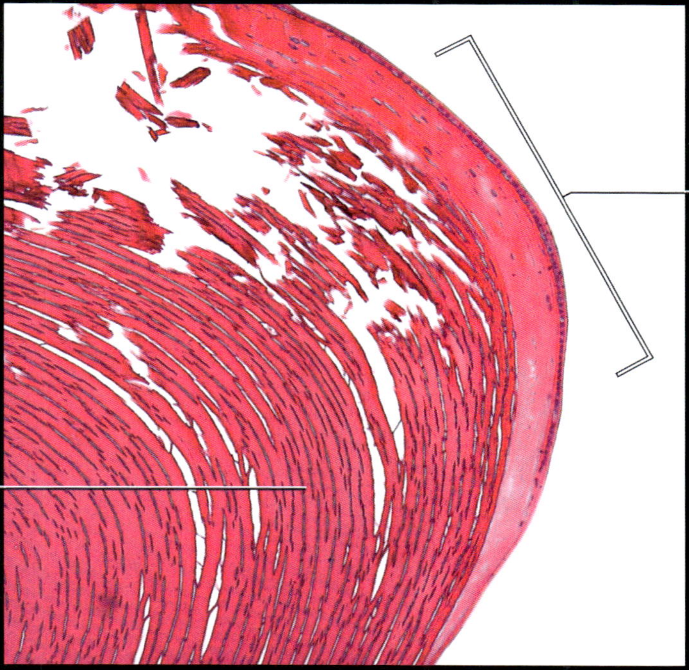

(Top) *This diagram demonstrates the location of the lens within the eye, just posterior to the iris, dividing the anterior and posterior chambers. The lens contains a centralized nucleus, surrounded by peripheral cortex, all contained within a thin capsule measuring roughly 8-14 μm anteriorly and 2-3 μm posteriorly. The lens is attached to the ciliary body by 360° of zonules, which attach to the lens capsule. When the ciliary body contracts during accommodation, tension on the zonules is released, which allows the lens to assume a more spherical shape and increases the lens curvature and the strength/power of the lens. Lens fibers are produced by cells that originate in the anterior or posterior "Y" sutures as they migrate toward the lens periphery. A cataract is an opacification of the lens.* ***(Bottom)*** *This histopathologic image of a hematoxylin and eosin-stained lens equator demonstrates the lens capsule epithelial cells on the anterior surface of the lens and lens cortex.*

CATARACT TYPES

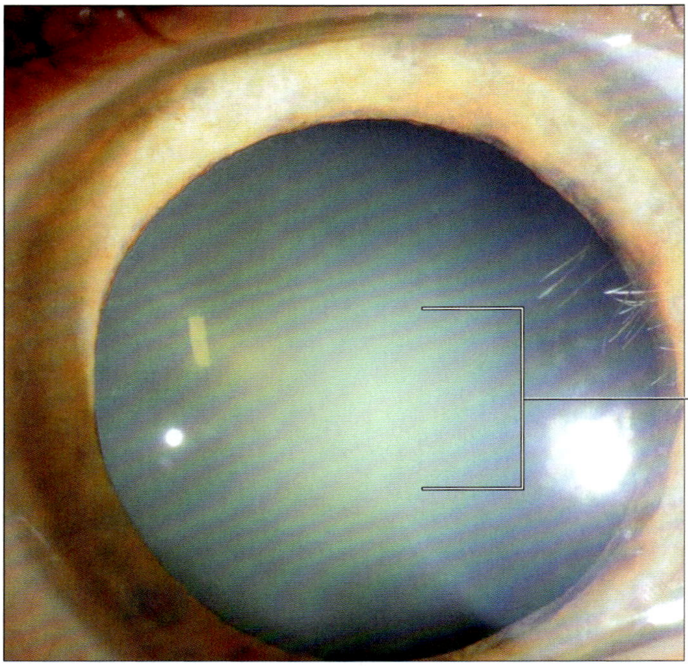

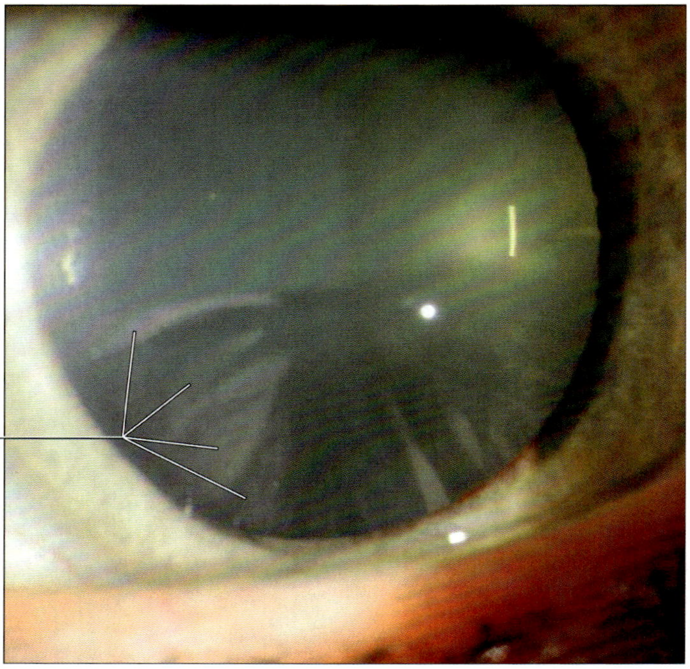

(Top) *A nuclear sclerosis cataract forms within the center of the lens, in the nucleus. As the equatorial epithelial cells of the lens continue to divide, they crowd the central fibers and cause sclerosis and lens darkening. The brown coloration is due to a urochrome pigment. This is the most common type of cataract and it is associated with aging. Patients often complain of difficulty with distance vision with preservation of reading vision. In young patients, these cataracts are associated with high myopia.* ***(Bottom)*** *A cortical cataract is characterized by white, wedge-shaped opacities in the periphery of the lens that extend towards the central nucleus in a spoke-like fashion as the cataract ages. As its name suggests, this cataract occurs in the peripheral cortex of the lens.*

CATARACT TYPES

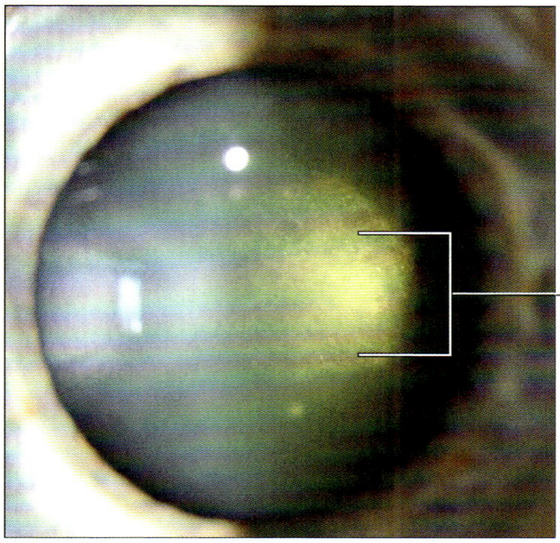

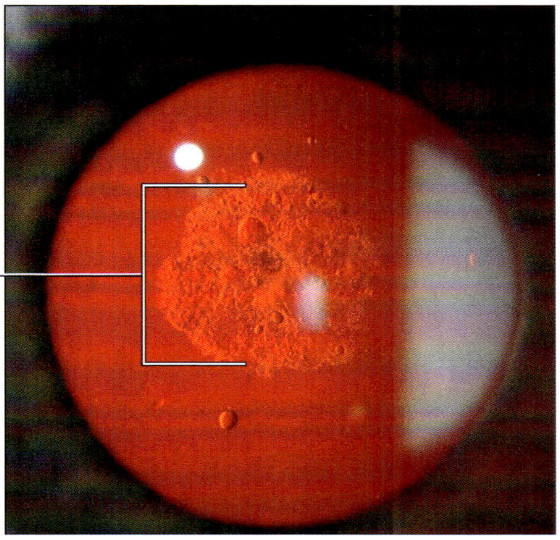

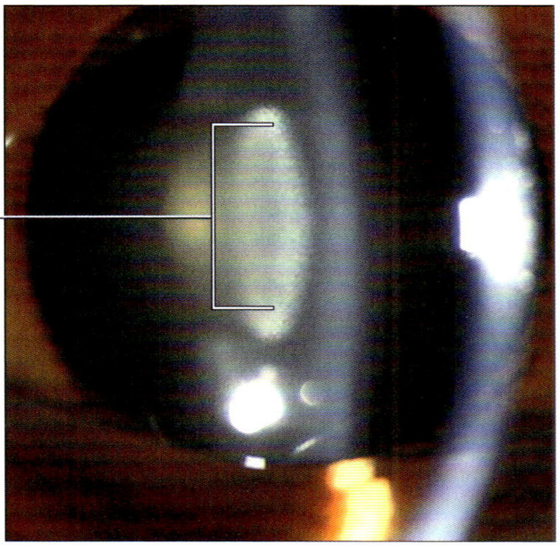

(Top) *A posterior subcapsular cataract occurs at the back of the lens just within the posterior capsule. This cataract is common in people with diabetes mellitus, those taking high-dose corticosteroids, or those with uveitis.* ***(Middle)*** *This posterior subcapsular cataract is viewed at the slit lamp with retroillumination. Patients with posterior subcapsular cataracts often complain of blurred reading vision, problems with glare, and poor vision in brightly lit situations with better functioning in dim lighting.* ***(Bottom)*** *The cortex of the lens is created in layers, like an onion. A lamellar cataract is characterized by a ring-like opacification within 1 layer of the cortex between the central nucleus and lens periphery. It is centered around the nucleus and may have cortical riders, which are linear opacities that wrap around the edge of the cataract. A lamellar cataract is associated with developmental and nutritional factors, seen in diabetes, rubella infection, galactosemia, and hypocalcemia.*

MYOTONIC DYSTROPHY

Key Facts

Introduction
- Inherited progressive multisystem disorder characterized by myotonia, muscle atrophy, cardiac dysfunction, endocrine abnormalities, & cataracts
- Most common muscular dystrophy of adults

Demographics
- Autosomal dominant inheritance
- Demonstrates genetic anticipation: Phenotype worsens in severity with each generation
- Often diagnosed in young adulthood
- Unstable expansion of CTG trinucleotide repeat (DM1) or CCTG tetranucleotide repeat (DM2)

Presentation
- Myotonia
- Facial, neck, pharyngeal, palatal weakness
- Frontal baldness
- Visual impairment in later stages
- "Masked facies" appearance
- Christmas tree cataract
  - Polychromatic iridescent crystals in anterior and posterior lens cortex
  - May be initial presenting sign
- Posterior subcapsular cataract
  - Stellate pattern
  - Often visually debilitating by mid life

Differential Diagnosis
- Idiopathic
- Drug induced
- Hypocalcemia

Treatment
- Cataract extraction and intraocular lens placement for visually significant opacities
- Premature death often from pulmonary infection, complete heart block, congestive heart failure

__(Left)__ Magnified slit-lamp photo demonstrates classic polychromatic iridescent crystals of Christmas tree cataract in the lens cortex, characteristic of myotonic dystrophy. Colors displayed vary according to the angle of illumination. __(Right)__ Slit-lamp photo shows retroillumination of a Christmas tree cataract.

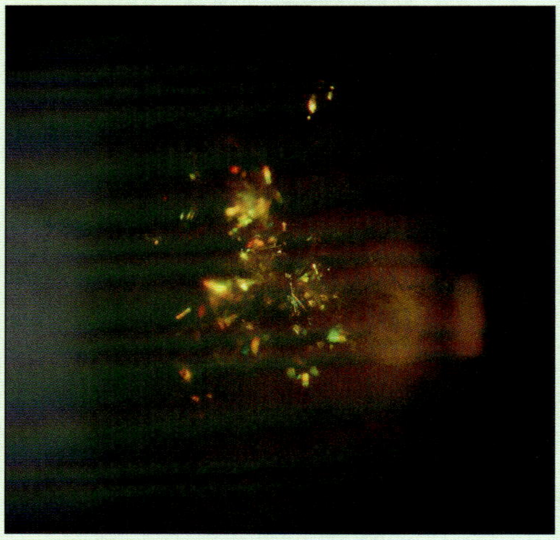

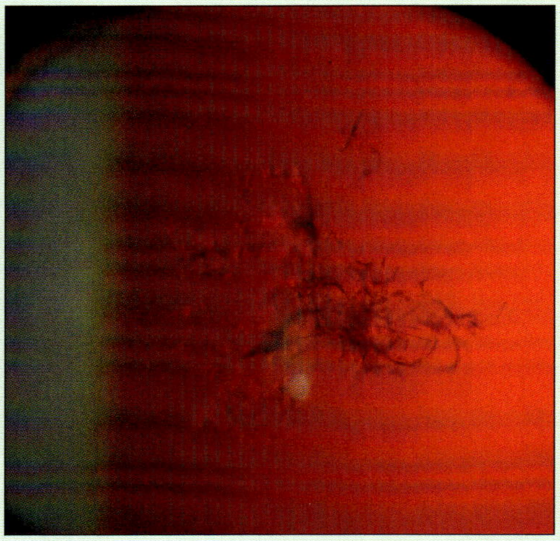

__(Left)__ This is another example of a multicolored Christmas tree cataract. Though it is visually insignificant early in its course, this is often the initial presenting sign for myotonic dystrophy. Similar cataracts can occur idiopathically, as an adverse drug effect or due to hypocalcemia. __(Right)__ Slit-lamp photo shows a retroilluminated cataract. Iridescent crystals are only visible with oblique illumination.

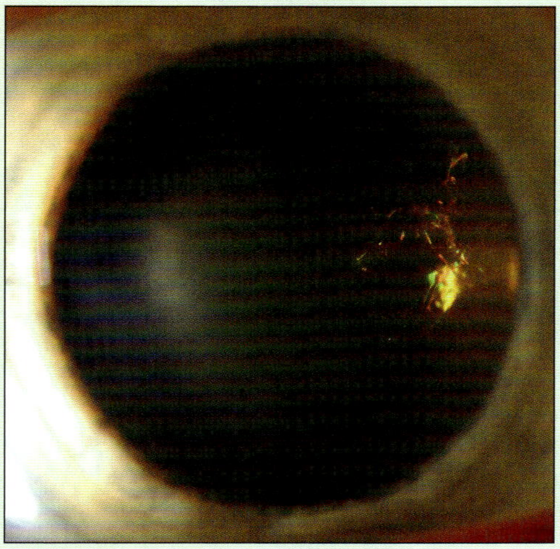

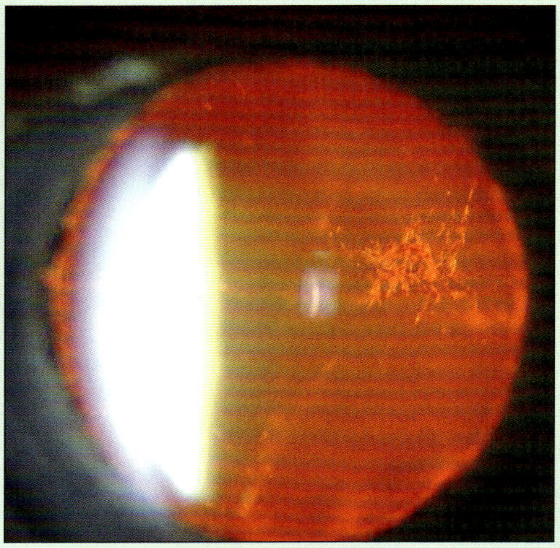

MYOTONIC DYSTROPHY

INTRODUCTION

Synonyms
- Dystrophia myotonica (DM)

Definitions
- Inherited progressive multisystem disorder characterized by myotonia, muscle atrophy, cardiac dysfunction, endocrine abnormalities, and cataracts

Subtypes
- Type 1 (DM1), also known as Steinert disease
  - More severe, 98% of myotonic dystrophy cases
- Type 2 (DM2), also known as proximal myotonic myopathy (PROMM)

DEMOGRAPHICS

Etiology/Risk Factors
- Autosomal dominant inheritance
- Unstable expansion of CTG trinucleotide repeat (DM1) or CCTG tetranucleotide repeat (DM2)
- Demonstrates genetic anticipation: Phenotype worsens in severity with each generation

Epidemiology
- Prevalence estimates range between 1 in 10,000 and 1 in 100,000
- Often diagnosed in young adulthood
- May present at any stage of life

PRESENTATION

Symptoms
- Myotonia
  - Slow relaxation of muscle after voluntary contraction
  - Commonly presents in childhood
  - May precede weakness by many years
- Distal > proximal limb muscle weakness and atrophy
- Facial, neck, pharyngeal, palatal weakness
  - Ptosis
  - Dysarthria, nasal voice
  - Dysphagia
- Frontal baldness
- Intellectual impairment
- Gonadal atrophy, hypogonadism
- Visual impairment in later stages

Exam Findings
- "Masked facies" appearance
  - Due to masseter and temporalis atrophy
- Ocular manifestations
  - Christmas tree cataract
    - Polychromatic iridescent crystals in anterior and posterior lens cortex
    - Highly refractile; blue, blue-green, red, yellow colors
    - May be initial presenting sign
    - Visually insignificant in early stages
  - Posterior subcapsular cataract
    - Develops progressively throughout course
    - Stellate pattern
    - Often visually debilitating by mid life
  - Ophthalmoplegia
  - Light-near dissociation

DIFFERENTIAL DIAGNOSIS

Other Myotonic Syndromes
- Paramyotonia
- Congenital myotonia
- Mild tetanus

Polychromatic Iridescent Crystals in Lens
- Idiopathic
- Drug induced
- Hypocalcemia

EVALUATION/WORK-UP

Labs
- Serum CK may be slightly elevated

Pathology
- Muscle biopsy: Atrophic & necrotic muscle fibers

Studies
- EMG often reveals evidence of myotonia
- EKG may demonstrate cardiac conduction deficits

TREATMENT

Medical
- No specific treatment warranted in most cases
- DM2 patients may desire treatment for muscle stiffness
  - Phenytoin and mexiletine are preferred

Surgical
- Cardiac pacemaker for advanced conduction abnormalities
- Cataract extraction and intraocular lens placement for visually significant opacities

Follow-Up
- Genetic counseling warranted if children desired
- Increased risk of respiratory depression and pneumonia following general anesthesia

Prognosis
- Most patients wheelchair bound within 15-20 years of diagnosis
- Premature death often from pulmonary infection, complete heart block, congestive heart failure

SELECTED REFERENCES

1. Bird TD: Myotonic Dystrophy Type 1. 1999 Sep 17 [updated 2011 Feb 08]. In: Pagon RA et al: GeneReviews. Seattle: University of Washington. 1993-. http://www.ncbi.nlm.nih.gov/books/NBK1165. Accessed July 1, 2013
2. Turner C et al: The myotonic dystrophies: diagnosis and management. J Neurol Neurosurg Psychiatry. 81(4):358-67, 2010
3. Reiter C et al: [Anticipation in patients with iridescent multicoloured posterior capsular lens opacities ("Christmas tree cataract") : The Role in the diagnosis of myotonic dystrophy.] Ophthalmologe. 106(12):1116-20, 2009

LENS SUBLUXATION

Key Facts

Introduction
- Malposition of lens due to congenital or acquired causes; also known as ectopia lentis
- Subluxation: Disruption of some zonular support leading to partial dislocation with lens still visible in pupillary area
- Luxation: Disruption of all zonular attachments leading to complete dislocation and displacement of lens from pupil

Demographics
- Ocular trauma is most common cause of subluxated lens
- Congenital ectopia lentis can be associated with
  - Marfan syndrome
  - Homocystinuria
  - Familial ectopia lentis
  - Ectopia lentis et pupillae
  - Aniridia
  - Ehlers-Danlos syndrome
  - Sulfite oxidase deficiency
  - Weill-Marchesani syndrome, which frequently causes microspherophakia with lens subluxation

Presentation
- Marfanoid habitus: Tall and thin stature, long limbs, arachnodactyly, kyphoscoliosis
- Superotemporal lens dislocation most common in Marfan syndrome
- Inferonasal dislocation most common in homocystinuria

Treatment
- Correction of refractive error is often sufficient
- Lens extraction may be indicated for failed refractive therapy, amblyopia, cataract, lens-induced glaucoma, uveitis, endothelial touch

__(Left)__ Slit-lamp photo shows superotemporal and bilateral lens subluxation in a patient with Marfan syndrome. Bilateral direction is the most common for subluxation in Marfan syndrome patients. It is estimated that > 50% of Marfan syndrome patients have some degree of subluxation. __(Right)__ This magnified slit-lamp photo shows the inferior edge of the dislocated lens. A clear zonular defect can be seen. In Marfan syndrome, a mutation in FBN-1 leads to zonular weakness and stretching.

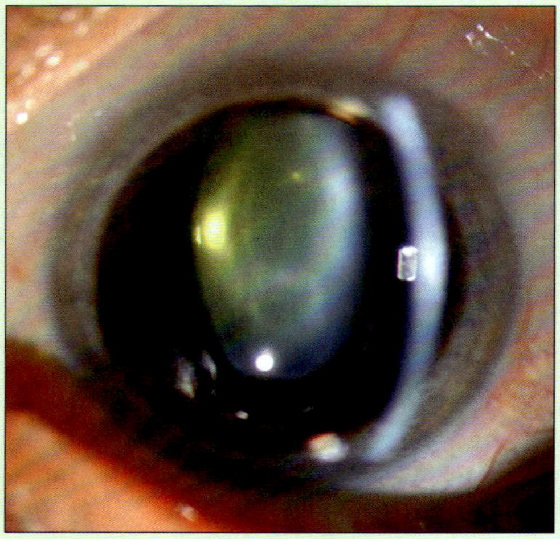

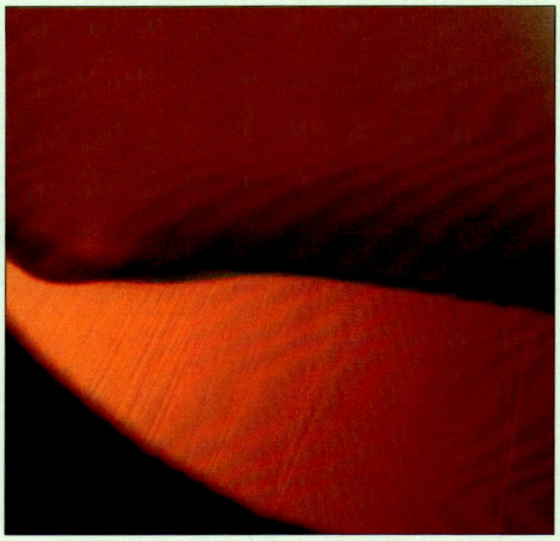

__(Left)__ This slit-lamp photo shows another example of superior lens subluxation in a 5-year-old patient. The most common cause of acquired lens dislocation is trauma; the differential for congenital lens subluxation includes Marfan syndrome, homocystinuria, familial ectopia lentis, Ehlers-Danlos syndrome, and sulfite oxidase deficiency, among others. __(Right)__ Slit-lamp photo shows retroillumination of the inferior lenticular border ➔. Individual zonules can be seen.

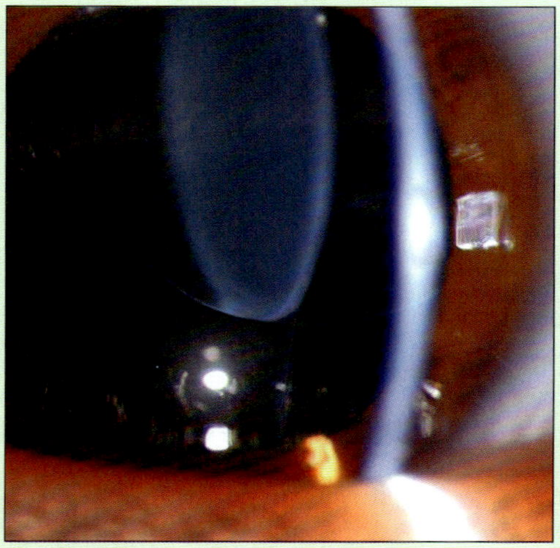

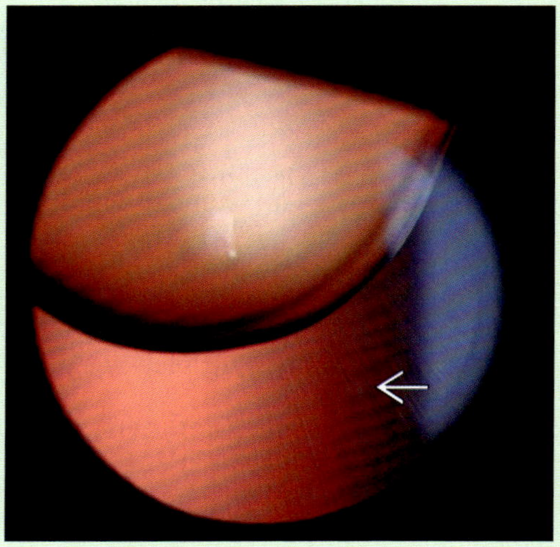

LENS SUBLUXATION

INTRODUCTION

Definitions

- Malposition of lens due to congenital or acquired causes

Subtypes

- Subluxation: Disruption of some zonular support leading to partial dislocation with lens still visible in pupillary area
- Luxation: Disruption of all zonular attachments leading to complete dislocation and displacement of lens from pupil

DEMOGRAPHICS

Etiology/Risk Factors

- Ocular trauma is most common cause of subluxated lens
- Other acquired causes include buphthalmos, high myopia, anterior uveal tumor
- Congenital ectopia lentis can be associated with many conditions

Epidemiology

- 50-80% of Marfan syndrome patients
- 80% of homocystinuria patients over age 15
- 50% of Weill-Marchesani patients

PRESENTATION

Symptoms

- Poor vision
- Significant astigmatism
- Monocular diplopia
- High myopia in Marfan patients

Exam Findings

- Marfanoid habitus: Tall and thin stature, long limbs, arachnodactyly, kyphoscoliosis
- Superotemporal lens dislocation most common in Marfan syndrome
- Inferonasal dislocation most common in homocystinuria
- Iridodonesis, phacodonesis

DIFFERENTIAL DIAGNOSIS

Congenital Ectopia Lentis

- Marfan syndrome
  - Inherited disorder of fibrillin glycoprotein leading to cardiovascular, musculoskeletal, ophthalmic anomalies
- Homocystinuria
  - Autosomal recessive defect in methionine metabolism
- Familial ectopia lentis
  - Autosomal dominant; may present at birth or later
- Ectopia lentis et pupillae
  - Autosomal recessive; pupil and lens are displaced in opposite directions
- Aniridia
- Congenital glaucoma
- Ehlers-Danlos syndrome
- Sulfite oxidase deficiency
  - Autosomal recessive; leads to ectopia lentis, seizures, mental retardation
- Weill-Marchesani syndrome frequently causes microspherophakia with lens subluxation
  - Lens is small and spherical, leading to high myopia and easy dislocation
    - Autosomal recessive condition
  - Short stature, small digits, reduced joint mobility, mental handicap

EVALUATION/WORK-UP

Labs

- Genetic testing if inherited disorder suspected

Imaging

- Life-threatening cardiovascular anomalies should be ruled out or managed before surgery

TREATMENT

Medical

- Correction of refractive error is often sufficient
- Bifocals are often helpful as subluxated lens has difficulty accommodating

Surgical

- Lens extraction may be indicated for failed refractive therapy, amblyopia, cataract, lens-induced glaucoma, uveitis, endothelial touch
- Standard IOL placement is not often feasible; options include aphakic contact lenses, scleral-sutured capsular tension ring with IOL, scleral-sutured IOL, iris-sutured IOL
- Increased surgical risk in Marfan syndrome and homocystinuria patients
  - Higher rate of vitreous loss, retinal detachment

Prognosis

- Potential complications of lens subluxation
  - Cataract development
  - Anterior lens displacement into anterior chamber
    - Pupillary block
    - Angle-closure glaucoma
  - Posterior lens displacement into vitreous
- Microspherophakia may lead to pupillary block, angle-closure glaucoma
  - Treat with cycloplegics or laser iridotomy
- Marfan syndrome patients have increased risk of lattice degeneration, retinal detachment, and glaucoma

SELECTED REFERENCES

1. American Academy of Ophthalmology: Trauma. American Academy of Ophthalmology: Lens and Cataract, AAO Basic and Clinical Science Course, Section 11. San Francisco: American Academy of Ophthalmology. 53-54, 2011
2. Yuan SM et al: Marfan's syndrome: an overview. Sao Paulo Med J. 128(6):360-6, 2010
3. Blecher MH et al: Surgical strategies for the management of zonular compromise. Curr Opin Ophthalmol. 19(1):31-5, 2008
4. Dureau P: Pathophysiology of zonular diseases. Curr Opin Ophthalmol. 19(1):27-30, 2008

POST-TRAUMATIC CATARACT

Key Facts

Demographics

- Cataract may develop following penetrating or nonpenetrating trauma, electric shock, or after exposure to ionizing or infrared radiation
- Cataract may occur acutely following trauma or have delayed presentation months to years later
- Coup and contrecoup injuries to the lens may lead to anterior or posterior lens damage
- Cataract formation and lens damage is thought to occur in 27-65% of cases of ocular trauma

Presentation

- Decreased visual acuity
- Monocular diplopia or reduced accommodation in case of lens subluxation
- Characteristic rosette cataract pattern in blunt trauma

Differential Diagnosis

- Age-related cataract
- Congenital cataract
- Cataract secondary to systemic disease
- Drug-induced cataract

Treatment

- May be managed conservatively in some cases to preserve accommodative function, especially in younger patients
- Cataract extraction with IOL placement if indicated
- Additional surgical complications may be present, including posterior capsule rupture, zonular defect, pupillary abnormalities
- Traumatic cataracts may self resolve, persist, or progress over months to years
- Overall prognosis variable depending on type and severity of injury, morphology of traumatic cataract

*(**Left**) The cataract shown in this slit-lamp photo developed secondary to blunt trauma. This cataract displays the characteristic rosette pattern seen in this type of injury. This pattern is thought to develop from absorption of fluid and subsequent swelling of lens fiber cells along suture lines. (**Right**) External photo shows traumatic cataract with lens dislocation ➲. Note the area of zonular injury, which led to dislocation. Zonular injury is thought to result from equatorial expansion of the globe secondary to anterior-posterior compression.*

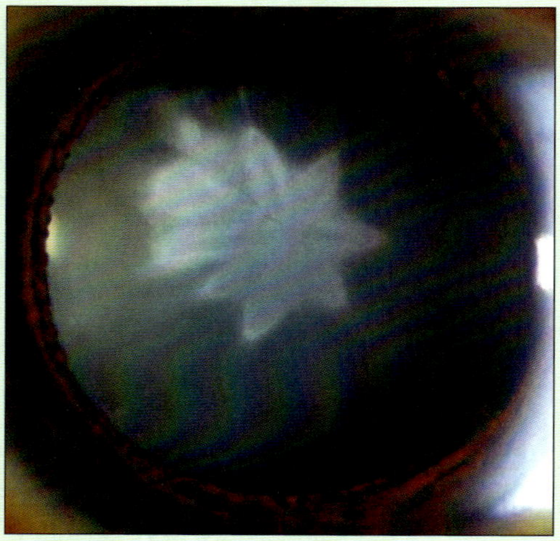

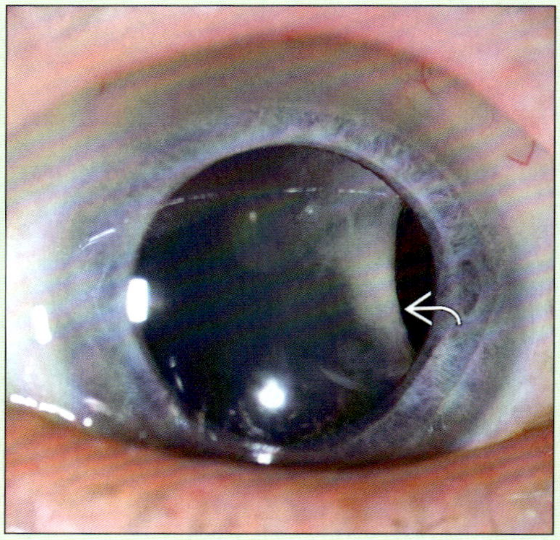

*(**Left**) External photo shows a cortical cataract that has developed secondary to trauma. Cortical cataracts often form in response to perforating lenticular injury and tend to progress rapidly. (**Right**) Slit-lamp photo shows retroillumination of a post-traumatic cataract. Although the exact etiology is unclear, post-traumatic cataracts are thought to form as a result of both direct lens fiber injury and microperforations in the lens capsule, leading to aqueous influx and edematous and opacified lens fibers.*

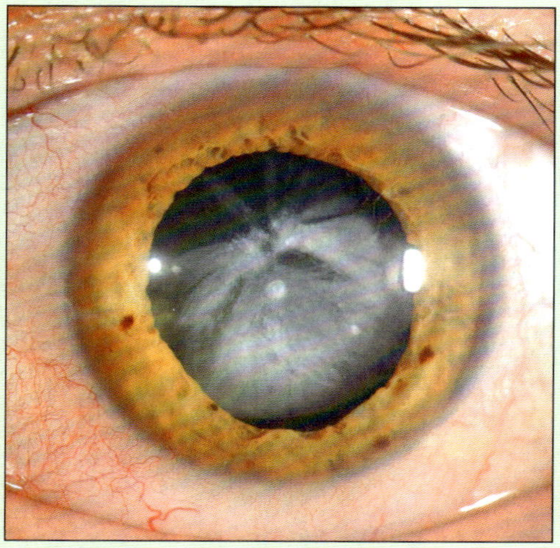

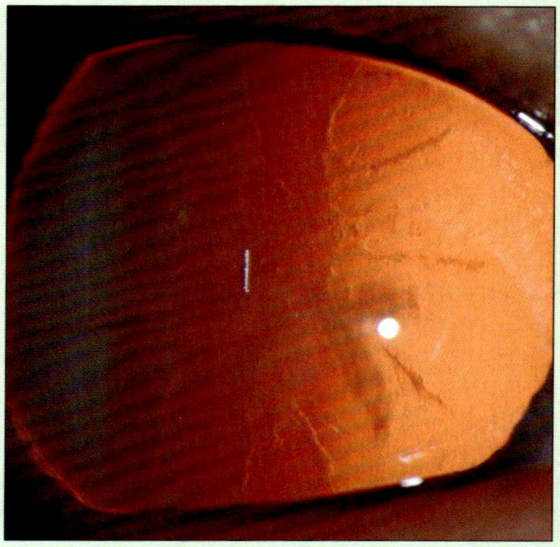

POST-TRAUMATIC CATARACT

INTRODUCTION

Definitions

- Cataract formation occurring secondary to penetrating or nonpenetrating ocular trauma

DEMOGRAPHICS

Etiology/Risk Factors

- Cataract may develop following penetrating or nonpenetrating trauma, electric shock, or after exposure to ionizing or infrared radiation
- Iatrogenic traumatic cataract may result from surgical trauma (i.e., peripheral iridectomy or vitrectomy)
- Exact pathophysiology of traumatic cataract unclear; multiple hypotheses exist, true pathophysiology likely a combination of these
  - Direct injury to lens fibers causing edema
  - Small perforations in lens capsule causing influx of aqueous humor and subsequent edematous, opacified lens fibers
- Lens capsule often ruptures posteriorly, leading to rapid hydration of lens and formation of white cataract, which causes complete opacification
- Cataract may occur acutely following trauma or have delayed presentation months to years later
- Coup and contrecoup injuries to lens may lead to anterior or posterior lens damage
- Perforating lenticular injury frequently leads to cortical cataract at perforated site with rapid progression to complete opacity

Epidemiology

- Cataract formation and lens damage is thought to occur in 27-65% of cases of ocular trauma

PRESENTATION

Symptoms

- Decreased visual acuity
- Monocular diplopia or reduced accommodation in the case of lens subluxation

Exam Findings

- Characteristic rosette cataract pattern in blunt trauma
  - Pattern is attributed to absorption of fluid and subsequent swelling of cells along lenticular sutural lines
- Associated findings
  - Vossius ring
    - Pigment from internal pupillary margin of iris becomes imprinted on anterior lenticular surface with accompanying transient miosis
  - Lens dislocation or subluxation
    - Zonular injury occurs secondary to equatorial expansion of anterior-posteriorly compressed eye; may see iridodonesis or phacodonesis on eye movement
  - Corneal or iris injuries
  - Vitreous in anterior chamber
- Ionizing radiation
  - Significant posterior subcapsular cataracts, which may develop after a several-year latency period
- Infrared radiation
  - Leads to "glassblowers" cataract due to exfoliation of lens capsule, associated cortical cataract

DIFFERENTIAL DIAGNOSIS

Other Causes of Cataract

- Age-related cataract
- Congenital cataract
- Cataract secondary to systemic disease
- Drug-induced cataract

TREATMENT

Surgical

- May be managed conservatively in some cases to preserve accommodative function especially in younger patients
- Indications for cataract extraction with IOL placement
  - Severe vision loss
  - Intraocular inflammation
  - Phacolytic or phacomorphic glaucoma
  - Intraocular foreign body
  - Perforating injury with obvious lens damage
    - Cataract extraction may be performed at time of laceration repair or deferred if lens damage is minimal
- Repair may be complicated by injury to additional structures
  - Posterior capsule rupture
    - May require anterior vitrectomy
    - Scleral fixated or anterior chamber IOL if capsular bag will not support IOL placement
  - Zonular defect
  - Pupillary abnormalities

Prognosis

- Traumatic cataracts may self resolve, persist, or progress over months to years
- Overall prognosis variable depending on type and severity of injury, morphology of traumatic cataract
- Postsurgical prognosis may be limited if other ocular structures sustained damage in initial injury

SELECTED REFERENCES

1. Shah MA et al: Morphology of traumatic cataract: does it play a role in final visual outcome? BMJ Open. 1(1):e000060, 2011
2. Agarwal A et al: Cataract surgery in the setting of trauma. Curr Opin Ophthalmol. 21(1):65-70, 2010
3. American Academy of Ophthalmology: Trauma. American Academy of Ophthalmology: Lens and Cataract, AAO Basic and Clinical Science Course, Section 11. San Francisco: American Academy of Ophthalmology. 53-58, 2010
4. Yanoff M et al: Ophthalmology. 3rd ed. Philadelphia: Mosby Elsevier, 2009
5. Dannenberg AL et al: Penetration eye injuries in the workplace. The National Eye Trauma System Registry. Arch Ophthalmol. 110(6):843-8, 1992

SENILE CATARACT

Key Facts

Introduction
- Subtypes: Nuclear sclerosis (NS), cortical cataract, posterior subcapsular cataract (PSC)

Demographics
- NS: Bilateral hardening and yellowing of lens nuclei
- Cortical cataract: Caused by disruption of lens fiber cell membranes, leading to cortical protein oxidation
- PSC: Due to migration and enlargement of lens epithelial cells from equator to inner posterior capsule
- Risk factors: Age, African American race, smoking, low education level, diabetes, ultraviolet exposure
- Estimated 17% of Americans > age 40 are affected

Presentation
- Myopic shift in early stages of nuclear sclerosis
- Decreased visual acuity; NS tends to affect distance vision, PSC affects near
- "Glare" from oncoming headlights due to light scattering, most striking in PSC
- NS: Yellow to brown appearance of lens nucleus
- Cortical cataract: Subcapsular vacuoles & water clefts, radial spoke-like opacities
- PSC: Granular, plaque-like appearance adjacent to posterior capsule on oblique illumination

Evaluation/Work-Up
- Thorough ophthalmic exam to assess factors that may limit prognosis
- Glare testing (brightness acuity testing)
- Biometry and IOL power calculation

Treatment
- Cataract extraction with IOL is mainstay of treatment
- Roughly 95% of otherwise healthy eyes attain 20/40 or better vision

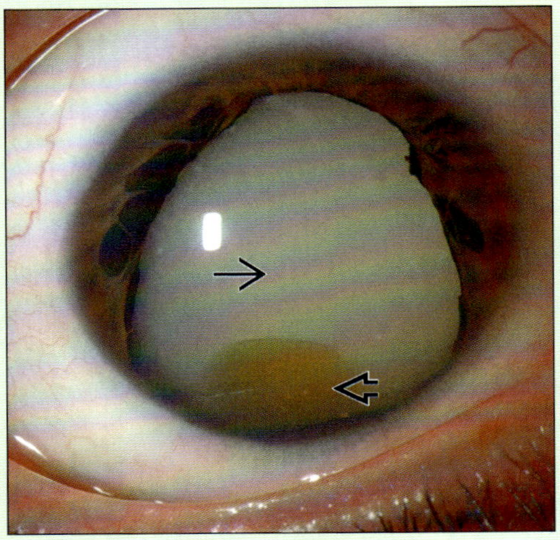
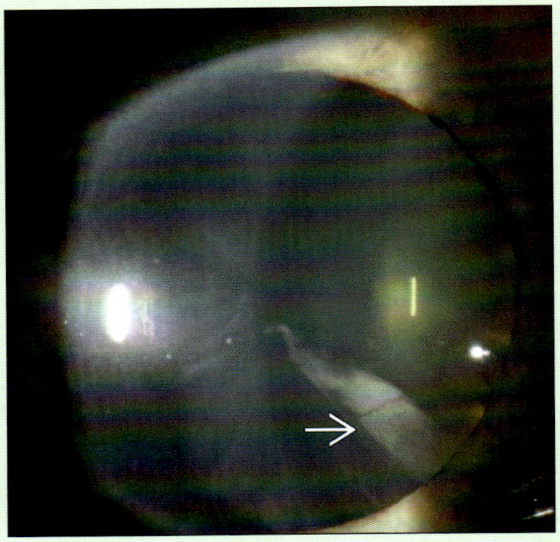

(Left) *External photo shows a Morgagnian cataract. In this extreme example, a hypermature nuclear cataract has progressed to the point of complete liquefaction of the lens cortex →, causing the brunescent lens nucleus to fall inferiorly in the lens capsule ⇨. This eye is at risk for phacomorphic glaucoma and angle closure as the lens capsule bulges anteriorly.* ***(Right)*** *This slit-lamp photo shows a cortical cataract ➡. Early subcapsular vacuoles and water clefts give rise to these radial spoke-like opacities.*

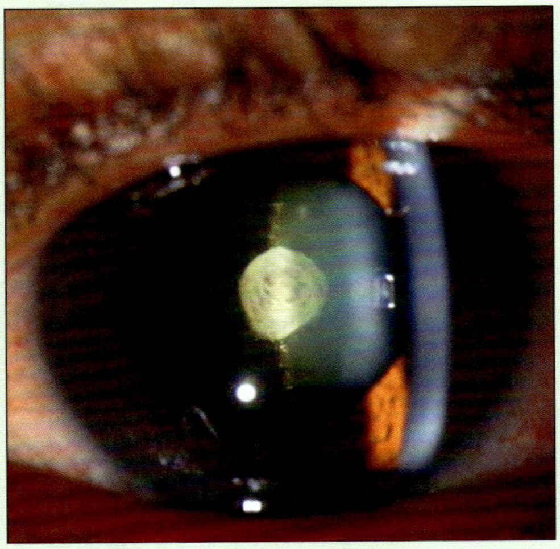
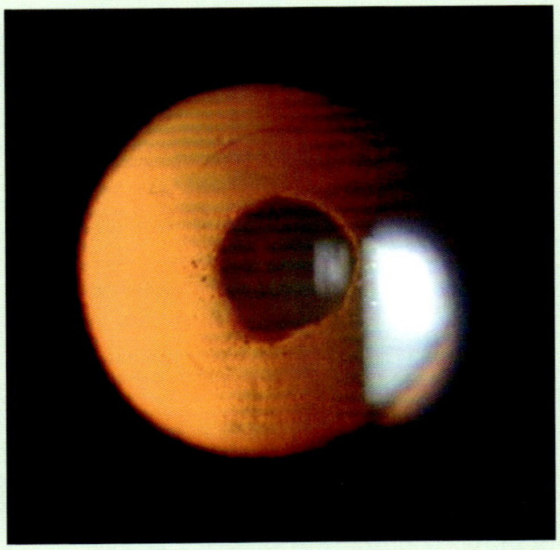

(Left) *Slit-lamp photo shows a posterior subcapsular cataract (PSC). PSCs frequently develop centrally in visual axis, causing early visual impairment and significant "glare" due to diffraction of oncoming light.* ***(Right)*** *Slit-lamp photo demonstrates retroillumination of a PSC. The mechanism of PSC development is thought to involve the migration and enlargement of lens epithelial cells from the equator to the inner posterior capsule.*

SENILE CATARACT

INTRODUCTION

Subtypes
- Nuclear sclerosis (NS)
- Cortical cataract
- Posterior subcapsular cataract (PSC)

DEMOGRAPHICS

Etiology/Risk Factors
- NS
  - Bilateral hardening and yellowing of lens nuclei
- Cortical cataract
  - Caused by disruption of lens fiber cell membranes, leading to protein oxidation in lens cortex
- PSC
  - Due to migration and enlargement of lens epithelial cells from equator to inner posterior capsule
- Risk factors
  - Age, African-American race, smoking, low education level, diabetes, ultraviolet exposure

Epidemiology
- Cataracts are the leading cause of blindness worldwide
- Senile or age-related cataract is most common form
- Estimated 17% of Americans > age 40 are affected
- 2,500,000 cataract surgeries performed in United States in 2004
- Prevalence higher in women

PRESENTATION

Symptoms
- Myopic shift in early stages of NS
  - May result in "2nd sight" of previously presbyopic patients
- Decreased visual acuity; NS tends to affect distance vision, PSC affects near
- Diminished color discrimination, especially in blue spectrum
- "Glare" from oncoming headlights due to light scattering, most striking in PSC
- Monocular diplopia can be seen in some patients

Exam Findings
- Slit-lamp biomicroscopy
  - NS
    - Yellow to brown appearance of lens nucleus on oblique illumination
  - Cortical cataract
    - Early: Subcapsular vacuoles & water clefts
    - Later: Radial spoke-like opacities
  - PSC
    - Granular, plaque-like appearance adjacent to posterior capsule on oblique illumination
    - Dark central opacity on retroillumination
- Cataract maturity
  - Immature: Partial lens opacity; multiple grading systems exist for further subclassification
  - Mature: Complete lens opacity
  - Hypermature: Wrinkled, shrunken lens capsule due to leakage of degenerated capsule material
  - Morgagnian: Further progression of hypermature cataract in which lens nucleus becomes freely mobile in liquified cortex

EVALUATION/WORK-UP

Testing
- Thorough ophthalmic exam to assess factors that may limit prognosis
- Glare testing (brightness acuity testing)
- Contrast sensitivity testing
- Potential acuity estimation
- Biometry and IOL power calculation
  - Keratometry: Manual and automatic methods available
  - Axial length measurement using optical coherence or A-scan ultrasonography

TREATMENT

Medical
- Ongoing research aimed at medical therapy for cataract; no current treatment has proven effective

Surgical
- Cataract extraction with IOL is mainstay of treatment
  - Indications: Expected visual improvement, disabling anisometropia, phacolytic or phacomorphic glaucoma, phacoantigenic uveitis, lens dislocation, poor fundus view for management of retinal disease
  - Phacoemulsification
    - 2-3 mm incision size = less corneal astigmatism, rapid wound healing
    - Requires complex and expensive machinery
  - Small incision extracapsular cataract surgery
    - Faster & cheaper alternative, used frequently in developing world
    - Low complication rate; less predictable but generally good results

Follow-Up
- Regular follow-up beginning at postoperative day 1 to assess possible complications
  - IOL dislocation
  - Endophthalmitis
  - Suprachoroidal hemorrhage
  - Posterior capsular opacification (PCO)

Prognosis
- Roughly 95% of otherwise healthy eyes attain 20/40 or better vision

SELECTED REFERENCES

1. American Academy of Ophthalmology: Aging Changes. American Academy of Ophthalmology: Lens and Cataract, AAO Basic and Clinical Science Course, Section 11. San Francisco: American Academy of Ophthalmology. 43-51, 2011
2. Kanski J et al: Clinical Ophthalmology: A Systematic Approach. 7th ed. Philadelphia: Elsevier Saunders, 2011
3. Allen D et al: Cataract and surgery for cataract. BMJ. 333(7559):128-32, 2006

Key Facts

Introduction

- Retina and glaucoma surgeries are accompanied by their respective risks and complications including
  - Glaucoma surgery: Overfiltration with hypotony, flat anterior chamber, bleb leak, choroidal detachment, choroidal hemorrhage, elevated IOP, blebitis, endophthalmitis, sterile uveitis, early or late failure of filtering bleb, aqueous misdirection, pupillary block, endothelial damage and corneal edema, hyphema, macular edema, RD, cataract, ptosis
  - Retina surgery: RD, choroidal detachment, choroidal hemorrhage, endophthalmitis, sterile uveitis, cataract, bleeding, macular edema, retina laser/ instrument damage, vitreous hemorrhage, diplopia, elevated IOP (includes silicone oil-related or overexpansion of intraocular gas), ptosis
  - Complications of anesthesia such as retrobulbar hemorrhage with retrobulbar block

Presentation

- Blebitis: Pain, injected eye, white bleb with inflammatory debris, no evidence of A/C cell
- Endophthalmitis: Decreased vision, A/C cell, hypopyon, vitritis, fibrin, retinitis, corneal edema, conjunctival injection, eyelid edema, possible RD
- Aqueous misdirection: High IOP with anterior movement of iris-lens diaphragm and shallowing of entire anterior chamber
- Pupillary block: High IOP with moderately deep central anterior chamber and bowing of the peripheral iris
- Choroidal effusion: Hypotonous eye with detached choroid on fundus exam
- Suprachoroidal hemorrhage: Severe pain, shallow anterior chamber, and elevated IOP

Treatment

- Directed at underlying condition

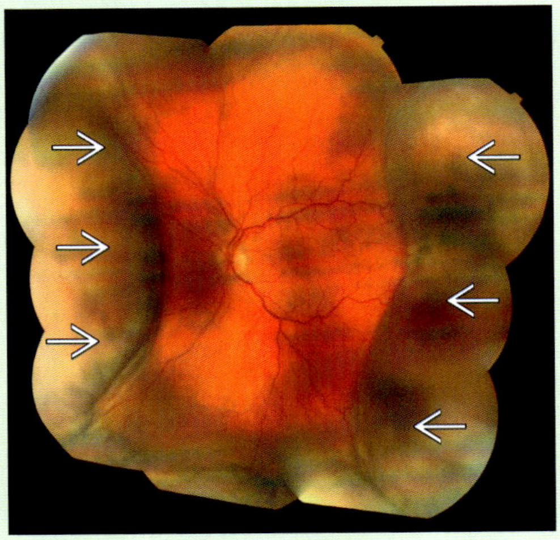

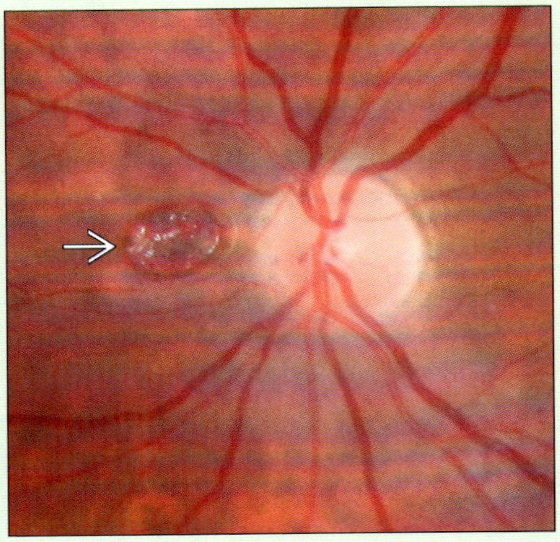

(Left) *This fundus photo mosaic shows a large serous choroidal effusion ➔ following intraocular surgery. Hypotony during or after surgery may lead to choroidal detachments, as is sometimes seen with overfiltration following glaucoma surgery. This patient's effusion resolved, and vision was 20/20. (Courtesy A. Schadlu, MD.)* ***(Right)*** *Fundus photo demonstrates subretinal migration of Perfluoron ➔, which was used during the patient's vitrectomy surgery 18 months prior. (Courtesy S. Cohen, MD.)*

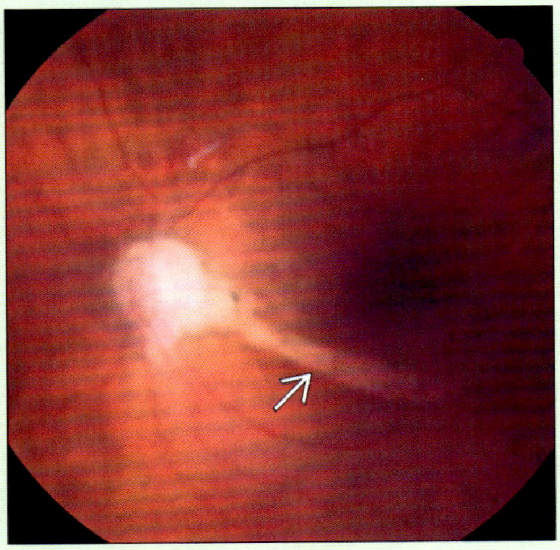

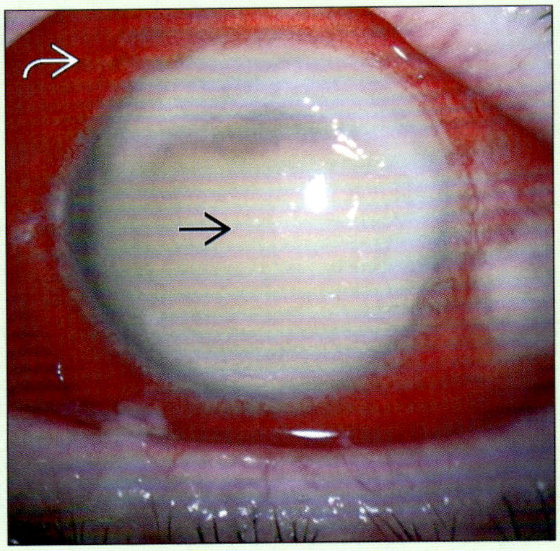

(Left) *This fundus photo shows a macular scar ➔ resulting from needle injury during retrobulbar anesthesia prior to vitrectomy surgery. This emphasizes the importance of discussing the risk of surgery, as well as that of anesthesia, with patients. (Courtesy S. Cohen, MD.)* ***(Right)*** *External photo depicts one of the most feared complications of intraocular surgery: Endophthalmitis. Note the intensely inflamed sclera ➔ and dense hypopyon ➔ filling the anterior chamber. (Courtesy J. Calhoun.)*

POSTSURGICAL COMPLICATIONS (RETINA AND GLAUCOMA SURGERY)

INTRODUCTION

Definitions

- Iatrogenic adverse events arising from retina and glaucoma surgery

Subtypes

- Glaucoma surgery: Overfiltration with hypotony, flat anterior chamber, bleb leak, choroidal detachment, choroidal hemorrhage, elevated IOP, blebitis, endophthalmitis, sterile uveitis, early or late failure of filtering bleb, aqueous misdirection, pupillary block, endothelial damage and corneal edema, hyphema, macular edema, retinal detachment (RD), cataract, ptosis
- Retina surgery: RD, choroidal detachment, choroidal hemorrhage, endophthalmitis, sterile uveitis, cataract, bleeding, macular edema, retina laser/instrument damage, vitreous hemorrhage, diplopia, elevated IOP (includes silicone oil-related or overexpansion of intraocular gas), ptosis
- Complications of anesthesia, such as retrobulbar hemorrhage with retrobulbar block

DEMOGRAPHICS

Etiology/Risk Factors

- Intraocular surgery

Epidemiology

- Intravitreal injection-related endophthalmitis
  - Intravitreal triamcinolone (Kenalog): 1.4% per injection
  - Ranibizumab (Lucentis): 0.2% per injection
- Pars-plana vitrectomy (PPV)-related endophthalmitis: 0.03-0.046%
- Glaucoma surgery-related endophthalmitis: 0.12-1.2% per year (increased risk with antifibrotic agent use)
- Aqueous misdirection: Affects ~ 2% of glaucoma cases

PRESENTATION

Symptoms

- Pain, decreased or blurred vision, red eye, swollen eyelid, floaters, flashes, veils, photophobia, visual field defects, diplopia

Exam Findings

- Blebitis: Pain, injected eye, white bleb with inflammatory debris, no evidence of anterior chamber (A/C) cell
- Endophthalmitis: Decreased vision, A/C cell, hypopyon, vitritis, fibrin, retinitis, corneal edema, conjunctival injection, eyelid edema, possible RD
- Aqueous misdirection: High IOP with anterior movement of iris-lens diaphragm and shallowing of entire anterior chamber
- Pupillary block: High IOP with moderately deep central anterior chamber and bowing of the peripheral iris
- Choroidal effusion: Hypotonous eye with detached choroid on fundus exam
- Suprachoroidal hemorrhage: Severe pain, shallow anterior chamber, and elevated IOP

EVALUATION/WORK-UP

Labs

- Gram stain and culture aqueous or vitreous

Imaging

- Ocular ultrasound: Performed for inadequate fundus view to rule out RD

TREATMENT

Medical

- IOP-lowering drops for ocular hypertension
- Digital ocular pressure may be tried for low-functioning bleb as early as day 1 postop
- Mydriatics are first-line treatment for aqueous misdirection
- Topical steroids and cycloplegics for postoperative inflammation
- Systemic and local (topical or intravitreal) antibiotics for blebitis and endophthalmitis per endophthalmitis vitrectomy study (EVS) guidelines

Surgical

- PPV or scleral buckle for RD
- PPV for endophthalmitis per EVS guidelines in light perception or worse vision
- Bleb needling ± mitomycin C or 5-fluorouracil may be attempted for refractory high IOP and evidence of episcleral fibrosis after glaucoma filtering surgery
- Laser suture lysis of scleral flap sutures may be attempted 1-2 weeks postop if IOP is still high
- Laser peripheral iridectomy for pupillary block
- Nd:YAG laser may be used to disrupt anterior hyaloid face and break aqueous misdirection
- Reformation of anterior chamber with sodium hyaluronate, air, or SF6 if there is risk of cornea-lens touch in overfiltration cases
- Sclerectomies may be used to drain choroidal hemorrhages

Follow-Up

- Daily for high-risk conditions

Prognosis

- Guarded to good depending on condition

SELECTED REFERENCES

1. Debrouwere V et al: Outcomes of different management options for malignant glaucoma: a retrospective study. Graefes Arch Clin Exp Ophthalmol. 250(1):131-41, 2012
2. Wu L et al: Endophthalmitis after pars plana vitrectomy: results of the Pan American Collaborative Retina Study Group. Retina. 31(4):673-8, 2011
3. Ang GS et al: Postoperative infection in penetrating versus non-penetrating glaucoma surgery. Br J Ophthalmol. 94(12):1571-6, 2010
4. Results of the Endophthalmitis Vitrectomy Study: a randomized trial of immediate vitrectomy and of intravenous antibiotics for the treatment of postoperative bacterial endophthalmitis. Endophthalmitis Vitrectomy Study Group. Arch Ophthalmol. 113(12):1479-96, 1995

IATROGENIC CATARACT

Key Facts

Introduction

- New formation or increased rate of progression of nuclear sclerotic, cortical, or subcapsular cataract following steroid therapy or intraocular surgery

Demographics

- Any intraocular surgery can accelerate cataract formation
- Most common is post-vitrectomy cataract
  - Vitrectomy induces or accelerates nuclear sclerosis
- Pathogenesis hypothesized to be due to increased oxygen tension
- Incidence varies with age
  - 80% of post-vitrectomy eyes > age 50 will likely develop cataract within 2 years
  - 7% of post-vitrectomy eyes < age 50 will develop cataract over same time frame
- Long-term corticosteroids cause or worsen cataracts; most notable is PSC formation

Differential Diagnosis

- Age-related cataract
- Diabetic cataract
- Traumatic cataract
- Retinal detachment
- Retinal tear
- Vitreous hemorrhage

Treatment

- Cataract extraction with IOL implantation
  - Phacoemulsification may be more difficult compared to extraction of nuclear cataracts in nonvitrectomized eyes
- Patient should be seen regularly after cataract extraction to assess for postsurgical complications
- Prognosis generally worse than nonvitrectomy cataract surgery as patients are likely to have underlying retinal disorder, which may limit visual potential

*(**Left**) This slit-lamp photo shows a nuclear sclerotic cataract. Cataracts such as this are common following intraocular surgery, particularly vitrectomy. The mechanism of cataract formation is hypothesized to be due to increased intraocular oxygen tension following vitrectomy. The vitreous normally acts as a barrier to oxygen diffusion toward the lens. Oxidative damage to lens fiber proteins leads to cataract. (**Right**) Slit-lamp photo shows a posterior subcapsular cataract (PSC), a common finding following steroid treatment.*

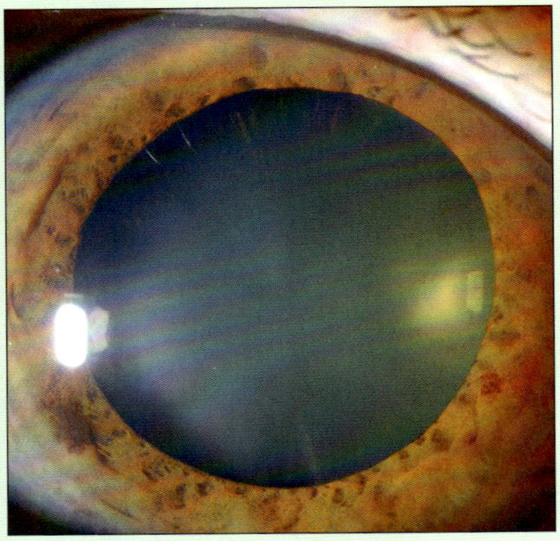

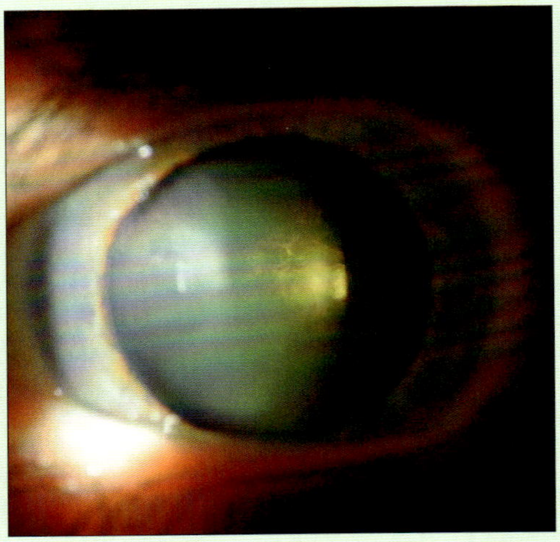

*(**Left**) This slit-lamp photo shows a dense PSC. PSC formation is a common adverse effect of steroids and can follow intraocular, topical, systemic, or inhaled corticosteroid therapy. The exact mechanism of PSC development in response to steroids is largely unknown, and these PSCs are identical in appearance to senile PSCs. (**Right**) Slit-lamp photo shows retroillumination of PSC. PSCs are frequently central in the visual axis and are symptomatic from early in their course.*

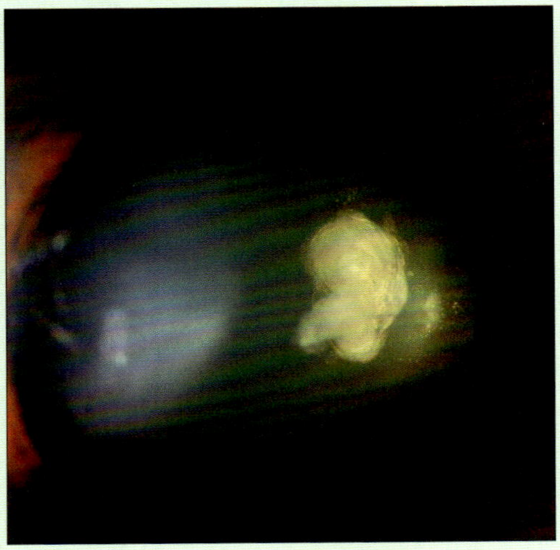

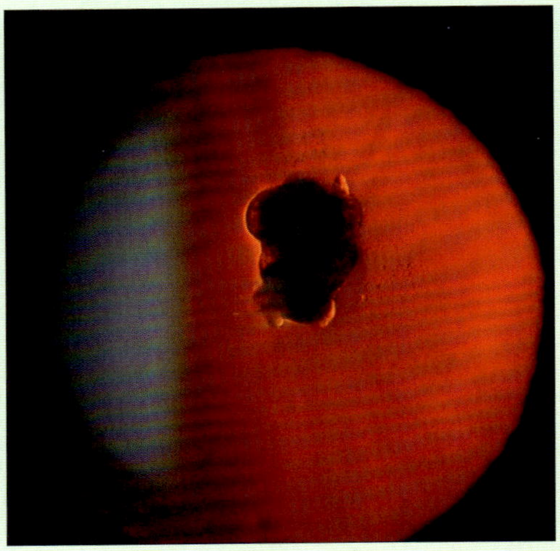

IATROGENIC CATARACT

INTRODUCTION

Definitions

- New formation or increased rate of progression of nuclear sclerotic, cortical, or subcapsular cataract following any intraocular procedure or surgery or corticosteroid administration

DEMOGRAPHICS

Etiology/Risk Factors

- Any intraocular surgery can accelerate cataract formation
- Most common is post-vitrectomy cataract
  - Vitrectomy induces or accelerates nuclear sclerosis (NS)
  - Most common complication following vitrectomy
  - Pathogenesis hypothesized to be due to increased oxygen tension
    - Oxygen tension is maintained at a gradient across vitreous with lower oxygen tension adjacent to lens compared to posterior vitreous
    - Vitreous acts as barrier to oxygen diffusion from choroid to lens
    - Intraocular oxygen tension is greatly increased post vitrectomy due to loss of barrier function of vitreous
    - NS forms as a result of increased oxidative damage to lens
      - Oxidation of lens proteins
      - Reactive oxygen species formation
  - Other causes/hypotheses
    - Use of intraocular gas frequently leads to posterior subcapsular cataract (PSC)
    - Silicone oil induced
    - Light toxicity
- Long-term corticosteroids cause or worsen cataracts; most notable is PSC formation
  - May occur following intraocular, topical, systemic, or even inhaled corticosteroids
  - IOP steroid responders are also more likely to develop PSC in response to steroids
  - Steroid-induced PSC is identical in appearance and histopathology to senile PSC

Epidemiology

- Incidence of post-vitrectomy cataract varies with age
  - 80% of post-vitrectomy eyes > age 50 will likely develop cataract within 2 years
  - 7% of post-vitrectomy eyes < age 50 will develop cataract over same time frame
- In 1 study, significant PSCs developed in 45% of eyes treated with intravitreal triamcinolone

PRESENTATION

Symptoms

- Decreased visual acuity despite apparent successful vitrectomy or following corticosteroid therapy

Exam Findings

- Slit-lamp exam: New or progressed nuclear sclerotic, cortical, or subcapsular cataract
- Contrast sensitivity testing, brightness acuity testing, and potential acuity meter testing may help differentiate cataract from noncataract causes of decreased visual acuity

DIFFERENTIAL DIAGNOSIS

Other Causes of Cataract

- Age-related cataract
- Diabetic cataract
- Traumatic cataract
- Cataract secondary to systemic disease
- Congenital cataract

Recurrent Retinal Pathology

- Retinal detachment
- Retinal tear
- Vitreous hemorrhage

TREATMENT

Surgical

- Cataract extraction with intraocular lens implantation
  - Retrospective studies have demonstrated 87-97.6% of cases had improved or unchanged visual acuity following post-vitrectomy cataract extraction, though all cases had < 2 Snellen lines gained
  - Phacoemulsification may be more difficult compared to extraction of nuclear cataracts in nonvitrectomized eyes
    - Nucleus often more dense, requiring longer phacoemulsification
    - Lack of vitreous increases risk for posterior capsular rupture
    - Zonular loosening increases anterior chamber depth

Follow-Up

- Patient should be seen regularly after cataract extraction to assess for potential postsurgical complications

Prognosis

- Variable
- Vitrectomized eyes generally have worse prognosis following cataract surgery as patients are likely to have underlying retinal disorder, which may limit visual potential

SELECTED REFERENCES

1. Do DV et al: Surgery for post-vitrectomy cataract. Cochrane Database Syst Rev. (3):CD006366, 2008
2. Thompson JT: Cataract formation and other complications of intravitreal triamcinolone for macular edema. Am J Ophthalmol. 141(4):629-37, 2006
3. Holekamp NM et al: Vitrectomy surgery increases oxygen exposure to the lens: a possible mechanism for nuclear cataract formation. Am J Ophthalmol. 139(2):302-10, 2005
4. Biró Z et al: Results of cataract surgery in previously vitrectomized eyes. J Cataract Refract Surg. 28(6):1003-6, 2002
5. Melberg NS et al: Nuclear sclerotic cataract after vitrectomy in patients younger than 50 years of age. Ophthalmology. 102(10):1466-71, 1995

DIABETES-INDUCED CATARACT

Key Facts

Demographics

- Hyperglycemia increases levels of metabolic products of glycolysis, which suppress hexokinase activity, driving reaction toward aldose reductase pathway
- Lens is poorly permeable to sorbitol, causing intralenticular sorbitol accumulation
- Degree of lens swelling is directly proportional to degree of hyperglycemia
- Cataract is primary cause of legal blindness in adult-onset diabetes and second most common cause in early-onset disease
- Prevalence of cataract is 3-4x higher in diabetics < age of 65, 2x higher in diabetics > age of 65

Presentation

- Diminished visual acuity, which may fluctuate with level of glycemic control
- Frequent glasses prescription changes owing to fluctuation of lens refractive power
- Frequent myopic shifts may be presenting sign for diabetes
- Diabetic cataract: Bilateral cortical and subcapsular opacities with "snowflake" appearance
- Age-related cataract occurs at higher frequency and at younger age in diabetics compared to nondiabetics

Evaluation/Work-Up

- Fluorescein angiography
- Macular ocular coherence tomography
- Macular photostress test or potential acuity test

Treatment

- Cataract extraction with IOL implantation
- May be associated with postoperative worsening of retinopathy or macular edema; current area of controversy
- Postsurgical prognosis may be limited by underlying diabetic retinopathy or diabetic macular edema

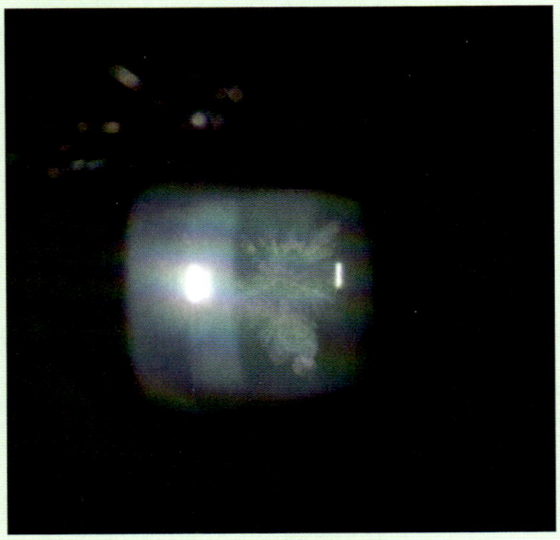

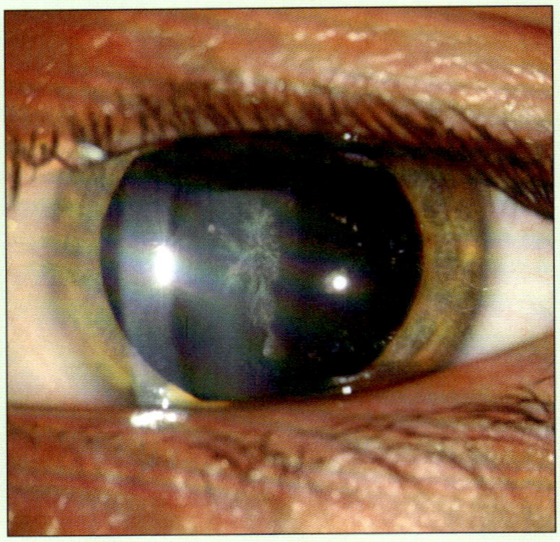

(Left) *This slit-lamp photo shows a classic "snowflake" cataract in the right eye of a 22-year-old diabetic patient. Though not commonly seen, these diabetes-induced cataracts can be found in young patients with poorly controlled diabetes and are usually bilateral.* ***(Right)*** *Slit-lamp photo shows another example of a diabetes-induced "snowflake" cataract in the left eye of a young diabetic patient. These cortical and subcapsular opacities may resolve spontaneously or rapidly progress.*

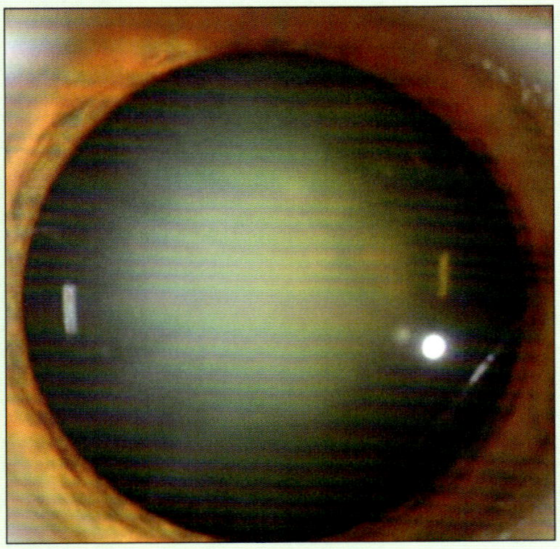

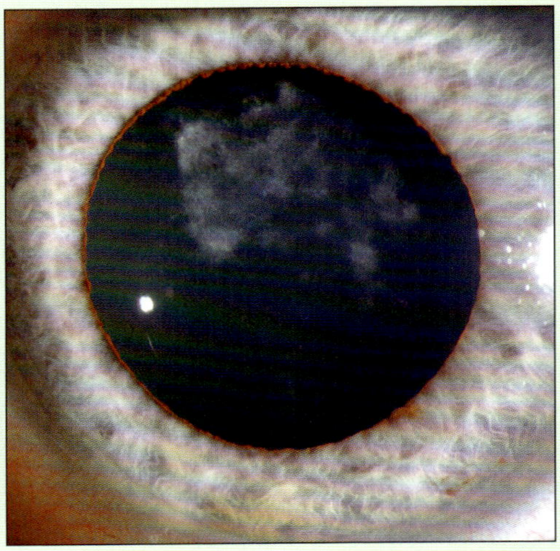

(Left) *This slit-lamp photo shows a mature nuclear cataract. Much more common than the characteristic "snowflake" diabetes-induced cataracts, nuclear cataracts and other senile cataracts have earlier onset, higher incidence, and faster progression in diabetics as compared to nondiabetics.* ***(Right)*** *Slit-lamp photo shows irregular subcapsular opacities and demonstrates another example of a diabetes-induced cataract.*

DIABETES-INDUCED CATARACT

DEMOGRAPHICS

Etiology/Risk Factors

- Biochemistry involves aldose reductase pathway
  - Under normal circumstances, only 4% of lens glucose is converted to sorbitol by aldose reductase
  - Hyperglycemia increases levels of metabolic products of glycolysis, which suppress hexokinase activity, driving reaction toward aldose reductase pathway
  - Lens is poorly permeable to sorbitol, causing intralenticular sorbitol accumulation and swelling
  - Degree of lens swelling is directly proportional to degree of hyperglycemia
- Similar pathogenesis in galactosemia
  - Enzyme deficiency leads to failure of galactose metabolism
  - Aldose reductase pathway forms galactitol in lens fiber cell cytoplasm
  - Accumulation of galactitol causes osmotic swelling, cell damage, opacification

Epidemiology

- Estimated 23.6 million people in USA suffer from diabetes (7.8% of population)
- 3.3 million with diabetes report visual impairment
- Cataract is primary cause of legal blindness in adult-onset diabetes and second most common cause in early-onset disease
- 10-year cumulative incidence of cataract surgery is > 27% in patients with early-onset diabetes, > 44% in adult-onset diabetics
- Galactosemia: Most common form occurs in 1/30,000-60,000 newborns

PRESENTATION

Symptoms

- Diminished visual acuity, which may fluctuate with level of glycemic control
- Frequent glasses prescription changes owing to fluctuation of lens refractive power
- Diminished accommodative function, early presbyopia
- Symptoms of galactosemia include failure to thrive, lethargy, vomiting, diarrhea, and mental handicap, all beginning in infancy

Exam Findings

- Frequent myopic shifts may be presenting sign for diabetic lens changes &/or cataract onset
- Diabetic cataract
  - Bilateral cortical and subcapsular opacities with "snowflake" appearance
  - Acute onset, often in young patients with poorly controlled diabetes
  - May mature rapidly over days or resolve spontaneously
  - Not commonly seen
- Age-related cataract
  - Occurs at higher frequency and at younger age in diabetics compared to nondiabetics
  - Tends to have more rapid progression than nondiabetic senile cataracts
- Galactosemia: Bilateral congenital cataracts found in 75% of patients
  - Characteristic central "oil droplet" opacities

DIFFERENTIAL DIAGNOSIS

Cataract

- Age related
- Medication induced

Other Diabetes-Related Ocular Pathology

- Diabetic retinopathy (DR)
- Diabetic macular edema (DME)

EVALUATION/WORK-UP

Labs

- Serum glucose, HbA1c

Imaging

- Fluorescein angiography
- Macular ocular coherence tomography
- Macular photostress test or potential acuity test

TREATMENT

Medical

- Prevention or prolongation of cataract development by good glycemic control throughout diabetic course
- Galactosemia: Immediate lifetime galactose-free diet

Surgical

- Cataract extraction with IOL implantation
  - Indications: Reduced visual function, poor view of retina
  - May be associated with postoperative worsening of retinopathy or macular edema; current area of controversy
    - Some evidence exists that perioperative sub-Tenon triamcinolone or intravitreal bevacizumab may improve outcomes in DR or DME patients
    - Panretinal photocoagulation for proliferative or severe nonproliferative DR improves outcomes; unclear benefit of performing before vs. after surgery
  - Surgery may be complicated by prior vitrectomy

Prognosis

- Postsurgical prognosis may be limited by underlying diabetic retinopathy or diabetic macular edema
- Galactosemia: Many symptoms, including cataracts, may be reversible with early treatment; however, long-term symptoms often persist

SELECTED REFERENCES

1. Shah AS et al: Cataract surgery and diabetes. Curr Opin Ophthalmol. 21(1):4-9, 2010
2. Suto C et al: Management of type 2 diabetics requiring panretinal photocoagulation and cataract surgery. J Cataract Refract Surg. 34(6):1001-6, 2008
3. Bosch AM: Classical galactosaemia revisited. J Inherit Metab Dis. 29(4):516-25, 2006
4. Dowler J et al: Cataract surgery in diabetes. Curr Opin Ophthalmol. 12(3):175-8, 2001

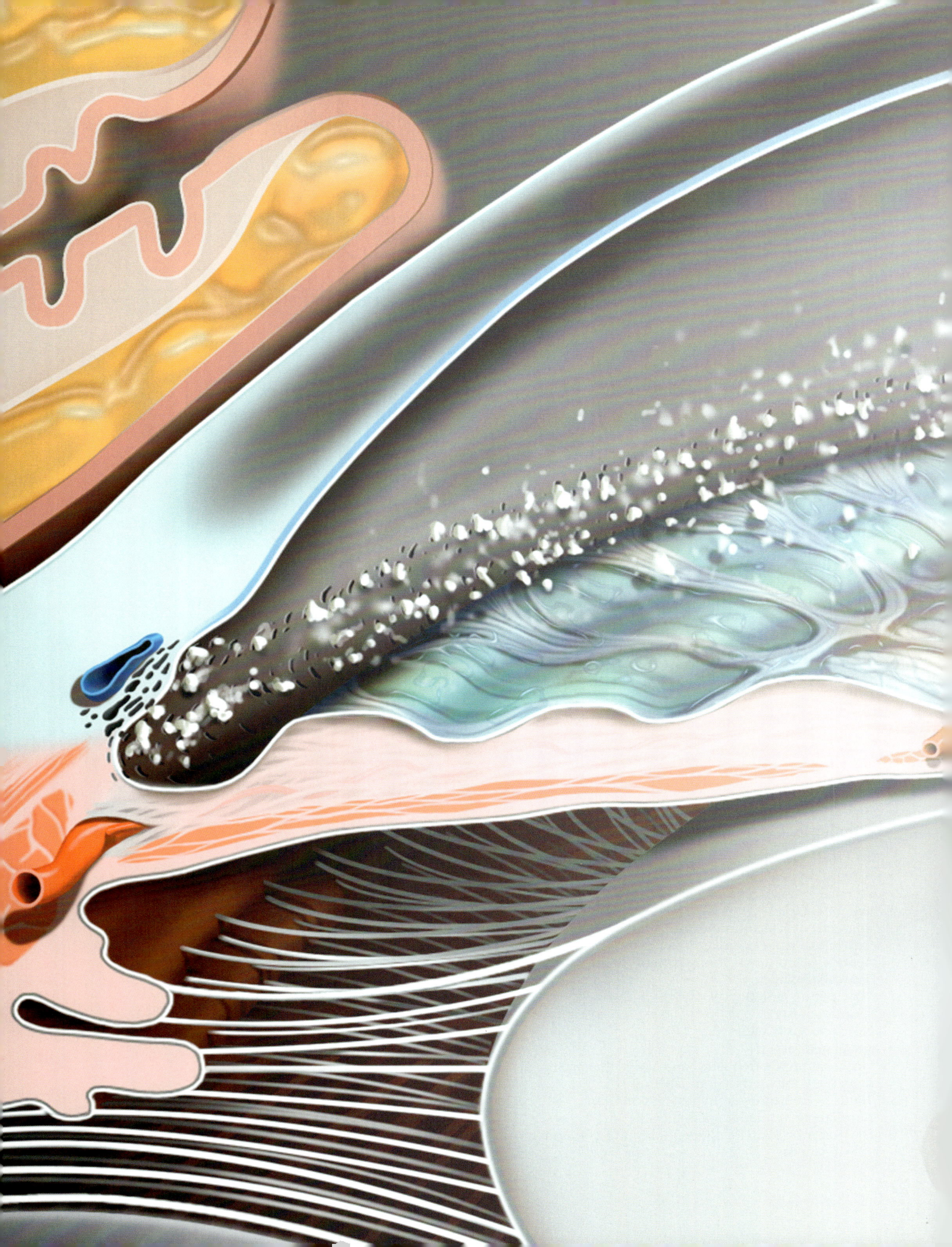

SECTION 1
Open-Angle Glaucoma

MAJOR CLINICAL STUDIES: OPEN-ANGLE GLAUCOMA

TERMINOLOGY

Abbreviations

- Open-angle glaucoma (OAG)

OCULAR HYPERTENSION TREATMENT STUDY (OHTS)

Objectives and Principal Conclusion

- Determine if reduction of intraocular pressure (IOP) prevents or delays onset of glaucomatous visual field loss &/or optic disc damage in patients at moderate risk for developing OAG
- Determine and quantify risk factors for developing OAG in patients with ocular hypertension
- Reducing IOP by ≥ 20% or to reach goal of ≤ 24 mm Hg delays or prevents OAG

Inclusion Criteria

- IOP 24-32 mm Hg in at least 1 eye and 21-32 mm Hg in other eye
- Normal visual fields and optic discs
- Best corrected visual acuity (BCVA) of 20/40 or better in both eyes
- Exclusion criteria
  - Prior intraocular surgery
  - Life-threatening or debilitating disease
  - Secondary causes of elevated IOP, angle-closure glaucoma, narrow angles
  - Presence of disease known to cause visual field loss, background retinopathy, optic disc abnormalities that can produce visual field loss or obscure interpretation of optic disc exam
  - Unwillingness to undergo random assignment

Randomization Method

- Patients randomly assigned to a stepped medical regimen or to no treatment with observation only

Results

- Risk factors for primary OAG: Older age, African American race, male gender, larger vertical or horizontal cup to disc ratio, high IOP, greater Humphrey visual field pattern standard deviation, cardiovascular disease, thinner central cornea
- Topical ocular antihypertensive medication delays or prevents onset of primary OAG in patients with elevated IOP
- Medical therapy can be considered for individuals with ocular hypertension who are at moderate or high risk for developing primary OAG

GLAUCOMA LASER TRIAL (GLT)/ GLAUCOMA LASER TRIAL FOLLOW-UP STUDY (GLTFS)

Objective and Principal Conclusion

- Compare safety and efficacy of argon laser trabeculoplasty (ALT) of trabecular meshwork with standard medical treatment for primary open-angle glaucoma (POAG); ALT was equivalent to medical therapy

Inclusion Criteria

- Age 35 or older
- IOP ≥ of 22 mm Hg in each eye
- Evidence of optic nerve damage in at least 1 eye

Randomization Method

- Patients received ALT in 1 eye and medical treatment in other eye
- Eye assigned to ALT was randomly selected

Results

- Initial treatment with ALT was at least as efficacious as initial treatment with topical medication
- Eyes initially treated with ALT had lower IOP, better visual field testing, and better optic disc status than those treated initially with topical medication
  - 1.2 mm Hg greater reduction in IOP if treated with ALT
  - 0.6 dB greater improvement in visual field from entry into trial
  - Cup to disc ratio changed by 0.01 in eyes treated with medication compared to eyes undergoing ALT, meaning slightly more optic nerve cupping

EARLY MANIFEST GLAUCOMA TRIAL (EMGT)

Objective and Principle Conclusion

- Compare early, late, and no treatment in progression of visual field loss and optic disc changes in newly detected OAG
  - Quantify expected IOP reduction with treatment, determine what factors influence glaucoma progression, and characterize disease progression
- Early treatment reduced glaucoma progression

Inclusion Criteria

- Age 50-80
- Newly detected and untreated chronic open-angle glaucoma diagnosed with repeatable visual field deficits on Humphrey perimetry
- Excluded for visual acuity < 0.5 in either eye, advanced visual field loss with mean deviation ≤ 16 dB or a threat to fixation, mean IOP > 30 mm Hg or any IOP > 35 mm Hg in 1 or more eyes, any condition that may obscure visual field or fundus photo results, inability for 4-year follow-up

Randomization Method

- Patients randomly assigned to therapy with Betaxolol and ALT or no initial treatment and followed for minimum 4 years

Results

- Treatment of early open-angle glaucoma results in significantly delayed progression of glaucoma
  - Average IOP reduction in treatment group 5.1 mm Hg or 25%
  - Progression of glaucoma was less frequent in treatment group

COLLABORATIVE INITIAL GLAUCOMA TREATMENT STUDY (CIGTS)

Objectives and Principal Conclusion

- Compare long-term effect of treating newly diagnosed OAG with standard medical treatment vs. filtration surgery

- Filtration was more effective at reducing IOP but had more risks

Inclusion Criteria

- Age 25-75
- IOP of 20 mm Hg or higher with evidence of optic nerve damage or visual field loss in 1 or both eyes
- No evidence of secondary causes of glaucoma on exam with exception of primary OAG, pigmentary glaucoma, or pseudoexfoliation glaucoma

Randomization Method

- Patients randomized to either stepped medication treatment regimen or filtration surgery
- Patients randomized to medical therapy
  - Typically started with a β-blocker with additional medications added for lack of IOP control or progressive visual field loss
  - If medications failed to control OAG, patients received ALT and then trabeculectomy
- Patients randomized to surgical therapy
  - Immediate trabeculectomy
  - If failure, ALT and then medical therapy
- If both eyes qualified for the study, both eyes underwent same treatment course

Results

- Both treatment groups had reduction in IOP from baseline
- Surgical group had IOPs 2-3 mm Hg lower than medical group
- Surgical group had more visual field loss and more visual acuity loss in first 3 years of follow-up, but after 4-5 years, this difference disappeared
- Surgical group had more cataract extractions than medical group
- Both groups were satisfied with quality of life and treatment, based on patient questionnaires

ADVANCED GLAUCOMA INTERVENTION STUDY (AGIS)

Objective and Principal Conclusion

- Determine long-term outcomes of trabeculectomy and ALT in eyes that have failed initial medical therapy for glaucoma
  - In such patients, next step should be trabeculectomy in whites and ALT in blacks

Inclusion Criteria

- Men and women aged 35-80 years
- Diagnosis of OAG not successfully controlled with medication

Randomization Method

- Eligible eyes were randomly assigned to 1 of 2 intervention sequences
  - Trabeculectomy, followed by ALT if trabeculectomy failed, followed by another trabeculectomy if ALT failed
  - ALT, followed by trabeculectomy if ALT failed, followed by another trabeculectomy if initial trabeculectomy failed
- Antifibrotic agents were used as an adjunct to trabeculectomy in eyes with previous history of invasive surgery
- Eyes that failed entire treatment sequence were managed at discretion of AGIS study physician and patient
- Patients were followed for 5 years to determine visual function loss, failure rates of interventions, complication rates, and need for supplemental therapy
  - Follow-up occurred after initial intervention at 1 week, 4 weeks, 3 months, 6 months, and every 6 months thereafter
  - After 2nd and 3rd interventions, follow-up occurred at 1 and 4 weeks, with additional visits scheduled as necessary

Results

- Black patients with advanced OAG should begin a treatment regimen that starts with ALT
  - Vision in eyes of black patients with advanced OAG was better preserved in those who started with ALT
  - Average % of eyes in black patients with decreased vision was 28% in those starting with ALT and 37% in those starting with trabeculectomy
- White patients with advanced OAG who have no life-threatening health problems should begin a treatment regimen that starts with trabeculectomy
  - In first 4 years of follow-up, vision in eyes of white patients with advanced OAG was better preserved in those who started with ALT, but after 7 years, the reverse was true
  - Average % of eyes in white patients with decreased vision after 7 years was 31% in those starting with trabeculectomy and 35% in those starting with ALT

RELATED REFERENCES

1. National Institutes of Health, National Eye Institute: Advanced Glaucoma Intervention Study (AGIS). http://www.nei.nih.gov/neitrials/static/study49.asp. Updated January 29, 2002. Accessed September 6, 2013
2. National Institutes of Health, National Eye Institute: Collaborative Initial Glaucoma Treatment Study (CIGTS). http://www.nei.nih.gov/neitrials/static/study50.asp. Updated June 3, 2003. Accessed September 6, 2013
3. National Institutes of Health, National Eye Institute: Early Manifest Glaucoma Trial (EMGT). Http://www.nei.nih.gov/neitrials/static/study31.asp. Updated December 6, 2002. Accessed September 6, 2013
4. National Institutes of Health, National Eye Institute: Glaucoma Laser Trial (GLT) Glaucoma Laser Trial Followup Study (GLTFS). http://www.nei.nih.gov/neitrials/static/study43.asp. Updated October 23, 1999. Accessed September 6, 2013
5. National Institutes of Health, National Eye Institute: Ocular Hypertension Treatment Study (OHTS). http://www.nei.nih.gov/neitrials/static/study24.asp. Updated June 13, 2002. Accessed September 6, 2013

OPEN-ANGLE GLAUCOMA OVERVIEW

TERMINOLOGY

Abbreviations

- Intraocular pressure (IOP)
- Cup to disc ratio (CDR)
- Optic nerve head (ONH)

Definitions

- Glaucoma: Diverse set of chronic optic neuropathies characterized by progressive retinal ganglion cell loss and declining visual function, often associated with increased IOP
- Iridocorneal angle: Anatomic angle between iris and cornea
- Primary open-angle glaucoma (POAG): Open-angle glaucoma (OAG) with no identified causative pathology
- Secondary open-angle glaucoma (SOAG): OAG secondary to an identifiable cause
- Gonioscopy: Goniolens used in conjunction with slit lamp or operative microscope to examine iridocorneal angle
- Applanation tonometry: Slit-lamp-based method to measure IOP based upon force required to flatten (applanate) specified area of cornea

PATHOPHYSIOLOGY

Overview

- Thought to involve poor outflow through trabecular meshwork (TM)
- High IOP worsens outcome
- Controlling IOP improves symptoms and is mainstay of treatment
- Symptoms often persist despite adequate pressure control

Anatomy

- High IOP thought to cause mechanical damage to retinal nerve fiber layer (ganglion cell axons) at level of lamina cribrosa
- Laminar organization of ONH leads to predominately peripheral axon loss before central axon loss

IOP-Related Pathophysiology

- TM obstruction (pigment, red blood cells)
- Trabecular endothelial cell death
- Dysfunction of trabecular endothelial phagocytic activity
- Schlemm canal changes (↓ pore size, ↓ vacuoles)

Non-IOP-Related Pathophysiology

- Reduced ocular perfusion pressure (hypertension, diabetes)
- Autoimmunity
- Loss of trophic growth factors
- Neuronal excitotoxicity
- Loss of retinal glial cells
- Dysregulation of choroidal and retinal vasculature

Secondary Causes of Open-Angle Glaucoma

- Pseudoexfoliation, pigmentary glaucoma, lens-associated glaucoma, tumors, uveitis, glaucomatocyclitic crisis, Fuchs heterochromic iridocyclitis, iris recession, hyphema, UGH syndrome, aphakia, steroid associated

CLINICAL PRESENTATION

Symptoms

- Patient often unaware of vision loss on presentation
- Usually painless with no acute attacks

Exam Findings

- Relative afferent pupillary defect
- Visual field exam
  - Slowly progressive loss of peripheral vision
  - Humphrey visual field; microperimetry
- Slit-lamp exam
  - Iris defect/pigment granules
  - Keratitic precipitates
  - Blood cells (traumatic/hemolytic glaucoma)
  - Synechiae
- Tonometry
  - IOP frequently high (> 21 mm Hg)
- Measure central corneal thickness (CCT)
- Gonioscopy
  - Open (wide) iridocorneal angle
- Funduscopy
  - **Confirm open iridocorneal angle prior to dilation to avoid inducing acute angle closure crisis**
  - ↑ CDR with cupping of ONH
  - Optic nerve pallor
  - Notching of optic disc rim
- Other imaging modalities
  - Ultrasound biomicroscopy (UBM)
  - Anterior segment OCT (AS-OCT)
  - Nerve fiber layer imaging (Heidelberg retinal nerve fiber layer [RNFL]; GDX)

EPIDEMIOLOGY

Prevalence

- ~ 1% in United States
- Accounts for > 90% of glaucoma in United States
- Leading cause of blindness in African Americans
- 2nd leading cause of blindness, after cataract

Risk Factors

- Thin CCT (< 555 μm), increasing age, elevated IOP, family history
- ↑ risk in blacks relative to whites (3-4x)
- ↑ risk with 1 affected sibling (2-4x)
- Several genetic causes identified, but most cases not associated with known genetic cause

RELATED REFERENCES

1. Boland MV et al: Comparative effectiveness of treatments for open-angle glaucoma: a systematic review for the U.S. Preventive Services Task Force. Ann Intern Med. 158(4):271-9, 2013
2. Burr J et al: Medical versus surgical interventions for open angle glaucoma. Cochrane Database Syst Rev. 9:CD004399, 2012
3. Gemenetzi M et al: Current concepts on primary open-angle glaucoma genetics: a contribution to disease pathophysiology and future treatment. Eye (Lond). 26(3):355-69, 2012
4. Liu Y et al: Molecular genetics in glaucoma. Exp Eye Res. 93(4):331-9, 2011
5. Sena DF et al: Neuroprotection for treatment of glaucoma in adults. Cochrane Database Syst Rev. (2):CD006539, 2010

KEY STRUCTURES INVOLVED IN GLAUCOMA

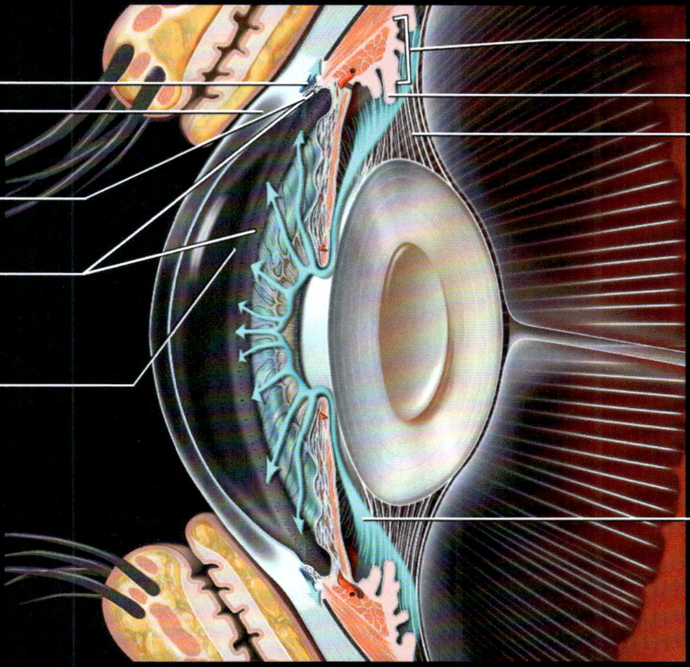

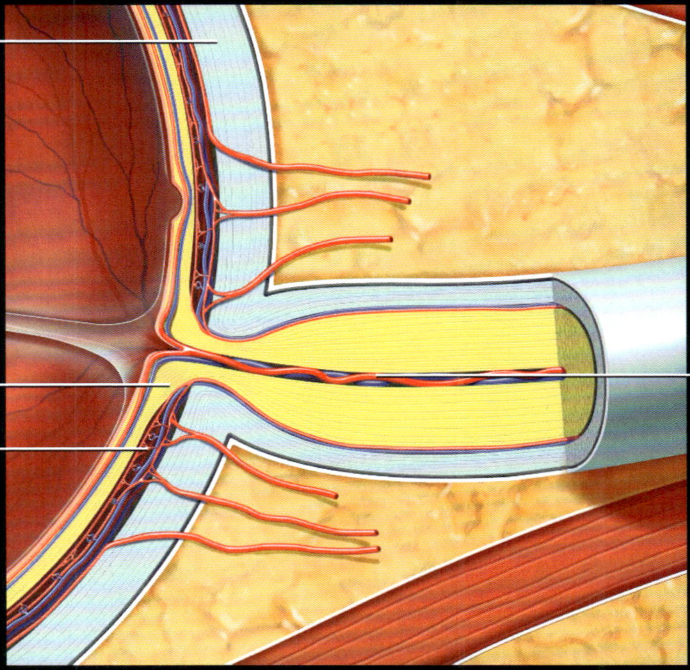

*(**Top**) This illustration depicts a normal angle. The blue arrows show the normal flow of the aqueous, which is produced by the ciliary body, flows through the pupil, and drains into the trabecular meshwork. From the trabecular meshwork, aqueous drains into Schlemm canal and then to the aqueous veins. Open-angle glaucoma is defined as progressive damage to the optic nerve that is associated with increased intraocular pressure with an open angle. There are many causes for open-angle glaucoma. Primary open-angle glaucoma is OAG in addition to the absence of another systemic or local disease that could lead to the elevation of intraocular pressure. One theory for the pathogenesis of primary open-angle glaucoma is that there is decreased outflow of aqueous through the trabecular meshwork. (**Bottom**) This illustration depicts a normal optic nerve. The hallmark of glaucoma is thinning of the nerve fiber layer. The nerve fiber layer is made up of the axons of ganglion cells.*

OCULAR HYPERTENSION

Key Facts

Introduction

- Increase in intraocular pressure (IOP) above normal range of 11-21 mm Hg without detectable glaucomatous damage

Demographics

- Risk factors for progression of ocular hypertension (OHT) to primary open-angle glaucoma (POAG) as determined by the Ocular Hypertension Treatment Study (OHTS)
  - Older age
  - Larger cup-disc ratio
  - Greater pattern standard deviation in visual fields
  - Higher IOP
  - Thinner central cornea thickness
- 3-6 million people in United States have OHT

Presentation

- Typically asymptomatic
- Exam findings
  - Tonometry: Increased IOP (> 21 mm Hg)
  - Gonioscopy: Open iridocorneal angle
  - Perimetry: No visual field deficits
  - Funduscopy: No evidence of optic nerve damage or glaucomatous cupping

Differential Diagnosis

- Undiagnosed glaucoma: Characteristic optic nerve damage and corresponding visual field deficits

Treatment

- Similar to medical treatment for POAG but with less aggressive IOP-lowering goals
  - Should likely treat if IOP consistently > 26 mm Hg
- Early treatment of patients is important for better outcomes

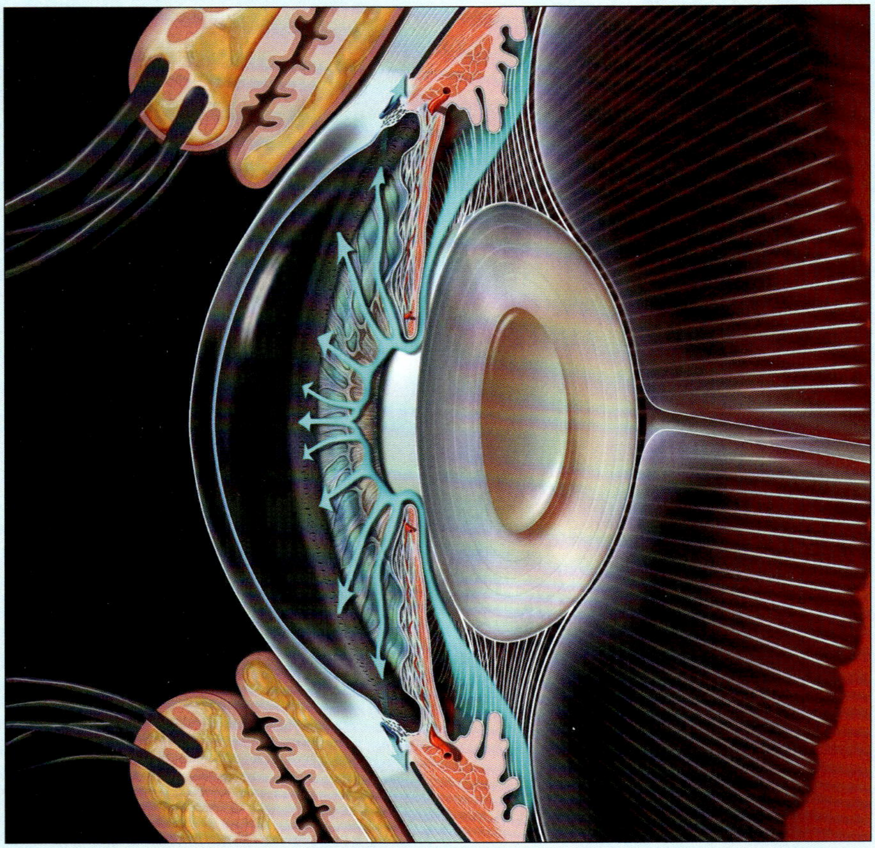

Ocular hypertension is an increase in intraocular pressure (IOP) above normal range of 11-21 mm Hg without detectable glaucomatous damage in the setting of a normal angle. This illustration depicts a normal angle. The blue arrows show the normal flow of the aqueous, which is produced by the ciliary body, flows through the pupil, and drains into the trabecular meshwork. From the trabecular meshwork, it drains into Schlemm canal and then to the aqueous veins. One theory for the pathogenesis of ocular hypertension is that there is decreased outflow of aqueous through the trabecular meshwork. Ocular hypertension may progress to primary open-angle glaucoma.

OCULAR HYPERTENSION

INTRODUCTION

Definitions

- Increase in intraocular pressure (IOP) above normal range of 11-21 mm Hg without detectable glaucomatous damage
  - Average IOP may be higher in elderly population
  - No evidence of ocular or systemic causes for increased IOP
  - Essentially, diagnosis of exclusion

DEMOGRAPHICS

Etiology/Risk Factors

- Prevalence of ocular hypertension (OHT) varies among ethnic groups and increases with age
- Risk factors for progression of OHT to primary open-angle glaucoma (POAG) as determined by the Ocular Hypertension Treatment Study (OHTS)
  - Older age
  - Larger cup to disc ratio
  - Greater pattern standard deviation in visual fields confirmed by standard automated perimetry
  - Higher IOP
    - Accepted IOP average is 15.5 mm Hg with standard deviation of 2.6 mm Hg
  - Thinner central cornea thickness
    - Eyes with a thinner central corneal thickness (< 556 μm) tended to progress to glaucoma as compared to eyes with a thicker central corneal thickness (>588 μm)
    - Powerful predictor of progression of disease
  - Risk factors not significant in OHTS (though other studies have shown them to be important risk factors in development of glaucoma)
    - Race (African race)
    - Family history of glaucoma
    - Myopia
    - Diabetes mellitus

Epidemiology

- 3-6 million people in United States have OHT
  - 4-7% of the population > 40 years old have OHT

PRESENTATION

Symptoms

- Typically asymptomatic

Exam Findings

- Tonometry: Increased IOP (> 21 mm Hg)
  - Important to perform pachymetry as tonometry measurements are influenced by central corneal thickness
  - Thinner central cornea thickness is a powerful predictor of progression of disease
- Gonioscopy
  - Open iridocorneal angle
- Perimetry
  - No visual field deficits
- Funduscopy
  - No evidence of optic nerve damage or glaucomatous cupping

DIFFERENTIAL DIAGNOSIS

Undiagnosed Glaucoma

- OHT may progress to glaucoma
- Characteristic optic nerve damage and corresponding visual field deficits are necessary to diagnose glaucoma

TREATMENT

Medical

- OHTS showed a reduction of progression of OHT to POAG from 9.5% to 4.4% when patients were treated with a topical hypotensive medication over a 5-year period
  - Goals were to reduce IOP by 20% or less than 24 mm Hg
- Similar to medical treatment for POAG but with less aggressive IOP-lowering goals
  - Closely monitoring low-risk patients may be an option
- IOP-lowering agents
  - Topical β-blockers
  - α-agonists
  - Prostaglandin analogues
  - Carbonic anhydrase inhibitors

Prognosis

- Early treatment of patients is important for better outcomes

SELECTED REFERENCES

1. Friedman DS et al: Prevalence of open-angle glaucoma among adults in the United States. Arch Ophthalmol. 122(4):532-8, 2004
2. Gordon MO et al: The Ocular Hypertension Treatment Study: baseline factors that predict the onset of primary open-angle glaucoma. Arch Ophthalmol. 120(6):714-20; discussion 829-30, 2002
3. Kass MA et al: The Ocular Hypertension Treatment Study: a randomized trial determines that topical ocular hypotensive medication delays or prevents the onset of primary open-angle glaucoma. Arch Ophthalmol. 120(6):701-13; discussion 829-30, 2002

PRIMARY OPEN-ANGLE GLAUCOMA

Key Facts

Introduction

- Open (unobstructed) iridocorneal angle with characteristic optic nerve damage

Demographics

- Etiology: Increase in intraocular pressure (IOP) due to increased outflow resistance and decreased outflow of aqueous humor
- Risk factors
  - Demographic: African race, increased age, family history
  - Ocular: Increased IOP, central cornea thickness (< 556 μm), myopia
  - Systemic: Diabetes, hypertension, steroid use
- Epidemiology
  - Most common form of glaucoma and 2nd leading cause of blindness in USA
  - Most patients diagnosed with primary open-angle glaucoma will not progress to blindness

Presentation

- Typically asymptomatic, although vision loss may be present with advanced disease

Differential Diagnosis

- Acute angle-closure glaucoma
- Iatrogenic glaucoma
- Normal tension glaucoma
- Ocular hypertension

Treatment

- IOP-lowering agents: Topical β-blockers, α-2 agonists, prostaglandin analogues, carbonic anhydrase inhibitors, and cholinergic agonists
- Laser trabeculoplasty
- Trabeculectomy
- Tube or microtube shunts

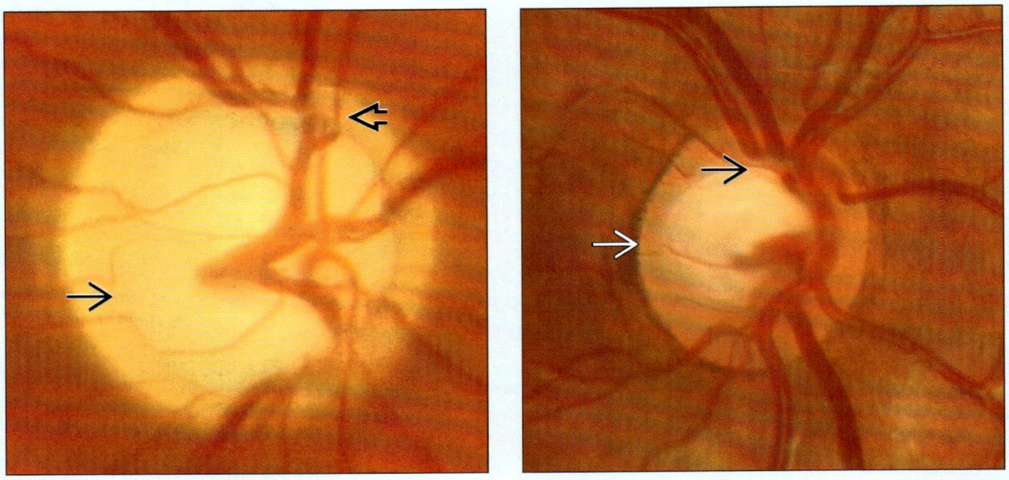

(Left) *This fundus photograph depicts a typical example of an optic disc demonstrating glaucomatous cupping ⇨. Note how the vessels appear to dive upon entry ⇨. Disc cupping is a physical exam finding suggestive of damage to the optic nerve.* ***(Right)*** *This fundus photograph is an example of a typical cupped disc. Note how the vessels dive upon entry into the cup →. The thinning is more pronounced temporally ➔. Optical coherence tomography is used to document glaucomatous cupping.*

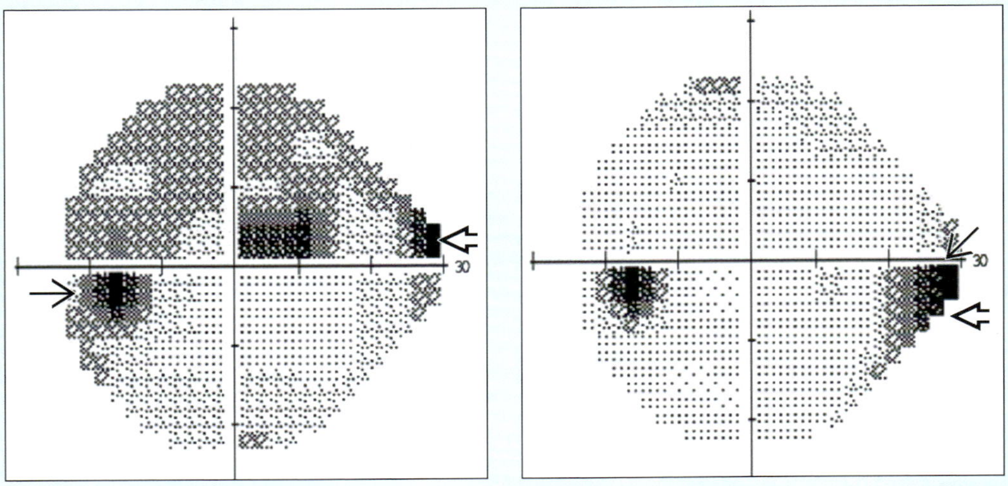

(Left) *This Humphrey visual field of the left eye is an example of a superior arcuate scotoma, which is typical of glaucoma. Arcuate scotomas typically start near the blind spot →, arch over the nasal fields, and terminate at the nasal horizontal midline ⇨.* ***(Right)*** *This Humphrey visual field of the left eye is typical of a nasal step defect ⇨. Note how the scotoma respects the horizontal midline →. Visual field loss secondary to glaucoma is irreversible.*

PRIMARY OPEN-ANGLE GLAUCOMA

INTRODUCTION

Definitions

- Open (unobstructed) iridocorneal angle with characteristic optic nerve damage
- Absence of secondary glaucoma or nonglaucomatous cause for optic neuropathy

DEMOGRAPHICS

Etiology/Risk Factors

- Etiology: ↑ in intraocular pressure (IOP) due to ↑ outflow resistance of uncertain etiology
  - Elevated IOP is considered a causative factor of POAG, but there is a variant of POAG with normal IOP (normal tension glaucoma)
  - Relationship between ↑ IOP and retinal ganglion apoptosis is still speculative but may be attributed to ischemic or mechanical injury
  - *GLC1A* gene and *TIGR*/myocilin mutations have been associated with open-angle glaucoma
- Risk factors
  - Demographic: African race, ↑ age, family history
  - Ocular: ↑ IOP, central cornea thickness (< 556 μm), myopia
  - Systemic: Diabetes mellitus, hypertension, steroid use

Epidemiology

- Most common form of glaucoma and 2nd leading cause of blindness in USA
- > 50% of persons with POAG are unaware that they are affected
- ↑ prevalence in USA due to aging population

PRESENTATION

Symptoms

- Typically asymptomatic, although vision loss may be present with advanced disease
  - Possible early symptomatic central visual field defects
- Late development of glaucomatous cupping with corresponding visual field deficits

Exam Findings

- Tonometry: Often reveals elevated IOP
- Gonioscopy: Open iridocorneal angle
- Perimetry: Characteristic visual field deficits corresponding to optic nerve damage
  - Early changes include variability of response or asymmetry between eyes
  - Small paracentral defects that terminate at horizontal midline
  - Arcuate scotomas representing a loss of arcuate nerve fibers that start near blind spot, arch over nasal fields, and terminate at nasal horizontal midline
  - Nasal step defects that respect horizontal midline
- Funduscopy: Glaucomatous cupping (especially verticalization of cup), can be confirmed by imaging techniques such as optical coherence tomography
  - Cup-to-disc ratio of > 0.3 in Caucasians and > 0.5 in African Americans is worrisome for glaucoma
- Pachymetry: Corneal thinning is independent risk factor for POAG
  - Accuracy of tonometry is related to central corneal thickness (readings are based on an average corneal thickness of 520 μm)
  - Especially important to perform pachymetry in laser-assisted in situ keratomileu (LASIK) patients

DIFFERENTIAL DIAGNOSIS

Acute Angle-Closure Glaucoma

- Closed angle, fixed pupil, microcystic corneal edema

Iatrogenic Glaucoma

- Primary elevated IOP with characteristic optic nerve damage secondary to medical treatment

Normal Tension Glaucoma

- Open anterior chamber angle with normal IOP and optic nerve damage

Ocular Hypertension

- Primary elevated IOP without optic nerve damage

EVALUATION/WORK-UP

Imaging

- Retinal nerve fiber layer thickness OCT and Humphrey visual field testing are important structural and functional markers

TREATMENT

Medical

- IOP-lowering agents: Topical β-blockers (timolol, betaxolol), α-2 agonists (brimonidine), prostaglandin analogues (latanoprost, travoprost, bimatoprost, tafluprost), carbonic anhydrase inhibitors (dorzolamide, brinzolamide), cholinergics (pilocarpine)
  - First-line therapy typically prostaglandin analogue, with addition of other medical therapies as needed
  - Side-effect profile and comorbid diseases should be taken into account (e.g., betaxolol is cardioselective as it is a β-1 blocker and safer for COPD patients)
  - Follow-up in 4-8 weeks to assess IOP response; consider laser or surgery if inadequate response

Surgical

- Laser trabeculoplasty: Laser application to trabecular meshwork to increase aqueous outflow and lower IOP
- Trabeculectomy: Fistula formation to increase aqueous outflow and lower IOP
- Tube shunts (Ahmed, Molteno) or recent microtube shunts (e.g., Express shunt, iStent) are useful if trabeculectomy fails or is contraindicated

Prognosis

- Avg time from onset to blindness if untreated: ~ 20 yrs
- Most patients diagnosed with POAG will not progress to blindness

SELECTED REFERENCES

1. Heijl A et al: Reduction of intraocular pressure and glaucoma progression: results from the Early Manifest Glaucoma Trial. Arch Ophthalmol. 120(10):1268-79, 2002

Key Facts

Introduction

- Spectrum of congenital disorders that result in bilateral abnormal development of iris and trabecular meshwork with presence of posterior embryotoxon
- Posterior embryotoxon: Prominent Schwalbe line that is displaced anteriorly

Demographics

- Autosomal dominant inheritance, occasional sporadic cases
- Abnormality in neural crest cells

Presentation

- Dental and facial abnormalities
- Posterior embryotoxon
- Iridocorneal adhesions to Schwalbe line, no other corneal abnormalities
- Iris hypoplasia
- Iris defects
  - Polycoria
  - Corectopia
- Glaucoma (~ 50% of cases)
- Systemic manifestations
  - Dental and facial abnormalities
  - Abnormalities of cardiac outflow tract
  - Hypospadias
  - Pituitary dysfunction

Treatment

- Medical management of glaucoma (preferred over surgical)
  - Drugs targeting production of aqueous humor (carbonic anhydrase inhibitors, β-blockers) preferred over those targeting outflow (pilocarpine, prostaglandin analogs)
- Surgical management of glaucoma
  - Trabeculectomy or goniotomy

*(**Left**) Slit-lamp photograph shows iris abnormalities ⇨ and iridocorneal adhesions ➡ associated with Axenfeld-Rieger spectrum (ARS). The iridocorneal adhesions are attached to the posterior embryotoxon. The posterior embryotoxon ➡ is a prominent Schwalbe line that is displaced anteriorly. (**Right**) Slit-lamp photograph shows iris abnormalities found in ARS →. Full thickness iris abnormalities are part of the definition of Rieger anomaly.*

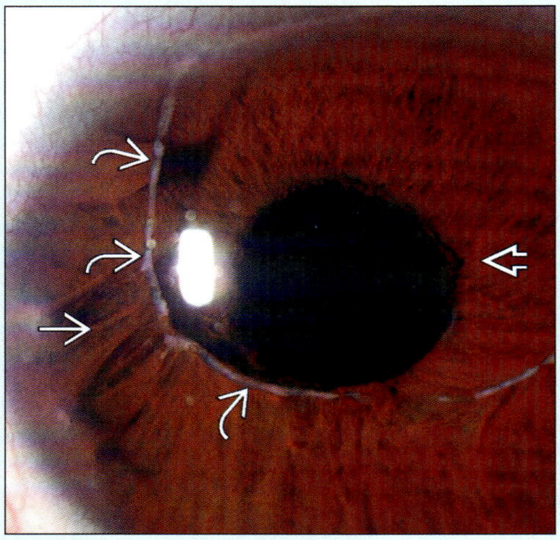

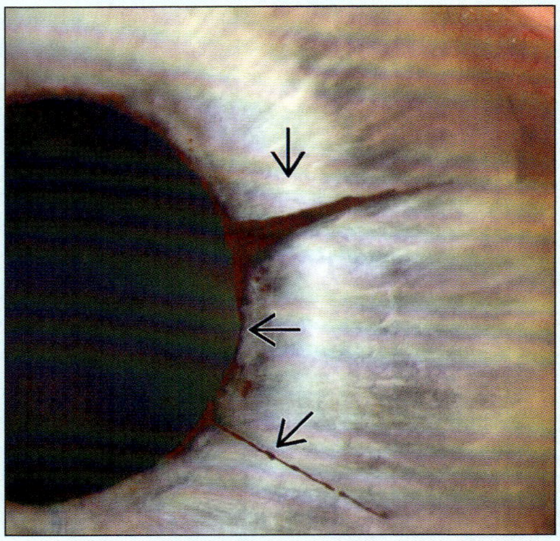

*(**Left**) Slit-lamp photograph shows transillumination of the iris of a patient with ARS. This image shows iris atrophy and defects ➡. Iris hypoplasia, polycoria, and corectopia are common iris defects seen in ARS. (**Right**) Gonioscopy of image shows iridocorneal adhesions to Schwalbe line ➡. These adhesions can be surgically repaired if they significantly impact iris function or are associated with uncontrollable glaucoma.*

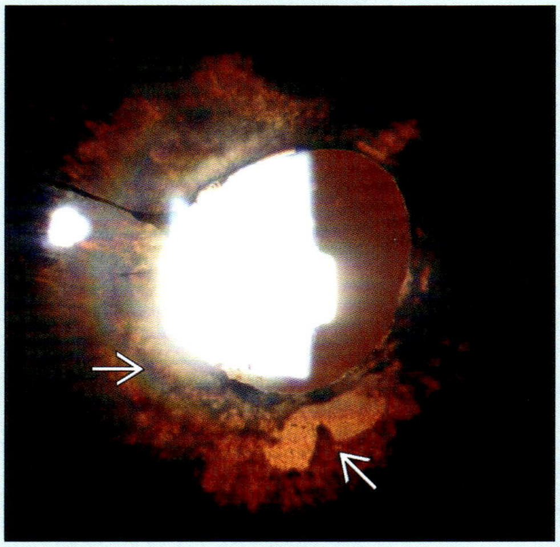

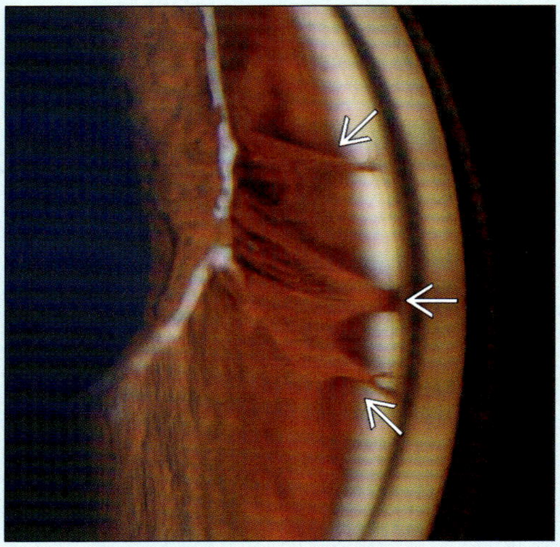

AXENFELD-RIEGER SPECTRUM

INTRODUCTION

Abbreviations
- Axenfeld-Rieger spectrum (ARS)

Definitions
- Spectrum of congenital disorders that result in bilateral abnormal development of iris and trabecular meshwork with presence of posterior embryotoxon
- Posterior embryotoxon: Prominent Schwalbe line that is displaced anteriorly

Subtypes
- Historically, ARS has been divided into 4 subtypes
  - Axenfeld anomaly: Posterior embryotoxon + iridocorneal adhesions to Schwalbe line
  - Axenfeld syndrome: Axenfeld anomaly + glaucoma
  - Rieger anomaly: Axenfeld anomaly + iris hypoplasia + full-thickness iris defects
  - Rieger syndrome: Rieger anomaly + dental abnormalities (small teeth, few teeth) + facial abnormalities (maxillary hypoplasia)

DEMOGRAPHICS

Etiology/Risk Factors
- Autosomal dominant inheritance, occasional sporadic cases
  - Implicated genes include *PITX2* at 4q25 and *FOXC4* at 6p25
- Abnormality in neural crest cells

Epidemiology
- Rare; patients most frequently have family history

PRESENTATION

Symptoms
- Abnormal iris
- Dental and facial abnormalities
- Vision loss secondary to glaucoma

Exam Findings
- Posterior embryotoxon
- Iridocorneal adhesions to Schwalbe line, no other corneal abnormalities
- Iris hypoplasia
- Iris defects
  - Polycoria (> 1 pupillary opening in iris)
  - Corectopia (noncentral location of pupil)
- Abnormal angle tissue
- Glaucoma (~ 50% of ARS patients develop glaucoma)
- Systemic manifestations
  - Dental and facial abnormalities
  - Abnormalities of cardiac outflow tract
  - Hypospadias
  - Pituitary dysfunction

DIFFERENTIAL DIAGNOSIS

Iridocorneal Endothelial Syndrome
- Affects corneal endothelium; ARS does not
- Affects middle-aged patients; ARS is present congenitally
- Typically unilateral; ARS typically is bilateral

Posterior Embryotoxon in Patients Without ARS
- Present in ~ 8-15% of population
- No signs of glaucoma or iris anomalies

EVALUATION/WORK-UP

Referral
- Cardiac evaluation due to associated abnormalities of cardiac outflow tract
- Hearing evaluation due to associated sensorineural hearing loss
- Evaluation for difficult airway, if anesthesia is necessary for surgery or exams under anesthesia

TREATMENT

Medical
- Medical management of glaucoma (preferred over surgical)
  - Drugs targeting production of aqueous humor (carbonic anhydrase inhibitors, β-blockers) preferred over those targeting outflow (pilocarpine, prostaglandin analogs)
- Early identification and treatment in pediatric patients is important due to risk of amblyopia

Surgical
- Surgical management of glaucoma
  - Trabeculectomy or goniotomy
  - Insertion of tubes for aggressive glaucoma
- Closure of iris defects
- Patients are at high risk for choroidal hemorrhage during intraocular surgery

Follow-Up
- Yearly if no glaucoma
- Every 1-3 months if glaucoma is present
- Primary care provider should be aware of risk of glaucoma; refer to ophthalmologist for pupillary abnormalities, eye enlargement, cloudy cornea, or photophobia

Prognosis
- ~ 50% of patients with ARS develop glaucoma

SELECTED REFERENCES

1. Chang TC et al: Axenfeld-Rieger syndrome: new perspectives. Br J Ophthalmol. 96(3):318-22, 2012
2. Berenstein-Aizman G et al: Axenfeld-Rieger syndrome: dentofacial manifestation and oral rehabilitation considerations. Pediatr Dent. 33(5):440-4, 2011
3. Kelberman D et al: Digenic inheritance of mutations in FOXC1 and PITX2: correlating transcription factor function and Axenfeld-Rieger disease severity. Hum Mutat. 32(10):1144-52, 2011
4. Tümer Z et al: Axenfeld-Rieger syndrome and spectrum of PITX2 and FOXC1 mutations. Eur J Hum Genet. 17(12):1527-39, 2009
5. Idrees F et al: A review of anterior segment dysgeneses. Surv Ophthalmol. 51(3):213-31, 2006

INFLAMMATORY GLAUCOMA

Key Facts

Introduction

- Inflammatory glaucoma: Secondary glaucoma associated with uveitis, a.k.a. uveitic glaucoma
- Open-angle inflammatory glaucoma
- Angle-closure inflammatory glaucoma

Demographics

- Any form of uveitis can result in glaucoma, though rheumatoid arthritis, pars planitis, herpes zoster iridocyclitis, herpes simplex keratouveitis, and toxoplasmosis are thought to be more commonly associated
- Glaucoma secondary to uveitis is present in 7-20% of patients with uveitis

Presentation

- History of uveitis
- Ocular pain
- Photophobia
- IOP increased above baseline
- Peripheral anterior synechiae, posterior synechiae, iris bombé may be present
- Optic nerve cupping and visual field deficits typical of glaucoma my develop as disease progresses

Treatment

- Continue treatment of uveitis as this will improve elevated IOP
- Treat with mydriatic/cycloplegic, such as cyclopentolate, atropine, or scopolamine
- Treat with pressure-lowering agents
- Laser iridotomy is used in cases of pupillary block to allow flow of aqueous from posterior to anterior chamber
- Trabeculectomy is typically first-line procedure; may consider drainage tubes in refractory cases

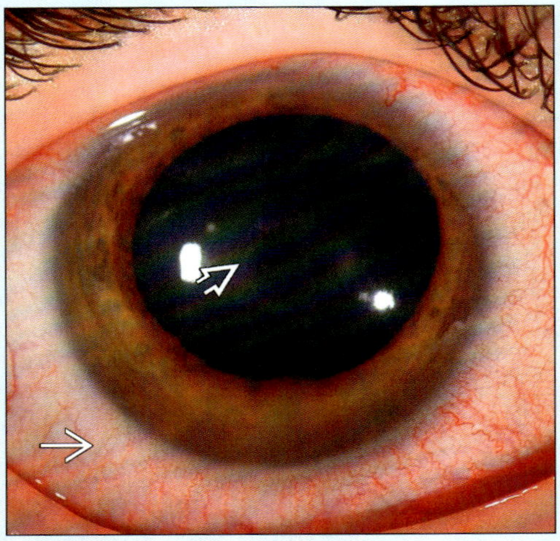

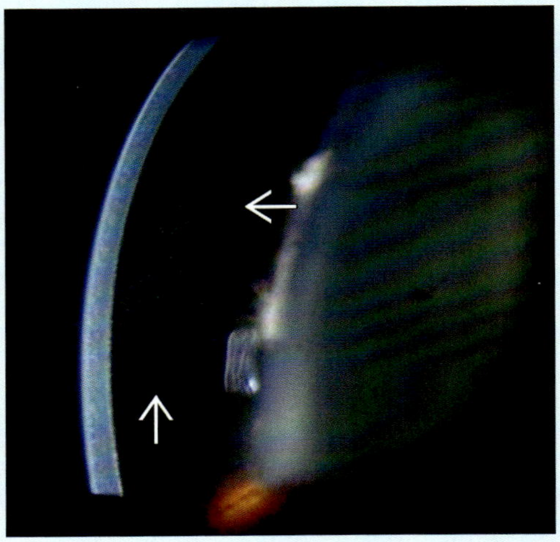

(Left) *Image shows an external view of an eye typical for inflammatory glaucoma. Note the injected conjunctiva ➔ and the inflammatory debris and fibrin ring in the anterior chamber ➔. Inflammatory debris may settle in the angle and reduce the functioning of the trabecular meshwork, leading to increased IOP.* ***(Right)*** *This slit-lamp photograph shows anterior chamber cell and flare ➔. Anterior chamber inflammation is seen in inflammatory glaucoma.*

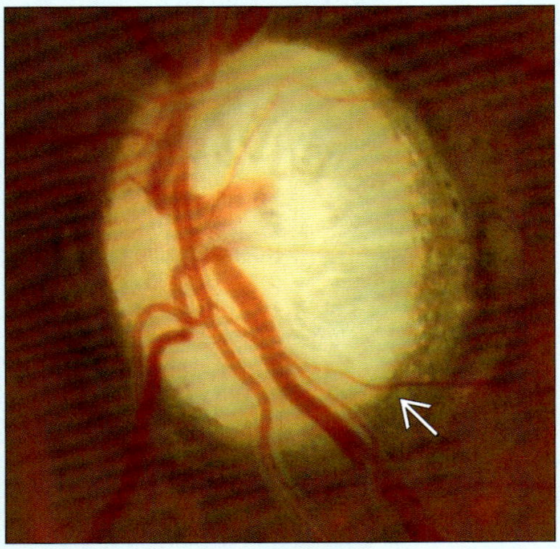

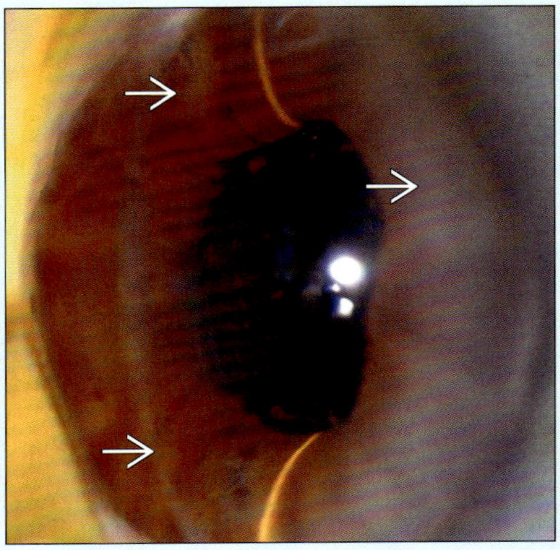

(Left) *This fundus photograph demonstrates optic disc cupping ➔. If not appropriately diagnosed and treated, inflammatory glaucoma can lead to progressive disc cupping and irreversible vision loss.* ***(Right)*** *Slit-lamp photograph shows iris bombé ➔. Iris bombé is a forward bowing of the iris caused by a buildup of fluid in the posterior chamber and associated with posterior synechiae. Iris bombé can be seen in advanced cases of inflammatory glaucoma.*

INFLAMMATORY GLAUCOMA

INTRODUCTION

Synonyms
- Uveitic glaucoma

Definitions
- Secondary glaucoma associated with uveitis

Subtypes
- Open-angle inflammatory glaucoma
- Angle-closure inflammatory glaucoma

DEMOGRAPHICS

Etiology/Risk Factors
- Any form of uveitis can result in glaucoma, though rheumatoid arthritis, pars planitis, herpes zoster iridocyclitis, HSV keratouveitis, and toxoplasmosis are more commonly associated
- Uveitis can cause both ciliary body hyposecretion and trabecular dysfunction; when trabecular dysfunction is more significant, glaucoma may occur
- Angle-closure inflammatory glaucoma caused by formation of synechia (both peripheral anterior synechiae [PAS] and posterior synechiae [PS])
- Open-angle inflammatory glaucoma caused by trabecular meshwork dysfunction from edema, inflammation, and obstruction by cellular debris

Epidemiology
- Glaucoma secondary to uveitis is present in 7-20% of patients with uveitis

PRESENTATION

Symptoms
- History of uveitis
- Ocular pain
- Photophobia
- Possible decrease in vision

Exam Findings
- IOP increased above baseline
- Slit-lamp examination
  - Uveitis (can be anterior, intermediate, posterior, panuveitis, or keratouveitis)
  - Cell and flare in anterior chamber
  - PAS, posterior synechiae, iris bombé may be present
- Gonioscopy
  - Evaluate for angle closure
  - Subtle inflammatory cell precipitates in trabecular meshwork
- Optic nerve cupping and visual field deficits typical of glaucoma my develop as the disease progresses

DIFFERENTIAL DIAGNOSIS

IOP Increase Due to Active Inflammation
- Active inflammation from uveitis may cause IOP increase
- Patients typically present with active inflammation and with no PAS, posterior synechiae, angle closure, or trabecular meshwork precipitates

IOP Increase Due to Corticosteroid Therapy
- Patients with uveitis often take corticosteroids, which can lead to steroid-response glaucoma
  - These patients typically have history of prolonged, large doses of steroids
  - IOP may decrease after cessation of steroids

Neovascular Glaucoma
- Can also be associated with chronic uveitis; distinguished by presence of anterior chamber neovascularization on gonioscopy

EVALUATION/WORK-UP

Labs
- Evaluate for systemic disease, especially if there have been previous attacks: HLA-B27, rheumatoid factor, antinuclear antibodies, angiotensin-converting enzyme, RPR or VDRL, HIV, ELISA

Imaging
- X-ray based on clinical suspicion for ankylosing spondylitis (sacroiliac joint films), sarcoidosis (chest x-ray), rheumatoid arthritis (joint films)

TREATMENT

Medical
- Continue treatment of uveitis (this will improve elevated IOP)
- Treat with mydriatic/cycloplegic, such as cyclopentolate, atropine, or scopolamine
- Treat with pressure-lowering agents; target IOP depends on severity of optic nerve damage (more severe damage requires lower target IOP)
  - First-line: Topical β-blocker (e.g., timolol)
  - Second-line: Systemic acetazolamide for higher IOP, α-adrenergic agonists for moderate IOP
  - Use of prostaglandin analogs historically discouraged due to risk of aggravating patient's uveitis
  - Miotics are contraindicated

Surgical
- Laser iridotomy is used in cases of pupillary block; may be followed by surgical iridectomy and synechiolysis
- Trabeculectomy is first-line procedure, may consider drainage tubes in refractory cases
  - Control of uveitis prior to surgery is desired

Follow-Up
- Follow-up appointments should occur every 1-7 days early in course of disease
- Treatment of elevated IOP may be discontinued as IOP returns to normal and inflammation subsides

Prognosis
- Good prognosis depends upon early diagnosis of elevated IOP and adequate treatment

SELECTED REFERENCES

1. Bodh SA et al: Inflammatory glaucoma. Oman J Ophthalmol. 4(1):3-9, 2011
2. Horsley MB et al: The use of prostaglandin analogs in the uveitic patient. Semin Ophthalmol. 26(4-5):285-9, 2011

HYPHEMA

Key Facts

Introduction

- Defined as blood in anterior chamber
  - Microhyphema: Suspended and free-floating red blood cells
  - Larger hyphemas cause layering of blood and may partially or completely (commonly referred to as an 8-ball hyphema) fill anterior chamber

Demographics

- Traumatic: Commonly secondary to blunt trauma
- Spontaneous: May be secondary to iris/angle neovascularization, juvenile xanthogranuloma, intraocular tumor, herpetic uveitis, coagulopathies, or anticoagulants

Presentation

- May have increased intraocular pressure
- When secondary to trauma, may have associated angle recession or cyclodialysis visible on gonioscopy
- May cause corneal blood staining, which clears peripherally before clearing centrally
  - Important concern in patients of amblyogenic age
  - ↑ IOP makes corneal blood staining more likely

Treatment

- Medical treatment
  - Includes bed rest and elevation of head of bed while protecting affected eye with eye shield
  - Topical mydriatic, topical and systemic medications for IOP control, and frequent follow-up
  - Topical steroids for anterior chamber inflammation
- Surgical treatment
  - Anterior chamber (AC) washout usually considered after 4 days and reserved for nonclearing hemorrhage, corneal blood staining, and elevated IOP refractory to medical treatment
  - AC paracentesis for transient IOP reduction in refractory cases while awaiting surgical evacuation

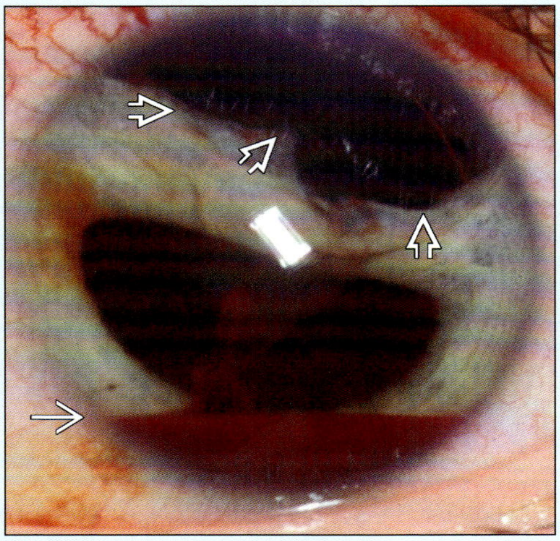

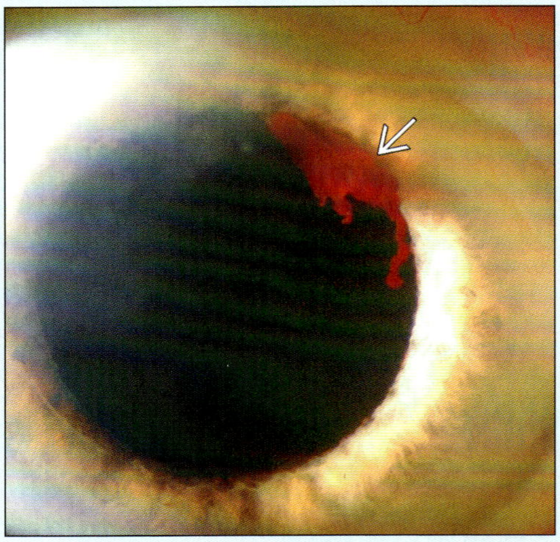

(Left) *This grade I hyphema demonstrates layering blood inferiorly ➔ with filling of < 1/3 of the anterior chamber. Note superior iridodialysis ➔. Smaller hyphemas without associated corneal blood staining or other ocular injury have a good prognosis.* ***(Right)*** *Slit-lamp photo shows a recent active bleed ➔ into the anterior chamber. Spontaneous hyphemas may be caused by anticoagulants, coagulopathies, juvenile xanthogranuloma, neovascularization of the iris or angle, and herpetic keratouveitis.*

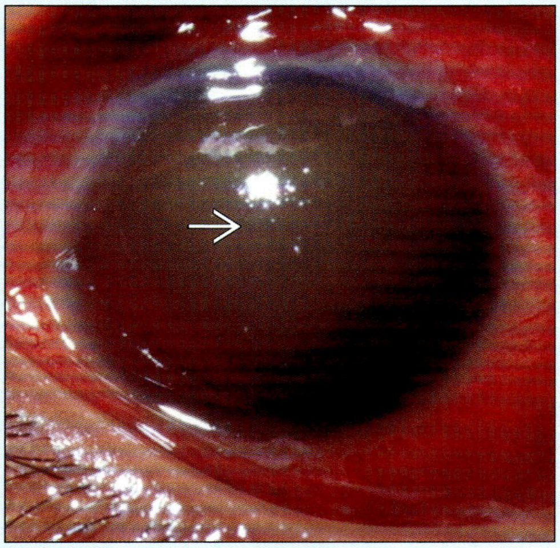

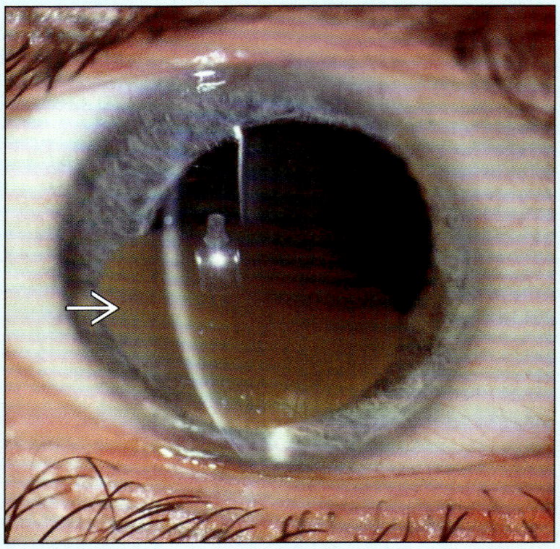

(Left) *This external photo shows a traumatic complete hyphema, commonly referred to as an 8-ball hyphema. The view into the anterior chamber is completely blocked by the dense blood clot ➔.* ***(Right)*** *Slit-lamp photo depicts corneal blood staining ➔ resulting from a prior hyphema. Blood staining clears from the periphery to the center and may take up to 3 years to clear, causing significant amblyopic concerns in young patients. High intraocular pressure with hyphema increases the chance of blood staining.*

HYPHEMA

INTRODUCTION

Definitions
- Blood in anterior chamber

Subtypes
- Microhyphema: Suspended red blood cells in anterior chamber
- **Grade 1**
  - Blood filling < 1/3 of anterior chamber
- **Grade 2**
  - Blood filling 1/3 to 1/2 of anterior chamber
- **Grade 3**
  - Blood filling 1/2 to subtotal filling of anterior chamber
- **Grade 4**
  - Total filling of anterior chamber with clotted blood (also known as 8-ball hyphema)

DEMOGRAPHICS

Etiology/Risk Factors
- Traumatic: Commonly secondary to blunt trauma
- Spontaneous: May be secondary to iris/angle neovascularization, juvenile xanthogranuloma, intraocular tumor, herpetic uveitis, coagulopathies, or anticoagulants
- Postsurgical

Epidemiology
- 20 cases per 100,000 people per year

PRESENTATION

Symptoms
- Decreased vision, floaters, pain, photophobia

Exam Findings
- Suspended red blood cells visible at slit lamp or layering blood or clot
- May have increased intraocular pressure
- May have associated angle recession or cyclodialysis visible on gonioscopy (wait several weeks for traumatic hyphemas before attempting)

EVALUATION/WORK-UP

Labs
- Sickle cell screen in patients of African or Mediterranean heritage
  - Sickling may lead to obstruction of trabecular meshwork and intraocular pressure spikes

Imaging
- Rarely necessary
  - Anterior segment fluorescein angiography may be used to look for iris neovascularization in ischemic or diabetic hyphemas
  - Ultrasonography may be used to rule out intraocular tumors or when view is limited
  - CT scan to rule out intraocular foreign body if open globe suspicion

TREATMENT

Medical
- Bed rest and elevate head of bed
- Discontinue aspirin or NSAIDs; if rebleeding occurs, e-aminocaproic acid can be used (antifibrinolytic agent)
- Protect affected eye with eye shield
- Topical scopolamine or atropine
- Treat increase in IOP with topical β-blocker or α-agonist
- May add systemic carbonic anhydrase inhibitor or hyperosmotic; avoid treating sickle cell patients with acetazolamide
- Topical steroids (prednisolone 6x/day) to prevent synechiae and minimize inflammation
- Antiemetics for nausea/vomiting, and avoid Valsalva/straining

Surgical
- Surgical evacuation of hyphema is usually considered after 4 days and is reserved for
  - Corneal blood staining
  - IOP ≥ 50 mm Hg for 4 days to prevent optic atrophy
  - IOP ≥ 25 mm Hg for > 6 days, with hyphemas filling > 75% of anterior chamber, to prevent corneal blood staining
  - IOP ≥ 35 mm Hg for > 24 hours in patients with sickle cell trait or disease and any hyphema
  - Hyphemas filling ≥ 50% of anterior chamber for > 8-9 days to prevent peripheral anterior synechiae
- Anterior chamber paracentesis may be used as temporizing measure for high IOP refractory to medical treatment

Follow-Up
- Daily for first 5-7 days, then every few days to a week, depending on severity
  - Rebleed is most likely to occur at 5-7 days after injury
- Gonioscopy and dilated fundus exam with depression at 4 weeks

Prognosis
- Depends on severity of injury and presence of secondary hemorrhage, glaucoma or optic atrophy, corneal blood staining, and damage to other structures such as posterior segment injury
- Recovery of visual acuity is good in ~ 75% of patients

SELECTED REFERENCES

1. Gharaibeh A et al: Medical interventions for traumatic hyphema. Cochrane Database Syst Rev. (1):CD005431, 2011
2. Papaconstantinou D et al: Contemporary aspects in the prognosis of traumatic hyphemas. Clin Ophthalmol. 3:287-90, 2009
3. Weiss JS et al: Surgical therapy of traumatic hyphema. Ophthalmic Surg. 14(4):343-5, 1983
4. Read J: Traumatic hyphema: surgical vs medical management. Ann Ophthalmol. 7(5):659-62, 664-6, 668-70, 1975
5. Yasuna E: Management of traumatic hyphema. Arch Ophthalmol. 91(3):190-1, 1974

NEOVASCULAR GLAUCOMA

Key Facts

Introduction

- Common, aggressive form of glaucoma caused by neovascularization and a fibrovascular membrane covering the angle; impaired function of the angle structures can lead to increased intraocular pressure
  - Secondary angle-closure may also develop
- 3 basic stages of neovascular glaucoma (NVG) are recognized
  - Iris neovascularization
  - Open-angle NVG: Iris neovascularization + glaucoma
  - Angle-closure NVG: Fibrovascular membrane contraction can lead to development of peripheral anterior synechiae (PAS) and secondary closure of angle

Demographics

- Most common causes of retinal ischemia associated with NVG are
  - Central retinal vein occlusion (CRVO)
  - Diabetic retinopathy
  - Carotid occlusive disease
  - Central retinal artery occlusion

Presentation

- Ocular pain, photophobia, conjunctival injection
- Small vascular tufts on iris at pupil margin
- Fibrovascular membrane covering trabecular meshwork

Treatment

- Reduce intraocular pressure
- Treat inflammation with corticosteroids, cycloplegics
- Treat retinal ischemia with panretinal photocoagulation (PRP) early in course of disease
- Consider treatment glaucoma with filtration surgery (glaucoma drainage devices or trabeculectomy with adjunctive mitomycin C)

*(**Left**) This slit-lamp photograph demonstrates early iris neovascularization. Note the neovascular rim surrounding the pupil margin ➡. (**Right**) This slit-lamp photograph demonstrates advanced iris neovascularization with the development of a fibrovascular membrane ➡. This patient's neovascular glaucoma (NVG) was a result of central retinal vein occlusion (CRVO), one of the most common causes of NVG.*

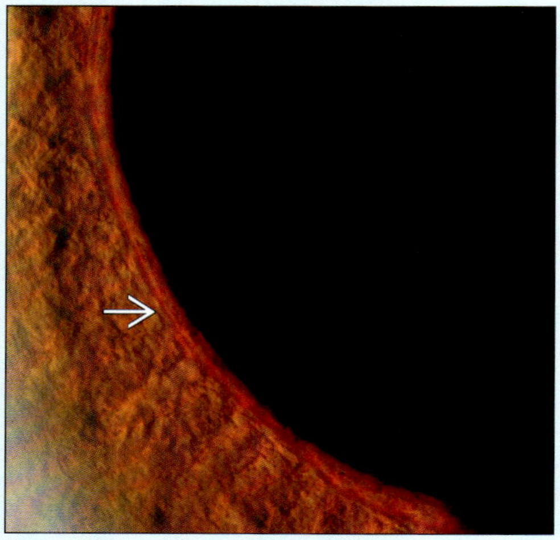

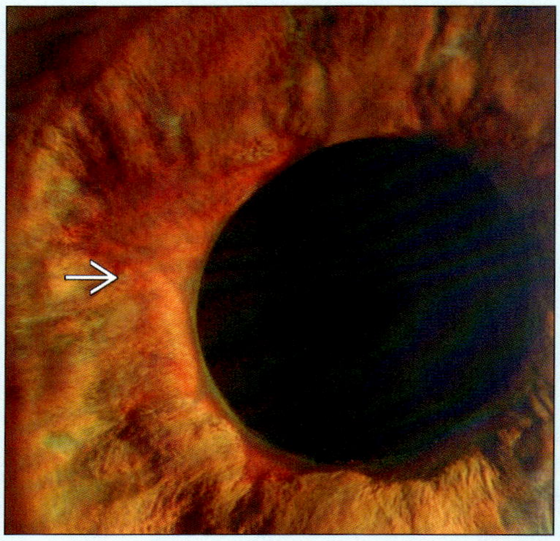

*(**Left**) This slit-lamp photograph demonstrates iris neovascularization ➡ in a patient with NVG. Note that a glaucoma shunt ➡ has been placed in an attempt to treat the elevated intraocular pressure. (**Right**) This photograph demonstrates the fundus of a patient with NVG caused by proliferative diabetic retinopathy. Note that the patient has been treated with panretinal photocoagulation ➡ in an attempt to reduce the proangiogenic signals that lead to iris neovascularization and subsequent NVG.*

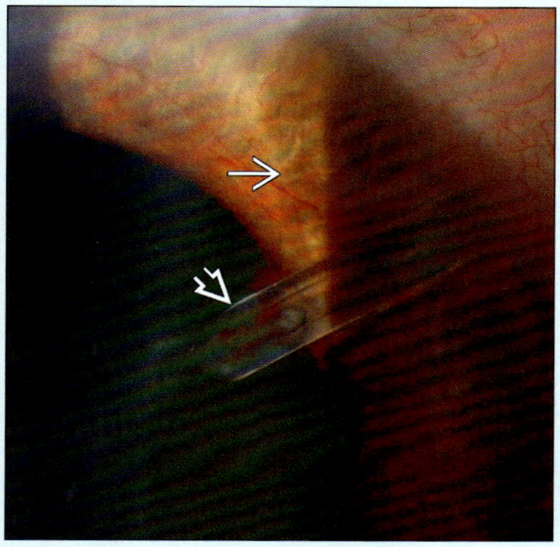

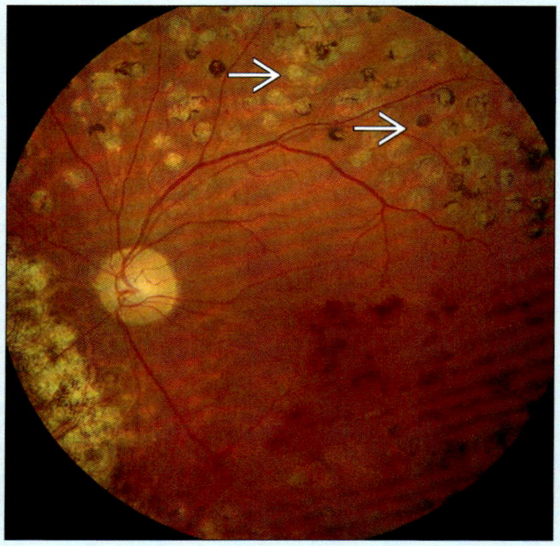

NEOVASCULAR GLAUCOMA

INTRODUCTION

Abbreviations
- Neovascular glaucoma (NVG)

Definitions
- Common, aggressive form of glaucoma caused by neovascularization (NV) and fibrovascular membrane covering the angle
- Impaired function of angle structures can lead to increased intraocular pressure (IOP)
- Secondary angle-closure glaucoma may also develop

Subtypes
- 3 basic stages of NVG are recognized
  - Iris NV
    - Typically develops in this order: Small vascular tufts on iris at pupil margin → radial growth of these vessels → angle NV
    - Occasionally, angle NV may develop without iris NV
  - Open-angle NVG: Iris NV + glaucoma
  - Angle-closure NVG: Fibrovascular membrane contraction leads to development of peripheral anterior synechiae (PAS) and secondary angle closure

DEMOGRAPHICS

Etiology/Risk Factors
- Any cause of severe retinal ischemia can result in NVG
- Most common causes of retinal ischemia associated with NVG are
  - Central retinal vein occlusion (CRVO) or central retinal artery occlusion (CRAO)
  - Diabetic retinopathy
  - Carotid occlusive disease
- Other rare causes of NVG: Uveal melanoma, retinoblastoma, retinopathy of prematurity

Epidemiology
- ~ 10% of patients with CRVO develop angle NV

PRESENTATION

Symptoms
- Ocular pain
- Photophobia
- Conjunctival injection
- Vision loss
- May be asymptomatic

Exam Findings
- Slit lamp
  - Small vascular tufts on iris at pupil margin
  - Radial vessel growth on iris
  - Microcystic corneal edema
- Gonioscopy
  - Fibrovascular membrane covering trabecular meshwork
  - NV of the trabecular meshwork
  - Angle closure
  - PAS
- Increased IOP
- Disc cupping and visual field deficits typical to glaucoma in later stages of disease

DIFFERENTIAL DIAGNOSIS

Primary Angle-Closure Glaucoma (PACG)
- Can be confused with angle-closure NVG
- PACG does not have iris and angle NV, nor does it have a fibrovascular membrane covering the trabecular meshwork

Pigmentary Glaucoma (PG)
- Shows increased trabecular meshwork pigment and iris defects
- Does not have iris and angle NV nor a fibrovascular membrane covering the trabecular meshwork

EVALUATION/WORK-UP

Imaging
- Fluorescein angiography (FA) to evaluate for possible retinal disease causing ischemia
- When no ocular cause of NVG is identified, carotid imaging to rule out carotid artery occlusive disease

TREATMENT

Medical
- Reduce IOP
  - Topical α-2 agonists (brimonidine), topical β-blockers (timolol), systemic carbonic anhydrase inhibitors
- Treat inflammation with corticosteroids, cycloplegics
- Consider reduction of NV with intravitreal VEGF inhibitor injection

Surgical
- Treat retinal ischemia with peripheral panretinal photocoagulation (PRP) early in course of disease
- Consider treatment of glaucoma with filtration surgery (glaucoma drainage devices or trabeculectomy with adjunctive mitomycin C)
- Consider treatment of angle NV with goniophotocoagulation

Follow-Up
- Treat iris NV within 1-2 days

Prognosis
- Poor unless NV is identified and treated early

SELECTED REFERENCES

1. Chan CK et al: SCORE Study report #11: incidences of neovascular events in eyes with retinal vein occlusion. Ophthalmology. 118(7):1364-72, 2011
2. Tolentino M: Systemic and ocular safety of intravitreal anti-VEGF therapies for ocular neovascular disease. Surv Ophthalmol. 56(2):95-113, 2011
3. Shazly TA et al: Neovascular glaucoma: etiology, diagnosis and prognosis. Semin Ophthalmol. 24(2):113-21, 2009
4. Sivak-Callcott JA et al: Evidence-based recommendations for the diagnosis and treatment of neovascular glaucoma. Ophthalmology. 108(10):1767-76; quiz1777, 1800, 2001

LENS-ASSOCIATED GLAUCOMA

Key Facts

Demographics

- Phacolytic glaucoma: Secondary open-angle glaucoma caused by protein that has leaked from a mature cataract, resulting in obstruction of drainage of aqueous humor through trabecular meshwork
- Phacomorphic glaucoma: Secondary angle-closure glaucoma caused by an enlarged, dense cataract that pushes iris anteriorly and closes angle
- Lens particle glaucoma: Secondary open-angle glaucoma caused by deposition of lens particles in angle after trauma or surgery, which leads to obstruction of the angle

Presentation

- Phacolytic glaucoma: Photophobia, pain, tearing with open angle in presence of advanced cataract
- Phacomorphic glaucoma: Photophobia, pain, tearing with closed angle/fixed pupil in presence of advanced cataract
- Lens particle glaucoma: Decreased vision, photophobia, pain, tearing with open angle and history of recent cataract surgery or trauma

Treatment

- Medical treatment to decrease IOP and reduce inflammation is 1st step in treating all forms of lens-associated glaucoma
- Removal of cataract after control of IOP is definitive treatment for both phacolytic and phacomorphic glaucoma
- Removal of lens particles is often necessary to treat lens particle glaucoma

Prognosis

- Majority of patients will have long-term improvement of visual acuity and IOP after removal of cataract

(Left) This slit-lamp photograph shows an example of an advanced, late-stage cataract. Both phacolytic and phacomorphic glaucoma are associated with advanced cataracts such as the one demonstrated. ***(Right)*** *This illustration depicts schematically the pathogenesis of phacolytic glaucoma. Protein that has leaked from a mature cataract may obstruct the drainage of aqueous humor through the trabecular meshwork ➔. Inflammation caused by macrophages digesting the lens protein also contributes to obstruction.*

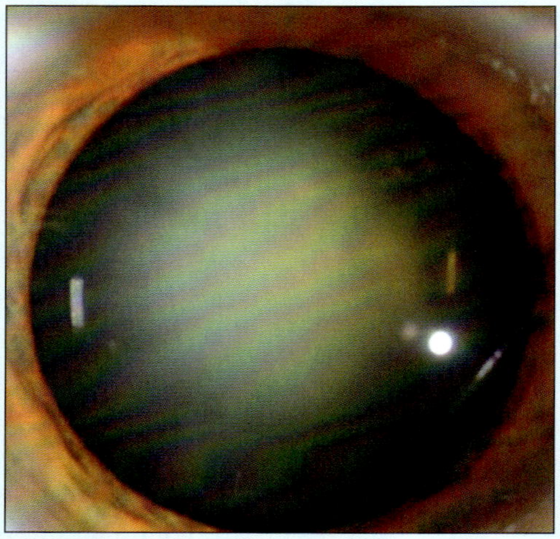

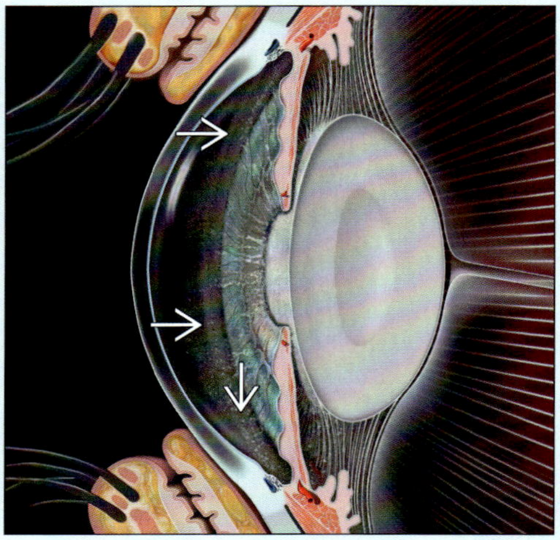

(Left) This illustration depicts schematically the pathogenesis of phacomorphic glaucoma. Phacomorphic glaucoma results when an enlarged, dense cataract pushes the iris anteriorly and closes the angle, leading to obstruction of aqueous humor flow. ***(Right)*** *This illustration depicts schematically the pathogenesis of lens particle glaucoma. Lens particle glaucoma occurs when lens particles released after trauma or surgery are deposited in the angle, leading to obstruction of aqueous drainage.*

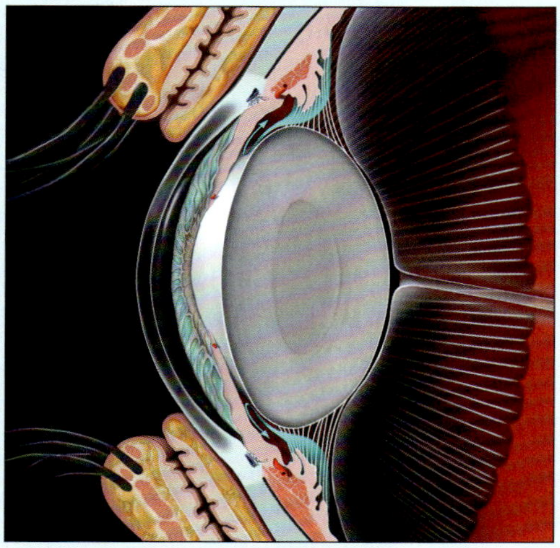

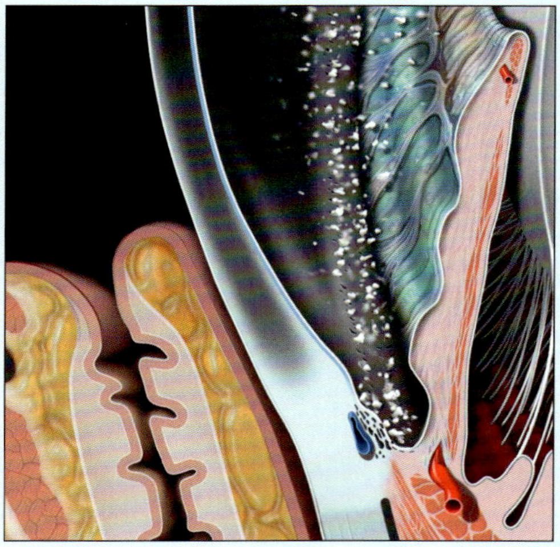

LENS-ASSOCIATED GLAUCOMA

INTRODUCTION

Subtypes
- Phacolytic glaucoma
- Phacomorphic glaucoma
- Lens particle glaucoma

DEMOGRAPHICS

Etiology/Risk Factors
- Both phacolytic and phacomorphic glaucomas are associated with hyperdense, mature cataracts
- Phacolytic glaucoma
  - Secondary open-angle glaucoma
  - Protein that has leaked from a mature cataract may obstruct drainage of aqueous humor through trabecular meshwork
  - Inflammation caused by macrophages digesting lens protein also contributes to obstruction
  - Obstruction of trabecular meshwork leads to increased IOP and glaucoma
- Phacomorphic glaucoma
  - Secondary angle-closure glaucoma
  - Caused by enlarged, dense cataract that pushes iris anteriorly and closes angle
- Lens particle glaucoma
  - Secondary open-angle glaucoma
  - Caused by deposition of lens particles in angle after trauma or surgery, which leads to obstruction of angle

Epidemiology
- Lens-associated glaucomas are more common in populations with limited access to care, as these populations are more likely to develop hyperdense cataracts prior to treatment

PRESENTATION

Symptoms
- Phacolytic glaucoma: Photophobia, pain, tearing, with open angle in presence of advanced cataract
- Phacomorphic glaucoma: Photophobia, pain, tearing with closed angle/fixed pupil in presence of advanced cataract
- Lens particle (formerly known as phacoanaphylactic) glaucoma: Decreased vision, photophobia, pain, tearing, with open angle and history of recent cataract surgery or trauma

Exam Findings
- Phacolytic glaucoma: Advanced cataract, increased IOP, open angle, with possible visible white material in anterior chamber and flare
- Phacomorphic glaucoma: Advanced cataract, increased IOP, closed angle, shallow anterior chamber, dilated pupil
- Lens particle glaucoma: Increased IOP, open angle, presence of white lenticular matter in anterior chamber

DIFFERENTIAL DIAGNOSIS

Inflammatory Glaucoma
- Associated with uveitis
- Presents with cell and flare in anterior chamber with possible peripheral anterior synechiae &/or posterior synechiae
- Not necessarily associated with advanced cataract

Pigmentary Glaucoma
- Shows increased trabecular meshwork pigment and iris transillumination defects
- Not necessarily associated with advanced cataract and findings of lens particles or visible white material in anterior chamber

TREATMENT

Medical
- Medical treatment to decrease IOP and reduce inflammation is 1st step in treating all forms of lens-associated glaucoma
- Treatment options to control pressure include
  - Topical brimonidine, timolol, or dorzolamide
  - Systemic acetazolamide
- Treatment options to reduce inflammation and pain include
  - Topical prednisolone
  - Topical scopolamine or atropine

Surgical
- Removal of the cataract after control of IOP is definitive treatment for both phacolytic and phacomorphic glaucoma
- Removal of lens particles is often necessary to treat lens particle glaucoma

Prognosis
- Majority of patients will have long-term improvement of visual acuity and IOP after removal of cataract

SELECTED REFERENCES

1. Lee JW et al: Retrospective analysis of the risk factors for developing phacomorphic glaucoma. Indian J Ophthalmol. 59(6):471-4, 2011
2. Lee JW et al: Retrospective case series on the long-term visual and intraocular pressure outcomes of phacomorphic glaucoma. Eye (Lond). 24(11):1675-80, 2010
3. Lee SJ et al: Long-term therapeutic efficacy of phacoemulsification with intraocular lens implantation in patients with phacomorphic glaucoma. J Cataract Refract Surg. 36(5):783-9, 2010
4. Ramakrishanan R et al: Visual prognosis, intraocular pressure control and complications in phacomorphic glaucoma following manual small incision cataract surgery. Indian J Ophthalmol. 58(4):303-6, 2010
5. Venkatesh R et al: Safety and efficacy of manual small incision cataract surgery for phacolytic glaucoma. Br J Ophthalmol. 91(3):279-81, 2007
6. Lim MC et al: Late onset lens particle glaucoma as a consequence of spontaneous dislocation of an intraocular lens in pseudoexfoliation syndrome. Am J Ophthalmol. 132(2):261-3, 2001

MALIGNANT GLAUCOMA

Key Facts

Introduction

- Rise in intraocular pressure accompanied by flattening or shallowing of anterior chamber, usually following ocular surgery

Demographics

- Etiology
  - Anterior rotation of ciliary body
  - Accumulation of aqueous in posterior segment
  - Increased intraocular pressure
- Rare; patients typically have history of ocular surgery

Presentation

- Anterior displacement of lens-iris diaphragm without iris bombé or choroidal detachment
- Normal posterior segment exam
- Pain, redness, change in visual acuity
- ↑ intraocular pressure (although pressure can be normal or even low)
- ↓ in anterior chamber depth centrally, peripherally

Treatment

- Medical: Mydriatics to pull lens posteriorly; acetazolamide IV or p.o., topical β-blockers or α-agonists, or osmotic agents to reduce intraocular pressure
- Surgical: Yttrium aluminium garnet (YAG) laser capsulotomy and disruption of anterior hyaloid face (pseudophakic or aphakic), lens extraction with intraocular lens placement, posterior capsulotomy, disruption of anterior hyaloid, and vitrectomy
- Prophylactic peripheral iridectomy treatment of fellow eye
- Continue control of intraocular pressure and use of atropine postoperatively
- Prognosis: Good when malignant glaucoma is identified early and intraocular pressure remains controlled

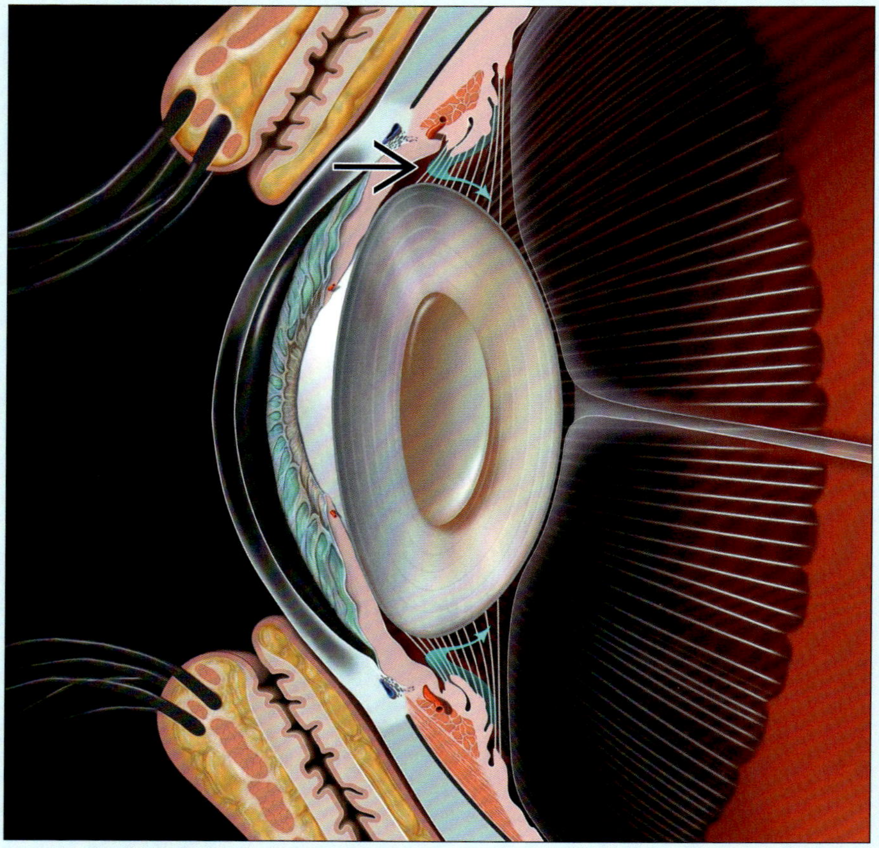

This illustration depicts an eye with malignant glaucoma, also termed aqueous misdirection syndrome. Note the anterior displacement of lens-iris diaphragm ⇒ with resulting angle closure and pupillary block. The pathogenesis of malignant glaucoma is thought to involve anterior rotation of the ciliary body; accumulation of aqueous in posterior segment; anterior displacement of the lens, intraocular lens, or hyaloid face; and increase in intraocular pressure results.

MALIGNANT GLAUCOMA

INTRODUCTION

Synonyms
- Also referred to as aqueous misdirection syndrome, ciliary block glaucoma, posterior aqueous diversion syndrome

Definitions
- Rise in intraocular pressure accompanied by flattening or shallowing of anterior chamber

Subtypes
- Classical: Usually follows ocular surgery in a patient with a history of angle closure of peripheral anterior synechia (PAS)
- Spontaneous: Very rare, consists of isolated case reports

DEMOGRAPHICS

Etiology/Risk Factors
- Poorly understood; thought to involve
  - Anterior rotation of ciliary body
  - Accumulation of aqueous in posterior segment
  - Anterior displacement of lens, intraocular lens, or hyaloid face
  - Increased intraocular pressure
- Small anterior segment (as in hyperopia or nanophthalmos)
- Surgery for primary open-angle glaucoma
  - Trabeculectomy
  - Tube-shunt procedure
  - Iridectomy
- Additional intraocular procedures
  - Cataract surgery
  - Cyclophotocoagulation
  - Retinal procedures
- Nonsurgical
  - Initiation of miotic agents or cessation of cycloplegic agents

Epidemiology
- Rare; patients typically have history of ocular surgery

PRESENTATION

Symptoms
- Pain, redness, change in visual acuity

Exam Findings
- Increased intraocular pressure (although pressure can be normal or even low)
  - In presence of patent iridectomy
- Decrease in anterior chamber depth centrally and peripherally
- Anterior displacement of lens-iris diaphragm
- Ultrasound biomicroscopy can show anterior displacement of ciliary body, thus pressing against lens equator or anterior hyaloid face, preventing anterior drainage of aqueous
- Normal posterior segment exam
- Note: Iris bombé and choroidal detachment must not be present for diagnosis

DIFFERENTIAL DIAGNOSIS

Pupillary Block Glaucoma
- Iris bombé and iris adhesions may be present
- Typically relieved by presence of patent peripheral iridectomy

Suprachoroidal Hemorrhage
- Elevated intraocular pressure
- Abnormal posterior segment exam

Choroidal Effusion
- Low intraocular pressure
- Typically painless
- Abnormal posterior segment exam

TREATMENT

Medical
- Cycloplegics to pull lens posteriorly
  - Atropine and phenylephrine
- Reduce intraocular pressure
  - Acetazolamide IV or p.o.
  - Topical β-blockers (timolol)
  - Topical α-agonists (apraclonidine or brimonidine)
  - Osmotic agents (mannitol or glycerin)
- Anti-inflammatory
  - Topical steroids

Surgical
- Peripheral iridectomy (PI)
  - Perform PI if one is not already present or is blocked to rule out pupillary block
- Aphakic or pseudophakic
  - YAG laser capsulotomy and disruption of anterior hyaloid face
  - Laser ciliary body ablation
  - Vitrectomy
- Phakic
  - Lens extraction with intraocular lens placement, posterior capsulotomy, disruption of anterior hyaloid, and vitrectomy

Follow-Up
- Prophylactic peripheral iridectomy treatment of fellow eye
- Continue control of intraocular pressure and use of atropine postoperatively
- Avoid use of miotics

Prognosis
- 50% of patients can be managed with medical therapy alone
- Good when malignant glaucoma is identified early and intraocular pressure remains controlled

SELECTED REFERENCES

1. Debrouwere V et al: Outcomes of different management options for malignant glaucoma: a retrospective study. Graefes Arch Clin Exp Ophthalmol. 250(1):131-41, 2012
2. Shahid H et al: Malignant glaucoma: a review of the modern literature. J Ophthalmol. 2012:852659, 2012
3. Ruben S et al: Malignant glaucoma and its management. Br J Ophthalmol. 81(2):163-7, 1997

IATROGENIC GLAUCOMAS

Key Facts

Introduction

- Iatrogenic glaucoma: Increase in intraocular pressure (IOP) associated with optic nerve damage caused by medical treatment

Subtypes

- Steroid-response glaucoma
  - Definition: IOP ↑ with possible development of glaucoma in patients using topical steroids
  - Etiology: ↓ drainage of aqueous humor through trabecular meshwork through unverified mechanism that likely involves extracellular matrix deposition
  - Prevention: Use least potent steroid that is appropriate, with lowest dose frequency that is appropriate
  - Treatment: IOP-lowering agents: Topical β-blockers, α-agonists, carbonic anhydrase inhibitors, prostaglandin agonists
- Postoperative glaucoma
  - Definition: IOP ↑ with possible vision loss in patient in postoperative period
  - Etiology: Retained viscoelastic material, inflammation, hyphema, steroid-response, lens material in anterior chamber (AC), vitreous in AC
  - Treatment: IOP-lowering agents: Topical β-blockers, α-agonists, carbonic anhydrase inhibitors (prostaglandin analogues are typically not used as they may increase inflammation)
- Uveitis, glaucoma, hyphema syndrome (UGH)
  - Anterior segment inflammation resulting in uveitis, hyphema, and ↑ IOP
  - Etiology: Anterior segment inflammation as a result of poorly placed intraocular lens (IOL)
  - Treatment: IOP-lowering agents: Topical β-blockers, α-agonists, carbonic anhydrase inhibitors
  - Surgical treatment: IOL repositioning or exchange is often necessary

*(**Left**) Slit-lamp photograph demonstrates an IOL haptic ➔ that has been displaced outside of the bag. A poorly positioned IOL haptic is a risk factor for the development of uveitis, glaucoma, hyphema syndrome (UGH). (**Right**) Slit-lamp photograph depicts an anterior chamber intraocular lens (AC IOL) ➔. AC IOLs are a risk factor for the development of UGH. Complicated cataract surgery, including posterior capsule rupture, is also a risk factor for the development of UGH.*

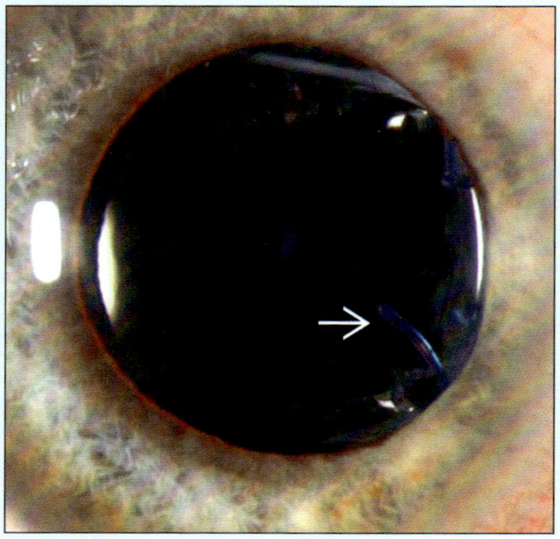

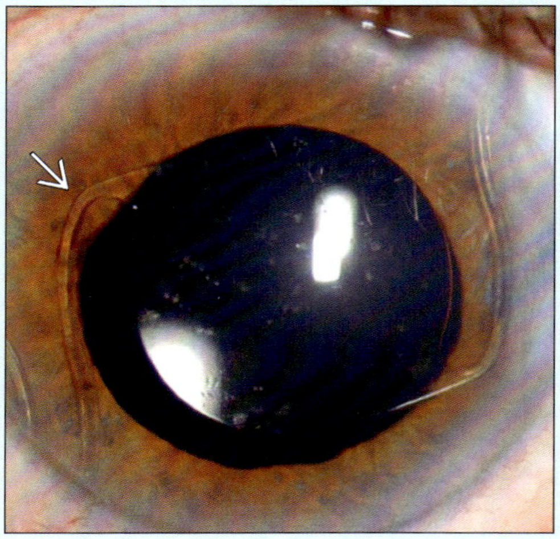

*(**Left**) Slit-lamp photograph shows the eye of a patient with UGH. Note the signs of anterior chamber inflammation, fibrin ➔, and poorly positioned IOL ➔. The patient also demonstrated microhyphema and optic nerve damage (not shown). (**Right**) Fundus photograph depicts optic nerve cupping ➔. Damage to the optic nerve is a late sequela of steroid-response glaucoma, postoperative glaucoma, and UGH.*

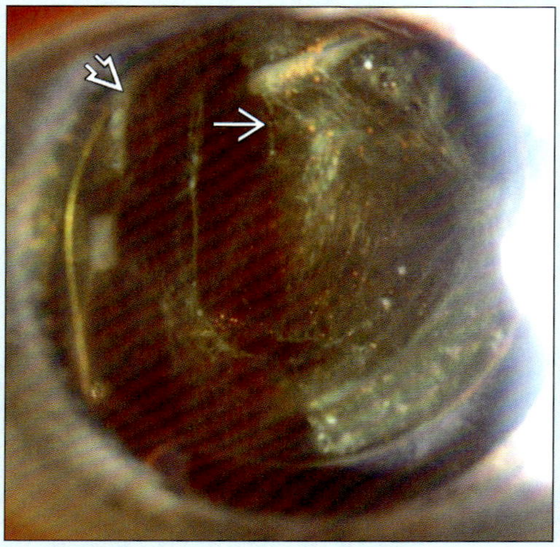

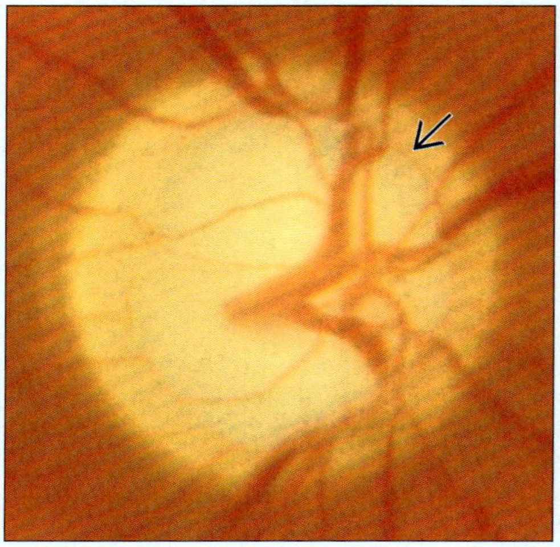

IATROGENIC GLAUCOMAS

INTRODUCTION

Definitions

- Increase in intraocular pressure (IOP) associated with optic nerve damage caused by medical treatment

Subtypes

- Steroid-response glaucoma
  - IOP ↑ with possible development of glaucoma in patients using topical steroids
- Postoperative glaucoma
  - IOP ↑ with possible vision loss in patient in postoperative period
- Uveitis, glaucoma, hyphema syndrome (UGH)
  - Anterior segment inflammation resulting in uveitis, hyphema, and ↑ IOP

DEMOGRAPHICS

Etiology/Risk Factors

- Steroid-response glaucoma
  - Etiology: ↓ drainage of aqueous humor through trabecular meshwork by unverified mechanism that likely involves extracellular matrix deposition
  - Risk factors: Primary open-angle glaucoma (POAG), glaucoma suspect, family history of POAG, older age, connective tissue disease, increased dose frequency of steroid, use of higher-potency steroids
- Postoperative glaucoma
  - Etiology: Retained viscoelastic material, inflammation, hyphema, steroid response, lens material in anterior chamber (AC), vitreous in AC
  - Risk factors: Underlying glaucoma, complicated surgery, prolonged steroid use
- UGH
  - Etiology: Anterior segment inflammation as a result of poorly placed intraocular lens (IOL)
  - Risk factors: Anterior chamber IOL, older style of IOL, complicated surgery, posterior capsule rupture

Epidemiology

- Steroid-response glaucoma
  - 5-10% of patients treated with topical steroids will have an IOP ↑ of 16 mm Hg or more
- Postoperative glaucoma
  - 2-8% of phacoemulsification patients will experience ↑ IOP during postop period
- UGH
  - Uncommon with modern IOLs, though it still rarely occurs

PRESENTATION

Symptoms

- Steroid-response glaucoma
  - Asymptomatic or symptoms of ↑ IOP (pain, decreased vision, nausea, headache)
- Postoperative glaucoma
  - Asymptomatic or symptoms of increased IOP
- UGH
  - Decreased vision, deep ocular pain, transient vision loss

Exam Findings

- Steroid-response glaucoma
  - ↑ IOP with history of steroid use
    - Typically no IOP elevation before 2 weeks, with maximum risk at 4-6 weeks
    - Rare reports of patients with an acute IOP elevation
- Postoperative glaucoma
  - ↑ IOP with history of recent ocular surgery
  - Microcystic edema of cornea
  - Identify signs of possible causes: Inflammation, vitreous in AC, lens fragments, angle closure
- UGH
  - ↑ IOP with cell and flare, hyphema/microhyphema, improperly positioned IOL

DIFFERENTIAL DIAGNOSIS

Primary Open-Angle Glaucoma (POAG)

- Risk factor for development of steroid-response glaucoma and postoperative glaucoma
- Patients with POAG are more sensitive to increases in IOP in setting of steroid-response glaucoma and postoperative glaucoma

Acute Angle-Closure Glaucoma (AACG)

- Shows fixed pupil, closed angle, and microcystic corneal edema

TREATMENT

Steroid-Response Glaucoma

- Prevention
  - Use least potent steroid that is appropriate, with lowest dose frequency that is appropriate
  - When starting steroids: Check IOP initially, then 2 weeks later, then every 4 weeks for 3 months, then every 6 months
- Stop steroid if possible
  - If not, reduce potency &/or dose frequency
- IOP-lowering agents: Topical β-blockers, α-agonists, carbonic anhydrase inhibitors, prostaglandin agonists

Postoperative Glaucoma

- IOP-lowering agents: Topical β-blockers, α-agonists, carbonic anhydrase inhibitors
  - Prostaglandin analogues are typically not used as they may increase inflammation

Uveitis, Glaucoma, Hyphema Syndrome

- IOP-lowering agents: Topical β-blockers, α-agonists, carbonic anhydrase inhibitors
- IOL repositioning or exchange is often necessary

SELECTED REFERENCES

1. Jones R 3rd et al: Corticosteroid-induced ocular hypertension and glaucoma: a brief review and update of the literature. Curr Opin Ophthalmol. 17(2):163-7, 2006
2. Kersey JP et al: Corticosteroid-induced glaucoma: a review of the literature. Eye (Lond). 20(4):407-16, 2006
3. McKellar MJ et al: The early complications of cataract surgery: is routine review of patients 1 week after cataract extraction necessary? Ophthalmology. 108(5):930-5, 2001
4. Mamalis N: Explantation of intraocular lenses. Curr Opin Ophthalmol. 11(4):289-95, 2000

PUPILLARY BLOCK

Key Facts

Introduction
- Elevation in intraocular pressure (IOP) due to blockage of aqueous flow through pupil, causing forward bowing of peripheral iris and blockage of aqueous drainage through trabecular meshwork
- Most frequent cause of acute angle-closure glaucoma

Demographics
- Phakic pupillary block: Contact between lens and iris blocks aqueous flow
- Pressure builds up in posterior chamber
- Iris bows forward, blocking aqueous drainage through trabecular meshwork (acute angle closure)
- Postoperative aphakic pupillary block: Contact between hyaloid face, air, gas, or silicone and iris blocks aqueous flow

Presentation
- Painful red eye, change in visual acuity, halos
- Headache, nausea, and vomiting
- Pupil often in mid-dilated position, iris bombé

Differential Diagnosis
- Suprachoroidal hemorrhage
- Malignant glaucoma (aqueous misdirection syndrome)

Treatment
- Yttrium aluminum garnet (YAG) laser peripheral iridotomy or argon laser peripheral iridoplasty
  - Medically manage only when cornea is too hazy to perform peripheral iridotomy
- Consider prophylactic peripheral iridotomy of opposite eye
- Prompt treatment with IOP returning to normal range will result in cessation of ocular and physical symptoms and normalization of visual acuity

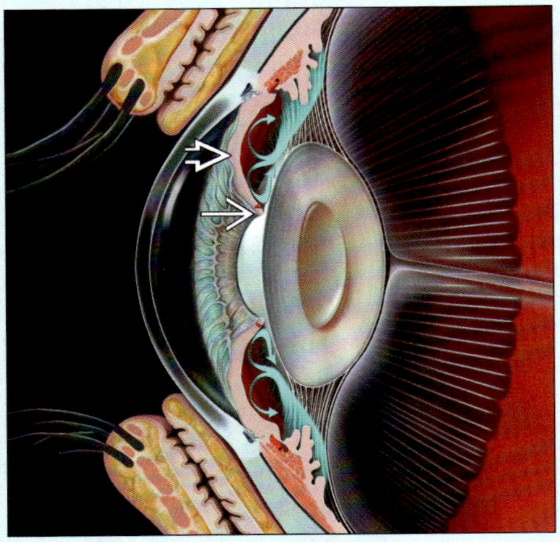

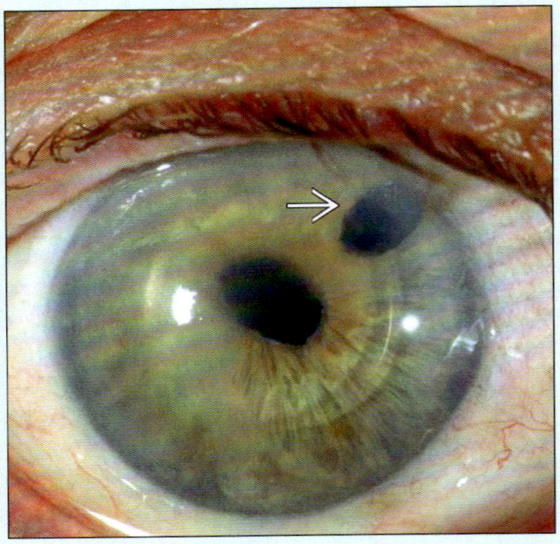

(Left) *This graphic illustrates the mechanism of pupillary block. Note how the peripupillary portion of the iris is pressed up against the body of the lens, blocking the flow of aqueous ➔. This causes the iris to bellow forward ➔ and results in increased intraocular pressure.* ***(Right)*** *This image shows the eye of a patient who underwent surgical iridectomy ➔ at the time of cataract surgery with anterior chamber lens implantation in order to prevent pseudophakic pupillary block.*

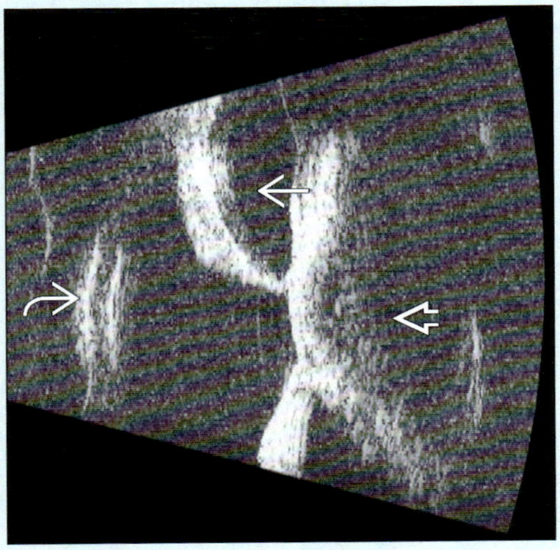

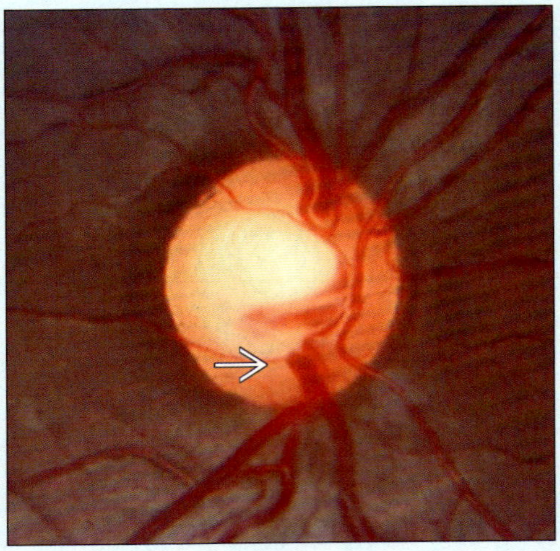

(Left) *This ocular ultrasound demonstrates iris bombé during pupillary block. The cornea ➔ is on the left side of the image. The lens is blocking ➔ the pupil, causing the iris ➔ to bow forward from pressure buildup posteriorly.* ***(Right)*** *This fundus photo shows the typical appearance of a glaucomatous optic disc, demonstrating an excavated disc with kinking of blood vessels along the rim of the optic disc ➔.*

PUPILLARY BLOCK

INTRODUCTION

Definitions
- Elevation in intraocular pressure (IOP) due to blockage of aqueous flow through pupil, causing forward bowing of peripheral iris and blockage of aqueous drainage through trabecular meshwork
- Most frequent cause of acute angle-closure glaucoma

DEMOGRAPHICS

Etiology/Risk Factors
- Phakic pupillary block: Contact between lens and iris blocks aqueous flow
  - Pressure builds up in posterior chamber, iris bows forward, blocking aqueous drainage through trabecular meshwork (acute angle closure)
  - Results in overall increase in intraocular pressure
- Predisposition to any of the preceding steps increases risk of pupillary block
  - Elderly: Larger lens with greater curvature
  - Trauma: Swollen and enlarged lens
  - Hypertropic: Smaller eye with smaller anterior chamber
  - Females: Narrow angle
  - Use of certain local and systemic medications: Mydriatics, α-adrenergics, anticholinergics, antidepressants, antianxiety medications
  - Systemic disorders (e.g., Marfan syndrome, homocystinuria, Weill-Marchesani syndrome)
    - Ectopia lentis
- Postoperative aphakic pupillary block: Contact between hyaloid face, air, gas, or silicone and iris blocks aqueous flow
  - Air or gas bubble displacing iris causing flow blockage or independently blocking aqueous flow
  - Vitreous can extrude forward and plug pupil
  - Silicone oil injection

PRESENTATION

Symptoms
- Painful red eye, change in visual acuity, halos
- Headache, nausea, and vomiting

Exam Findings
- Shallow anterior chamber, increased IOP
- Conjunctival injection, corneal edema
- Pupil often in mid-dilated position, iris bombé
- Loss of iridocorneal angle structures on gonioscopy

DIFFERENTIAL DIAGNOSIS

Suprachoroidal Hemorrhage
- Abnormal posterior segment exam

Malignant Glaucoma (Aqueous Misdirection Syndrome)
- Flattening or shallowing of anterior chamber
- Iris bombé not present

EVALUATION/WORK-UP

Imaging
- Optical coherence tomography of optic nerve head
  - Ultrasound biomicroscopy is helpful to distinguish pupillary block from plateau iris or other angle abnormalities
- Visual field testing

TREATMENT

Medical
- Typically only used when cornea is too hazy to perform peripheral iridectomy
- Topical glycerin to assist in clearing corneal edema
- Reduce inflammation with topical steroids (prednisolone acetate)
- Pull lens posteriorly with mydriatics (cyclopentolate and phenylephrine)
- Reduce IOP

Surgical
- Phakic pupillary block
  - Yttrium aluminum garnet (YAG) laser peripheral iridotomy
  - Argon laser peripheral iridoplasty
  - Lensectomy if appropriate
- Postoperative aphakic pupillary block
  - YAG peripheral iridotomy or Argon laser peripheral iridoplasty
  - Hyaloid face incision
  - Capsulotomy
  - Pars plana vitrectomy or placement of tube shunt can be options

Follow-Up
- Continue use of IOP reduction medications; check 1 hour after surgery
- 1-day postoperative check
- Consider prophylactic peripheral iridotomy of opposite eye

Prognosis
- Possible complications include hyphema from laser procedures or wound infection if surgery is required
- Prompt treatment with IOP returning to normal range will result in cessation of ocular and physical symptoms and normalization of visual acuity

SELECTED REFERENCES

1. Boey PY et al: Conventional and emerging treatments in the management of acute primary angle closure. Clin Ophthalmol. 6:417-24, 2012
2. Tarongoy P et al: Angle-closure glaucoma: the role of the lens in the pathogenesis, prevention, and treatment. Surv Ophthalmol. 54(2):211-25, 2009
3. Jackson TL et al: Pupil block glaucoma in phakic and pseudophakic patients after vitrectomy with silicone oil injection. Am J Ophthalmol. 132(3):414-6, 2001
4. Ellant JP et al: Lens-induced glaucoma. Doc Ophthalmol. 81(3):317-38, 1992

ANGLE-RECESSION GLAUCOMA

Key Facts

Introduction
- Secondary glaucoma caused by recession of anterior chamber angle and damage to trabecular meshwork, usually secondary to blunt ocular trauma

Demographics
- May affect > 75% of patients with history of blunt ocular trauma

Presentation
- Usually asymptomatic

Differential Diagnosis
- Cyclodialysis cleft: Will frequently cause dramatic decrease in intraocular pressure, with sudden increase and spontaneous closure of cyclodialysis cleft
- Iridodialysis: Visible dehiscence of iris root from ciliary body, causing polycoria and possible diplopia

Evaluation/Work-Up
- Tear between longitudinal and circular ciliary body muscle fibers
- Appears as widening of ciliary body band on gonioscopy
- Usually has asymmetric intraocular pressure &/or optic nerve cupping

Treatment
- First-line medical treatment includes topical prostaglandin analogues, β-blockers, α-adrenergic agents, &/or carbonic anhydrase inhibitors
- Trabeculectomy and tube-shunt devices are surgical procedures of choice for glaucoma refractory to medical treatment
- Laser trabeculoplasty is not effective for this condition

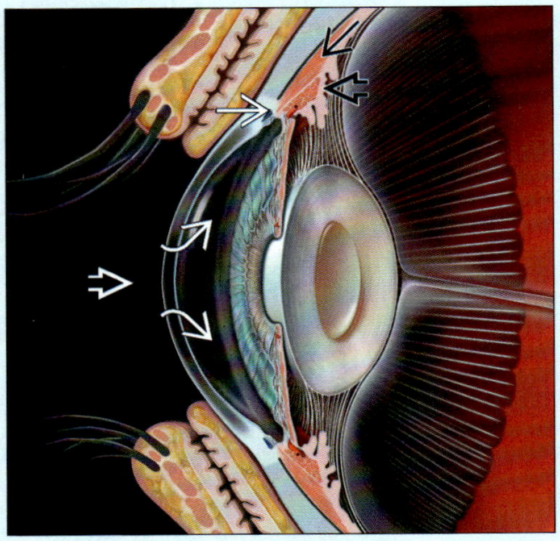

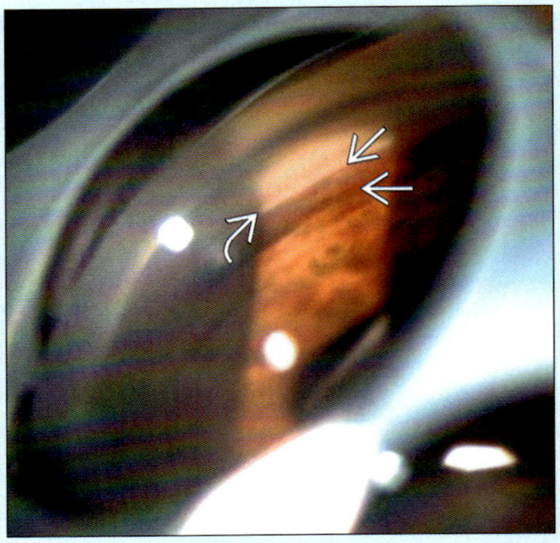

(Left) *Graphic illustrates the area of angle recession, which produces a cleavage plane between the longitudinal and circular fibers of the ciliary muscle. Anteroposterior compressive forces on the globe cause equatorial displacement of aqueous that may lead to angle recession.* ***(Right)*** *Gonioscopic image shows characteristic widening of the ciliary body band posterior to the scleral spur.*

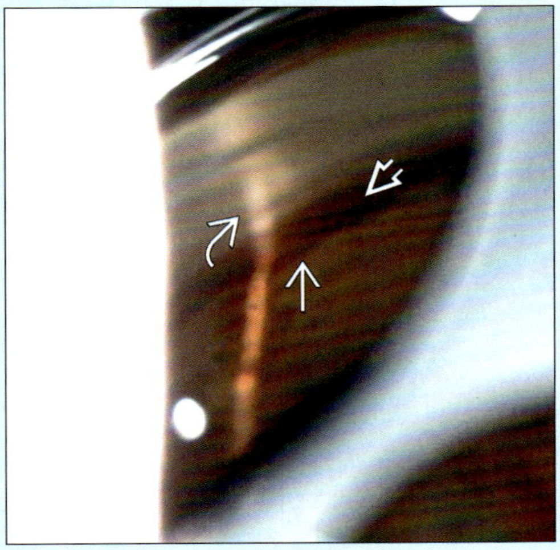

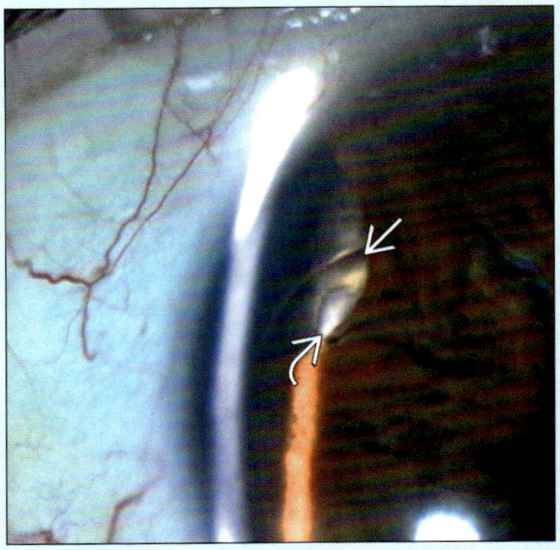

(Left) *Gonioscopy shows posterior displacement of circular muscle fibers and iris root, with visible longitudinal muscle fibers. Concurrent damage to the trabecular meshwork causes increase in intraocular pressure.* ***(Right)*** *Slit-lamp photo depicts iridodialysis and angle recession (not visible) following blunt trauma. Note the pseudophakic lens visible through the iris defect. Angle recession may be associated with other traumatic findings, such as iridodialysis, cyclodialysis, and hyphema.*

ANGLE-RECESSION GLAUCOMA

INTRODUCTION

Definitions

- Traumatic secondary open-angle glaucoma
  - Caused by recession of anterior chamber angle and damage to trabecular meshwork, with resultant decrease in outflow capacity

DEMOGRAPHICS

Etiology/Risk Factors

- Most commonly caused by blunt ocular trauma
  - May have remote or forgotten blunt trauma history not elicited on routine questioning
  - Compressive forces on globe cause anterior to posterior axial compression followed by equatorial expansion
  - Aqueous is rapidly forced laterally, causing a tear of ciliary body between longitudinal and circular muscle fibers
  - Damage to trabecular meshwork leads to decreased outflow and eventual glaucoma if untreated
  - Glaucoma is more commonly seen in angle recession > 180°

Epidemiology

- May affect > 75% of patients with history of blunt ocular trauma
- Up to 20% of eyes with angle recession may develop glaucoma

PRESENTATION

Symptoms

- Usually asymptomatic

Exam Findings

- Unilateral increased intraocular pressure
- Angle recession on gonioscopy
- Asymmetric optic nerve cupping
- Visual field deficits and nerve fiber layer thinning on optical coherence tomography (OCT)
- May be associated with other signs of ocular trauma
  - Cataract
  - Cyclodialysis/iridodialysis
  - Hyphema
  - Chorioretinal scars/rupture
  - Retinal tears/detachment
  - Iris atrophy

DIFFERENTIAL DIAGNOSIS

Cyclodialysis Cleft

- Will frequently cause dramatic decrease in intraocular pressure, with sudden increase and spontaneous closure of cyclodialysis cleft

Iridodialysis

- Visible dehiscence of iris root from ciliary body, causing polycoria and possible diplopia

EVALUATION/WORK-UP

Pathology

- Tear between longitudinal and circular ciliary body muscle fibers

Imaging

- Normally, gonioscopy is only modality necessary for diagnosis
  - Anterior segment OCT and ultrasound biomicroscopy may also be used
- Retinal nerve fiber layer OCT, disc photos, and visual field testing are used for glaucoma monitoring

TREATMENT

Medical

- Medical treatment is reserved for eyes with high intraocular pressures or evidence of glaucoma
- Prostaglandin analogues have theoretical benefit due to increased uveoscleral outflow in a setting of damaged trabecular outflow
- May also use β-blockers, α-adrenergic agents, &/or carbonic anhydrase inhibitors
- Avoid miotics because of decreased uveoscleral outflow associated with their use

Surgical

- Reserved for eyes with glaucomatous damage and intraocular pressure refractory to medical treatment
- Selective laser trabeculoplasty and argon laser trabeculoplasty have decreased effectiveness due to trabecular meshwork scarring
- Trabeculectomy and tube-shunt devices are surgical procedures of choice for refractory glaucoma

Follow-Up

- Due to risk of progression, routine follow-up is recommended for eyes with evidence of angle recession even without evidence of glaucoma
- Eyes with evidence of glaucoma should be followed closely depending on severity

Prognosis

- Good prognosis with appropriate follow-up

SELECTED REFERENCES

1. Bai HQ et al: Causes and treatments of traumatic secondary glaucoma. Eur J Ophthalmol. 19(2):201-6, 2009
2. Manners T et al: Trabeculectomy with mitomycin C in the treatment of post-traumatic angle recession glaucoma. Br J Ophthalmol. 85(2):159-63, 2001
3. Canavan YM et al: Anterior segment consequences of blunt ocular injury. Br J Ophthalmol. 66(9):549-55, 1982
4. Wolff SM et al: Chronic secondary glaucoma. Associated with retrodisplacement of iris root and deepening of the anterior chamber angle secondary to contusion. Am J Ophthalmol. 54:547-63, 1962

EXFOLIATIVE GLAUCOMA

Key Facts

Introduction

- Classic exfoliation of iris occurred in glassblowers
- Systemic deposition of white fibrillary (exfoliative) material on multiple organs throughout the body, specifically, the anterior segment of the eye and trabecular meshwork, resulting in increase in intraocular pressure and optic nerve damage

Demographics

- Associated with pseudoexfoliation syndrome
- Risk increases with age

Presentation

- Asymptomatic or decreased visual acuity from optic nerve damage
- Often asymmetric clinical findings
- Distinct target-like pattern of white protein material deposits on the anterior capsule
- Iris transillumination defects likely caused by pigment dispersion from scraping of pseudoexfoliative material during iris movement
- Excavated, cupped optic discs that can present ± elevated intraocular pressure

Evaluation/Work-Up

- Optical coherence tomography (OCT) shows and tracks changes in thickness of optic disc and retinal nerve fiber layer

Treatment

- Relative to POAG, PES glaucoma is resistant to medical therapy with poorer prognosis
- Typical late presentation and rapid progression generally results in a worse prognosis than POAG
- Surgical procedures have higher efficacy: Argon laser trabeculoplasty, selective laser trabeculoplasty, trabeculectomy

__(Left)__ This slit-lamp photo shows the hallmark target-like sign of pseudoexfoliation. White, fibrillary proteinaceous material can be observed on the lens surface. This area ➡ is clear of the deposits due to the wiper movement of the pupil from dilation and constriction. __(Right)__ This is a slit-lamp photo demonstrating the central iris. Note the loss of the normal pupillary ruff ➡. Jagged deposits of exfoliative material can be observed on the lens surface ➡.

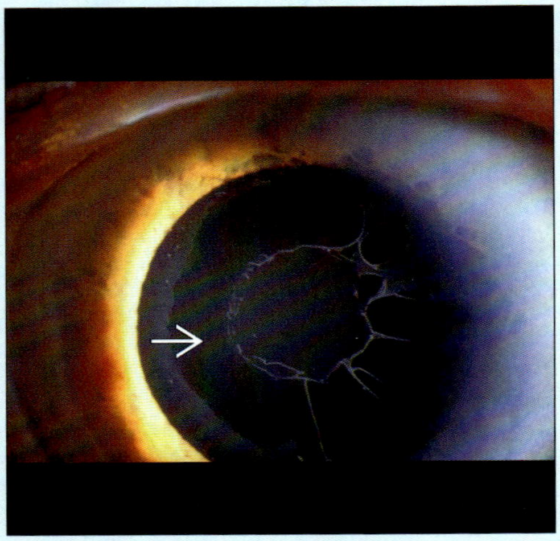

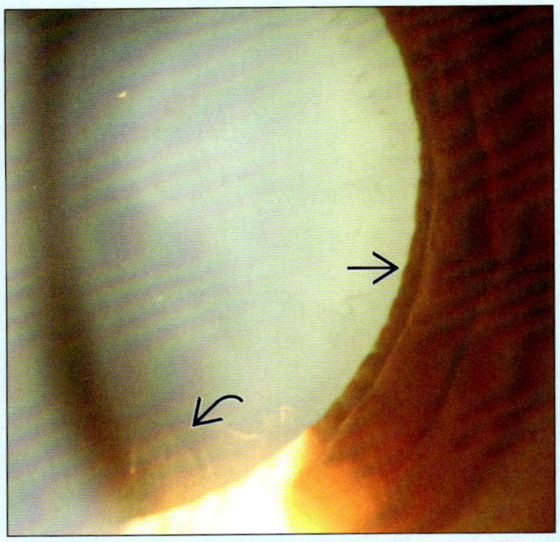

__(Left)__ Another slit-lamp photo demonstrates the target-like pattern of exfoliation material. __(Right)__ This is a histopathology slide of the anterior lens capsule. The lens capsule is stained blue and lined internally by lens epithelial cells ➡. The external surface is lined with pink-staining exfoliative material ➡, classically described as having an "iron-filing" orientation.

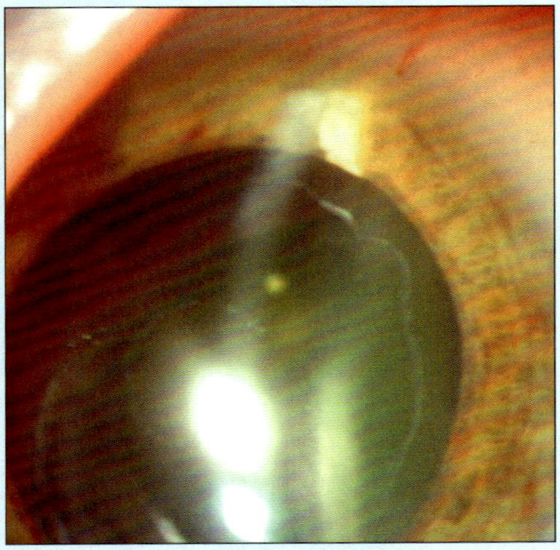

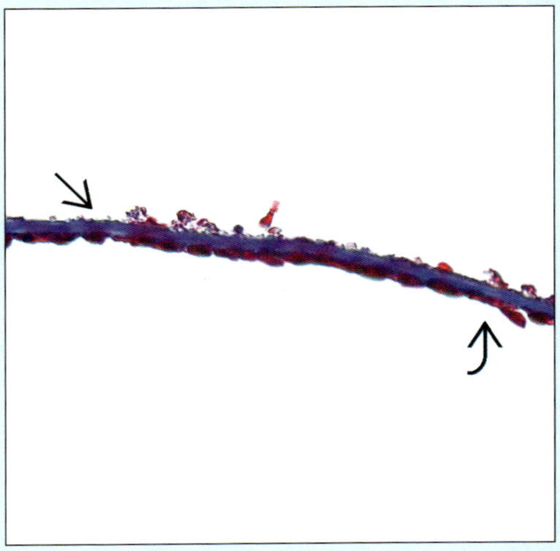

EXFOLIATIVE GLAUCOMA

INTRODUCTION

Definitions

- Classic exfoliation of iris occurred in glassblowers
- Exfoliative (pseudoexfoliative) syndrome (PES or PXF) is systemic deposition of white fibrillary (exfoliative) material on multiple organs throughout the body
  - Specifically, anterior segment of eye and trabecular meshwork
  - Often results in increase in intraocular pressure (IOP) and optic nerve damage

DEMOGRAPHICS

Etiology/Risk Factors

- Associated with pseudoexfoliation syndrome
- Risk increases with age
- Genetics: Mutations in lysyl oxidase-like protein 1 (*LOXL1*) gene have been shown to be strongly associated with PES

Epidemiology

- Previously thought to be prevalent in only Scandinavian populations, PES has been found to occur worldwide
- 3x more common in females

PRESENTATION

Symptoms

- Asymptomatic or decreased visual acuity from optic nerve damage
- Larger diurnal IOP fluctuations than primary open-angle glaucoma (POAG)
- Greater inflammatory response due to defective blood-aqueous barrier

Exam Findings

- Often asymmetric clinical findings, with initial unaffected eye often eventually presenting with symptoms
- Distinct target-like pattern of white protein material deposits on anterior capsule
  - Central disc of material deposited on lens
  - Pericentral clear area thought to be formed by iris movement
  - Scalloped deposition of white material on the periphery observed with a dilated pupil
- Poor mydriasis, along with zonular weakness, makes cataract extraction riskier
- Iris transillumination defects ("moth-eaten" pupil margin) likely caused by pigment dispersion from scraping of pseudoexfoliative material during iris movement
- On gonioscopic exam, increased pigmentation of iridocorneal angle may be observed
- Posterior synechiae
- Excavated, cupped optic discs that can present ± elevated intraocular pressure

DIFFERENTIAL DIAGNOSIS

Uveitis

- Splotchy pigment in trabecular meshwork
- Anterior synechiae may be present

Pigmentary Glaucoma

- Affects younger and more myopic individuals
- Heavier, more diffusely distributed pigment (Sampoelesi line visible on gonioscopy), Krukenberg spindle on corneal endothelium

True Exfoliation

- Exposure to extreme heat/infrared radiation
- Splitting of lens capsule

Primary Amyloidosis

- Amyloid can deposit in same pattern as exfoliation material, on lens capsule, iris, and trabecular meshwork

EVALUATION/WORK-UP

Pathology

- Histopathology has shown that capillary density does not change with decrease in axon thickness in PES vs. primary open-angle glaucoma (POAG), which shows increase in connective tissue and decrease in capillary density

Imaging

- Visual field testing, funduscopy, retroillumination, gonioscopy
- Optical coherence tomography (OCT) shows and tracks changes in thickness of optic disc and retinal nerve fiber layer

TREATMENT

Medical

- Same as POAG (prostaglandin analogues, β-blockers, α-2 agonists, carbonic anhydrase inhibitors)
- PES glaucoma is often resistant to medical therapy with a poorer prognosis

Surgical

- Argon laser or selective laser trabeculoplasty
- Trabeculectomy
- Cataract surgeons should be wary of capsule instability

Follow-Up

- Generally over 4-6 months

Prognosis

- Typical late presentation and rapid progression generally results in worse prognosis than POAG

SELECTED REFERENCES

1. Sein J et al: Exfoliation syndrome: new genetic and pathophysiologic insights. Curr Opin Ophthalmol. 24(2):167-74, 2013
2. Ritch R: Exfoliation syndrome: beyond glaucoma. Arch Ophthalmol. 126(6):859-61, 2008
3. Ritch R: The management of exfoliative glaucoma. Prog Brain Res. 173:211-24, 2008

GLAUCOMATOCYCLITIC CRISIS

Key Facts

Introduction

- Also known as Posner-Schlossman syndrome (PSS)
- Characterized by recurrent attacks of markedly increased intraocular pressure (IOP) with mild anterior inflammation of unknown etiology

Demographics

- No current consensus on its etiology
- Glaucomatocyclitic crisis is a very rare occurrence in the United States

Presentation

- Unilateral blurred vision and mild pain
- Asymptomatic between attacks
- Elevated IOP (40-60 mm Hg) lasting from several hours to multiple weeks
- Mild inflammation in anterior chamber
- Gonioscopy will show an open angle

Differential Diagnosis

- Acute angle-closure glaucoma: Angle will be closed on gonioscopy
- Chronic angle-closure glaucoma: Peripheral anterior synechiae on gonioscopy
- Primary open-angle glaucoma: Consistently high IOP with cupped optic disc

Treatment

- Medically reduce IOP
- Medically reduce inflammation
- Evaluated on a case-by-case basis, certain patients can be qualified to self-administer medications when they sense an acute attack
- Due to the intermittent nature of glaucomatocyclitic crisis, medication is not necessary between attacks
- Filtering procedures may help regulate IOP but do not prevent recurrent attacks
- Traditionally thought of as a benign disease

__(Left)__ This slit-lamp photograph shows anterior chamber cell and flare ➔. Mild anterior chamber inflammation is an important finding in glaucomatocyclitic crisis. __(Right)__ This slit-lamp photograph depicts keratic precipitates ➔, which are a common finding in glaucomatocyclitic crisis. The defining features of glaucomatocyclitic crisis are an elevated IOP in the setting of mild anterior chamber inflammation of unknown etiology.

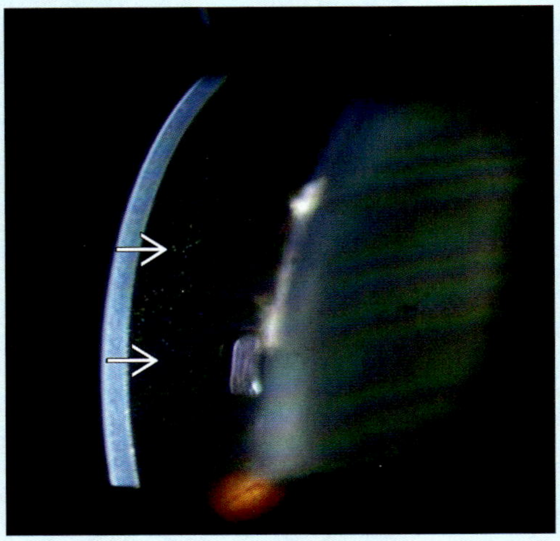

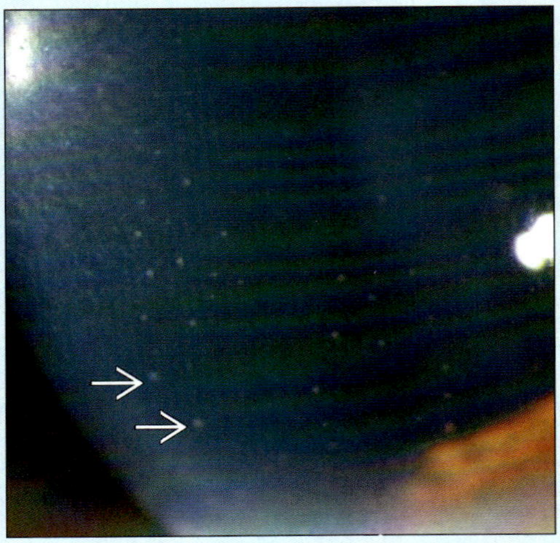

__(Left)__ This gonioscopic image demonstrates a normal angle. Patient with glaucomatocyclitic crisis presents with elevated IOP in the setting of a normal, open angle. Confirming an open angle is necessary for the diagnosis of glaucomatocyclitic crisis. __(Right)__ This gonioscopic image demonstrates a closed angle ➔. When making the diagnosis of glaucomatocyclitic crisis, it is necessary to rule out angle-closure glaucoma.

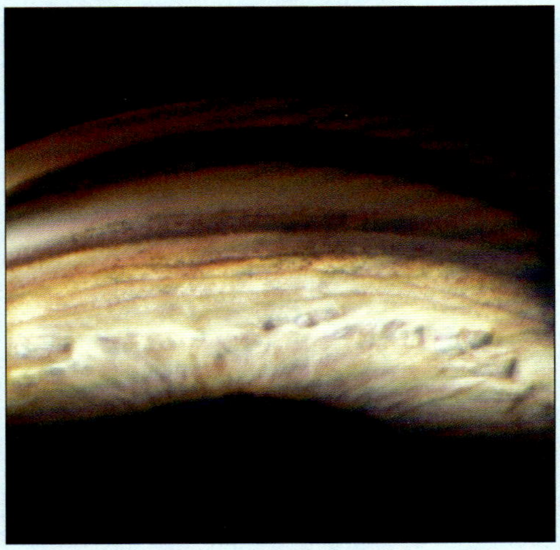

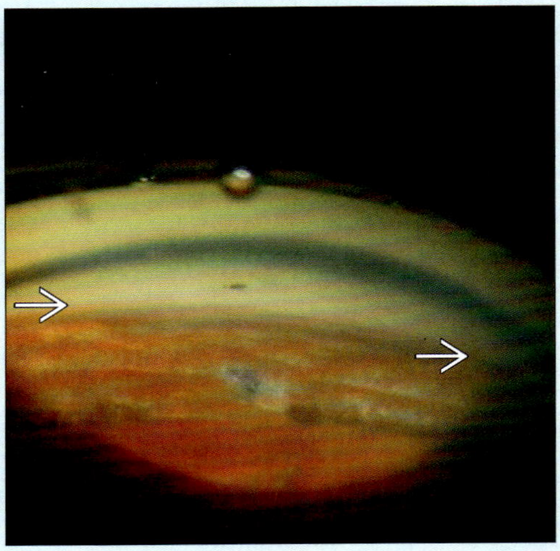

GLAUCOMATOCYCLITIC CRISIS

INTRODUCTION

Synonyms
- Posner-Schlossman syndrome (PSS)

Definitions
- Characterized by recurrent attacks of markedly increased intraocular pressure (IOP) with mild anterior inflammation of unknown etiology

DEMOGRAPHICS

Etiology/Risk Factors
- No current consensus on etiology of glaucomatocyclitic crisis; HLA-Bw54 is associated
- Prominent theories
  - Vascular endothelial dysfunction: Dysregulation results in reduced ocular blood flow
  - Autoimmune: Increased prostaglandins may have a role in increasing the production of aqueous while simultaneously decreasing the outflow
  - Infection with the following pathogens may be associated with PSS
    - Herpes simplex
    - Cytomegalovirus
    - *Helicobacter pylori*

Epidemiology
- Glaucomatocyclitic crisis is a very rare occurrence in the United States
- Typically occurs in individuals between 20 and 50 years old

PRESENTATION

Symptoms
- Unilateral blurred vision and mild pain
- Asymptomatic between attacks

Exam Findings
- Elevated IOP (40-60 mm Hg) lasting from several hours to multiple weeks
- Corneal edema
- Mild inflammation in anterior chamber
- Small, round, self-resolving keratic precipitates
- Gonioscopy will show an open angle
- Normal-appearing optic disc

DIFFERENTIAL DIAGNOSIS

Acute Angle-Closure Glaucoma
- Shallow anterior chamber on exam
- Angle will be closed on gonioscopy

Chronic Angle-Closure Glaucoma
- Peripheral anterior synechiae on gonioscopy

Primary Open-Angle Glaucoma
- Consistently high IOP with cupped optic disc

Ocular Hypertension
- Consistently high IOP with normal optic disc

Uveitic Glaucoma
- More severe and chronic inflammation in anterior chamber

EVALUATION/WORK-UP

Pathology
- Histopathology of trabecular meshwork biopsies during an attack have shown inflammation consisting of mononuclear cell infiltrate
- Specular microscopy of the keratic precipitates show clustering with pseudopods

TREATMENT

Medical
- Reduce IOP
  - Topical β-blockers (timolol)
  - Topical α-agonists (apraclonidine or brimonidine)
  - Carbonic anhydrase inhibitors (dorzolamide or acetazolamide)
  - Prostaglandin inhibitors
- Anti-inflammatory
  - Steroids (prednisolone acetate)
  - Topical nonsteroidal anti-inflammatory drugs (NSAIDs)
  - Oral NSAIDs
- Evaluated on a case-by-case basis, certain patients can be qualified to self-administer medications when they sense an acute attack
- Due to the intermittent nature of glaucomatocyclitic crisis, medication is not necessary between attacks

Surgical
- Filtering procedures may help regulate IOP but do not prevent recurrent attacks
- Laser trabeculoplasties have not been shown to be efficacious

Follow-Up
- Annual examinations to monitor optic nerve health and potential development of primary open angle glaucoma given association between the 2 diseases

Prognosis
- Traditionally thought of as a benign disease
- Patients that have prolonged, recurrent attacks may suffer permanent optic nerve damage

SELECTED REFERENCES

1. Shazly TA et al: Posner-Schlossman glaucomatocyclitic crisis. Semin Ophthalmol. 26(4-5):282-4, 2011
2. Van Gelder RN: Idiopathic no more: clues to the pathogenesis of Fuchs heterochromic iridocyclitis and glaucomatocyclitic crisis. Am J Ophthalmol. 145(5):769-71, 2008
3. Hirose S et al: HLA-Bw54 and glaucomatocyclitic crisis. Arch Ophthalmol. 103(12):1837-9, 1985
4. Posner A et al: Syndrome of unilateral recurrent attacks of glaucoma with cyclitic symptoms. Arch Ophthal. 39(4):517-35, 1948

PIGMENTARY GLAUCOMA

Key Facts

Introduction

- Form of open-angle glaucoma in which iris pigment epithelium deposits on the corneal endothelium or trabecular meshwork and obstructs aqueous flow, leading to ↑ intraocular pressure

Etiology

- Sloughing of iris pigment epithelium and deposition in the trabecular meshwork
- Male gender; myopia
- Incidence decreases with age

Presentation

- Gradual visual loss, blurred vision
- May present with eye pain after exercise
- Redness
- Iris transillumination shows slit-like transparency/thinning from loss of pigmented epithelium of mid peripheral iris
- Krukenberg spindle is pigment deposition on posterior surface of central inferior cornea

Evaluation/Work-Up

- Melanin pigment deposition in trabecular meshwork and corneal endothelium
    - Decreased aqueous drainage secondary to increased aqueous humor outflow resistance, leading to glaucoma
- Transillumination defects

Treatment

- β-blockers, prostaglandin analogues, cholinergic agents; laser iridotomy is important

Prognosis

- Can lead to visual field loss &/or optic disc cupping
- Iris transillumination and trabecular meshwork pigmentation may normalize with time

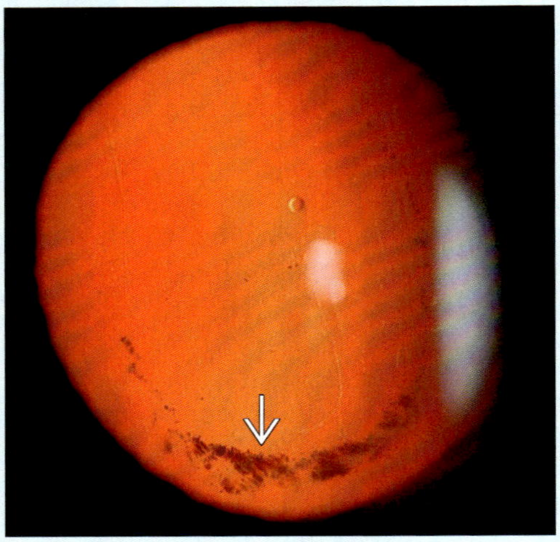
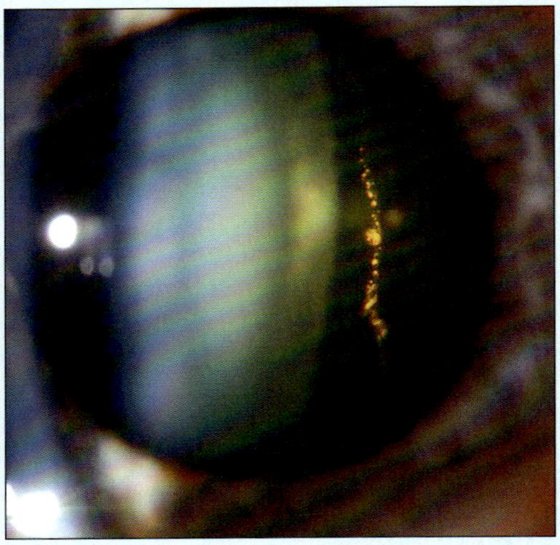

(Left) *This slit-lamp photo shows pigmented iris cells ➔ deposited on the anterior lens capsule, a characteristic finding in pigment dispersion syndrome.* ***(Right)*** *This image shows pigmentation granules deposited on the corneal endothelium. Fine pigment deposited in a spindle configuration in the central cornea is commonly referred to as Krukenberg spindle. The pigment in this image is viewed by reflected light rather than direct illumination.*

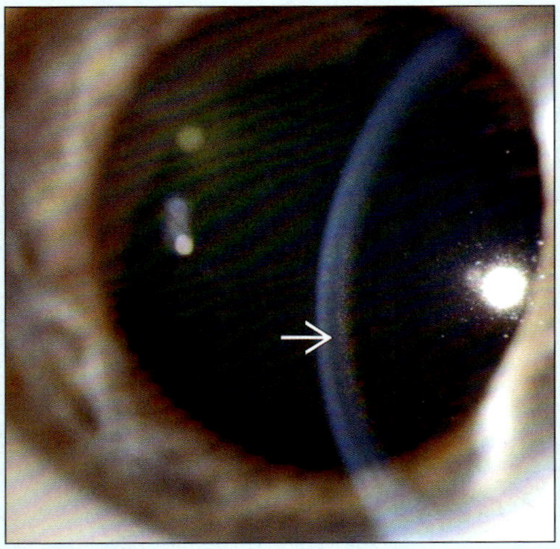
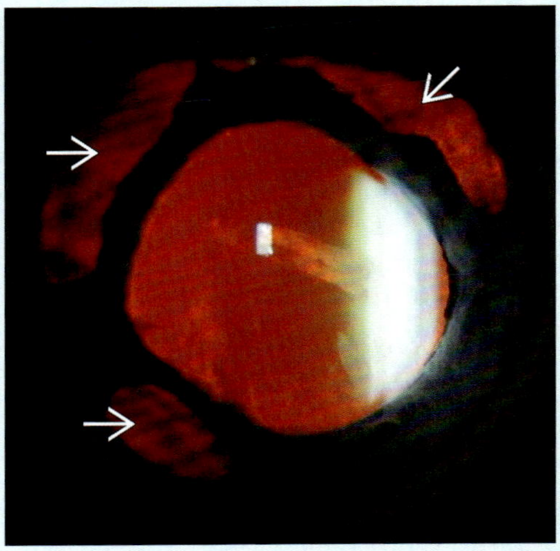

(Left) *This slit-lamp photograph shows pigment deposition ➔ on the endothelial surface of the cornea.* ***(Right)*** *This slit-lamp photograph shows patchy iris transillumination defects (TIDs) viewed by retroillumination ➔. TIDs are a common finding in pigmentary glaucoma. However, the TIDs seen in pigmentary glaucoma typically follow a radial or spoke-like pattern whereas the patchy TIDs seen in this image typically occur after trauma or surgery.*

PIGMENTARY GLAUCOMA

INTRODUCTION

Definitions

- Form of open-angle glaucoma in which iris pigment epithelium deposits on corneal endothelium or trabecular meshwork and obstructs aqueous flow leading to ↑ intraocular pressure

Subtypes

- Pigmentary dispersion syndrome: Increased pigmentation deposition without glaucoma

DEMOGRAPHICS

Etiology/Risk Factors

- Thought to be caused by anterior lens zonules in contact with pigmentary layer of the iris → sloughing of iris pigment epithelium and deposition in the trabecular meshwork
- Myopia
- Male gender
- Commonly diagnosed in 30s or 40s
  - Incidence decreases with age

Epidemiology

- ~ 1.4/100,000, likely higher but undiagnosed

PRESENTATION

Symptoms

- Asymptomatic
- Gradual visual loss, blurred vision
- May present with eye pain & pressure spikes after exercise
- Halos
- Redness
- Photophobia

Exam Findings

- Iris transillumination shows slit-like radial defects
- Krukenberg vertical spindle pigment deposition on posterior surface of cornea
- Visual field changes
- Glaucomatous optic disc atrophy
- Sampaoelesi line (pigment line on trabecular meshwork visible on gonioscopy)

DIFFERENTIAL DIAGNOSIS

Pseudoexfoliation Syndrome

- Typically seen in older patients

Inflammatory Open-Angle Glaucoma

- May or may not have transillumination defects

Iris Melanoma

- Iris mass
- Heavy pigmentation

Acute Anterior Uveitis

- Like pigmentary dispersion, may present with eye pain, redness, photophobia, or loss of vision
- Floating pigment may be mistaken for inflammation

EVALUATION/WORK-UP

Labs

- None

Pathology

- Melanin pigment deposition in trabecular meshwork and corneal endothelium
  - Degeneration of trabecular meshwork
  - Increased sclerotic tissue
  - Decreased aqueous drainage secondary to increased aqueous humor outflow resistance, leading to glaucoma

Imaging

- Slit-lamp examination
  - Look for transillumination defects
- Use of gonioscope
- Ultrasound biomicroscopy

TREATMENT

Medical

- β-blocker
  - If increased IOP persists, prostaglandin analogues or cholinergic agents may be added

Surgical

- If medical treatment fails, laser trabeculoplasty can be effective
- When reverse pupillary block is present, laser iridotomy is indicated

Follow-Up

- 1-6 months, with formal visual field testing every 6-12 months, depending on severity
  - Monitor intraocular pressures

Prognosis

- Can lead to visual field loss &/or optic disc cupping
- Iris transillumination and trabecular meshwork pigmentation may normalize with time

SELECTED REFERENCES

1. Gonzalez-Gonzalez LA et al: Pigment dispersion syndrome masquerading as acute anterior uveitis. Ocul Immunol Inflamm. 19(3):158-66, 2011
2. Mora P et al: Ultrasound biomicroscopy and iris pigment dispersion: a case--control study. Br J Ophthalmol. 94(4):428-32, 2010
3. Siddiqui Y et al: What is the risk of developing pigmentary glaucoma from pigment dispersion syndrome? Am J Ophthalmol. 2003 Jun;135(6):794-9. Erratum in: Am J Ophthalmol. 136(3):592, 2003
4. Campbell DG: Pigmentary dispersion and glaucoma. A new theory. Arch Ophthalmol. 97(9):1667-72, 1979

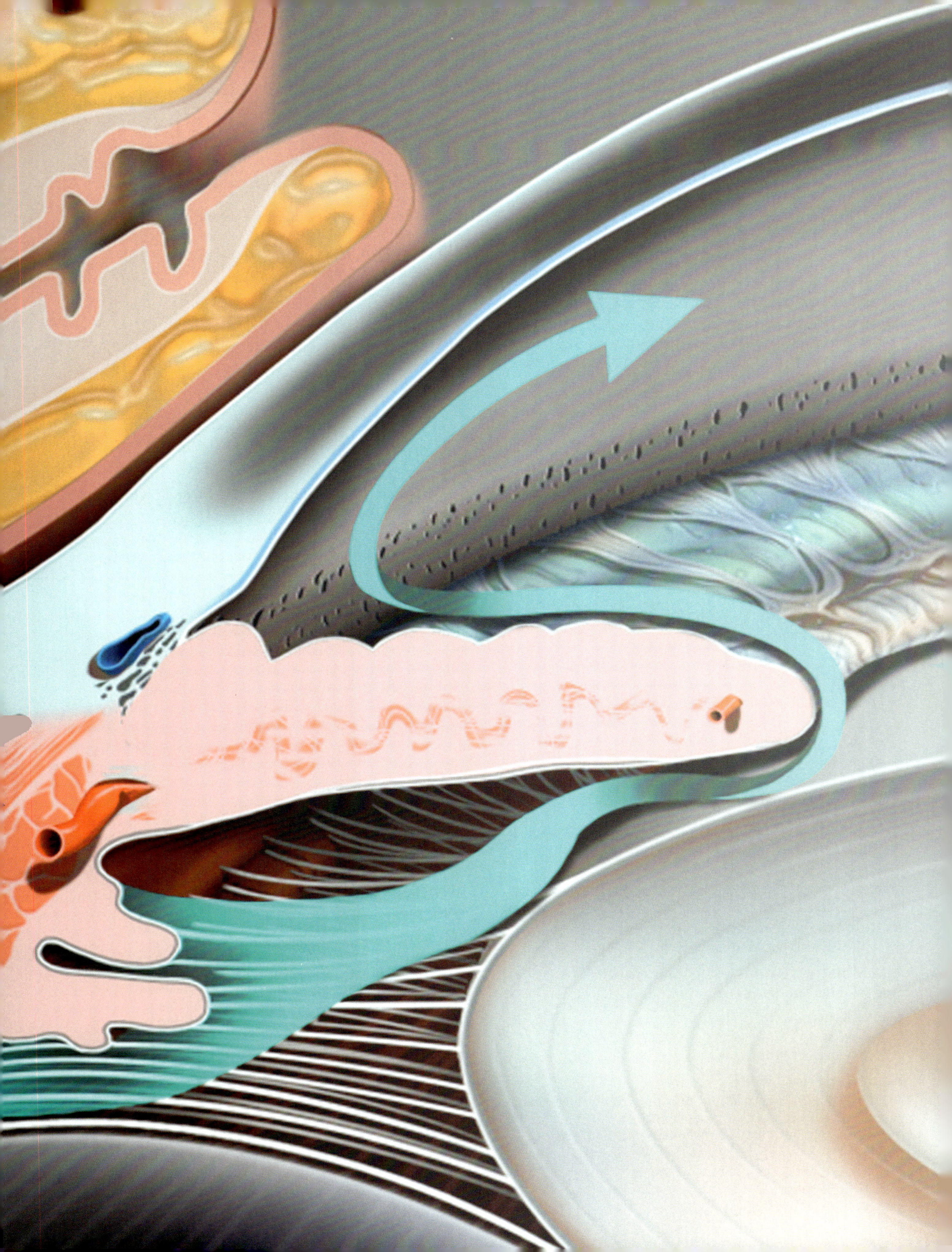

SECTION 2
Closed-Angle Glaucoma

Introduction and Overview

Miscellaneous

CLOSED-ANGLE GLAUCOMA OVERVIEW

TERMINOLOGY

Abbreviations

- Primary angle-closure glaucoma (PACG)
- Intraocular pressure (IOP)
- Cup to disc ratio (CDR)
- Optic nerve head (ONH)
- Central corneal thickness (CCT)
- Peripheral anterior synechiae (PAS)
- Disc damage likelihood scale (DDLS)

Definitions

- Iridocorneal angle: Angle between iris and cornea
- Glaucoma: Diverse set of chronic optic neuropathies with progressive ganglion cell loss and declining visual function, often associated with ↑ IOP
- Closed-angle glaucoma (narrow-angle glaucoma): Glaucoma with closed or narrowed iridocorneal angle
- Gonioscopy: Goniolens used in conjunction with slit lamp or operative microscope to examine iridocorneal angle
- Indentation gonioscopy: Gonioscopy used in conjunction with direct corneal pressure to examine reversibility of iridocorneal angle block
- Applanation tonometry: Slit-lamp-based method to measure IOP based upon force required to flatten (applanate) specified area of cornea
- Anterior synechiae: Condition in which iris adheres anteriorly to cornea
- Posterior synechiae: Condition in which iris adheres posteriorly to lens capsule

PATHOPHYSIOLOGY

Normal Anatomy

- Normal aqueous humor flow: Ciliary body → posterior chamber → pupil → anterior chamber → iridocorneal angle → trabecular meshwork → Schlemm canal → aqueous veins

Primary Angle Closure

- Pupillary block: Apposition of lens and posterior iris → obstruction of aqueous humor outflow from posterior chamber → ↑ posterior chamber pressure → forward displacement of iris → closure of iridocorneal angle
  - Typically occurs in individuals with anatomic predisposition (narrow iridocorneal angle, hyperopia, shallow anterior chamber, abnormal iris anatomy)
  - Often precipitated by pupillary accommodation (e.g., reading, low-light environments)
  - Often precipitated by medications (anticholinergics, adrenergic, topiramate)
- Plateau iris: Aqueous humor flows through the pupil but is blocked at the trabecular meshwork
  - Angle is closed by the iris, but the iris comes off flat (plateau) so that the anterior chamber depth is normal

Secondary Angle Closure

- Posterior pressure → anterior displacement of iris
  - Ciliary or choroidal swelling (uveitis, postoperative inflammation, topiramate, panretinal photocoagulation (PRP), central retinal vein occlusion (CRVO), scleral buckle)
  - Tumor: Melanoma or retinoblastoma
  - Lens block
  - Retrolenticular tissue contraction (retinopathy of prematurity, persistent fetal vasculature)
- Anterior traction → anterior displacement of iris
  - Contracting inflammatory or fibrovascular membranes
  - Corneal endothelial migration

CLINICAL PRESENTATION

Symptoms

- **Acute angle-closure glaucoma is a medical emergency requiring immediate vision-saving intervention**
- Sudden-onset eye pain
- Rapidly progressive visual field loss
- Halos surrounding objects
- Conjunctival injection
- Nausea, vomiting, headache

Exam Findings

- Visual field exam
  - Profound visual field deficit
- Slit-lamp exam
  - Fixed or sluggish, mid-dilated pupil
  - Corneal edema
  - Iris atrophy on retroillumination
  - Cell in anterior chamber
  - Peripheral anterior synechiae
  - Relative afferent pupillary defect
  - Exam contralateral eye for narrow angle
- Tonometry
  - Frequently very high; eye can feel hard
- Gonioscopy
  - Narrow or closed iridocorneal angle
  - Neovascularization of iridocorneal angle is secondary angle closure
  - May have anterior synechiae
  - Indentation gonioscopy may break an acute attack
- Funduscopy
  - **Do not dilate patients with narrow iridocorneal angle to avoid inducing acute angle-closure crisis**
  - Notching of optic disc rim
  - ↑ CDR

EPIDEMIOLOGY

Prevalence

- < 10% of glaucoma in United States

Risk Factors

- Increasing age
- Hyperopia (short axial length)
- Shallow anterior chamber depth (< 2.5 mm)
- Family history
- Increased risk in women relative to men (3-4x) due to shallower anterior chamber depth
- Increased risk in Asians relative to whites (30-40x in Inuits) due to shallower anterior chamber depth

RELATED REFERENCES

1. Morgan WH et al: Surgical management of glaucoma: a review. Clin Experiment Ophthalmol. 40(4):388-99, 2012
2. Ng WS et al: Laser peripheral iridoplasty for angle-closure. Cochrane Database Syst Rev. 2:CD006746, 2012

ANATOMIC FEATURES

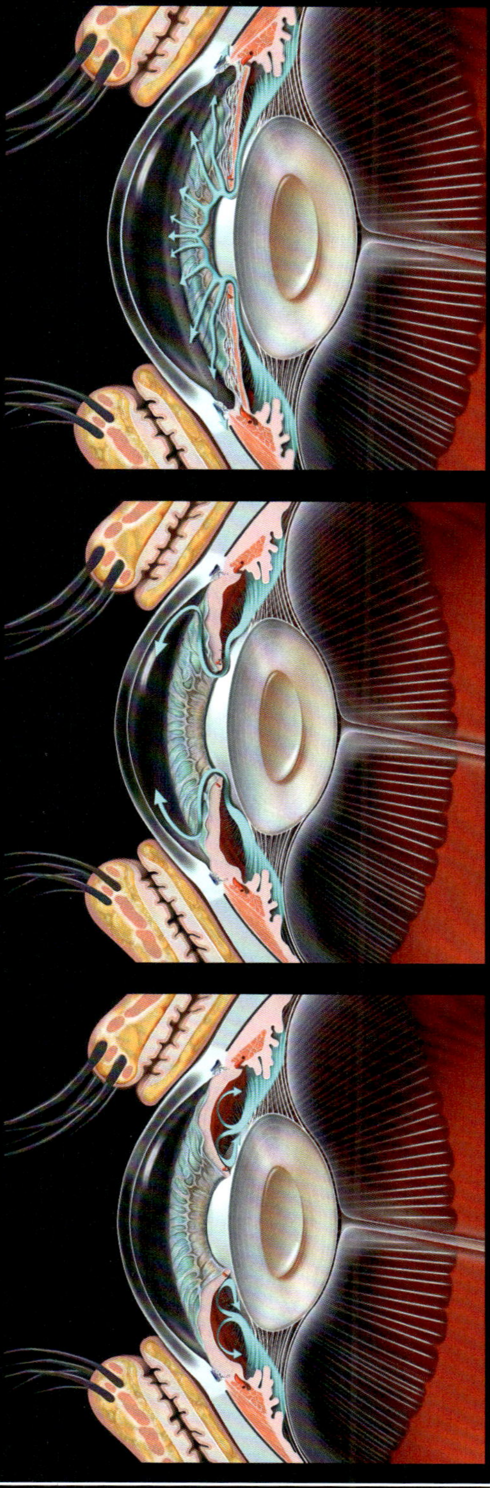

(Top) *This illustration shows a normal iridocorneal angle. The blue arrows show the normal flow of the aqueous, which is produced by the ciliary body, flows through the pupil, and drains into the trabecular meshwork. From the trabecular meshwork, it drains into the Schlemm canal and then to the aqueous veins.* ***(Middle)*** *This illustration shows a closed iridocorneal angle. Forward displacement of the iris blocks the trabecular meshwork, preventing outflow of aqueous humor from the anterior chamber, resulting in increased intraocular pressure.* ***(Bottom)*** *This illustration shows a closed iridocorneal angle with pupillary block. Apposition of the posterior iris to the anterior lens capsule prevents forward movement of aqueous humor from the posterior chamber, resulting in increased pressure in the posterior chamber. This increased pressure leads to forward displacement of the iris and subsequent obstruction of the iridocorneal angle, causing a global increase in intraocular pressure.*

ACUTE ANGLE-CLOSURE GLAUCOMA

Key Facts

Introduction

- **Acute angle-closure glaucoma is a medical emergency requiring immediate vision-saving intervention**
- Primary angle closure
  - Relative pupillary block: Apposition of lens and posterior iris → obstruction of aqueous humor outflow from posterior chamber → ↑ posterior chamber pressure → forward displacement of iris → closure of iridocorneal angle
  - Often acutely precipitated by pupillary accommodation (e.g., reading, low-light environments)
  - Often acutely precipitated by medications (anticholinergics, adrenergics, topiramate)
- Secondary angle closure
  - Posterior pressure → anterior displacement of iris
  - Anterior traction → anterior displacement of iris

Demographics

- Increased risk in women relative to men (3-4x) due to shallower anterior chamber depth
- Increased risk in Inuits (30-40x) and Asians relative to Caucasians due to shallower anterior chamber depth
- Other risk factors
  - Increasing age
  - Hyperopia
  - Family history

Treatment

- **Do not dilate patients with narrow iridocorneal angle to avoid inducing acute angle-closure crisis**
- Primary goal of therapy: ↓ IOP
  - Medical and surgical treatments available
- Indentation gonioscopy may reduce obstruction
- Laser peripheral iridotomy is mainstay; if view is poor, can use topical glycerin to improve view

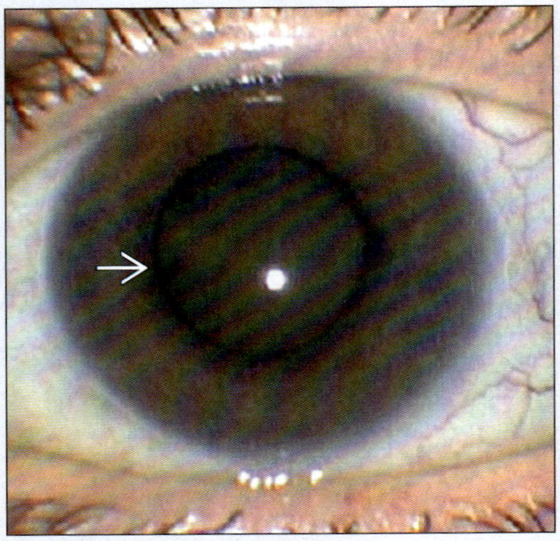

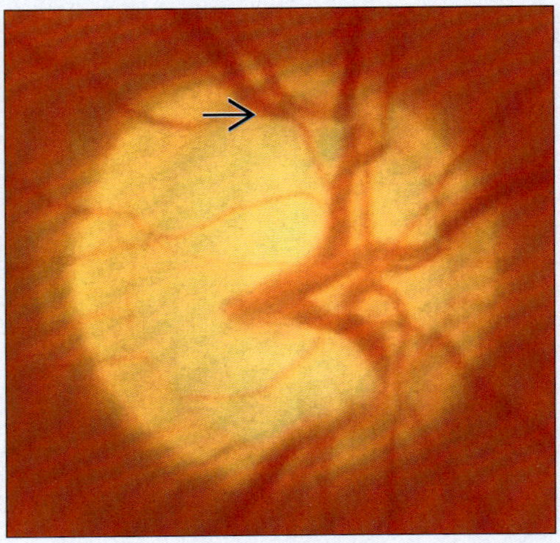

*(**Left**) This external photograph depicts an eye with acute angle-closure glaucoma. Note how the pupil is found in a fixed, mid-dilated position ➔. Patients with acute angle-closure glaucoma often have a narrow angle in the other eye as well, which predisposes them to the development of acute angle closure. (**Right**) This photograph of the optic disc demonstrates severe cupping →. Acute angle-closure glaucoma can lead to optic nerve damage and cupping.*

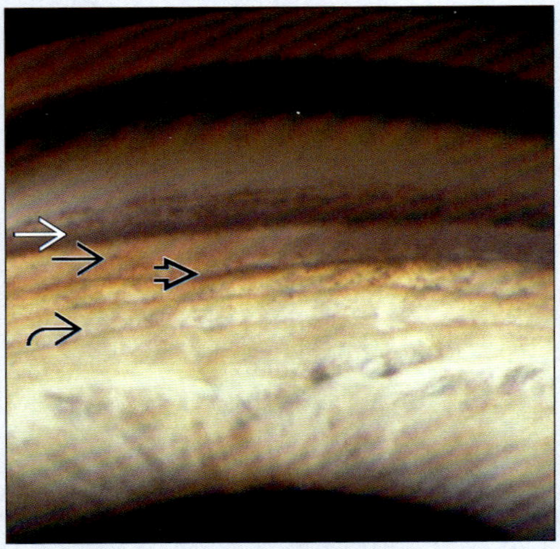

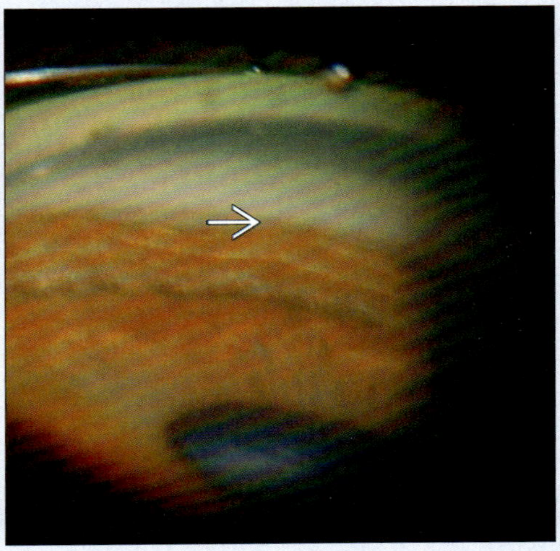

*(**Left**) This gonioscopic image demonstrates a normal angle. Note the iris →, the ciliary body ➔, the scleral spur →, and trabeculum ➔. (**Right**) This gonioscopic image depicts an eye with angle-closure glaucoma ➔. Note that the structures identified on the previous image of a normal angle are not visible.*

ACUTE ANGLE-CLOSURE GLAUCOMA

INTRODUCTION

Definitions
- Closed-angle glaucoma (narrow-angle glaucoma): Glaucoma with a closed or narrowed iridocorneal angle
- Iridocorneal angle: Angle between iris and cornea

Subtypes
- Primary angle closure
  - Relative pupillary block: Apposition of lens and posterior iris → obstruction of aqueous humor outflow from posterior chamber → ↑ posterior chamber pressure → forward displacement of iris → closure of iridocorneal angle
    - Often acutely precipitated by pupillary accommodation (e.g., reading, low-light environment)
    - Often acutely precipitated by medications (anticholinergics, adrenergics, topiramate)
- Secondary angle closure
  - Posterior pressure → anterior displacement of iris
    - Ciliary or choroidal swelling
    - Traumatic retrobulbar hemorrhage
  - Anterior traction → anterior displacement of iris
    - Inflammatory or fibrovascular membranes
    - Corneal endothelial migration

DEMOGRAPHICS

Etiology/Risk Factors
- Increasing age, hyperopia (short axial length), family history, race, anterior chamber depth < 2.5 mm

Epidemiology
- Increased risk in women relative to men (3-4x) and in Inuits (30-40x) and Asians relative to Caucasians due to shallower anterior chamber depth

PRESENTATION

Symptoms
- Sudden-onset eye pain with conjunctival injection
- Rapidly progressing vision loss with halos
- Nausea, vomiting, headache

Precipitating Events
- Accommodation (reading, low-light environments)
- Medications
- Trauma
- Inflammation (uveitis, recent surgery)

Exam Findings
- Slit-lamp exam
  - Corneal edema
  - Fixed or sluggish, mid-dilated pupil
  - Iris atrophy, pigment in anterior chamber
- Tonometry
  - IOP frequently very high (> 21 mm Hg)
  - Measure central corneal thickness
- Gonioscopy
  - Narrow or closed iridocorneal angle
- Funduscopy
  - Optic nerve head (ONH) hyperemic, edematous
- Narrow angle in fellow eye

DIFFERENTIAL DIAGNOSIS

Acute Increase in Posterior Pressure
- Pupillary block
- Retrobulbar hemorrhage

Acute Increase in Anterior Traction
- History of chronic angle-closure glaucoma
- History of peripheral anterior synechiae

EVALUATION/WORK-UP

Imaging
- Urgent treatment should take precedent over extensive studies, which may be performed later, after normalization of IOP
- Slit-lamp exam, tonometry, gonioscopy, funduscopy
- B-scan ultrasound or anterior segment OCT to evaluate iris configuration
- Visual field exam

TREATMENT

Medical
- β-blockers (timolol, levobunolol, betaxolol), ↓ aqueous humor production
- α-agonists (brimonidine, apraclonidine), ↓ aqueous humor production, ↑ uveoscleral outflow
- Parasympathomimetics (pilocarpine), pupillary dilation → opening trabecular meshwork
- Carbonic anhydrase inhibitors (topical dorzolamide, brinzolamide; oral acetazolamide), ↓ aqueous humor production
- Prostaglandin analogs (latanoprost, bimatoprost, travoprost), ↑ uveoscleral outflow of aqueous humor
- Supportive therapy (pain relief, antiemetics)
- Oral glycerin and IV mannitol are vitreous desiccants that can be used if nothing else is working

Surgical
- Laser peripheral iridotomy: Creation of an opening in iris without removal of iris tissue (done typically superiorly)
  - If view is poor, use topical glycerin to dehydrate the cornea (after topical anesthesia)
  - Consider prophylactic peripheral iridotomy in fellow eye
- Filtering procedures (e.g., trabeculectomy, tube shunts), cataract surgery, ciliary body ablation, goniosynechiolysis
- Iridectomy: Creation of an opening in iris through removal of iris tissue
- Laser iridoplasty/gonioplasty
- Canaloplasty: Catheter augmentation of outflow tract

SELECTED REFERENCES

1. Friedman DS et al: Angle closure and angle-closure glaucoma: what we are doing now and what we will be doing in the future. Clin Experiment Ophthalmol. 40(4):381-7, 2012
2. Morgan WH et al: Surgical management of glaucoma: a review. Clin Experiment Ophthalmol. 40(4):388-99, 2012

CHRONIC ANGLE-CLOSURE GLAUCOMA

Key Facts

Introduction

- Form of angle-closure glaucoma with presence of permanent PAS
  - May develop after a single episode of acute angle closure with persistent synechial closure, or more commonly as a gradual "creeping angle closure" in which PAS slowly advances circumferentially
- Posterior pressure → anterior displacement of iris
  - Ciliary or choroidal swelling (uveitis, postoperative inflammation)
  - Tumor, relative pupillary block, phacomorphic
- Anterior traction → anterior displacement of iris
  - Contracting inflammatory or fibrovascular membranes
  - Can occur following primary angle closure (permanent synechiae)
  - Corneal endothelial migration (ICE, PPCD)

Demographics

- Increased risk in women relative to men (3-4x) due to shallower anterior chamber depth (ACD)
- Increased prevalence in Chinese (1.26%) relative to Caucasians (0.25%)
- Lowest risk in blacks
- Other risk factors
  - Increasing age, hyperopia, family history, shallow ACD (< 2.5 mm)

Presentation

- Angle closes slowly, frequently asymptomatic
- Chronic eye pain
- Slowly progressive visual field deficits

Treatment

- Primary goal of therapy: ↓ intraocular pressure
  - Medical and surgical treatments available

(Left) This illustration depicts what occurs in chronic angle-closure glaucoma. The aqueous is produced in the ciliary body, flows toward the anterior chamber, but is unable to drain through the trabecular meshwork because of narrowing of the angle ➡. (Right) This gonioscopy image shows a closed angle with the iris approximating the cornea ➡.

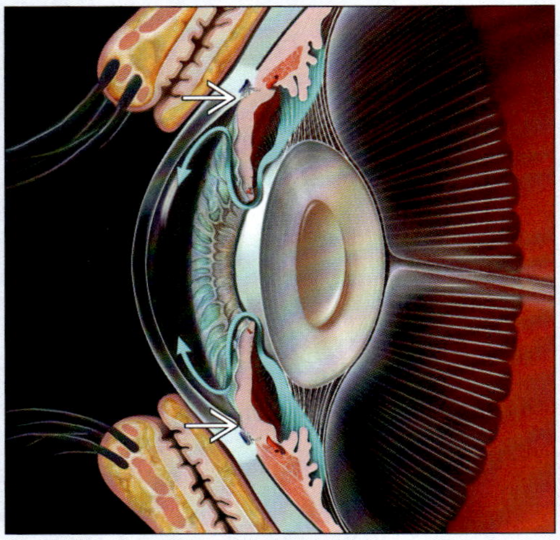

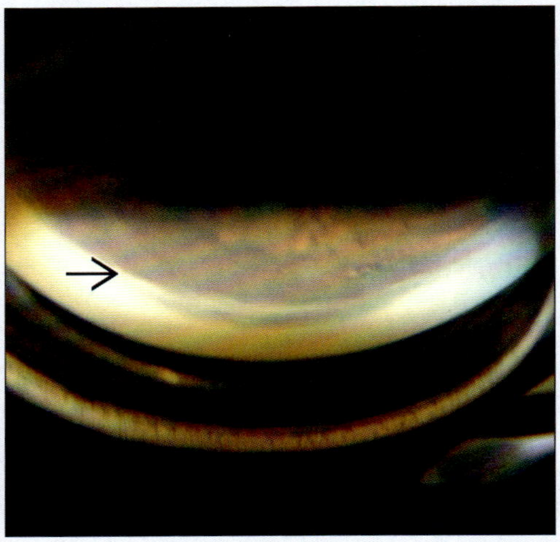

(Left) This gonioscopy image shows peripheral anterior synechiae (PAS) ➡. PAS is common with chronic angle-closure glaucoma. (Right) This fundus photograph shows cupping of the optic disc ➡. Chronic angle closure can lead to extended periods of elevated intraocular pressure and damage of the optic nerve and cupping.

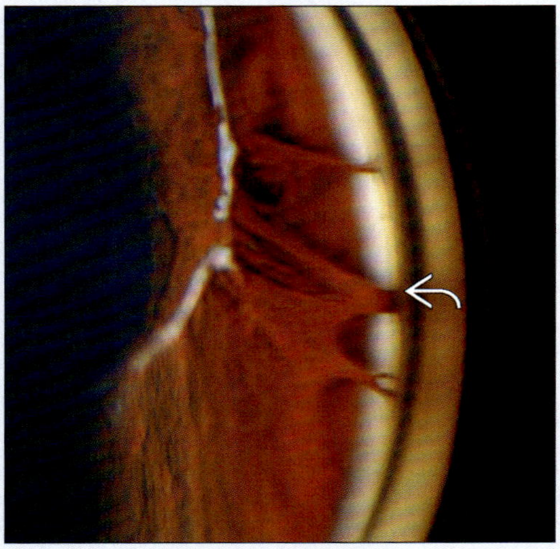

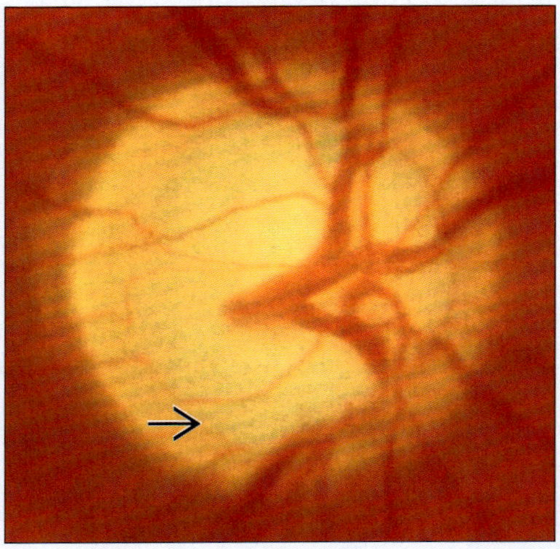

CHRONIC ANGLE-CLOSURE GLAUCOMA

INTRODUCTION

Abbreviations
- Chronic angle-closure glaucoma (CACG)

Definitions
- Form of angle-closure glaucoma with presence of permanent peripheral anterior synechiae (PAS)
  - May develop after a single episode of acute angle closure with persistent synechial closure, or more commonly as a gradual "creeping angle closure" in which PAS slowly advances circumferentially
  - May prove difficult to determine what caused PAS to form

Subtypes
- Posterior pressure → anterior displacement of iris
  - Relative pupillary block
  - Ciliary or choroidal swelling (uveitis, postoperative inflammation, tumor, medications [e.g., Topamax])
  - Phacomorphic glaucoma
- Anterior traction → anterior displacement of iris
  - Contracting inflammatory or fibrovascular membranes
  - Can occur following primary angle closure (permanent synechiae)
  - Corneal endothelial migration as in iridocorneal endothelial syndrome (ICE) and posterior polymorphous corneal dystrophy (PPCD)

DEMOGRAPHICS

Etiology/Risk Factors
- Increasing age
- Hyperopia
- Family history and race
- Shallow ACD (< 2.5 mm)

Epidemiology
- Increased risk in women relative to men (3-4x) due to shallow anterior chamber depth (ACD)
- Increased prevalence in Chinese (1.26%) relative to Caucasians (0.25%)
- Lowest risk in blacks

PRESENTATION

Symptoms
- Angle closes slowly, frequently asymptomatic
- Slowly progressive vision loss with halos; may resemble open-angle glaucoma
- Can be associated with acute angle-closure attacks

Exam Findings
- Slit-lamp exam: Iris atrophy, glaukomflecken (lens opacities associated with epithelial infarct from prior angle closure episodes)
- Tonometry: IOP usually elevated (> 21 mm Hg)
- Measure central corneal thickness (CCT) for more accurate IOP interpretation
- Gonioscopy
  - Narrow or closed iridocorneal angle, PAS present
- Funduscopy
  - ↑ cup-to-disc ratio (CDR), notching of optic nerve head (ONH)

DIFFERENTIAL DIAGNOSIS

Primary Open-Angle Glaucoma (POAG)
- No angle narrowing or PAS on gonioscopy

Acute Angle-Closure Glaucoma (AACG)
- Mid-dilated fixed pupil
- Acute pain and ciliary flush
- Patients with CACG may have intermittent attacks of AACG

EVALUATION/WORK-UP

Imaging
- Visual field exam
- Slit-lamp exam
  - Funduscopy, gonioscopy, tonometry
- Ultrasound biomicroscopy (UBM) or anterior segment OCT to evaluate angle/iris configuration

TREATMENT

Medical
- Primary goal of therapy: ↓ IOP
- β-blockers (timolol, levobunolol, betaxolol), ↓ aqueous humor production
- α-agonists (brimonidine, apraclonidine), ↓ aqueous humor production, ↑ uveoscleral outflow
- Parasympathomimetics (pilocarpine), pupillary constriction → opening the trabecular meshwork (TM)
- Carbonic anhydrase inhibitors (dorzolamide, brinzolamide, acetazolamide), ↓ aqueous humor production
- Prostaglandin analogs (latanoprost, bimatoprost, travoprost), ↑ uveoscleral and TM outflow

Surgical
- Treat underlying cause of secondary angle closure
- Peripheral iridotomy: Creation of peripheral iris opening with a laser; consider fellow eye
- Iridectomy: Creation of opening in the iris through surgical removal of iris tissue
- Laser iridoplasty/gonioplasty
- Filtering procedures (e.g., trabeculectomy, tube shunts)
- Canaloplasty: Microcatheterization of outflow tract
- Cataract surgery for phacomorphic involvement
- Ciliary body ablation
- Goniosynechiolysis

SELECTED REFERENCES

1. Friedman DS et al: Angle closure and angle-closure glaucoma: what we are doing now and what we will be doing in the future. Clin Experiment Ophthalmol. 40(4):381-7, 2012
2. Morgan WH et al: Surgical management of glaucoma: a review. Clin Experiment Ophthalmol. 40(4):388-99, 2012
3. Salmon JF: Predisposing factors for chronic angle-closure glaucoma. Prog Retin Eye Res. 18(1):121-32, 1999

IRIDOCORNEAL ENDOTHELIAL SYNDROME

Key Facts

Introduction
- Syndrome characterized by irregular corneal endothelium resulting in glaucoma, corneal edema, and iris destruction
- 3 clinical variations: Chandler syndrome, progressive iris atrophy, and Cogan-Reese syndrome

Demographics
- Generally unilateral; more common in women with onset between ages 20 and 50

Presentation
- Corectopia; corneal edema (decreased vision is more noticeable in the morning), iris atrophy, and secondary angle-closure glaucoma
- Gonioscopy shows peripheral anterior synechiae extending above Schwalbe line
- Chandler syndrome: Greater degree of corneal edema with minimal changes to the iris
- Progressive iris atrophy: Corectopia with marked atrophy of the iris characterized by numerous stretch holes or melting holes (polycoria)
- Cogan-Reese syndrome: Iris atrophy associated with multiple, pigmented, pedunculated iris nodules

Evaluation/Work-Up
- Specular microscopy to evaluate the corneal endothelium for asymmetric endothelial cell loss or morphology
- Gonioscopy to evaluate peripheral anterior synechiae and glaucoma progression

Treatment
- Topical eyedrops to reduce intraocular pressure
- Trabeculectomy with antifibrotic agents, mitomycin C, or 5-fluorouracil to decrease IOP
- Descemet-stripping endothelial keratoplasty (DSEK) generally effective to replace endothelium

*(**Left**) This external photograph demonstrates pupillary irregularity ➔. Pupil irregularity is a common early finding in iridocorneal endothelial syndrome. It is important to evaluate intraocular pressure in these patients. (**Right**) In this slit-lamp photograph, corectopia (malposition of the pupil) is present ➔. Corectopia is a common finding in patients with iridocorneal endothelial (ICE) syndrome. A patient with ICE syndrome can also develop pseudopolycoria (false pupils on an iris with no previous deformity).*

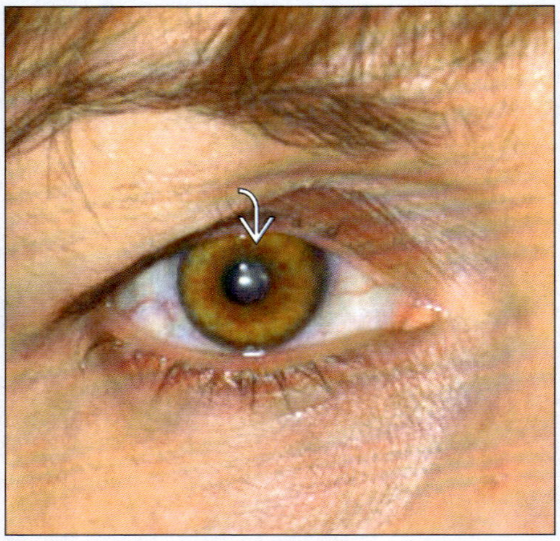

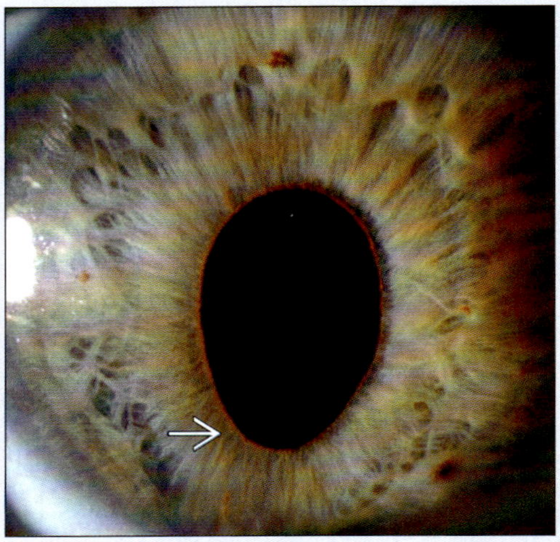

*(**Left**) This slit-lamp photograph demonstrates iris atrophy ➔. Progressive iris atrophy is a typical finding in iridocorneal endothelial syndrome. (**Right**) This slit-lamp photograph demonstrates a pigmented lesion on the iris ➔. These lesions are found in iridocorneal endothelial syndrome. Cogan-Reese syndrome is a subset of iridocorneal endothelial syndrome.*

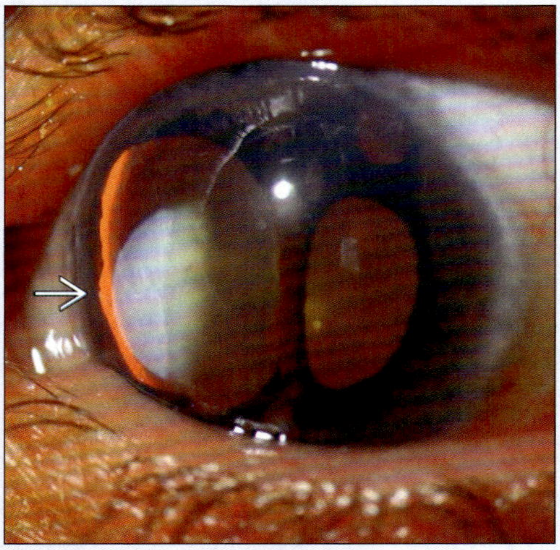

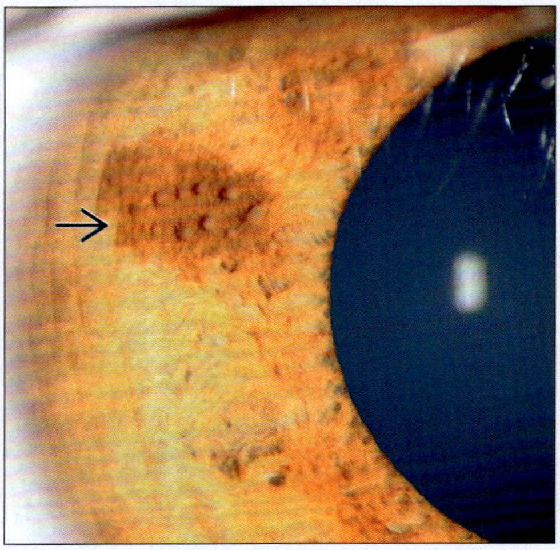

IRIDOCORNEAL ENDOTHELIAL SYNDROME

INTRODUCTION

Abbreviations
- Iridocorneal endothelial (ICE) syndrome

Definitions
- Syndrome characterized by irregular corneal endothelium resulting in glaucoma, corneal edema, and iris destruction

Subtypes
- 3 clinical subtypes
  - Chandler syndrome (most common subtype)
  - Progressive iris atrophy
  - Cogan-Reese syndrome (a.k.a. iris-nevus syndrome)

DEMOGRAPHICS

Etiology/Risk Factors
- Unknown etiology though recent studies suggest viral infection (i.e., EBV or HSV) may play an inciting role
- Endothelium displays epithelial-like characteristics
  - Proliferates and migrates to trabecular meshwork and iris, resulting in characteristic findings

Epidemiology
- Unilateral disease is more commonly seen in women, with onset between ages 20 and 50

PRESENTATION

Symptoms
- Acquired change in shape or position of the pupil (corectopia)
  - Decreased vision is more noticeable in the morning and improves throughout the day
- Monocular pain due to increased intraocular pressure and corneal edema

Exam Findings
- Corneal edema, iris atrophy, and secondary angle-closure glaucoma
- Fine, hammered-silver appearance of posterior cornea indicating corneal endothelial irregularity
- Gonioscopic exam shows peripheral anterior synechiae extending above Schwalbe line, which is classic for ICE syndrome
- Chandler syndrome: Greater degree of corneal edema with minimal changes to the iris
- Progressive iris atrophy: Corectopia with marked atrophy of the iris characterized by numerous stretch holes or melting holes (polycoria)
- Cogan-Reese syndrome: Iris atrophy associated with multiple, pigmented, pedunculated iris nodules

DIFFERENTIAL DIAGNOSIS

Posterior Polymorphous Dystrophy
- Bilateral, inherited disorder with autosomal dominant inheritance pattern
- Endothelial cell dystrophy with vesicles and bands on specular microscopy

Aniridia
- Bilateral, congenital disease characterized by absence of the iris, cataracts, glaucoma, and corneal pannus
- Bilaterality and lack of corneal endothelial changes distinguishes aniridia from ICE syndrome

Axenfeld-Rieger Syndrome
- Commonly a bilateral, congenital presentation with autosomal dominant and sporadic inheritance
- Younger age at presentation, bilaterality, and a lack of corneal endothelial findings distinguish from ICE syndrome

EVALUATION/WORK-UP

Imaging
- Specular microscopy or confocal corneal microscopy to evaluate the corneal endothelium for asymmetric endothelial cell loss or morphology
- Gonioscopy to evaluate peripheral anterior synechiae and glaucoma progression

TREATMENT

Medical
- Medical management aims to reduce intraocular pressure and prevent secondary angle-closure glaucoma
- Topical β-blockers, α-agonists, and carbonic anhydrase inhibitors help reduce aqueous secretions
- Topical hypertonic saline solutions and gels help reduce corneal edema
- Miotics are generally ineffective since the trabecular meshwork is obstructed

Surgical
- Trabeculectomy with antifibrotic agents, mitomycin C, or 5-fluorouracil to decrease intraocular pressure (IOP)
- Aqueous shunts can also be used to decrease IOP when medical management fails
- Ciliary body destruction with diode laser cyclophotocoagulation (diode CPC) may be successful in cases of refractory glaucoma
- Large-diameter endothelial keratoplasty (Descemet-stripping endothelial keratoplasty) can be tried to replace abnormal corneal endothelium; penetrating keratoplasty (PK) rarely needed

Prognosis
- Most patients present with subtle disease and respond well with adequate control of intraocular pressure
- If surgical intervention is required, prognosis is poor

SELECTED REFERENCES

1. Levy SG et al: The histopathology of the iridocorneal-endothelial syndrome. Cornea. 15(1):46-54, 1996
2. Laganowski HC et al: Glaucoma and the iridocorneal endothelial syndrome. Arch Ophthalmol. 110(3):346-50, 1992
3. Campbell DG et al: The corneal endothelium and the spectrum of essential iris atrophy. Am J Ophthalmol. 86(3):317-24, 1978

PLATEAU IRIS

Key Facts

Introduction
- Condition in which ciliary body is enlarged or anteriorly displaced, causing iris root to appose and narrow trabecular meshwork
- Crowding of trabecular meshwork can lead to blockage of aqueous outflow and acute or chronic angle-closure glaucoma

Demographics
- Can occur spontaneously and in situations that cause the pupil to dilate
- Typically occurs in individuals < 50 years old and is more common in females

Presentation
- Headache, ocular pain, nausea, vomiting, and blurred vision
- Normal anterior chamber depth with a flat or minimally forward-bowing iris
- Gonioscopy will show an extremely narrow or closed angle and the double-hump sign

Evaluation/Work-Up
- Ultrasound biomicroscopy can show the configuration of the iris root and angle

Treatment
- Primary treatment is surgical, but miotics may be used in cases when surgical treatment fails
- Peripheral iridotomy is typically first-line of treatment with peripheral iridoplasty in refractive or recurrent cases
- Regular serial gonioscopy and glaucoma screenings should be performed due to potential for repeat closure of the angle following surgical procedures
- Outlook is good when plateau iris is diagnosed early and prior to vision loss

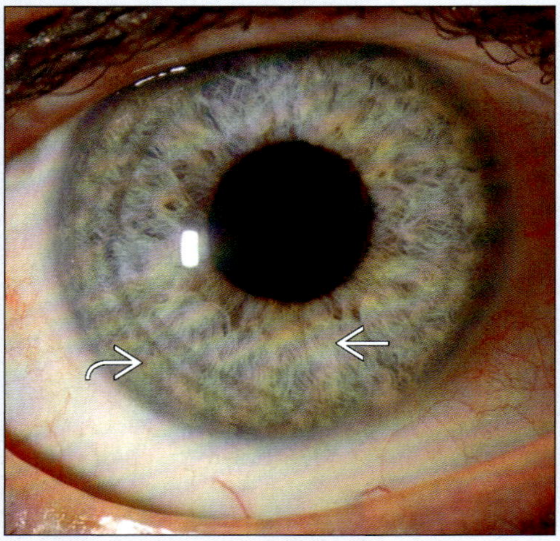

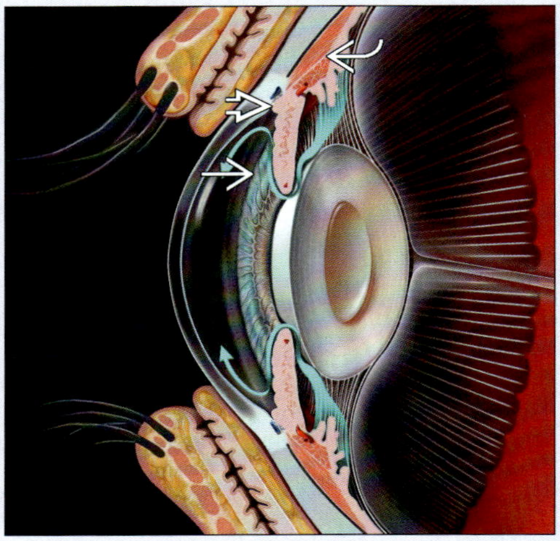

(Left) *This is an external photograph of a patient with plateau iris. The peripheral iris approximates the cornea* ➔ *while the central iris forms a plateau (levels off)* ➔. ***(Right)*** *This graphic illustration depicts an eye with plateau iris. The hallmark finding of plateau iris is a closed angle* ➔ *with a deep anterior chamber* ➔ *because the iris comes off flat in a plateau configuration. The ciliary body* ➔ *is typically enlarged and the iris is positioned more anteriorly.*

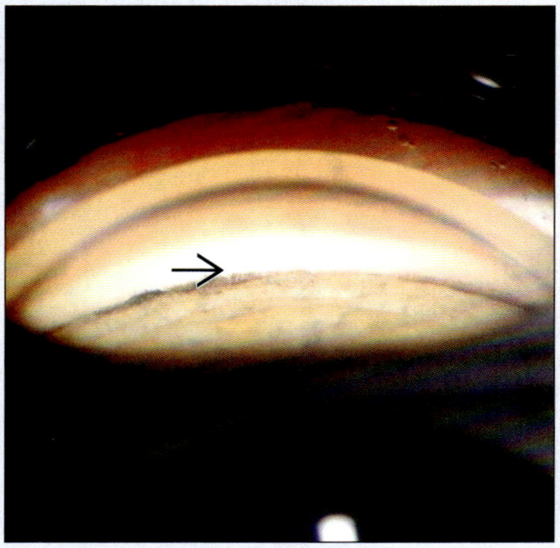

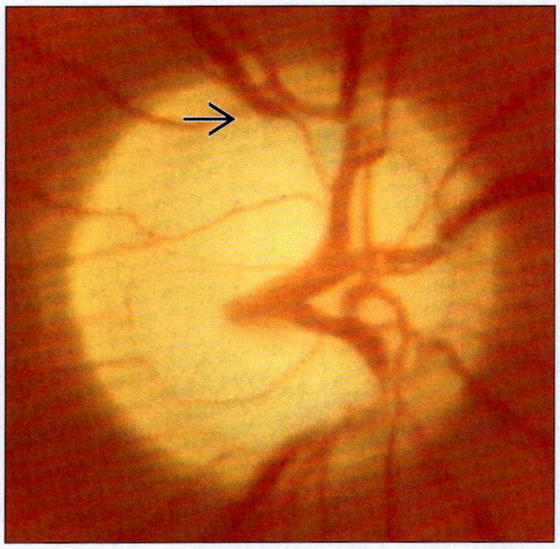

(Left) *This gonioscopic image shows narrowing of the angle. Note how the iris approaches the cornea* ➔. ***(Right)*** *This photograph of the optic disc shows cupping from a glaucomatous nerve head* ➔. *Plateau iris can lead to acute and chronic angle-closure glaucoma.*

PLATEAU IRIS

INTRODUCTION

Definitions

- Condition in which ciliary body is enlarged or anteriorly displaced, causing iris root to appose and narrow trabecular meshwork
- Crowding of the trabecular meshwork can lead to blockage of aqueous outflow and acute or chronic angle-closure glaucoma

Subtypes

- Plateau iris configuration: Preoperative condition with gonioscopically confirmed closed angles but a flat iris and deep anterior chamber
- Plateau iris syndrome: Postoperative persistent occludable angle after a peripheral iridotomy has been performed
- Complete: Involves entire trabecular meshwork causing intraocular pressure to rise
- Incomplete: Involves only posterior trabecular meshwork without rise in intraocular pressure
  - May develop peripheral anterior synechiae, increasing risk for increase in intraocular pressure in following years

DEMOGRAPHICS

Etiology/Risk Factors

- Can occur spontaneously
- In dark environments or with the use of mydriatics, dilation of the pupil can cause the iris to bunch at the periphery and further narrow or close the angle
- May be genetically inherited in an autosomal dominant pattern with incomplete penetrance
- Component of pupillary block is commonly present

Epidemiology

- Typically occurs in individuals < 50 years old
- More commonly seen in females

PRESENTATION

Symptoms

- Headache and ocular pain
- Nausea and vomiting
- Blurred vision

Exam Findings

- Normal anterior chamber depth with a flat or minimally forward-bowing iris
- Gonioscopy will show an extremely narrow or closed angle
  - Double-hump sign: Peripheral hump from ciliary process, central hump from lens

DIFFERENTIAL DIAGNOSIS

Pupillary Block

- Will present with iris bombé
- Treat pupillary block component of plateau iris with peripheral iridectomy

Iridociliary Cysts (Pseudoplateau Iris)

- Common and often clinically insignificant
- Can be identified with the use of ultrasound biomicroscopy

Peripheral Anterior Synechiae

- Caused by physical apposition of the iris to the trabecular meshwork (including plateau iris configuration)
- Also caused by inflammation and cellular proliferative disorder
- Synechiae can be visualized during gonioscopic exam

EVALUATION/WORK-UP

Imaging

- Ultrasound biomicroscopy can be used to visualize anterior chamber angle and iris root
- Anterior segment optical coherence tomography can also show the configuration of the iris root and angle

TREATMENT

Medical

- Primary treatment is surgical, but miotics may be used in cases when surgical treatment fails
  - Pilocarpine can thin the iris and assist in opening the angle

Surgical

- Peripheral iridotomy to treat any component of pupillary block
- Argon laser peripheral iridoplasty is the preferred treatment and can be effective for years
- If refractive to the above therapies, trabeculectomy or tube shunt procedures may be necessary

Follow-Up

- Serial gonioscopy is imperative due to potential for repeat closure of the angle following surgical procedures
- Routine, periodic screening for glaucoma is also recommended given the potential for recurrence and permanent vision loss

Prognosis

- Outlook is good when plateau iris is diagnosed early and prior to vision loss

SELECTED REFERENCES

1. Kumar RS et al: Prevalence of plateau iris in primary angle closure suspects an ultrasound biomicroscopy study. Ophthalmology. 115(3):430-4, 2008
2. Ritch R et al: Long-term success of argon laser peripheral iridoplasty in the management of plateau iris syndrome. Ophthalmology. 111(1):104-8, 2004
3. Ritch R et al: Angle closure in younger patients. Ophthalmology. 110(10):1880-9, 2003
4. Pavlin CJ et al: Plateau iris syndrome: changes in angle opening associated with dark, light, and pilocarpine administration. Am J Ophthalmol. 128(3):288-91, 1999
5. Pavlin CJ et al: Ultrasound biomicroscopy in plateau iris syndrome. Am J Ophthalmol. 113(4):390-5, 1992
6. Wand M et al: Plateau iris syndrome. Trans Sect Ophthalmol Am Acad Ophthalmol Otolaryngol. 83(1):122-30, 1977

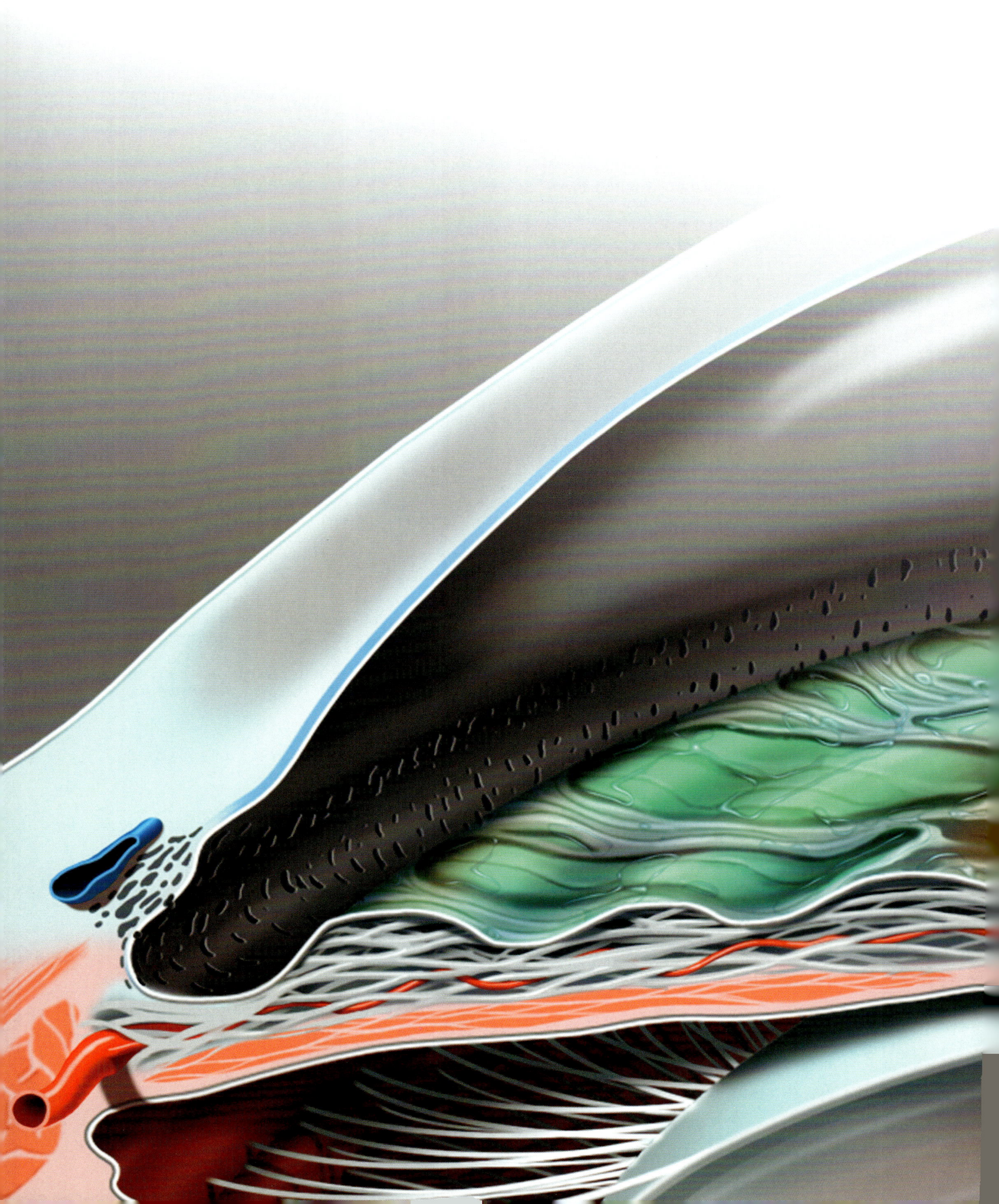

SECTION 1
Iris

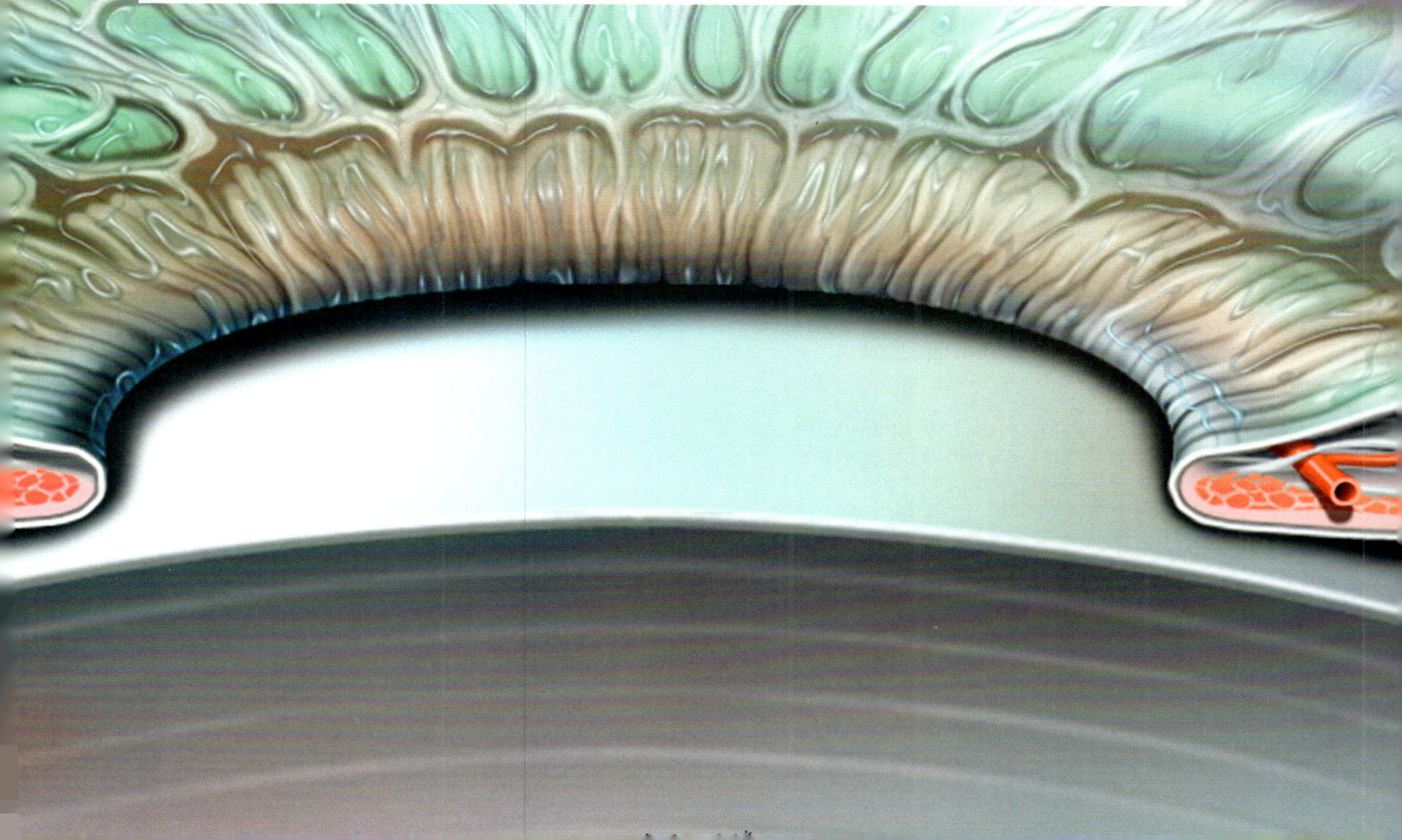

IRIS OVERVIEW

TERMINOLOGY

Definitions

- Diaphragm that controls pupil size and thus the amount of light entering the eye
  - Can be divided into pupillary, mid, and root zones
- Divides anterior and posterior chambers
- Considered part of uveal tract, which consists of iris, ciliary body, and choroid
- Persistent pupillary membrane: Strands of mesodermal tissue cross the pupil
  - Occurs when tissue and lenticular fetal vasculature do not completely reabsorb during development
- Mutations in *PAX6* on band p13 of chromosome 11 can cause aniridia
  - Majority of cases are familial (66%) but can have sporadic cases
  - Autosomal dominant inheritance
  - Mutation in both *PAX6* and *WT1* lead to WAGR syndrome (Wilms tumor, aniridia, genitourinary abnormalities, and mental retardation)
  - Aniridia also associated with aniridia-associated keratopathy due to lack of limbal stem cells, glaucoma due to drainage angle abnormalities, cataracts, and optic nerve hypoplasia

GROSS ANATOMY

Histology

- Stroma
  - Anterior surface with many folds, ridges, and crypts
  - Collarette is thickest portion of iris
  - Blood vessels
    - Anterior and long posterior ciliary arteries provide blood supply
    - Tight endothelial junctions
    - Thick vascular walls
    - Course radially toward pupil
    - Minor vascular circle: Venous and arterial anastomoses that occur near collarette
    - Major circle is located in ciliary body
  - Melanocytes
    - Determine iris color
    - Melanocytes in darker-colored eyes contain more pigment granules than those with lighter-colored eyes
    - Atypical melanocytes can give rise to iris nevus or melanoma
    - Most iris melanomas arise from iris nevi
    - Nevi should be monitored for growth, as it can be difficult to distinguish between iris spindle cell nevus and iris melanoma
    - Iris melanoma is less likely to metastasize than choroidal melanoma and has a better prognosis
  - Collagen, fibroblasts, mucopolysaccharides make up loose extracellular matrix
  - Lymphocytes
- Muscles
  - Made of smooth muscle, derived from neuroectoderm
  - Sphincter muscle
    - Found in pupillary zone
    - Circular smooth muscle
    - Primarily innervated by short ciliary nerve, which is parasympathetic; fibers originate from nucleus of CN3
    - Also has sympathetic innervation for sphincter relaxation
  - Dilator muscle
    - Innervated by both sympathetic and parasympathetic systems
    - Innervated by long ciliary nerve, which is sympathetic and causes contraction
    - Also has parasympathetic innervation for inhibition
    - Those with sympathetic lesions can develop Horner syndrome with dilation lag
    - Horner syndrome is characterized by ptosis, anhydrosis (lack of perspiration), and miosis (pupil constriction)
    - Runs along base of iris toward ciliary zone
- Epithelium
  - 2 pigmented epithelium layers posteriorly
    - Helps prevent extraneous light from entering
    - Pigment granules from pigmented epithelium can deposit onto other tissues in a process known as pigment dispersion syndrome; can lead to development of pigmentary glaucoma if aqueous flow is obstructed, causing increase in intraocular pressure
    - Zonules of lens or haptics from a posterior chamber intraocular lens implant rub posterior iris surface, leading to sloughing of pigmented epithelium
    - Can deposit onto corneal endothelium, trabecular meshwork, or anterior iris surface
  - Cells are apex to apex
    - Fluid can infiltrate virtual space between cells, causing iris cysts

IMAGING ANATOMY

Overview

- Typically imaged using slit lamp
- Newer instruments, such as anterior segment optical coherence tomography, have been gaining popularity
- Ultrasound biomicroscopy gives excellent resolution of iris, angle, ciliary body, and anterior lens

RELATED REFERENCES

1. Davis-Silberman N et al: Iris development in vertebrates; genetic and molecular considerations. Brain Res. 1192:17-28, 2008
2. Lee H et al: Aniridia: current pathology and management. Acta Ophthalmol. 86(7):708-15, 2008
3. Shields CL et al: Iris melanoma: risk factors for metastasis in 169 consecutive patients. Ophthalmology. 108(1):172-8, 2001

IRIS ANATOMY

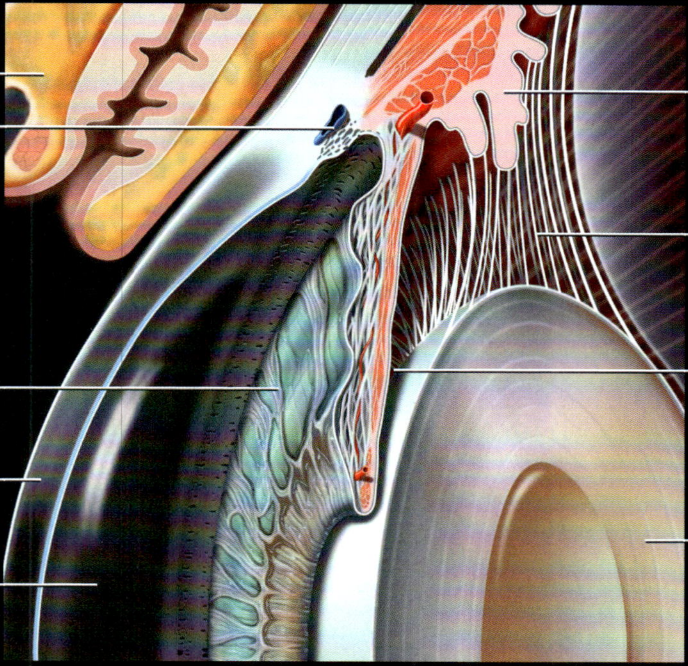

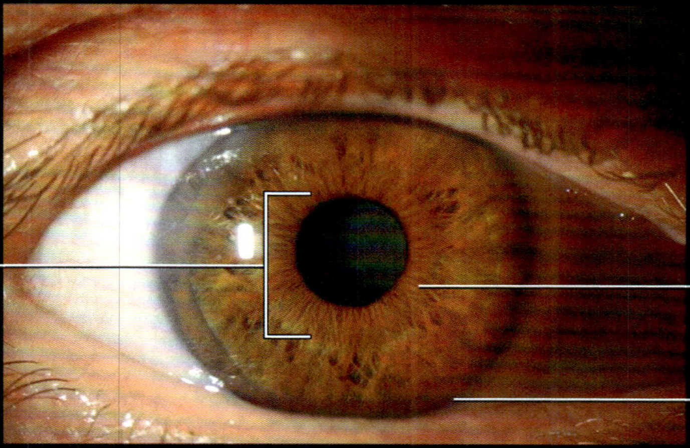

(Top) *This illustration of the anterior segment shows normal anatomy. The anterior chamber can be seen between the iris and cornea and is typically 3 mm deep. The posterior chamber can also be seen between the posterior surface of the iris and the anterior surface of the lens. Notice the folds, ridges, and crypts present on the anterior surface of the iris.* ***(Bottom)*** *This external photograph shows a normal iris.*

ANIRIDIA

Key Facts

Introduction

- Bilateral iris tissue hypoplasia due to mutation or absence of *PAX6* gene
- *PAX6* is involved in regulating transcription in cornea, lens, ciliary body, and retina

Demographics

- Autosomal dominant inheritance in 66-85% of cases
- Sporadic mutations associated with WAGR syndrome (Wilms tumor, aniridia, genitourinary abnormalities, mental retardation)

Presentation

- Diagnosis made on slit-lamp examination
- Cataract, glaucoma, keratopathy, hypoplastic optic nerve and fovea, retinal tears, or retinal detachment
- Nystagmus, small or absent irides, dilated and nonreactive pupils, poor vision, photophobia, dry eyes

Treatment

- Iris reconstruction, implant, corneal tattoo, or colored contact lens for cosmesis and glare suppression
- Limbal stem cell transplant + amniotic membrane for keratopathy (requires systemic immunosuppression to prevent rejection)
- Treat secondary glaucoma with goniotomy procedure or trabeculectomy; trabeculotomy if under age 20
- Cataract extraction ± IOL implantation for secondary cataract formation
- Patients require regularly scheduled eye exams to monitor for astigmatism, amblyopia, elevated IOP
- Abdominal ultrasound every 3 months until age 10, then annually until age 16 to screen for Wilms tumor
- Vision typically no better than 20/200; however, limbal stem cell transplant has shown improved visual acuity beyond 20/200

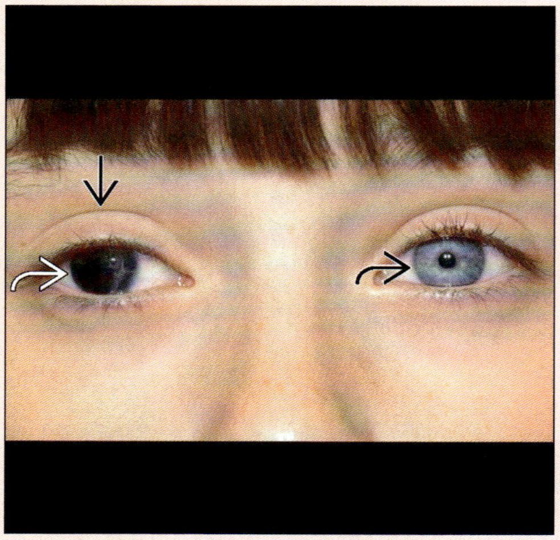

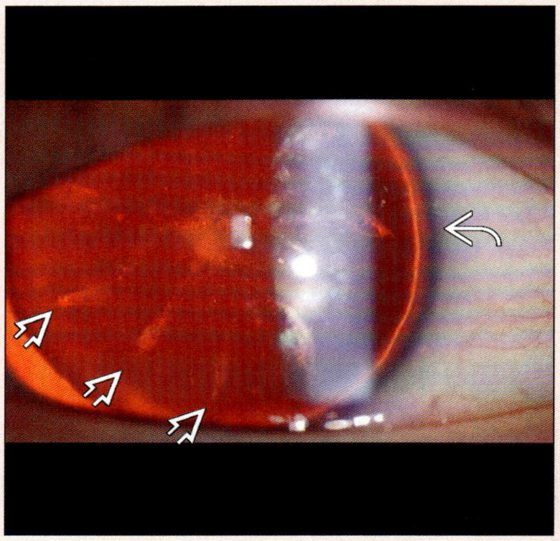

(Left) *External photo of a child with traumatic aniridia shows the difference in appearance between the affected right iris ➔ and the normal left iris ➔. There is also slight ptosis of the affected right eye ➔.* ***(Right)*** *This slit-lamp photo demonstrates a cataract ➔ in a case of congenital aniridia, seen as radially oriented opacities surrounding a central lenticular opacity. The iris is partially absent, and a thin sliver of iris tissue is seen at the limbus ➔.*

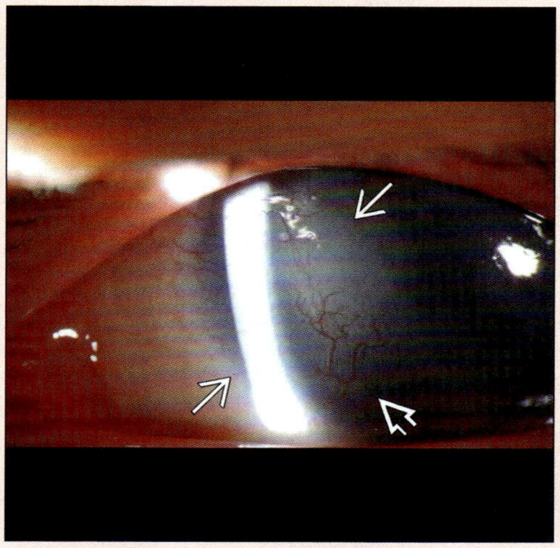

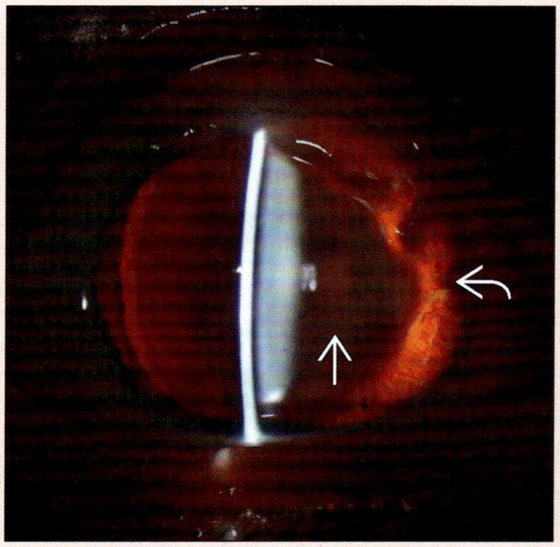

(Left) *Slit-lamp photo shows aniridia with corneal pannus ➔. Overgrowth of fibrovascular connective tissue causes a thickened and opaque cornea. Absence of the PAX6 gene leads to reduced vision, spontaneous corneal neovascularization ➔, abnormal corneal cytokeratin, and poor cell adhesion.* ***(Right)*** *This slit-lamp photo shows retroillumination of an aniridic eye. Some peripheral iris tissue ➔ has developed in front of the visible ciliary body and a cataract ➔ is present posteriorly.*

ANIRIDIA

INTRODUCTION

Definitions
- Bilateral iris tissue hypoplasia due to mutation or absence of *PAX6* gene on chromosome 11p13
- *PAX6* is involved in regulating transcription in cornea, lens, ciliary body, and retina
- Iris tissue may be partially or completely absent

DEMOGRAPHICS

Etiology/Risk Factors
- Family history of aniridia

Epidemiology
- Prevalence: 1.8 per 100,000
- Familial congenital aniridia
  - Autosomal dominant, complete penetrance, variable expressivity
  - 66-85% of aniridia cases
- Miller syndrome
  - Sporadic congenital aniridia
  - 13-33% of aniridia cases
- Gillespie syndrome
  - Autosomal recessive
  - 1-2% of aniridia cases

PRESENTATION

Symptoms
- Complete or partial absence of irides bilaterally
- Disparity between pupil sizes
- Photophobia
  - Severity related to iris involvement
  - Child may hide head under blanket or into caregiver's chest
- Nystagmus
- Dry eye and excess tearing
- Glare

Exam Findings
- Diagnosis is made clinically based on characteristic findings
  - Hypoplastic iris tissue on slit lamp and gonioscopy
  - Dilated, nonreactive pupils
  - Decreased visual acuity
  - Cataract (50-85%)
  - Glaucoma (6-75%)
  - Aniridia-associated keratopathy (20%)
  - Optic nerve hypoplasia ± foveal aplasia (10%)
  - Retinal detachment
- Diagnostic testing: Tonometry, pachymetry, optic nerve exam with visual field testing for optic nerve damage

DIFFERENTIAL DIAGNOSIS

WAGR Syndrome
- Wilms tumor (nephroblastoma), bilateral aniridia, genitourinary abnormalities, mental retardation
- Cranial facial abnormalities including long narrow face, prominent stubby nose, low-set ears, down-slanting palpebral fissures, long philtrum, thin upper lip, delayed closure of anterior fontanelle
- Absence of both *PAX6* and *WT1* genes, both located on chromosome 11p13

Bardet-Biedl Syndrome
- Autosomal recessive, causing peripheral retinal pigment atrophy, renal failure, hypogenitalism, and polydactyly
  - Parafoveal macular atrophy causing decreased central vision
- Ocular findings may or may not include aniridia with zonular cataract

EVALUATION/WORK-UP

Labs
- Genetic testing for *PAX6* mutation

Pathology
- Arrested neuroectodermal tissue development
- Small iris stump lacking iris musculature
- Iris stroma continuous with trabecular meshwork and Schlemm canal

TREATMENT

Medical
- Colored contact lenses with dark periphery, filter lenses, or photogray transition glasses for photophobia
  - Prevent excessive light from entering eye
- Preservative-free artificial tears for aniridia-associated keratopathy and dry eye syndrome

Surgical
- Iris reconstruction, implant
  - Prosthetic iris-lens diaphragm inserted into capsular bag or ciliary sulcus
- Corneal tattoo for cosmesis
- Limbal stem cell transplant with amniotic membrane
  - For aniridia-associated keratopathy
  - Prevents corneal pannus and scarring

Follow-Up
- Regularly scheduled eye exams
  - Monitor for astigmatism, amblyopia, elevated IOP
- Abdominal ultrasound every 3 months until age 10, then annually until age 16 to screen for Wilms tumor

Prognosis
- Vision typically no better than 20/200
- Limbal stem cell transplant with systemic immunosuppression has been shown to improve visual acuity beyond 20/200

SELECTED REFERENCES

1. Mikhail M et al: Traumatic aniridia in a pseudophakic patient 6 years following surgery. Clin Ophthalmol. 6:237-41, 2012
2. Wolff J: [Prosthetic iris devices.] Ophthalmologe. 108(8):714-9, 2011
3. Kokotas H et al: Clinical and molecular aspects of aniridia. Clin Genet. 77(5):409-20, 2010
4. Lee H et al: Aniridia: current pathology and management. Acta Ophthalmol. 86(7):708-15, 2008

CYTOMEGALOVIRUS

Key Facts

Introduction

- Chronic or recurrent infection of anterior chamber with cytomegalovirus (CMV), causing an anterior segment inflammation, secondary glaucoma, and iris atrophy

Demographics

- Risk factors: HIV/AIDS with low CD4 T-cell count, immunosuppression, female gender, foreign born, low economic status, low education, multiple sexual partners, history of prior sexually transmitted infection

Presentation

- Blurred vision, halos, and painful eye
- Decreased visual acuity, increased IOP, cells and debris in anterior chamber, iris atrophy, keratic precipitates, granulomatous inflammation of optic disc, retinitis

Evaluation/Work-Up

- Screen with real-time PCR for CMV DNA in aqueous humor
- Confirm CMV with presence of serum CMV antigen (pp65) and anti-CMV (pp65) IgG antibodies
- Histology shows localized iris infiltration of inflammatory cells infected with CMV
- Negative serologic testing does not exclude virus as inciting pathogen

Treatment

- Combined therapy with antiviral agent (ganciclovir, valganciclovir), anti-inflammatory agent (prednisolone acetate), and antiglaucoma agent (β-blocker, α-2 agonist, acetazolamide)
- Foscarnet and cidofovir are alternatives

__(Left)__ Slit-lamp photo demonstrates peripupillary iris atrophy from cytomegalovirus. Thinning of the iris stroma is apparent circumferentially, and iris discoloration can be seen at 1-o'clock ➡ and 6-o'clock ⇨ positions. __(Right)__ Color fundus photo shows early CMV retinitis in a patient with AIDS. The white spots to the left of the optic nerve ➦ is an area of retinitis, which expands as the retinitis progresses. Venous sheathing ➡ is present along the vasculature.

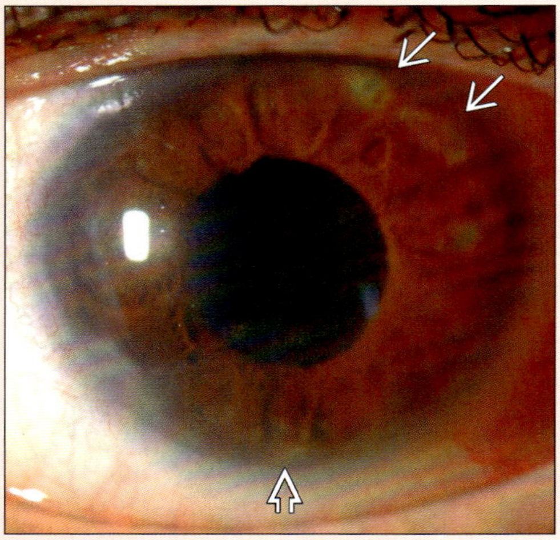

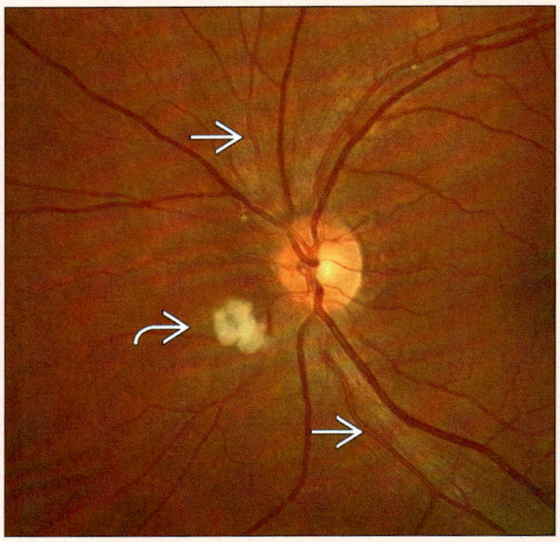

__(Left)__ This color fundus photo illustrates diffuse retinal whitening from CMV retinitis in a patient with AIDS. CMV retinitis is an AIDS-defining lesion, typically seen in patients with CD4(+) cell count ≤ 50. These lesions are treated with oral, topical, or intravitreal ganciclovir or valganciclovir for a minimum of 6 weeks. __(Right)__ Color fundus photo shows multiple black foci of necrotic retina ➡ in CMV retinitis. Areas of necrosis are larger in the peripheral retina in this patient.

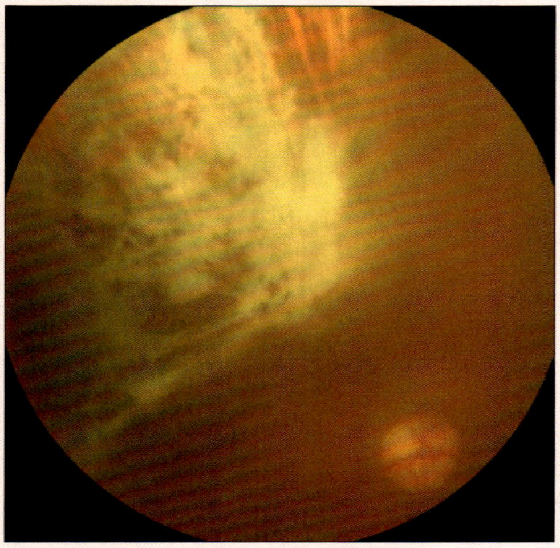

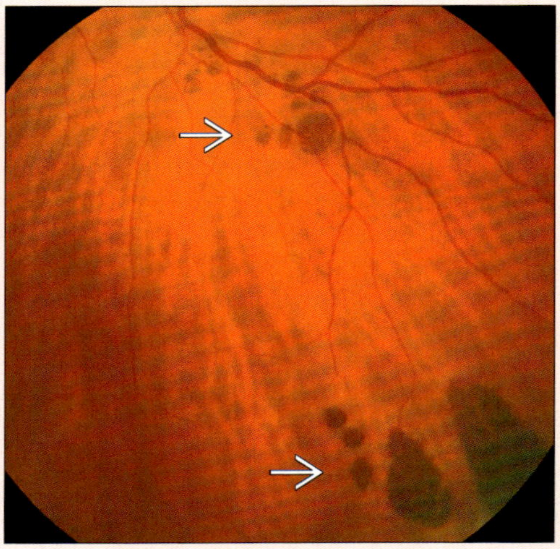

CYTOMEGALOVIRUS

INTRODUCTION

Abbreviations
- Cytomegalovirus (CMV)

Definitions
- Chronic or recurrent infection of anterior chamber with CMV, causing anterior segment inflammation, secondary glaucoma, and iris atrophy
  - CMV infects smooth muscle cells of iris, ciliary body, and endothelial lining of Schlemm canal
  - Infection of trabecular meshwork cells causes swelling and obstruction of aqueous humor outflow path, which increases IOP

DEMOGRAPHICS

Etiology/Risk Factors
- HIV/AIDS with low CD4 T-cell count, immunosuppression, female sex, low economic status, low education, multiple sex partners, history of prior sexually transmitted infection
- Incidence of ocular CMV infection is increasing
  - New strains of CMV
  - Better diagnostic testing with PCR identifies cases otherwise classified as unknown in origin

Epidemiology
- 40-100% of adults are seropositive for CMV
  - Seropositivity for CMV increases with age
  - Inverse correlation between seropositivity and economic development
    - Highest rates of CMV in developing countries in Africa and Asia
    - In USA, CMV is more common in Mexican Americans and African Americans
- Average age of onset is 40 years

PRESENTATION

Symptoms
- Blurred vision
- Halos
- Painful eye

Exam Findings
- Decreased visual acuity
- Elevated IOP
- Corneal haze or edema
- Cells within anterior chamber
  - Typically ≥ 2 cells with rare flare
  - Debris within anterior chamber angle
- Peripupillary iris atrophy
  - Anisocoria or difference in color between irides may be present
- Keratic precipitates along corneal endothelium
  - Large collections associated with granulomatous inflammation
  - Small collections associated with leukocytic inflammation
- Diffuse retinal whitening
- Granulomatous inflammation of optic disc ± disc cupping
- Retinal hemorrhages or venous infarcts
- "Pizza pie" appearance to fundus with CMV retinitis

DIFFERENTIAL DIAGNOSIS

Posner-Schlossman Syndrome
- Recurrent mild iritis with increased IOP
- Fine keratic precipitates
- Corneal epithelium edema

Fuchs Heterochromic Iridocyclitis
- Chronic, asymptomatic mild iritis with stellate keratic precipitates
- Patients present with diffuse iris atrophy and absence of posterior synechiae
- Associated with peptic ulcers, allergies, gastrointestinal distress

Herpes Simplex Virus (HSV) Uveitis
- Epithelial or stromal keratitis
- Endotheliitis
  - Linearly arranged inflammation at former surgical incision sites or corneal wounds
- Mild to moderate anterior uveitis
- Aqueous humor analysis with PCR positive for herpes virus

Varicella Zoster Virus (VZV) Uveitis
- Double-stranded DNA virus causing chicken pox, which remains dormant in nerve roots and upon reactivation causes herpes zoster ophthalmicus
- Patients present with eyelid involvement, conjunctivitis, keratitis, anterior uveitis with patchy iris atrophy, scleritis, acute retinal necrosis, optic neuritis
- Diagnosis is made from aqueous humor analysis with PCR positive for varicella virus DNA

Sarcoidosis
- Systemic disease characterized by granulomatous inflammation of lung
- More common in African American women in their 3rd or 4th decade
- Patients present with uveitis, cough, dyspnea, erythema nodosum, bilateral hilar lymphadenopathy on chest x-ray

Syphilis
- Systemic sexually transmitted disease caused by *Treponema pallidum* with primary, secondary, and tertiary disease stages
  - Primary syphilis: Ulcer and painless chancre at site of infection
  - Secondary syphilis: Rash, mucocutaneous lesions, and generalized lymphadenopathy
  - Tertiary syphilis: Neurologic symptoms, gummas, and cardiovascular symptoms
- Neurosyphilis presents with loss of peripheral vision, loss of hearing, and tinnitus
- VDRL and RPR are screening tests; FTA-ABS is used to confirm disease

Tuberculosis (TB)
- Multisystemic disease caused by *Mycobacterium tuberculosis*, an acid-fast bacillus

- Patients present with hemoptysis, night sweats, weight loss, and apical chest x-ray findings in reactivation TB
- Ocular TB can cause granulomatous keratitis, iridocyclitis, intermediate uveitis, retinitis, scleritis, and orbital cellulitis, with choroidal tubercles and choroiditis as the most common presentations
  - Patients present with blurry vision, painful and red eye, proptosis, double vision, or restricted extraocular muscle motility

EVALUATION/WORK-UP

Labs

- Screening test
  - Aqueous humor analysis with real-time PCR for CMV DNA
- Confirmatory test
  - Presence of serum CMV antigen (pp65) and anti-CMV (pp65) IgG antibodies
    - Negative serologic testing does not exclude virus as inciting pathogen
    - Aqueous and serologic viral counts may differ significantly
- Goldmann-Witmer coefficient
  - (Aqueous anti-CMV-Ig)/(serum anti-CMV-IgG) x (total serum IgG)/(total aqueous IgG)
  - Value > 3 correlates to CMV uveitis infection
- Characteristic profiling
  - Profile 1
    - Non-herpes simplex virus, non-varicella zoster virus corticosteroid-resistant inflammatory ocular hypertensive syndrome
    - Positive predictive value: 94.7%
  - Profile 2
    - Corneal endotheliitis with specific coin-shaped keratic precipitates
    - Positive predictive value: 90.9%

Pathology

- Localized iris infiltration of inflammatory cells infected with CMV
- Extensive atrophy of retina with infiltration of giant cells
- Characteristic "owl's eye" cells have intranuclear and intracytoplasmic inclusions that represent CMV
- Electron microscopy of organisms shows viral particles with dense central cores surrounded by thick capsule

TREATMENT

Medical

- Antiviral: Indicated if positive aqueous humor analysis for CMV or during recurrent episodes of uveitis despite therapy with steroids
  - Ganciclovir
    - 5 mg/kg body weight IV b.i.d. for 6 weeks followed by 1 g p.o. t.i.d. for 6 weeks
    - Intravitreal: 2 mg/0.1 mL injection weekly for 3 months
    - Topical: 0.15% q.i.d.
  - Valganciclovir
    - 900 mg p.o. b.i.d. for 6 weeks, followed by 450 mg p.o. b.i.d. for 6 weeks
  - Duration of therapy is not well established
  - Treat until symptoms are absent and viral load is negative
  - Foscarnet and cidofovir are alternatives
- Treat inflammation with corticosteroids and raised IOP with antiglaucoma medications
  - Anti-inflammatory
    - Topical: Prednisolone acetate 1%
    - Taper dose as inflammation resolves
    - Use of steroids without concomitant antiviral therapy can result in severe scarring of cornea
  - Antiglaucoma
    - Topical: β-blocker, α-2 agonist, acetazolamide
    - Oral: Acetazolamide
      - Indicated if IOP > 40 mm Hg
    - Target IOP is ≤ 25 mm Hg

Surgical

- Secondary glaucoma
  - Trabeculotomy, trabeculectomy for uncontrolled IOP resistant to medical therapy
- Secondary cataracts
  - Complication of long-term steroid therapy
  - Cataract extraction with intraocular lens implantation

Follow-Up

- During treatment, monitor CBC and serum creatinine with CMP every 2 weeks to evaluate for nephrotoxicity and bone marrow suppression
- Average follow-up is 2 years
- Recurrence occurs in 77% of patients within 8 months of discontinuation of therapy
  - Monitor for anterior segment inflammation on slit-lamp exam and elevated IOP

Prognosis

- Anterior chamber inflammation should resolve within a few weeks of oral or intravenous antiviral therapy
- With treatment of virus and IOP control, visual acuity of 20/20 can be achieved

SELECTED REFERENCES

1. Kongyai N et al: Viral causes of unexplained anterior uveitis in Thailand. Eye (Lond). 26(4):529-34, 2012
2. Hwang YS et al: The validity of clinical feature profiles for cytomegaloviral anterior segment infection. Graefes Arch Clin Exp Ophthalmol. 249(1):103-10, 2011
3. Chee SP et al: Clinical features of cytomegalovirus anterior uveitis in immunocompetent patients. Am J Ophthalmol. 145(5):834-40, 2008
4. van Boxtel LA et al: Cytomegalovirus as a cause of anterior uveitis in immunocompetent patients. Ophthalmology. 114(7):1358-62, 2007
5. Westeneng AC et al: Infectious uveitis in immunocompromised patients and the diagnostic value of polymerase chain reaction and Goldmann-Witmer coefficient in aqueous analysis. Am J Ophthalmol. 144(5):781-5, 2007
6. De Groot-Mijnes JD et al: Polymerase chain reaction and Goldmann-Witmer coefficient analysis are complimentary for the diagnosis of infectious uveitis. Am J Ophthalmol. 141(2):313-8, 2006

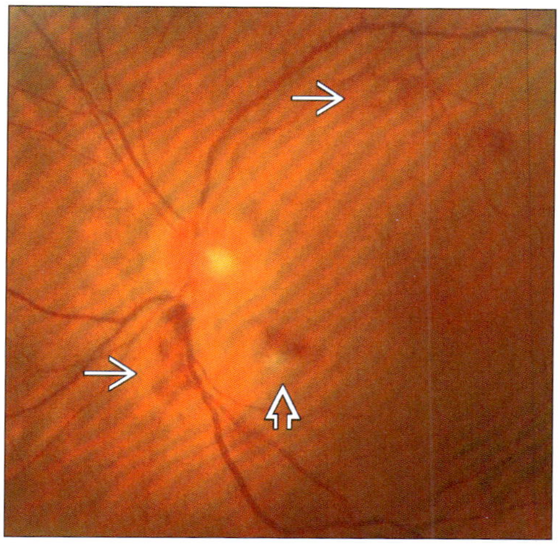

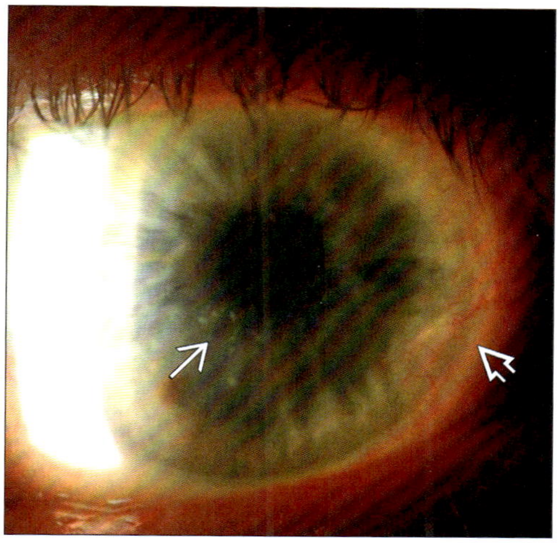

(Left) *Color fundus photo shows CMV retinitis with multiple sites of retinal hemorrhage. One focus of hemorrhage is juxtaposed to a small focus of early retinitis from CMV.* **(Right)** *Slit-lamp photo shows corneal neovascularization and round keratic precipitates within the corneal endothelium in an eye infected with CMV.*

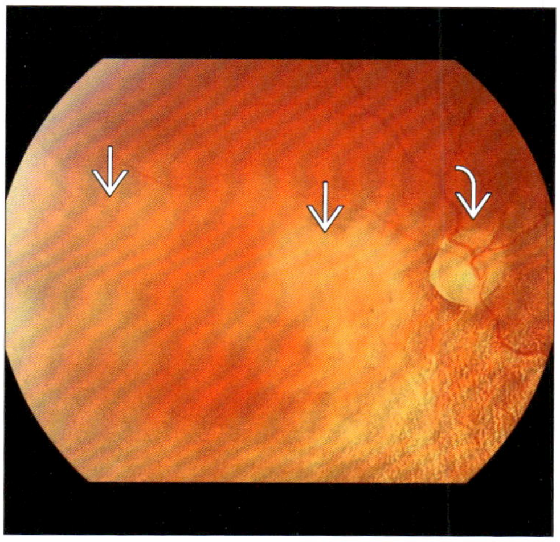

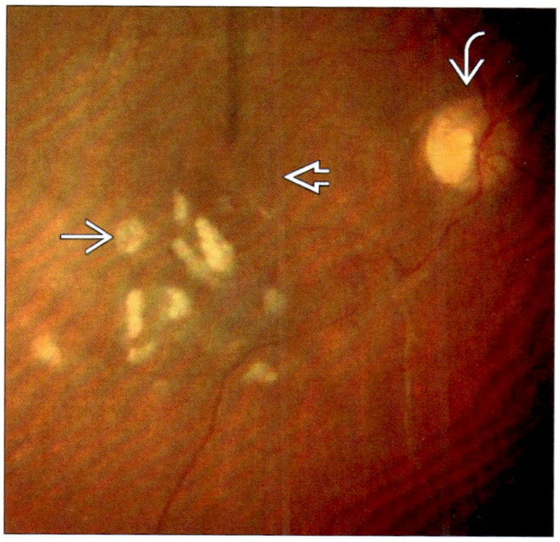

(Left) *Fundus photo shows white patchy areas of retinal inflammation in a patient with CMV retinitis. The optic nerve head is affected by granulomatous inflammation.* **(Right)** *This fundus photo shows a branched retinal vein occlusion secondary to CMV infection. Discrete white lesions represent vascular inflammation and infarcts from CMV infection. There is also cystoid macular edema and swelling of the optic nerve head due to venous occlusion.*

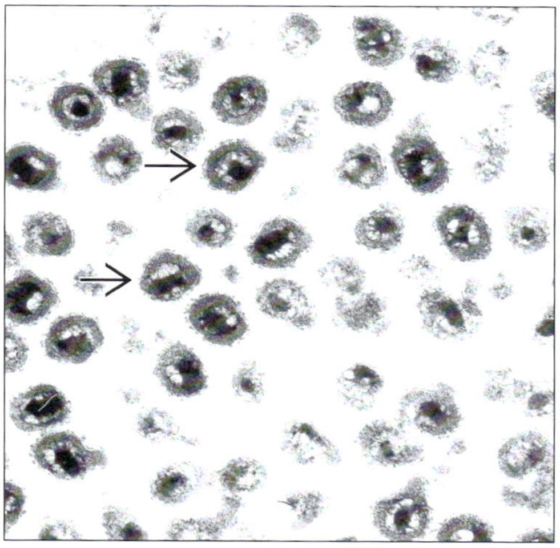

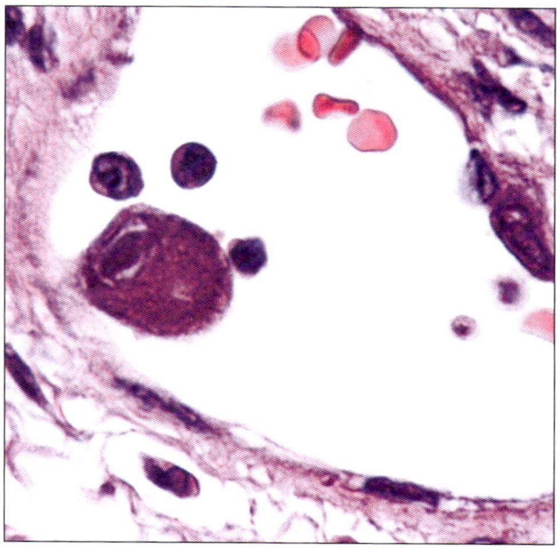

(Left) *Electron microscopy shows individual viral particles measuring approximately 150-200 nm in diameter with dense central cores surrounded by a thick capsule, which is characteristic of CMV. (Courtesy J. Taxy, MD.)* **(Right)** *Hematoxylin & eosin stain shows the characteristic "owl's eye" CMV inclusion within the endothelium of a vessel. In the retina, these cells are found adjacent to sites of former retinal necrosis. (Courtesy M. Scott, MD.)*

HERPES SIMPLEX VIRUS UVEITIS

Key Facts

Introduction

- Unilateral infection of iris with herpes simplex virus (HSV) type 1 or type 2, triggering granulomatous inflammatory response and elevated intraocular pressure, often associated with herpetic keratitis
- Transmitted via direct or indirect contact to mucous membrane droplets (typically saliva or ocular secretions) from person shedding the virus
- Anterior uveitis is due to 1 of the following
  - Extension of virus from cornea into anterior chamber and subsequent immune response
  - Secondary inflammatory reaction in response to keratitis
  - Anti-HSV antibodies cross-reacting with host antigens

Demographics

- Prevalence in USA: 400,000
- Incidence in USA: 20,000 per year

Presentation

- Patients complain of injected, painful red eye with photophobia, foreign-body sensation, and decreased vision
- Characteristic findings on exam: Anterior uveitis, sectoral iris atrophy, keratitis, secondary glaucoma

Evaluation/Work-Up

- Viral culture with PCR of aqueous humor
- Histology shows infiltration of lymphocytes and plasma cells within iris stroma
- Slit-lamp biomicroscopy with transillumination identifies iris atrophy, and administration of fluorescein dye may show dendritic corneal ulcers in epithelium; IOP elevation is common

Treatment

- Oral antivirals ± topical steroids, cycloplegics, antiglaucoma agents

*(**Left**) Slit-lamp photo shows a dendritic corneal scar ➔, which usually occurs in cases complicated by recurrent epithelial keratitis. It causes a branched lesion of the corneal epithelium, resembling a tree with dilated terminal bulbs that stain with fluorescein. Corneal neovascularization ➔ is due to irritation from viral particles within the cornea. (**Right**) This slit-lamp photo shows a dendritic corneal lesion highlighted by fluorescein staining ➔.*

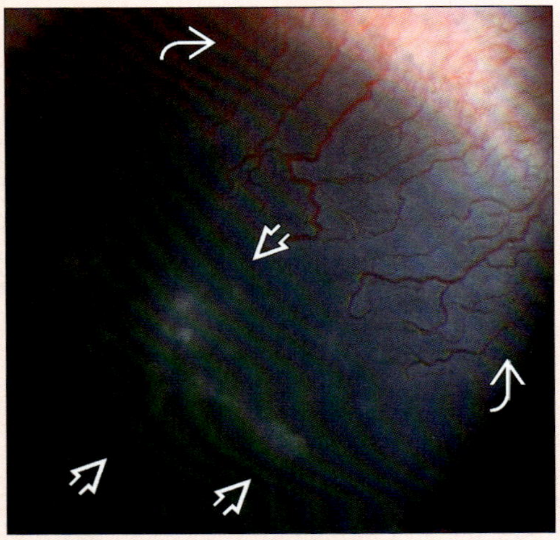

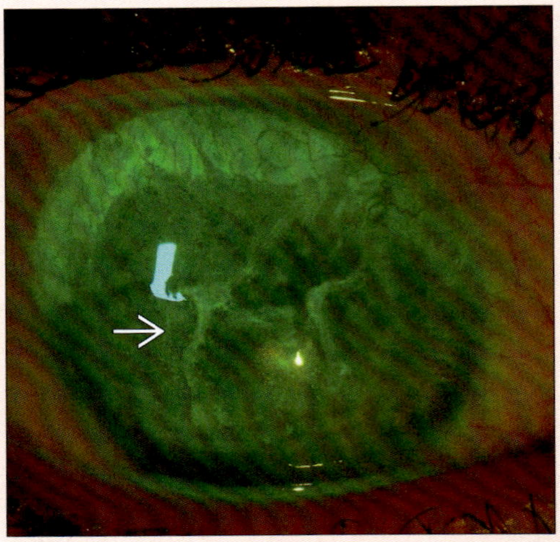

*(**Left**) Slit-lamp photo shows a herpes simplex virus infection complicated by disciform keratitis ➔, a central disc-shaped corneal opacity within the corneal stroma with anterior uveitis. This immunologic response to the virus causes pain and vision loss. Keratic precipitates ➔ are present inferiorly. (**Right**) This slit-lamp photo shows corneal neovascularization ➔ and irregularities in corneal thickness due to a semitransparent scar ➔ in the superficial layers of the cornea.*

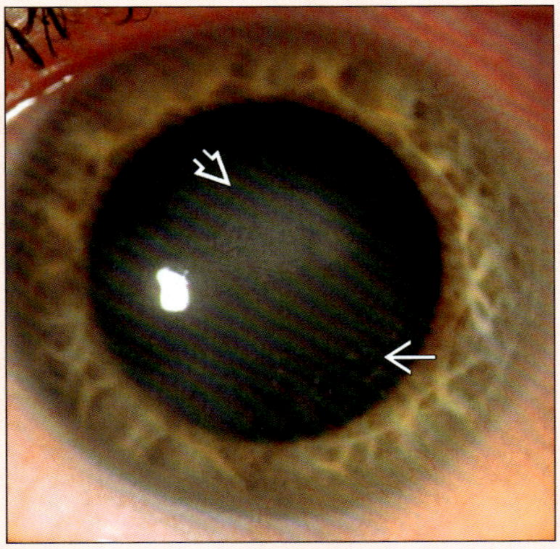

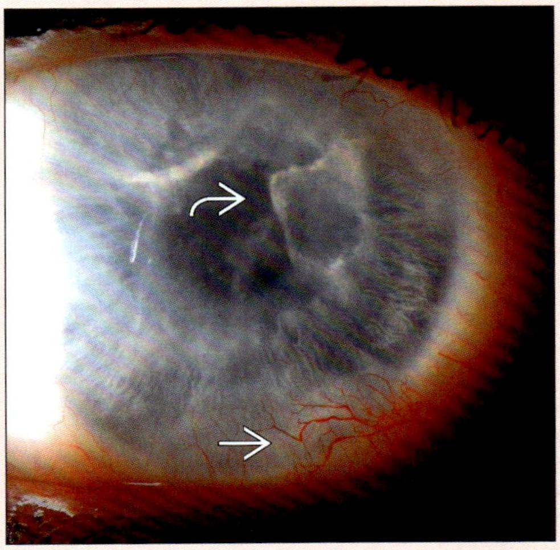

HERPES SIMPLEX VIRUS UVEITIS

INTRODUCTION

Definitions

- Herpes simplex virus (HSV): Double-stranded DNA virus
- Infection of iris with HSV type 1 or type 2 triggers a T-cell-mediated granulomatous inflammatory response within anterior chamber

Subtypes

- HSV1
  - Transmitted through contact with oral or ocular secretions
  - Affects children or adults
  - May cause keratoconjunctivitis, uveitis, or secondary glaucoma
- HSV2
  - Transmitted through contact with genital secretions
  - Affects adults; can also affect fetus as it passes through vaginal canal
  - Causes severe keratoconjunctivitis with uveitis and typically secondary glaucoma

DEMOGRAPHICS

Epidemiology

- Prevalence in United States: 400,000
- Incidence of new HSV keratitis: 20,000 per year
- Total cases of acute HSV keratitis (either initial or recurrent infection): 48,000 per year

PRESENTATION

Symptoms

- Injected, painful red eye with photophobia, foreign body sensation, reflex tearing, and decreased vision
- Pain in dermatomal distribution in involved area
- History may include previous herpetic keratitis

Exam Findings

- Characteristic dendritic corneal ulcer with anterior uveitis, ↑ IOP, and keratitis
  - Dendritic corneal ulcer stains with fluorescein
- Cells and flare in anterior chamber
  - Can lead to trabecular debris or trabeculitis, which can increase IOP acutely
- Mutton-fat keratic precipitates
- Disciform corneal edema and opacification
- Descemet folds
- Iris atrophy
- Iridocyclitis, hypopyon, hyphema, synechiae
- Persistently dilated pupil, anisocoria
- Acute retinal necrosis (ARN) or progressive outer retinal necrosis (PORN) can be seen with posterior segment involvement

DIFFERENTIAL DIAGNOSIS

Herpes Zoster Ophthalmicus

- Painful dermatomal forehead rash and painful inflammation of anterior ± posterior segment(s) of eye
  - Conjunctivitis, episcleritis, uveitis
- Conjunctival, episcleral, and circumlimbal hyperemia
- Corneal edema, epithelial and stromal keratitis
- Uveitis, glaucoma, and pain

Interstitial Keratitis

- Chronic, nonulcerative inflammation of corneal mid stroma ± uveitis
- Photophobia, pain, tearing, progressive visual deterioration
- Slit-lamp exam shows neovascularization of cornea with ground-glass opacification obscuring view of iris
- Anterior uveitis, choroiditis may be present

Adult Inclusion Conjunctivitis

- Chronic unilateral conjunctivitis resulting after sexual contact with person with genital *Chlamydia trachomatis*
- Hyperemia and mucopurulent discharge
- Follicles on palpebral conjunctiva
- Swollen preauricular lymph nodes

EVALUATION/WORK-UP

Labs

- Culture with PCR of aqueous fluid to determine infectious etiology and rule out bacterial keratitis

Pathology

- Lymphocytes and plasma cells within iris stroma

Imaging

- Slit-lamp biomicroscopy
  - Dendritic ulcer of corneal epithelium seen with fluorescein dye and filtered cobalt blue light
  - Transillumination identifies iris atrophy
- Dilated fundus exam to identify posterior uveitis

TREATMENT

Medical

- Topical antiviral agents
- Oral antiviral agents
- Cycloplegics: Decrease eye pain and prevent synechiae
- Antiglaucoma medication: If IOP is elevated
- Topical steroids: Stromal keratitis, iritis, trabeculitis
  - Contraindicated if epithelial defects/keratitis

Prognosis

- Delayed diagnosis if no history of prior infection
  - Leads to chronic inflammation, corneal hypoesthesia, ulceration, and scaring
  - Severe glaucoma with poor visual outcome
- Morbidity increases in immunosuppressed patients and in bacterial superinfection
- Recurrent infections result in neurotrophic keratopathy
- Chronic iris and trabecular meshwork inflammation results in glaucoma with vision loss if untreated

SELECTED REFERENCES

1. Jap A et al: Viral anterior uveitis. Curr Opin Ophthalmol. 22(6):483-8, 2011
2. Wensing B et al: Necrotizing and nonnecrotizing variants of herpetic uveitis with posterior segment involvement. Arch Ophthalmol. 129(4):403-8, 2011
3. Yang SY et al: Cytomegalovirus and herpes simplex virus as causes of bilateral anterior uveitis in an immunocompetent patient. J Chin Med Assoc. 74(1):48-50, 2011

VARICELLA ZOSTER VIRUS

Key Facts

Introduction
- Varicella zoster virus (VZV): Human herpesvirus 3, double-stranded DNA virus belonging to herpes family
  - Causes chicken pox with fever, myalgia, malaise, anorexia, sore throat, and vesicular rash
- Herpes zoster (shingles): Reactivation of latent VZV in sensory spinal or cerebral ganglia
  - Patients present with unilateral pain in dermatomal distribution with vesicular rash
- Herpes zoster ophthalmicus (HZO): Reactivation of latent VZV in trigeminal ganglia, causing infection along ophthalmic branch of trigeminal nerve

Demographics
- Estimated ≥ 1 million cases per year in USA
- Incidence of varicella ↓ by 90% after initiation of widespread varicella vaccination in 1995
  - ↓ incidence of VZV and postherpetic neuralgia; ↓ severity and duration of HZO

Presentation
- Punctate keratopathy, dendritic keratitis, neurotrophic keratopathy with ↓ corneal sensation, poor wound healing, and corneal ulcers
  - Multiple, isolated lesions seen on slit-lamp exam that stain with rose bengal or fluorescein dye

Evaluation/Work-Up
- Diagnosis is clinical, and routine laboratory testing is not necessary

Treatment
- Oral antiviral agents: Acyclovir, valacyclovir, famciclovir
  - Melts require careful corneal protective therapy with vitamin C, doxycycline, medroxyprogesterone, bandage contact lens, &/or amniotic membrane
- Systemic corticosteroids indicated in cases of severe pain, cranial nerve palsies, or CNS involvement

__(Left)__ Pseudodendritic staining ➔ is a characteristic finding in herpes zoster virus (HZV) infection. Pseudodendrites are found in varicella zoster virus, whereas dendrites are seen in HSV epithelial keratitis. A key distinguishing factor present in dendrites but not in pseudodendrites is the presence of terminal bulbs at the tips of the dendrites. __(Right)__ This slit-lamp photograph is another example of pseudodendritic epithelial keratitis ➔ seen in a case of reactivated herpes zoster virus.

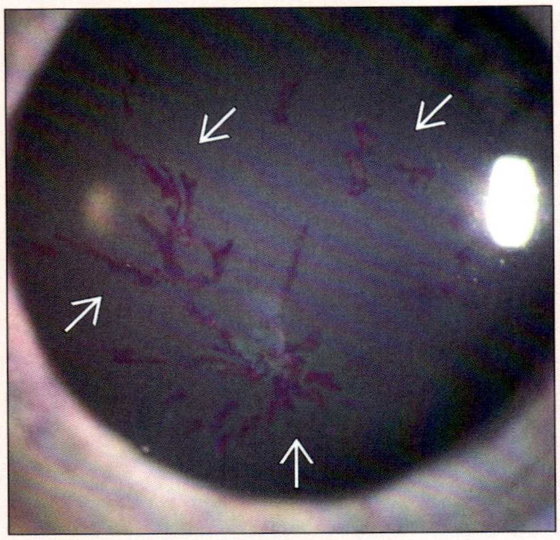

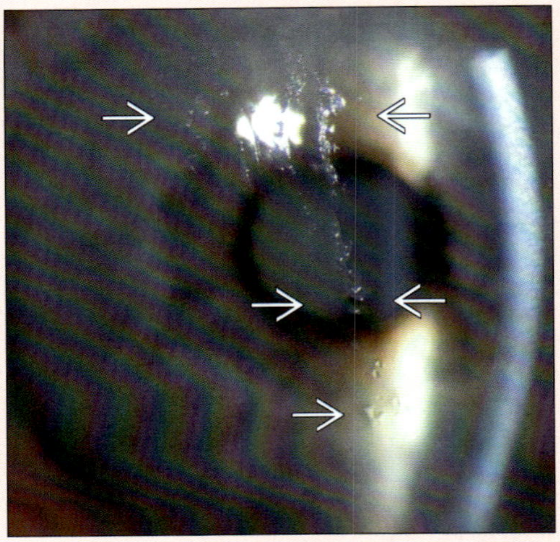

__(Left)__ This image demonstrates peripapillary atrophy ➔ in a patient with varicella zoster virus infection. Prompt diagnosis and antiviral therapy are important due to rapid disease progression and poor visual outcome if untreated. Retinal detachment occurs within the 1st weeks to months following the onset of retina involvement. __(Right)__ This retroillumination slit-lamp photo shows small pseudodendritic lesions ➔, which are creating indentations in the corneal epithelium.

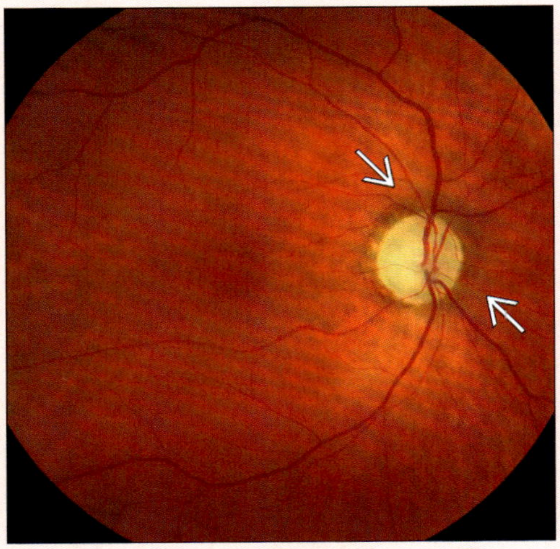

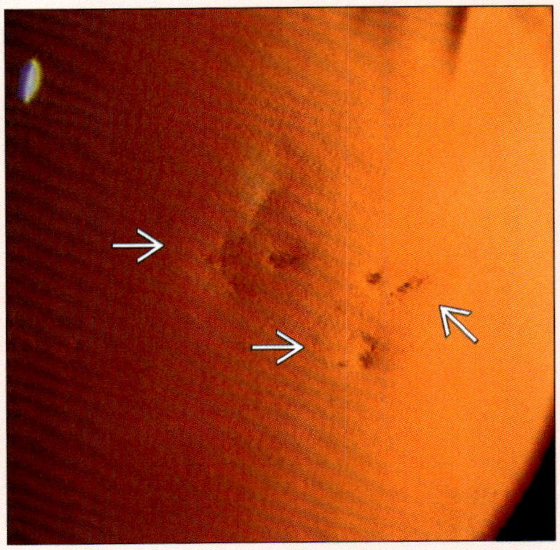

VARICELLA ZOSTER VIRUS

INTRODUCTION

Definitions

- Varicella zoster virus (VZV): Human herpesvirus 3, a double-stranded DNA virus belonging to herpes family
  - Causes chicken pox, spread via respiratory droplets
  - Patients present with fever, myalgia, malaise, anorexia, sore throat, vesicular rash
- Herpes zoster (shingles): Reactivation of latent VZV in sensory spinal or cerebral ganglia
  - Patients present with unilateral pain in dermatomal distribution with vesicular rash
- Herpes zoster ophthalmicus (HZO): Reactivation of latent VZV in trigeminal ganglia, causing infection along ophthalmic branch of trigeminal nerve
  - Ophthalmic branch of trigeminal nerve divides into nasociliary, frontal, and lacrimal nerves; of these, frontal nerve is most commonly involved
- Postherpetic neuralgia (PHN): Persistent, severe pain after resolution of dermatologic VZV lesion, seen in 50% of patients
- Ocular zoster sine herpete: VZV infection with ophthalmic involvement without dermatologic manifestations
  - Neuralgic pain along distribution of trigeminal nerve, severe pain in and around eye radiating to side of nose, external eye muscle involvement
- VZV causes primary chicken pox infection, then remains dormant in dorsal nerve root ganglia
- Reactivation causes HZO years later when host immune system is stressed

Subtypes

- Orbital apex syndrome
  - Can present with ptosis, pain, and double vision, due to involvement of 3rd, 4th, or 6th cranial nerves from either vasculitis or brain stem infection
- Transplacental VZV infection
  - Affects fetus when mother acquires VZV during pregnancy
  - Congenital varicella: Microcephaly, scaring of skin with areas of hypopigmentation, underdeveloped lungs, autonomic nervous system damage

DEMOGRAPHICS

Etiology/Risk Factors

- Immunosuppression, HIV or AIDS, defects in cellular immune system, advanced age, poor nutritional status, emotional or physical stress, and fatigue

Epidemiology

- Estimated ≥ 1 million cases per year in USA
- 95-99% of adults in USA > age 50 show serologic evidence of VZV exposure
- 33% of USA population will be affected by HZV
  - 10-25% of those affected by HZV will have ocular involvement (HZO)
  - 5-20% of those with HZO will develop PHN
- Incidence of varicella ↓ by 90% after initiation of widespread varicella vaccination in 1995

PRESENTATION

Symptoms

- History of prodromal phase with low-grade fever, headache, malaise, paresthesia, or hyperesthesia of involved dermatome surrounding eye
- 3-5 days later: Painful, unilateral, vesicular rash in dermatomal distribution overlying ophthalmic division of trigeminal nerve
  - Progresses from erythema to macules, papules, vesicles, pustules, and crusting lesions
- Inflammatory destruction of nerves leads to corneal hypoesthesia, increased susceptibility to injury, and neurotrophic keratopathy with poor corneal healing

Exam Findings

- Hutchinson sign: VZV skin lesions involving the top of the nose during prodromal phase, which increases likelihood of ocular involvement
- Eyelid involvement
  - Blepharitis, ptosis, eyelid scaring, loss of eyelid pigmentation, entropion, or ectropion
    - Due to edema and inflammation of upper eyelid
- Conjunctivitis with conjunctival injection and petechial hemorrhages
  - Patient may develop secondary *Staphylococcus aureus* conjunctivitis that persists after 1 week, requiring antibiotic treatment
- Epithelial keratitis
  - Multiple, isolated lesions seen on slit-lamp exam that stain with rose bengal or fluorescein dye
  - Lesions spontaneously resolve or progress to pseudodendritic keratitis
    - Pseudodendrites of VZV present as elevated plaques in a dendritic pattern without presence of terminal bulbs, which differentiates them from dendrites of HSV
  - Corneal findings may include stromal, nummular, disciform, mucous plaque, or exposure keratitis; corneal ulcers, perforations, edema, or scaring; punctate keratopathy
- Neurotrophic keratopathy: Decreased corneal sensation and poor wound healing
- Anterior uveitis with inflammation of iris and ciliary body, iris atrophy, or phthisis bulbi
  - Isolated herpetic uveitis without herpetic keratitis can be seen
  - Findings include keratic precipitates, posterior synechiae, sectoral iris atrophy
  - May cause secondary glaucoma or cataract formation
- Scleritis or episcleritis: Diffuse redness and swelling of conjunctiva and episclera with deep eye pain
- Acute retinal necrosis (ARN) or progressive outer retinal necrosis (PORN)
  - Blurry vision, eye pain, occlusive retinal vasculitis, inflammation of vitreous, and retinal detachment
  - Unilateral or bilateral involvement may occur
- Optic neuritis
  - May appear up to 10 weeks after dermatomal rash
  - Normal or swollen optic nerve with eventual optic atrophy
  - Decreased visual acuity with central field defects
- Orbital myositis or orbital apex syndrome

VARICELLA ZOSTER VIRUS

DIFFERENTIAL DIAGNOSIS

Herpes Simplex Keratitis

- Infection of anterior chamber with herpes simplex virus strain 1 or 2, without cutaneous findings
- Corneal epithelium shows terminal end bulbs that stain with fluorescein and rose bengal
- Dendrites cannot be peeled off and have an epithelial defect ± heaped-up edges
- Patients are typically younger

Trigeminal Neuralgia/Tic Douloureux

- Severe unilateral pain in sensory distribution of 5th cranial nerve, typically maxillary or mandibular branches

Ramsay Hunt Syndrome

- VZV infection of trigeminal nerve with facial paralysis

Corneal Abrasion

- Disruption of corneal epithelium due to trauma, toxins that disrupt corneal integrity, severe dry eye syndrome, contact lens wear abuse
- Eye pain, worse with eye opening or extraocular movement, foreign body sensation, photophobia, blurred vision, excessive tearing, corneal edema
- Epithelial defect stains with fluorescein

EVALUATION/WORK-UP

Labs

- Diagnosis is clinical; routine labs are not necessary
- Viral culture, PCR, or direct immunofluorescence assay differentiates herpes zoster from herpes simplex
- Cell-mediated immunity testing: VZV antigen skin test, VZV lymphocyte proliferation
- Serology for anti-VZV antibodies: Neutralizing or complement-fixing antibody tests, ELISA, radioimmunoassay, membrane antigen immunofluorescence, immune adherence hemagglutination
- Test for HIV in patients < 50 years of age with HZV involving the face or eyelids

Pathology

- Tzanck smear and Wright stain of vesicular lesions show multinucleated giant cells and acidophilic intranuclear antibodies
- Ganglionic inflammation and hemorrhagic necrosis of trigeminal ganglion

TREATMENT

Medical

- Oral antiviral agents: Acyclovir, valacyclovir, famciclovir
  - Improve healing time and decrease pain, ↓ incidence, severity, and duration of PHN (if given within 72 hours of onset)
- Topical antiviral agents: 3% acyclovir
  - Indicated in the setting of corneal epithelial involvement
  - Decrease complications, duration of viral shedding, healing time, pain severity
  - Best if started within 72 hours of symptom onset
    - Start medical therapy after 72 hours if formation of new vesicles, advanced age, severe pain, or ocular, neuro, or motor complications
- Systemic corticosteroids: Prednisone with slow taper
  - Use with antiviral agent in immunocompetent only
  - Indicated in cases of severe pain, cranial nerve palsies, or CNS involvement
- Topical corticosteroids: For corneal infection, episcleritis, scleritis, iritis, or uveal inflammation
  - Avoid steroids if epithelial defects, as steroids inhibit healing
- Intravenous or intravitreal injection of antiviral in severe retinal necrosis
- Lubricants: Artificial tears for dry eye syndrome, keratopathy
- Cold compress, 5% lidocaine cream, systemic NSAIDs, and antidepressants for severe, chronic pain and depression
- For postherpetic neuralgia: Desipramine, nortriptyline
  - Opioids: Oxycodone, tramadol if needed
  - Anticonvulsant: Gabapentin, pregabalin
  - Topical analgesic: Lidocaine ointment or patch, 0.075% capsaicin cream, calamine

Surgical

- Deep corneal scarring: Penetrating keratoplasty, Descemet stripping endothelial keratoplasty
- Superficial corneal scarring: Lamellar keratoplasty, keratectomy with microkeratome, excimer laser phototherapeutic keratectomy
- Keratoprostheses for patients with corneal scaring and multiple donor graft rejections (high risk for corneal melt)

Follow-Up

- Periodic funduscopic examination to identify posterior segment inflammation

Prognosis

- Varicella zoster vaccine (Zostavax) approved for ages ≥ 60 years
  - ↑ immunity and ↓ incidence of VZV infection
  - ↓ severity and duration of VZV ophthalmia
  - ↓ incidence of PHN
  - Adverse effects include erythema, swelling, and tenderness at injection site
- Relapse of HZO may occur up to 10 years after onset
- Corneal involvement can result in chronic epithelial keratitis

SELECTED REFERENCES

1. Hamrah P et al: Unilateral herpes zoster ophthalmicus results in bilateral corneal nerve alteration: an in vivo confocal microscopy study. Ophthalmology. 120(1):40-7, 2013
2. Arda H et al: Orbital apex syndrome in herpes zoster ophthalmicus. Case Rep Ophthalmol Med. 2012:854503, 2012
3. Wang TJ et al: Increased risk of anterior uveitis following herpes zoster: a nationwide population-based study. Arch Ophthalmol. 130(4):451-5, 2012
4. Sanjay S et al: Herpes zoster ophthalmicus. Curr Treat Options Neurol. 13(1):79-91, 2011
5. Kaufman SC: Anterior segment complications of herpes zoster ophthalmicus. Ophthalmology. 115(2 Suppl):S24-32, 2008

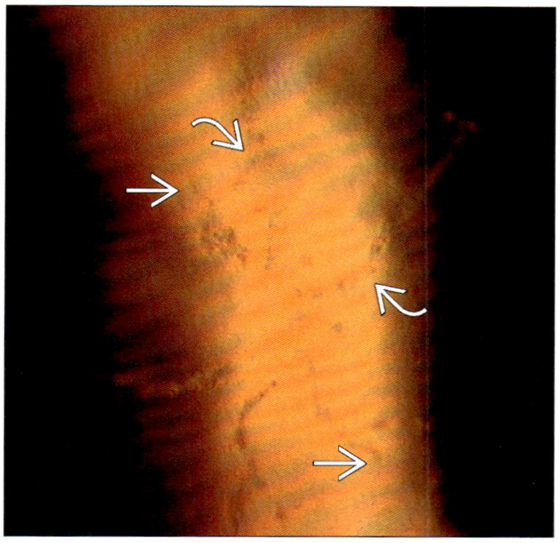

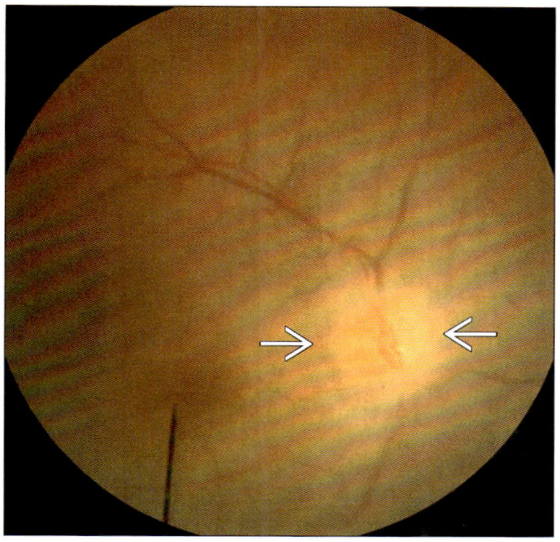

(Left) *Retroillumination reveals a large pseudodendritic lesion on the corneal epithelium, seen in varicella zoster virus infection. Note the absence of terminal bulbs at the tips of the pseudodendrites.* ***(Right)*** *Color fundus photograph shows optic nerve edema in the eye of a patient with herpes zoster ophthalmicus. This finding is concerning for an active papillitis, which can be an early finding of acute retinal necrosis.*

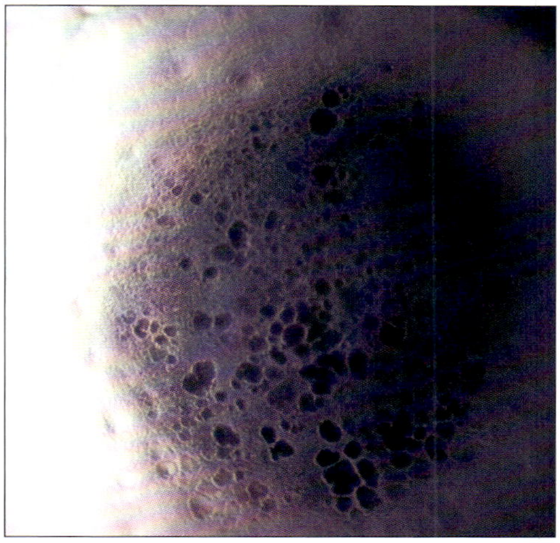

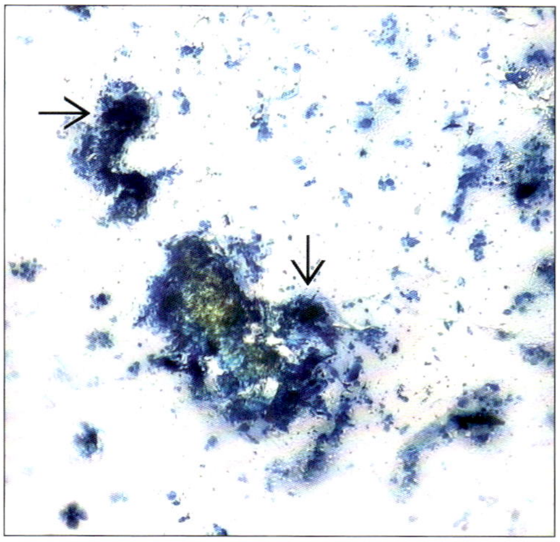

(Left) *Stellate keratic precipitates (KPs), seen in patients with anterior uveitis from varicella zoster virus infection, are distributed over the entire cornea as opposed to the usual distribution in the inferior 1/3 of the cornea. Though diffuse KPs are suggestive of the diagnosis, they are not diagnostic as a stand-alone finding.* ***(Right)*** *Tzanck smear shows multinucleated giant cells, which are characteristic of herpes simplex virus or varicella zoster virus. (Courtesy B. Hall, MD.)*

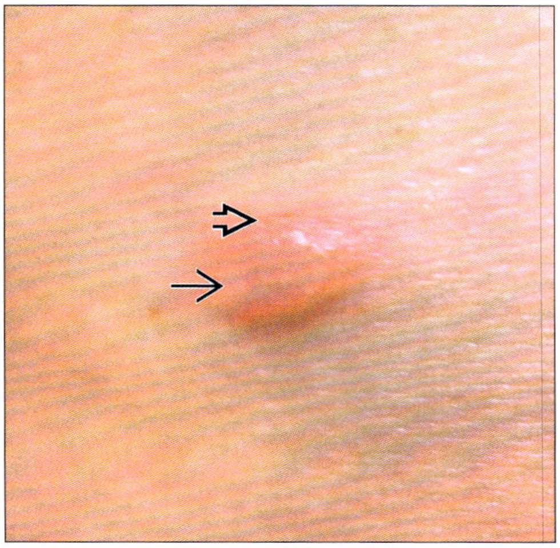

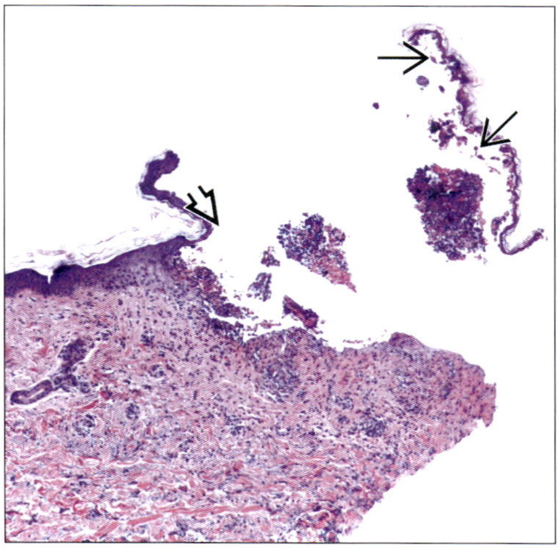

(Left) *A small vesicle with clear fluid on an erythematous base, a.k.a. "dew drop on a rose petal," is the characteristic skin lesion of chickenpox with varicella infection. Lesions progress from erythematous macules to raised papules, vesicles, pustules, and, finally, crusting lesions. (Courtesy A. Lipworth, MD.)* ***(Right)*** *At scanning magnification, an intraepidermal blister and acantholytic cells are noted in this biopsy of primary varicella. (Courtesy H. Sidhu, MD.)*

IRITIS/IRIDOCYCLITIS

Key Facts

Introduction
- Intraocular inflammation of iris only (iritis) or iris and ciliary body (iridocyclitis)

Demographics
- Uveitis causes 10% of blindness worldwide
- Incidence of anterior uveitis: 8-12 per 100,000

Presentation
- Classic triad of pain, photophobia, and blurred vision
- Redness around limbus, miosis, irregular pupils due to posterior synechiae, keratic precipitates, iris nodules (Koeppe, Busacca), hypopyon
- Complications: Synechiae and secondary glaucoma, cataract, cystoid macular edema, neovascularization of ora serrata or optic disc with vitreous or retinal hemorrhage, retinal detachment, retinoschisis

Evaluation/Work-Up
- Fluorescein angiography shows leakage from small perifoveal capillaries into adjacent retina during late vessel filling or abnormal leakage throughout fundus
- PCR of aqueous humor aspirate: Herpes simplex virus keratouveitis; Cytomegalovirus or varicella zoster virus are also possibilities

Treatment
- 4 major complications: Band keratopathy, cataract, glaucoma, cystoid macular edema
- Topical corticosteroids are primary initial treatment for noninfectious anterior uveitis
- Topical antibiotics for infectious etiology
- Mydriatics and cycloplegics ↓ pain from ciliary spasm
- Nongranulomatous uveitis may last days to weeks
- Granulomatous uveitis may last months to years

*(**Left**) Slit-lamp photo shows cells (white blood cells) ➔ and flare (plasma protein) in the anterior chamber, a common finding in anterior uveitis. (**Right**) Band keratopathy ➔ is calcific degeneration of the superficial cornea that involves Bowman layer and can be seen in chronic inflammation.*

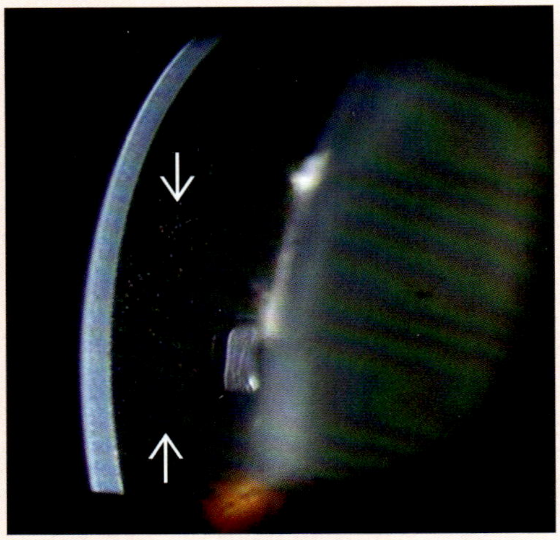

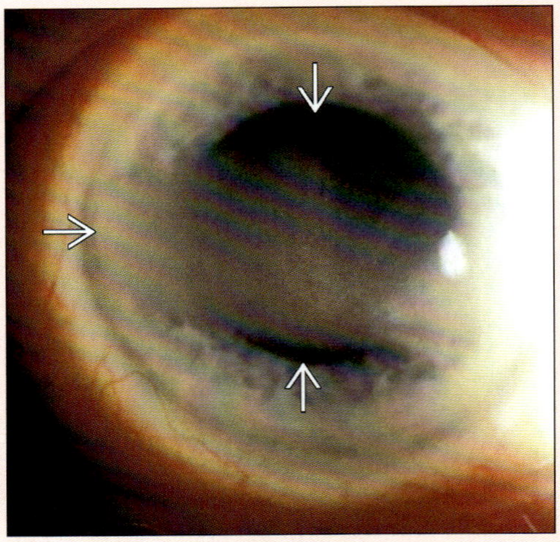

*(**Left**) Slit-lamp photo shows hypopyon in a patient with anterior uveitis. Hypopyon ⇨ is the collection of white blood cells in the anterior chamber, which pool inferiorly due to the effect of gravity. (**Right**) This image shows iris bombé, a complication of severe iritis. Adhesions develop between the pupillary margin and anterior lens capsule, tethering the pupillary margin to the lens capsule ➔. Accumulation of fluid within iris stroma from severe inflammation causes the iris stroma to bow forward ➔. Aggressive control of inflammation is required.*

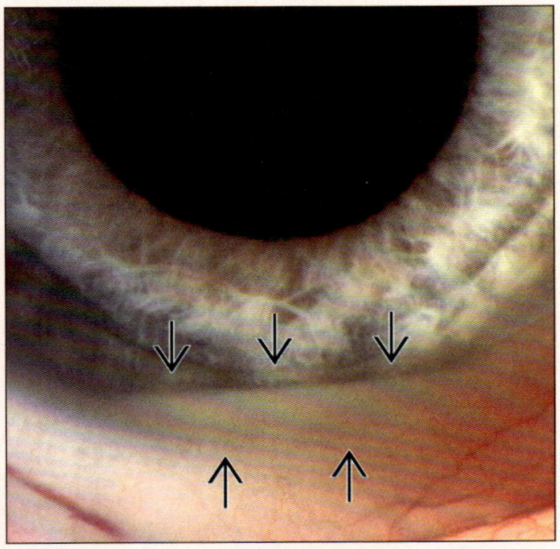

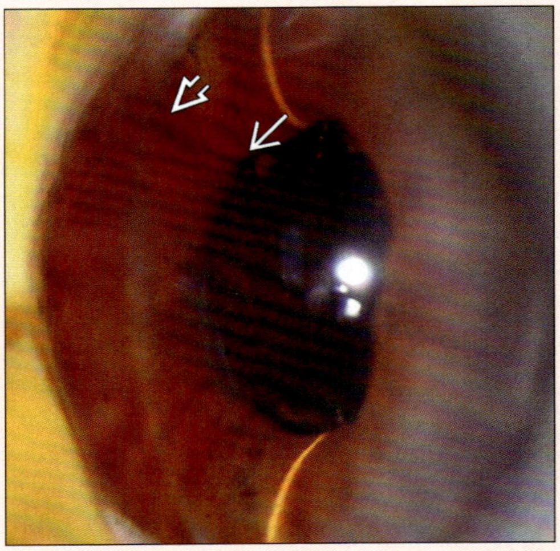

IRITIS/IRIDOCYCLITIS

INTRODUCTION

Synonyms

- Anterior uveitis: Inflammation of iris (iritis) &/or ciliary body (iridocyclitis)
- Chronic iridocyclitis: Pars planitis or peripheral uveitis

Subtypes

- Classification system: Standardization of Uveitis Nomenclature (SUN) criteria
  - Duration
    - Limited: ≤ 3 months (acute: < 6 weeks)
    - Persistent: > 3 months (chronic: > 6 weeks)
  - Pattern
    - Acute: Sudden onset with limited duration
    - Recurrent: Repeated inflammatory episodes with periods of disease quiescence lasting > 3 months in duration without treatment
    - Chronic: Persistent disease with relapse occurring ≤ 3 months after discontinuing treatment
  - Etiology
    - Autoimmune: Ocular, systemic
    - Infectious: Viral, bacterial, fungal, protozoal
    - Malignant or masquerade syndromes
  - Inflammation
    - Nongranulomatous
      - Small, fine keratic precipitates of neutrophils, lymphocytes, and epithelioid cells
      - No inciting pathogen found in most cases
    - Granulomatous
      - Large mutton-fat keratic precipitates with mononuclear macrophages, giant cells, and epithelioid cells
      - Seen with active microbial invasion
      - Posterior uveitis is common

DEMOGRAPHICS

Etiology/Risk Factors

- Caucasian
- Age range: 20-50 years; peak at 20-30 years
- History of iritis, intraocular injection, or surgery
- Blunt ocular trauma
- HLA-B27

Epidemiology

- Incidence of anterior uveitis: 8-12 per 100,000
  - Incidence increases to 220 per 100,000 in those aged 65 years or older
- Uveitis causes roughly 10% of blindness worldwide
  - Among various types of uveitis, anterior uveitis (including iritis and iridocyclitis) is most common
- Equal prevalence in males and females

PRESENTATION

Symptoms

- Acute disease: Unilateral eye pain, photophobia, redness, irritation, ↑ tearing, ↓ vision, floaters
- Chronic disease: Insidious onset of gradually ↓ vision with blurriness and diffuse redness, photophobia, and minimal pain
  - History of recurring symptoms and trials of topical or systemic medications with multiple ophthalmology consults
- Rule out exposure to histoplasmosis, toxoplasmosis, tuberculosis, and syphilis

Exam Findings

- Nongranulomatous anterior uveitis
  - Dilated circumferential blood vessels at limbus, keratic precipitates, band keratopathy, cells and flare in anterior chamber, hypopyon, rubeosis iridis, peripheral anterior synechiae, posterior synechiae, anterior lens capsule fibrin ring, anterior vitreous cells
- Granulomatous anterior uveitis
  - Circumferential corneal flush, abnormally constricted irregular pupil, mutton-fat keratic precipitates, anterior chamber cells and flare, Koeppe nodules at pupillary margin, Busacca nodules on the iris surface, anterior vitreous cells, chorioretinitis
  - Chorioretinitis presents as yellow-white patches seen with direct ophthalmoscope through hazy vitreous
- Aqueous cells and flare are graded on 0-4+ scale, indicating active inflammation
  - Iritis: Cells appear mostly in aqueous fluid
  - Iridocyclitis: Cells distributed equally within aqueous fluid and vitreous
- Severe uveitis: Hypopyon, fibrin clot in anterior chamber, posterior synechiae, acute angle-closure glaucoma, iris bombe, fixed pupil
- Chronic iridocyclitis: Band keratopathy, iris atrophy, cyclitic membrane formation, ciliary body detachment, exudate overlaying ora serrata and inferior pars plana, hypotony, phthisis bulbi
- Intraocular pressure (IOP) may be increased or decreased
  - Increased IOP: Trabecular meshwork inflammation and plugging with inflammatory cell debris, anterior synechiae, pupillary block from posterior synechiae, iris neovascularization, chronic glucocorticoids
  - Decreased IOP: Inflammation of ciliary body or cyclitic membrane formation decreases aqueous humor production

DIFFERENTIAL DIAGNOSIS

Posterior Uveitis With Spread to Anterior Chamber

- Patient may complain of floaters
- Optic nerve head edema/hyperemia, perivascular exudates, vascular sheathing, cystoid macular edema, pars planitis, choroiditis, retinitis, retinal detachment, loss of foveal light reflex, macular degeneration

Panophthalmitis

- Inflammation of all segments of eye
- Often due to sepsis or perforating eye injury
- Extreme eye pain, eye congestion, periorbital edema
- May require enucleation or evisceration

Acute Angle-Closure Glaucoma

- Nonreactive, mid-dilated pupil
- "Steamy" or cloudy cornea
- No posterior synechiae

IRITIS/IRIDOCYCLITIS

Conjunctivitis
- Ocular discharge, redness, papillae or follicles, ± preauricular lymphadenopathy
- Normal pupillary reaction
- Absent pain, photophobia, ciliary body injection

Pars Planitis
- Idiopathic intermediate bilateral uveitis
- Painless decrease in visual acuity, anterior vitreous cells, vitreous condensation, peripheral retinal vasculitis

Keratitis/Keratoconjunctivitis
- Vision may be blurred with pain and photophobia
- Some causes of keratitis can lead to and overlap with anterior uveitis

EVALUATION/WORK-UP

Labs
- Tailor work-up to individual patient based on history, review of symptoms (ROS), and clinical exam
  - Refer patient to internist to rule out associated systemic diseases based on history and ROS
- Systemic work-up is indicated if anterior uveitis is unresponsive to treatment
  - CBC: Leukocytosis
  - ESR: Nonspecific marker of inflammation
  - Mantoux test, skin PPD, quantiferon gold, CXR: Tuberculosis exposure
  - Venereal disease research laboratories, *Treponema pallidum* hemagglutination test: Syphilis
  - HLA-B27, ANA: Associated with recurrent bilateral uveitis and collagen vascular disease
  - Serum ACE, CXR, CT scan of chest: Sarcoidosis
  - PCR of aqueous humor aspirate: HSV keratouveitis
    - ANCA, Lyme titer, *Bartonella*, antiphospholipid antibody, and lysozyme are other serologies for rarer conditions that can be assessed

Imaging
- Fluorescein angiography shows leakage from small perifoveal capillaries into adjacent retina during late vessel filling or abnormal leakage throughout fundus
  - Leakage near peripapillary retina presents as papilledema
- Gonioscopy for anterior synechiae, angle closure
- Fluorescein angiography to rule out cystoid macular edema (CME), serous retinal detachment, choroiditis, vascular changes
- B-scan ultrasonography to rule out posterior segment pathology, especially if lens opacity prevents adequate funduscopic exam
- Ocular coherence tomography to rule out CME

TREATMENT

Medical
- Corticosteroids: Topical, periocular, or systemic
  - Primary initial treatment for noninfectious uveitis
  - ↓ inflammation and prevent structural damage to eye
    - ↓ exudate leakage into eye, ↑ cell wall stability, inhibit lysozyme release from granulocytes, inhibit lymphocyte circulation
  - Concomitant NSAIDs may allow for decreased therapeutic corticosteroid dosing
- Immunomodulators
  - Antimetabolites: Methotrexate, azathioprine, mycophenolate mofetil
  - Alkylating agents: Cyclophosphamide, chlorambucil
  - T-cell inhibitors: Ciclosporin, tacrolimus
  - Biologic agents: Etanercept, infliximab, daclizumab
- Antimicrobials: Antibacterials, antivirals, antifungals, antiprotazoals
- Mydriatics and cycloplegics: Atropine
- Symptomatic therapy
  - Analgesics for pain from inflammation
  - Shaded glasses for photophobia
  - Glaucoma medications to decrease IOP

Surgical
- Treat pupillary block with iridectomy
- Surgically remove cataracts and implant posterior capsular intraocular lens
- Laser or surgery for retinal detachment

Follow-Up
- Frequency depends on severity of initial disease presentation
- ↑ interval between follow-up appointments as frequency of inflammation flare-ups ↓ with treatment

Prognosis
- Ranges from self-limiting in mild disease to loss of vision in recalcitrant cases
  - Decreased vision secondary to corneal edema, anterior chamber cells or flare, CME
- Most patients with mild or moderate inflammation improve with treatment
- Damaged blood vessels may leak, causing recurrent, severe disease, requiring aggressive therapy
- Cataracts can develop in eyes with vitritis, posterior inflammation, and long-term corticosteroid use
- Glaucoma
  - Anterior synechiae block trabecular meshwork outflow tract
  - Posterior synechiae create build-up of aqueous humor behind iris, pushing iris tissue forward and blocking trabecular meshwork
- Neovascularization of ora serrata or optic disc
- Retinal detachment
  - Due to vitritis and strand formation → retinal traction
- Nongranulomatous uveitis may last days to weeks
- Granulomatous uveitis may last months to years

SELECTED REFERENCES

1. Mozayan A et al: Acute anterior uveitis following intravitreal injection of bevacizumab. Ophthalmic Surg Lasers Imaging Retina. 44(1):25-7, 2013
2. Agrawal RV et al: Current approach in diagnosis and management of anterior uveitis. Indian J Ophthalmol. 58(1):11-9, 2010
3. Zheng YZ et al: [The diagnosis and treatment analysis of anterior uveitis.] Zhonghua Yan Ke Za Zhi. 46(1):25-8, 2010
4. Holland GN et al: Chronic anterior uveitis in children: clinical characteristics and complications. Am J Ophthalmol. 147(4):667-678, 2009
5. Khan AA et al: Acute anterior uveitis. BMJ. 339:b2986, 2009

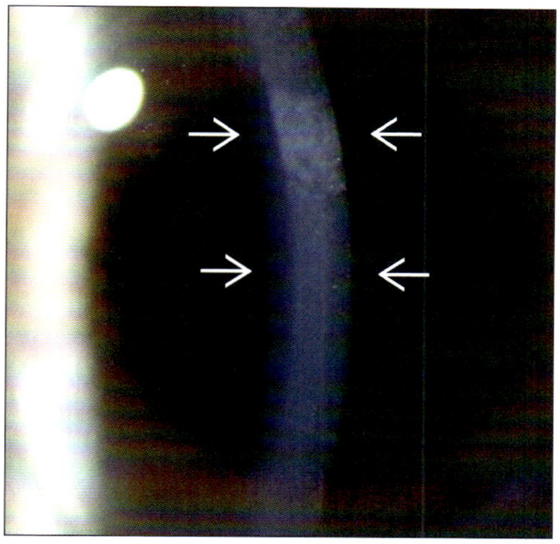

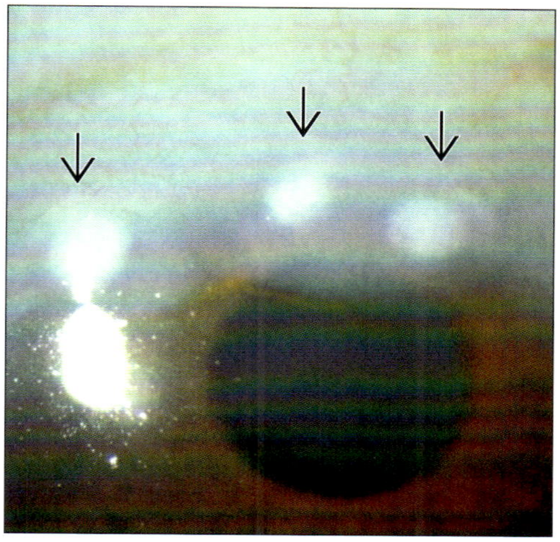

(Left) *This image displays fine keratic precipitates (KPs) ➔ along the endothelial surface of the cornea, a characteristic finding in anterior uveitis caused by iritis and iridocyclitis. KPs are best seen using optical section illumination with the slit-lamp beam. Dysfunction of the endothelium leads to acute corneal edema.* ***(Right)*** *Image displays mutton-fat KPs →, seen in granulomatous iritis and iridocyclitis. Mutton-fat KPs form as a result of deposition of macrophages on the posterior surface of Descemet membrane.*

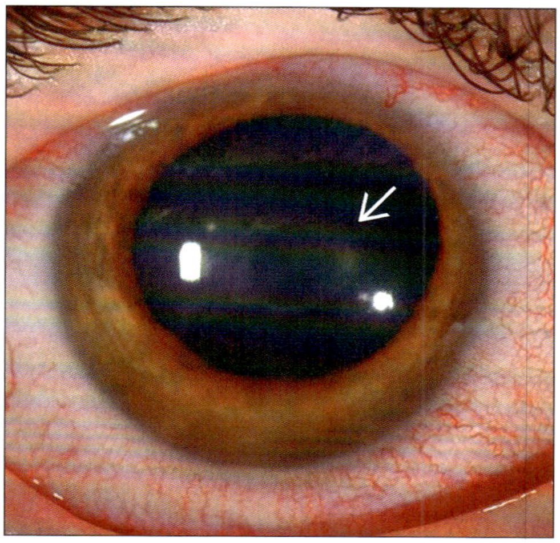

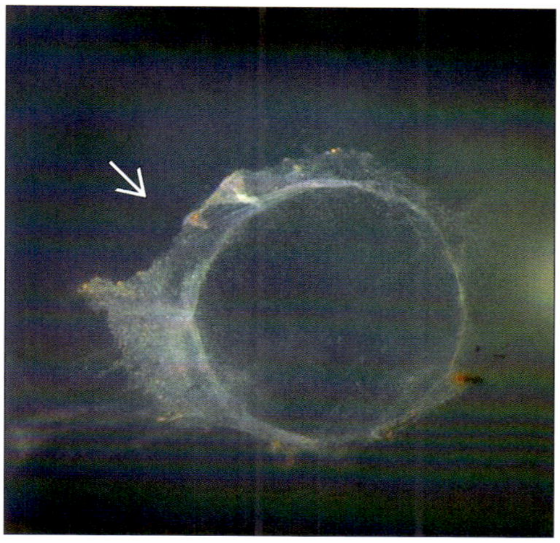

(Left) *Slit-lamp photo of severe iritis demonstrates circumlimbal conjunctival injection, due to decreased oxygen to the iris, and a fibrin ring ➔ on the anterior lens capsule. Circumlimbal injection leads to rubeosis iridis, extension of new vessels into the anterior chamber angle, and angle-closure glaucoma.* ***(Right)*** *Image shows a fibrin ring ➔ that has developed on the anterior lens capsule in a case of severe iritis. The pigmented fibrin ring derives from clotting factors.*

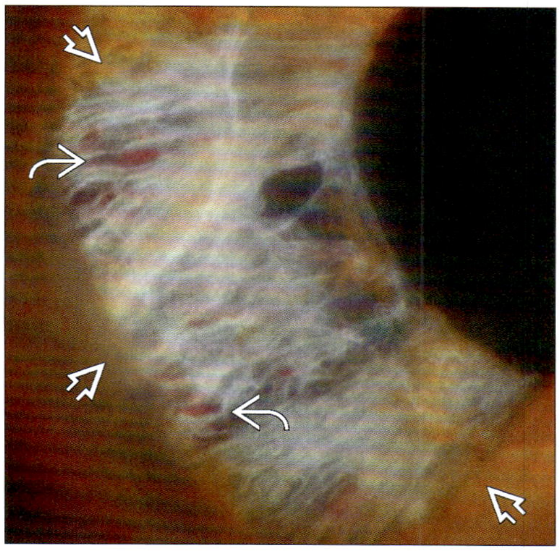

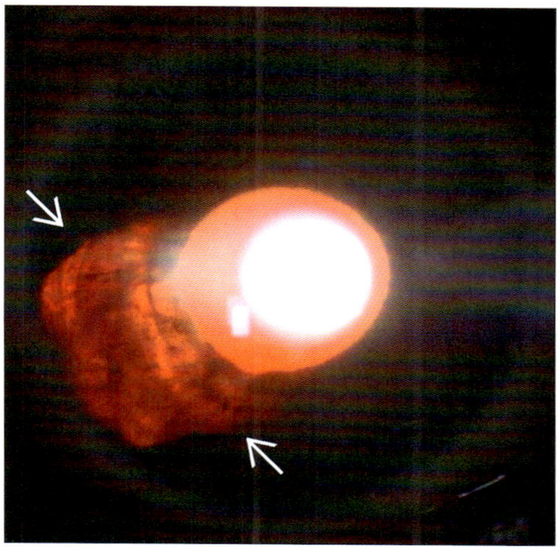

(Left) *Slit-lamp photo demonstrates sectoral iris atrophy ➔ in severe iritis. Dilated blood vessels ➔ are seen within the atrophied and inflamed iris stroma.* ***(Right)*** *Iris atrophy ➔ seen in iritis or iridocyclitis can be viewed with retroillumination on slit-lamp exam. Iris atrophy may be patchy or sectoral (as in this case) and is usually described in terms of clock hours involved.*

TRAUMATIC IRITIS/IRIDOCYCLITIS

Key Facts

Introduction

- Inflammation of iris or anterior uvea due to contusion injury to iris or electric shock
- Causes include blunt force with contusion injury, foreign body (FB), retained cataractous lens material following cataract extraction, electrical injury
- Post-traumatic iridocyclitis: Inflammatory reaction of uvea and iris with onset ≤ 3 days of eye trauma
- Corneal edema causes posterior displacement of anterior chamber, which places stress on iris root, triggering inflammatory response

Presentation

- Watering red eye with blurry vision, photophobia, and pain
- Scattering of iris pigment onto corneal endothelium, trabecular meshwork, anterior lens capsule, or vitreous
- Cells and flare in anterior chamber or hypopyon
- Iridodialysis or cyclodialysis: Base of iris separates from iris root
- Rupture or tear of iris sphincter
- Anisocoria or poorly reactive pupil

Treatment

- Spontaneous recovery usually occurs
- Mild traumatic iritis usually resolves spontaneously and can be managed without medical intervention
- Topical cycloplegic or mydriatic agents provide symptomatic pain relief

Complications

- Damage to corneal epithelium by FB provides pathway for infectious agents to enter eye
- Metallic FBs may remain inside eye for years without causing inflammatory response
- Sympathetic ophthalmia is vision-threatening complication following trauma to eye

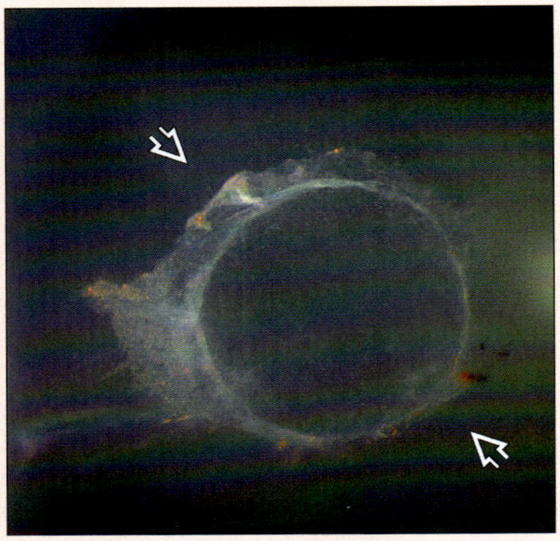

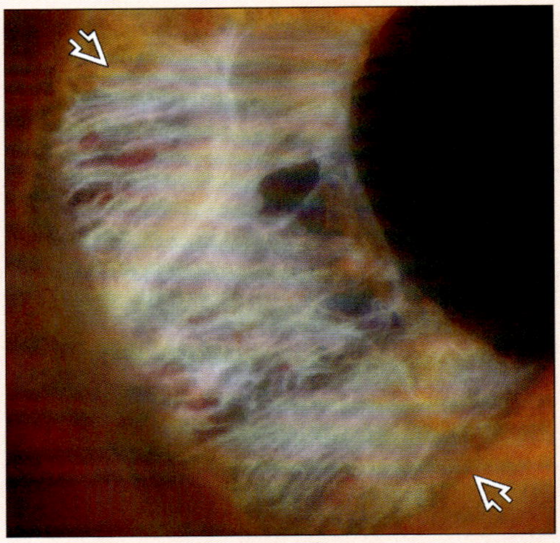

(Left) *The Vossius lenticular ring forms when dislodged iris pigment deposits onto the anterior lens capsule after blunt trauma. Iris pigment may also deposit onto the posterior corneal endothelium and cause cloudy vision or onto the trabecular meshwork, raising the intraocular pressure.* ***(Right)*** *Slit-lamp photo demonstrates iridoschisis after blunt ocular trauma. A portion of the anterior iris stroma has detached from the posterior iris stroma, leaving sections of the iris thin and depigmented.*

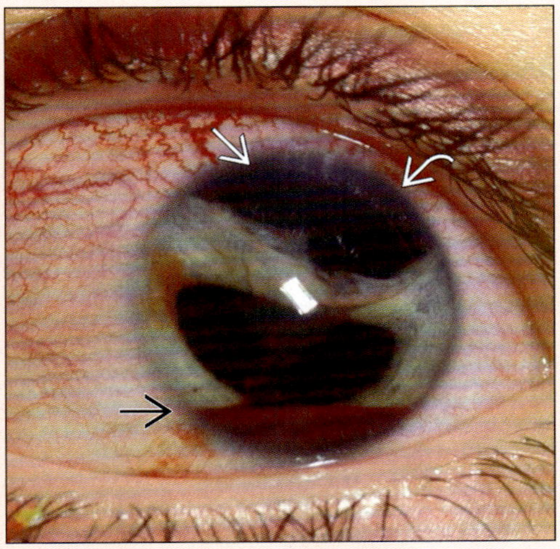

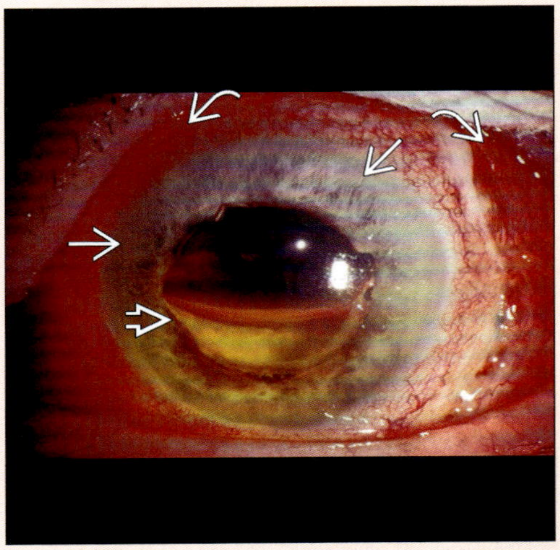

(Left) *Photo shows iridodialysis and hyphema in the anterior chamber after blunt trauma. The iris stroma has separated from the iris root, creating an accessory pupil. A pressure wave following blunt injury strikes the lens, and the blunt force is redirected peripherally to the iris root.* ***(Right)*** *Slit-lamp photo shows severe traumatic iritis after a bottle-rocket injury to the eye. Acutely injected conjunctiva, small iris stromal tears, and edematous fluid within the anterior chamber are seen.*

TRAUMATIC IRITIS/IRIDOCYCLITIS

INTRODUCTION

Definitions

- Traumatic iridocyclitis: Inflammation of iris or anterior uvea, usually developing within 3 days of blunt eye trauma or following intraocular surgery or electric shock

Subtypes

- Blunt ocular injury or contusion
  - May be coup or contrecoup injury
  - Corneal edema causes posterior displacement of anterior chamber, which places stress on iris root, triggering inflammatory response
  - Pressure wave following blunt injury strikes lens, and blunt force is redirected peripherally to iris root
  - Disrupts ability of ciliary body to secrete aqueous humor, leading to ocular hypotony
- Foreign body (FB) penetrating injury
  - Penetrating eye injury or corneal abrasion from a fingernail "poke" to eye, metal object, organic material, contact lens abuse, or insect (e.g., bee) sting
- Electrical shock injury
  - Due to electric shock, lightening strike, Taser gun

DEMOGRAPHICS

Epidemiology

- Continuous ↑ in ocular trauma incidence has been seen

PRESENTATION

Symptoms

- Watering red eye with blurry vision
- Constant aching or throb radiating to brow or temple
- Photophobia with pain upon direct illumination into uninjured contralateral eye
- History of symptom onset within 3 days after blunt eye injury

Exam Findings

- Ocular contusion injury
  - Decreased visual acuity
  - Scattering of iris pigment onto corneal endothelium, trabecular meshwork, anterior lens capsule (Vossius lenticular ring), or into the vitreous
  - Cells and flare in anterior chamber &/or hypopyon
  - Ciliary or perilimbal injection
  - Iridodialysis or cyclodialysis
  - Iridoschisis
  - Rupture or tear of iris sphincter
  - Anisocoria or poorly reactive pupil
  - Anterior chamber angle recession
    - Separated strands of uveal meshwork
    - Seen with hyphema, though degree of angle recession does not correlate to amount of bleeding
  - Rupture of anterior lens capsule or cataract formation
  - Self-limiting hyphema, miosis, mydriasis, or iridoplegia
  - Decreased intraocular pressure (IOP) initially due to ciliary body injury &/or inflammatory mediators
  - Absence of cells in anterior vitreous
- Electrical shock injury
  - Iritis, bilateral cataracts, and macular cysts

DIFFERENTIAL DIAGNOSIS

Microhyphema

- Bleeding into anterior chamber due to trauma to vasculature of iris or angle
- Microscopic red blood cells floating in anterior chamber seen only on slit-lamp exam
  - These disappear with green light whereas traumatic iritis white cells still persist with green light
- Complications include increased IOP, rebleeding, corneal blood staining in presence of endothelial dysfunction
- Treat with topical corticosteroids and antiglaucoma agents, shield eye, and rest

Ophthalmia Nodosa

- Delayed granulomatous inflammation of iris, cornea, conjunctiva, or retina caused by hairs from certain insects
- Inflammatory iris nodules &/or hypopyon
- Treat with local corticosteroids and remove hair with keratectomy, keratoplasty, iridectomy, or vitrectomy

TREATMENT

Medical

- Spontaneous recovery can occur in mild cases
- Topical cycloplegic or mydriatic agents provide symptomatic pain relief
  - Scopolamine, cyclopentolate, homatropine
  - Prevents painful reflex spasm of ciliary muscle and iris sphincter
- Topical steroids relieve pain and speed recovery time
  - Prednisolone acetate 1%

Prognosis

- Contusion injury may permanently alter globe structure
- Contralateral eye may also be damaged in severe blunt trauma
- Damage to corneal epithelium by FB provides pathway for infectious agents to enter eye
  - Antibiotic treatment may be necessary
- Metallic FBs may remain inside eye for years without causing inflammatory response
  - Manage conservatively until inflammation or visually significant cataract develops
- Sympathetic ophthalmia is vision-threatening complication following trauma to eye

SELECTED REFERENCES

1. Limaïem R et al: An unusual clinical presentation of ocular trauma in a child. Int Ophthalmol. 33(1):87-9, 2013
2. Heiner JD et al: Eye pain after blunt ocular trauma. Traumatic mydriasis with hyphema. Ann Emerg Med. 59(6):456, 468, 2012
3. Dezhagah H: Circular anterior lens capsule rupture caused by blunt ocular trauma. Middle East Afr J Ophthalmol. 17(1):103-5, 2010

MALIGNANT MELANOMA OF IRIS

Key Facts

Introduction

- Malignant neoplasm derived from neuroectodermal melanocytes within iris stroma

Demographics

- Incidence of 0.4-1.2 in 1,000,000 per year
- Risk factors: Increased age, light-colored irides, fair skin tone, UV light exposure

Presentation

- Grossly visible dark brown or yellow elevated lesion on inferior half of iris or diffuse iris discoloration that does not disturb vision, noted by patient or by examiner on routine eye exam
- Tension on iris from tumor causes pupillary peaking, ectropion irides, and failure to dilate with pharmacologic agents at site of lesion (iris splinting)
- Increased likelihood of metastasis: Choroid or ciliary body involvement, tumor diameter > 3 mm & depth > 1 mm, epithelioid cell type, secondary glaucoma from sloughing of tumor cells, extrascleral involvement, prominent vasculature

Evaluation/Work-Up

- Slit-lamp biomicroscopy, anterior segment photography, B-scan ultrasonography, anterior segment OCT, incisional biopsy

Treatment

- Conservative management with close observation of nevus size and growth rate when mass is likely a nevus
- After excision with iridectomy, follow-up every 6 months for 2-3 years, then annually for recurrence
- Evaluate for and treat hematogenous metastasis to liver, lung, bone, or other organs

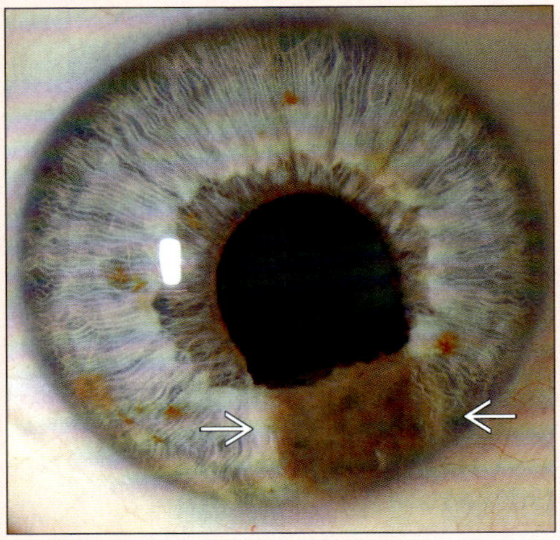

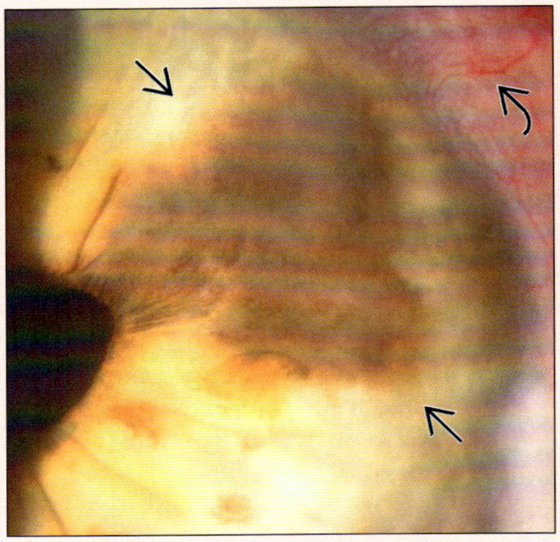

(Left) *Malignant iris melanoma → is more common in lighter irides. A nodular mass is grossly visible on the iris surface and is clearly demarcated from the iris stroma by its dark brown pigmentation.* ***(Right)*** *This slit-lamp photo illustrates a malignant melanoma of the iris. A lesion typically presents in middle-aged or elderly patients as a brown nodular mass → within the iris stroma and is well vascularized, with a large vessel from the conjunctiva feeding the mass ↷, as seen here.*

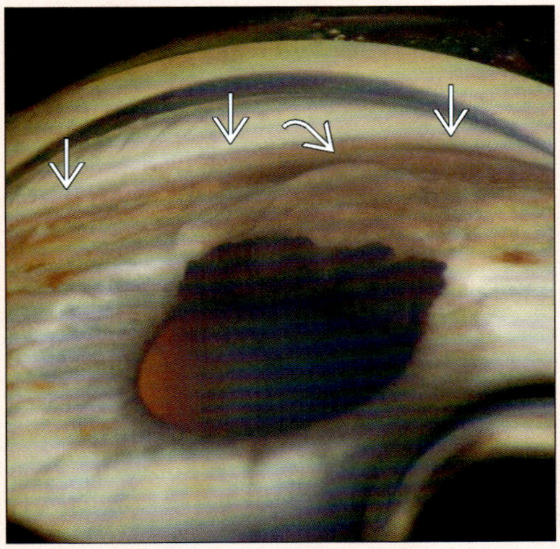

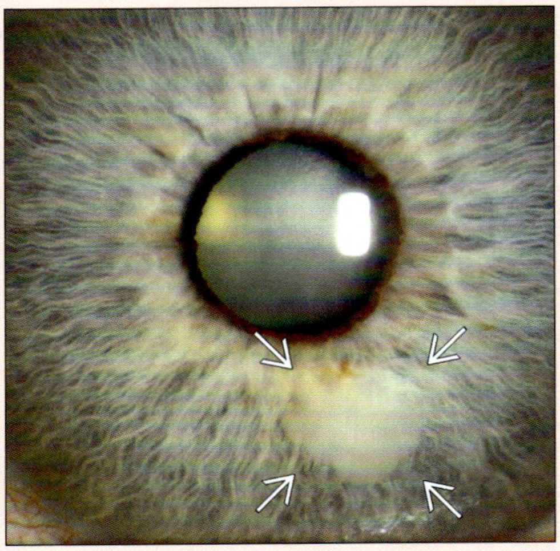

(Left) *Gonioscopy image shows a malignant melanoma of the iris through a gonioscope lens. The raised lesion → creates traction on the iris stroma and distorts the pupillary margin, causing characteristic pupillary peaking. Gonioscopy allows the examiner to view the depth of the mass and the involvement of the anterior chamber angle →.* ***(Right)*** *Slit-lamp photo shows an amelanotic "tapioca" melanoma →. This rare lesion owes its name to the resemblance of its granular surface to tapioca pudding.*

MALIGNANT MELANOMA OF IRIS

INTRODUCTION

Definitions

- Malignant proliferation of neuroectodermally derived melanocytes located in iris stroma
- Consists of epithelioid cells, spindle cells, or both
- Often causes unilateral glaucoma when tumor cells shed into aqueous humor or directly invade angle
- Shields criteria for clinical diagnosis
  - Size > 3 mm in diameter and 1 mm in thickness
  - Lesion replaces iris stroma
  - 3 of the following 5 features
    - Photographic documentation of growth
    - Secondary glaucoma
    - Secondary cataract
    - Prominent vasculature
    - Ectropion irides

Subtypes

- Circumscribed iris melanoma: Elevated tumor with distinct margins
- Diffuse iris melanoma: 10% of iris melanomas
  - Presents as slow-growing tumor with multiple patchy flat foci or diffuse, continuous pattern of tumor cell distribution within iris stroma
  - Measures ≥ 6 clock hours in size
  - Causes unilateral hyperchromic heterochromia and secondary glaucoma
- Tapioca (amelanotic) melanoma: Nonpigmented nodules resembling tapioca in pudding that may cause secondary glaucoma or hyperpigmented hyperchromic iris
  - These are malignant even without pigment
- Iris metastasis: Yellow, white, or pink nodules within iris stroma that may cause secondary glaucoma or pseudohypopyon when tumor cells shed into aqueous humor

DEMOGRAPHICS

Etiology/Risk Factors

- Risk factors: Increased age, blue or green irides, fair skin tone that sunburns easily, UV light exposure, congenital ocular melanocytosis, dysplastic nevus syndrome
  - Rare in darker pigmented irides, though prognosis is same among various races
- No strong familial inheritance pattern exists, but likelihood of metastasis or melanoma-related death increases in cases associated with
  - Monosomy of chromosome 3
  - Partial duplication of chromosome 8q
  - Complementary gains of material on chromosome 6p and loss of material from chromosome 6q

Epidemiology

- Most common primary malignancy of iris; 50-70% of all iris tumors
- Incidence: 0.4-1.2 in 1,000,000 per year; increases with age
- 5% of all uveal melanomas
  - > 80% involve choroid; ~ 10% involve ciliary body
- 98% of cases occur in whites
- Average age at diagnosis is 40-50 years
  - Diagnosed 10-20 years earlier than other uveal melanomas due to visibility of lesion

PRESENTATION

Symptoms

- Often asymptomatic other than visible lesion on iris
  - Most commonly located on inferior half of iris due to UV light exposure
- Patient may complain of poor vision or eye pain if there is secondary glaucoma

Exam Findings

- Grossly visible, dark brown or yellow elevated lesion or diffusely discolored iris, noted by patient or by examiner on routine eye exam
  - Lesion can be amelanotic or maximally pigmented with jagged or smooth border
  - Size of lesion varies with growth rate; average size at diagnosis is 6 mm in diameter and 2 mm in depth
  - Prominent blood vessels supplying tumor may cause spontaneous hyphema
- Hyperpigmented heterochromic iridum occurs when melanoma of anterior chamber seeds into iris, causing diffusely pigmented iris and often secondary glaucoma
- Tension on iris from tumor causes pupillary peaking, ectropion iridis, and failure to dilate with pharmacologic agents at site of lesion (iris splinting)
- Increased likelihood of metastasis: Choroid or ciliary body involvement, tumor size > 3 mm and depth > 1 mm with rapid growth, epithelioid cell type, secondary glaucoma from sloughing of tumor cells, extrascleral involvement, prominent vasculature
- Majority of patients have visual acuity of 20/40 or better
- Secondary glaucoma
  - Invasion of malignant cells into trabecular meshwork
  - Decreased aqueous outflow due to pigment-ingesting macrophages blocking angle
  - Angle closure
  - Neovascularization

DIFFERENTIAL DIAGNOSIS

Benign Iris Nevus

- Localized pigmented melanotic lesion < 3 mm in diameter and < 0.5 mm in depth
- Located within iris stroma between pupillary margin and iris root
- May cause pupillary peaking or ectropion iridis, but rarely contains intrinsic vasculature

Epithelioid Cyst

- Globe transillumination on slit-lamp exam transmits light
- Cystic lesion on B-scan ultrasound

Congenital Ocular Melanocytosis

- Thickened choroidal stroma infiltrated with pigmented benign melanocytes
- Iris heterochromia, retinal pigment epithelium abnormalities with drusen on surface of choroid, patchy areas of pigmentation within sclera

MALIGNANT MELANOMA OF IRIS

- Darkly pigmented melanotic uveal tissue blocks light transillumination on slit-lamp exam

Heterochromia

- Congenital: 1 iris has different color than the other due to excessive pigmentation of iris stroma
- Partial: Section of iris has different color than the rest
- Acquired heterochromia: Secondary to trauma, inflammation, pharmaceuticals, tumors
- No elevated iris mass or increased vasculature supplying discolored area
- No association with glaucoma

Pigmentary Glaucoma

- Increased trabecular meshwork pigment that obstructs trabecular meshwork and increases IOP, causing bilateral secondary open-angle glaucoma
- Iris defects that transilluminate in spoke-like pattern
- Seen in young adults with myopia

EVALUATION/WORK-UP

Labs

- Incisional biopsy or fine-needle aspiration for questionable lesions suspicious for malignancy
- Systemic evaluation for tumors suspicious of metastasis includes physical exam, liver function tests, US or CT of liver, CXR

Pathology

- Histology shows atypical melanocytes with high nuclear to cytoplasmic ratio replacing iris stroma and frequent mitotic figures
  - Spindle melanoma cells: Fusiform or cigar-shaped cells with mildly atypical features
    - Most common type seen in iris melanoma with better prognosis
  - Epithelioid melanoma cells: Spherical shape with pronounced anaplasia
    - Rare in iris melanoma

Imaging

- Slit-lamp biomicroscopy, gonioscopy, and fundus exam to show progressive growth and rule out involvement of ciliary body or choroid
- Transillumination of globe
  - If tumor is confined to iris, will not project a shadow in pars plicata
  - If tumor involves iris and ciliary body, will project a shadow into pars plicata &/or pars plana region(s)
- Photography of anterior segment and angle (goniophotography) to follow size, location, growth rate, color, surface texture, vasculature, and extent of iris involvement prior to biopsy or treatment
- B-scan ultrasonography to rule out involvement of choroid or ciliary body and differentiate solid melanocytic tumor from cystic lesion
- Anterior and posterior segment optical coherence tomography (OCT) to rule out involvement of choroid or optic nerve

TREATMENT

Medical

- Conservative management with close observation of size and growth rate when lesion is nevus limited to iris
- Control IOP with topical or oral medications, laser trabeculoplasty, or ciliary body ablation; bevacizumab (Avastin) can reduce neovascularization
  - Avoid trabeculectomy or other open-eye procedures to avoid extraocular tumor spread
- Sunitinib (Sutent) is emerging therapy

Surgical

- Iridectomy, iridocyclectomy, iridogoniocyclectomy: Smaller lesions limited to iris, ciliary body, or angle (respectively) with minimal tumor seeding
- Plaque radiotherapy or proton beam irradiation: Residual tumor after excision or tumors too large for local resection
- Enucleation: Large lesions that cannot be resected, diffuse iris melanomas with seeding into aqueous, iris melanomas extending through sclera, painful and blind eye

Follow-Up

- Prior to treatment, follow tumor size, growth rate, color, vasculature, extent of iris involvement
- After excision, follow-up every 6 months for 2-3 years, then annually to observe for recurrence

Prognosis

- Melanoma of iris has better prognosis with less likelihood to metastasize compared to melanoma of choroid or ciliary body
  - 95% 10-year survival rate; 4-5% 10-year metastasis rate
- Hematogenous metastasis to liver, lung, bone, or other organs (need chest and abdomen CT)
- Risk factors for metastasis or death from primary iris melanoma
  - Increased age at diagnosis
  - Larger tumor size: Diameter > 3 mm or depth > 1 mm
  - Elevated IOP: Tumors that shed cells or pigment can cause secondary glaucoma with increased likelihood of metastasis
  - Location of tumor: Near iris root, ciliary body involvement, extrascleral tumor extension
  - Diffuse or ring growth pattern
  - Epithelioid cell type
  - Extrascleral tumor extension
- Complications: Glaucoma, cataract, heterochromia irides, ectropion uveae, extension into uvea with retinal detachment, hemangioma, spontaneous hyphema

SELECTED REFERENCES

1. Shields CL et al: Iris melanoma: features and prognosis in 317 children and adults. J AAPOS. 16(1):10-6, 2012
2. Demirci H et al: Iris melanocytoma: clinical features and natural course in 47 cases. Am J Ophthalmol. 139(3):468-75, 2005
3. Shields CL et al: Iris melanoma: risk factors for metastasis in 169 consecutive patients. Ophthalmology. 108(1):172-8, 2001
4. Batioğlu F et al: Malignant melanomas of the iris. Jpn J Ophthalmol. 42(4):281-5, 1998

MALIGNANT MELANOMA OF IRIS

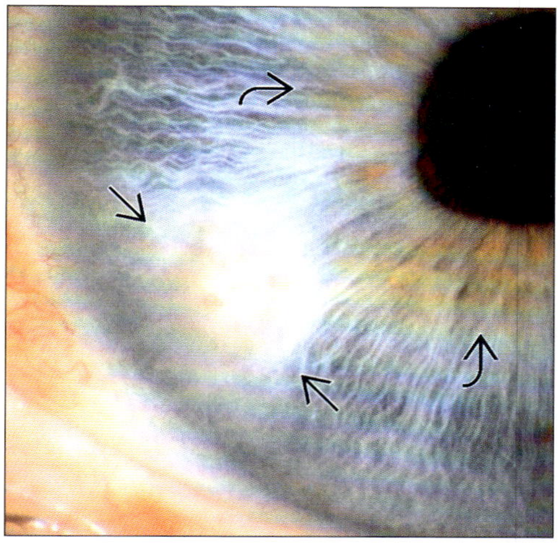

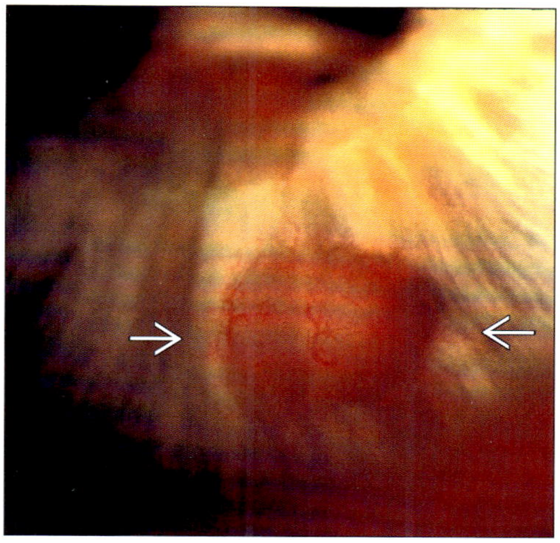

(Left) *"Tapioca" melanomas → cause hyperpigmented hyperchromic iridum → when malignant cells seed into the iris stroma. If tumor cells block the trabecular meshwork, a secondary glaucoma may result. "Tapioca" melanomas are quite rare and have a granular surface* ***(Right)*** *This slit-lamp image shows a highly vascularized malignant melanoma of the iris →. Iris melanomas are characteristically elevated off the iris surface and have a dark brown pigment. Feeder blood vessels course through the mass.*

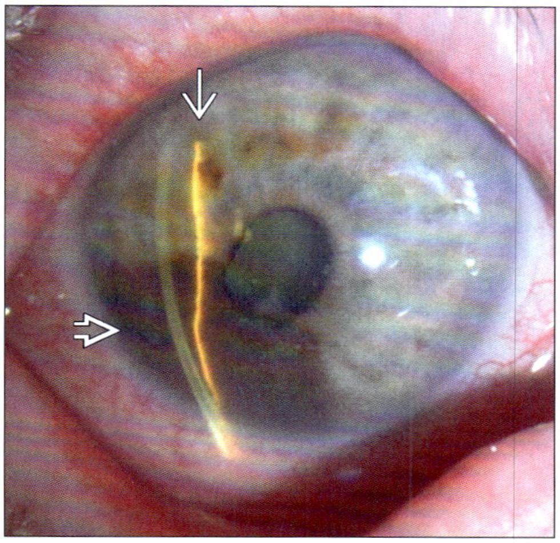

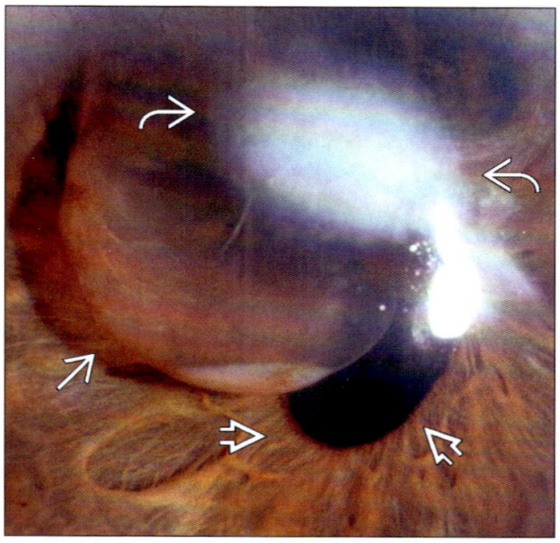

(Left) *Slit-lamp photo shows a dark brown malignant melanoma of the iris →, causing distortion of the pupil known as pupillary peaking. The raised lesion alters the contour of the iris stroma, seen as a bend in the slit-lamp light beam →.* ***(Right)*** *This slit-lamp photo shows a well-vascularized, benign epithelioid iris cyst → pushing on the corneal endothelium, which disrupts corneal deturgescence resulting in corneal edema →. Tension from the iris cyst creates pupillary peaking →.*

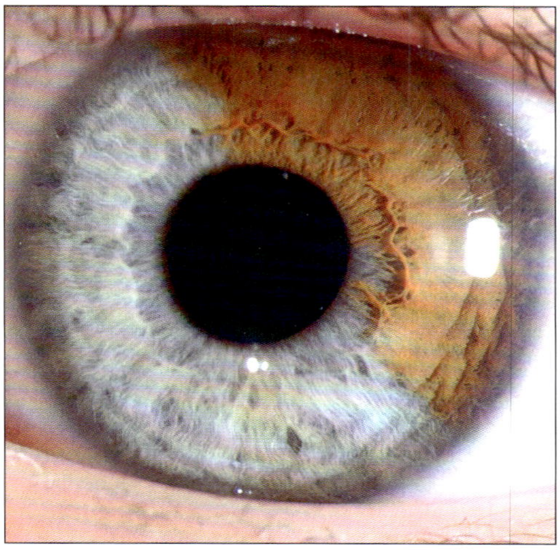

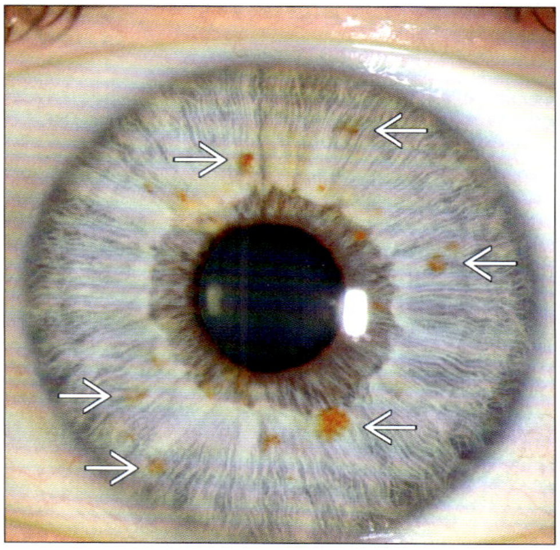

(Left) *Heterochromia can be mistaken for malignant melanoma. In complete heterochromia, 1 iris is of a different color than the other. In partial heterochromia, as seen here, a section of the iris is of a different color.* ***(Right)*** *Slit-lamp photo shows multiple benign iris nevi →. These lesions are typically first noticed at puberty, are < 3 mm in diameter and 0.5 mm in depth, and are not well vascularized, which differentiates them from malignant melanoma.*

IRIDODIALYSIS/CYCLODIALYSIS

Key Facts

Introduction
- Iridodialysis: Tear in iris root resulting in separation of iris from ciliary body and scleral spur, creating secondary pupil at limbus
- Cyclodialysis: Complete separation of longitudinal ciliary body muscle fibers from scleral spur, forming pathway for aqueous humor to drain from anterior chamber into suprachoroidal space

Presentation
- Iridodialysis: Monocular diplopia, glare, photophobia
- Cyclodialysis: Visible white sclera posterior to scleral spur, ocular hypotension, shallow anterior chamber, ciliary choroidal effusion, anterior or posterior displacement of iris in complete detachments
  - Macular hypotony is rare complication due to aqueous humor flow into suprachoroidal space

Evaluation/Work-Up
- Gonioscopy, ultrasound biomicroscopy, or anterior segment OCT

Treatment
- Iridodialysis: No treatment required for small defects unless patient is symptomatic
- If large iridodialysis, suture iris to sclera or suspend iris by suture from iris insertion site under limbus
- Cyclodialysis: Cycloplegic agent for 6-8 weeks for cyclodialysis clefts < 3 clock hours in size
- Injection of high-viscosity viscoelastic into anterior chamber to close cyclodialysis cleft and prevent communication between anterior chamber and suprachoroidal space
- Surgical closure of cyclodialysis cleft > 3 clock hours in size or if hypotonic maculopathy is present

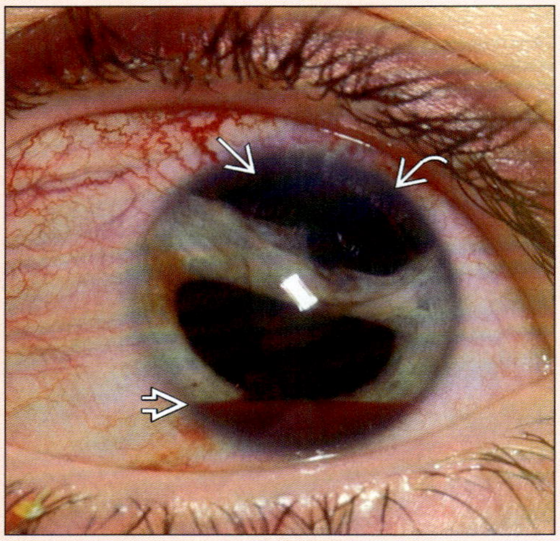
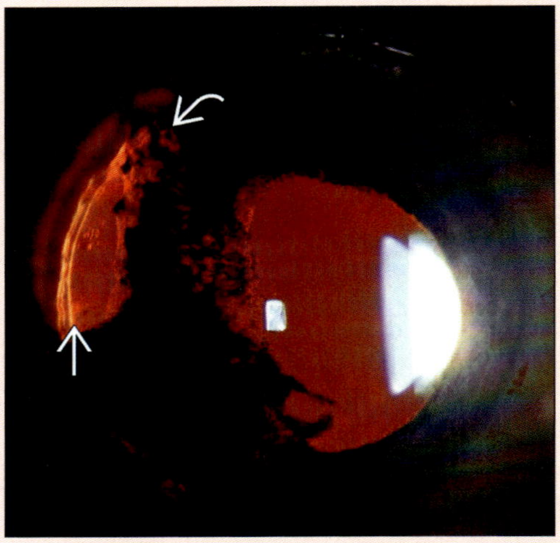

(Left) *This slit-lamp photo shows an eye with iridodialysis and hyphema ➔ in the anterior chamber after blunt trauma. The iris stroma has separated from the iris root ➔, creating a large peripheral iris defect ➔.* ***(Right)*** *Retroillumination on slit-lamp examination shows an iridodialysis defect ➔. The examiner can also see the edge of the crystalline lens through the iris defect ➔.*

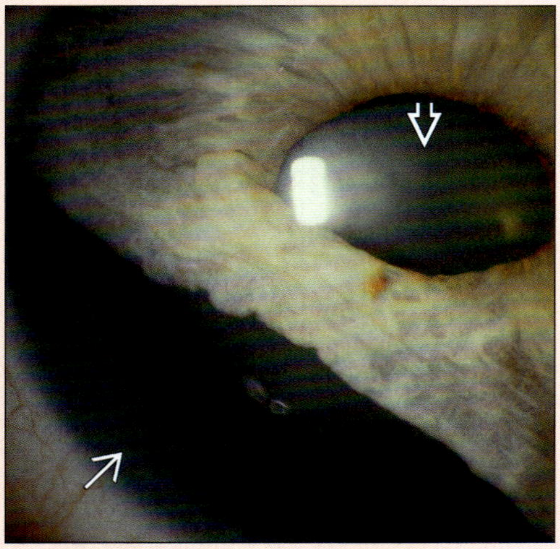
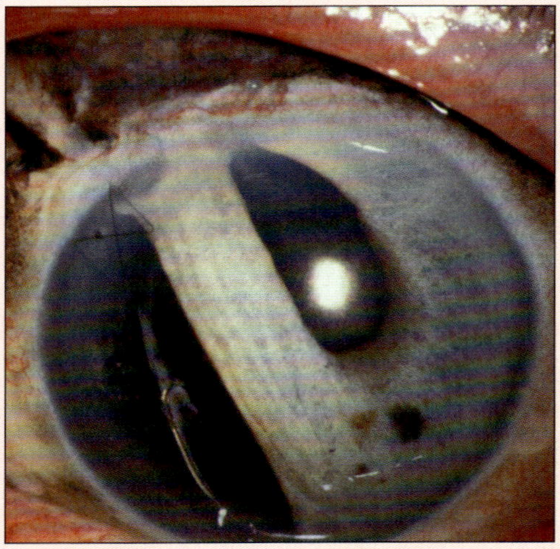

(Left) *Slit-lamp photo shows cyclodialysis. The ciliary body has completely separated from its attachment site to the scleral spur and sclera ➔ and is visible posterior to the scleral spur through the iris defect. A cataract ➔ is also seen.* ***(Right)*** *This slit-lamp photo was taken intraoperatively during surgical closure of a peripheral iris defect in iridodialysis. The iris is sutured to the normal iris insertion site under the limbus. Surgical closure is required for defects > 3 clock hours in size.*

IRIDODIALYSIS/CYCLODIALYSIS

INTRODUCTION

Definitions

- Iridodialysis: Tear in iris root resulting in separation of iris from ciliary body and scleral spur, creating secondary pupil at limbus
- Cyclodialysis: Complete separation of longitudinal ciliary body muscle fibers from scleral spur, forming new drainage pathway of aqueous humor from anterior chamber into suprachoroidal space

DEMOGRAPHICS

Etiology/Risk Factors

- Severe concussive injuries after blunt trauma to eye
- Occasionally occurs after eye surgery
- Intentional surgical cyclodialysis has been used in treatment of glaucoma

PRESENTATION

Symptoms

- Iridodialysis: Monocular diplopia, glare, photophobia
  - Defects in superior iris may be less bothersome if covered by upper eyelid

Exam Findings

- Iridodialysis: Peripheral iris defect on slit-lamp exam
  - Large hyphema may block examiner's view of iris
- Cyclodialysis: Seen with gonioscopy
  - Visible white sclera posterior to scleral spur
  - Decreased visual acuity
  - ↓ IOP, often < 10 mm Hg, may have high IOP following closure
  - Shallow anterior chamber
  - Ciliary choroidal effusion
  - Optic nerve head edema
  - Retinal folds with retinal vein stasis and dilation
  - Complete (360°) ciliary and choroidal detachment shifts iris-lens diaphragm and ciliary body posteriorly or anteriorly
- Slit-lamp exam with gonioscopy
  - Limited use in patients with hyphema, corneal opacity, excessive hypotonia, distorted anatomy

DIFFERENTIAL DIAGNOSIS

Angle Recession

- Separation between circular and longitudinal fibers of ciliary body
- Seen on gonioscopy or ultrasound biomicroscopy
- ↑ IOP directly related to degrees of angle recession
  - May occur up to 10 years after initial trauma, requiring annual follow-up

EVALUATION/WORK-UP

Imaging

- Ultrasound biomicroscopy or anterior ocular coherence tomography (OCT)

TREATMENT

Medical

- Iridodialysis: No treatment required for small defects unless patient experiences symptoms or if lesion is aesthetically displeasing
- Cyclodialysis: Noninvasive management with cycloplegic agent for 6-8 weeks for clefts < 3 clock hours in size
  - Topical atropine approximates ciliary body to sclera and assists with closure
  - Avoid topical corticosteroids, which increase IOP and prevent scar formation, inhibiting closure
  - Spontaneous closure of small cyclodialysis clefts
  - If medical management does not close cyclodialysis cleft within 3-6 months, proceed with surgical repair

Surgical

- Surgical closure of iridodialysis
  - Suture iris to sclera or suspend iris by double-armed 9-0 Prolene suture on CIF-4 needle (dividing iridodialysis in 3rds) placed at normal iris root 1 mm posterior to limbus
    - Docking 30-gauge needle often very helpful
- Surgical closure of cyclodialysis cleft
  - Initial management for clefts > 3 clock hours in size or if hypotonic maculopathy is present
  - Suture cyclopexy reattaches ciliary body to sclera
  - Vitrectomy with pars plana cryotherapy and gas tamponade
- Injection of high-viscosity viscoelastic into anterior chamber to close cyclodialysis cleft
  - Prevents communication between anterior chamber and suprachoroidal space

Follow-Up

- Ultrasound biomicroscopy or anterior OCT to observe cyclodialysis closure under conservative management

Prognosis

- Complications of iridodialysis repair: Corectopia, hyphema, damage to lens capsule, postoperative glaucoma
- Complications of cyclodialysis repair: Erosion of intraocular suture material through scleral flaps, infection, epithelial ingrowth along suture tract, sympathetic ophthalmia
- Hypotonic maculopathy is rare, vision-threatening complication of cyclodialysis
  - Due to aqueous humor flow into suprachoroidal space seen with scleral transillumination and ultrasonography
  - OCT shows increased retinal thickness

SELECTED REFERENCES

1. Romano MR et al: Management of cyclodialysis cleft associated to hypotonic maculopathy. Graefes Arch Clin Exp Ophthalmol. 251(3):1023-4, 2013
2. Kumar M et al: Post-traumatic cyclodialysis cleft with hypotonic maculopathy. Clin Exp Optom. 94(5):481-3, 2011
3. Snyder ME et al: Nonappositional repair of iridodialysis. J Cataract Refract Surg. 37(4):625-8, 2011
4. Corrales G et al: Eye trauma in boxing. Clin Sports Med. 28(4):591-607, vi, 2009

JUVENILE XANTHOGRANULOMA

Key Facts

Introduction

- Juvenile xanthogranuloma (JXG): Self-limiting dermatologic and intraocular inflammatory disease consisting of painless small pink, yellow, or brown nodules of multinucleated giant cells and histiocytes
- Ocular involvement occurs in < 1% of cases of JXG
- Affects the eyelids, orbit, iris, conjunctiva, choroid, retina, skin, and viscera; can cause spontaneous hyphema

Demographics

- Typically afflicts children < 2 years old, though similar lesions have been found in adults

Presentation

- Iris involvement can result in hyphema or heterochromia iridis
- May present as a yellow-colored solitary nodule in the eyelid or on hairy body surfaces
- Conjunctival mass with orange-pink coloration is more common in young adults but can be seen in adults

Differential Diagnosis

- Langerhans cell histiocytosis, dermatofibroma, molluscum contagiosum

Evaluation/Work-Up

- Well-circumscribed nodules consisting of Touton giant cells surrounded by histiocytes, lymphocytes, plasma cells, and eosinophils seen on hematoxylin and eosin stain
- Stains positive for CD68 and HAM-56
- Stains negative for S100

Treatment

- Often resolves spontaneously
- Treat with corticosteroids, chemotherapy, or radiation therapy

*(**Left**) Slit-lamp photo shows heterochromia, which can occur in juvenile xanthogranuloma (JXG) when foamy histiocytes infiltrate diffusely through the iris. (**Right**) Touton giant cells ⇒ are characteristic histologic findings of JXG. They are identified by a central pink area surrounded by a wreath of nuclei and an outer foamy rim of cytoplasm. There are also foamy (xanthomatized) histiocytes ⇨. Biopsy of the iris shows fewer histiocytes and Touton giant cells than a skin biopsy. (Courtesy C. Ko, MD.)*

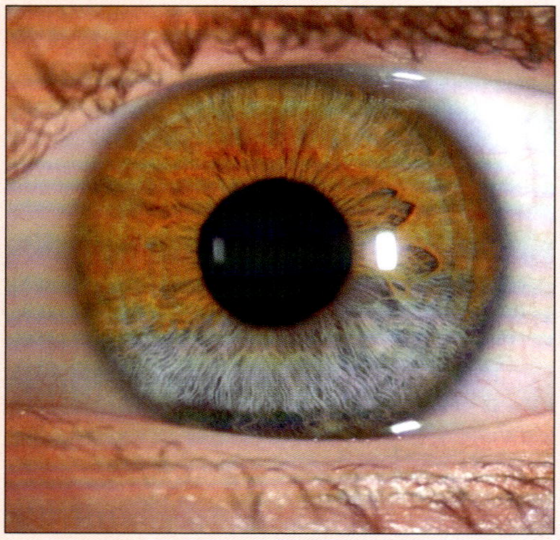

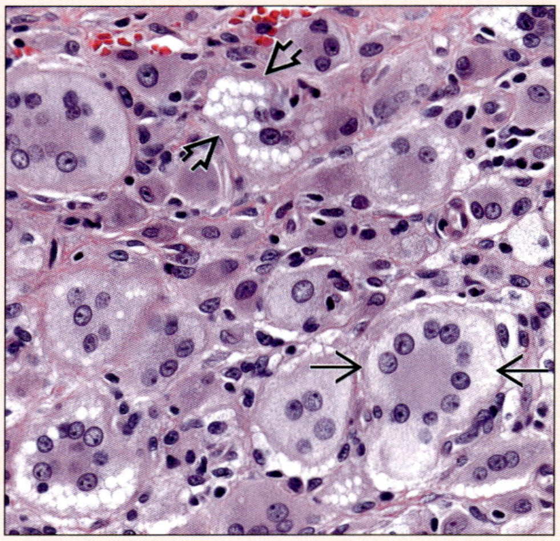

*(**Left**) Fundus photo shows an optic nerve that has had damage resulting in cupping. Note how vessels are abruptly redirected ⇒, delineating the edge of the optic cup and revealing an enlarged cup to disc ratio. Secondary glaucoma with raised IOP and vision loss can occur in JXG. (**Right**) Skin-colored to slightly erythematous dome-shaped papules with central umbilication ⇒ are the hallmark of molluscum contagiosum, which is included in the differential for JXG. (Courtesy T. Whang, MD.)*

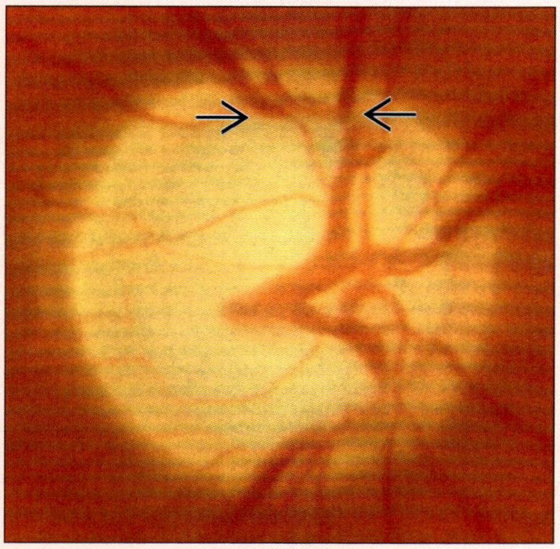

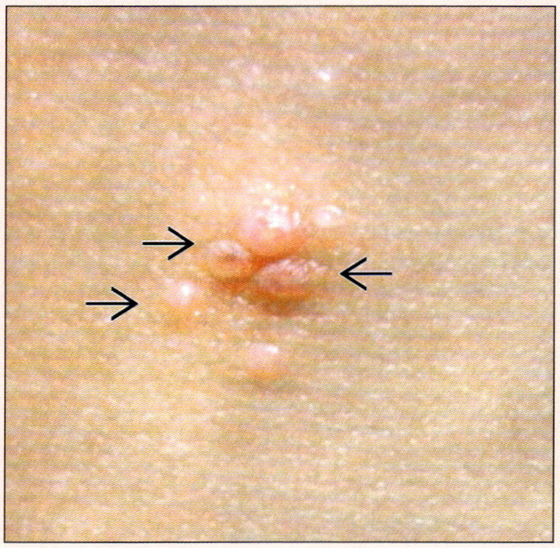

JUVENILE XANTHOGRANULOMA

INTRODUCTION

Abbreviations
- Juvenile xanthogranuloma (JXG)

Definitions
- Self-limiting cutaneous and intraocular inflammation
  - Affects eyelids, orbit, iris, conjunctiva, skin, viscera
  - Painless small pink, yellow, or brown nodules of multinucleated giant cells and histiocytes representing vascular lesions of the iris
- Xanthogranuloma: Benign, usually asymptomatic nodules of non-Langerhans cell histiocytes and multinucleated giant cells ± cytoplasmic lipid deposits

Subtypes
- Cutaneous JXG
  - ≥1 cutaneous nodule(s) ± soft tissue or visceral lesions
  - Affects the head, neck, and trunk most commonly
  - Other sites affected include eyelids, genitourinary tract, toenails, palms, soles, and lips
- Extracutaneous JXG (~ 4% of cases)
  - Ocular involvement in < 1% of JXG cases
    - Most common site: Iris
    - Other sites: Choroid, retina, eyelid, conjunctiva, optic nerve, and orbit
  - Visceral involvement: Lung, liver, and bone

DEMOGRAPHICS

Etiology/Risk Factors
- Associated with Niemann-Pick disease, urticaria pigmentosa, neurofibromatosis type 1, juvenile chronic myelogenous leukemia

Epidemiology
- Children < 2 years, lesions rarely seen in adults
  - 35% of cases occur at birth
  - 70% of cases during 1st year of life
  - 10% of cases occur in adulthood
- Caucasian to African American ratio is 10:1
- Childhood male to female ratio is 1.4:1

PRESENTATION

Symptoms
- Pain, photophobia, vision loss if glaucoma develops

Exam Findings
- Iris involvement is always unilateral
  - Spontaneous bleeding of iris lesion with hyphema
  - May be small, localized fleshy lesion or distributed throughout the entire iris, creating heterochromia
- Other findings: Conjunctivitis, conjunctival chemosis, scleritis, corneal perforation, uveitis, orbital mass
- Orange-pink conjunctival mass can be seen in adults

DIFFERENTIAL DIAGNOSIS

Langerhans Cell Histiocytosis
- Abnormal clonal proliferation of Langerhans cells
- Stains positive for CD1a, langerin, and S100
- Histology shows Birbeck granules

Dermatofibroma
- Superficial benign fibrous histiocytoma of the skin, bone, orbit, airway, gastrointestinal tract, genitourinary tract, or intracranium
- Asymptomatic presentation or pruritic or tender lesions
- Remove tumor if there is pain or diagnosis is uncertain

Molluscum Contagiosum
- Infectious papules on the skin or mucous membranes
- Does not affect the iris
- Caused by poxvirus
- Seen primarily in children
- Pearly, dome-shaped papules with central umbilication, ranging from 3-5 mm in diameter

EVALUATION/WORK-UP

Pathology
- Well-circumscribed nodules of Touton giant cells surrounded by foamy histiocytes, lymphocytes, plasma cells, & eosinophils seen on hematoxylin & eosin stain
  - Lipid-laden macrophage with multiple foamy cytoplasmic vacuoles
  - Yellow discoloration of optic nerve
  - Touton giant cells and histiocytes are less commonly present in iris biopsy compared to skin biopsy
  - Touton giant cells can occur in the rare Erdheim-Chester disease
- Electron microscopy shows organelles within cells
  - Dense bodies, worm-like bodies, "popcorn" bodies
- Stains positive for CD68 and HAM-56, and negative for S100 (a marker for Langerhans cell histiocytosis)

TREATMENT

Medical
- Treatment is reserved for ocular involvement
  - Topical, periocular, or systemic corticosteroids are treatment of choice
  - Antiglaucoma medications for elevated IOP
  - Low-dose radiation or immunomodulators for intraocular inflammation and intractable glaucoma
  - If spontaneous hyphema is persistent, topical e-aminocaproic acid (antifibrinolytic) can be used q.i.d.

Surgical
- Local excision for resistant intraocular lesions
- Excise dermatologic lesions for aesthetic or diagnostic purposes

Prognosis
- Often resolves by age 5
- Hyperpigmented or atrophic scar may remain

SELECTED REFERENCES

1. Papagoras C et al: Periocular xanthogranuloma: A forgotten entity? Clin Ophthalmol. 4:105-10, 2010
2. Cypel TK et al: Juvenile xanthogranuloma: case report and review of the literature. Can J Plast Surg. 16(3):175-7, 2008
3. Casteels I et al: Early treatment of juvenile xanthogranuloma of the iris with subconjunctival steroids. Br J Ophthalmol. 77(1):57-60, 1993

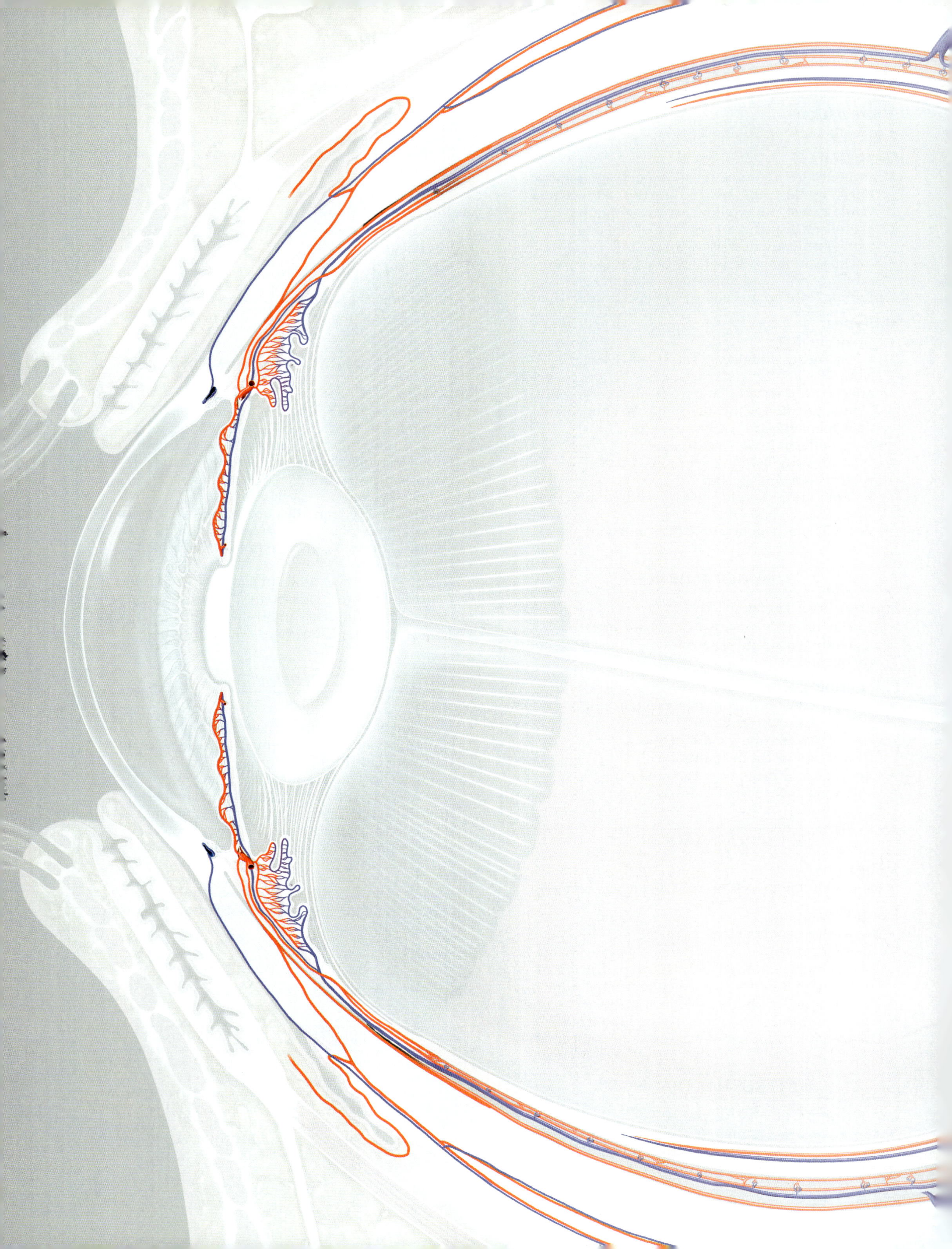

SECTION 2
Uveal Tract

Introduction and Overview

Infectious Disorders

Autoimmune Disorders

Trauma

Treatment-Related Disorders

Miscellaneous

MAJOR CLINICAL STUDIES: UVEAL TRACT

TERMINOLOGY

Abbreviations

- Early treatment for diabetic retinopathy study (ETDRS)
- Multicenter uveitis steroid treatment (MUST) trial
- National Eye Institute 25-item visual function questionnaire (NEI-VFQ 25)

RANDOMIZED TRIAL OF ACETAZOLAMIDE FOR UVEITIS-ASSOCIATED CME

Objective and Principal Conclusion

- To study the effect of acetazolamide on cystoid macular edema (CME) in patients with uveitis
- Acetazolamide improves macular edema, but showed no significant ↑ in best corrected visual acuity (BCVA) and should be used on a case-by-case basis

Inclusion Criteria

- Males/females age 8 or older, weighing at least 77 lbs
- BCVA of 20/40 or worse in at least 1 eye with CME seen on fluorescein angiography (FA)

Exclusion Criteria

- Current use of acetazolamide as part of therapy for uveitis
- History of hypersensitivity to acetazolamide, sulfonamides, or angiography dye
- Unclear ocular media obscuring fluorescein angiography
- Macular subretinal neovascularization
- Macular hole
- Inability to take acetazolamide for medical reasons

Randomization Method

- 37 patients randomized into a masked, cross-over trial comparing acetazolamide with placebo
- Patients received an initial 4-week course of either acetazolamide or placebo, followed by a 4-week washout period, and then a 4-week course of the opposite study medication
  - Patients taking acetazolamide received 500 mg every 12 hours for 4 weeks
  - Children ≥ 8 years received a weight-based dose of acetazolamide

Results

- Acetazolamide resulted in a 0.5-disc area decrease in CME over placebo seen on FA ($P = .01$)
- No statistically significant effect of acetazolamide on visual acuity studied on standardized ETDRS charts ($P = .61$)
- Possible adverse drug reactions were reported by 34/37 study participants during acetazolamide therapy
- Since acetazolamide is associated with adverse effects, patients should be closely monitored and drug discontinued if no clinical benefit is documented

MUST TRIAL

Objective and Principal Conclusion

- Compare systemic therapy with fluocinolone acetonide implant therapy for treatment of vision-threatening, noninfectious intermediate uveitis, posterior uveitis, or panuveitis
- Treatment of severe, vision-threatening uveitis with local intraocular implant resulted in similar changes in BCVA and macular edema, ↓ uveitis activity, ↑ self-reported visual function on NEI-VFQ 25, greater ↑ in IOP, greater incidence of glaucoma requiring medical and surgical therapy, greater incidence of cataract, and similar rates of systemic adverse effects

Inclusion Criteria

- Age ≥ 13 years
- BCVA of hand motions or better in at least 1 eye with uveitis
- IOP ≤ 24 mm Hg in all eyes with uveitis

Exclusion Criteria

- Inadequately controlled diabetes
- Uncontrolled glaucoma or advanced glaucomatous optic nerve injury
- History of scleritis
- Presence of ocular toxoplasmosis scar
- HIV infection or other immunodeficiency disease for which corticosteroid use would be contraindicated

Randomization Method

- Patients were randomly assigned to treatment with systemic corticosteroid + immunosuppressive agents PRN or to fluocinolone acetonide intraocular implant

Results

- Change in BCVA on ETDRS chart at 24 months
  - Those treated with intraocular fluocinolone acetate gained a mean 6.0 ± 1.4 letters vs. 3.2 ± 1.4 letters in group treated with systemic therapy ($P = .16$)
- Macular edema at 24 months
  - 22% of eyes receiving implant therapy vs. 30% of eyes receiving systemic therapy had macular edema with macular thickness ≥ 240 µm on ocular coherence tomography (OCT) ($P = .071$)
- Uveitis activity at 24 months
  - 12% of eyes receiving implant therapy vs. 29% of eyes receiving systemic therapy showed evidence of active uveitis on examination ($P = .001$)
- IOP at 24 months
  - 32.8% of eyes receiving implant therapy vs. 6.3% of eyes receiving systemic therapy had IOP ≥ 30 mm Hg ($P < .0001$)
  - 53.1% of eyes receiving implant therapy vs. 18.7% of eyes receiving systemic therapy had IOP ≥ 24 mm Hg ($P < .0001$)
  - 51.8% of eyes receiving implant therapy vs. 15.5% of eyes receiving systemic therapy had IOP ≥ 10 mm Hg above baseline ($P < .0001$)
- Glaucoma-related findings at 24 months
  - 16.5% of eyes receiving implant therapy vs. 4.0% of eyes receiving systemic therapy had glaucoma based on visual field testing, clinical data, and fundus photography ($P = .0008$)
  - 61.1% of eyes receiving implant therapy vs. 20.1% of eyes receiving systemic therapy required topical or systemic treatment for elevated IOP at any time during 24-month follow-up and were not on IOP-lowering therapy at baseline ($P < .0001$)

 - 26.2% of eyes receiving implant therapy vs. 3.7% of eyes receiving systemic therapy required IOP-lowering surgery during 24-month follow-up period ($P < .0001$)
- Cataract at 24 months
  - 90.7% of eyes receiving implant therapy vs. 44.9% of eyes receiving systemic therapy developed cataract ($P < .0001$)
- Change in self-reported vision-related function (as measured by NEI-VFQ 25) from baseline
  - Patients who received implant therapy reported mean improvement in vision-related function score by 11.44 ± 1.67 points vs. gain of 6.80 ± 1.58 points in those receiving systemic therapy ($P = .043$)
  - Patients who received implant therapy reported mean improvement in mental component score by 2.55 ± 1.11 points vs. loss of 1.1 ± 1.15 points in those receiving systemic therapy ($P = .023$)
  - Patients who received implant therapy reported mean improvement in physical component score by 1.15 ± 0.83 points vs. loss of 1.8 ± 0.90 points in those receiving systemic therapy ($P = .016$)
- Adverse systemic effects at 24 months
  - Incidence of hyperlipidemia was 9.8% vs. 11.0% in patients receiving implant vs. systemic therapy, respectively ($P = .84$)
  - Incidence of hypertension requiring treatment was 4.6% vs. 10.5% in patients receiving implant vs. systemic therapy, respectively ($P = .13$)
  - Incidence of diabetes mellitus was 1.0% vs. 3.6% in patients receiving implant vs. systemic therapy, respectively ($P = .24$)

PROSPECTIVE TRIAL OF INFLIXIMAB THERAPY FOR REFRACTORY UVEITIS

Objective and Principal Conclusion

- Determine safety & efficacy of infliximab in patients with refractory uveitis
- Infliximab is effective at treating refractory uveitis in all patients able to complete 50 weeks of therapy with retention rates similar to standard immunosuppressives in initial responders

Inclusion Criteria

- Age ≥ 9 years
- Vision-threatening, noninfectious uveitis
- Failure or intolerance of prednisone therapy and ≥ 1 other systemic immunosuppressive therapy
- No evidence of malignancy or systemic infection and general good health
  - Based on history, physical exam, chest x-ray, and purified protein derivative skin testing
- MRI of brain showing no evidence of demyelination for patients with pars planitis

Exclusion Criteria

- Recent serious, chronic or recurrent infectious disease
  - Tuberculosis, hepatitis, HIV
- Congestive heart failure
- Multiple sclerosis or other central demyelinating disease
- Known malignancy within previous 5 years (except excised and cured skin cancer)
- Transplanted organ (except cornea)
- Substance abuse within 3 years
- Enrollment in other investigative clinical trial
- Previous treatment with infliximab or other monoclonal antibody, or known allergy to murine or chimeric proteins

Randomization Method

- Patients received 3 infusions of infliximab 5 mg/kg at weeks 0, 2, and 6 and were followed for 2 years
- Patients showing clinical improvement at week 10 were allowed to receive infliximab every 8 weeks, starting at week 14
- Patients with continued inflammation at maximal doses were removed from study

Results

- 18 (78%) of 23 patients met criteria for clinical success at week 10
  - Criteria based on BCVA, control of intraocular inflammation, ability to taper concomitant medication therapy, improvement in inflammatory signs on FA or OCT
  - 8 (44%) patients had improved BCVA of ≥ 2 lines on Snellen chart
  - 9 (50%) had control of intraocular inflammation with ↓ anterior chamber cells or vitreous haze by 2 steps in ≥ 1 eye, using Nussenblatt criteria
  - 10 (56%) patients were able to ↓ their medication therapy by ≥ 50% with maintained control of inflammation
  - 11 (61%) showed improvement in inflammatory signs on FA or OCT
- Serious adverse events included pulmonary embolus, congestive heart failure, lupus-like reaction, vitreous hemorrhage

RELATED REFERENCES

1. National Institutes of Health, National Eye Institute: Randomized Trial of Acetazolamide for Uveitis-Associated Cystoid Macular Edema. http://www.nei.nih.gov/neitrials/static/study11.asp. Updated September 22, 1999. Accessed September 6, 2013
2. National Institutes of Health: Multicenter Uveitis Steriod Treatment (MUST) Trial. ClinicalTrials.gov. http://clinicaltrials.gov/ct2/show/NCT00132691. Published August 19, 2005. Updated June 22, 2013. Accessed September 6, 2013
3. Comparison of Age-related Macular Degeneration Treatments Trials (CATT) Research Group et al: Ranibizumab and bevacizumab for treatment of neovascular age-related macular degeneration: two-year results. Ophthalmology. 119(7):1388-98, 2012
4. Suhler EB et al: Infliximab therapy for refractory uveitis: 2-year results of a prospective trial. Arch Ophthalmol. 127(6):819-22, 2009
5. Suhler EB et al: A prospective trial of infliximab therapy for refractory uveitis: preliminary safety and efficacy outcomes. Arch Ophthalmol. 123(7):903-12, 2005

UVEAL TRACT OVERVIEW

TERMINOLOGY

Definitions

- Primary vascular compartment in the eye and is composed of
  - Iris
  - Ciliary body
  - Choroid

UVEAL TRACT ANATOMY AND CLINICAL IMPLICATIONS

Iris

- Anterior portion of uveal tract, made up of blood vessels, connective tissue, and pigmented cells
- Stroma
  - Composed of pigmented (melanocytes) and nonpigmented cells, collagen fibrils, and a matrix containing hyaluronic acid
  - Overall structure of iris is similar in all individuals, though variation in eye color is due to density of pigmented cells within iris stroma
    - Light-pigmented eyes contain low density of pigmented cells
    - Dark-pigmented eyes contain high density of pigmented cells
  - Blood vessels make up the majority of the stroma, arising from major arterial circle at apex of ciliary body and running radially toward pupil
- Muscles of iris allow for pupillary constriction and dilation
  - Dilator muscle: Contracts in response to sympathetic stimulation and relaxes in response to parasympathetic stimulation
    - Pathologic interruption of parasympathetic stimulation results in pupillary constriction seen in Horner syndrome
  - Sphincter muscle: Circularly oriented muscle fibers around pupil enable pupillary constriction upon stimulation from CN3

Ciliary Body

- Bridge between anterior and posterior uveal tract, functioning primarily in aqueous humor production and lens accommodation
- Shaped triangularly in cross section, apex directed posteriorly toward ora serrata, and consists of 2 components
  - Pars plana: ~ 4 mm wide and relatively avascular, providing a safe route through which to achieve surgical access to vitreous cavity
  - Pars plicata: Highly vascular region with ~ 70 radial folds called ciliary processes, providing attachment for zonular lens fibers
    - Ciliary processes produce aqueous humor
- Ciliary muscle attaches to the trabecular meshwork, contributing to regulation of aqueous humor outflow

Choroid

- Posterior portion of uveal tract, which lies between sclera and retina, and functions primarily as vascular supply to outer rod and cone layers of retina
  - Defects in Bruch membrane (formed by fusion of retinal pigment epithelium with choriocapillaris) due to trauma, inflammation, or ischemia may lead to development of neovascularization
  - Degree of fundus pigmentation is based on density of pigmented melanocytes in choroid
  - Near fovea, only vascular supply to retina is via choriocapillaris
    - In the case of a central retinal artery occlusion, "cherry-red spot" represents continued blood supply to fovea (choroidal supply) despite blockage to remainder of the retina

INFLAMMATION OF UVEAL TRACT

Anterior Uveitis

- Iritis: Inflammation of iris
- Iridocyclitis: Inflammation of iris and ciliary body
- Anterior cyclitis: Inflammation of anterior ciliary body
- Symptoms include pain, photophobia, redness, and blurred vision

Intermediate Uveitis

- Posterior cyclitis: Inflammation of posterior ciliary body
- Pars planitis: Inflammation of pars plana
- Hyalitis: Inflammation of vitreous body
- Symptoms include
  - Floaters due to shadows of vitreous cells on retina
  - Blurred vision due to cystoid macular edema (CME) or vitreous opacities in visual axis

Posterior Uveitis

- Focal, multifocal, or diffuse choroiditis: Inflammation of choroid
- Retinochoroiditis or chorioretinitis: Inflammation of retina and choroid
- Retinitis: Inflammation of retina
- Neuroretinitis: Inflammation of optic nerve and retina
- Symptoms include
  - Painless decreased vision, flashes, floaters, blind spots
  - Blurred vision may be due to inflammation, CME, epiretinal membrane, choroidal neovascularization, refractive error, or opacities in visual axis

Panuveitis

- Inflammation of anterior chamber, vitreous, and retina or choroid

Other Classifications of Uveitis

- Infectious vs. noninfectious
- Granulomatous vs. nongranulomatous
- Acute vs. chronic vs. recurrent

RELATED REFERENCES

1. Barsky D: Anatomy of the Uveal Tract. In Duane's Foundations of Clinical Ophthalmology. 2006 ed. Philadelphia: Lippincott Williams & Wilkins; 2006. http://www.oculist.net/downaton502/prof/ebook/duanes/pages/v4/v4c031.html. Accessed June 12, 2013
2. American Academy of Ophthalmology: Fundamentals and Principles of Ophthalmology. In American Academy of Ophthalmology: Basic and clinical science course 2007-2008 San Francisco: The Academy; 2:61-71: 2007
3. Bonfioli AA et al: Intermediate uveitis. Semin Ophthalmol. 20(3):147-54, 2005

UVEAL TRACT

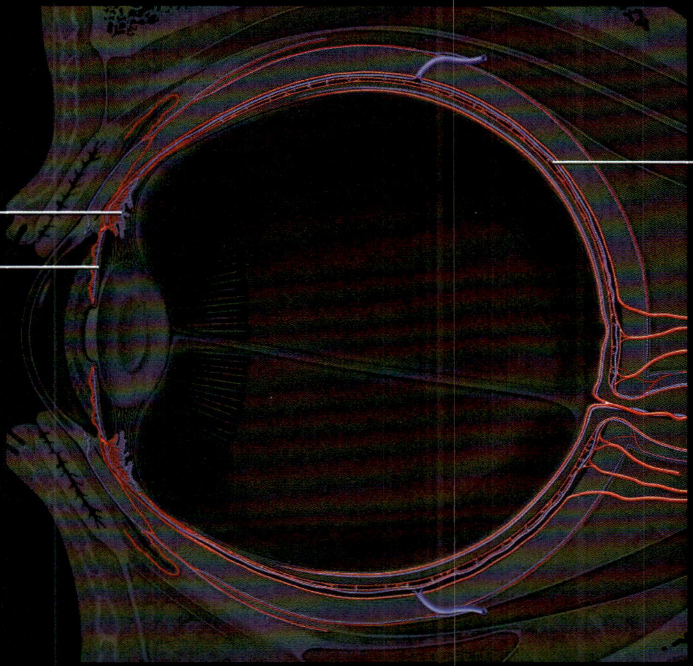

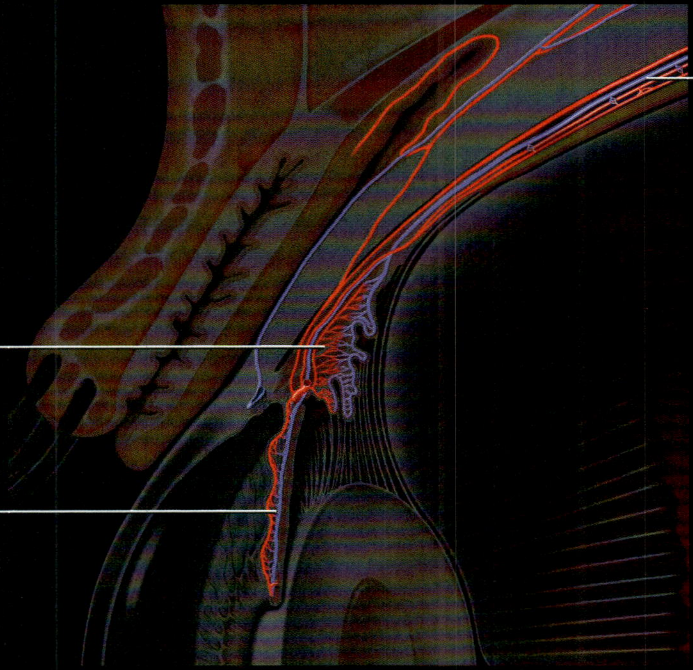

*(**Top**) The uveal tract is the primary vascular compartment in the eye and is composed of the iris, the ciliary body, and the choroid. This illustration shows the normal globe with the uveal tract highlighted. Any portion of the uveal tract can become inflamed in uveitis. This can lead to anterior uveitis, intermediate uveitis, posterior uveitis, or panuveitis. (**Bottom**) This illustration shows a magnified view of the uveal tract in the region of the angle. Anterior uveitis affects the structures depicted in this illustration. Anterior uveitis includes iritis (inflammation of the iris), iridocyclitis (inflammation of the iris and ciliary body), and anterior cyclitis (inflammation of the anterior portion of the ciliary body). The hallmark finding of anterior uveitis is anterior chamber cell and flare. Anterior uveitis is the most common location of uveitis.*

ACUTE RETINAL NECROSIS

Key Facts

Introduction
- Bilateral or unilateral progressive necrosis of retina caused by reactivation of herpes simplex virus (HSV) type 1 or 2, or varicella zoster virus (VZV)
- Results in uveitis ± retinal detachment and blindness
- May result in vitreous opacification

Demographics
- 5.5% of uveitis cases over 10-year period
- Bimodal age distribution that peaks at 20 and 50 years
  - Median age: 20 (HSV2), 47 (HSV1), and 57 (VZV)

Presentation
- White, well-demarcated lesions in peripheral retina
- Lesions spread rapidly in circumferential pattern and form 1 confluent lesion
- Occlusive vasculitis of retinal & choroidal vasculature
- Acute panuveitis, vitreous opacities, necrotizing retinitis, retinal detachment, optic neuritis
- Injected conjunctiva, pain around orbit, blurry vision, history of primary varicella or herpes zoster infection

Evaluation/Work-Up
- Acute retinal necrosis is clinical diagnosis, and laboratory tests may be limited in diagnostic value
- Viral titers or PCR analysis of viral DNA in vitreous aspirate
- Fluorescein angiography (FA), ocular ultrasound (US), CT scan, MRI

Treatment
- Medical treatment with antiviral, anti-inflammatory, and antithrombotic agents
- Initially, daily follow-up, then monthly for 1st year to observe for retinal tears, RD, and optic neuropathy
- Vision loss is due to vasculitis and necrosis of blood vessels supplying macula and optic nerve

__(Left)__ Color fundus photo shows small, white, fluffy lesions ➔ within the retina in a case of acute retinal necrosis (ARN). Early lesions are focal with well-demarcated margins, and they begin to coalesce with time. __(Right)__ This color fundus photo demonstrates ARN lesions ⇨ that have spread in a circumferential pattern to create 1 confluent, ring-shaped lesion in the peripheral retina.

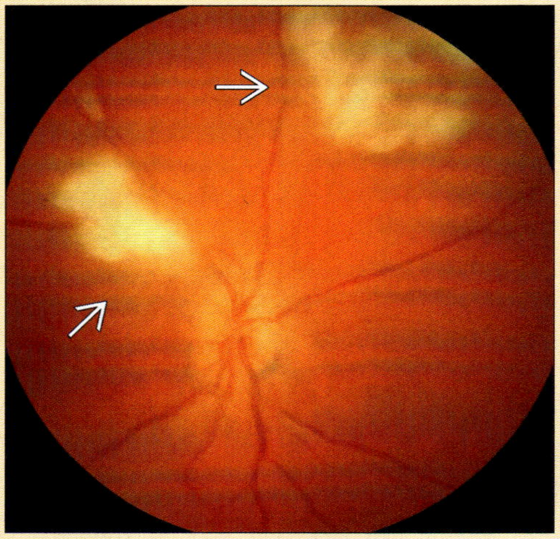

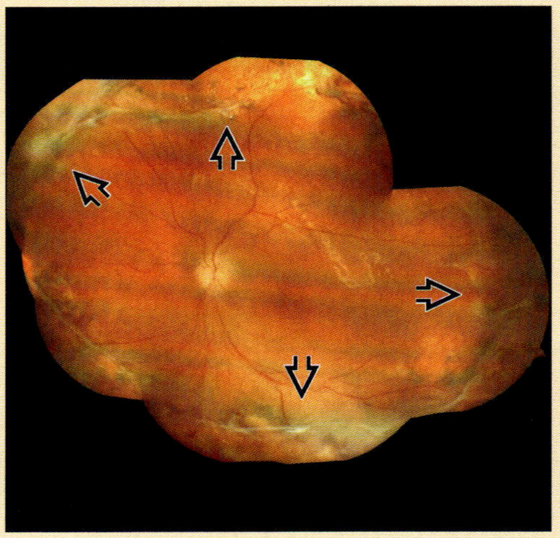

__(Left)__ Color fundus photo of a patient with ARN demonstrates multiple small, fluffy, white lesions ➔ in the peripheral retina. Occlusive vasculitis is a common finding in ARN and results in vitreous hemorrhage ➚. __(Right)__ This slit-lamp photo shows keratic precipitates → on the cornea in an eye with ARN. Keratic precipitates can be fine or granulomatous, and they represent collections of white blood cells on the endothelial corneal surface. (Courtesy R. Nosé, MD.)

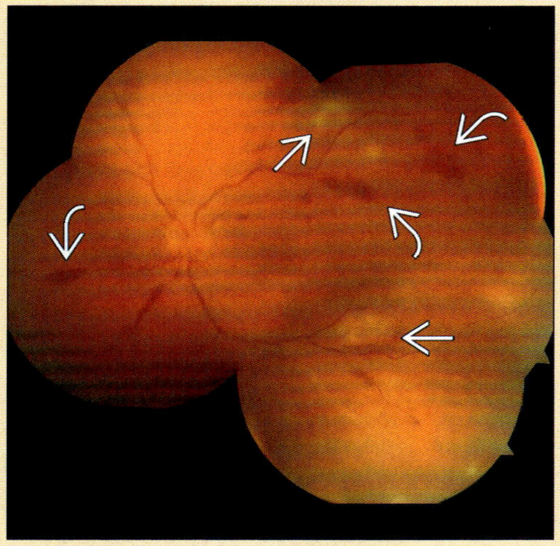

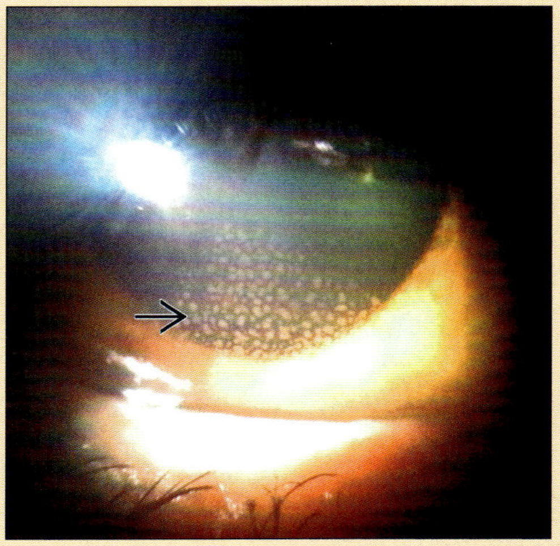

ACUTE RETINAL NECROSIS

INTRODUCTION

Abbreviations
- Acute retinal necrosis (ARN)

Definitions
- Bilateral or unilateral progressive necrosis of retina caused by herpes simplex virus (HSV) type 1 or 2, or varicella zoster virus (VZV)
- Results in uveitis, retinal detachment (RD), blindness

Subtypes
- Stage 1: Necrotizing retinitis
- Stage 2: Vitreous opacification
- Stage 3: Regression of retinal necrosis with pigmentary changes of retinal lesions
- Stage 4: RD
  - Stage 4a: Acute retinal tears or detachment with traction or vitreal inflammation
  - Stage 4b: Chronic RD

DEMOGRAPHICS

Etiology/Risk Factors
- Etiologic agents: VZV, HSV1, HSV2
  - Cytomegalovirus (CMV) is rare cause seen in immunocompromised patients
- Occurs almost always in immunocompetent hosts with history of primary VZV or HSV infections

Epidemiology
- 5.5% of uveitis cases over 10-year period
- Bimodal age distribution, peaking at 20 and 50 years
  - Median age: 20 (HSV2), 47 (HSV1), and 57 (VZV)
- Males are affected more frequently than females

PRESENTATION

Symptoms
- Injected conjunctiva, pain around orbit, blurry vision, photophobia, floaters

Exam Findings
- ≥ 1 focal area of peripheral retinal inflammation and necrosis
  - White lesions with well-demarcated margins
  - ± retinal breaks, RD, and optic nerve head edema
- Lesions spread rapidly in circumferential pattern and form 1 confluent lesion
- Occlusive vasculitis of retinal and choroidal vasculature
  - → neovascularization and vitreous hemorrhage
- Significant panuveitis with white blood cells in vitreous and aqueous
- Associated findings: Fine or granulomatous keratic precipitates, episcleritis or scleritis, anterior uveitis, vitreitis, RD, optic neuritis

DIFFERENTIAL DIAGNOSIS

Progressive Outer Retinal Necrosis (PORN)
- Herpetic retinitis in immunocompromised or HIV-positive patient with CD4(+) count ≤ 100/mm³
- Peripheral lesions of outer retinal layers
- Absence of vitreous or aqueous humor inflammation
- Absence of retinal vasculitis or vasculopathy

CMV Retinitis
- Painless loss of vision in a patient with AIDS
- Fluffy, white retinal infiltrates in absence of vitreitis
- Retinal vasculitis in frosted branch angiitis pattern with multiple retinal hemorrhages

Ocular Toxoplasmosis
- Vitritis creating "headlight in fog" appearance
- Single retinal lesion without retinal hemorrhage
- Moderate ocular pain

EVALUATION/WORK-UP

Labs
- ARN is clinical diagnosis
- Lab tests may be of limited diagnostic value
  - Viral titers of serum of vitreous aspirate
  - PCR analysis of viral DNA in vitreous biopsy sample

Imaging
- FA: ↓ choroidal perfusion, late arterial filling, hypofluorescence in areas of active lesions
- Ocular US: Detached retina, enlarged optic nerve sheath
- CT scan: Optic nerve sheath enlargement
- MRI: Lesions of optic tract indicating axonal spread

TREATMENT

Medical
- Antiviral therapy: Acyclovir, valacyclovir, famciclovir, foscarnet
- Anti-inflammatory therapy: Prednisone
- Antithrombotic therapy: Aspirin

Surgical
- Prophylactic argon laser treatment directed around necrotic retinal lesions to prevent RD
- Vitrectomy for vitreous hemorrhage

Follow-Up
- Initially, daily follow-up, then monthly for 1 year
- Scleral depression for retinal tears or detachment
- Test pupils and color vision for optic neuropathy

Prognosis
- Clinical manifestations of infection range from typical rapidly progressing retinal necrosis to slowly progressing inflammation ± necrosis
- Vision-threatening complications: Macular hole, macular pucker, RD, hypotony, cataract, glaucoma, optic atrophy

SELECTED REFERENCES

1. Wiertz K et al: Intraocular and serum levels of vascular endothelial growth factor in acute retinal necrosis and ocular toxoplasmosis. Retina. 30(10):1734-8, 2010
2. Lau CH et al: Acute retinal necrosis features, management, and outcomes. Ophthalmology. 114(4):756-62, 2007
3. Muthiah MN et al: Acute retinal necrosis: a national population-based study to assess the incidence, methods of diagnosis, treatment strategies and outcomes in the UK. Br J Ophthalmol. 91(11):1452-5, 2007

CANDIDA RETINITIS/UVEITIS/ENDOPHTHALMITIS

Key Facts

Introduction
- Hematogenous spread or direct introduction of *Candida* species into eye
- Results in granulomatous or suppurative inflammation, which progresses from chorioretinitis to vitreitis and endophthalmitis

Etiology
- *C. albicans, C. parapsilosis, C. glabrata, C. krusei*

Demographics
- History of eye surgery, broad spectrum antibiotic use, diabetes mellitus, premature birth (associated with retinopathy of prematurity)
- Incidence of ocular candidiasis: 2-9% of inpatients with candidemia

Presentation
- Subacute onset of blurry vision, floating scotomas ("floaters"), flashes, low-grade eye pain (bulbar pain with extension into anterior chamber), light sensitivity, conjunctival injections
- Destruction of Bruch membrane results in choroidal neovascularization and membrane formation

Treatment
- Oral fluconazole 100-200 mg p.o. b.i.d.
- Intravitreal antifungal for vitreitis or endophthalmitis; IV amphotericin can be used
- Pars plana vitrectomy and surgical removal of epiretinal or choroidal neovascular membrane
- Repeat eye exam 2 weeks after initial exam to avoid misdiagnosis
- 13% of patients with benign eye exam on presentation have been misdiagnosed
- If left untreated, will progress to fungal endophthalmitis with irreversible vision loss
- If treated early, resolution of visual acuity is likely

*(**Left**) Fundus photo shows a characteristic chorioretinal lesion ⇨ of Candida endophthalmitis. Lesions are white, distinct, single or multiple and < 1 mm in diameter. They are located in the posterior or peripheral retina and do not involve the vitreous. A small retinal hemorrhage ➡ is also seen. (**Right**) Fundus photo shows multiple chorioretinal lesions ➡ in a patient with Candida retinitis. These lesions do not form in neutropenic patients.*

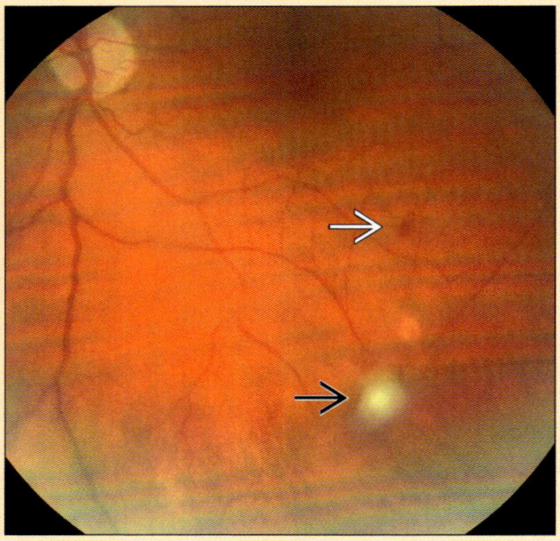

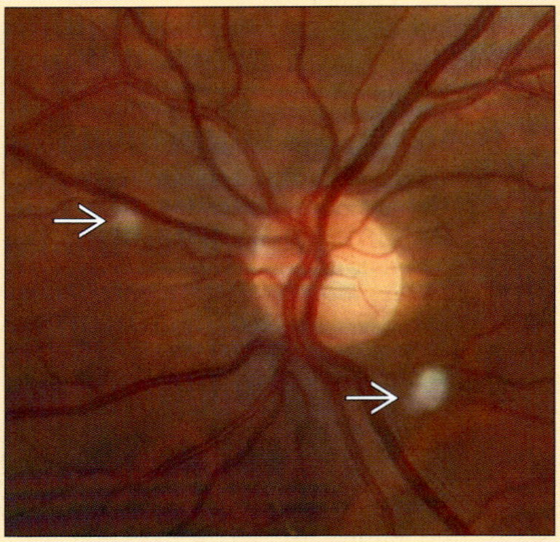

*(**Left**) Fundus photo shows an eye with Candida endophthalmitis. The most common infectious agents include Candida albicans, Candida parapsilosis, Candida glabrata, and Candida krusei. (**Right**) Fundus photo shows Candida endophthalmitis. Characteristic "fluff ball" intravitreal abscesses ➡ contain Candida organisms and neutrophils. The cloudy vitreous obstructs the view of the fundus and obscures the intravitreal lesion margins.*

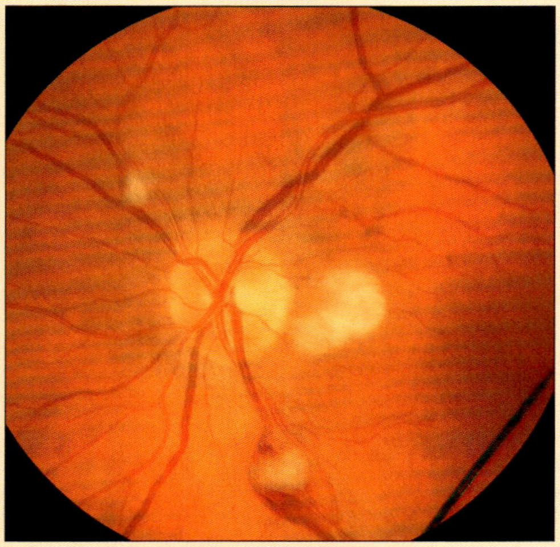

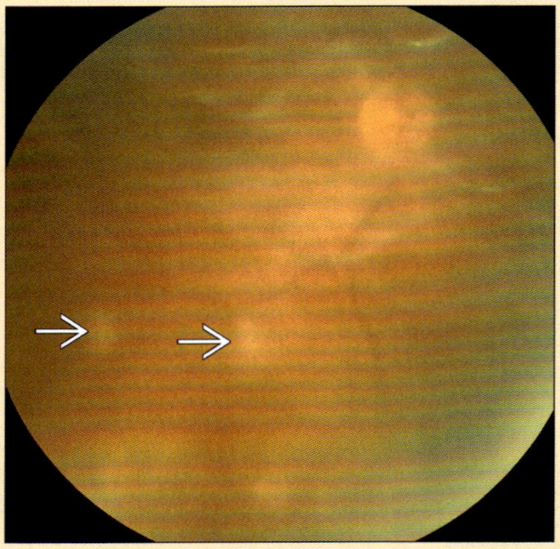

CANDIDA RETINITIS/UVEITIS/ENDOPHTHALMITIS

INTRODUCTION

Definitions

- Hematogenous spread or direct introduction of *Candida* species into eye, resulting in granulomatous or suppurative inflammation that progresses from chorioretinitis to vitreitis and eventually to endophthalmitis

DEMOGRAPHICS

Etiology/Risk Factors

- *Candida albicans*, *Candida parapsilosis*, *Candida glabrata*, *Candida krusei*
- Recent eye surgery, broad spectrum antibiotics, diabetes mellitus, premature birth (associated with retinopathy of prematurity)
- Risk factors for ocular disease: Visual symptoms or inability to verbalize ocular symptoms due to comorbid conditions such as intubation or delirium
- Risk factors for disseminated candidemia
  - ICU admission, long-term indwelling catheter, parenteral nutrition, trauma, intraabdominal surgery, IV drug abuse
  - Immunosuppression, malignancy, debilitation, diabetes mellitus, HIV infection, recent childbirth/abortion

Epidemiology

- 4th leading cause of nosocomial infection
- Increased incidence in ICU patients
- Incidence of ocular candidiasis has been decreasing since 1998 despite rise in candidemia
  - Seen in 2-9% of inpatients with candidemia
  - Decreasing incidence attributed to earlier recognition and treatment, though outpatients tend to present with more advanced disease

PRESENTATION

Symptoms

- Blurry vision, floating scotomas ("floaters"), flashes, low-grade eye pain (bulbar pain with extension into anterior chamber), light sensitivity, injected conjunctiva
- Lack of ocular symptoms carries strong negative predictive value

Exam Findings

- Posterior uveitis with chorioretinal lesions
- Retinal hemorrhage, vitreous inflammation obscuring view of fundus, iridocyclitis, hypopyon
- Epiretinal neovascular membrane secondary to chronic retinal inflammation and ischemia
- Nonspecific findings in patients with confirmed fungemia: Roth spots, cotton wool spots, superficial retinal hemorrhages
- *Candida* endophthalmitis occurs when infection extends into vitreous
  - Cloudy vitreous with "fluff ball" intravitreal abscesses
  - Signs on exam: Hypopyon, scleritis, optic neuritis

DIFFERENTIAL DIAGNOSIS

Cytomegalovirus (CMV) Retinitis

- Chronic or recurrent infection of anterior chamber with CMV, causing anterior segment inflammation, secondary glaucoma, and iris atrophy
- Patients present with blurred vision, halos, eye pain, elevated intraocular pressure, corneal edema, and anterior chamber cells with rare flare

Toxoplasmosis Retinochoroiditis

- Focal necrosis of retina and choroid due to recurrent infection with *Toxoplasma gondii,* leaving patients with permanent retinal scar and vision loss
- Patients present with eye pain & decreased vision along with systemic complaints of fever, night sweats, malaise, myalgias, sore throat, lymphadenopathy, and maculopapular rash sparing palms and soles

EVALUATION/WORK-UP

Labs

- Positive blood culture for *Candida* species
- Positive culture, smear, or PCR of pars plana vitrectomy fluid or vitreous aspirate for *Candida* species

Pathology

- *Candida* organisms surrounded by granulomatous or suppurative inflammation

TREATMENT

Medical

- Oral fluconazole is preferred for chorioretinitis
- Intravenous voriconazole or amphotericin B for fluconazole-resistant *Candida* species ± 5-flucytosine
- Intravitreal voriconazole for vitritis or endophthalmitis

Surgical

- Pars plana vitrectomy
- Removal of epiretinal or choroidal membrane

Follow-Up

- Repeat eye exam 2 weeks after initial exam to avoid misdiagnosis
- 13% of patients with benign eye exam on presentation have been misdiagnosed
- Endophthalmitis warrants systemic work-up to identify involvement of vital organs, e.g., heart or kidneys

Prognosis

- If untreated, results in irreversible vision loss
- If treated early, vision can be restored

SELECTED REFERENCES

1. Shah CP et al: Ocular candidiasis: a review. Br J Ophthalmol. 92(4):466-8, 2008
2. Mehta S et al: Ocular lesions in disseminated candidiasis. J Assoc Physicians India. 55:483-5, 2007
3. Jang GJ et al: Treatment of candida chorioretinitis with voriconazole. Korean J Ophthalmol. 19(1):73-6, 2005
4. Jampol LM et al: Choroidal neovascularization secondary to Candida albicans chorioretinitis. Am J Ophthalmol. 121(6):643-9, 1996

ENDOGENOUS BACTERIAL ENDOPHTHALMITIS

Key Facts

Introduction

- Breakdown of blood-eye barrier allows for endogenous bacteria to enter eye, leading to infection and destructive intraocular inflammation

Demographics

- Etiology: *Staphylococcus aureus*, *Escherichia coli*, *Streptococcus* species
- Risk factors: Sepsis, debilitated state, indwelling catheter, endocarditis, UTI, meningitis, IV drug abuse, immunocompromised state
- Makes up 2-8% of all cases of endophthalmitis

Presentation

- Decreased vision, red eye, deep ocular pain, floater, ocular discharge, no history of recent eye surgery
- Decreased visual acuity, eyelid swelling, injected conjunctiva, corneal edema, cells and flare in anterior chamber, hypopyon, keratic precipitates, fibrin membrane formation, vitreitis obstructing view of retina, loss of red reflex, retinal periphlebitis

Evaluation/Work-Up

- Culture and sensitivities of aqueous and vitreous samples to determine etiology and antibiotic choice
- Cultures of blood, sputum, and urine to determine source of endogenous infection

Treatment

- Ocular emergency requiring urgent treatment to avoid complete vision loss
- Broad spectrum coverage with vancomycin + ceftriaxone or vancomycin + amikacin until culture results are known
- Vitrectomy with intravitreal antibiotic injection reduces bacterial load
- Outcome depends on virulence of bacteria, presenting visual acuity, and time until diagnosis and treatment

__(Left)__ The eye in this photo is affected by endogenous bacterial endophthalmitis. A choroidal lesion is seen superior to the optic nerve. __(Right)__ Fundus photo shows a case of endogenous bacterial endophthalmitis. Characteristic collections of vitreous cells and debris are seen here and represent severe disease. The patient may experience floaters in addition to an acute blurring and decrease in vision.

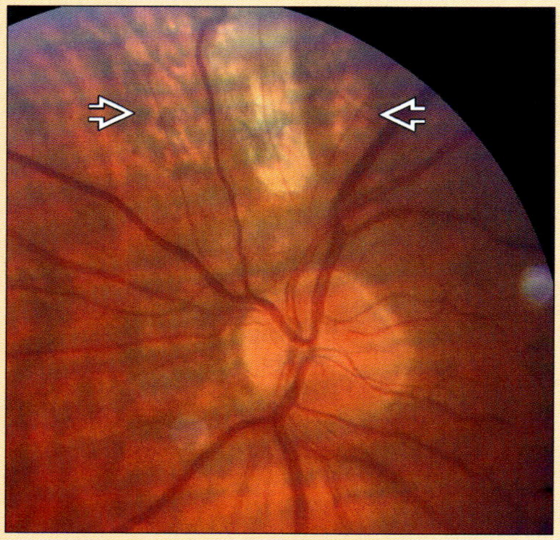

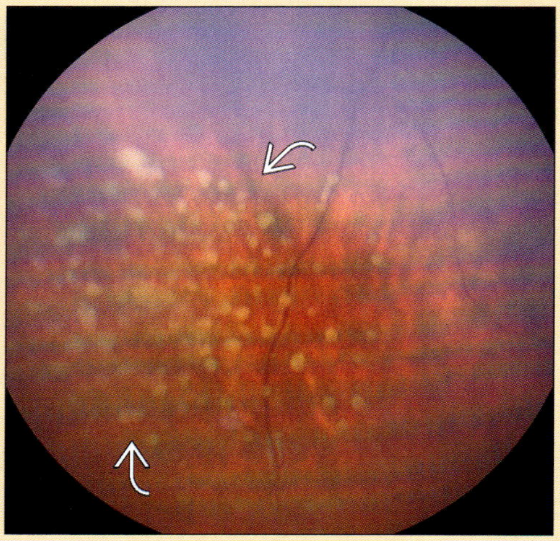

__(Left)__ This fundus photo shows a subretinal abscess temporal to the optic nerve, a complication in a severe case of endogenous bacterial endophthalmitis. __(Right)__ This external photo shows hypopyon and hazy vitreous viewed through the pupil in a case of endogenous bacterial endophthalmitis that has progressed into panophthalmitis with possible extension into the orbit. Conjunctival erythema and injection are also seen. Note the fibrinous inflammatory membrane.

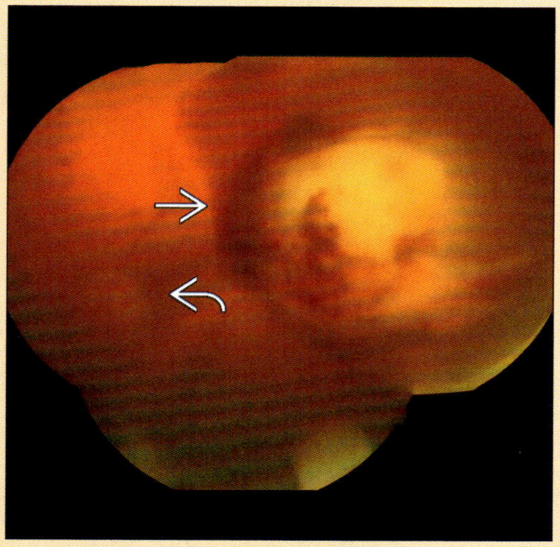

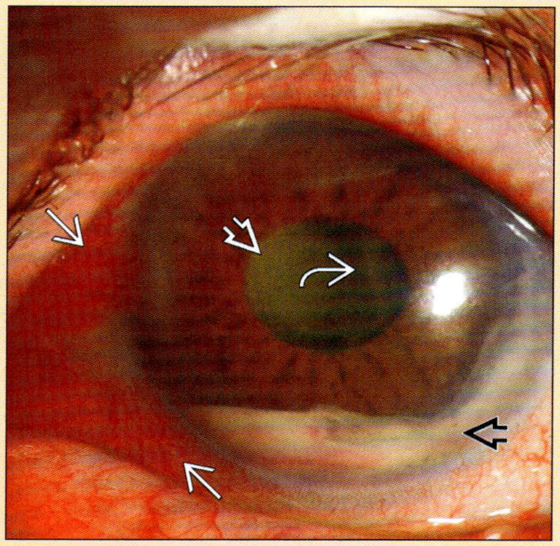

ENDOGENOUS BACTERIAL ENDOPHTHALMITIS

INTRODUCTION

Definitions
- Hematogenous spread of bacteria into eye due to damage of ocular vasculature
  - Breakdown of blood-eye barrier allows for endogenous bacteria to enter eye
  - As neutrophils release digestive enzymes and bacteria release toxins within eye, further intraocular damage occurs
- Intraocular infection and destructive inflammatory response in a patient without history of recent ocular trauma or intraocular surgery

DEMOGRAPHICS

Etiology/Risk Factors
- *Staphylococcus aureus, Escherichia coli, Streptococcus* species, *Bacillus cereus, Neisseria meningitidis, Haemophilus influenzae, Klebsiella*
- Sepsis, IV drug use, immunocompromised/debilitated state, extensive GI surgery, endoscopy, dental surgery
  - Identifiable sources of infection: Indwelling catheter, endocarditis, intraabdominal abscess, meningitis, UTI, GI/hepatic abscess
- Diabetes mellitus, sickle cell anemia, systemic lupus erythematosus, HIV increase risk

Epidemiology
- Makes up 2-8% of all forms of endophthalmitis
  - Most cases of endogenous endophthalmitis are fungal
- M:F = 1.5-2:1
- Bilateral involvement in 25% of cases
- Can occur in newborns/infants < 6 months of age

PRESENTATION

Symptoms
- ↓ vision, pain, photophobia, floaters, ocular discharge

Exam Findings
- Systemic illness or constitutional symptoms
- Eyelid edema, conjunctival injection, chemosis, corneal edema, keratic precipitates, fibrin membrane on lens capsule
- Retinal hemorrhage, abscess, periphlebitis
- Severe disease: Hypopyon, anterior chamber cell/flare, vitreitis obstructing view of retina, loss of red reflex
- Panophthalmitis: Inflammation of all 3 coats of the eye (retina, choroid, sclera/cornea)
  - May be associated with orbital extension

DIFFERENTIAL DIAGNOSIS

Exogenous Bacterial Endophthalmitis (EBE)
- Postoperative EBE after complicated intraocular surgery
- Delayed-onset or chronic pseudophakic postop EBE
  - Onset 6 months postop, followed by chronic disease
- Vision loss greater than expected for typical postoperative state, deep eye pain in addition to typical symptoms of endophthalmitis
- ± white plaque on center of remaining lens capsule

Acute Retinal Necrosis
- Syndrome of uveitis, vitreitis, retinal vasculitis, and necrotizing retinitis

Fungal Endophthalmitis
- Risk factors: IV drug abuse, surgery, malignancy, IV hyperalimentation
- Etiology: *Candida, Aspergillus*
- Characteristic chorioretinal infiltrates with white vitreous opacities resembling string of pearls

EVALUATION/WORK-UP

Labs
- Culture and sensitivities of aqueous and vitreous samples to determine etiology and antibiotic choice
  - Anterior chamber tap, vitreous chamber tap, or vitrectomy with vitreous biopsy
- Cultures of blood, sputum, urine, and indwelling catheters to determine source of infection

Imaging
- B-scan ultrasound (US) if view of fundus is obstructed
  - Thickened choroid, US echoes in anterior and posterior vitreous support diagnosis
  - Identifies vitreous debris or retinal detachment

TREATMENT

Medical
- Topical, intravitreal, and systemic antibiotics determined by culture and sensitivities
  - Broad spectrum coverage with vancomycin and ceftriaxone or vancomycin and amikacin
  - Aminoglycoside and clindamycin for *Bacillus cereus* in patients with history of IV drug abuse
  - Treat with IV antibiotics for ≥ 2 weeks
  - Start systemic antibiotics prior to culture results
- Systemic, topical, and periocular steroids
  - Prednisolone acetate, dexamethasone, triamcinolone
- Cycloplegics
  - Atropine 1% t.i.d.
  - Prevents ciliary spasm and synechiae formation

Surgical
- Vitrectomy with intravitreal antibiotic injection
  - Reduces intraocular bacterial load and provides fluid for culture and pathology

Prognosis
- Ocular emergency requiring urgent treatment intervention to avoid complete vision loss or death
- Outcome is related to virulence of bacteria, presenting visual acuity, and time until diagnosis and treatment
- Full recovery occurs slowly over many months
- 32-40% of patients will have visual acuity of counting fingers or better

SELECTED REFERENCES

1. Durand ML: Bacterial endophthalmitis. Curr Infect Dis Rep. 11(4):283-8, 2009
2. Smith SR et al: Endogenous bacterial and fungal endophthalmitis. Int Ophthalmol Clin. 47(2):173-83, 2007

TOXOPLASMOSIS

Key Facts

Introduction

- Necrotizing retinitis caused by protozoan *Toxoplasma gondii*, with chorioretinal scaring, vitritis, retinal vasculitis, optic neuritis, and anterior uveitis
- Congenital toxoplasmosis: Transmission to fetus occurs in utero and manifests as chorioretinitis, hydrocephalus, intracranial calcifications
- Acquired toxoplasmosis occurs after ingestion of undercooked meat, dairy products, or cat feces and manifests as necrotizing chorioretinitis ± anterior uveitis, vitritis, or retinal vasculitis

Demographics

- Infects roughly 33% of world's population and 10-15% of USA population, but active disease only occurs in small portion of those infected

Presentation

- Blurred vision, floaters, and scotomas
- Retinal lesions appear as fluffy, white discrete areas of necrosis lacking well-defined borders, often located adjacent to healed chorioretinal scar
- Classic "headlight in the fog" appearance when viewed by indirect ophthalmoscopy in dense vitritis

Evaluation/Work-Up

- Fluorescein angiography and optical coherence tomography
- Serum *Toxoplasma*-specific IgG, IgM, and IgA
- Fetal ultrasound in utero may detect congenital disease

Treatment

- Systemic pyrimethamine, sulfadiazine, and folinic acid; clindamycin for sulfa allergy
- Follow-up every 2 weeks until stable, then every month while on medical treatment
- Resolution of active chorioretinitis occurs in 3-4 weeks
- Steroids can minimize scarring

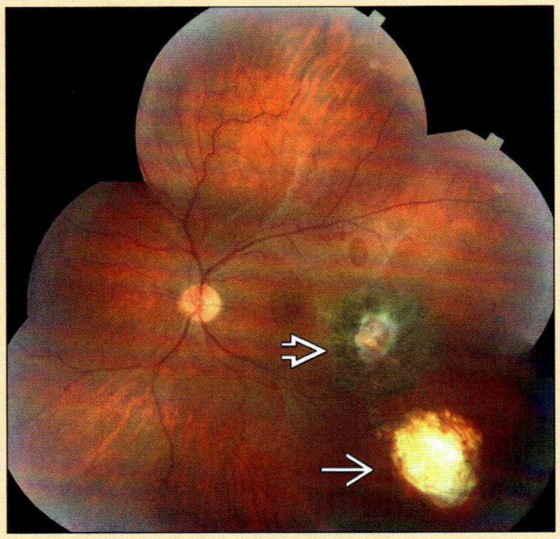

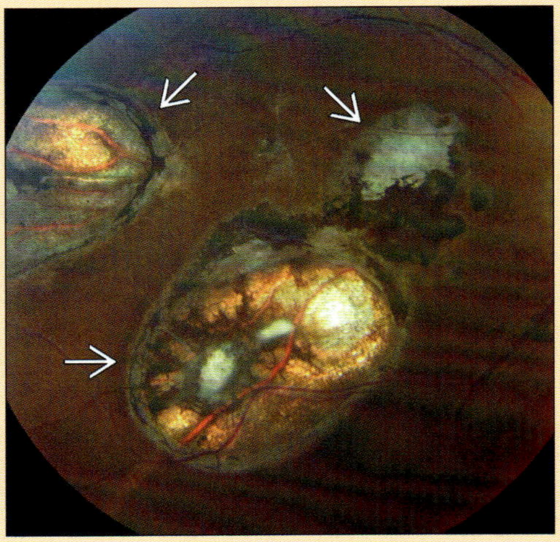

(Left) *Photo shows a recently acquired large, nonpigmented necrotizing lesion ➔ of toxoplasmosis adjacent to a chorioretinal scar ➔ from a prior lesion. Small lesions in the peripheral retina resolve spontaneously without treatment, but large lesions near the optic disc, retinal vascular arcades, or macula require treatment to decrease the size of retinal scarring and preserve vision.* ***(Right)*** *Color fundus photo shows multiple hyperpigmented congenital toxoplasmosis macular scars ➔.*

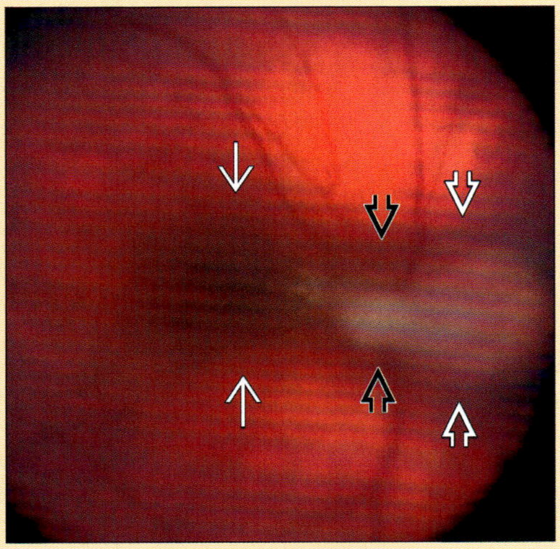

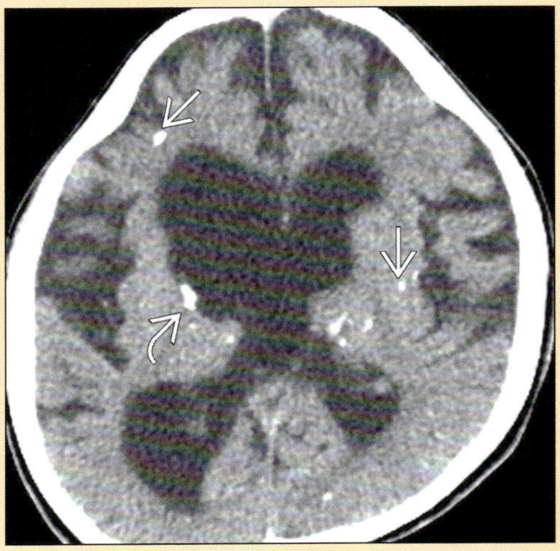

(Left) *Photo shows the characteristic white, fluffy lesion ➔ of early toxoplasmosis, located between the macula ➔ and optic nerve ➔. As the lesion begins to regress with time, the borders will atrophy and become more defined. Papillitis blurs the optic disc margins.* ***(Right)*** *Axial NECT shows punctate calcifications in an infant with congenital toxoplasmosis. Calcifications may be either periventricular ➔ or scattered throughout the parenchyma ➔. Ventriculomegaly is also present.*

TOXOPLASMOSIS

INTRODUCTION

Definitions

- Necrotizing retinitis caused by protozoan *Toxoplasma gondii*, with chorioretinal scaring, vitritis, retinal vasculitis, optic neuritis, and anterior uveitis

Subtypes

- Congenital toxoplasmosis
  - Transmission to fetus occurs in utero or during passage through birth canal during maternal parasitemia
  - Chorioretinitis, hydrocephalus, intracranial calcifications
  - Reactivation disease in adults is often bilateral
- Acquired toxoplasmosis
  - Ingestion of undercooked meat, dairy products, or cat feces
  - Necrotizing chorioretinitis ± anterior uveitis, vitritis, or retinal vasculitis
  - Lesions are more commonly unilateral
  - Occurs in ages 10-40 years

DEMOGRAPHICS

Etiology/Risk Factors

- Risk factors: T-lymphocyte immunodeficiency, bone marrow or organ transplant recipient, contact with cat feces

Epidemiology

- Infects roughly 33% of world's population and 10-15% of USA population
  - Disease manifests in only a small portion of those infected
- Causes 30-50% of posterior uveitis cases in USA
- Most common cause of posterior uveitis in immunocompetent patients

PRESENTATION

Symptoms

- Blurred vision, floaters, and scotomas

Exam Findings

- Retinal lesions appear as fluffy, white discrete areas of necrosis lacking well-defined borders
  - Often adjacent to pigmented or atrophic scars from previous lesions that have healed; in late evolution, scars can become very hyperpigmented and dark
- Other findings include anterior uveitis, cataracts, vitritis, glaucoma; inflammation is very common, and absence of vitritis points toward other conditions

DIFFERENTIAL DIAGNOSIS

Herpes Simplex Virus

- Yellow areas of localized or diffuse necrotizing retinitis, keratoconjunctivitis, and optic neuritis
- Dense vitritis, retinal vasculitis, and persistent fetal vasculature (causing a white reflex) may occur
- Skin lesions, chorioretinitis, and brain abnormalities in a neonate suggest disease was acquired during passage through birth canal
- May result in disseminated or central nervous system disease

Varicella Zoster Virus

- Necrotizing retinitis characterized by occlusive vasculitis and vitritis
- Occurs in neonates whose mother had chickenpox during 1st 20 weeks of pregnancy
- Skin scarring, chorioretinitis, cataracts, microphthalmia, skeletal abnormalities, microcephaly, neurologic defects

EVALUATION/WORK-UP

Labs

- Serum *Toxoplasma*-specific IgG, IgM, and IgA
- Immunoblot or PCR testing of aqueous for *Toxoplasma*-specific IgG and IgA

Imaging

- Fluorescein angiography
  - Early-phase blocking at site of lesion followed by hyperfluorescence starting at periphery of lesion and filling centrally
- Ocular coherence tomography
  - Shows retinal thinning at sites of chorioretinal scars, as well as edema of active lesions

TREATMENT

Medical

- Antiparasitic medications
  - Vision-threatening lesions located near macula or optic nerve head, or severe peripheral lesions
  - Pyrimethamine, sulfadiazine, and folinic acid; for sulfa-allergy, clindamycin is substituted for sulfadiazine
  - Intravitreal injection of clindamycin ± dexamethasone if no response to antibiotics

Surgical

- Local treatment to lesions with photocoagulation, cryotherapy, or surgical vitrectomy

Follow-Up

- Every 2 weeks until stable, then every month while on medical treatment
  - CBC every week for 1st month, then every 2 weeks

Prognosis

- Disease is self-limited in immunocompetent patients
- Resolution of active chorioretinitis occurs in 3-4 weeks
- Vision loss results from tractional distortion of macula, optic nerve atrophy, cataract, and retinal detachment

SELECTED REFERENCES

1. Delair E et al: Clinical manifestations of ocular toxoplasmosis. Ocul Immunol Inflamm. 19(2):91-102, 2011
2. Soheilian M et al: Randomized trial of intravitreal clindamycin and dexamethasone versus pyrimethamine, sulfadiazine, and prednisolone in treatment of ocular toxoplasmosis. Ophthalmology. 118(1):134-41, 2011
3. Vasconcelos-Santos DV et al: Review for disease of the year: differential diagnosis of ocular toxoplasmosis. Ocul Immunol Inflamm. 19(3):171-9, 2011

POSTERIOR UVEITIS

Key Facts

Introduction

- Inflammation involving the retina, choroid, or both

Demographics

- Large series of 2,619 patients reported that 18.3% of cases were posterior uveitis

Presentation

- Floaters
- Blurred &/or decreased vision
- Retinitis or choroiditis
- Retinal vasculitis
- Retinal neovascularization and hemorrhages

Differential Diagnosis

- Toxoplasmosis is most common cause of infectious posterior uveitis in immunocompetent
- Parasites: Toxoplasmosis, toxocariasis
- Bacteria: Tuberculosis, syphilis
- Virus: Herpes simplex, varicella zoster, cytomegalovirus
- Other: Presumed histoplasmosis
- Sarcoidosis
- White dot syndromes: Multiple evanescent white dot syndrome, birdshot choroidopathy, multifocal choroiditis, acute posterior multifocal placoid pigment epitheliopathy, serpiginous choroidopathy
- Vogt-Koyanagi-Harada syndrome
- B-cell lymphoma
- Behçet disease

Treatment

- Treatment depends on etiology
  - Corticosteroids
  - Immunosuppressives
  - Anti-infective treatments
- Recurrent inflammation can lead to permanent visual loss, even blindness

*(**Left**) Fundus photo shows yellowish exudates around the optic disc in a patient with sarcoid uveitis. The fluorescein angiograms show an elevated edematous lesion superior to the optic disc and later shows a hyperfluorescent optic disc. (**Right**) Fundus photo shows round yellow-orange lesions deep to the retina in a patient with birdshot chorioretinopathy.*

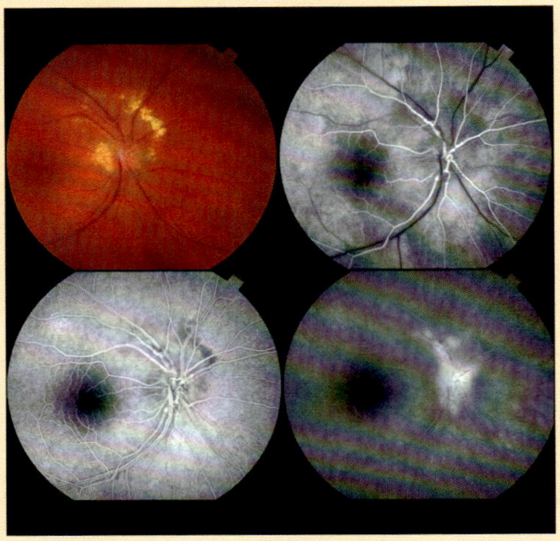

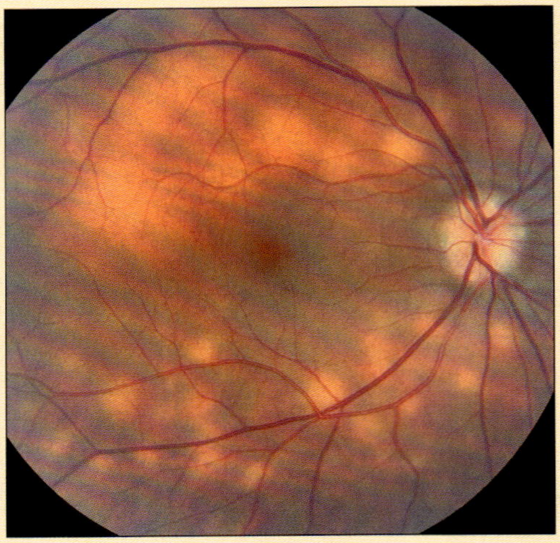

*(**Left**) Fundus photo shows a variety of lightly and darkly pigmented lesions in the deep retina with flame-shaped hemorrhages superior to the optic disc in a patient with acute posterior multifocal placoid pigment epitheliopathy. (**Right**) OCT shows subretinal fluid and cystoid macular edema in a patient with persistent uveitis.*

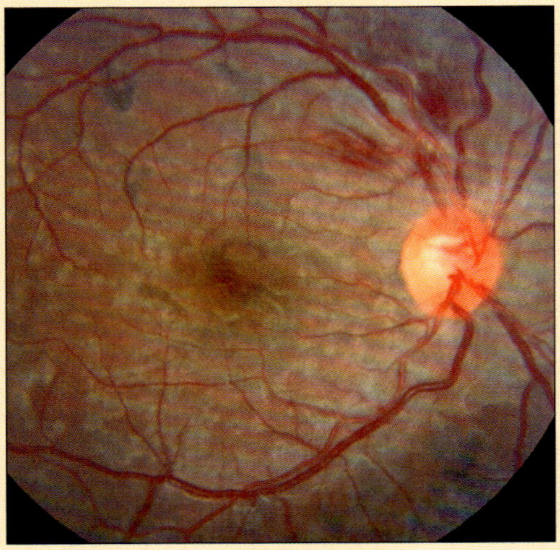

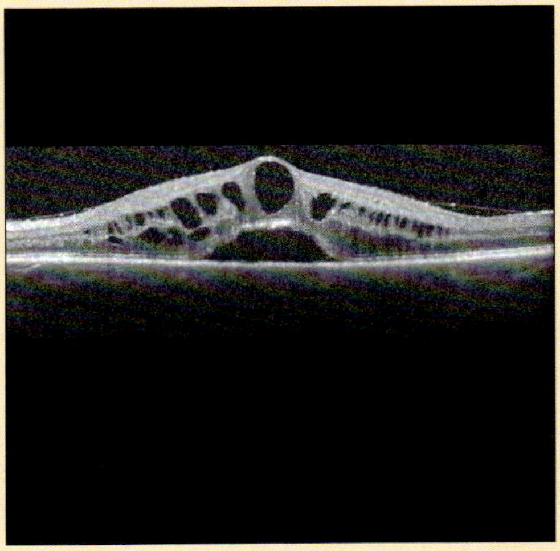

POSTERIOR UVEITIS

INTRODUCTION

Definitions
- Inflammation involving the retina, choroid, or both

Subtypes
- Focal
- Multifocal
- Diffuse choroiditis
- Chorioretinitis
- Retinochoroiditis
- Retinitis
- Neuroretinitis

DEMOGRAPHICS

Epidemiology
- For all uveitis: 38 cases per 100,000 people
- In a large series of 2,619 patients, 18.3% of cases were posterior uveitis

PRESENTATION

Symptoms
- Insidious onset typically
- Floaters
- Blurred vision
- Decreased vision

Exam Findings
- Retinitis
- Choroiditis
- Retinal vasculitis
- Retinal neovascularization and hemorrhages
- Retinal detachment
- Macular edema
- Retinal scars

DIFFERENTIAL DIAGNOSIS

Infectious
- Parasites
  - ○ Toxoplasmosis, toxocariasis
    - ▪ Toxoplasmosis is most common cause of infectious posterior uveitis in immunocompetent
      - – Typically unilateral with history of contact with dogs or cats, eating undercooked meat, or contaminated water
      - – Often occurs at posterior pole
      - – May see focal necrotizing retinitis or retinochoroidal scars
- Bacteria
  - ○ Tuberculosis, syphilis
    - ▪ Tuberculosis typically presents with disseminated choroiditis, with lesions often occurring at posterior pole
      - – Ring of fire appearance in granuloma on angiography
- Viruses
  - ○ Herpes simplex, varicella zoster, cytomegalovirus
    - ▪ May see acute retinal necrosis with herpetic viruses
      - – Vitritis, arteritis, periphlebitis, and retinal necrosis
    - ▪ Cytomegalovirus retinitis usually occurs in immunocompromised
      - – Granular appearance
      - – Brushfire spread along blood vessels
- Other
  - ○ Presumed histoplasmosis

Noninfectious
- Sarcoidosis
- Retinal pigment epithelitis
- White dot syndromes
  - ○ Multiple evanescent white dot syndrome, birdshot choroidopathy, multifocal choroiditis, acute posterior multifocal placoid pigment epitheliopathy, serpiginous choroidopathy
- Vogt-Koyanagi-Harada syndrome
- B-cell lymphoma
- Behçet disease

EVALUATION/WORK-UP

Labs
- PCR & antibody testing
- ELISA

Imaging
- Ultrasound (B scan)
  - ○ Useful with media that is hazy or has opacities
- Fluorescein angiography
  - ○ Identify macular edema, active choroiditis, or neovascularization
- OCT
  - ○ Identify macular edema or epiretinal membrane

TREATMENT

Medical
- Treatment depends on etiology
  - ○ Corticosteroids
  - ○ Immunosuppressives
  - ○ Anti-infective treatments

Follow-Up
- Patients will need to be followed for underlying etiology and to monitor for development of associated complications

Prognosis
- Recurrent inflammation can lead to permanent visual loss, even blindness

SELECTED REFERENCES

1. Mandelcorn ED: Infectious causes of posterior uveitis. Can J Ophthalmol. 48(1):31-9, 2013
2. Barisani-Asenbauer T et al: Uveitis- a rare disease often associated with systemic diseases and infections- a systematic review of 2619 patients. Orphanet J Rare Dis. 7:57, 2012
3. Sudharshan S et al: Current approach in the diagnosis and management of posterior uveitis. Indian J Ophthalmol. 58(1):29-43, 2010
4. Tabbara KF: Clinical diagnosis of posterior uveitis. Int Ophthalmol Clin. 35(3):1-19, 1995

SARCOIDOSIS

Key Facts

Introduction

- Multisystem inflammatory disorder of undetermined etiology, characterized by noncaseating granulomas
- Etiology: Occupational exposure, infectious, immunologic, familial

Presentation

- Adnexa: Granulomas of orbit and eyelids, lacrimal gland inflammation, exophthalmos, proptosis
- Conjunctiva: Bulbar or palpebral conjunctival nodules
- Cornea: Band keratopathy, keratoconjunctivitis sicca, mutton-fat keratic precipitates, endothelial opacification
- Anterior chamber: Synechiae, iris nodules, iridocyclitis, iris bombé, angle-closure glaucoma, cataract
- Posterior segment: Vitreous inflammation, perivascular sheathing, periphlebitis, branched or central retinal vein occlusion, granulomas
- Children present with erythema nodosum, uveitis, and polyarthritis with rare pulmonary findings and elevated serum ACE level or elevated serum lysozyme

Evaluation/Work-Up

- CXR and chest CT show hilar adenopathy or pulmonary fibrosis
- Biopsy of skin or conjunctival lesions confirms diagnosis
- Characteristic epithelioid cells, multinucleated giant cells encircled by lymphocytes

Treatment

- Goal: Minimize inflammation to prevent ocular tissue destruction
- Topical, periocular, or systemic corticosteroids
- Cycloplegics prevent synechiae formation

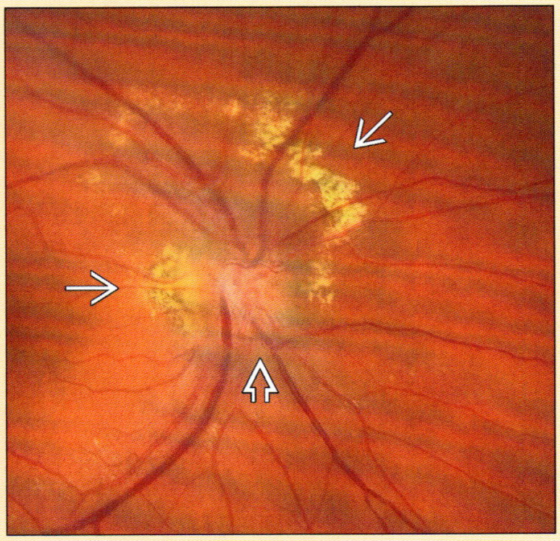
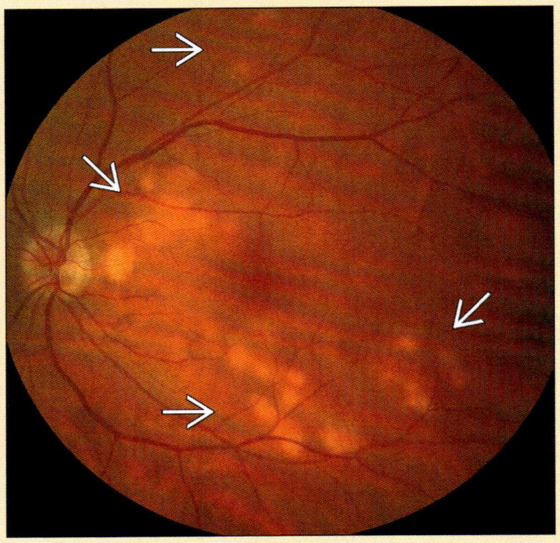

*(**Left**) Fundus photo shows the characteristic candlewax dripping lesions → of sarcoidosis, which appear as nodular yellow-white granulomas in the choroid. There is also optic disc swelling and papillitis → seen as obscured disc margins. (**Right**) Color fundus photograph shows multiple retinal and choroidal nodular granulomas → in a patient with posterior segment involvement in sarcoidosis. Posterior segment involvement occurs in roughly 20% of patients with ocular sarcoidosis.*

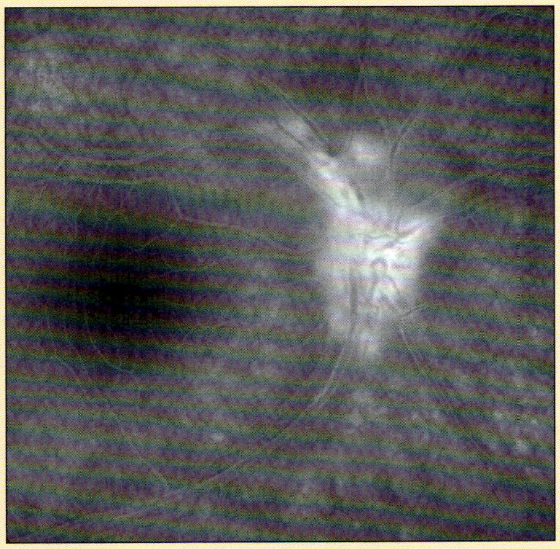
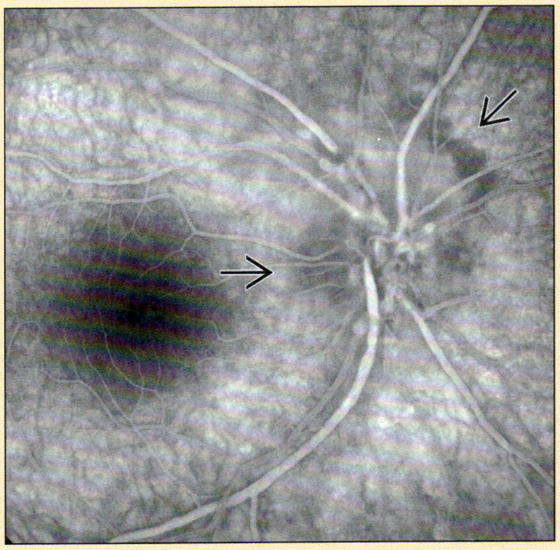

*(**Left**) This fluorescein angiography (FA) of a patient with sarcoidosis shows early hypofluorescence. The characteristic FA staining pattern of sarcoidosis is early blocking with late staining and hyperfluorescence throughout the posterior globe. (**Right**) Late-stage FA in sarcoidosis shows hyperfluorescence except in areas of candlewax dripping lesions →, where hypofluorescence remains due to poor perfusion.*

SARCOIDOSIS

INTRODUCTION

Definitions
- Multisystem inflammatory disorder of undetermined etiology, characterized histologically by noncaseating granulomas

Subtypes
- Heerfordt syndrome: Uveitis, parotitis, chronic fever, facial nerve palsy
- Löfgren syndrome: Erythema nodosum, febrile arthropathy, bilateral hilar adenopathy, iritis
- Chronic sarcoidosis: Symptomatic disease with duration > 2 years
- Mikulicz syndrome: Involvement of lacrimal gland

DEMOGRAPHICS

Etiology/Risk Factors
- Etiology
  - Occupational exposure: Clay, metal dusts, insecticide, pine pollen, mold, mildew, musty odors
  - Genetic predisposition: 5x increased risk of developing disease if sibling has sarcoidosis
  - Infectious: Atypical mycobacteria, propionibacterium acnes, certain fungi or viruses
  - Immunologic: HLA-DRB1, HLA-DQ1
  - Exposure to IFN-α for treatment of hepatitis C infection
- Risk factors: Family history of disease, African American heritage, female gender, age 20-50 years

Epidemiology
- Prevalence in USA: 40 per 100,000
- Ocular sarcoidosis seen in 25-80% of cases of sarcoidosis
  - Makes up 10-20% of uveitis cases
  - Ocular sarcoidosis is more common in African Americans and the elderly

PRESENTATION

Symptoms
- Acute uveitis: Decreased vision, loss of color vision, red eye, photophobia, glare, aching eye pain, excessive tearing, dry eyes, or patient may be asymptomatic
- Chronic uveitis: Progressive pain and blurry vision

Exam Findings
- Presence of definite, probable, or possible findings in absence of causal condition other than sarcoidosis
  - Definite: Uveitis, lacrimal gland swelling, optic neuritis
  - Probable: Blindness (visual acuity < 20/200 with correction)
  - Possible: Cataract, glaucoma
- Findings based on age
  - < 5 years: Uveitis, arthritis, skin rash
    - May resemble juvenile idiopathic arthritis
  - 20-40 years: Bilateral chronic granulomatous iritis or panuveitis, hilar adenopathy
  - > 40 years: Multifocal choroiditis or birdshot chorioretinitis-like lesions, interstitial lung disease
- Acute increase in intraocular pressure
- Adnexa: Granulomatous nodules on eyelids or within orbit, lacrimal gland inflammation
- Conjunctiva: Bulbar or palpebral conjunctival granulomas
- Cornea: Endothelial mutton-fat precipitates, band keratopathy, keratoconjunctivitis sicca, endothelial opacification
- Anterior chamber
  - Anterior uveitis: More common in African Americans with sudden onset of pain, red eye, and blurry vision, which may progress to fibrosis, glaucoma, and blindness
  - Anterior or posterior synechiae, Koeppe (pupil margin) or Busacca (mid peripheral iris) iris nodules, iridocyclitis, iris bombé, angle-closure glaucoma, cataract, mutton-fat keratic precipitates
- Posterior segment
  - Posterior uveitis is more common in whites
    - Gradual worsening
  - Retinal vasculitis: Nodular granulomas along retinal vasculature with candlewax dripping (taches des bougie) appearance
  - Vitritis presents as yellow-white nodular aggregates of inflammatory cells termed "snowball" lesions or arranged in linear distribution termed "string of pearls"
  - Choroidal granulomas
  - Cystoid macular edema
  - Optic nerve granulomas → optic neuritis or atrophy
    - Optic neuritis presents as papilledema with focal scotoma in absence of demyelinating disease process
    - Optic nerve head edema seen in patients with neurosarcoidosis
- Children present with erythema nodosum, uveitis, and polyarthritis with rare pulmonary findings and elevated serum ACE level

DIFFERENTIAL DIAGNOSIS

Tuberculosis
- Caseating granulomatous posterior uveitis caused by *Mycobacterium*
- Patient presents with blurry vision and red eye
- Mutton-fat keratic precipitates, iris nodules, localized yellow mass of retina, vitreous haze

Vogt-Koyanagi-Harada Syndrome
- Bilateral or unilateral uveitis associated with alopecia, poliosis, vitiligo, and hearing defects
- Prodrome of headache, dysacusis, tinnitus, vertigo
- Recurrent iridocyclitis, patchy choroiditis, and serous exudative retinal detachment
- Women aged 20-40 are most commonly affected

Toxoplasmosis
- Eye inflammation caused by *Toxoplasma gondii*, an obligate intracellular protozoan
- Patients present with floaters, blurred vision, and photophobia
- Active lesions appear as fluffy, white areas of necrotic chorioretinitis adjacent to chorioretinal scars
- Retinal vasculitis with hemorrhage, iridocyclitis, and vitreitis

SARCOIDOSIS

- Positive serum anti-*Toxoplasma* immunoglobulin

Behçet Disease

- Relapsing uveitis, aphthous ulcers, and either genital ulcers, positive Behçetine pathergy test, erythema nodosum, or dermatographia
- Ocular manifestations: Severe anterior uveitis with hypopyon, retinal vasculitis, papillitis
- Individuals 20-40 years of age of Japanese, Turkish, or Middle Eastern descent

Birdshot Chorioretinopathy

- Granulomatous panuveitis characterized by focal cream-colored hypopigmented lesions throughout retina
- Lesions located in retina pigment epithelium and choroid
- Associated with HLA-A29 and retinal S-antigen

EVALUATION/WORK-UP

Labs

- No definitive laboratory testing confirms disease
- Order: Serum ACE, lysozyme, calcium, liver function tests, and urine calcium level
- Findings
  - Elevated ACE produced by epithelioid cells of granulomas
  - Elevated lysozyme produced by macrophages and epithelioid cells
  - Hypercalcemia due to production of 1,25 dihydroxyvitamin D3
  - Soluble serum IL-2 receptors produced by activated T cells in lungs

Pathology

- Biopsy confirms diagnosis
  - Biopsy site: Cutaneous nodules, conjunctiva, sclera, eyelid, lacrimal or parotid gland, palpable lymph nodes, pulmonary tissue
  - Characteristic epithelioid cells, multinucleated giant cells encircled by lymphocytes; noncaseating granulomas
    - Multinucleated giant cells contain cytoplasmic inclusions: Schaumann (or lamellar) bodies and asteroid bodies
- Pars plana vitrectomy with vitreous fluid analysis showing noncaseating granulomatous inflammation

Imaging

- Systemic imaging
  - CXR and chest CT scan show hilar adenopathy or pulmonary fibrosis
  - Gallium scan shows panda sign: Increased uptake of gallium into parotid and lacrimal glands
  - Ultrasound-guided biopsy to exclude lymphoma if parotid gland swelling or Heerfordt syndrome
  - Gadolinium-enhanced MRI of brain to rule out neurosarcoidosis
- Ocular imaging
  - Slit-lamp examination regardless of ocular symptoms
  - Fluorescein angiography if posterior uveitis is suspected
  - Optical coherence tomography (OCT) to identify cystoid macular edema or involvement of macula
  - Electroretinography to determine severity of retinal disease

TREATMENT

Medical

- Topical or intraocular/subconjunctival/sub-tenon corticosteroid injection and topical cycloplegics for mild ocular inflammation
  - Cycloplegics prevent synechiae formation; atropine or 10% phenylephrine might be necessary for synechialysis
- Systemic corticosteroids for refractory inflammation, posterior uveitis, retinal neovascularization, optic nerve involvement
- Immunomodulator therapy allows for decreased corticosteroid dosing
  - Methotrexate, azathioprine, cyclosporine, mycophenolate mofetil, infliximab, tacrolimus
- Topical NSAIDs and acetazolamide can be helpful for cystoid macular edema

Surgical

- Iris nodule excision if nodules persist after trial of medical therapy
- Cataract extraction
- Implanted glaucoma drainage device
- Vitreoretinal surgery
  - Indicated for epiretinal membranes, tractional or rhegmatogenous retinal detachment, vitreous hemorrhages, debris, or inflammation
- Laser photocoagulation or cryopexy
  - For neovascularization of retina or optic nerve head
  - Panretinal photocoagulation for recurrent vitreous hemorrhage

Prognosis

- Disease severity ranges from asymptomatic to lethal
  - 20% of patients without ocular complaints are noted to have ocular involvement on slit-lamp examination
  - 5% mortality rate; 10% if CNS is involved
- Poor prognostic indicators: CNS involvement, lupus pernio, nephrocalcinosis
- Poor visual outcome occurs associated with eye involvement, posterior uveitis, cystoid macular edema, optic neuritis, secondary glaucoma
  - Posterior uveitis may lead to blindness
- Visual acuity is worse than 20/200 in 2-25% of cases

SELECTED REFERENCES

1. Haimovic A et al: Sarcoidosis: a comprehensive review and update for the dermatologist: part II. Extracutaneous disease. J Am Acad Dermatol. 66(5):719, 2012
2. Scott AW et al: Diagnostic yield of vitreous biopsy in presumed sarcoidosis-related posterior segment inflammation. Graefes Arch Clin Exp Ophthalmol. 250(9):1379-85, 2012
3. Baughman RP et al: A concise review of pulmonary sarcoidosis. Am J Respir Crit Care Med. 183(5):573-81, 2011
4. Demirci H et al: Orbital and adnexal involvement in sarcoidosis: analysis of clinical features and systemic disease in 30 cases. Am J Ophthalmol. 151(6):1074-1080, 2011

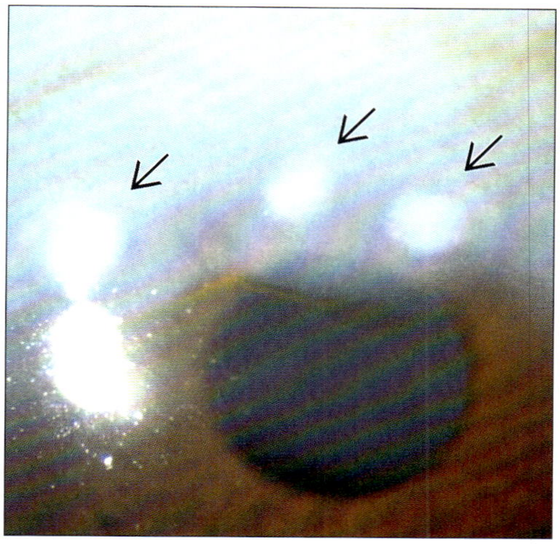

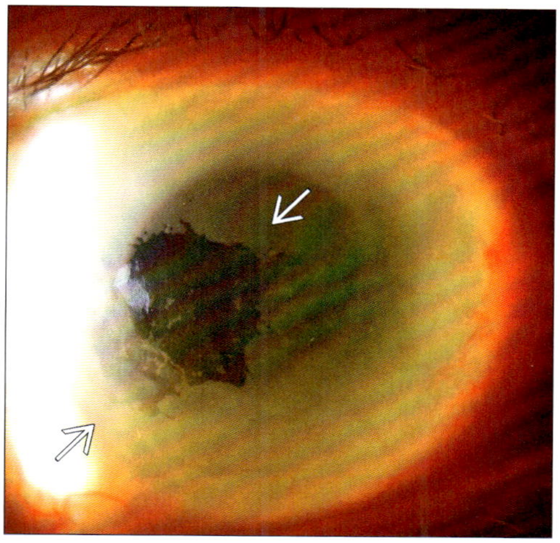

(Left) *Gray mutton-fat keratic precipitates ⇨ are associated with ocular sarcoidosis. These granulomatous lesions are located on the posterior surface of the Descemet membrane. Large granulomas involving the cornea can lead to posterior synechiae, iris bombé, and angle-closure glaucoma.* ***(Right)*** *Slit-lamp photo demonstrates band keratopathy ➡ seen in a case of ocular sarcoidosis. Band keratopathy is the result of calcium deposition and develops as a sequela to chronic uveitis or hypercalcemia.*

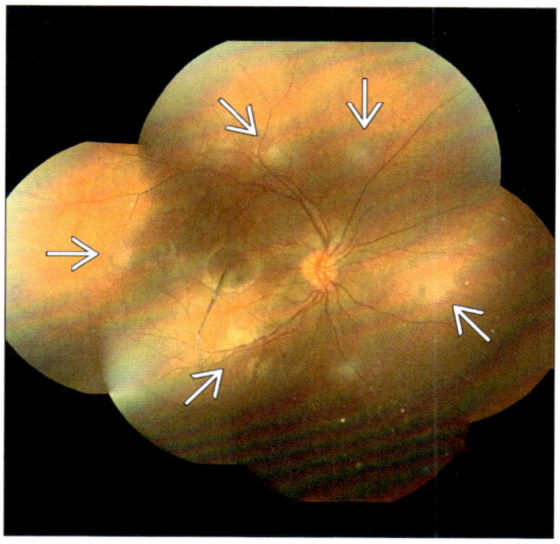

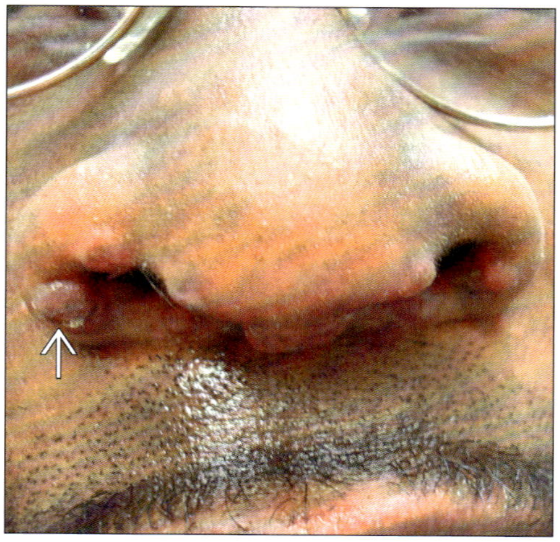

(Left) *This image demonstrates sarcoidosis with involvement of the posterior segment. Multiple characteristic "snowball" lesions ➡ are white or yellow in color and represent vitreous inflammation. These nodules can be diffuse, resembling a snow globe, as seen here, or arranged in a linear fashion and termed "string of pearls."* ***(Right)*** *Sarcoidosis presented as apple jelly-colored, slightly pink discrete papules ➡ on the rim of the nose of an African American man. (Courtesy J. Hall, MD.)*

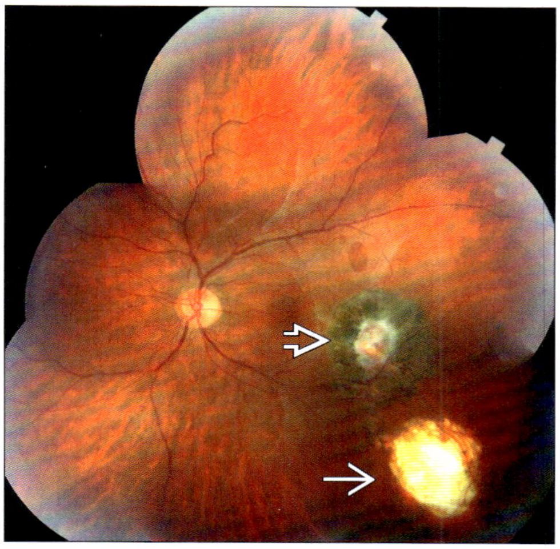

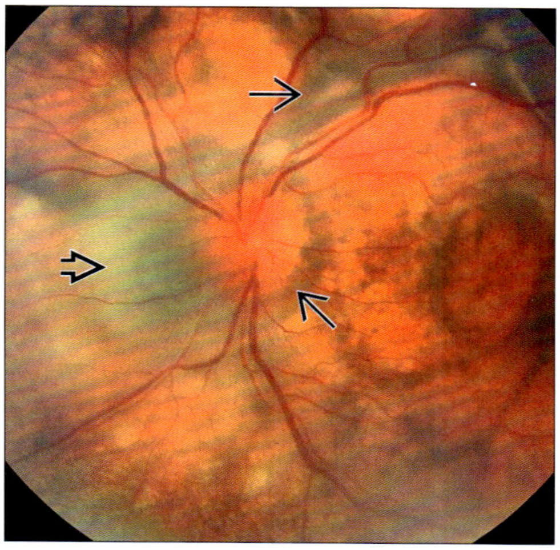

(Left) *This fundus photograph shows a recently acquired, large, nonpigmented necrotizing lesion ➡ of toxoplasmosis adjacent to a chorioretinal scar from a prior lesion ➡. Toxoplasmosis is in the differential for sarcoidosis.* ***(Right)*** *This fundus photograph shows an example of Vogt-Koyanagi-Harada syndrome, which is in the differential diagnosis for sarcoidosis. Note the vitreous haze ⇨ and pigment clumping ⇨.*

BEHÇET SYNDROME

Key Facts

Introduction

- Current diagnostic criteria requires 3 episodes over a 12-month period of recurrent oral aphthous ulcers and ≥ 2 of the following
  - Genital ulcers, skin lesions, uveitis, or positive pathergy test

Demographics

- Correlation with HLA-B51, HLA-B5, and factor V Leiden mutation
- Most often occurs in adults between ages 20 and 40, with typical age of onset in 30s

Presentation

- Symptoms present in recurrences and remissions
- Aphthous ulcers on mucous membranes: Oral, genital, gastrointestinal
- Vasculitis
- Ocular
  - Anterior uveitis: Hypopyon, flare, and cells
  - Retinal perivasculitis
- Later complications: Iris neovascularization, optic nerve atrophy, phthisis bulbi, posterior synechiae

Evaluation/Work-Up

- Pathergy test to detect hyperreactivity
- Histopathologic evaluation shows acute neutrophil infiltration or chronic plasma cell or lymphocyte infiltration
- Fundus fluorescein angiography to examine retinal vessels
- Optical coherence tomography to evaluate for cystoid macular edema

Treatment

- Corticosteroids, immunotherapy, vitreoretinal surgery
- Recurrent attacks of uveitis lead to cumulative ocular damage

*(**Left**) Fundus photograph shows the fundus of a patient with Behçet eye disease. The optic nerve has begun to develop pallor, suggestive of a chronic disease process ➦. Gliotic sheathing is also present ➡. (**Right**) External photograph shows hypopyon, a typical finding in Behçet disease ➡. Hypopyon is a common finding in many forms of ocular inflammation.*

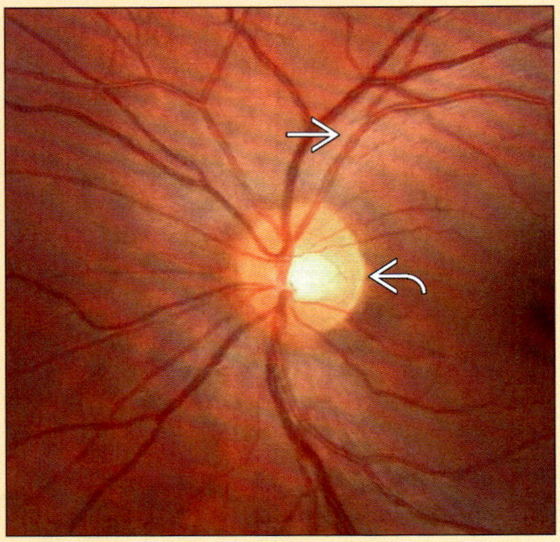

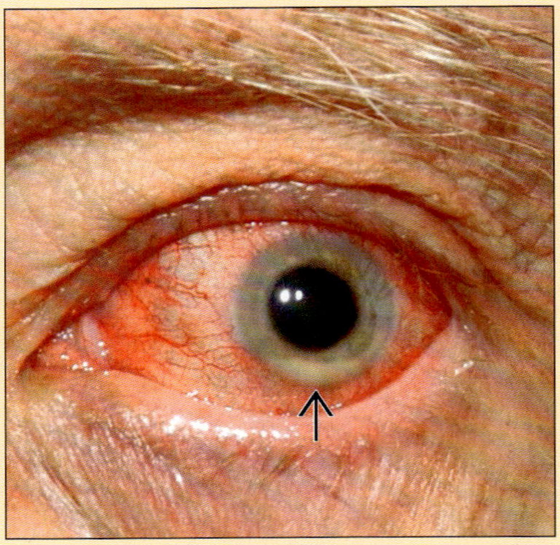

*(**Left**) OCT image shows cystoid macular edema in a patient with Behçet disease ➡. (**Right**) This fundus photograph depicts retinal vasculitis, which can be seen in Behçet disease ➡. The overall haziness of the image suggests inflammation.*

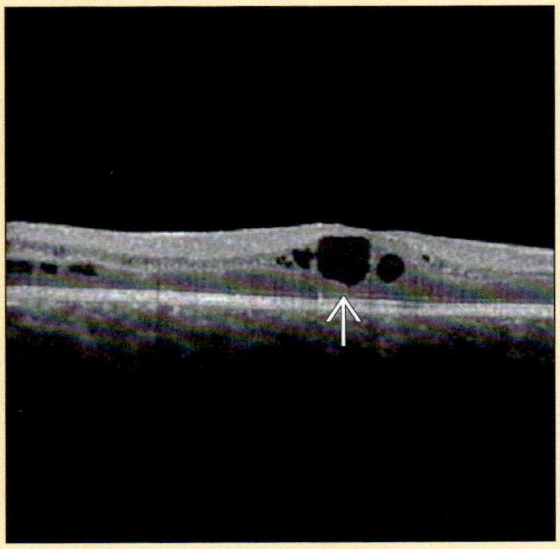

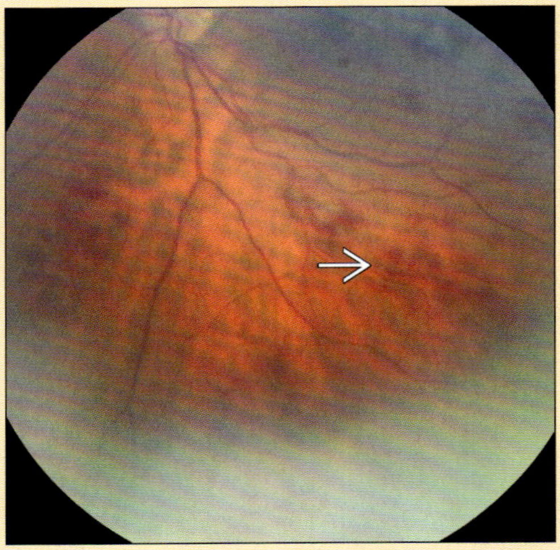

BEHÇET SYNDROME

INTRODUCTION

Definitions

- Current diagnostic criteria requires 3 episodes over a 12-month period of recurrent oral aphthous ulcers and ≥ 2 of the following
  - Genital ulcers, skin lesions, uveitis, or positive pathergy test

DEMOGRAPHICS

Etiology/Risk Factors

- Correlation with HLA-B51, HLA-B5 genotype and factor V Leiden mutation

Epidemiology

- Most often occurs in adults between ages 20 and 40, with typical age of onset in 30s
- 1 case/100,000 in USA
  - More common in males in countries along historical Silk Road trading route, especially Turkey and Japan

PRESENTATION

Symptoms

- Present in recurrences and remissions
- Systemic: Oral or genital ulcers, skin lesions, joint pain, swelling or redness, gastrointestinal disturbances
- Ocular: Vision loss, redness, pain, floaters, photophobia

Exam Findings

- Systemic
  - Aphthous ulcers on mucous membranes: Oral, genital, gastrointestinal
  - Skin manifestations: Erythema nodosum, pseudofolliculitis
  - Arthralgias, joint swelling, or redness
  - Vasculitis
    - Thrombosis, migratory thrombophlebitis
    - Aneurysms: Pulmonary (rare), aortic
  - Central nervous system manifestations: Meningoencephalitis, parenchymal lesions, stroke
- Ocular
  - Typically bilateral exam findings but can be unilateral initially
  - Inflammation (most common ocular manifestation)
    - Anterior uveitis: Possible hypopyon, flare, and cells
    - Posterior uveitis
    - Retinal perivasculitis, may lead to branched retinal artery or vein occlusion
    - Necrotizing retinitis with yellow-white infiltrate
  - Retinal hemorrhage
  - Ischemic optic neuropathy
  - Later complications: Iris neovascularization, optic nerve atrophy, phthisis bulbi
    - Posterior synechiae
      - Secondary angle closure glaucoma due to pupillary block

DIFFERENTIAL DIAGNOSIS

HLA-B27-Related Uveitis

- Exam findings: Unilateral, acute anterior uveitis (iridocyclitis), ± posterior synechiae, keratic precipitates, fibrinous exudates
- May also have symptoms of other HLA-B27-associated diseases, such as ankylosing spondylitis, etc.

Sarcoidosis (Multisystem Inflammatory Disease)

- Noncaseating granulomas, bilateral hilar lymphadenopathy, cutaneous lesions, cardiomyopathy, arthralgias
- Uveitis (anterior or posterior), iris nodules, mutton-fat keratic precipitates, vitreitis, lacrimal gland swelling, optic nerve involvement

Syphilis (Treponema pallidum Infection)

- Ocular exam findings: Argyll Robertson pupil, interstitial keratitis, iritis, chorioretinitis, cataracts
- Systemic exam findings: Chancres, rash, gummas

EVALUATION/WORK-UP

Labs

- Pathergy test to detect hyperreactivity

Pathology

- Evidence of vasculitis: Can be acute or chronic

Imaging

- Chest CT to detect evidence of thoracic involvement or possible MRI to detect intracranial lesions
- Fundus fluorescein angiography to examine retinal vessels
- Optical coherence tomography to evaluate for cystoid macular edema

TREATMENT

Medical

- Systemic corticosteroids are useful for acute attacks but not for preventing recurrences
- Immunotherapy (useful for severe attacks); need rheumatology comanagement
  - Cytoxic agents: Methotrexate, azathioprine, cyclophosphamide, chlorambucil
  - Cyclosporin A, tacrolimus
    - Decreases frequency of uveitis
    - Not used for those with neurologic involvement
  - Interferon-α for skin, joint manifestations
  - Infliximab

Prognosis

- Mortality ranging from 3-4%, up to 25% with blindness
- Recurrent attacks of uveitis lead to cumulative damage

SELECTED REFERENCES

1. Evereklioglu C: Current concepts in the etiology and treatment of Behçet disease. Surv Ophthalmol. 50(4):297-350, 2005

ENDOPHTHALMITIS

Key Facts

Introduction
- Inflammation limited to inside of eye, typically infectious
- Can be exogenous or endogenous

Etiology
- Acute post cataract: Coagulase-negative staphylococci most commonly but also *Staphylococcus aureus* and streptococci
- Post traumatic: Staphylococci and *Bacillus cereus*
- Bleb related: *Pneumococcus* and *Haemophilus influenzae*
- Chronic/delayed onset: *Propionibacterium acnes*

Presentation
- Symptoms present 2-10 days after surgery
- Hypopyon, injected conjunctiva, eyelid swelling
- Deep pain not improved by topical anesthesia or cycloplegia
- May have difficulty viewing retina due to white cell infiltrate in aqueous and vitreous
- Decreased visual acuity

Evaluation/Work-Up
- Culture of intraocular fluids, either from fine-needle aspirate or vitrectomy, with Gram and Giemsa stains

Treatment
- Intravitreal antibiotics, typically vancomycin plus ceftazidime for bacteria or amphotericin for mold/yeast
- IV antibiotics (e.g., vancomycin + ceftazidime) or oral antibiotics (moxifloxacin 400 mg/day for 1 week), depending on cause
- Vitrectomy

(Left) *Slit-lamp photograph of a patient with endophthalmitis shows the formation of a plaque ➔, obscuring the view to the posterior chamber.* ***(Right)*** *This B-scan ultrasound of a patient with endophthalmitis shows cellular debris in the vitreous ➔ and no evidence of retinal detachment. Evaluation with ultrasound plays an important role in cases of endophthalmitis as the view to the posterior chamber may often be obscured.*

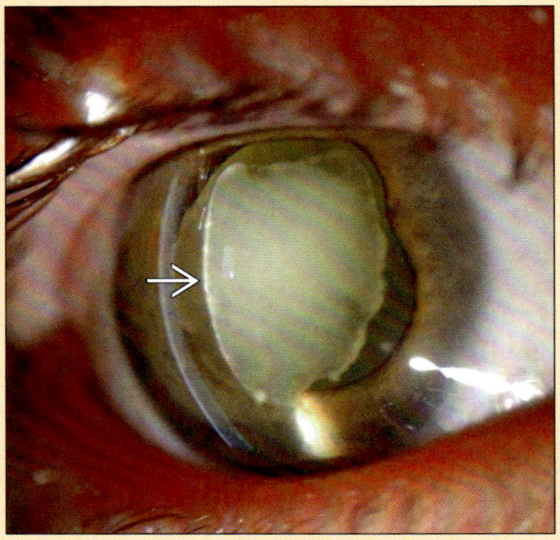

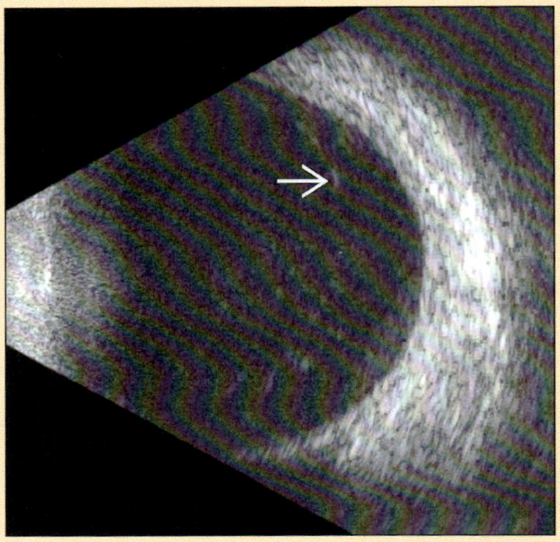

(Left) *External photo of a patient with endophthalmitis shows hypopyon ➔ and severe ocular injection.* ***(Right)*** *This fundus photo shows a patient with endophthalmitis. Note the local areas of increased inflammation ➔ within the retina and overall haziness of view due to inflammatory cells in the vitreous.*

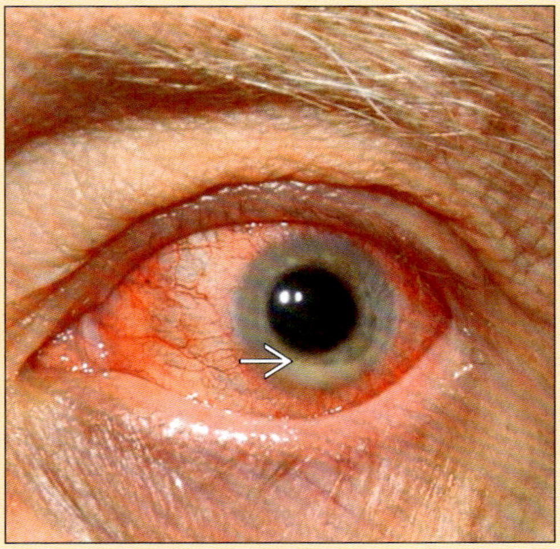

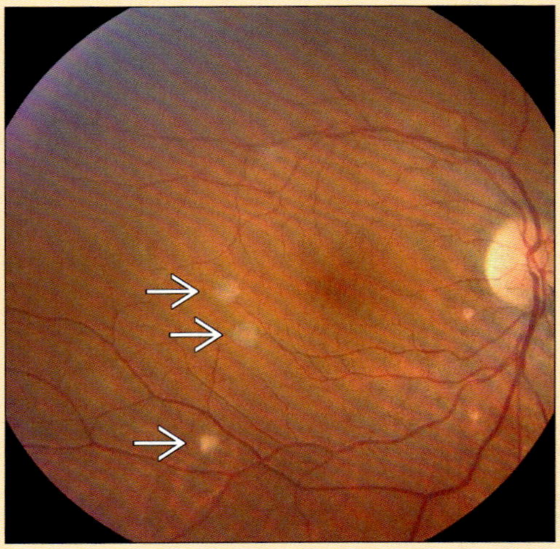

ENDOPHTHALMITIS

INTRODUCTION

Definitions
- Inflammation limited to inside of eye, typically infectious
- Can be exogenous or endogenous
  - Exogenous: Infection from outside source such as surgery or trauma
  - Endogenous: Infection from bloodstream

Subtypes
- Acute post-cataract-related endophthalmitis
- Post-traumatic endophthalmitis
- Mold (*Aspergillus*) or *Candida* endophthalmitis
- Bleb-related endophthalmitis
- Chronic post-cataract-related endophthalmitis
- Endogenous bacteremia can cause endophthalmitis
- Other intraocular procedures such as intravitreal injections can cause endophthalmitis

DEMOGRAPHICS

Etiology/Risk Factors
- Acute post cataract: Coagulase-negative staphylococci most commonly but also *Staphylococcus aureus* and streptococci
- Post traumatic: *Staphylococcus* is most common, but *Bacillus cereus* is very frequent
  - Increase risk of *Bacillus cereus* if wound is contaminated by soil
- Bleb related: *Streptococcus pneumoniae* and *Haemophilus influenzae* are common
- Endogenous: 40% due to endocarditis (*S. aureus, Streptococcus*) but also UTI, gastrointestinal bacteria, and fungi
- Chronic post cataract/delayed onset: *Propionibacterium acnes*

Epidemiology
- Acute post cataract: ~ 0.1-0.2% of cataract cases
  - Increased risk with clear corneal incision
- Post traumatic: 3-10% after penetrating trauma to eye
- Bleb related: ~ 1.3% per patient year

PRESENTATION

Symptoms
- Typically present 2-10 days after surgery
- Decreased vision, red eye, pain not improved by topical anesthesia or cycloplegia

Exam Findings
- Decreased visual acuity
- Hypopyon, conjunctival injection, eyelid edema
- May have difficulty viewing retinal vessels due to anterior &/or posterior chamber cell
- Corneal edema; loss of red reflex
- White plaque on posterior lens capsule in chronic post cataract related

DIFFERENTIAL DIAGNOSIS

History of Intraocular Procedure
- Toxic anterior segment syndrome (TASS)
  - Presents 24-48 hours after surgery
  - Inflammation limited to anterior segment
- Sterile intraocular inflammation
  - Typically presents on day 1 post cataract surgery

Retinitis or Chorioretinitis
- Initially, can be painless or asymptomatic
- Typically caused by virus or *Candida* infection

EVALUATION/WORK-UP

Labs
- Culture of intraocular fluids, either from fine-needle aspirate or vitrectomy, with Gram and Giemsa stains
- Some studies have found PCR to be more sensitive

Pathology
- Acute inflammation markers: Neutrophils
- Chronic inflammation markers: Lymphocytes, possible granulomas

Imaging
- Ultrasound can be useful since initial views may be obstructed

TREATMENT

Medical
- Intravitreal antibiotics, typically vancomycin plus ceftazidime for bacteria or amphotericin for mold/yeast
  - Vancomycin: 1 mg/0.1 mL normal saline
  - Ceftazidime: 2.25 mg/0.1 mL
  - Systemic antibiotics for post-traumatic and endogenous subtypes; oral or intravenous depending on agent
    - Consider moxifloxacin 400 mg/day or vancomycin + ceftazidime IV

Surgical
- Vitrectomy has been found useful in patients with endophthalmitis after cataract surgery presenting with light-perception-only or worse visual acuity

Follow-Up
- Considered ophthalmic emergency, requires daily follow-up

Prognosis
- 53% with acute post cataract subtype returned to 20/40 visual acuity after 1 year
  - Streptococci, *B. cereus,* and mold associated with poorer visual outcomes than coagulase-negative staphylococci

SELECTED REFERENCES

1. Durand ML: Endophthalmitis. Clin Microbiol Infect. 19(3):227-34, 2013
2. Results of the Endophthalmitis Vitrectomy Study: A randomized trial of immediate vitrectomy and of intravenous antibiotics for the treatment of postoperative bacterial endophthalmitis. Endophthalmitis Vitrectomy Study Group. Arch Ophthalmol. 113(12):1479-96, 1995

CHRONIC POSTOPERATIVE UVEITIS

Key Facts

Introduction
- Mild to moderate inflammation of intraocular fluid and tissues with onset > 6 weeks postoperatively

Etiology
- Retained lens fragments or contamination of IOL or surgical instruments
- Improper use or abrupt cessation of steroids
- Most commonly due to *Propionibacterium acnes*, *Candida*, and *Staphylococcus epidermidis*

Presentation
- Indolent and often recurring episodes of decreased vision, ± pain or discomfort
- Cellular white opacity covering IOL, often coating posterior lens capsule
- Large granulomatous precipitates on cornea
- Fluffy white vitreous infiltrates ("fluff balls" or "string of pearls") suggestive of fungal infection

Evaluation/Work-Up
- Acquire aqueous and vitreous samples for Gram stain, fungal stain, culture, and antibiotic sensitivity testing

Treatment
- If bacterial infection suspected, consider intravitreal vancomycin injection (intravitreal steroids optional)
  - If inflammation does not resolve with antibiotics alone, perform pars plana vitrectomy and central capsulotomy and continue intravitreal antibiotics (may need to remove IOL if it is colonized)
- If fungal infection suspected, consider intravitreal injection with amphotericin B or voriconazole
  - If inflammation does not resolve, consider total capsulectomy and IOL removal or exchange

Prognosis
- 54% experience visual impairment; 46% have visual outcome of 20/40 or better following treatment

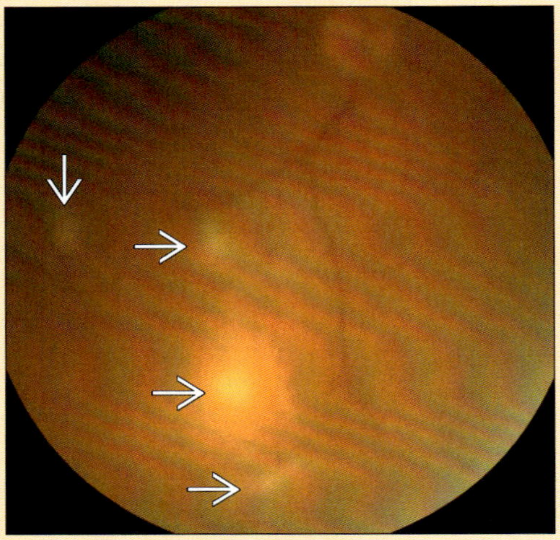

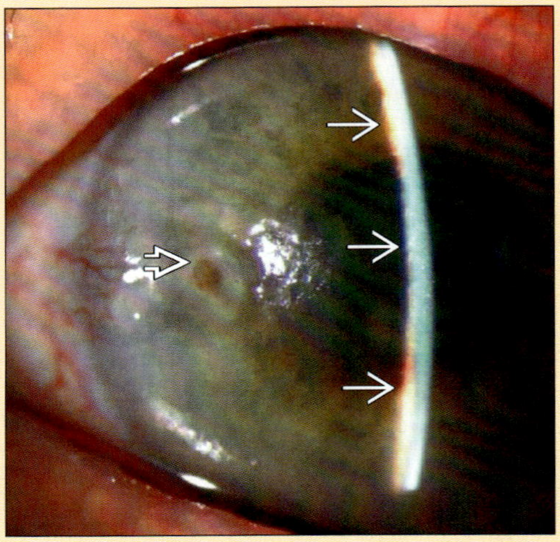

(Left) *Fundus photo shows several fluffy white vitreous infiltrates ("fluff balls") ➡ and diffuse vitreous haze suggestive of a chronic postoperative uveitis of fungal etiology.* ***(Right)*** *This slit-lamp photo shows a flat anterior chamber ➡ and possible endophthalmitis following corneal perforation ⇨.*

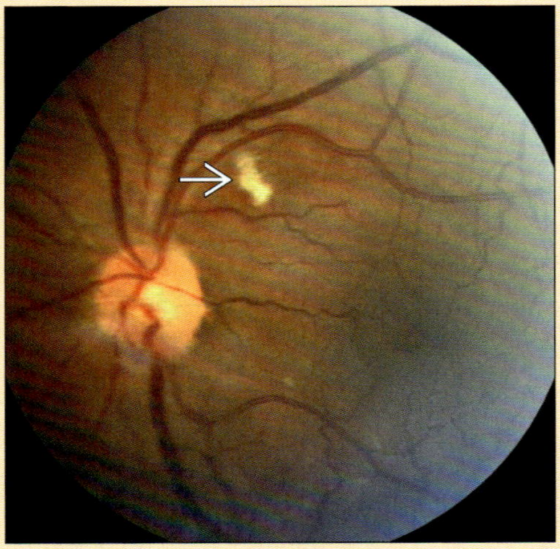

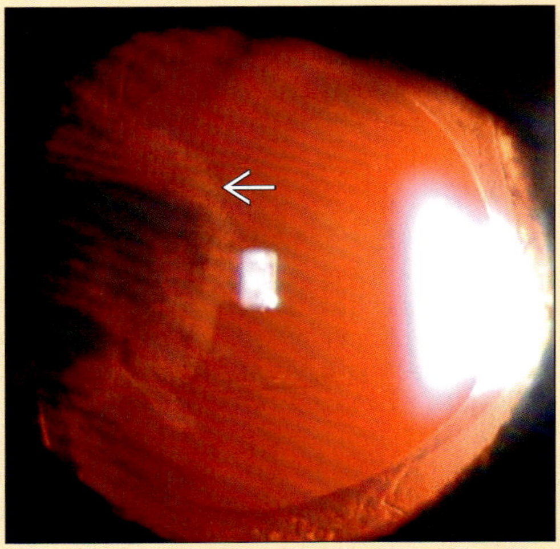

(Left) *Fundus photo shows a chorioretinal scar ➡ characteristic of chronic postoperative uveitis due to Aspergillus endophthalmitis.* ***(Right)*** *This slit-lamp photo shows retained lens fragments ➡ following cataract surgery, a common nidus for growth of Propionibacterium acnes and subsequent chronic postoperative uveitis.*

CHRONIC POSTOPERATIVE UVEITIS

INTRODUCTION

Definitions

- Mild to moderate postoperative inflammation of intraocular fluid and tissues
  - Onset > 6 weeks following surgery but may present months or years after inciting surgical event

DEMOGRAPHICS

Etiology/Risk Factors

- Retained lens fragments
- Persistent postoperative bacterial endophthalmitis
- Contamination of IOL or instruments
- Improper use or abrupt cessation of steroids

Epidemiology

- Most commonly due to *Propionibacterium acnes*, *Candida*, and *Staphylococcus epidermidis*
- Incidence of 0.017% following cataract surgery
  - Ratio of acute to chronic postoperative endophthalmitis estimated between 2:1 and 5:1

PRESENTATION

Symptoms

- Indolent and often recurring episodes of decreased vision, ± pain or discomfort

Exam Findings

- Cellular white opacity covering IOL and often coating posterior lens capsule
- Large granulomatous corneal precipitates, often without frank hypopyon, but microhypopyon visible by gonioscopy
- Fluffy white vitreous infiltrates ("fluff balls" or "string of pearls") near capsular remnant suggestive of fungal infection
- Presence of white blood cells, red blood cells, persistent lens material, or vitreous in anterior chamber
- Increased IOP

DIFFERENTIAL DIAGNOSIS

Acute Postoperative Endophthalmitis

- Severe inflammation with onset < 6 weeks following surgery; infectious etiology from exogenous or endogenous source

Uveitis-Glaucoma-Hyphema (UGH) Syndrome

- Scattering of light beam and presence of individual cells seen on slit-lamp exam of anterior chamber, elevated IOP, and hyphema due to irritation of iris by IOL, but not due to infectious etiology

Epithelial Downgrowth

- Growth of corneal or conjunctival epithelium into eye through corneal wound resulting in elevated IOP and inflammation
- Confirm with appearance of white spots following treatment with argon laser

Sympathetic Ophthalmia

- Inflammation of uninvolved eye following unilateral ocular surgery or trauma

EVALUATION/WORK-UP

Labs

- Acquire aqueous and vitreous samples for Gram stain, fungal stain, culture, and antibiotic sensitivity testing

Imaging

- Perform gonioscopy for presence of retained lens fragments or microhypopyon
- B-scan ultrasound if view of fundus is obscured

TREATMENT

Medical

- Antibiotics
  - If bacterial infection suspected, consider empiric intravitreal injection with vancomycin
  - If fungal infection suspected, consider intravitreal injection with amphotericin B or voriconazole
    - Continue systemic antifungal for 6 weeks to 6 months
- Corticosteroids
  - Use of intravitreal steroids is optional
  - Inflammation initially improves with steroids but often recurs upon steroid tapering

Surgical

- If bacterial infection suspected or inflammation is refractory to antibiotics alone, perform pars plana vitrectomy and central capsulotomy, with possible IOL removal or exchange
- If fungal infection refractory to intravitreal antifungals, consider capsulectomy and IOL removal or exchange

Follow-Up

- Weekly and then monthly for complete resolution of symptoms without signs of recurrent inflammation

Prognosis

- Decreased recurrence rate with aggressive treatment
- 54% experience visual impairment; 46% have visual outcome of 20/40 or better following treatment
- Poor prognosis with chronic fungal postop uveitis

SELECTED REFERENCES

1. Maalouf F et al: Chronic postoperative endophthalmitis: a review of clinical characteristics, microbiology, treatment strategies, and outcomes. Int J Inflam. 2012:313248, 2012
2. Shirodkar AR et al: Delayed- versus acute-onset endophthalmitis after cataract surgery. Am J Ophthalmol. 153(3):391-398, 2012
3. Al-Mezaine HS et al: Incidence, clinical features, causative organisms, and visual outcomes of delayed-onset pseudophakic endophthalmitis. Eur J Ophthalmol. 19(5):804-11, 2009
4. Ciulla TA: Update on acute and chronic endophthalmitis. Ophthalmology. 106(12):2237-8, 1999
5. Fox GM et al: Delayed-onset pseudophakic endophthalmitis. Am J Ophthalmol. 111(2):163-73, 1991

POSTOPERATIVE ENDOPHTHALMITIS

Key Facts

Introduction
- Severe inflammation of intraocular fluid and tissues
  - Onset < 6 weeks following ocular surgery

Subtypes
- Exogenous: Infectious source found outside the body such as from skin or contaminated instruments
- Endogenous: Infection reaches eye via hematologic seeding; most commonly in immunocompromised

Demographics
- Incidence: 0.12-0.7%
- Roughly 90% of cases occur following cataract surgery

Presentation
- Pain, red eye, blurred vision, and swollen eyelids

Exam Findings
- Increased anterior chamber flare and cell, corneal infiltrates, fibrin, ± hypopyon
- Vitreous inflammation, lens opacity, retinal vasculitis, posterior hypopyon, and hemorrhage

Evaluation/Work-Up
- Aqueous, vitreous, and systemic blood samples for Gram stain, culture, and antibiotic sensitivity testing

Treatment
- Prompt empiric antibiotic treatment with intravitreal vancomycin and either ceftazidime or amikacin with modification according to antibiotic sensitivities; IV vancomycin &/or moxifloxacin
- Pars plana vitrectomy in light perception only or nonresponsive eyes to remove infectious organisms, toxins, inflammatory materials, and opacities
- Topical or subconjunctival steroids to modulate inflammatory response and reduce secondary damage
- Improvement by 48 hours after initiation of treatment
- Prognosis based on presenting acuity and virulence

*(**Left**) External photo demonstrates findings consistent with postoperative endophthalmitis, including multiple foci of involvement → and marked palpebral ➡ and bulbar ➡ conjunctival injection. Also note the loss of iris detail ➡, possibly due to corneal infiltrates and anterior chamber cell and flare. (**Right**) This slit-lamp photograph demonstrates anterior chamber fibrin ➡ in a patient with recent cataract surgery who was found to have endophthalmitis.*

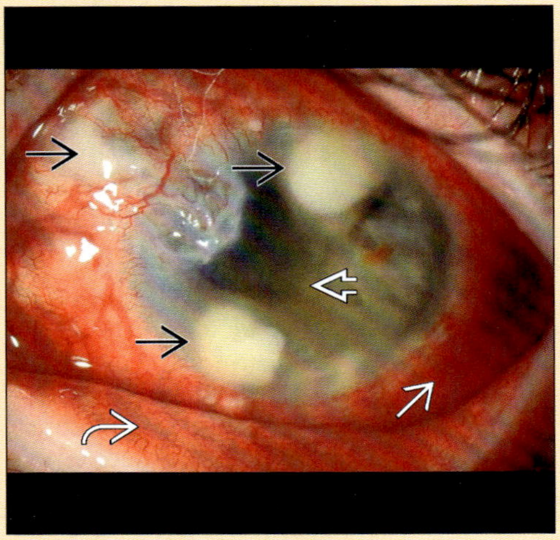

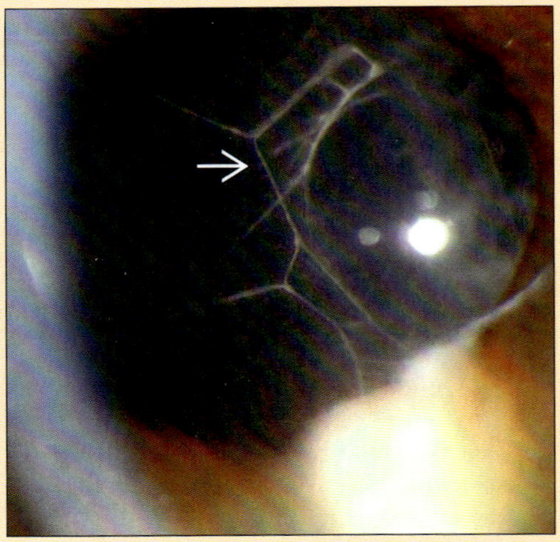

*(**Left**) Fundus photo shows posterior hypopyon ➡ and a diffuse haze that obscures clear visualization of the retina and optic nerve, consistent with an associated inflammatory vitritis possibly due to postoperative endophthalmitis. (**Right**) This external photo shows marked inflammatory chemosis ➡ of the conjunctiva and obscuration of any details of the normally white sclera following keratoprosthesis implantation.*

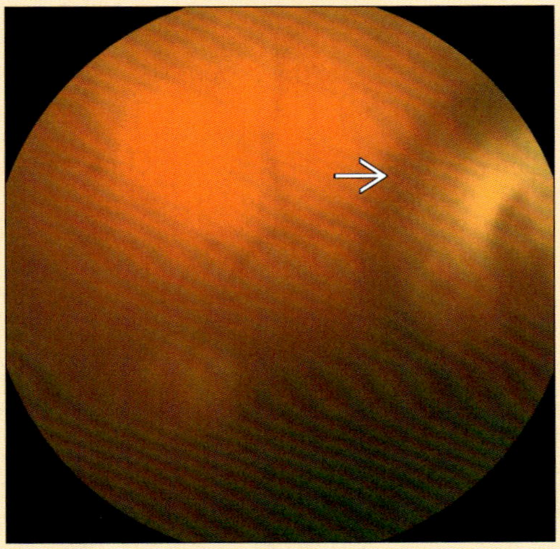

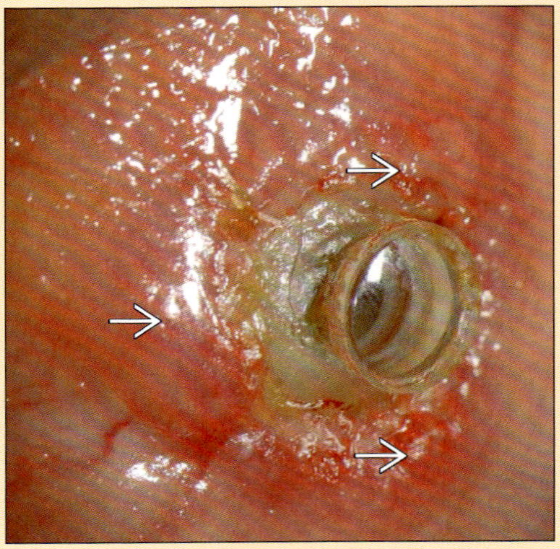

POSTOPERATIVE ENDOPHTHALMITIS

INTRODUCTION

Definitions

- Severe inflammation of intraocular fluid and tissues
  - Onset < 6 weeks following ocular surgery

Subtypes

- Exogenous
  - Infectious source found outside the body such as from skin or contaminated surgical instruments
  - More common than endogenous
- Endogenous
  - Infectious source found within the body and reaches eye via hematologic seeding
  - Most commonly in immunocompromised individuals

DEMOGRAPHICS

Etiology/Risk Factors

- Most frequently caused by coagulase-negative *Staphylococcus*, *Staphylococcus aureus*, *Streptococcus* species, and gram-negative organisms
- Preoperative risk factors include
  - Diabetes mellitus, blepharitis, lacrimal duct obstructions, contact lens wear
- Operative and postoperative risk factors include
  - Conjunctival filtering bleb, wound dehiscence, vitreous wick, or following suture removal

Epidemiology

- Incidence of 0.12-0.7%
  - Roughly 90% of cases occur following cataract surgery (although trabeculectomies may pose a higher proportional risk)
  - Increasing incidence with intravitreal injections

PRESENTATION

Symptoms

- Pain
- Blurred vision
- Red eye
- Increased exudate
- Swollen eyelids

Exam Findings

- Increased anterior chamber flare and cell, corneal infiltrates, ± hypopyon
- Vitreous inflammation, lens opacity, retinal vasculitis, posterior hypopyon, and hemorrhage
- Infection with more virulent organisms may present earlier and with increased chemosis, exudate, lid edema, afferent pupillary defect, and loss of red reflex

DIFFERENTIAL DIAGNOSIS

Chronic Postoperative Uveitis

- Onset > 6 weeks postoperatively

Sterile Endophthalmitis

- Due to retained lens fragments or vitreous hemorrhage

Toxic Anterior Segment Syndrome

- Inflammatory reaction to noninfectious agents that enter the eye intraoperatively

EVALUATION/WORK-UP

Labs

- Acquire aqueous, vitreous, and systemic blood samples for Gram stain, culture, and antibiotic sensitivity testing
  - Culture with chocolate agar, 5% sheep blood agar, thioglycollate broth, anaerobic blood agar, and Sabouraud agar

Imaging

- Consider B-scan ultrasound if significant media opacification prevents adequate view of fundus to rule out retinal or choroidal detachment, dislocated lens material, or retained foreign bodies

TREATMENT

Medical

- Prompt empiric antibiotic treatment with intravitreal vancomycin 1.0 mg/0.1 mL and either ceftazidime 2.25 mg/0.1 mL or amikacin 400 μg/0.1 mL
  - Be very cautious with aminoglycosides as their therapeutic window is small and can be toxic to the retina
  - Modify treatment according to results of sensitivity testing
- While endophthalmitis vitrectomy study did not show benefit to systemic antibiotics, many ophthalmologists would still use vancomycin &/or moxifloxacin systemically (which were not studied in the trial)
- Topical or subconjunctival steroids to modulate inflammatory response and reduce secondary damage can be considered

Surgical

- Pars plana vitrectomy to remove infectious organisms, toxins, inflammatory material, and opacities
  - Particularly beneficial in eyes with light perception only, diabetes mellitus, and cases refractory to culture and intravitreal antibiotic ("tap and inject") treatment

Follow-Up

- Monitor every 12 hours for decreased inflammation, pain relief, and resolution of hypopyon
- Expect improvement by 48 hours following initiation of antibiotic and steroid treatment
- Adjust antibiotic regimen according to culture and sensitivity results
- Taper steroid regimen after 48 hours if improvement in signs and symptoms

Prognosis

- Depends largely on visual acuity at presentation and virulence of causative organism

SELECTED REFERENCES

1. Kernt M et al: Endophthalmitis: Pathogenesis, clinical presentation, management, and perspectives. Clin Ophthalmol. 4:121-35, 2010

Key Facts

Introduction
- Granulomatous inflammation of entire uveal tract with lymphocytic and epithelial cell infiltration involving both inciting and sympathizing eye

Demographics
- Follows penetrating injury to eye: Trauma or intraocular surgery
- Males affected more than females if following trauma

Presentation
- Decreased visual acuity, photophobia, bilateral eye pain or generalized headache, & dysacusis or tinnitus
- Disease onset ranges between 5 days and ≥ 60 years
- Majority of cases occur between 10 days and 2 months
- Mild anterior to bilateral panuveitis
- Dalen-Fuchs nodules in midperiphery
- Anterior chamber: Cell and flare, ciliary flush, infiltration of iris with iris nodule formation, iris neovascularization, peripheral anterior synechiae, posterior synechiae, cataract
- Posterior chamber: Vitreous cell and haze, retinal detachment, chorioretinal scarring, papillitis

Treatment
- Medical: Corticosteroids + immunomodulators
- Surgical: Enucleation of inciting eye
- 50% of patients experience relapse after SO is controlled, requiring long-term follow-up
- Blindness secondary to macular edema and chorioretinal scarring/neovascularization
- 60% will have visual acuity of 20/50 or better
- Poor prognostic factors: Trauma as cause, exudative retinal detachment, active inflammation
- Complications include band keratopathy, subretinal fibrosis and scarring, retinal detachment, hypotony, phthisis bulbi

__(Left)__ External photograph shows an eye in a patient with sympathetic ophthalmia. The eye initially suffered a penetrating corneal injury ➔. Both this eye and the sympathizing eye developed inflammation and vision loss. __(Right)__ This fundus photograph depicts multifocal infiltrates ➔ at the level of the choroid in the sympathizing eye of a patient with sympathetic ophthalmia. Often, the sympathetic eye develops worse vision than the inciting eye.

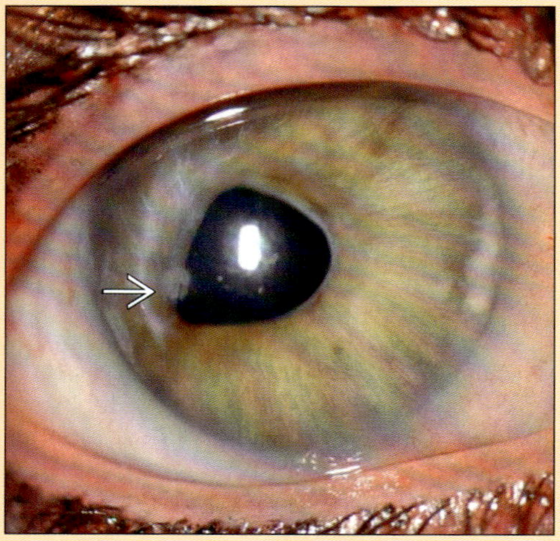

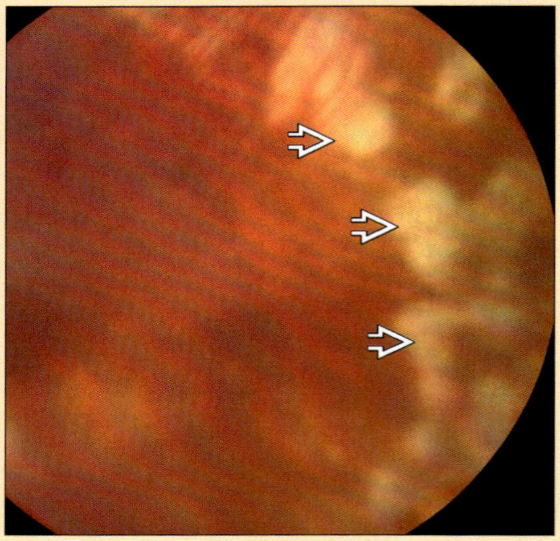

__(Left)__ Fundus photograph shows an eye with sympathetic ophthalmia demonstrated by multifocal choroidal infiltrates ➔. A history of ocular injury in the inciting eye is necessary to make a diagnosis of sympathetic ophthalmia. __(Right)__ This fundus photograph depicts a serous retinal detachment in a patient with sympathetic ophthalmia. Note how the course of the vessels changes as they travel over the detachment ➔.

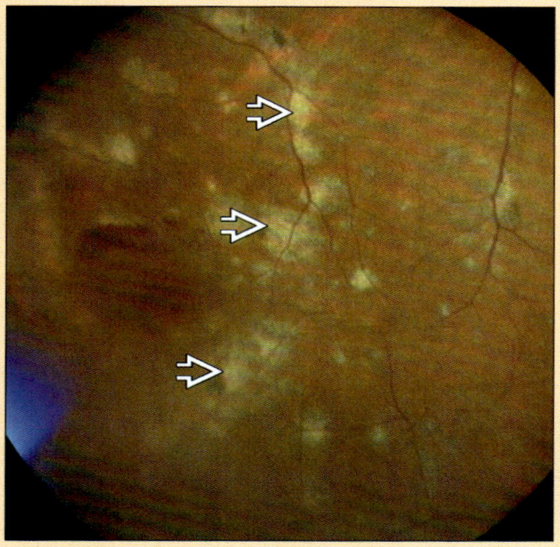

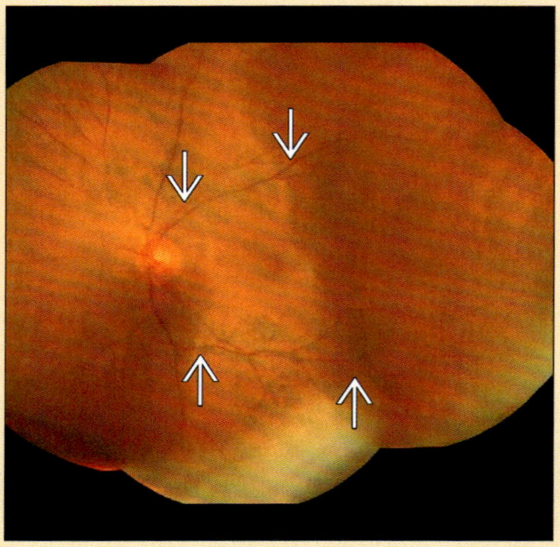

SYMPATHETIC OPHTHALMIA

INTRODUCTION

Abbreviations

- Sympathetic ophthalmia (SO)

Definitions

- Granulomatous inflammation of entire uveal tract with lymphocytic and epithelial cell infiltration involving both inciting and sympathizing eye
  - Inciting eye: Eye sustaining penetrating injury
  - Sympathizing eye: Contralateral eye

DEMOGRAPHICS

Etiology/Risk Factors

- Follows penetrating injury to eye
  - 0.2% incidence following penetrating ocular trauma
  - 0.007% incidence following intraocular surgery

Epidemiology

- Average age of presentation is 45 years

PRESENTATION

Symptoms

- Decreased visual acuity, photophobia, bilateral eye pain or generalized headache, and dysacusis or tinnitus
- Disease onset: Time period between injury and SO
  - Ranges from 5 days to ≥ 60 years
  - 65% of cases occur between 10 days and 2 months
  - 90% of cases occur within 1st year

Exam Findings

- Uveitis: Mild anterior to bilateral panuveitis
  - Persists after original wound heals
  - Mutton-fat keratic precipitates
  - Choroidal inflammation, thickening, and scarring
- Dalen-Fuchs nodules
  - Yellow-white infiltrates 60-700 μm in diameter
  - Within retinal pigment epithelium (RPE) and Bruch membrane, at midperiphery
- Anterior chamber: Cell and flare, ciliary flush, infiltration of iris, iris neovascularization, peripheral anterior synechiae, posterior synechiae, cataract
- Posterior chamber: Vitreous cell and haze, retinal detachment, chorioretinal scarring, papillitis

DIFFERENTIAL DIAGNOSIS

Bilateral Phacoanaphylactic Endophthalmitis

- Autoimmune complex reaction to lens protein placed inside lens capsule after cataract extraction
- Patient presents with a severe anterior uveitis

Vogt-Koyanagi-Harada (VKH) Syndrome

- Bilateral or unilateral uveitis in young adults associated with alopecia, poliosis, vitiligo, and hearing defects
- Prodrome of headache, dysacusis, and vertigo
- Acute iridocyclitis, patchy choroiditis, and serous retinal detachment
- No history of penetrating ocular injury
- On pathology, VKH inflammation involves choriocapillaris, unlike SO, which spares it

Multifocal Choroiditis

- Panuveitis in women aged 10-60
- Decreased visual acuity, enlarged blind spot, photopsias, anterior/posterior uveitis, disruption of peripapillary RPE, peripapillary or macular choroidal neovascular membranes
- Yellow-gray lesions in RPE appear as linear clusters or as streaks

EVALUATION/WORK-UP

Labs

- CBC, rapid plasmin reagin, FTA-Abs treponemal test for syphilis, PPD, Quantiferon gold, angiotensin-converting enzyme (ACE) level

Pathology

- Nonnecrotizing choroidal inflammation with epithelioid cells and pigment-containing giant cells
  - Absence of choriocapillaris or retinal involvement

Imaging

- Fluorescein angiogram: Early hypofluoresence followed by multiple hyperfluorescent focal dots representing leakage within RPE layer
- Ultrasonography: Thickened choroid
- CXR to rule out tuberculosis, sarcoidosis

TREATMENT

Medical

- Corticosteroids
  - Not effective in preventing SO in sympathizing eye
  - Topical + oral prednisone 1.5-2 mg/kg with slow taper for several months is usually therapeutic
- Concomitant immunomodulator therapy allows for decreased corticosteroid dosing

Surgical

- Enucleation of inciting eye
  - Enucleation within 2 weeks of injury is preventative
  - If useful vision is possible in inciting eye, enucleation is not recommended because SO may occur even after enucleation

Follow-Up

- 50% of patients experience relapse many years after SO is controlled, so long-term follow-up is required

Prognosis

- Blindness secondary to macular edema and chorioretinal scarring/neovascularization
- 30% will have visual acuity worse than 20/200
- Poor prognostic factors: Trauma as cause, exudative retinal detachment, active inflammation

SELECTED REFERENCES

1. Chaithanyaa N et al: Sympathetic ophthalmia: a review of literature. Oral Surg Oral Med Oral Pathol Oral Radiol. 113(2):172-6, 2012
2. Chang GC et al: Sympathetic ophthalmia. Semin Ophthalmol. 26(4-5):316-20, 2011
3. Sen HN et al: Sympathetic ophthalmia: what have we learned? Am J Ophthalmol. 148(5):632-3, 2009

VOGT-KOYANAGI-HARADA SYNDROME

Key Facts

Introduction
- Autoimmune disorder with bilateral, chronic granulomatous posterior or panuveitis
  - T lymphocytes attack self antigens in melanocytes found in uveal tract, skin, meninges, and cochlea
- Fluid accumulates beneath retina → RD
- 4 disease stages: Prodromal, acute uveitis, convalescent, chronic recurrent

Demographics
- Associated with HLA-DR4 and HLA-DR1 alleles
- Common in Asian, Asian Indian, Hispanic, Native American, and Middle Eastern populations
- Women aged 20-50 are most commonly affected

Presentation
- Characteristic: Bilateral granulomatous panuveitis, multifocal choroiditis, serous RD, Dalen-Fuchs nodules, sunset-glow fundus
- Cutaneous: Patchy vitiligo on eyelids, back, buttocks; poliosis; alopecia
- Neurologic: Tinnitus, vertigo, headache, meningismus
- Skin: Alopecia, poliosis, vitiligo

Evaluation/Work-Up
- Inflammatory infiltrate of lymphocytes, macrophages, epithelioid cells, multinucleated giant cells
- Ultrasound: Thickening of posterior choroid and sclera/episclera, exudative retinal detachment, vitreous opacities
- OCT: Peripapillary choroidal thickening and elevation

Treatment
- Acute uveitic stage: Topical, periocular, or systemic corticosteroids ± cycloplegics, mydriatics
- Chronic recurrent stage: Immunomodulators
  - Cyclosporine, azathioprine, mycophenolate mofetil, chlorambucil, cyclophosphamide, infliximab

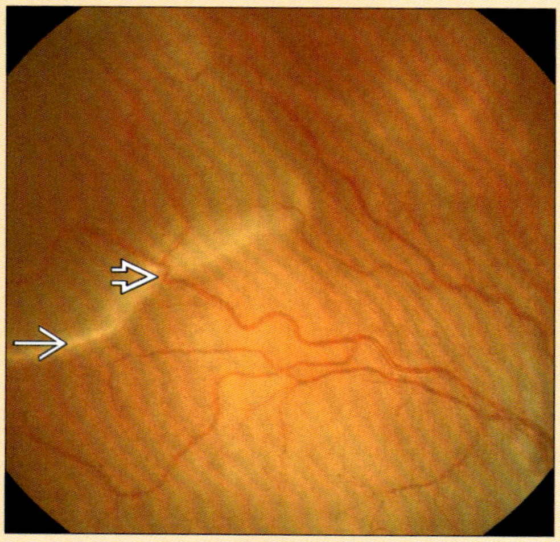
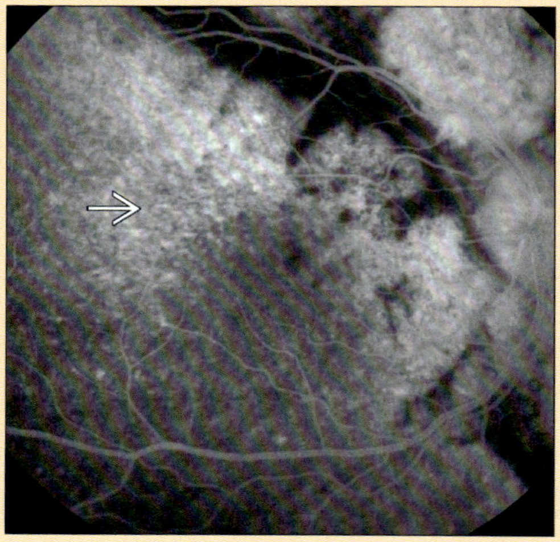

(Left) *Fundus photograph of the eye of a Vogt-Koyanagi-Harada (VKH) syndrome patient shows serous retinal detachment. Notice that the course of the vessel changes as it reaches the point of detachment ➡. The demarcation line clearly marks the extent of detachment ➡.* ***(Right)*** *This fluorescein angiography image shows the eye of a patient with VKH. Note the multiple pinpoint areas of leakage of fluorescein dye ➡.*

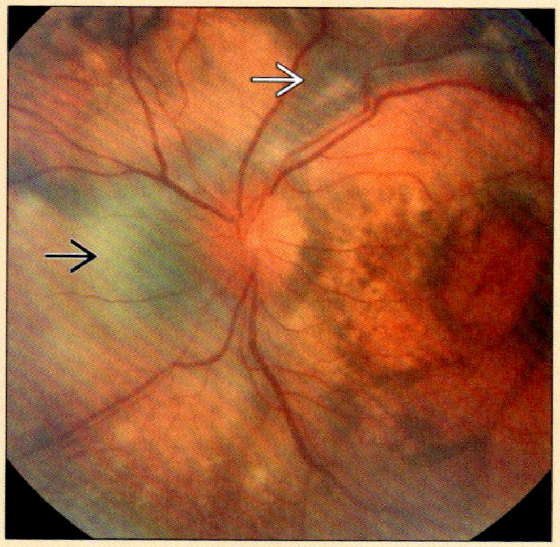
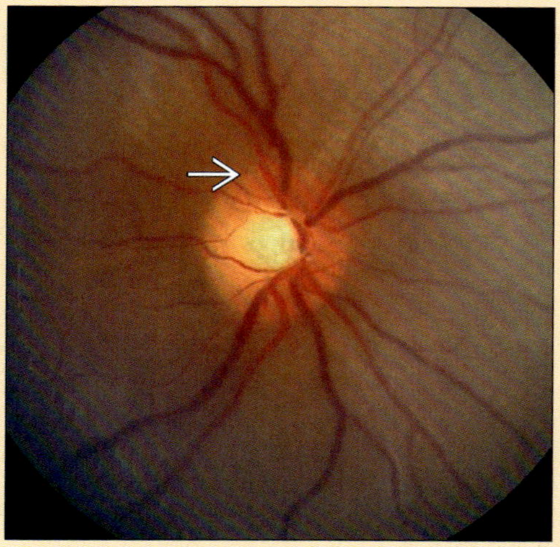

(Left) *This fundus photograph is of a patient with VKH. Note the haziness from inflammation of the posterior chamber ➡. There is also pigment clumping ➡ just nasal to the optic disc.* ***(Right)*** *Fundus photograph shows an eye of a patient with VKH. There is optic disc edema ➡ and generalized haziness, suggestive of inflammation.*

VOGT-KOYANAGI-HARADA SYNDROME

INTRODUCTION

Definitions

- Autoimmune disorder with bilateral, chronic granulomatous posterior or panuveitis with systemic involvement of skin, nervous, and auditory systems
  - T lymphocytes attack self antigens in melanocytes found in uveal tract, skin, meninges, and cochlea
- Fluid accumulates beneath retina → retinal detachment (RD)

Subtypes

- Prodromal stage
  - Early flu-like constitutional symptoms: Headache, meningismus, dysacusis, tinnitus, fever
  - Neurologic symptoms: Orbital pain, photophobia, hypersensitivity to touch of skin and hair
- Acute uveitic stage
  - Blurry vision 1-2 days after prodromal phase
  - Diffuse, nonnecrotizing, granulomatous uveitis
  - Dalen-Fuchs nodules
  - Multiple serous RDs
  - Mutton-fat keratic precipitates, iris nodules, ↑ IOP
- Convalescent stage
  - Occurs several weeks after acute uveitic stage
  - Nongranulomatous inflammation of the uvea
  - Resolution of RD
  - Sunset-glow fundus
- Chronic recurrent stage
  - Recurrent granulomatous panuveitis
  - Destruction of choriocapillaris with overlaying RD
  - Keratic precipitates, posterior synechiae, iris nodules, iris depigmentation, and stromal atrophy

DEMOGRAPHICS

Etiology/Risk Factors

- Associated with HLA-DR4 and HLA-DR1 alleles

Epidemiology

- Common in Asian, Asian Indian, Hispanic, Native American, and Middle Eastern populations
- Uncommon in whites and blacks
- Women aged 20-50 are most commonly affected
- 1.5-6 per 1 million patients in USA

PRESENTATION

Symptoms

- Neurologic: Tinnitus, vertigo, headache, meningismus
- Skin: Alopecia, poliosis, vitiligo
- Ocular: Vague complaints, may have good visual acuity

Exam Findings

- Characteristic: Bilateral granulomatous panuveitis, multifocal choroiditis (involving choriocapillaris), serous exudative RD, choroidal effusions, Dalen-Fuchs nodules, sunset-glow fundus
- Cutaneous: Patchy vitiligo on eyelids, back, buttocks; poliosis; alopecia
- CSF: Pleocytosis

DIFFERENTIAL DIAGNOSIS

Sympathetic Ophthalmia

- Penetrating ocular trauma → rapid bilateral vision loss
- Anterior segment inflammation, optic disc edema, choroidal thickening, and serous RDs
- Intact choriocapillaris underlying areas of RD (sympathetic ophthalmia spares choriocapillaris)
- Absence of systemic features

Uveal Effusion Syndrome

- Abnormal collection of fluid in suprachoroidal space
- Seen in middle-aged men
- Chronic effusion → RPE changes and ↓ visual acuity
- Treatment requires full-thickness sclerotomy

EVALUATION/WORK-UP

Pathology

- Inflammatory infiltrate of lymphocytes, macrophages, epithelioid cells, multinucleated giant cells

Imaging

- Fluorescein angiography
  - Acute uveitic stage
    - Multiple hyperfluorescent dots at level of RPE
    - Late pooling of dye in subretinal space in areas of RD
  - Convalescent/chronic recurrent stage
    - Hyperfluorescence at areas of focal retinal pigment epithelial loss and atrophy
- Ultrasound
  - Thickening of posterior choroid and sclera/episclera, exudative retinal detachment, vitreous opacities
- Ocular coherence tomography
  - Peripapillary choroidal thickening and elevation

TREATMENT

Medical

- Acute uveitic stage
  - Topical, periocular, or systemic corticosteroids
- Chronic recurrent stage
  - Immunomodulator therapy

Prognosis

- 70% of patients with visual acuity of 20/40 or better
- Complications: Cataract, glaucoma, choroidal neovascularization, subretinal fibrosis

SELECTED REFERENCES

1. Fang W et al: Vogt-koyanagi-harada syndrome. Curr Eye Res. 33(7):517-23, 2008
2. Read RW et al: Complications and prognostic factors in Vogt-Koyanagi-Harada disease. Am J Ophthalmol. 131(5):599-606, 2001
3. Moorthy RS et al: Vogt-Koyanagi-Harada syndrome. Surv Ophthalmol. 39(4):265-92, 1995
4. Rubsamen PE et al: Vogt-Koyanagi-Harada syndrome. Clinical course, therapy, and long-term visual outcome. Arch Ophthalmol. 109(5):682-7, 1991

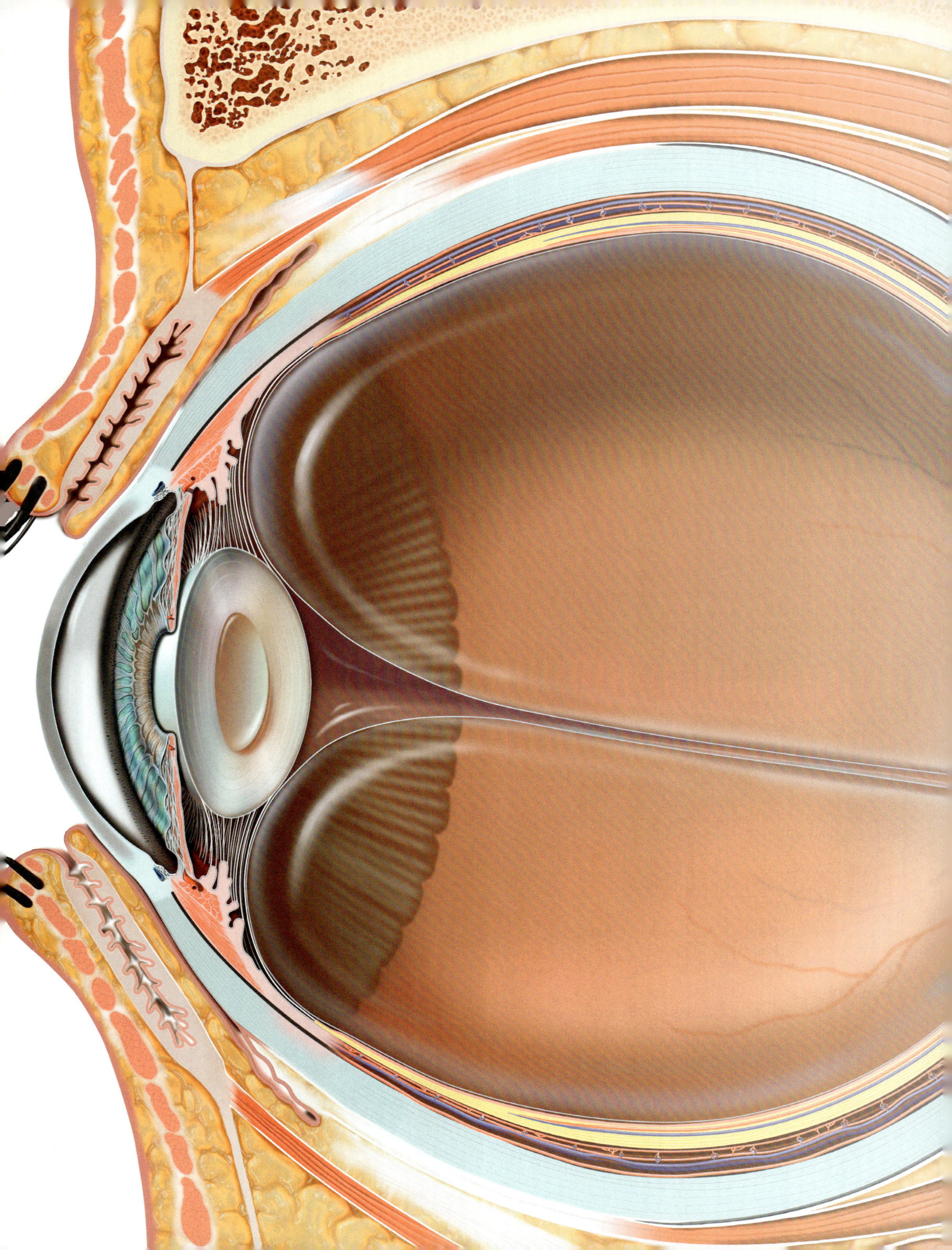

SECTION 1
Vitreous

Introduction and Overview

Trauma

Degenerations

MAJOR CLINICAL STUDIES: ANTI-VEGF IN AGE-RELATED MACULAR DEGENERATION

TERMINOLOGY

Abbreviations

- Age-related macular degeneration (ARMD)
- Fluorescein angiography
- Minimally classic/occult trial of anti-VEGF antibody ranibizumab in treatment of neovascular ARMD (MARINA)
- Anti-VEGF antibody for the treatment of predominantly classic choroidal neovascularization in ARMD (ANCHOR)
- 7-year outcomes in ranibizumab-treated patients in ANCHOR, MARINA, and HORIZON (SEVEN-UP)
- Vascular endothelial growth factor trap-eye: Investigation of efficacy and safety in wet ARMD (VIEW)
- Variable-dosing regimen with intravitreal ranibizumab for neovascular ARMD: Year 2 (PRONTO)
- Comparison of ARMD treatments trials (CATT)

MARINA TRIAL

Objective and Principal Conclusions

- Evaluate safety/efficacy of repeated intravitreal injections of ranibizumab to treat choroidal neovascularization (CNV) associated with ARMD
- Ranibizumab improved vision in CNV, outperforming prior treatments (laser and pegaptanib)

Inclusion Criteria

- Age ≥ 50
- Best corrected visual acuity (BCVA) of 20/40 to 20/320
- ARMD with active primary or recurrent subfoveal lesions
- Maximum lesion size of 12 optic disc areas
- CNV composing ≥ 50% of total lesion area

Randomization Method

- Randomized to 1 of 3 monthly injections for 2 years
  - Ranibizumab 0.3 mg, 0.5 mg, or sham injection

Results

- After 24 months, 92.0% of patients receiving 0.3 mg ranibizumab and 94.6% receiving 0.5 mg had lost < 15 letters from baseline vs. 52.9% in sham-injection group
  - $P < .001$ for comparison of each dose with sham-injection group

ANCHOR TRIAL

Objective and Principal Conclusions

- Compare repeated intravitreal injections of ranibizumab with photodynamic therapy using verteporfin in patients with CNV lesions due to ARMD
- Ranibizumab was better than photodynamic therapy in preventing vision loss, improving VA, and decreasing CNV and had a similar safety profile

Inclusion Criteria

- Age ≥ 50
- BCVA of 20/40 to 20/320
- Maximum lesion size 5,400 μm in greatest diameter
- No permanent structural damage to central fovea
- No previous therapy

Randomization Method

- Patients randomized to receive 1 of 3 treatments
  - 0.3 mg of ranibizumab + sham verteporfin photodynamic therapy
  - 0.5 mg of ranibizumab + sham verteporfin photodynamic therapy
  - Sham intravitreal injection + active verteporfin photodynamic therapy
- All injections were given monthly for 1 year
- Either verteporfin or sham verteporfin was given on day 0 and repeated p.r.n. at 3, 6, 9, or 12 months

Results

- Efficacy
  - 94.3% of patients in 0.3 mg group and 96.4% in 0.5 mg group lost < 15 letters from baseline VA vs. 64.3% in verteporfin group ($P < .001$ for each comparison)
- Safety
  - Rates of intraocular inflammation (e.g., iritis, iridocyclitis, vitritis, uveitis, anterior-chamber inflammation) was 10.2% in 0.3 mg group, 15% in 0.5 mg group, and 2.8% in verteporfin group
  - Ocular safety profiles for the 3 treatment groups showed no overall imbalance in serious and nonserious adverse events

SEVEN-UP TRIAL

Objective and Principal Conclusions

- Study ARMD progression and long-term visual changes 7-8 years after intensive ranibizumab treatment in ARMD patients
- Even 7 years from initiation of ranibizumab treatment, patients with exudative ARMD are at risk for substantial vision loss
- Anti-VEGF therapy is associated with a high risk of long-term geographic atrophy and subretinal fibrosis

Inclusion Criteria

- Patients with exudative ARMD who were treated with ranibizumab in ANCHOR or MARINA and HORIZON trials

Results

- After average of 7.3 years following entry into ANCHOR or MARINA trials
  - 37% had BCVA of 20/70 or better
  - 37% had BCVA of 20/200 or worse

VIEW TRIAL

Objective and Principal Conclusions

- Determine efficacy and safety of aflibercept in patients with neovascular ARMD
- Aflibercept was equivalent to ranibizumab in treatment efficacy but showed increased risk of cerebrovascular events in patients age ≥ 85 years

Inclusion Criteria

- Age ≥ 50
- BCVA of 20/40 to 20/320
- Active subfoveal CNV lesions due to ARMD

Randomization Method

- Patients were randomly assigned to 1 of 4 groups

- Ranibizumab 0.5 mg q. 4: Intravitreal ranibizumab 0.5 mg monthly for 1 year, then every 4-12 weeks
- Aflibercept 2 mg q. 4: Intravitreal aflibercept 2 mg monthly for 1 year, then every 4-12 weeks
- Aflibercept 0.5 mg q. 4: Intravitreal aflibercept 0.5 mg monthly for 1 year, then every 4-12 weeks
- Aflibercept 2 mg q. 8: Intravitreal injections of aflibercept 2 mg every 8 weeks (with 1 additional 2.0 mg dose at week 4) for 1 year with sham injections at interim monthly visits, and every 4-12 weeks thereafter

Results

- Percentage of patients who lost < 15 letters in ETDRS letter score at 52 weeks
  - Ranibizumab 0.5 mg q. 4: 94.42%
  - Aflibercept 2 mg q. 4: 95.62%
  - Aflibercept 0.5 mg q. 4: 96.27%
  - Aflibercept 2 mg q. 8: 95.56%
- In patients age ≥ 85, rate of cerebrovascular events was 7.1% in aflibercept group vs. 1.1% in ranibizumab group at year 1 and 9.5% and 3.4% at year 2, respectively

PRONTO TRIAL

Objective and Principal Conclusions

- Determine long-term outcome of 3 consecutive monthly intraocular injections of ranibizumab followed by p.r.n. dosing for 2 years
- OCT-guided variable-dosing of ranibizumab resulted in visual outcomes comparable with monthly dosing and decreased number of injections by 1/2 over 2 years

Inclusion Criteria

- ARMD with CNV involving central fovea
- CRT ≥ 300 μm on OCT

Randomization Method

- All participants received 0.5 mg intraocular injection at baseline, week 4 and 8, then p.r.n. if patient met retreatment criteria without control comparison

Results

- Visual acuity at 24 months improved by mean of 11.1 letters, median 14 letters on ETDRS chart
- OCT showed ↓ in CRT by mean 212 μm, median 209 μm
- Intravitreal ranibizumab improved VA and rapidly decreased amount of macular fluid in most patients with ARMD
  - ↓ in retinal thickness was seen within 1 day after 1st injection through month 3 and maintained to month 24
- No correlation between number of reinjections and baseline VA or lesion size
- No correlation between VA and OCT-CRT at 24 months, but did correlate at months 2, 3, and 12
- OCT-CRT measurement correlated with changes in VA at months 2, 3, 12, and 24 ($P < .05$)

CATT STUDY

Objectives and Principal Conclusions

- Compare ranibizumab with bevacizumab given monthly or p.r.n. for 2 years
- Determine effects of switching to p.r.n. dosing after 1 year of monthly treatment
- Monthly ranibizumab or bevacizumab had better visual outcomes than p.r.n. and were equal to each other

Inclusion Criteria

- Active CNV due to ARMD
- VA of 20/25 to 20/320
- Neovascularization, fluid, or hemorrhage under fovea
- No history of previous treatment

Randomization Method

- Patients were randomly assigned to 1 of 4 groups
  - Monthly ranibizumab
  - p.r.n. ranibizumab
  - Monthly bevacizumab
  - p.r.n. bevacizumab
- At 1 year, patients assigned to monthly treatment were randomly reassigned to p.r.n. or monthly, without changing the drug assignment

Results

RELATED REFERENCES

1. National Institutes of Health: A Study of Ranibizumab Administered Monthly or on an As-needed Basis in Patients With Subfoveal Neovascular Age-related Macular Degeneration (HARBOR). ClinicalTrials.gov. http://clinicaltrials.gov/ct2/show/NCT00891735. Published April 29, 2009. Updated December 11, 2012. Accessed September 6, 2013
2. National Institutes of Health: Comparison of Age-Related Macular Degeneration Treatment Trials: Lucentis-Avastic Trial. ClinicalTrials.gov. http://clinicaltrials.gov/ct2/show/study/NCT00593450?term=CATT+trial&rank=1&sect=X9876015. Published January 3, 2008. Updated July 2, 2013. Accessed September 6, 2013
3. National Institutes of Health: Vascular Endothelial Growth Factor (VEGF) Trap-Eye: Investigation of Efficacy and Safety in Wet Age-Related Macular Degeneration (AMD) (VIEW 2). ClinicalTrials.gov. http://clinicaltrials.gov/show/NCT00637377. Published March 12, 2008. Updated March 12, 2013. Accessed September 6, 2013
4. Rofagha S et al: Seven-Year Outcomes in Ranibizumab-Treated Patients in ANCHOR, MARINA, and HORIZON: A Multicenter Cohort Study (SEVEN-UP). Ophthalmology. Epub ahead of print, 2013
5. Comparison of Age-related Macular Degeneration Treatments Trials (CATT) Research Group et al: Ranibizumab and bevacizumab for treatment of neovascular age-related macular degeneration: two-year results. Ophthalmology. 119(7):1388-98, 2012
6. Brown DM et al: Ranibizumab versus verteporfin photodynamic therapy for neovascular age-related macular degeneration: Two-year results of the ANCHOR study. Ophthalmology. 116(1):57-65, 2009
7. Lalwani GA et al: A variable-dosing regimen with intravitreal ranibizumab for neovascular age-related macular degeneration: year 2 of the PrONTO Study. Am J Ophthalmol. 148(1):43-58, 2009
8. Lalwani GA et al: A variable-dosing regimen with intravitreal ranibizumab for neovascular age-related macular degeneration: year 2 of the PrONTO Study. Am J Ophthalmol. 148(1):43-58, 2009
9. Rosenfeld PJ et al: Ranibizumab for neovascular age-related macular degeneration. N Engl J Med. 355(14):1419-31, 2006

VITREOUS OVERVIEW

TERMINOLOGY

Definitions

- Thick, gelatinous, clear substance that occupies center of eye
- Occupies 80% of globe volume
  - Roughly 2/3 of total volume of eye
- Has various functions
  - Maintains shape of eye
  - Light refraction
- Begins to liquify (syneresis) over time

ANATOMY

Structure

- Vitreous body
  - Central vitreous: Core or inner vitreous
  - Cortical vitreous: Outer vitreous
- Cloquet/hyaloid canal
  - Transverses central vitreous from lens (Berger space) to optic nerve (area of Martegiani)
  - Remnant lumen of embryogenic hyaloid artery
  - Devoid of collagen
  - 1-2 mm in diameter
- Wieger ligament
  - Also known as Egger line and hyaloideocapsular ligament
  - Serves as anterior attachment site for vitreous
  - Fuses with posterior group of zonular fibers

Vitreoretinal Attachments

- Vitreous base: Strongest retinal attachment
  - Straddles ora serrata; 3-4 mm wide
- Optic nerve: Strong attachment
- Macula: Weak attachment
  - Surrounds and attaches in annular fashion; 3-4 mm diameter
- Retinal vessels: Weak attachment

VITREOUS COMPOSITION AND FUNCTION

Composition

- Water (99%)
- Collagen (mainly type II, some type XI): Highest in concentration at vitreous base
- Hyaluronic acid (HA): Total molecular weight of HA estimated to be between 2-4 million
- Albumin accounts for ~ 60-70% of protein concentration of vitreous
- Mucopolysaccharide produced by nonpigmented epithelial cells of pars plana
- Contains volume just over 4 cm^3
- Mainly acellular except for phagocytes

Function

- Maintains shape of eyeball through process of vitreoretinal traction
  - Vitreoretinal traction is force that components of vitreous exert on surrounding retina
- Refraction of light
  - Index of refraction: 1.33

VITREOUS PATHOLOGY

Posterior Vitreous Detachment

- Cross-linking and loss vitreous collagen → destabilizes vitreous matrix
- Separation of vitreous from retina
- Can create floaters, also known as muscae volitantes (Latin for "flying flies")

Vitreous Hemorrhage

- Blood surrounds &/or penetrates into vitreous cavity
- Causes
  - Trauma, proliferative diabetic retinopathy, bleeding dysfunction, altitude retinopathy, posterior vitreous detachment, Terson syndrome, retinal tears, proliferative vitreoretinopathy, retinopathy of prematurity

Amyloidosis

- Bilateral vitreous opacification
- Yellowish-white, gold, or multicolored cholesterol crystals form in vitreous and anterior chamber

Syneresis

- Vitreous humor begins to liquefy
  - Liquefied vitreous termed as floaters often obscures vision and can even lead to posterior vitreous detachment
- Occurs with aging

Asteroid Hyalosis (Benson Disease)

- White opacities composed of calcium-containing phospholipids found in otherwise normal vitreous
- Cholesterolosis (hemophthalmos, synchysis scintillans)

Hereditary Vitreopathy

- Jansen disease
- Wagner disease
- Stickler syndrome

Persistent Fetal Vasculature

- Often other abnormalities in eye (e.g., microphthalmia)
  - Can cause leukocoria in children

IMAGING

Dark-Field Slit-Lamp Microscopy

- Avoids dehydration of vitreous and use of histologic fixatives
- Useful for in vitro imaging

Optical Coherence Tomography

- Useful for in vivo imaging of vitreoretinal interface
- Inability to see vitreous body

B-Scan Ultrasonography

- Can be useful to detect more advanced stages of PVD

Dynamic Light Scattering

- Useful to estimate average size of vitreous opacities and macromolecules

VITREOUS IMAGES

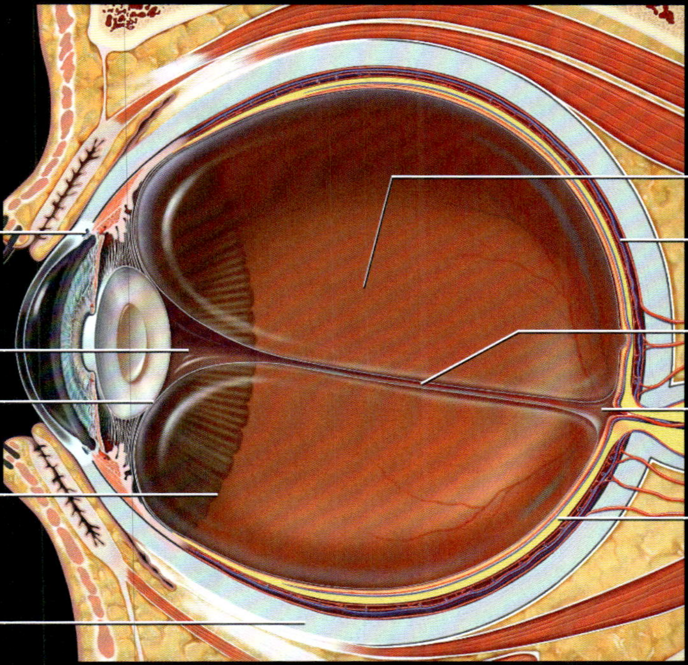

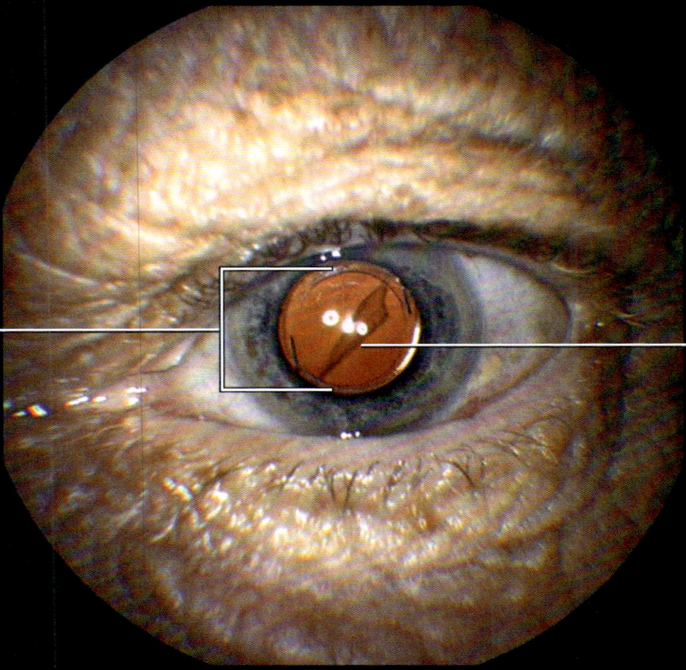

(Top) *This diagram outlines the basic anatomical structures and landmarks of the vitreous.* ***(Bottom)*** *This external photo depicts a posterior vitreous detachment. A useful way to visualize a posterior vitreous detachment is by eliciting the red reflex and viewing a flapping opacity in the fundus. This finding is commonly associated with increased age.*

INTRAOCULAR FOREIGN BODY

Key Facts

Demographics
- Penetrating injury to globe with retained foreign body
- Risk of endophthalmitis increases with delay in wound closure, retained intraocular foreign body (IOFB), rural setting, ruptured lens capsule
- IOFBs may be present in up to 41% of all open globe injuries

Presentation
- Decreased vision, eye pain, ocular hypotony, uveal prolapse, peaked pupil, corneal or scleral lacerations, subconjunctival hemorrhage, hyphema, vitreous hemorrhage, foreign body on slit-lamp or fundus exam

Evaluation/Work-Up
- Thorough history to determine mechanism, time of injury, vision before accident
- Slit-lamp and dilated fundus exam
- CT scan with axial and coronal fine cuts through the orbit; avoid MRI if any chance IOFB could be metallic
- Ultrasound may be used carefully with special attention to avoid pressure on globe
- Vitreous Gram stain and culture to help guide treatment

Treatment
- Tetanus prophylaxis if not current
- Systemic broad-spectrum antibiotic coverage with oral levofloxacin or moxifloxacin for endophthalmitis prophylaxis
- Topical fortified vancomycin and ceftazidime or fluoroquinolone every hour
- Primary surgical goal is comprehensive anatomical reconstruction of injured eye; secondary goal is removal of intraocular foreign body
- Up to 71% of patients achieve 20/40 or better vision

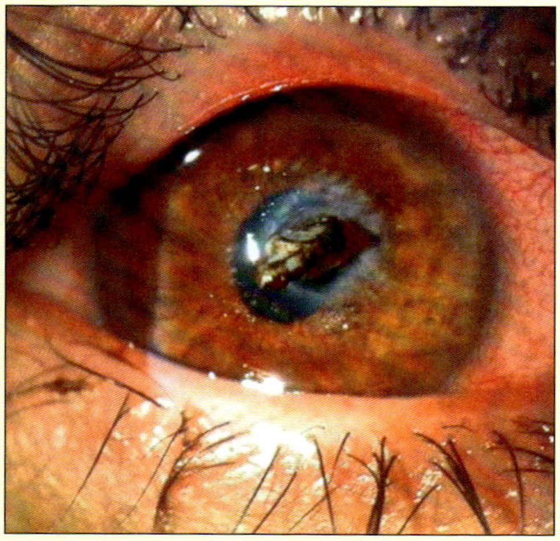
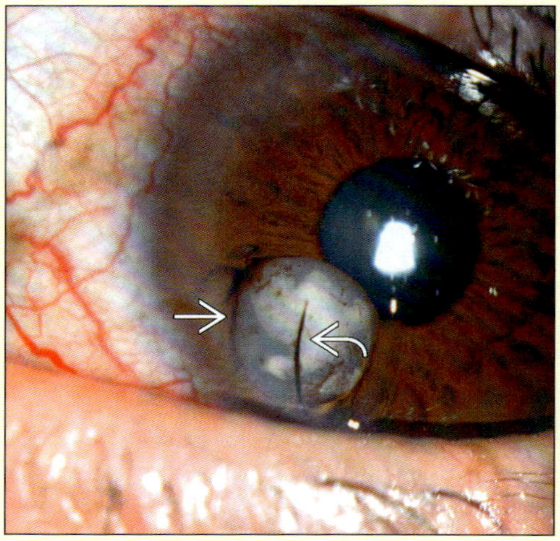

(Left) *External photo shows wooden intraocular foreign body embedded in the cornea. Some intraocular foreign bodies are obvious, as this photo depicts. Wood foreign bodies are often difficult to visualize on CT or MRI. (Courtesy R. Nosé, MD.)* ***(Right)*** *External photo shows intraocular cement and cilia. The patient was a construction worker jackhammering 3 months prior to presentation. The superior corneal wound is not visible on this image. (Courtesy K. Shah, MD.)*

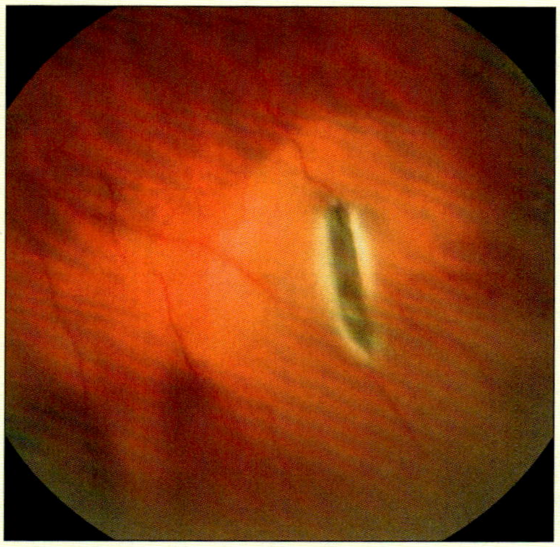
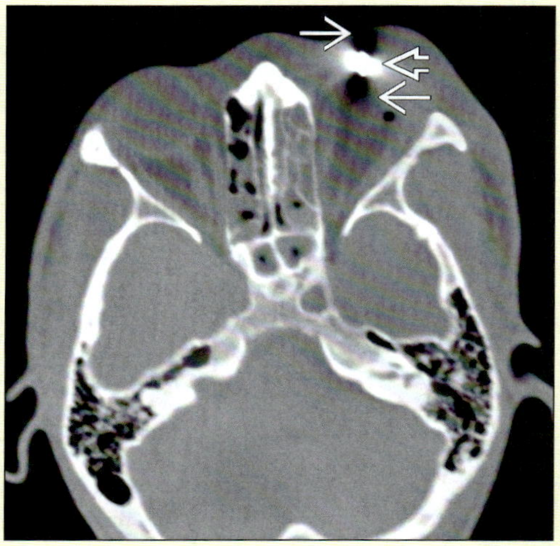

(Left) *Fundus photo depicts a subretinal intraocular foreign body visible on dilated fundus examination. Inert objects that would cause more harm to remove may be left in place. (Courtesy J. Perron.)* ***(Right)*** *CT shows intraocular metallic foreign body with characteristic metal artifact distorting the surrounding image. CT is ideal for intraocular foreign body localization, and newer CT scanners provide less artifact and increased resolution, further aiding surgical planning.*

INTRAOCULAR FOREIGN BODY

INTRODUCTION

Abbreviations
- Intraocular foreign body (IOFB)

Definitions
- Foreign body inside globe

DEMOGRAPHICS

Etiology/Risk Factors
- Penetrating injury to globe with retained foreign body
- 44.1% of eye injuries occur at home, 15.6% in industrial/office setting, 14.7% during sports or recreational activities, 11.4% in connection with motor vehicle accidents, and 14.2% elsewhere
- Combat, metalworking, hammering, lack of protective eyewear, and other high-risk activities are risk factors for IOFB
- Increased risk of endophthalmitis with
  - Delay in wound closure > 24 hours
  - Retained IOFB
  - Injury in a rural setting, attributed to higher incidence of soil contamination
  - Ruptured lens capsule
- Up to 13% of patients with IOFB may develop endophthalmitis

Epidemiology
- Incidence of 0.16 per 100,000 people
- Present in up to 41% of all open globe injuries

PRESENTATION

Symptoms
- Eye pain, decreased vision, floaters

Exam Findings
- Signs of open globe, including decreased vision, ocular hypotony, uveal prolapse, peaked pupil, corneal or scleral lacerations, subconjunctival hemorrhage, hyphema, asymmetric AC depth compared to fellow eye, vitreous hemorrhage, foreign body on slit-lamp or fundus exam

DIFFERENTIAL DIAGNOSIS

Orbital Foreign Body
- Intraocular vs. orbital location may be differentiated on imaging and exam

EVALUATION/WORK-UP

Labs
- Vitreous Gram stain and cultures for bacterial and fungal elements

Imaging
- CT scan with axial and coronal fine cuts through the orbit is study of choice
- Orbital ultrasound may help detect IOFB but should be avoided or used only with extreme caution in open globes due to pressure on the globe
- Avoid MRI if any chance IOFB could be metallic

TREATMENT

Medical
- Tetanus prophylaxis if not current
- Systemic broad-spectrum antibiotic coverage with oral levofloxacin or moxifloxacin for endophthalmitis prophylaxis
- For suspected fungal endophthalmitis, oral voriconazole or fluconazole may be used; amphotericin B is less commonly used due to toxicity
- Topical fortified vancomycin and ceftazidime or a fluoroquinolone every hour
- Intravitreal vancomycin (1 mg/0.1 mL) and ceftazidime (2.25 mg/0.1 mL) may be used in eyes with history of soil contamination, retinal periphlebitis, hypopyon, or exudation around IOFB due to high risk of endophthalmitis

Surgical
- Primary goal is comprehensive anatomical reconstruction of injured eye
- Secondary goal is removal of IOFB, either with pars plana wound or scleral tunnel incision, depending on size
- Early IOFB removal may decrease endophthalmitis rate; however, recent combat experience showed no endophthalmitis with delayed extraction (median of 21 days post injury) although this may be due to heat sterilization of shrapnel derived from improvised explosive devices
- For posterior segment IOFB, vitrectomy with fluid-gas exchange, silicone oil, or retinal detachment repair are usually necessary
- Magnets may be used to assist removal of metallic IOFB

Follow-Up
- Close follow-up is recommended to evaluate for development of endophthalmitis, retinal detachment, or proliferative vitreoretinopathy

Prognosis
- Depends on extent of injury; poor prognostic indicators include
  - Large entrance wound located posteriorly
  - Large, blunt, nonmetallic objects in posterior segment
  - Initial visual acuity of < 5/200
  - Relative afferent pupillary defect
  - Endophthalmitis
- Up to 71% of patients achieve 20/40 or better vision

SELECTED REFERENCES

1. Ahmed Y et al: Endophthalmitis following open-globe injuries. Eye (Lond). 26(2):212-7, 2012
2. Imrie FR et al: Surveillance of intraocular foreign bodies in the UK. Eye (Lond). 22(9):1141-7, 2008
3. Yeh S et al: Current trends in the management of intraocular foreign bodies. Curr Opin Ophthalmol. 19(3):225-33, 2008
4. Thach AB et al: Intraocular foreign body injuries during Operation Iraqi Freedom. Ophthalmology. 112(10):1829-33, 2005
5. Lit ES et al: Anterior and posterior segment intraocular foreign bodies. Int Ophthalmol Clin. 42(3):107-20, 2002

POSTERIOR VITREOUS DETACHMENT

Key Facts

Demographics
- Incidence of retinal complications in up to 24% of patients with symptomatic posterior vitreous detachment
- More common in older, myopic patients
- More common in patients with history of posterior vitreous detachment in fellow eye

Presentation
- Floaters and flashing lights
- Symptoms more common in dim light
- Weiss ring
  - Discrete vitreous opacity
- Detached posterior vitreous cortex
  - Detectable by slit-lamp biomicroscopy
- If Shaffer cells (pigmented vitreous cells) or mild vitreous hemorrhage are present, risk of an underlying retinal tear is much higher

Differential Diagnosis
- Migraine with aura, vitreitis, transient ischemic attack, retinal break or detachment

Evaluation/Work-Up
- Dilated funduscopy
- OCT image
- B-scan ultrasound

Treatment
- No treatment indicated
- If retinal break found
  - Laser or cryotherapy within 24-72 hours to avoid retinal detachment
- Immediate evaluation if there is a sudden increase in floaters or flashes of light as there may be retinal detachment, hole, or tear

*(**Left**) This external photograph of the eye demonstrates a posterior vitreous detachment. A useful way to visualize a posterior vitreous detachment is by eliciting the red reflex and viewing a flapping opacity in the fundus, as depicted here. (**Right**) This OCT image depicts a posterior vitreous detachment. The posterior hyaloid of the vitreous can be seen separated from the internal limiting membrane of the retina.*

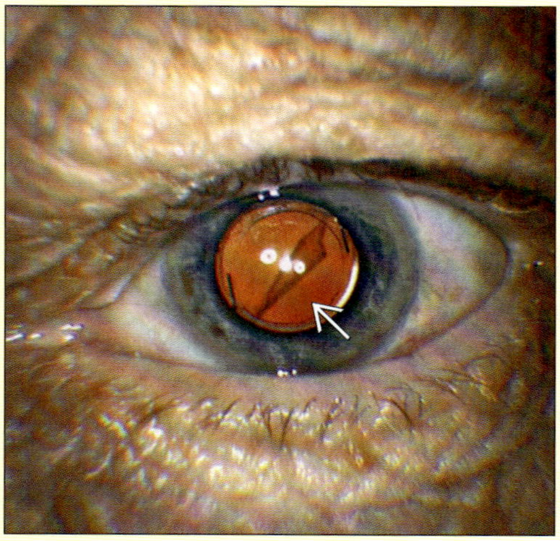

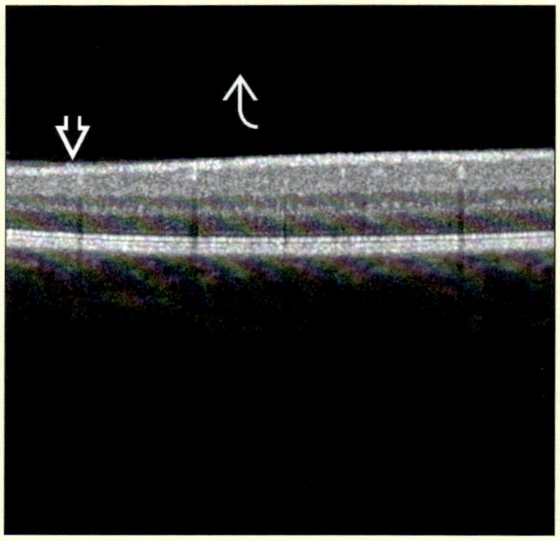

*(**Left**) This B-scan ultrasound demonstrates a posterior vitreous detachment. In the setting of poor visibility of the fundus, B-scan ultrasound is often necessary to identify the presence of a posterior vitreous detachment and rule out a retinal detachment. (**Right**) This fundus photograph shows a hemorrhagic posterior vitreous detachment. The blood in the vitreous is visible. Hemorrhagic posterior vitreous detachments are a possible complication of a PVD.*

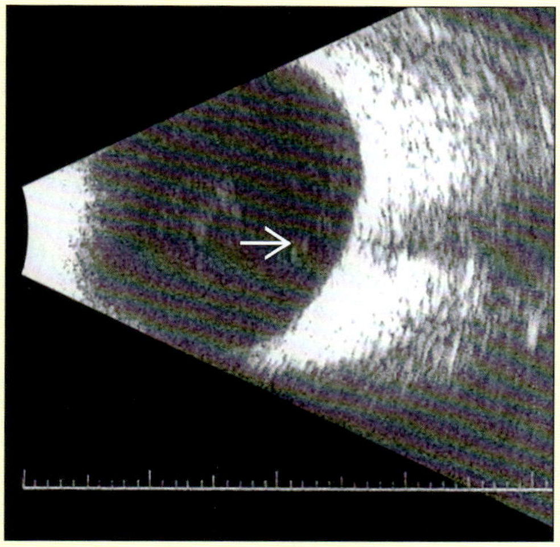

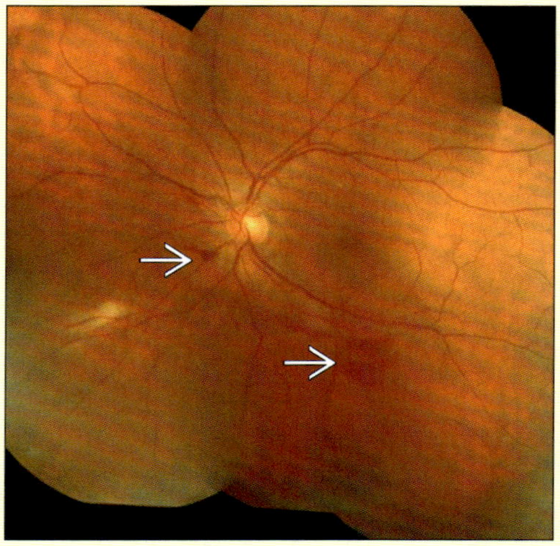

POSTERIOR VITREOUS DETACHMENT

INTRODUCTION

Abbreviations

- Posterior vitreous detachment (PVD)

Definitions

- Separation of the dense outer layer of type II collagen fibrils of vitreous (posterior vitreous cortex) from internal limiting lamina of retina

Subtypes

- PVD with collapse of detached vitreous
  - More common in older, myopic patients
- PVD without collapse
- Partial PVD with thickened posterior vitreous cortex
- Partial PVD without thickening

DEMOGRAPHICS

Etiology/Risk Factors

- Risk factors
  - Increased age
  - Myopia
  - Previous vitreous detachment in fellow eye
  - Trauma from decelerating injuries

Epidemiology

- Prevalence in population
  - Age 50-59: 24%
  - Age 80-89: 87%
- Incidence of retinal complications in up to 24% of patients with symptomatic PVD

PRESENTATION

Symptoms

- Floaters or flashing lights
- "Cobweb" effect across vision
- Symptoms more common in dim light

Exam Findings

- Weiss ring
  - Discrete vitreous opacity
  - Suspended over optic disc
- Detached posterior vitreous cortex
  - Detectable by slit-lamp biomicroscopy
- If Shaffer cells (pigmented vitreous cells) or mild vitreous hemorrhage are present, risk of underlying retinal tear is much higher

DIFFERENTIAL DIAGNOSIS

Optic Neuritis

- Photopsia
- Pain with eye movement

Migraine With Aura

- Bilateral flashing lights may precede a migraine headache
  - Last ~ 20 minutes
- No vitreous or retinal abnormalities found on dilated examination

Hypotension

- Photopsias upon standing

Vitreitis

- Bilateral photopsias

Vitreous Hemorrhage

- Must rule out using funduscopic exam
- May occur ± PVD

Transient Ischemic Attack

- Neurological findings

Retinal Break or Detachment

- Must rule out using funduscopic exam
- May occur ± PVD

EVALUATION/WORK-UP

Imaging

- Dilated funduscopy
- OCT image (can pick up vitreomacular adhesion or traction, epiretinal membranes, early macular holes, cystoid macular edema)
- B-scan ultrasound if view is poor

TREATMENT

Medical

- No treatment indicated
  - If retinal break found
    - Laser or cryotherapy within 24-72 hours to avoid retinal detachment (especially if horseshoe tears; operculated holes without fluid may be observed closely)

Surgical

- None needed in absence of complications; vitrectomy can be done if central PVD is occupationally disabling

Follow-Up

- Sudden increase in floaters or flashes of light in peripheral vision
  - Must see eye care professional immediately
  - Sign of
    - Macular hole
    - Retinal detachment
    - Retinal break

SELECTED REFERENCES

1. Retinal Detachment. In ADAM Medical Encyclopedia. Atlanta: ADAM. http://www.nlm.nih.gov/medlineplus/ency/article/001027.htm. Accessed March 22, 2013
2. Johnson MW: Posterior vitreous detachment: evolution and complications of its early stages. Am J Ophthalmol. 149(3):371-82, 2010
3. Chuo JY et al: Risk factors for posterior vitreous detachment: a case-control study. Am J Ophthalmol. 142(6):931-7, 2006
4. Margo CE et al: Posterior vitreous detachment. How to approach sudden-onset floaters and flashing lights. Postgrad Med. 117(3):37-42, 2005
5. Takahashi M et al: Biomicroscopic evaluation and photography of posterior vitreous detachment. Arch Ophthalmol. 98(4):665-8, 1980

SECTION 2
Retina and Choroid

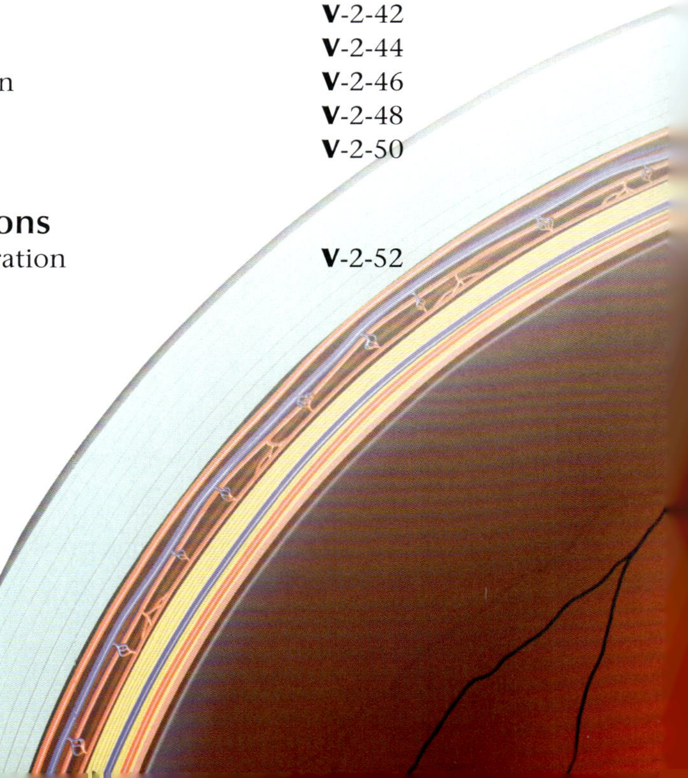

Malignant Neoplasms

Treatment-Related Disorders

Miscellaneous

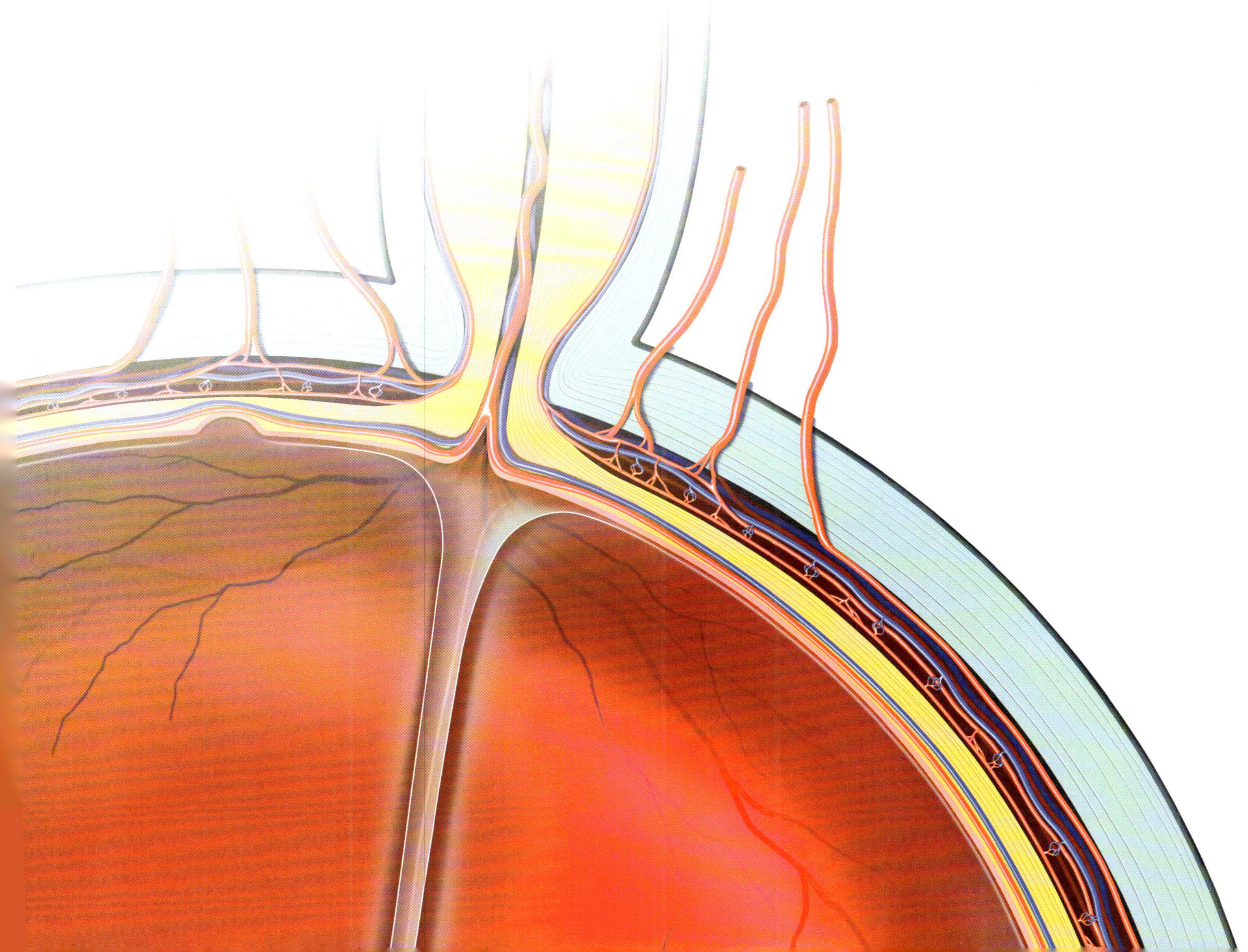

MAJOR CLINICAL STUDIES: OTHER RETINAL STUDIES

TERMINOLOGY

Definitions

- Major branched retinal vein occlusion (BRVO): On or outside arcade and > 5 disc diopters of retinal involvement

CENTRAL VEIN OCCLUSION STUDY (CVOS)

Objectives and Principal Conclusions

- Assess ability of laser photocoagulation in preventing neovascularization of the iris (NVI) in patients with retinal ischemia following central vein occlusion (CVO) and determine ability of grid-pattern laser photocoagulation in preventing central vision loss due to macular edema (ME) in patients with CVO
- Panretinal photocoagulation (PRP) should be reserved until NVI develops (unless monthly follow-up is not feasible)
- For bilateral CVO, young patients, or patients with other thrombotic history, do a hyperviscosity work-up
- Grid laser did not reduce vision loss
- Afferent pupillary defect (APD), < 20/200 vision, and > 10 disc areas of retinal perfusion were ischemic risk factors for progression to NVI

Inclusion Criteria

- Men and women age ≥ 21 years
- Patients with retinal vascular disease other than diabetic retinopathy were excluded
- Patients with macular disease other than that secondary to CVO were excluded from the grid-pattern photocoagulation portion of study

Randomization Method

- Patients were randomized to 3 groups based on initial presentation
  - Eyes with extensive retinal ischemia ≥ 10 disc areas of nonperfusion received PRP or observation
    - If NVI developed, patients in observation group were treated
  - Eyes with vision loss due to macular edema were assigned to receive grid-pattern photocoagulation or nontreatment
  - Eyes with relatively perfused retinas and eyes with retinas unable to visualize due to hemorrhage were followed to study natural disease course
- Green argon laser delivered at slit lamp was used for all photocoagulation treatments
- Patients were followed for at least 3 years and underwent fundus photography at entry, post-treatment, and at specific follow-up visits
- Visual acuity (VA) was measured with modified early treatment for diabetic retinopathy study (ETDRS) protocol

Results

- Grid-photocoagulation of macula
  - ↓ macular edema on fluorescein angiography (FA)
  - Did not ↑ visual acuity in eyes with ME due to CVO
- PRP for nonischemic CVO
  - Prophylactic PRP did not prevent NVI in eyes with ≥ 10 disc areas of retinal nonperfusion on FA
  - Safe to wait for early NVI prior to providing PRP

BRANCH VEIN OCCLUSION STUDY (BVOS)

Objective and Principal Conclusions

- Determine if scatter argon laser photocoagulation can prevent choroidal neovascularization (CNV) and vitreous hemorrhage in BRVO
- Determine if focal macular argon laser photocoagulation improves visual acuity in BRVOs with ME and VA ≤ 20/40
- Reserve laser until NV occurs &/or until vitreous hemorrhage clears
- Focal laser is useful in BRVO-related ME with vision < 20/40 but avoid in patients with macular nonperfusion
- If > 5 disc areas of nonperfusion, follow-up at least every 4 months

Inclusion Criteria

- Group inclusion criteria
  - Group 1: Major BRVO without CNV
  - Group 2: Major BRVO with CNV
  - Group 3: BRVO with ME and ↓ vision
  - Group X: BRVO without CNV with FA showing ≥ 5 disc diameters of nonperfusion
    - These patients were recruited only after group 1 recruitment was complete and could enter group 2 if they became eligible
- Other inclusion criteria
  - BRVO < 18 months before study participation
  - Vision of 5/200 or better
  - Clear ocular media, allowing fundus photography

Randomization Method

- Groups 1 and 2 were randomized to scatter argon laser photocoagulation or observation
- Group 3 was randomized to focal macular argon laser photocoagulation or observation
- Group X was observed

Results

- Laser photocoagulation should be done for patients with BRVO who develop CNV
  - Treated eyes had less CNV ($P = .009$)
  - CNV developed in 22% of controls vs. 12% of treated eyes (average follow-up at 3.7 years)
  - Peripheral scatter treatment should be applied after, rather than before, development of neovascularization (NV)
- Focal argon laser photocoagulation improves sight in patients with ↓ VA due to BRVO with ME

SILICONE STUDY

Objectives and Principal Conclusions

- Compare postoperative tamponade with intraocular silicone oil vs. intraocular gas (initially sulfur hexafluoride [SF6], later perfluoropropane [C3F8]) in management of retinal detachment (RD) with proliferative vitreoretinopathy (PVR)
- Silicone oil was > SF6 but = to C3F8
- Hypotony, keratopathy, glaucoma, and retinotomy were associated with poor outcome
- Posterior PVR patients had better prognosis than anterior PVR patients
- Inferior peripheral iridotomy was needed in patients treated with silicone oil due to increased IOP

Inclusion Criteria
- PVR of grade C-3 or greater (Retina Society classification)
- VA of light perception or better

Randomization Method
- All study patients underwent vitrectomy and were randomized intraoperatively either to intravitreal silicone oil or gas

Results
- IOP
  - Chronic ↑ in IOP was more prevalent in silicone oil eyes than in C3F8-filled eyes
    - Inferior peripheral iridotomy was needed in silicone oil eyes
  - Chronic hypotony was more prevalent in C3F8-filled eyes than in silicone oil eyes
- Retinotomy
  - Required more frequently in eyes undergoing repeat vitreous surgery for PVR
- Outcomes after silicone oil removal
  - ↑ in VA and ↓ in complications after silicone oil removal in eyes with attached retinas at time of silicone oil removal
  - ↑ risk of recurrent retinal detachment in silicone oil-removed eyes compared to silicone oil-retained eyes

COLLABORATIVE OCULAR MELANOMA STUDY

Objectives and Principal Conclusions
- Study disease progression and prognosis in patients with small choroidal melanomas (1.0-3.0 mm in apical height and at least 5.0 mm in basal diameter)
- Compare enucleation vs. brachytherapy with I-125 episcleral plaque in survival of patients with medium-sized choroidal melanoma
- Assess role of preoperative radiation in prolonging life in patients with large choroidal melanomas that undergo enucleation
- Radiation is a safe and effective alternative to immediate enucleation and can be attempted first

Inclusion Criteria
- Age ≥ 21 years
- Primary choroidal melanoma in only 1 eye
- No evidence of metastatic disease
- Accurate estimation of tumor size by ultrasound

Randomization Method
- Patients with small choroidal melanomas were followed for an average of 92 months
- Medium-sized tumor study: Patients were randomized to receive either enucleation or brachytherapy with I-125 episcleral plaque
- Preoperative radiation study: Patients randomized to receive enucleation alone or enucleation preceded by 20 Gy of external beam radiation

Results
- Small choroidal melanoma
  - 5-year all-cause mortality: 6% (2.7-9.3 95% confidence interval [CI])
  - 8-year all-cause mortality: 14.9% (9.6-20.2 95% CI)
- I-125 brachytherapy for medium choroidal melanoma
  - 5-year survival rate of patients treated with either brachytherapy or eye removal was 82%
  - Eyes treated with brachytherapy steadily lost vision, with 63% having visual acuity of 20/200 or worse by 3 years after treatment
- Pre-enucleation radiation for large choroidal melanoma
  - Similar survival rates between patients receiving external beam radiation prior to enucleation and those undergoing enucleation alone
  - 5-year survival rates were ~ 60% in both treatments
  - Patient who had pre-enucleation radiation had fewer local complications

RANIBIZUMAB FOR MACULAR EDEMA FOLLOWING BRVO

Objective and Principal Conclusions
- Determine efficacy of intraocular injections of 0.3 mg or 0.5 mg ranibizumab in ME following BRVO
- Intraocular injections of 0.3 mg or 0.5 mg ranibizumab were effective treatments for ME following BRVO with low rates of ocular and nonocular adverse events

Inclusion Criteria
- Age ≥ 18 years
- Foveal center-involved ME due to BRVO in prior 12 months
- BCVA 20/40 to 20/400 Snellen equivalent with ETDRS chart
- Mean central subfield thickness ≥ 250 μm from 2 ocular coherence tomography (OCT) measurements

Randomization Method
- Patients randomized to receive monthly intraocular injections of ranibizumab 0.3 mg, 0.5 mg, or sham injections

Results
- Mean (95% CI) change from baseline BCVA letter score was 16.6 (14.7-18.5) and 18.3 (16.0-20.6) in 0.3 mg and 0.5 mg ranibizumab groups vs. 7.3 (5.1-9.5) in sham injection group
  - $P < .001$ for each ranibizumab group vs. sham injection group

RELATED REFERENCES

1. National Institutes of Health, National Eye Institute: Branch Vein Occlusion Study. http://www.nei.nih.gov/neitrials/static/study64.asp. Updated October 23, 1999. Accessed September 9, 2013
2. National Institutes of Health, National Eye Institute: Central Vein Occlusion Study (CVOS). http://www.nei.nih.gov/neitrials/static/study30.asp. Updated October 21, 1999. Accessed September 9, 2013
3. National Institutes of Health, National Eye Institute: Collaborative Ocular Melanoma Study (COMS). http://www.nei.nih.gov/neitrials/static/study23.asp. Updated November 15, 2001. Accessed September 9, 2013
4. National Institutes of Health, National Eye Institute: The Silicone Study. http://www.nei.nih.gov/neitrials/static/study39.asp. Updated October 22, 1999. Accessed September 9, 2013
5. Campochiaro PA et al: Ranibizumab for macular edema following branch retinal vein occlusion: six-month primary end point results of a phase III study. Ophthalmology. 117(6):1102-1112, 2010

MAJOR CLINICAL STUDIES: DIABETIC RETINOPATHY

TERMINOLOGY

Abbreviations

- Diabetic retinopathy (DR)
- Insulin-dependent diabetes mellitus (IDDM)

DR STUDY (DRS)

Objective

- Role of photocoagulation in preventing severe vision loss from proliferative DR (PDR)
- Compare efficacy and safety of argon vs. xenon photocoagulation for PDR

Inclusion Criteria

- PDR in at least 1 eye, or severe nonproliferative DR (NPDR) in both eyes
- No prior treatment with photocoagulation or pituitary ablation
- Best corrected visual acuity (BCVA) of 20/100 or better in each eye
- Eyes determined to be suitable for photocoagulation
- Age < 70 years; estimated survival ≥ 5 years

Randomization Method

- 1 eye of each patient was randomly assigned to treatment with photocoagulation, while the other eye was assigned to follow-up without treatment
- Eye assigned to treatment with photocoagulation was randomly assigned to either argon laser or xenon arc photocoagulation

Results

- Photocoagulation with both argon and xenon ↓ risk of severe vision loss by > 50% compared to no treatment
- Benefits of photocoagulation outweighed risks in patients with high-risk PDR

EARLY TREATMENT OF DIABETIC RETINOPATHY STUDY (ETDRS)

Objective

- Role and efficacy of argon laser photocoagulation and aspirin in preventing or delaying progression of early DR to severe vision loss and blindness
- Determine ideal timing of photocoagulation in treatment of DR
- Describe impact of DM and photocoagulation on vision
- Determine risk factors and etiology for DR

Inclusion Criteria

- Age 18-70 years
- Moderate or severe NPDR or mild PDR in both eyes
- No previous treatment with photocoagulation
- Visual acuity (VA) of 20/40 or better if no macular involvement and 20/200 or better if DME present

Randomization Method

- Random assignment of 1 eye to immediate photocoagulation and other eye to delayed photocoagulation until high-risk PDR was present
- Aspirin treatment determined by clinical need

Results

- Aspirin
  - In patients with mild to severe NPDR or early PDR, aspirin did not prevent progression of DR
  - In eyes that delayed photocoagulation treatment, aspirin did not affect progression of retinopathy to high-risk proliferative stage
  - No increase risk of vitreous hemorrhage
  - No impact on vision
  - Associated with ↓ risk of cardiovascular disease
  - No ocular contraindications to aspirin use when required for cardiovascular disease or other systemic medical therapy
- Focal photocoagulation for macular edema
  - ↓ risk of moderate vision loss for eyes with macular edema involving or threatening central macula
  - Decreases retinal thickening
- Early scattered photocoagulation reduces severe vision loss, especially in non-insulin-dependent DM (IDDM)
- Scattered photocoagulation should be reserved for patients with severe NPDR or those with early PDR
- Early vitrectomy indicated for advanced PDR

DIABETES CONTROL AND COMPLICATIONS TRIAL

Objective and Principal Conclusion

- Determine if intensive glucose control slows or prevents DR and other complications in type 1 diabetics
- Intensive glucose control halts and reverses retinopathy in type 1 diabetics

Inclusion Criteria

- Primary prevention group: IDDM 1-5 years, no DR, VA ≥ 20/25, < 40 mg/day albuminuria
- Secondary prevention group: IDDM 1-15 years, mild to moderate DR, VA ≥ 20/32, < 200 mg/day albuminuria

Randomization Method

- Conventional insulin therapy: 1 or 2 daily injections
- Intensive insulin therapy: ≥ 3 daily injections or external pump; dose adjustments by self-monitoring

Results

- Intensive glucose control
  - ↓ DR progression by 50%
    - Benefit seen after 3 years
    - 9-year risk reduction of 76%
    - Initial worsening of DR in 1st year
  - 50% ↓ in development of severe NPDR, PDR, and need for photocoagulation
  - ↓ albuminuria in 54%
  - ↓ in clinical neuropathy in 60%
  - ↓ in macrovascular disease in 41%
  - 2-3x ↑ in severe hypoglycemia events and 33% ↑ risk of becoming overweight
- No glycemic threshold; keeping HbA1c < 8% was beneficial

2-YEAR OUTCOMES OF RANIBIZUMAB FOR EDEMA OF THE MACULA IN DIABETES STUDY (READ-2)

Objective and Principal Conclusion

- Determine long-term effects of ranibizumab in patients with diabetic macular edema (DME)

- Intraocular injections of ranibizumab benefit patients with DME for at least 2 years, reduce frequency of injections, and reduce residual edema when combined with grid or focal laser
- Suggested treatment approach to DME is to initiate aggressive treatment with intraocular ranibizumab followed by a period of giving ranibizumab p.r.n. with focal or grid laser to decrease number of ranibizumab injections

Inclusion Criteria

- BCVA of 20/40 to 20/320 from DME
- Subfoveal thickness on OCT ≥ 250 μm

Randomization Method

- Study participants were randomized into 1 of 3 groups
  - Group 1: 0.5 mg of ranibizumab at day 0, month 1, 3, and 5
  - Group 2: Focal or grid laser photocoagulation at baseline and month 3 if center subfoveal thickness ≥ 250 μm
  - Group 3: 0.5 mg ranibizumab + focal or grid laser at baseline and month 3
- At month 6, patients could be treated if center subfoveal thickness ≥ 250 μm
  - Group 1: Follow-up every 2 months with repeat ranibizumab 0.5 mg
  - Group 2: Follow-up every 2 months with injection of ranibizumab 0.5 mg or laser
  - Group 3: Follow-up every 3 months with either ranibizumab 0.5 mg injection ± laser within 5-9 days

Results

- BCVA of 20/40 or better at 24 months was achieved by 45% of group 1, 44% of group 2, and 35% of group 3
- Mean foveal thickness at 24 months was 340 μm in group 1, 286 μm in group 2, and 258 μm in group 3
- Unlikely optimal to use either focal or grid laser alone or ranibizumab alone in most patients

RANIBIZUMAB MONOTHERAPY OR COMBINED WITH LASER VS. LASER MONOTHERAPY FOR DME (RESTORE STUDY)

Objective and Principal Conclusion

- Determine whether ranibizumab monotherapy or combined with focal or grid laser is superior to laser alone based on changes in BCVA in patients with vision impairment due to diabetic macular edema (DME)
- Treatment with ranibizumab as monotherapy and combined with laser photocoagulation is superior to laser treatment alone in improving and maintaining VA in patients with vision impairment due to DME

Inclusion Criteria

- Age ≥18 years
- Diagnosis of type 1 or type 2 DM
  - Hemoglobin A1c ≤ 10%
- Eyes with focal or diffuse DME & visual impairment that are able to undergo laser therapy
- No changes to systemic medication for DM in prior 3 months with no expectations to change medications
- BCVA 79-39 on ETDRS chart at 4 m

Randomization Method

- 3 possible groups
  - R: Ranibizumab + sham laser
  - R + L: Ranibizumab + focal/grid laser
  - L: Sham injection + focal/grid laser
- Ranibizumab treatment
  - 3 injections of ranibizumab every 4 weeks then p.r.n. with monthly follow-up
  - Participants were retreated unless BCVA was ≥ 84 letters (20/20) at 2 consecutive visits or if investigator thought no further improvement in BCVA would be attributable to treatment
  - Injections were resumed for a ↓ in BCVA secondary to DME progression on fundus exam or OCT
- Laser therapy
  - Given at baseline but could be split into 2 treatments separated by 4 weeks
  - Retreatment based on ETDRS guidelines if ≥ 3 months since last laser treatment

Results

- Mean change in BCVA from baseline to month 12 (*P* value compared to L group)
  - R: 6.3 ± 8.3 ($P < .0001$)
  - R + L: 6.4 ± 11.8 ($P + .0004$)
  - L: 0.9 ± 11.4
- BCVA ≥ 73 (20/40 Snellen equivalent) in 53% of R, 44.9% of R + L, 23.6% of L
- Mean decrease in CRT from baseline to month 12: 118.7 μm (R, $P = .0002$), 128.3 μm (R + L, $P < .0001$), 61.3 μm (L)
- Resolution of leakage on fundus angiography: 19.4% of R ($P = .0002$), 13.7% of R + L ($P = .0114$), 2.2% of L
- Health-related quality of life questionnaire, change from baseline to month 12: ↑ by 5 (R, $P = .014$), ↑ by 5.4 (R + L, $P = .004$), decreased in L

RELATED REFERENCES

1. National Institutes of Health, National Eye Institute: Diabetic Retinopathy Study (DRS). http://www.nei.nih.gov/neitrials/static/study62.asp. Updated October 23, 1999. Accessed September 6, 2013
2. National Institutes of Health, National Eye Institute: Diabetic Retinopathy Vitrectomy Study (DRVS). http://www.nei.nih.gov/neitrials/static/study56.asp. Updated October 23, 1999. Accessed September 6, 2013
3. National Institutes of Health, National Eye Institute: Early Treatment Diabetic Retinopathy (ETDRS). http://www.nei.nih.gov/neitrials/static/study53.asp. Updated March 28, 2000. Accessed September 6, 2013
4. National Institutes of Health: Diabetes Control and Complications Trial (DCCT). ClinicalTrials.gov. http://clinicaltrials.gov/ct2/show/study/NCT00360815. Published August 2, 2007. Updated March 1, 2010. Accessed September 6, 2013
5. Mitchell P et al: The RESTORE study: ranibizumab monotherapy or combined with laser versus laser monotherapy for diabetic macular edema. Ophthalmology. 118(4):615-25, 2011
6. Nguyen QD et al: Two-year outcomes of the ranibizumab for edema of the mAcula in diabetes (READ-2) study. Ophthalmology. 117(11):2146-51, 2010

MAJOR CLINICAL STUDIES: MACULAR DISEASES

AGE-RELATED EYE DISEASE STUDY (AREDS)

Objective and Principal Conclusion

- Study effects of antioxidants and zinc on progression of age-related macular degeneration (ARMD) and antioxidants on development and progression of lens opacification
- AREDS found that nutritional supplementation with lutein + zeaxanthin reduced fellow eye risk of developing ARMD in patients with ARMD in 1 eye
- Patients at risk should eat dark, green, leafy vegetables and take nutritional supplements

Inclusion Criteria

- Men or women age 55-80
- Macula with no evidence of ARMD in either eye to relatively severe disease with vision loss in 1 eye and vision of 20/30 or better in other eye

Randomization Method

- Study participants were randomized to receive either placebo, antioxidants, zinc, or antioxidants + zinc and followed for a minimum of 5 years

Results

- Combination of antioxidants (i.e., vitamin C, vitamin E, beta carotene, lutein, and zeaxanthin) and zinc
  - ↓ risk for developing ARMD by 25% in patients with intermediate ARMD or advanced ARMD in 1 eye
  - ↓ risk of vision loss by 19%
  - No effect on development or progression of cataract

AGE-RELATED EYE DISEASE STUDY 2 (AREDS2)

Objectives and Principal Conclusion

- Study effects of lutein, zeaxanthin, docosahexaenoic acid, and eicosapentaenoic acid on progression to advanced ARMD &/or moderate vision loss in people at moderate to high risk for progression
- Study effects of eliminating beta carotene, lowering zinc doses, or both in original AREDS formulation on development and progression of ARMD
- Supplementation did not reduce progression of ARMD
- Omega-3 fatty acids did not affect ARMD course
- ↓ zinc dose and eliminating beta carotene did not affect progression
- Results in new AREDS2 formula, concentrating mainly on lutein + zeaxanthin to ↓ risk of developing ARMD in patients at risk

Inclusion Criteria

- Age 50-85
- Large drusen in both eyes or large drusen in 1 eye and advanced ARMD (neovascular ARMD or geographic atrophy) in fellow eye
- Ocular media clear enough for fundus photography

Randomization Method

- Double-masked, 2 x 2 factorial trial with 2 randomizations
  - Primary randomization of adding 1 of the following to AREDS formula (vitamin C [500 mg], vitamin E [400 IU], beta carotene [15 mg], zinc [80 mg as zinc oxide], copper [2 mg as cupric oxide])
    - Lutein (10 mg) + zeaxanthin (2 mg)
    - DHA (350 mg) + EPA (650 mg)
    - Lutein (10 mg) + zeaxanthin (2 mg) + DHA (350 mg) + EPA (650 mg)
    - No additional supplementation to AREDS formula
  - Secondary randomization of AREDS formula
    - Original AREDS supplement
    - AREDS supplement with no beta carotene
    - AREDS supplement with a lower zinc dose (25 mg)
    - AREDS supplement with no beta carotene and a lower zinc dose (25 mg)

Results

- Primary outcome measure
  - Addition of lutein + zeaxanthin, DHA + EPA, or lutein + zeaxanthin + DHA + EPA to original AREDS formula showed no statistically significant effect in advanced ARMD progression or visual acuity (VA) changes
    - Probability of progression to advanced ARMD by 5 years was 31% for placebo, 29% for lutein + zeaxanthin, 31% for DHA + EPA, 30% for lutein + zeaxanthin + DHA + EPA

ENZYMATIC VITREOLYSIS WITH OCRIPLASMIN FOR VITREOMACULAR TRACTION AND MACULAR HOLES

Objective and Principal Conclusions

- Determine benefits of intravitreal injections of ocriplasmin 125 μg vs. placebo in patients with symptomatic vitreomacular adhesion
- Ocriplasmin resolved vitreomacular traction and closed macular holes in more patients than injection of placebo and was associated with higher incidence of ocular adverse events, which were transient

Inclusion Criteria

- Age ≥ 18 years
- Focal vitreomacular adhesion
  - Vitreous adhesion to macula within a 6 mm central retinal field surrounded by elevation of posterior vitreous cortex seen on OCT
- Best corrected visual acuity (BCVA) of 20/25 or worse in study eye and 20/800 or better in nonstudy eye on early treatment for diabetic retinopathy study (ETDRS) charts

Randomization Method

- Patients were randomly assigned to a single intravitreal injection of ocriplasmin 125 μg or placebo

Results

- Resolution of vitreomacular adhesion occurred in 26.5% of ocriplasmin-injected eyes and in 10.1% of placebo-injected eyes ($P < .001$)
- PVD occurred in 13.4% of ocriplasmin-injected eyes vs. 3.7% of placebo-injected eyes ($P < .001$)
- Nonsurgical closure of macular hole occurred in 40.6% of ocriplasmin-injected eye vs. 10.6% of placebo-injected eyes ($P < .001$)
- BCVA was more likely to improve by ≥ 3 lines with ocriplasmin than placebo
- Adverse events occurred in 68.4% of ocriplasmin-injected eyes vs. 53.5% of placebo-injected eyes ($P < .001$)
  - Vitreous floaters, photopsia, injection-related eye pain, conjunctival hemorrhage

- Incidence of serious ocular adverse events was similar between groups ($P = .26$)

VITRECTOMY FOR PREVENTION OF MACULAR HOLE STUDY GROUP

Objective and Principal Conclusions

- Determine benefit of vitrectomy for eyes with stage 3 or 4 macular holes
- Significant benefits in VA and rates of hole closure from vitrectomy compared with observation alone

Inclusion Criteria

- Stage 3 or 4 macular hole
- Clear ocular media
- Pupil diameter ≥ 5 mm
- No retinal disease that could ↓ macular function or aphakic/pseudophakic cystoid macular edema
- VA < 20/50 with symptoms of ↓ central vision
- Loss of foveal tissue > 400 μm in diameter with a cuff of subretinal fluid
- Positive Watzke-Allen test (a break seen through a slit beam projected onto fovea)

Randomization Method

- Patients were randomized to 3 port pars plana vitrectomy or observation

Results

- Rate of hole closure was 69% in vitrectomy group vs. 4% in observation group ($P < .001$)
- Benefit from surgery was found in VA testing with Bailey-Lovie word reading chart ($P = .02$), potential acuity meter ($P < .01$), and ETDRS chart ($P = .05$)
- Eyes randomized to vitrectomy had higher nuclear sclerosis scores (2.4 vs. 1.3, $P < .001$)

MACULAR PHOTOCOAGULATION STUDY

Objective and Principal Conclusions

- Argon study: Determine whether argon photocoagulation of abnormal, leaky blood vessels in CNV membranes outside fovea prevents or delays central vision loss in patients with ARMD, presumed ocular histoplasmosis (POH), and idiopathic neovascular membranes (INM)
- Krypton study: Determine whether krypton red laser photocoagulation of CNV lesions bordering foveal avascular zone (FAZ) prevents or delays large amounts of vision loss in patients with ARMD, POH, and INM
- Foveal study: Determine whether laser photocoagulation prevents or delays vision loss in patients with new or recurrent CNV under center of FAZ
- Eyes with ARMD, POH, and INM with well-demarcated areas of classic CNV on fluorescein angiography (FA) that did not involve FAZ center had better visual outcomes when treated with laser photocoagulation compared to observation

Inclusion Criteria

- ARMD patients
  - Age ≥ 50 years
  - ↓ VA or Amsler grid distortion
  - Well-demarcated hyperfluorescence (CNV) on FA
  - Visible drusen in macula in at least 1 eye
- POH patients
  - Age ≥ 18 years
  - ≥1 characteristic histo spot in 1 or both eyes
- INM patients
  - Age ≥18 years
  - No evidence of ARMD, POH, angioid streaks, high myopia, diabetic retinopathy, or other conditions that might cause CNV
  - No large drusen or histo spots
- Argon study
  - Visible serous retinal detachment with leakage
  - Discrete CNV 200-2,500 μm from FAZ center
  - VA of 20/100 or better in study eye
- Krypton study
  - Neovascularization ± blood &/or pigment in the FAZ
  - Posterior border of CNV extending up to 1 μm to FAZ center
  - VA of 20/400 or better in study eye
- Foveal study
  - Only patients with ARMD
  - Leaking choroidal neovascular membrane on FA
    - Portion of leakage extending under FAZ center
  - Neovascular lesion consisting of an old laser treatment scar and contiguous leaking CNV within 150 μm of FAZ center
  - New, never-treated subfoveal lesions < 4 disc areas
  - Recurrent lesions < 6 disc areas in size
  - BCVA between 20/40 to 20/320

Randomization Method

- Patients in each study were randomly assigned to either argon laser photocoagulation or observation alone

Results

- Eyes with ARMD and subfoveal CNV benefited more from laser treatment than from observation
- Eyes receiving direct laser treatment to fovea for new CNV initially lost more VA than observed eyes, but by 12 months, eyes undergoing observation alone had greater VA loss than treated eyes
- Eyes with smaller lesions and worse initial VA had greater and earlier benefits of laser treatment
- Eyes with large subfoveal neovascular lesions and good initial VA are not good candidates for focal laser photocoagulation

RELATED REFERENCES

1. Age-Related Eye Disease Study 2 Research Group: Lutein + zeaxanthin and omega-3 fatty acids for age-related macular degeneration: the Age-Related Eye Disease Study 2 (AREDS2) randomized clinical trial. JAMA. 309(19):2005-15, 2013
2. National Institutes of Health, National Eye Institute: Age-Related Eye Disease Study (AREDS). http://www.nei.nih.gov/neitrials/static/study44.asp. Updated February 4, 2002. Accessed September 9, 2013
3. National Institutes of Health, National Eye Institute: Macular Photocoagulation Study (MPS). http://www.nei.nih.gov/neitrials/static/study60.asp. Updated November 27, 2001. Accessed September 9, 2013
4. Stalmans P et al: Enzymatic vitreolysis with ocriplasmin for vitreomacular traction and macular holes. N Engl J Med. 367(7):606-15, 2012
5. Freeman WR et al: Vitrectomy for the treatment of full-thickness stage 3 or 4 macular holes. Results of a multicentered randomized clinical trial. The Vitrectomy for Treatment of Macular Hole Study Group. Arch Ophthalmol. 115(1):11-21, 1997

RETINA AND CHOROID OVERVIEW

TERMINOLOGY

Definitions

- Retina: Light-sensitive tissue located in back of eye
- Choroid: Vascular layer of eye responsible for providing oxygen to outer layers of retina

ANATOMY AND PHYSIOLOGY

Anatomy

- Retina is composed of several layers of cells
  - Retinal pigment epithelium (RPE) is outermost cell layer
    - Responsible for vitamin A metabolism and regeneration for visual cycle and phagocytosis of outer segment discs
  - Outer nuclear layer is composed of cell bodies of photoreceptor cells (rods and cones)
    - Outer segments of photoreceptors contain visual pigment (e.g., rhodopsin), which starts the visual signal transduction pathway after light stimulus
    - Photoreceptors degenerate in several inherited retinal diseases (e.g., retinitis pigmentosa, Leber congenital amaurosis)
  - Inner nuclear layer is composed of cell bodies of bipolar, horizontal, amacrine, and Müller cells
  - Innermost layer is composed of cell bodies of ganglion cells
    - Axons of ganglion cells (nerve fiber layer) combine to make optic nerve
    - Ganglion cells die in glaucoma
- Vascular supply
  - Choroid (choriocapillaries) is responsible for vascular supply of RPE and photoreceptors
  - Branches of central artery and vein are vascular supply of inner nuclear layer and ganglion cells

Physiology

- Visual transduction
  - Rods are responsible for dim light vision; cones function in bright light and are responsible for color vision
  - Rod (rhodopsin) and cone (L-, M-, and S-) pigments absorb maximally at different wavelengths
  - Upon light absorption of visual pigment, pigment isomerizes and initiates biochemical cascade that is ultimately responsible for hyperpolarizing the photoreceptor

Retinal Anatomic Variations

- Macula
  - Located inferotemporally of optic disc
  - Distinguishable as yellow (due to lutein and zeaxanthin), capillary-free zone of retina
  - Age-related macular degeneration (ARMD): Disease of cells in macula leading to progressive loss of central vision
- Fovea
  - Region in macula with maximal cone density; responsible for central vision
  - Some inherited retinal diseases affect cone vision (central) before affecting rod vision (peripheral) (e.g., cone-rod dystrophies [CORDs])
- Ora serrata
  - Boundary between retina and ciliary body

Imaging and Other Tests

- Optical coherence tomography (OCT)
  - Noninvasive, 3D cross-section image of retina
- Fluorescein angiography (FA)
  - Used to image retinal and choroidal vasculature
  - Important test for diabetic neovascularization, vein and retinal artery occlusions, and optic disc edema
- Electroretinography (ERG)
  - Noninvasive test to measure electrical potentials of different cells in retina
  - Flash ERG: Dark-adapted eye (measures rod function); light-adapted eye (measures cone function)
  - Patter ERG: Measures ganglion cell function

DISEASES OF RETINA AND CHOROID

Common Diseases

- Inherited retinal disease
  - Retinitis pigmentosa
    - Loss of night vision and peripheral vision
  - Macular degeneration
    - Loss of central vision
  - CORD
  - Retinoblastoma
    - Most common cancer of eye
- Other retinal/choroidal diseases
  - Diabetic retinopathy
    - Neovascularization
  - Choroidal dystrophy
    - Degeneration of the choriocapillaris, RPE, and photoreceptors

Emergency Cases

- Central retinal artery occlusion (CRAO)
  - Usually from carotid artery atherosclerosis
  - Acute unilateral vision loss (presence of cherry-red spot in macula)
  - Can lead to permanent vision loss
- Chemical burns
- Endophthalmitis
  - Serious eye infection that may lead to rapid blindness
  - Symptoms include severe eye pain, redness, and loss of vision
  - Emergency intervention may include intravitreal antibiotics and pars plana vitrectomy
- Retinal detachment
  - Detachment of retina from RPE
  - Symptoms include sudden appearance of flashing lights (photopsia), floaters, and vision loss
  - Common surgical procedures include scleral buckle, pars plana vitrectomy, cryotherapy, laser photocoagulation, and pneumatic retinopexy

RELATED REFERENCES

1. Varma DD et al: A review of central retinal artery occlusion: clinical presentation and management. Eye (Lond). 27(6):688-97, 2013
2. Kreissig I: Surgical techniques for repair of primary retinal detachment: part I. Review of their development during the last 80 years. Folia Med (Plovdiv). 51(4):5-11, 2009

RETINA AND CHOROID ANATOMY AND HISTOLOGY

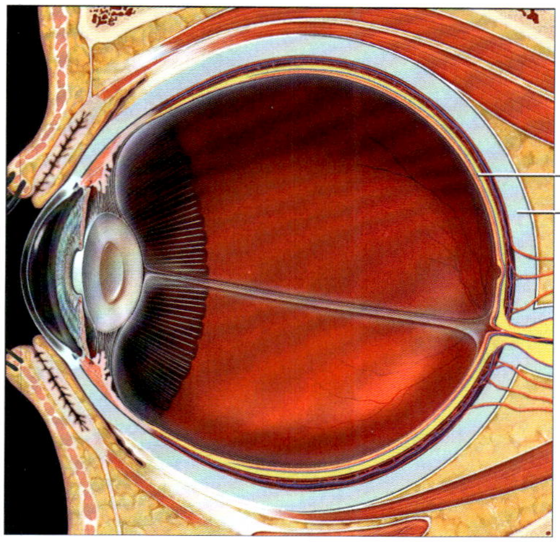

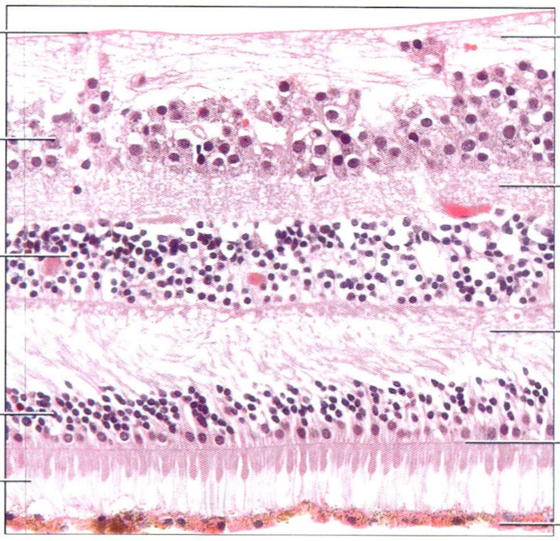

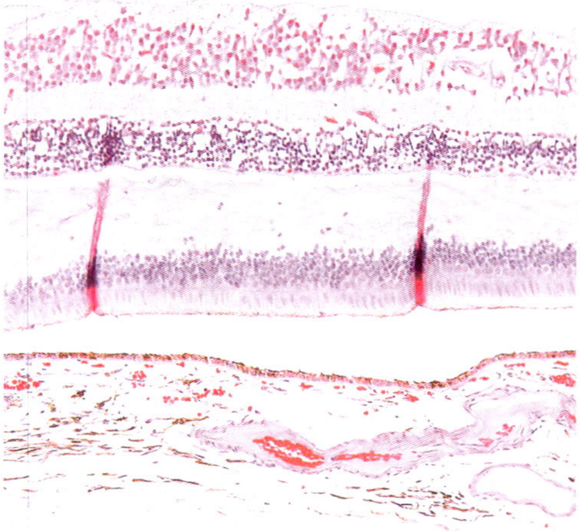

(Top) *The retina is a thin tissue lining the back of the eye (yellow). The choroid is the vascular supply of the outer retina, which is located between the retina and the sclera (white).* ***(Middle)*** *The 10 retinal layers are depicted: (1) Internal limiting membrane, (2) nerve fiber layer, (3) ganglion cell layer, (4) inner plexiform layer, (5) inner nuclear layer, (6) outer plexiform layer, (7) outer nuclear layer, (8) external limiting membrane, (9) rods and cones, and (10) retinal pigment epithelium. (Courtesy H. Brown, MD.)* ***(Bottom)*** *Grossly, the macula lutea appears as a yellow spot within the retina. The macula is a region of the retina that can be identified histologically when the ganglion cell layer is > 1 cell thick, as seen here. (Courtesy H. Brown, MD.)*

BEST DISEASE

Key Facts

Introduction
- Hereditary juvenile-onset vitelliform macular dystrophy

Demographics
- Caused by 1 of > 200 disease-causing mutations in *BEST1* (formerly known as *VMD2*) gene on chromosome 11q12-q13.1
- *BEST1* encodes bestrophin-1 protein, a calcium-sensitive chloride channel on basolateral plasma membrane of retinal pigment epithelium (RPE)
- Age of onset is variable, typically 5-10 years old
- Both autosomal dominant and autosomal recessive inheritance patterns exist

Presentation
- Decreased central visual acuity
- Typically, vision is relatively preserved in at least 1 eye throughout course
- Yellow, yolk-like macular lesion (lipofuscin deposit) early in course
- Eventual "scrambled egg" appearance that may progress to RPE atrophy, macular scarring, &/or choroidal neovascularization (CNV)
- Metamorphopsia

Evaluation/Work-Up
- Fluorescein angiogram (FA)
- Spectral domain optical coherence tomography (OCT)
- Electrooculogram is most specific test and detects disease in earliest stages
- Arden ratio, defined as the light-peak to dark-trough ratio, is decreased (< 1.5)

Treatment
- No effective treatment before CNV develops
- 20% of patients will develop CNV during course of disease

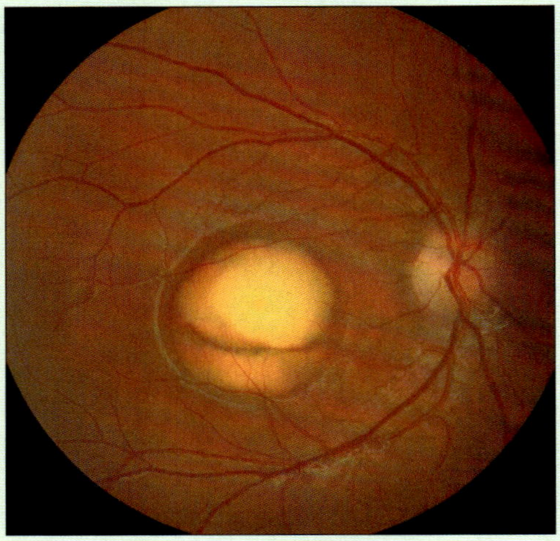
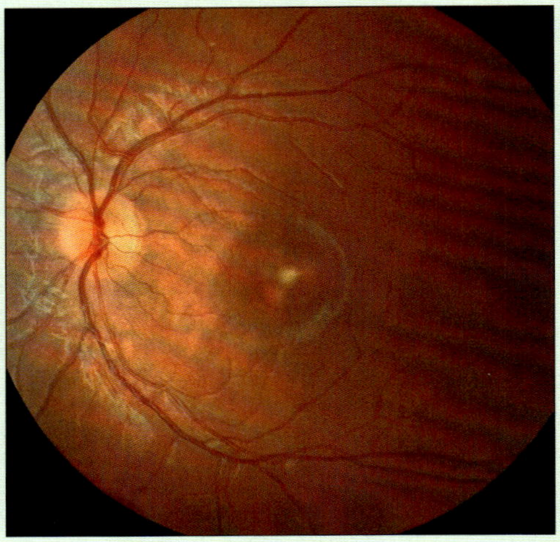

(Left) *Fundus photo shows the classic "egg yolk" appearance of a stage 2 vitelliform lesion. At this stage of disease, vision is often well preserved or only minimally affected.* ***(Right)*** *Fundus photograph in a patient with Best disease shows another example of a stage 2 vitelliform lesion. In the vitelliruptive stage of disease that follows, these cysts break apart and give more of a "scrambled egg" appearance.*

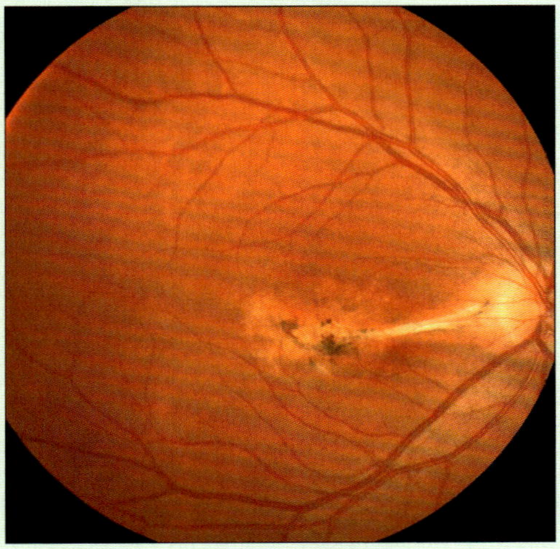
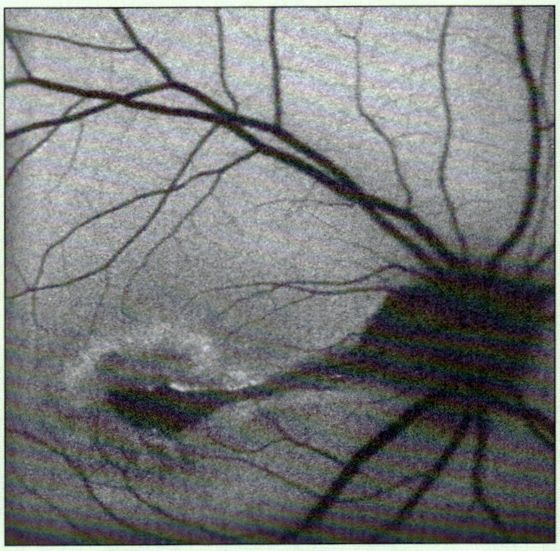

(Left) *Fundus photograph depicts a Best lesion in the pseudohypopyon stage. Typical Best patients have progressed to this stage by young adulthood and often still have only mild vision loss. Though it is more subtle in this image, a yellow fluid level can be seen as subretinal material layers out in the lesion.* ***(Right)*** *Fluorescein angiography image shows fundus autofluorescence of a Best lesion in pseudohypopyon stage. Signal is blocked in the area of the pseudohypopyon with hyperfluorescence above the area.*

BEST DISEASE

INTRODUCTION

Definitions

- Hereditary juvenile-onset vitelliform macular dystrophy
- Adult foveomacular vitelliform dystrophy is similar condition with later onset and better prognosis

DEMOGRAPHICS

Etiology/Risk Factors

- Caused by 1 of > 200 disease-causing mutations in *BEST1* (formerly known as *VMD2*) gene on chromosome 11q12-q13.1
  - Encodes bestrophin-1 protein, a calcium-sensitive chloride channel on basolateral plasma membrane of the retinal pigment epithelium (RPE)
  - Mutations can result in 1 or more of following
    - Accumulation of vitelliform material (lipofuscin) in subretinal space
    - Fibrotic sub-RPE nodules
    - Outer retina disruption and atrophy over intact RPE
  - Recent study found thickness of photoreceptor layer to be increased in Best disease patients compared to controls
  - Both autosomal dominant and autosomal recessive inheritance patterns exist

Epidemiology

- Age of onset is variable, typically 5-10 years old

PRESENTATION

Symptoms

- Decreased central visual acuity
  - Typically, vision is relatively preserved in at least 1 eye throughout course
- Metamorphopsia
- Color vision defects
- Central scotoma

Exam Findings

- Yellow, yolk-like macular lesion early in course
- Eventual "scrambled egg" appearance that may progress to RPE atrophy, macular scarring, &/or choroidal neovascularization (CNV)
- Up to 30% of patients have vitelliform lesions in extramacular areas

DIFFERENTIAL DIAGNOSIS

Other Macular Dystrophies

- Adult-onset foveomacular vitelliform dystrophy (normal electrooculogram [EOG])
- Vitelliform exudative macular detachment
- Pattern dystrophies
- Dominant drusen

EVALUATION/WORK-UP

Imaging

- Spectral domain optical coherence tomography (OCT)
  - Vitelliform material in subretinal space
  - Diffuse photoreceptor outer segment abnormalities
  - Sub-RPE fibrotic nodules
- Fluorescein angiogram (FA)
- Electrooculogram is most specific test and detects disease in earliest stages
  - Arden ratio, defined as the light-peak to dark-trough ratio, is decreased (< 1.5)
  - Signifies altered chloride ion conductance across RPE basolateral plasma membrane
  - Dark adaptation is normal
- Electroretinogram usually normal

Staging

- Stage 0: Previtelliform, normal-appearing macula and normal vision but abnormal EOG
- Stage 1: Previtelliform, normal vision, RPE defects visible on FA
- Stage 2: Vitelliform, macular "egg yolk" appearance, mild visual loss, abnormal FA
  - Stage 2a: Vitelliruptive, "scrambled egg" appearance, mild vision loss, FA blocking and hyperfluorescence
- Stage 3: Pseudohypopyon, subretinal vitelline material forms fluid level, FA blocking, and hyperfluorescence
- Stage 4a: Atrophic, increased visual loss, RPE atrophy
- Stage 4b: Cicatricial, macular scarring is present
- Stage 4c: Neovascular, CNV development; occurs in ~ 20% of patients

TREATMENT

Medical

- No effective treatment in earlier stages before CNV develops
- CNV can be treated with photodynamic therapy or laser; intravitreal bevacizumab has also been reported

Prognosis

- In 1 study, 47% of patients < age 40 retained 20/40 or better vision in at least 1 eye
  - 74% of patients > age 30 had 20/100 or worse vision in at least 1 eye
  - Only 20% of patients > age 40 and no patients > age 50 had 20/40 or better in either eye
- 20% of patients will develop CNV during course of disease

SELECTED REFERENCES

1. Kay CN et al: Three-dimensional distribution of the vitelliform lesion, photoreceptors, and retinal pigment epithelium in the macula of patients with best vitelliform macular dystrophy. Arch Ophthalmol. 130(3):357-64, 2012
2. American Academy of Ophthalmology: Vitelliform Degenerations. American Academy of Ophthalmology: Retina and Vitreous, AAO Basic and Clinical Science Course, Section 12. San Francisco: American Academy of Ophthalmology. 241-243, 2011
3. Friedman N et al: Retina and Choroid. In The Massachusetts Eye and Ear Infirmary Illustrated Manual of Ophthalmology. 3rd ed. Philadelphia: Saunders. 10:448-451, 2009
4. Petrukhin K et al: Identification of the gene responsible for Best macular dystrophy. Nat Genet. 19(3):241-7, 1998
5. Fishman GA et al: Visual acuity in patients with best vitelliform macular dystrophy. Ophthalmology. 100(11):1665-70, 1993

CHOROIDEREMIA

Key Facts

Introduction

- X-linked recessive disorder characterized by progressive, diffuse, bilateral chorioretinal dystrophy

Demographics

- Caused by a mutation in choroideremia gene (*CHM*) found on chromosome Xq21.1
- Visual loss begins after 1st or 2nd decade, but central visual acuity is retained until ~ 7th decade
- Chorioretinal degeneration in affected males
- Milder symptoms in carrier females
- Incidence: 1 per 50,000 men

Presentation

- Affected males present with night blindness
- Visual decline progresses to peripheral field loss
- Central visual acuity preserved until late in life
- Patchy areas of degeneration begin in midperiphery of fundus
- Visual field: Peripheral or mid peripheral ring scotoma
- Carrier females are typically asymptomatic
- Progresses to tunnel vision and often blindness

Evaluation/Work-Up

- Confirm diagnosis with western blot analysis against Rab escort protein-1 (REP-1) antibody
- Atrophy seen in RPE and photoreceptor layer
- Carrier females show normal photoreceptors in periphery, which contrasts with findings among males

Treatment

- Currently, there is no available medical treatment
- Useful vision is maintained until after 6th decade when vision loss is severe

*(**Left**) Funduscopic photograph shows the patchy degeneration of the retinal pigment epithelium (RPE), which begins in the midperiphery of the fundus ➔. Visual acuity in the periphery declines as the disease progresses. (**Right**) Macular sparing can be seen in this photo ➔. Degeneration of fundus results from degeneration of RPE and photoreceptors. The macula is spared until ~ the 7th decade. The disease then progresses to affect central vision and can cause complete blindness.*

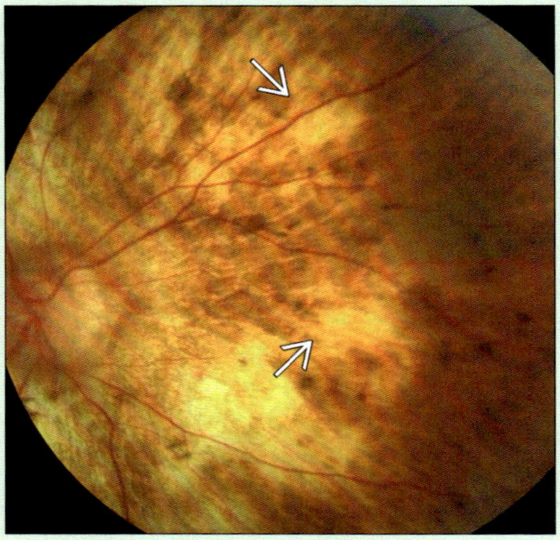

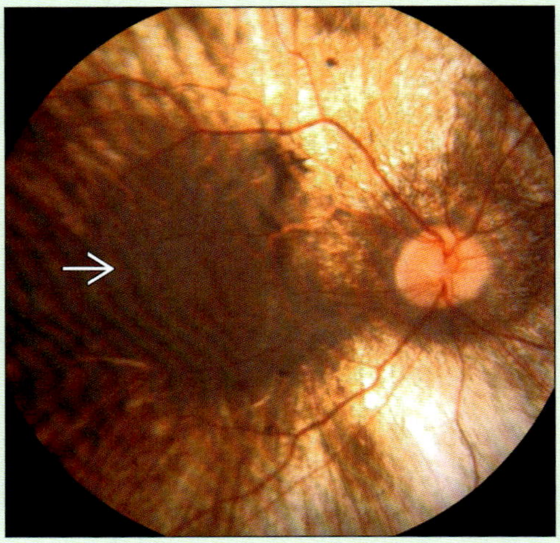

*(**Left**) Funduscopic photograph is an example of a female carrier of choroideremia. Compared with males affected by choroideremia, carriers have significantly less pigment change of the fundus. (**Right**) Fluorescence angiography demonstrates a loss of choriocapillaries ➔. The central macula shows relative hyperfluorescence as the choriocapillaries are spared in this area ➔. This type of imaging is not required for definitive diagnosis.*

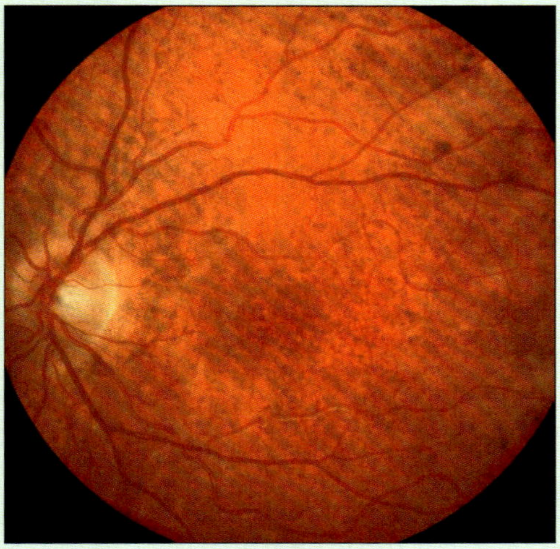

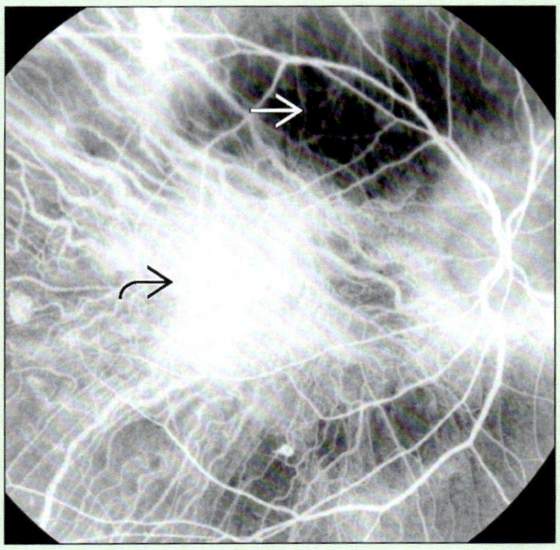

CHOROIDEREMIA

INTRODUCTION

Definitions

- X-linked recessive disorder characterized by progressive, diffuse, bilateral chorioretinal dystrophy

DEMOGRAPHICS

Etiology/Risk Factors

- X-linked recessive inheritance
- Caused by a mutation in choroideremia (*CHM*) gene found on chromosome Xq21.1
- *CHM* gene codes for Rab escort protein-1 (REP-1)
- Loss of REP-1 is compensated by REP-2 in rest of body except in eye
- Lack of REP-1 causes degeneration of retinal pigment epithelium (RPE) as well as rod photoreceptors

Epidemiology

- Chorioretinal degeneration in affected males
- Milder symptoms in carrier females
- Visual loss begins after 1st or 2nd decade
- Central visual acuity is retained until ~ 7th decade
- Incidence: 1 per 50,000 people

PRESENTATION

Symptoms

- Affected males present with night blindness
- Visual decline progresses to peripheral field loss
- Central visual acuity preserved until late in life
- Progresses to tunnel vision and often blindness
- Posterior subcapsular cataracts in 31% of males
- Carrier females are typically asymptomatic

Exam Findings

- Fundus exam
  - Patchy areas of degeneration begin in midperiphery of fundus
  - Hypopigmented fundus
  - RPE mottling
  - Progresses to RPE and choriocapillaris atrophy
  - Central macula spared until later in life
  - Carrier females show pigment changes in midperiphery of fundus similar to that seen in males during early disease
- Visual field
  - Peripheral or mid peripheral ring scotoma
  - Visual field loss corresponds to areas of chorioretinal atrophy
- Electroretinography (ERG)
  - Displays rod then cone degeneration
- Fluorescein angiography (unnecessary for diagnosis)
  - Choriocapillaris loss represented by areas of hypofluorescence

DIFFERENTIAL DIAGNOSIS

X-Linked Retinitis Pigmentosa

- Significant migration of pigment into retina
- Earlier loss of central acuity
- Bone spicule-like pigmentation
- Cystoid macular edema

Gyrate Atrophy

- Autosomal recessive inheritance
- Elevated plasma levels of ornithine
- Scalloped areas of chorioretinal atrophy

EVALUATION/WORK-UP

Labs

- Genetics
  - Confirm diagnosis with western blot analysis against Rab escort protein-1 (REP-1) antibody

Pathology

- Atrophy seen in RPE and photoreceptor layer
- RPE and photoreceptors degenerate independently
- Carrier females show normal photoreceptors in periphery, which contrasts with findings among males

Imaging

- ERG
  - Progressive reduction from childhood with delays in the B wave
  - Increased dark-adaptation thresholds
  - Reduced rod responses

TREATMENT

Medical

- Currently, there is no available medical treatment

Surgical

- Cataract removal is indicated if posterior subcapsular cataract develops

Follow-Up

- Periodic ophthalmologic examination is useful to determine extent of vision loss and to give advice regarding level of visual function

Prognosis

- Very poor
- Useful vision is maintained until after 6th decade
- Develops into tunnel vision and often blindness

SELECTED REFERENCES

1. MacDonald IM et al: Choroideremia: new findings from ocular pathology and review of recent literature. Surv Ophthalmol. 54(3):401-7, 2009
2. Mura M et al: Clinical and functional findings in choroideremia due to complete deletion of the CHM gene. Arch Ophthalmol. 125(8):1107-13, 2007
3. Tolmachova T et al: Independent degeneration of photoreceptors and retinal pigment epithelium in conditional knockout mouse models of choroideremia. J Clin Invest. 116(2):386-94, 2006
4. Preising M et al: Rab escort protein 1 (REP1) in intracellular traffic: a functional and pathophysiological overview. Ophthalmic Genet. 25(2):101-10, 2004

CONE DYSTROPHIES

Key Facts

Presentation

- Slowly progressing decrease in visual acuity in first 3 decades of life
- Dyschromatopsia
- Early disease presentation includes fine macular lesions
- Late disease presentation usually involves a symmetric bull's-eye pattern of central atrophy of macula and central atrophy of retinal pigment epithelium and choriocapillaris
- Additional findings also include spotty pigmentary deposits in macula, waxy pallor of optic disc, and tapetal-like retinal sheen

Demographics

- Frequently sporadic, hereditary forms are often autosomal dominant but can be X-linked
- 1 per 40,000 in general population

Evaluation/Work-Up

- Electroretinogram (ERG) will show
  - Implicit time shift at 30 Hz flicker responses and delayed a- and b-wave single-flash photopic response
  - Large decrease of a- and b-wave amplitude
  - Abnormal cone function: Reduced single-flash photopic response and reduced flicker response
- Complete family history
- Complete ophthalmic exam, with color plates and formal color testing

Treatment

- Palliative care involving vision and occupational therapists
- Poor visual prognosis including a continued decrease in visual and color acuity

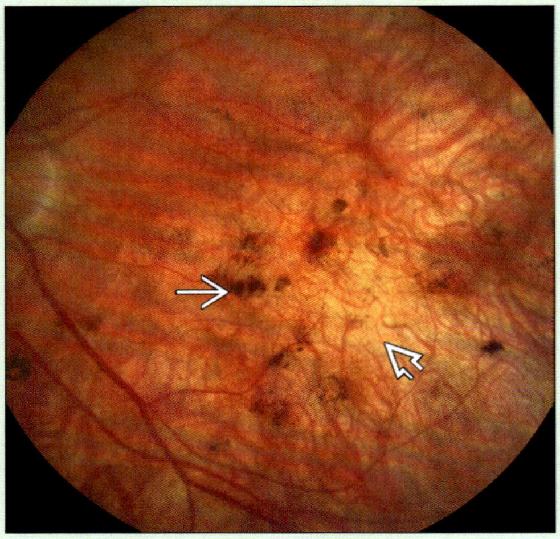

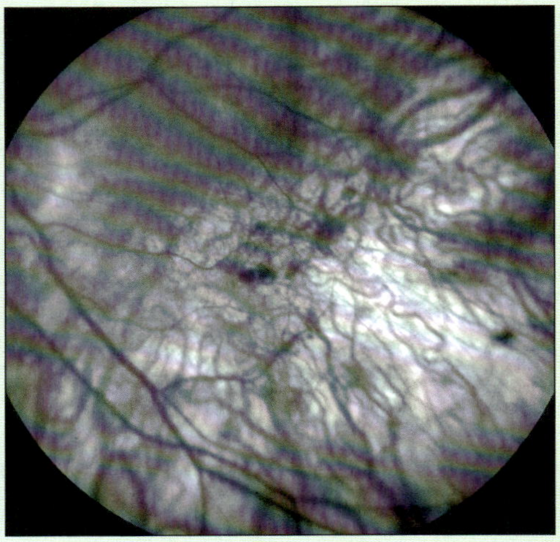

(Left) *Fundus photo shows pigment remodeling ➡ and a large area of atrophic retinal pigment epithelium ➡ in a patient with cone dystrophy. Patients may also have involvement of the rods, which is termed cone-rod dystrophy. Both cone dystrophy and cone-rod dystrophy have a poor visual prognosis.* ***(Right)*** *Red-free image of the same eye clearly shows choroidal vessels. The choroidal vessels are more easily visualized given the atrophic retinal pigment epithelium.*

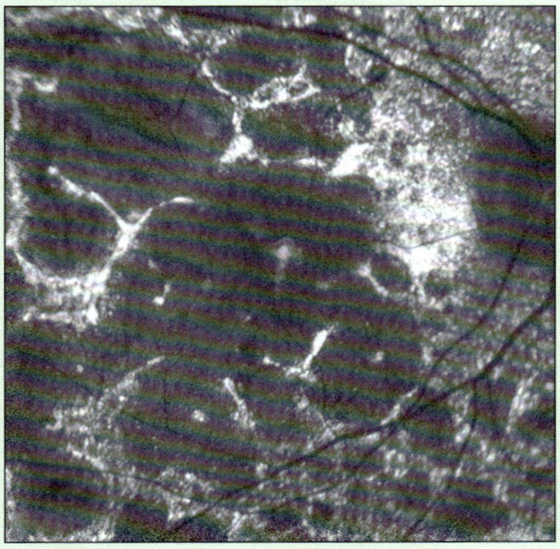

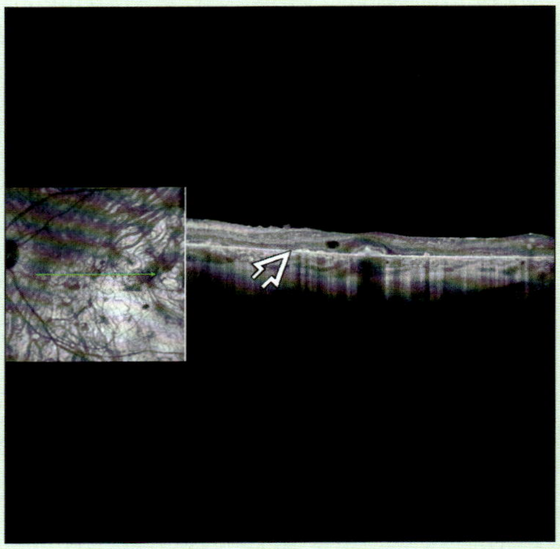

(Left) *Autofluorescence shows large areas of dark retinal pigment epithelium indicating poor metabolic activity. Bright areas indicate an accumulation of lipofuscin.* ***(Right)*** *Optical coherence tomography shows a disrupted photoreceptor line in a patient with cone dystrophy ➡. Cone dystrophy is frequently sporadic, though hereditary forms are also recognized. These hereditary forms are often autosomal dominant but can also be X-linked.*

CONE DYSTROPHIES

INTRODUCTION

Abbreviations
- Cone dystrophies (CDs)
- Cone-rod dystrophies (CRDs)

Definitions
- Retinal dystrophy that is a subcategory of pigmentary retinopathies

Subtypes
- CRDs
  - Loss of cone photoreceptors followed by the loss of rod photoreceptors; also possible to lose both photoreceptors concurrently

DEMOGRAPHICS

Etiology/Risk Factors
- Frequently sporadic
- Hereditary forms are usually autosomal dominant but can be X-linked

Epidemiology
- 1 per 40,000 in general population

PRESENTATION

Symptoms
- Slowly progressing decrease in visual acuity in first 3 decades
- Photophobia and hemeralopia (day blindness)
- Dyschromatopsia

Exam Findings
- Fundus exam
  - Early
    - Normal macula or fine macular lesions
  - Late
    - Symmetric bull's-eye pattern of central atrophy of the macula
    - Central atrophy of the retinal pigment epithelium and choriocapillaris
  - Additional findings
    - Spotty pigmentary deposits often in macular area
    - Waxy pallor of optic disc
    - Tapetal-like retinal sheen (glistening green-gold sheen)

DIFFERENTIAL DIAGNOSIS

Macular Dystrophies
- Stargardt disease, especially in early presentations of the disease
- Chloroquine/hydroxychloroquine maculopathy
  - May produce bull's-eye macula and poor color vision

Retinitis Pigmentosa
- Night blindness and peripheral visual field loss

Central Areolar Choroidal Dystrophy
- Atrophy of retinal pigment epithelium and normal photopic electroretinogram (ERG)

Congenital Color Blindness
- Onset at birth with normal visual acuity; easily ruled out by accurate history or color perception

EVALUATION/WORK-UP

Labs
- None

Pathology
- None

Imaging
- ERG
  - Implicit time shift (between a- and b-wave peaks) at 30 Hz flicker responses and delayed a- and b-wave single flash photopic (cone) response
  - Decrease of photopic a- and b-wave amplitude
  - Abnormal cone function: Reduced single-flash photopic response and reduced flicker response

Work-Up
- Complete family history
- Complete ophthalmic exam, with color plates and formal color testing

TREATMENT

Medical
- Palliative care
  - Help patient with social and psychological impact of blindness
  - Other heath care providers and social workers should be included in this process
    - Vision counselor or therapist to discuss what changes the patient will need to make in their home and daily routine
    - Occupational therapist to ensure patient is adjusting as vision decreases; will also help to provide the necessary tools and training to improve patient's quality of life
  - Sunglasses may help with photophobia
  - Miotic drops may help to improve vision/reduce photophobia

Surgical
- None

Follow-Up
- Once yearly to determine the progression of the disease and to determine what type of care and counseling the patient may need

Prognosis
- Poor visual prognosis
  - Care is only palliative at this time; patient will continue to lose visual acuity and color perception; can lead to blindness

SELECTED REFERENCES

1. Hamel CP: Cone rod dystrophies. Orphanet J Rare Dis. 2:7, 2007

GYRATE ATROPHY

Key Facts

Introduction
- Autosomal recessive chorioretinal dystrophy caused by inborn error of ornithine metabolism leading to night blindness, peripheral vision loss, and ultimately, blindness
- Caused by mutations in ornithine aminotransferase (*OAT*) gene

Demographics
- Rare disease: 200 cases reported since first described
- Highest prevalence in Finland

Presentation
- Night blindness, loss of peripheral vision, myopia, and cataracts by 10 years of age
- Macular sparing and central vision not affected early in disease
- Macular involvement during 4th and 5th decades
- Bilateral, sharply demarcated, rounded areas of chorioretinal atrophy in fundus midperiphery

Differential Diagnosis
- Chorioretinal atrophy
  - Diffuse choriocapillaris atrophy (autosomal dominant)
  - Choroideremia (X-linked)

Evaluation/Work-Up
- Plasma ornithine (elevated ornithine in gyrate atrophy [GA])
- Imaging
  - Fundus photos, fundus autofluorescence, optical coherence tomography (OCT), Humphrey visual fields, full-field electroretinography (ERG)

Treatment
- Arginine-restricted diet reduces serum ornithine levels and has been shown to slow disease progression

__(Left)__ Fundus photo shows classic appearance of gyrate atrophy (GA). Note rounded, sharply demarcated areas of chorioretinal atrophy ➡. These lesions are present in the 1st decade in the mid peripheral fundus and increase in size and number throughout life. There is also posterior spread of lesions with eventual macular involvement in the 5th to 6th decades. __(Right)__ This fundus photo shows choroideremia, a differential diagnosis consideration when GA is suspected.

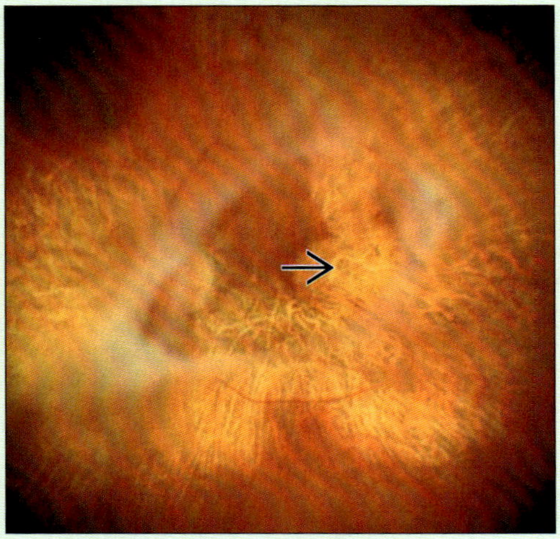

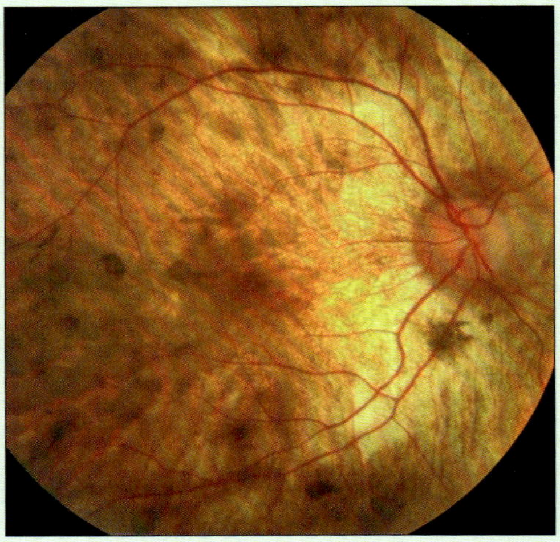

__(Left)__ Fundus photo shows retinitis pigmentosa, which is a differential diagnosis of GA. Both diseases present with night blindness and peripheral vision loss and often lead to blindness at age 40-50. Note multiple bone spicules in the nasal periphery. __(Right)__ Fundus photo shows retinoschisis, exemplified by separation within the neurosensory retina giving a blister appearance ➡. Retinoschisis is a consideration in the differential diagnosis of GA.

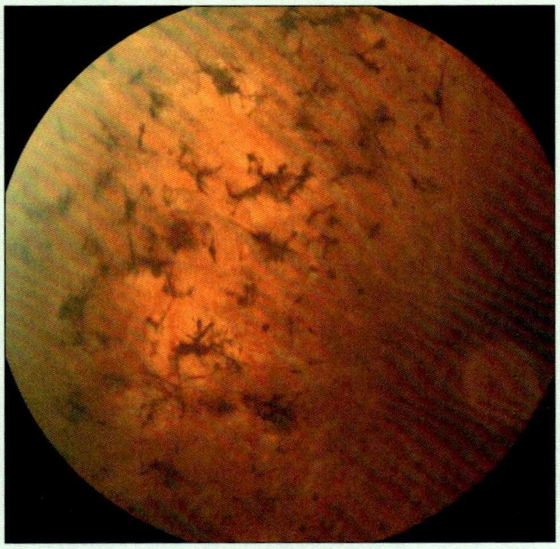

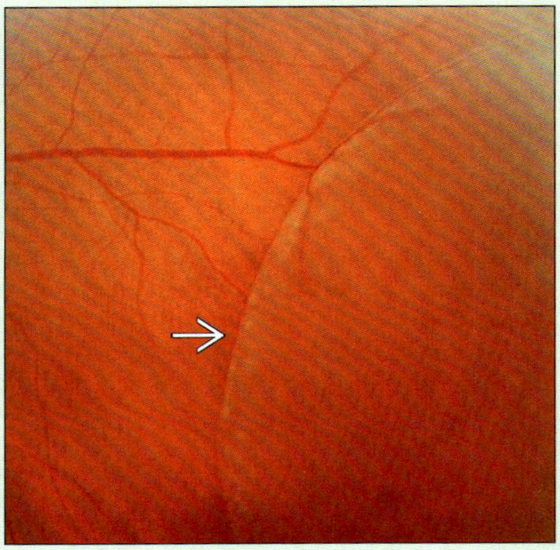

GYRATE ATROPHY

INTRODUCTION

Abbreviations
- Gyrate atrophy (GA)

Definitions
- Autosomal recessive chorioretinal dystrophy caused by inborn error of ornithine metabolism leading to night blindness, peripheral vision loss, and ultimately, blindness
- Caused by mutations in ornithine aminotransferase (*OAT*) gene

DEMOGRAPHICS

Etiology/Risk Factors
- Autosomal recessive
  - Most commonly implicated mutation: L402P mutation of *OAT* gene (10q26)
  - > 60 mutations in *OAT* gene have been identified
- Defect in *OAT*
  - Vitamin B-6 dependent mitochondrial matrix enzyme
    - Enzyme responsible for formation of ornithine from proline, also responsible for reverse reaction
  - Expressed in retinal pigment epithelium, thought to be primary cell type affected in GA but still unknown pathophysiology

Epidemiology
- Rare disease: 200 cases reported since first described
- Significant proportion of cases in Finland where prevalence is estimated to be 1 per 50,000 people

PRESENTATION

Symptoms
- Ocular
  - Symptoms present during 1st decade
  - Night blindness
  - Loss of peripheral vision
  - Myopia
  - Blindness by 4th-5th decades
- Systemic
  - Hyperornithinemia
    - 10-15x elevation in plasma ornithine concentrations
    - Develop ornithinuria
  - Reduction in plasma lysine, glutamate, glutamine, and creatinine

Exam Findings
- Characteristics
  - Myopia
  - Early cataracts, often posterior sutural
    - Common finding during 2nd decade
- Bilateral, sharply demarcated, rounded areas of chorioretinal atrophy in fundus midperiphery
  - Appear during 1st decade
  - Atrophic lesions increase in number and size, coalesce and spread posteriorly as disease progresses
- Macular involvement late in disease
  - Appears during 4th-5th decades
  - Central vision spared early in disease
  - Cystoid macular edema

DIFFERENTIAL DIAGNOSIS

Chorioretinal Atrophy
- Diffuse choriocapillaris atrophy (autosomal dominant)
- Choroideremia (X-linked)

EVALUATION/WORK-UP

Labs
- Plasma ornithine
- Plasma lysine, glutamate, glutamine, and creatinine
- Molecular identification of *OAT* mutations

Imaging
- Fundus autofluorescence
  - Highly circumscribed areas of increased or decreased autofluorescence
- Fluorescein angiography
  - Capillary leakage
  - Dye accumulation in central macula
- Optical coherence tomography (OCT)
  - Intraretinal cystoid spaces
  - Nerve fiber layer thinning
- Humphrey visual field
  - Visual field constriction with central sparring
- Full-field ERG
  - Absent photopic and scotopic responses

TREATMENT

Medical
- Arginine-restricted diet reduces serum ornithine levels and has been shown to slow disease progression
- Gene replacement therapy targeting RPE

Prognosis
- Slowly progressive disease with macular involvement leading to complete blindness by the 4th or 5th decade

SELECTED REFERENCES

1. Sergouniotis PI et al: Retinal structure, function, and molecular pathologic features in gyrate atrophy. Ophthalmology. 119(3):596-605, 2012
2. Fleury M et al: Myopathy with tubular aggregates and gyrate atrophy of the choroid and retina due to hyperornithinaemia. J Neurol Neurosurg Psychiatry. 78(6):656-7, 2007
3. Oliveira TL et al: Cystoid macular edema in gyrate atrophy of the choroid and retina: a fluorescein angiography and optical coherence tomography evaluation. Am J Ophthalmol. 140(1):147-9, 2005
4. Kaiser-Kupfer MI et al: Gyrate atrophy of the choroid and retina: further experience with long-term reduction of ornithine levels in children. Arch Ophthalmol. 120(2):146-53, 2002
5. Peltola KE et al: Ophthalmologic heterogeneity in subjects with gyrate atrophy of choroid and retina harboring the L402P mutation of ornithine aminotransferase. Ophthalmology. 108(4):721-9, 2001
6. Hayasaka S et al: Differential diagnosis of diffuse choroidal atrophies. Diffuse choriocapillaris atrophy, choroideremia, and gyrate atrophy of the choroid and retina. Retina. 5(1):30-7, 1985

RETINITIS PIGMENTOSA

Key Facts

Introduction
- Set of hereditary retinal diseases that feature degeneration of rod and cone photoreceptors

Demographics
- Progressive disease with exponential decline
- Worldwide prevalence of 1 in 4,000
- Age of onset can vary from infancy through late middle age

Presentation
- Highly variable symptoms
- Classic pattern
  - Night blindness in adolescence
  - Loss of mid peripheral visual field in young adulthood
  - Loss of far peripheral vision in adulthood
  - Loss of central vision by 60 years
- Most patients are legally blind by age 40
- Refractive errors (hyperopia/ myopia)
- Low contrast sensitivity
- Low color vision
- Bone spicule deposits in mid or far periphery
- Bilateral involvement

Evaluation/Work-Up
- Electroretinogram confirms clinical diagnosis

Treatment
- Currently, no established standard treatment
- Vitamin A palmitate supplementation
- Treat associated ocular manifestations
- Gene therapy for Leber congenital amaurosis (LCA), a type of RP

Differential Diagnosis
- Traumatic retinopathy is most common mimicker
- Infectious retinopathy
- Drug toxicity retinopathy

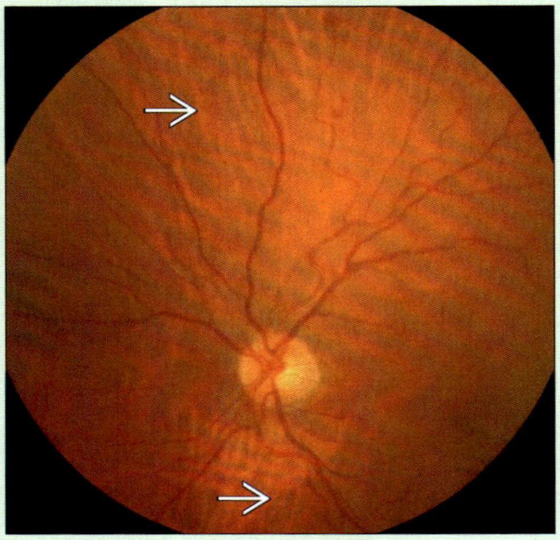
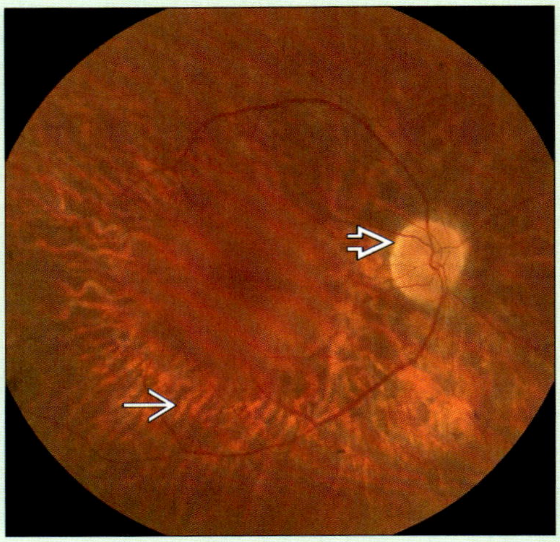

(Left) *This fundus photo shows loss of the retinal pigment epithelium and choriocapillaries, revealing underlying large choroidal vessels seen as orange stripes or lines throughout the fundus.* ***(Right)*** *Fundus photo shows a waxy optic disc and large choroidal vessels seen as orange stripes concentric to the macula.*

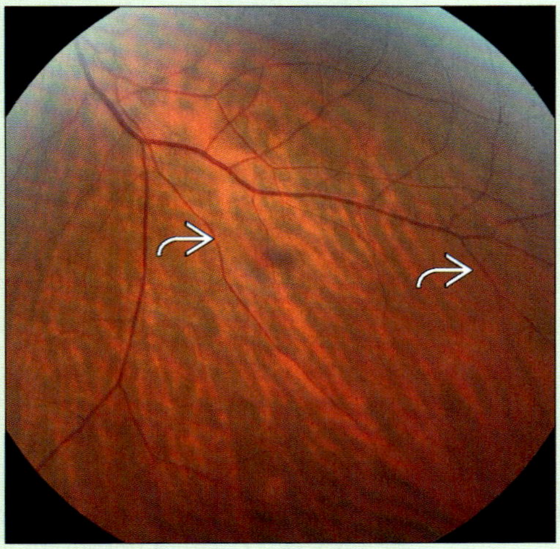
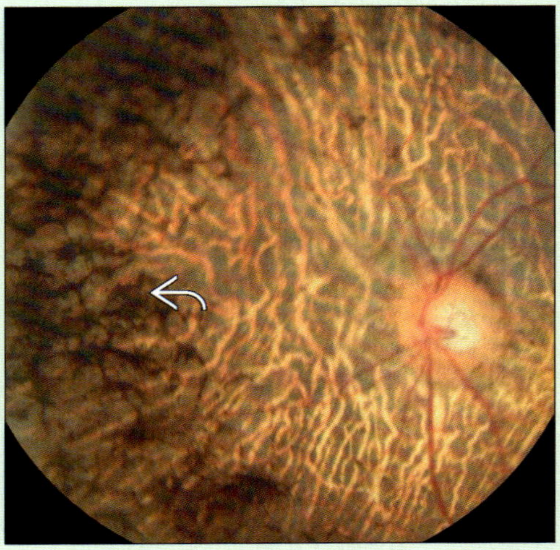

(Left) *This fundus photo shows attenuated arterioles along with the classic orange stripes of retinitis pigmentosa.* ***(Right)*** *Fundus photo shows bone spicules and a general mottled appearance of the retina. This demonstrates a more advanced case of retinitis pigmentosa.*

RETINITIS PIGMENTOSA

INTRODUCTION

Abbreviations
- Retinitis pigmentosa (RP)

Synonyms
- Pigmentary maculopathy
- Pigmentary retinopathy

Definitions
- Set of hereditary retinal diseases that feature degeneration of rod and cone photoreceptors

Subtypes
- Categorized by photoreceptor subtype
  - Rod-cone dystrophies
    - Loss of rod sensitivity followed by loss of cone sensitivity
  - Cone-rod dystrophies
    - Simultaneous loss of cone and rod function

DEMOGRAPHICS

Etiology/Risk Factors
- Progressive disease with exponential decline
- May be
  - Autosomal dominant (30-40% of cases)
  - Autosomal recessive (50-60% of cases)
  - X-linked (5-15% of cases)

Epidemiology
- Worldwide prevalence of 1 in 4,000
- Age of onset can vary

PRESENTATION

Symptoms
- Highly variable symptoms
- Classic pattern
  - Night blindness in adolescence
  - Loss of mid peripheral visual field in young adulthood
  - Loss of far peripheral vision in adulthood
  - Loss of central vision by 60 years
- Most patients are legally blind by age 40
- Bilateral involvement
- Photopsia in mid peripheral field of vision
- May find syndromic retinitis pigmentosa

Exam Findings
- Myopia
  - Related to X-linked retinitis pigmentosum
- Hyperopia
  - Related to dominant inheritance
- Low contrast sensitivity
- Low color vision
- Direct ophthalmoscopy shows intraretinal pigmentation
  - Bone spicule deposits in mid or far periphery
- Rod dysfunction measured by
  - Decreased dark adaptation
  - Electroretinogram (ERG)

DIFFERENTIAL DIAGNOSIS

Traumatic Retinopathy
- Most common mimic of RP
- RPE becomes dark several months after injury to eye
- Bone spicule pattern is very similar to RP

Acquired Retinal Degenerations
- Peripheral reticular pigmentary degeneration

Drug Toxicity Retinopathy
- Phenothiazine, chlorpromazine, chloroquine, deferoxamine, thioridazine

Infectious Retinopathy
- Rubella, syphilis

Vitamin A Deficiency
- Also presents with night blindness

Dystrophy of Choroid and Retina
- Gyrate atrophy
- Choroideremia

Cancer-Associated Retinopathy
- Vision loss occurs before malignancy is diagnosed
- Bilateral central vision loss

EVALUATION/WORK-UP

Imaging
- ERG confirms clinical diagnosis
- Gene testing

TREATMENT

Medical
- Currently, no established standard treatment
- Vitamin A palmitate supplementation and omega-3 fatty acids may slow retinal degeneration
- Reduction in exposure to light may slow rate of degeneration
- Treat associated ocular manifestations

Surgical
- Argus II retinal prosthesis may benefit some patients

Follow-Up
- Genetic counseling about hereditary nature of RP

Prognosis
- Autosomal dominant form has best prognosis
- Gene therapy (AAV.RPE6S) has benefited LCA

SELECTED REFERENCES

1. Shintani K et al: Review and update: current treatment trends for patients with retinitis pigmentosa. Optometry. 80(7):384-401, 2009
2. Hartong DT et al: Retinitis pigmentosa. Lancet. 368(9549):1795-809, 2006
3. Kalloniatis M et al: Retinitis pigmentosa: understanding the clinical presentation, mechanisms and treatment options. Clin Exp Optom. 87(2):65-80, 2004

SICKLE CELL DISEASE

Key Facts

Introduction

- Subtypes
  - Proliferative sickle retinopathy
  - Nonproliferative sickle cell ocular disease

Demographics

- Proliferative sickle retinopathy is the major cause of vision loss in sickle cell disease
- Worldwide, there are 250,000 children born with sickle cell disease every year

Presentation

- Early sickle cell disease does not result in visual symptoms
  - Vision loss may occur due to hemorrhage or retinal detachment
- Lesions seen in periphery initially
- Proliferative sickle cell retinopathy
  - Sea fans sign (retinal neovascularization)
- Retinal vessel occlusion
  - Vessels terminate as hairpin loops
- Retinal hemorrhage
  - Salmon patch: Superficial retinal hemorrhage
  - Sunburst: Retinal scarring
- Venous tortuosity
  - Due to arteriovenous anastomoses
- Evaluate with dilated ophthalmoscopy

Treatment

- Proliferative sickle retinopathy
  - Scatter photocoagulation
- Vitrectomy or scleral buckle for retinal detachment
- Treat underlying disease with hematologist

Prognosis

- Blindness may occur
- Spontaneous regression of neovascular proliferation may occur

__(Left)__ Fundus photo shows evidence of stage 3 sickle cell retinopathy, with neovascular and fibrous proliferation in the peripheral retina. Proliferative retinopathy is the major cause of visual loss in sickle cell disease. __(Right)__ This peripheral blood smear from a young woman with sickle cell disease shows anemia and prominent erythrocyte sickling. This crisis was precipitated by viral gastroenteritis with dehydration. (Courtesy K. Hunt, MD.)

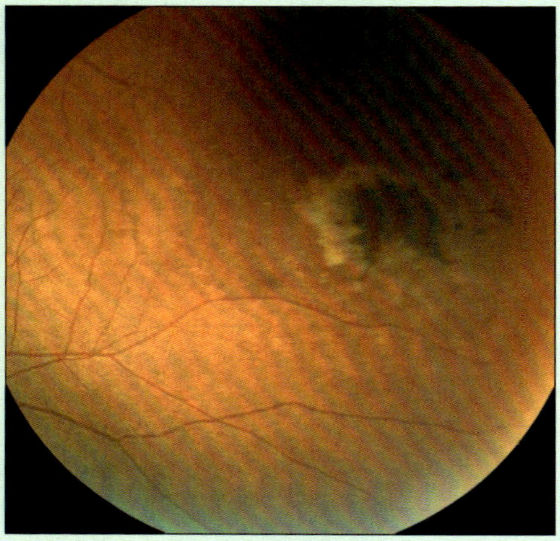

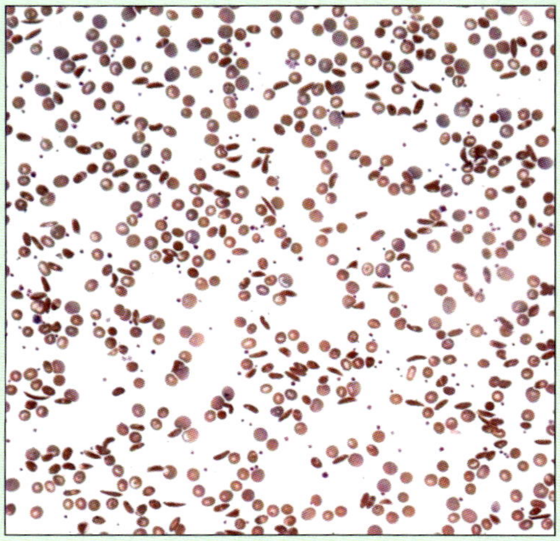

__(Left)__ Hemoglobin S is less soluble in deoxygenated conditions such as during infection or at high altitude. Rigid polymers form and distort the erythrocytes into the characteristic sickled shape. (Courtesy K. Hunt, MD.) __(Right)__ Fluorescein angiography demonstrates sea fan pattern of preretinal neovascularization in far periphery in proliferative sickle cell retinopathy ➔. Differential diagnosis of sickle cell retinopathy includes diabetic retinopathy, Eales disease, branch retinal vein occlusion, or lupus.

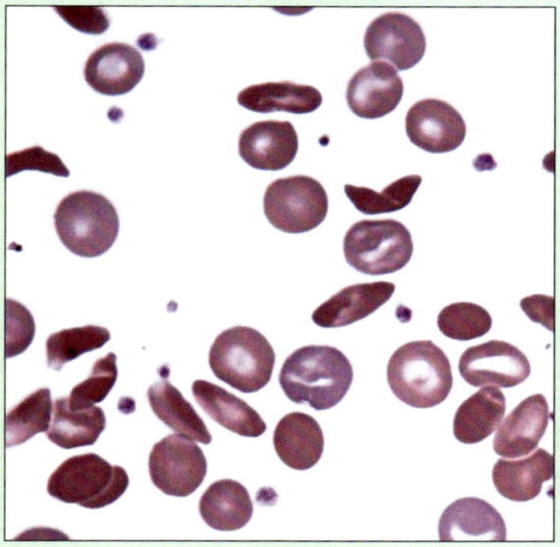

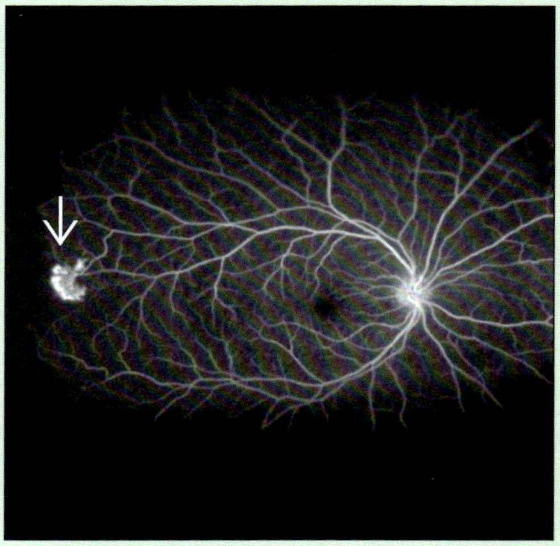

SICKLE CELL DISEASE

INTRODUCTION

Definitions
- Due to a single point mutation in the β-globin protein
- Autosomal recessive inheritance

Subtypes
- Proliferative sickle retinopathy (highest risk of SC disease vs. SS)
  - Stage 1: Peripheral arterial occlusion
  - Stage 2: Peripheral arteriovenous anastomoses (hairpin loop)
  - Stage 3: Neovascular and fibrous proliferations (sea fan sign)
  - Stage 4: Vitreous hemorrhage
  - Stage 5: Retinal detachment
- Nonproliferative sickle cell ocular disease

DEMOGRAPHICS

Etiology/Risk Factors
- Risk factors for developing proliferative sickle retinopathy
  - High hemoglobin in males
  - Low fetal hemoglobin in males and females
- Proliferative sickle retinopathy is the major cause of vision loss in sickle cell disease

Epidemiology
- Worldwide, there are 250,000 children born with sickle cell disease every year
  - One of the most prevalent genetic disorders
- 8% of black Americans have sickle cell trait
- Low prevalence of sickle cell disease among adults because of high childhood mortality

PRESENTATION

Symptoms
- Early sickle cell disease does not result in visual symptoms
- Vision loss results from advanced sickle disease

Exam Findings
- May see anterior segment changes
  - Conjunctival sign
    - Comma-shaped dilatations of conjunctival capillaries
- Lesions seen in periphery initially
  - Poor perfusion to retina
- Use dilated ophthalmoscopy
  - Evaluate retinal vessels with fluorescein angiography
- Proliferative sickle cell retinopathy
  - Sea fan sign
    - Preretinal neovasculature
    - Forms between perfused and nonperfused retina
  - White fibrous tissue found temporally
- Retinal vessel occlusion
  - Children
    - Only arterioles and capillaries are occluded
  - Adults
    - Arteries and veins are occluded
    - Submacular choroidal infarction is more common in adults
  - Vessels terminate as hairpin loops
- Retinal hemorrhage
  - Salmon patch
    - Superficial retinal hemorrhage
    - Pink appearance
    - Leave mottled brown appearance and iridescent deposits after they resolve
  - Sunburst
    - Retinal scarring following hemorrhage
    - Black appearance because of the retinal pigment epithelium involvement
- Venous tortuosity
  - Due to arteriovenous anastomoses

DIFFERENTIAL DIAGNOSIS

Proliferative Diabetic Retinopathy
- Dot-and-blot hemorrhages
- Cotton-wool spots

Eales Disease
- Vascular sheathing can cause occlusion
- Anterior chamber may have keratic precipitates

Branch Retinal Vein Occlusion
- Intraretinal hemorrhages

Systemic Lupus Erythematosus
- Retinal vasculitis

TREATMENT

Medical
- Hydration; treat underlying disease with hematology

Surgical
- Proliferative sickle retinopathy
  - Scatter photocoagulation
- Vitrectomy

Follow-Up
- Observation is indicated in nonproliferative sickle cell ocular disease

Prognosis
- Blindness may occur
  - Blood vessel hemorrhage may cause traction retinal detachments
  - Proliferative sickle retinopathy may cause retinal detachment
  - Occurs in 10-20% of eyes of patients with sickle cell disease
- Spontaneous regression of neovascular proliferation may occur
  - Occurs in 32% of proliferative sickle retinopathy eyes

SELECTED REFERENCES

1. Elagouz M et al: Sickle cell disease and the eye: old and new concepts. Surv Ophthalmol. 55(4):359-77, 2010
2. Downes SM et al: Incidence and natural history of proliferative sickle cell retinopathy: observations from a cohort study. Ophthalmology. 112(11):1869-75, 2005
3. Clarkson JG: The ocular manifestations of sickle-cell disease: a prevalence and natural history study. Trans Am Ophthalmol Soc. 90:481-504, 1992

STARGARDT DISEASE

Key Facts

Introduction

- Autosomal recessive retinal dystrophy caused by mutation of *ABCA4* gene
- *ABCA4* mutation causes lipofuscin to accumulate in retinal pigment epithelium (RPE), leading to changes in membrane permeability, lysosomal dysfunction, and cell death

Demographics

- *ABCA4* mutation is also found in age-related macular degeneration, fundus flavimaculatus, bull's-eye maculopathy, cone-rod dystrophy, retinitis pigmentosa, and many other visual disorders
- 1 per 8,000-10,000 affected with STGD

Presentation

- Age of onset ~ 10-20 years (may be highly variable due to mutation spectrum)
- Slowly progressive central vision loss
- Different phenotypic groups show variation of scotopic &/or photopic vision loss
- Fishman described 4 stages of disease using fundus analysis and electrophysiology testing
- Dyschromatopsia

Evaluation/Work-Up

- Accumulation of lipofuscin-like pigment throughout RPE
- ERG findings show a progressive decrease of photopic and scotopic response
- Dark choroid on fluorescein angiography: Choroidal fluorescence is blocked due to lipofuscin buildup

Treatment

- No known treatment exists
- Wide variability of outcomes are seen, with a decrease of visual acuity being the main symptom
- Acuity ranges between 20/50 and 20/200

*(**Left**) Fundus photograph depicts the fundus of a patient with Stargardt disease. Note the diffuse yellow-white flecks that are characteristic of the disease. Macular mottling is also present. (**Right**) Fundus photograph demonstrates diffuse yellow-white flecks in a patient with Stargardt disease. These flecks can be found in various shapes and sizes and are typically diffusely present. Resorption of the flecks may occur as the disease progresses.*

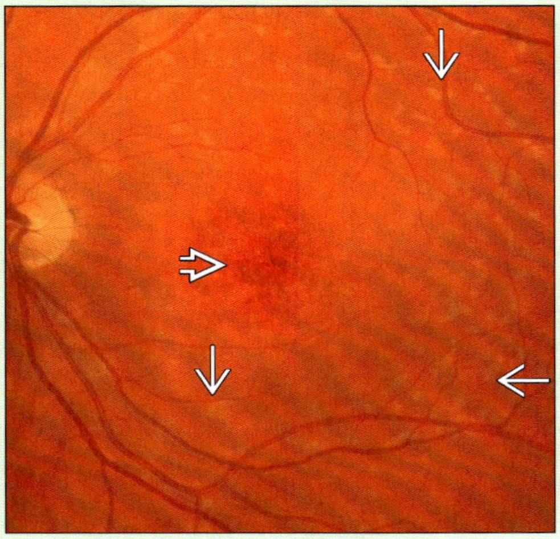

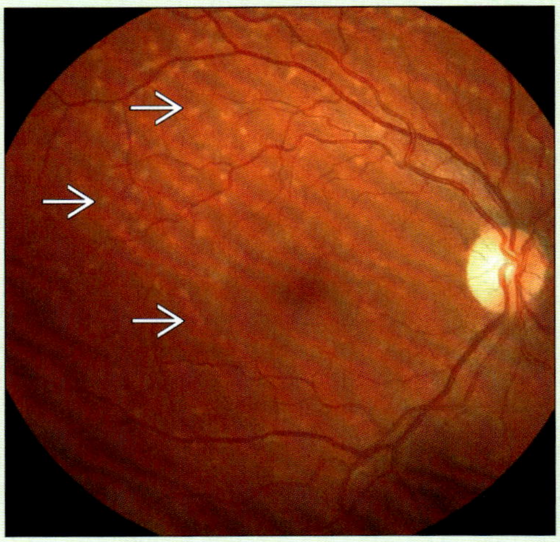

*(**Left**) Fundus photograph of a patient with Stargardt disease demonstrates macular degeneration in a bull's-eye pattern. Bull's-eye maculopathy has a differential diagnosis that includes Stargardt disease, chloroquine toxicity, and cone dystrophies in the late phases. (**Right**) This fluorescein angiography image demonstrates an eye with Stargardt disease with the classic finding of dark (or silent) choroid and macular hyperfluorescence. The typical choroidal fluorescence is blocked due to lipofuscin buildup.*

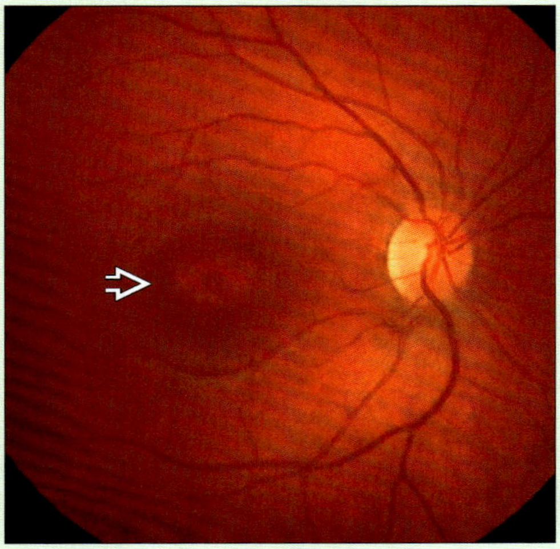

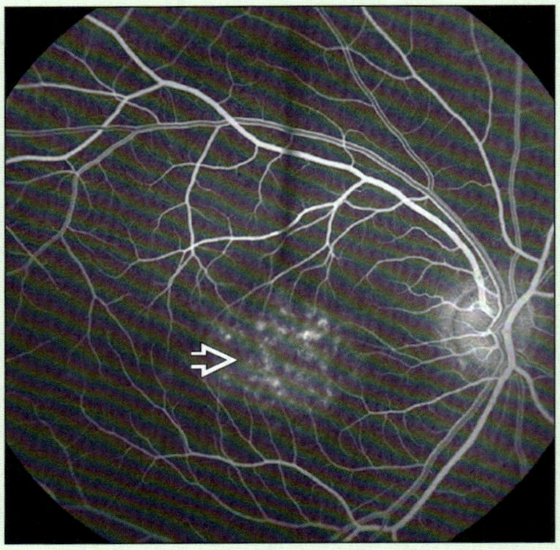

STARGARDT DISEASE

INTRODUCTION

Abbreviations

- Stargardt disease (STGD)

Definitions

- Autosomal recessive retinal dystrophy caused by mutation of *ABCA4* gene
  - Retinal changes include photoreceptor degeneration and retinal pigment epithelium (RPE) atrophy
- Scotopic vision: Vision in low light conditions
- Photopic vision: Vision in well-lit conditions
- Flecks: Yellowish-white lesions of various size in retina

Subtypes

- Autosomal dominant Stargardt-like disease
  - Phenotypically similar retinal dystrophy; however, caused by *ELOV4* mutation on chromosome 6q

DEMOGRAPHICS

Etiology/Risk Factors

- Autosomal recessive inheritance
  - *ABCA4* mutation on chromosome 1p21-22.1
    - STGD is 1 of several phenotypic presentations of *ABCA4* retinopathy
    - *ABCA4* mutation is also found in age-related macular degeneration, fundus flavimaculatus, bull's-eye maculopathy, cone-rod dystrophy, retinitis pigmentosa, and many other visual disorders
    - *ABCA4* mutation causes lipofuscin to accumulate in RPE, leading to changes in membrane permeability, lysosomal dysfunction, and cell death

Epidemiology

- 1 per 8,000-10,000 affected with STGD
- Difficult to determine prevalence of *ABCA4* but could be as high as 1:20 or higher

PRESENTATION

Symptoms

- Age of onset ~ 10-20 years (may be highly variable due to mutation spectrum)
- Slowly progressive central vision loss
- Different phenotypic groups show variation of scotopic &/or photopic vision loss
- Dyschromatopsia

Exam Findings

- Fishman described 4 stages of disease using fundus analysis and electrophysiology testing
  - Stage I
    - Disease confined to fovea or parafoveal region with or without flecks
  - Stage II
    - Flecks become more widespread
    - Subnormal cone and rod response observed
  - Stage III
    - Resorption of flecks with atrophy of choriocapillaris
  - Stage IV
    - Further resorptions of flecks with extensive atrophy of choriocapillaris
    - Large decrease in rod and cone response with ERG
- Best corrected visual acuity (BCVA) is a useful marker of progression of disease

DIFFERENTIAL DIAGNOSIS

Familial Drusen

- Inherited or sporadic disease presents with drusen deposits in RPE throughout macula that are present early in life
- Visual acuities tend to be better with familial drusen

Pattern Dystrophy

- Autosomal dominant group of dystrophies that present in midlife with a variety of patterns of deposits in macular area
- On fluorescein angiography, patterns of hyperfluorescence are more distinct and dark choroid is absent

EVALUATION/WORK-UP

Pathology

- Accumulation of lipofuscin-like pigment throughout RPE

Imaging

- Electroretinography (ERG) findings show a progressive decrease of photopic and scotopic response
- Fluorescein angiography (FA)
  - Dark (or silent) choroid: Choroidal fluorescence is blocked due to the lipofuscin buildup; this can occur in argyrosis as well
    - Central macula shows hyperfluorescent flecks on FA
- Fundus autofluorescence (FAF)
  - Examination of serial images allows analysis of rate of progression of disease

TREATMENT

Medical

- No known treatment exists

Prognosis

- Wide variability of outcomes are seen, with a decrease of visual acuity being the main symptom
- May appear as early as 1st decade of life or later into middle age
- Acuity ranges between 20/50 and 20/200

SELECTED REFERENCES

1. Burke TR et al: Allelic and phenotypic heterogeneity in ABCA4 mutations. Ophthalmic Genet. 32(3):165-74, 2011
2. Walia S et al: Natural history of phenotypic changes in Stargardt macular dystrophy. Ophthalmic Genet. 30(2):63-8, 2009
3. Klevering BJ et al: The spectrum of retinal phenotypes caused by mutations in the ABCA4 gene. Graefes Arch Clin Exp Ophthalmol. 243(2):90-100, 2005
4. Lois N et al: Phenotypic subtypes of Stargardt macular dystrophy-fundus flavimaculatus. Arch Ophthalmol. 119(3):359-69, 2001

OCULAR HISTOPLASMOSIS

Key Facts

Introduction
- Presumed ocular histoplasmosis syndrome (POHS)

Demographics
- No conclusive evidence for histoplasmosis as cause of POHS
- Occurs in ages 20-50
- Endemic to Ohio and Mississippi River valleys

Presentation
- Nonexudative POHS is asymptomatic
- Exudative POHS
  - Blurring of central vision
- Classic triad
  - Discrete atrophic choroidal scars in macula or midperiphery
  - Peripapillary atrophy
  - Choroidal neovascularization
- No signs of vitreous or aqueous inflammation

Evaluation/Work-Up
- Serological tests for antibodies to histoplasmosis are negative
- Antigen detection tests are negative
- OCT and fluorescein angiography
  - Use to observe choroidal neovascularization

Treatment
- Observation for inactive (without choroidal neovascularization) histoplasmosis scarring
- Corticosteroids
- Antiangiogenic compounds
- Photodynamic therapy
  - First-line treatment
- Submacular surgery
  - Use for subfoveal choroidal neovascularization
- Laser photocoagulation
  - Use for subfoveal choroidal neovascularization
- Not responsive to antifungal therapy

__(Left)__ This fundus photograph of a patient with early ocular histoplasmosis shows peripapillary scarring ➔. __(Right)__ This fluorescein angiography image of the same patient highlights an area of neovascularization ➔ characteristic of this disease process. OCT imaging can also be used to visualize neovascularization. Antiangiogenic compounds may be used to treat the neovascularization associated with ocular histoplasmosis.

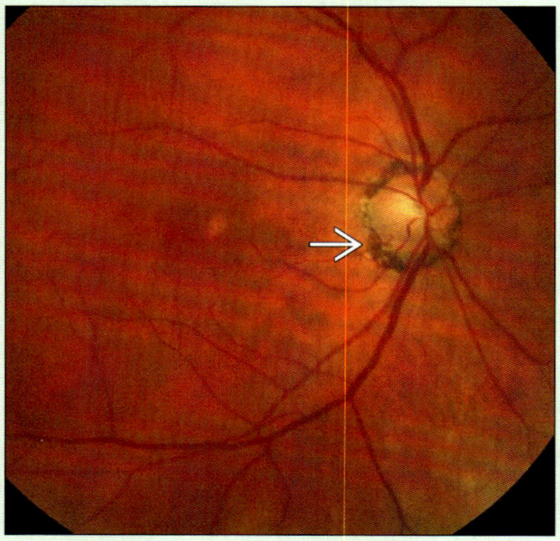

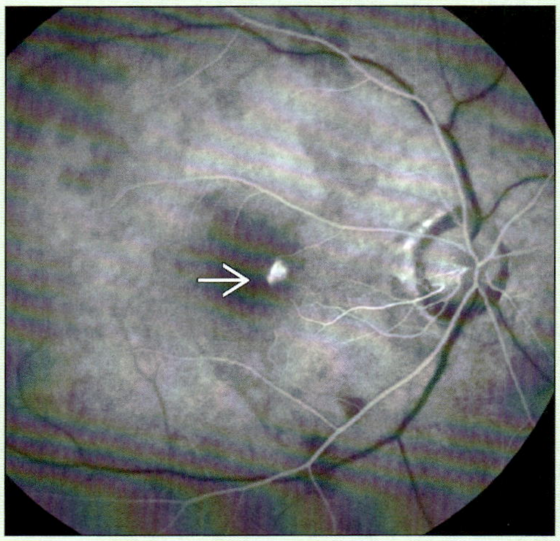

__(Left)__ This fundus photograph of a patient with ocular histoplasmosis shows both a yellow-white histo spot ➔, peripapillary scarring ➔, and scattered gray-green subretinal patches of blood or exudate ➔, representing multifocal choroiditis. __(Right)__ This fluorescein angiography image of the same patient with ocular histoplasmosis and multifocal choroiditis shows areas of choroidal neovascularization ➔ and peripapillary scarring.

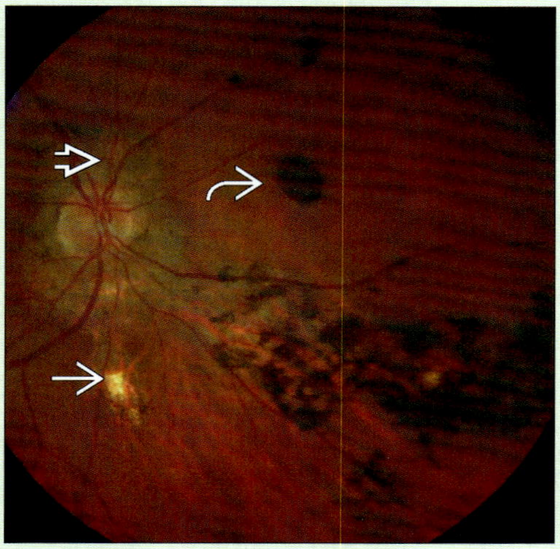

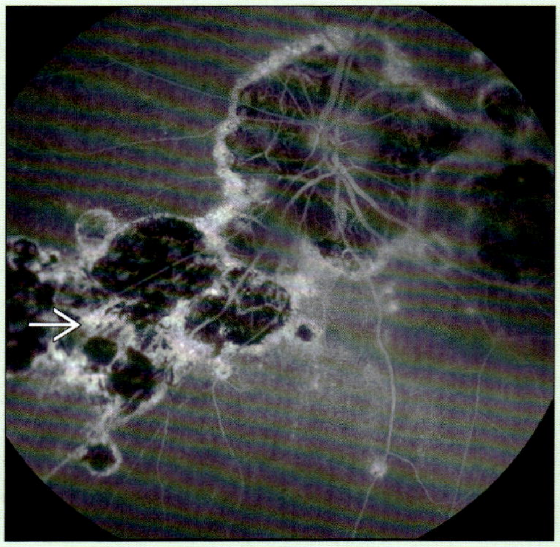

OCULAR HISTOPLASMOSIS

INTRODUCTION

Abbreviations
- Presumed ocular histoplasmosis syndrome (POHS)

DEMOGRAPHICS

Etiology/Risk Factors
- No conclusive evidence for histoplasmosis as cause of POHS
  - Hypothesized that *Histoplasma capsulatum* spreads to eye in childhood, causing scars to form that remain after systemic infection
  - Scars represent focal defects in Bruch membrane, which allows choroidal neovascularization
- Most patients do not have history of systemic histoplasmosis infection
- No clear occupational predisposition

Epidemiology
- Occurs in ages 20-50
- Endemic to Ohio and Mississippi River valleys
- Chorioretinal lesions (histo spots)
  - Present in 2.6% of population living in endemic areas
  - Present in 4.4% of population living in endemic areas with positive histoplasmosis skin test

PRESENTATION

Symptoms
- Nonexudative POHS is asymptomatic
- Exudative POHS
  - Blurring of central vision
  - Acute or insidious

Exam Findings
- Classic triad
  - Discrete atrophic choroidal scars in macula or midperiphery
    - Histo spots
    - Defects in Bruch membrane
  - Peripapillary atrophy
  - Choroidal neovascularization
    - Develops from histo spots
    - Yellow-green subretinal discoloration that may be surrounded by pigment ring
    - Lacy pattern seen with angiography
- No signs of vitreous or aqueous inflammation

DIFFERENTIAL DIAGNOSIS

Exudative Age-Related Macular Degeneration
- Older patients
- Without firm attachment of retinal pigment epithelium to Bruch membrane

Toxoplasmosis
- Usually painful
- May see floaters

EVALUATION/WORK-UP

Labs
- Serological tests for antibodies to histoplasmosis are negative
  - Antibodies decline to low levels 2-5 years after infection
- Histopathology is negative
- Culture tests are negative
- Antigen detection tests are negative

Imaging
- Optical coherence tomography (OCT)
- Fluorescein angiography

TREATMENT

Medical
- Observation for inactive (without choroidal neovascularization) histoplasmosis scarring
- Corticosteroids
  - Angiostatic properties
  - Inhibition of inflammatory cells
- Not responsive to antifungal therapy
- Antiangiogenic compounds
  - VEGF-specific antibodies

Surgical
- Laser photocoagulation
  - First-line treatment for POHS patients with choroidal neovascularization located in
    - Extrafoveal area
    - Juxtafoveal area
    - Peripapillary area
- Photodynamic therapy
  - Use when there is subfoveal choroidal neovascularization because laser photocoagulation would cause blinding central scotoma
  - Intravenous photosensitizing dyes that cause isolated vascular occlusion
    - Verteporfin
- Submacular surgery
  - Removal of subfoveal choroidal neovascularization

Prognosis
- 33% of patients who receive laser photocoagulation treatment will have recurrent choroidal neovascularization within 2 years
- On average, symptoms occur in 2nd eye 4 years after onset of symptoms in 1st eye
- 44% of eyes that receive submacular surgery develop recurrent choroidal neovascularization

SELECTED REFERENCES

1. Wheat LJ: Histoplasmosis: a review for clinicians from non-endemic areas. Mycoses. 49(4):274-82, 2006
2. Ciulla TA et al: Presumed ocular histoplasmosis syndrome: update on epidemiology, pathogenesis, and photodynamic, antiangiogenic, and surgical therapies. Curr Opin Ophthalmol. 12(6):442-9, 2001
3. McMillan TA et al: Ocular histoplasmosis. Int Ophthalmol Clin. 36(3):179-86, 1996

HIV AND ASSOCIATED CONDITIONS

Key Facts

Demographics
- Most common risk factors: Unprotected sexual contact, IV drug use
- In 2009, 1,148,200 persons 13 and older were living with HIV in USA alone

Presentation
- Most common symptom (up to 70% of patients): HIV-related microangiopathy of retina
- Multiple opportunistic infections and conditions
- Cytomegalovirus retinitis (screen every 3 months if CD4[+] cell count is < 200)
- Toxoplasma retinochoroiditis
- Kaposi sarcoma
  - Common finding on eyelid and anterior segment and an AIDS-defining condition
- Blepharitis
  - Common eyelid finding
- Keratitis
  - Common finding on anterior segment
- Posterior segment can show a myriad of conditions
  - Main subcategories: Retinal microangiopathy, HIV retinitis, or progressive retinal necrosis

Evaluation/Work-Up
- Serological testing for HIV done with ELISA screening test followed by Western blot confirmatory test
- CD4(+) T-cell counts every 3 months with primary care physician

Treatment
- HIV is a chronic manageable disease; with appropriate therapy, patients can have normal life expectancy
- Without treatment, HIV will progress to AIDS
- AIDS average life expectancy: 3 years

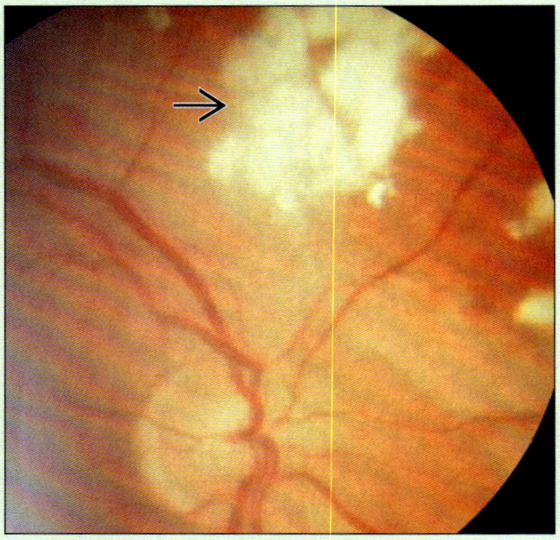
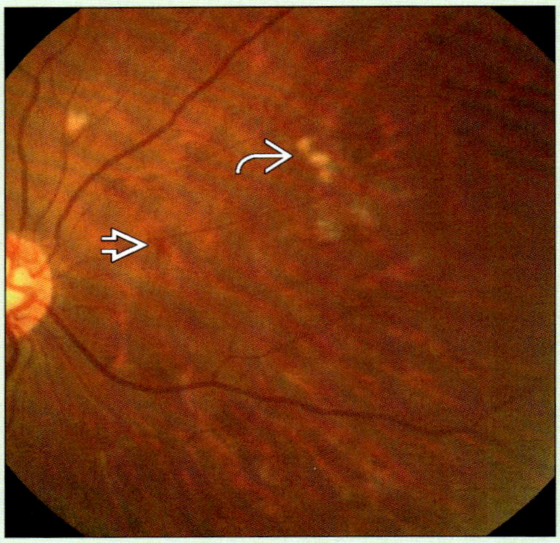

(Left) Progressive retinal necrosis is a vision-threatening complication of AIDS. This fundus photograph is an example of progressive retinal necrosis seen in a patient with HIV. The yellow-white infiltrates ➔ present in this image are characteristic. (Right) This fundus photograph of a patient with HIV is concerning for HIV microangiopathy. Characteristic signs include cotton-wool spots ➔ and retinal hemorrhages ➔.

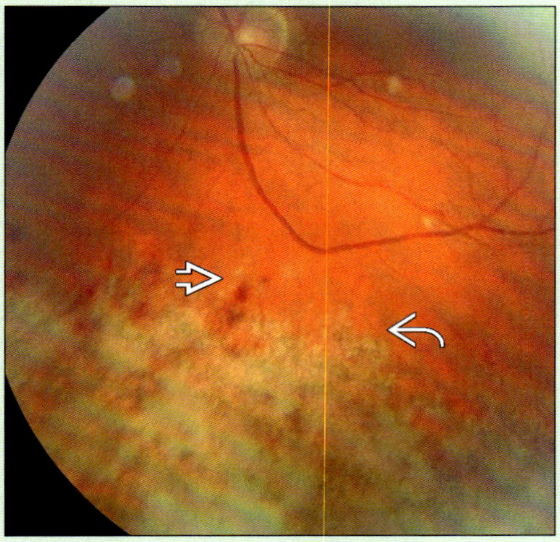
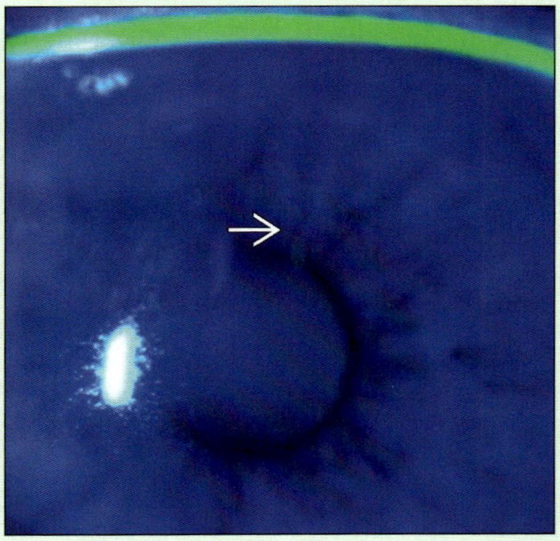

(Left) HIV patients are often infected by opportunistic bacterial, viral, and fungal pathogens. This fundus photograph shows Cytomegalovirus retinitis as evidenced by the granular opacifications ➔ and punctate hemorrhages ➔. (Right) Herpes zoster ophthalmicus (HZO) tends to afflict immunodeficient patients more severely than others. Infection may lead to conjunctivitis and epithelial keratitis. A pseudodendrite lesion ➔ is present in this fluorescein-stained eye.

HIV AND ASSOCIATED CONDITIONS

INTRODUCTION

Abbreviations
- Human immunodeficiency virus (HIV)
- Acquired immunodeficiency syndrome (AIDS)

DEMOGRAPHICS

Etiology/Risk Factors
- Most common risk factors: Unprotected sexual contact, IV drug use

Epidemiology
- In 2009, 1,148,200 persons 13 and older were living with HIV in USA alone

PRESENTATION

Symptoms
- Opportunistic infections and conditions
  - Cytomegalovirus (CMV) retinitis
  - Acute retinal necrosis (usually HSV or VZV)
  - Toxoplasma retinochoroiditis
  - Syphilitic chorioretinitis
  - *Pneumocystis jirovecii* choroiditis
  - *Cryptococcus neoformans* choroiditis
  - *Mycobacterium* (*M. tuberculosis* or *M. avium* complex) choroiditis and systemic dissemination
  - Kaposi sarcoma

Exam Findings
- Most common symptom (up to 70% of patients): HIV-related microangiopathy of retina (largely cotton-wool spots, which are nonspecific)
- Eyelid: Blepharitis, Kaposi sarcoma, multiple *Molluscum* lesions, herpes zoster ophthalmicus
- Orbit: Cellulitis
- Anterior segment
  - Conjunctival Kaposi sarcoma
  - Keratitis
  - Keratoconjunctivitis sicca
  - Anterior uveitis
- Posterior segment
  - Retinal microangiopathy
    - Retinal hemorrhages
    - Microaneurysms
    - Cotton-wool spots
    - Ischemic maculopathy (3% of patients)
  - HIV retinitis
  - Progressive outer retinal necrosis
    - Minimal anterior uveitis and vitreitis
    - Yellow-white retinal infiltrates
    - Retinal necrosis with macula being involved early
    - Late vitreal inflammation showing extensive retinal necrosis
  - Toxoplasmosis
  - Choroidal *Cryptococcus*; often there is vitreous involvement, disc edema
  - B-cell intraocular lymphoma
  - CMV retinitis most common opportunistic infection in AIDS patients

DIFFERENTIAL DIAGNOSIS

Drug-Induced Immunosuppression
- Review patient medications to determine long-term immunosuppressant use

New-Onset Systemic Lupus Erythematosus
- Distinguished by presence of antinuclear antibodies

EVALUATION/WORK-UP

Labs
- Serological testing for HIV should be done if suspicion based on 1 of the disease-defining illnesses or risky sexual history
  - Initially done with enzyme-linked immunosorbent assay (ELISA) screening test; if positive, secondary Western blot test required to make final diagnosis
- CD4(+) T-cell counts every 3 months with primary care physician

TREATMENT

Medical
- None specifically for eyes, but systemic antiviral treatment for HIV (e.g., highly active antiretroviral therapy [HAART]) that increases CD4 counts often improves eye symptoms
  - HAART regimen
    - 2 nucleoside reverse transcriptase inhibitors
    - 1 non-nucleoside reverse transcriptase inhibitor, 1 protease inhibitor, or 1 integrase inhibitor

Surgical
- None

Follow-Up
- Should be done every 3 months with patient's primary care physician to monitor antiviral drug regimen

Prognosis
- HIV is a chronic manageable disease; with appropriate therapy, patients can have normal life expectancy
  - HIV PCR viral load test determines amount of viral RNA within patient's plasma; high viral load is associated with worse prognosis
- Without treatment, HIV progresses to AIDS
  - AIDS average life expectancy: 3 years
  - HIV becomes AIDS when
    - CD4(+) cells/mm3 < 200
    - Patient diagnosed with AIDS-defining illness
    - CD4/CD8 ratio < 1.5

SELECTED REFERENCES

1. Centers for Disease Control and Prevention: Monitoring selected national HIV prevention and care objectives by using HIV surveillance data—United States and 6 U.S. dependent areas—2010. HIV Surveillance Supplemental Report 2012. 17(3), part A. http ://www.cdc.gov/hiv/topics/surveillance/resources/reports/. Published June 2012. Accessed August 12, 2013

RETINAL AND CHOROIDAL COMPLICATIONS OF TRAUMA

Key Facts

Introduction

- Commotio retinae (Berlin edema): Common occurrence following blunt injury
- Choroidal rupture: Tear in choroid, Bruch membrane, and retinal pigment epithelium (RPE) due to blunt or penetrating trauma
- Purtscher retinopathy: Bilateral retinal whitening and hemorrhage around optic discs associated with head and chest trauma

Presentation

- Commotio retinae: Whitening of retina
- Choroidal rupture: White crescent-shaped lesions situated concentrically from the optic nerve
- Purtscher retinopathy: Cotton-wool spots, Purtscher flecken, and retinal hemorrhage

Evaluation/Work-Up

- Commotio retinae: Photoreceptor outer segment disruption and damage to retinal pigment epithelium
- Purtscher retinopathy: Retinal arterioles and choroidal vessels show occluding material, positive for fibrin
- Choroidal rupture: Evaluate for possible associated choroidal neovascularization (CNV)

Treatment

- Commotio retinae: Mild cases have good prognosis with most patients recovering complete vision in ~ 6 weeks
- Purtscher retinopathy: Most show variable visual recovery without treatment within 1st few weeks
- Choroidal rupture: CNV may be treated with laser photocoagulation or intravitreal bevacizumab/ ranibizumab

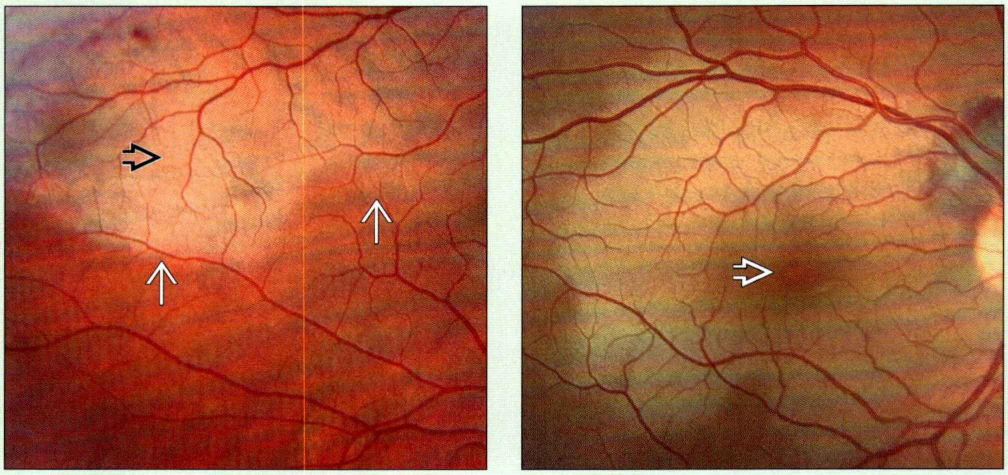

(Left) *This fundus photograph depicts commotio retinae involving the peripheral retina. The retina affected by the swelling appears gray. Also note the demarcation line between the healthy and swollen retina. The pathophysiology of commotio retinae is similar to that of a cerebral concussion.* ***(Right)*** *This fundus photograph shows commotio retinae involving the macula and the central portion of the retina. The macula remains markedly more red in color than the pale surrounding retina.*

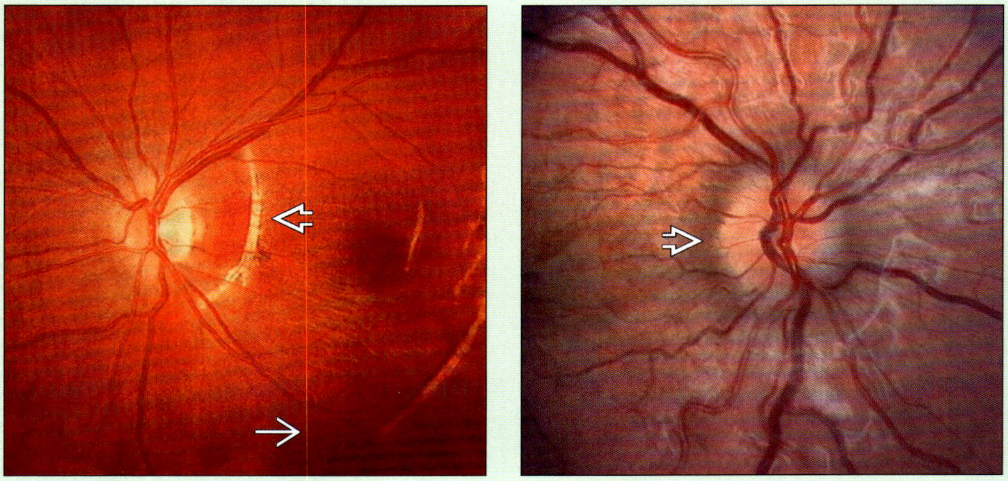

(Left) *This fundus photograph is an example of an eye after severe ocular trauma with resulting choroidal rupture. Note the subretinal blood that is a result of the disruption of the choroid, Bruch membrane, and retinal pigment epithelium (RPE).* ***(Right)*** *This fundus photograph shows Purtscher retinopathy with associated optic nerve edema. Purtscher retinopathy is particularly associated with head and chest trauma.*

RETINAL AND CHOROIDAL COMPLICATIONS OF TRAUMA

INTRODUCTION

Subtypes

- Commotio retinae (Berlin edema)
  - Acute vision loss
  - Disruption of photoreceptor layer and thinning of outer nuclear and plexiform layers
- Choroidal rupture
  - Tear in choroid, Bruch membrane, and retinal pigment epithelium (RPE) due to blunt or penetrating trauma
  - Sclera and retina are more resistant to rupture due to high tensile strength and elasticity, respectively
  - 5-10% of eyes develop choroidal neovascularization (CNV) that may cause delayed visual loss after rupture heals
- Purtscher retinopathy
  - Bilateral retinal whitening and hemorrhage around optic discs associated with head, chest, and long bone trauma
  - Medical causes include pancreatitis, systemic lupus erythematosus (SLE), thrombotic thrombocytopenic purpura, scleroderma, dermatomyositis, and chronic renal failure
  - Pathogenesis most likely involves embolic occlusion of precapillary arterioles

PRESENTATION

Exam Findings

- Commotio retinae
  - Acute vision loss
  - Whitening of retina
- Choroidal rupture
  - Visual loss is severe, especially if macula is involved
  - Fundus exam
    - White, crescent-shaped lesions situated concentrically from the optic nerve
  - Sclopetaria is combined retinal-choroid rupture (poor prognosis)
- Purtscher retinopathy
  - Bilateral or unilateral acute, painless loss of central vision
  - Fundus exam
    - Cotton-wool spots
    - Purtscher flecken
      - Located in peripapillary area and posterior pole
      - Areas of retinal whitening with typical polygonal shape
    - Retinal hemorrhage

DIFFERENTIAL DIAGNOSIS

Fat Embolism Syndrome

- Cotton-wool spots and small blot hemorrhages may occur anywhere in fundus
- Acutely, most patients are visually asymptomatic whereas Purtscher retinopathy patients are aware of visual problems

EVALUATION/WORK-UP

Pathology

- Commotio retinae
  - Photoreceptor outer segment disruption
  - Damage to retinal pigment epithelium
- Purtscher retinopathy
  - Retinal arterioles and choroidal vessels show occluding material, positive for fibrin

Imaging

- Commotio retinae
  - Spectral-domain optical coherence tomography (SD-OCT)
    - Mild injuries show hyperreflectivity underneath inner/outer segment junction
    - More severe injuries show a loss of inner/outer segment junction
- Choroidal rupture
  - CT scan and MRI to evaluate for further orbital trauma
  - Fluorescein angiography for possible CNV
- Purtscher retinopathy
  - Diagnosis is supported with fluorescein angiography, which shows blockage of choroidal fluorescence by retinal whitening

TREATMENT

Medical

- Purtscher retinopathy
  - Without treatment, majority of patients recover some visual function
  - Systemic steroids may improve visual outcome in some patients, but little evidence is available to support routine treatment

Surgical/Laser

- Choroidal rupture
  - CNV may be treated with laser photocoagulation or intravitreal bevacizumab/ranibizumab

Prognosis

- Commotio retinae
  - Mild cases have good prognosis with most patients recovering complete vision in ~ 6 weeks
  - More severe cases may include progressive pigmentary degeneration and macular hole formation
- Choroidal rupture
  - CNV typically occurs during the 1st year after trauma; if temporal rupture, observe macula closely and frequently
  - Schedule regular examinations to check for CNV during 1st year; if nasal rupture, then can stretch out longer as low probability of involving macula
- Purtscher retinopathy
  - Most show variable visual recovery without treatment within 1st few weeks
  - Initial extent of retinal vascular occlusion may influence visual prognosis

SELECTED REFERENCES

1. Agrawal A et al: Purtscher's and Purtscher-like retinopathies: a review. Surv Ophthalmol. 51(2):129-36, 2006

ANGIOID STREAKS

Key Facts

Introduction

- Fundus abnormality described as irregular blood vessel-like lines caused by breaks in Bruch membrane

Demographics

- Pseudoxanthoma elasticum (PXE) is most common systemic disease associated with angioid streaks
- Other causes: PEPSI (pseudoxanthoma elasticum, Ehlers-Danlos, Paget, sickle cell, idiopathic)
- Bruch membrane loses elasticity, and the stress put on the eye with intrinsic eye muscle movements causes cracks to develop

Presentation

- Most patients are asymptomatic
- If visual acuity (VA) is decreased, then it is most likely due to macular involvement, bleeding, or leakage
- Patients may complain of metamorphopsia when macula is involved
- Peripapillary ring from which irregularly radiating linear streaks spread out in all directions
- Typically, streaks taper and fade a few millimeters away from the optic disc but may continue further along the fundus

Evaluation/Work-Up

- Optical coherence tomography (OCT)
- Fluorescein angiography (FA)

Treatment

- Asymptomatic individuals with angioid streaks do not require treatment
- Photodynamic therapy and bevacizumab for choroidal neovascularization (CNV) treatment show initial VA stabilization but limited long-term benefit

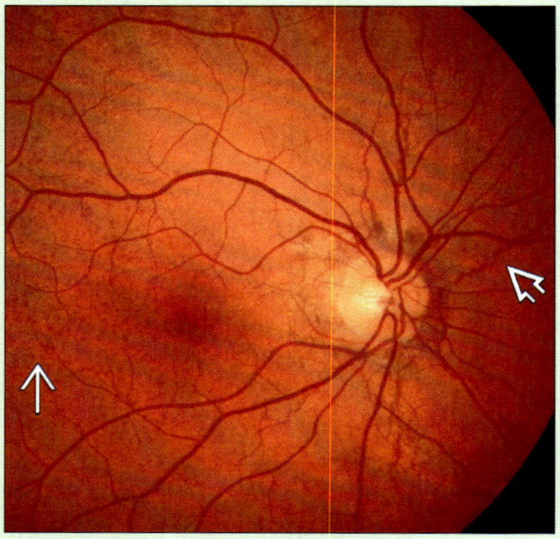

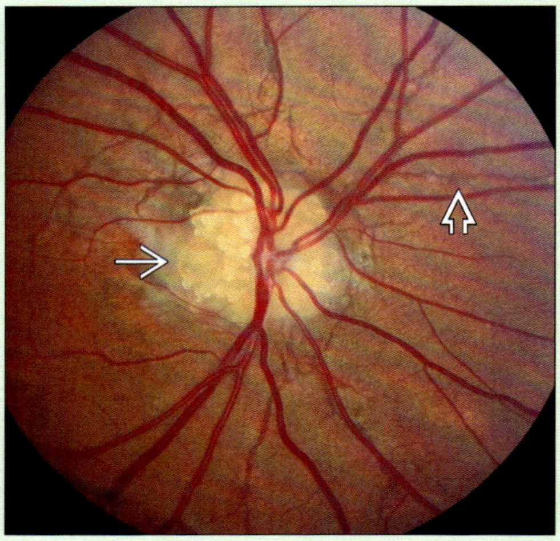

(Left) *Fundus photo shows angioid streaks ➡ as they extend outward from the optic disc. The patient also shows a peau d'orange texture ➡ to the temporal retina.* ***(Right)*** *Fundus photo shows a patient with angioid streaks ➡ and optic nerve head drusen ➡.*

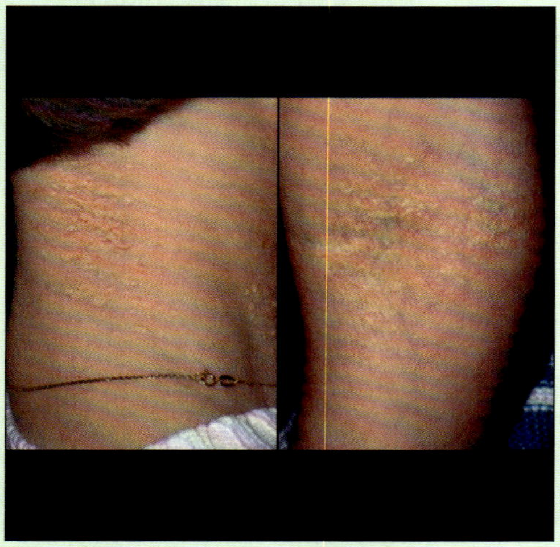

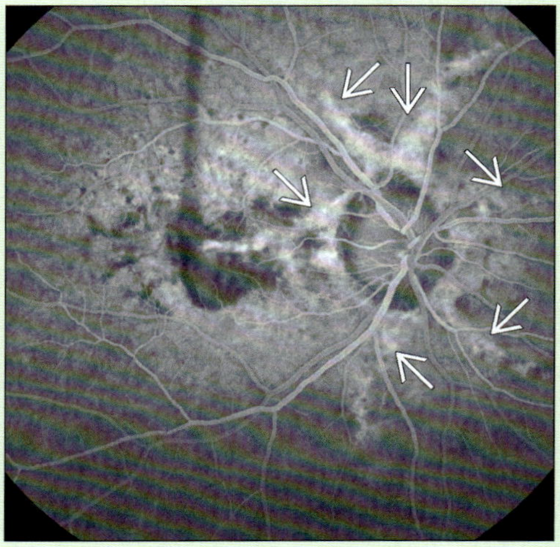

(Left) *External photo shows a patient with pseudoxanthoma elasticum on the neck and inside of the elbow. These areas are often described as "gooseflesh." These patients also have angioid streaks.* ***(Right)*** *Fluorescein angiography shows the angioid streaks as they stain with fluorescein ➡. The cracks in Bruch membrane can become opportune areas for choroidal neovascularization.*

ANGIOID STREAKS

INTRODUCTION

Definitions

- Fundus abnormality described as irregular blood vessel-like lines caused by breaks in Bruch membrane

DEMOGRAPHICS

Etiology/Risk Factors

- Systemic associations: PEPSI (pseudoxanthoma elasticum [PXE], Ehlers-Danlos, Paget, sickle cell, idiopathic)
  - PXE is most common systemic disease associated with angioid streaks
    - Autosomally inherited disorder associated with the accumulation of mineralized and fragmented elastic fibers in skin, Bruch membrane in retina, and vessel walls
  - Other, less common, systemic associations include diabetes, hemochromatosis, hypercalcinosis, lead poisoning, neurofibromatosis, Sturge-Weber syndrome, and tuberous sclerosis
- Pathogenesis
  - Bruch membrane loses elasticity, and the stress put on the eye with intrinsic eye muscle movements causes cracks to develop
  - PXE and Paget disease causes Bruch membrane to calcify and become brittle
  - Sickle hemoglobinopathies lead to iron deposition and may result in disturbance of elastin metabolism and structural deterioration of elastic fibers

Epidemiology

- Age at development depends on systemic disease involved

PRESENTATION

Symptoms

- Most patients are asymptomatic
- If visual acuity (VA) is decreased, then it is most likely due to macular involvement, bleeding, or leakage

Exam Findings

- Fundus exam
  - Peripapillary ring from which irregularly radiating linear streaks spread out in all directions
  - Typically occur bilaterally
  - Typically, streaks taper and fade a few millimeters away from optic disc but may continue further along the fundus
  - Angioid streak pigmentation depends on fundus pigmentation of individual
    - More pigment causes streaks to appear dark brown
    - Less pigment causes streaks to appear red
  - Some show a mottled retinal pigment epithelium (RPE) pigmentation referred to as peau d'orange or "skin of an orange"

DIFFERENTIAL DIAGNOSIS

Exudative Age-Related Macular Degeneration (ARMD)

- Patients experience a central scotoma that progresses over many years
- Fundus exam shows subretinal fluid, hemorrhage, or lipid deposits

Choroidal Rupture

- White curvilinear crescent-shaped streak concentric to the optic nerve
- History of blunt trauma

EVALUATION/WORK-UP

Pathology

- Basophilic staining from calcification of Bruch membrane
- Breaks in the membrane correspond to angioid streaks
- Choroidal neovascularization (CNV) penetrates the breaks; hemorrhage, exudation, and edema subsequently result

Imaging

- Fluorescein angiography (FA)
  - Angioid streaks show increased hyperfluorescence with thinning of RPE and an intact choriocapillaris
  - FA usually unnecessary for diagnosis but may be needed if fundus exam is unclear

TREATMENT

Medical

- Asymptomatic individuals with angioid streaks do not require treatment
- Trials using bevacizumab for individuals with CNV prove to have short-term benefits; however, after 1 year CNV recurred or developed in a new area

Surgical

- Photodynamic therapy may initially stabilize VA
  - Due to high recurrence rate and adverse effects on normal tissue, it provides no long-term visual benefit

Prognosis

- Untreated eyes with CNV generally have poor visual outcomes

SELECTED REFERENCES

1. Hu X et al: Pseudoxanthoma elasticum: a clinical, histopathological, and molecular update. Surv Ophthalmol. 48(4):424-38, 2003
2. Aessopos A et al: Elastic tissue abnormalities resembling pseudoxanthoma elasticum in beta thalassemia and the sickling syndromes. Blood. 99(1):30-5, 2002
3. Clarkson JG et al: Angioid streaks. Surv Ophthalmol. 26(5):235-46, 1982

BRANCH RETINAL ARTERY OCCLUSION

Key Facts

Demographics
- Embolus is most common cause
- Risk factors: Smoking, hypertension, hypercholesterolemia, diabetes, coronary artery or cerebrovascular disease, history of stroke or transient ischemic attack, hypercoagulable state
- 2.5x more likely in men than women
- 90% of cases involve temporal retinal arteries

Presentation
- Acute unilateral, painless, partial vision loss
- History of amaurosis fugax or neurologic loss due to previous episodes of emboli that quickly dislodge, allowing retinal reperfusion
- Partial visual field defect
- Intracellular edema → segmental whitening of retina along distribution of affected artery

Evaluation/Work-Up
- Erythrocyte sedimentation rate (ESR) in patients > 50 years to rule out giant cell arteritis
- Test for coagulopathies in patients < 50 years

Treatment
- No treatment with definitely proven benefit
- Antiplatelet therapy, hyperbaric oxygen, steroids, isovolemic hemodilution, intraarterial thrombolysis with recombinant tissue-type plasminogen activator, transluminal Nd:YAG laser embolysis
- 80-90% of patients will achieve visual acuity (VA) of 20/40 or better
- Usually, vision recovery occurs over 4-6 weeks
- Nonspecific visual field defects may persist based on occlusion location
- Retina begins to suffer irreversible damage after 97 minutes of complete occlusion to blood flow

*(**Left**) This fundus photo shows a typical cholesterol-emboli plaque ➡, a.k.a. Hollenhorst plaque, which appears as an iridescent, reflective, yellow plate dislodged in a retinal artery. Digital pressure on the eye can sometimes help the plaque dislodge, restoring blood flow. (**Right**) This fundus photo shows retinal whitening due to ischemia and edema following a branch retinal artery occlusion. Retinal whitening surrounds the area of distribution of the affected retinal artery branch ➡.*

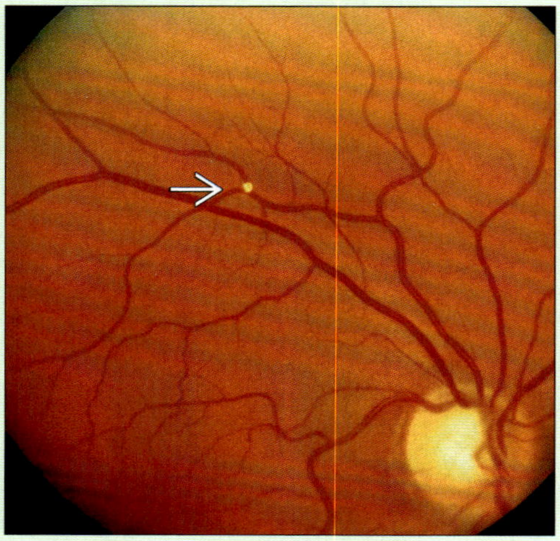

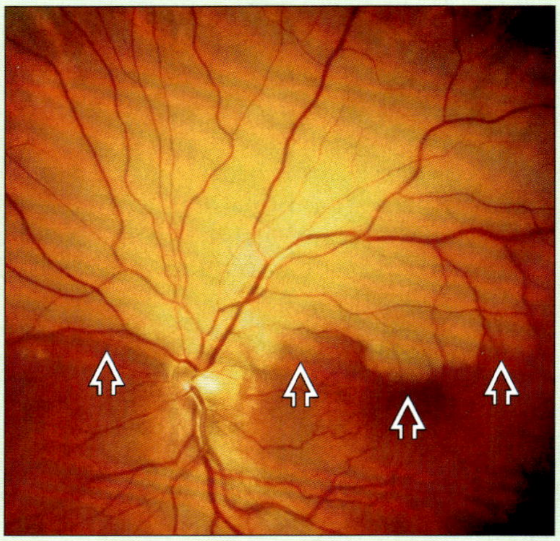

*(**Left**) This fundus photo shows a cholesterol emboli plate ➡ made up of rhomboid crystal. The thin size of these plates makes them translucent, and choroidal blood vessels laying behind these thin plates give them their yellow color. (**Right**) Fluorescein angiography shows poor circulation in a branch of the retinal artery ➡, represented by delayed filling of the retinal artery with fluorescein dye.*

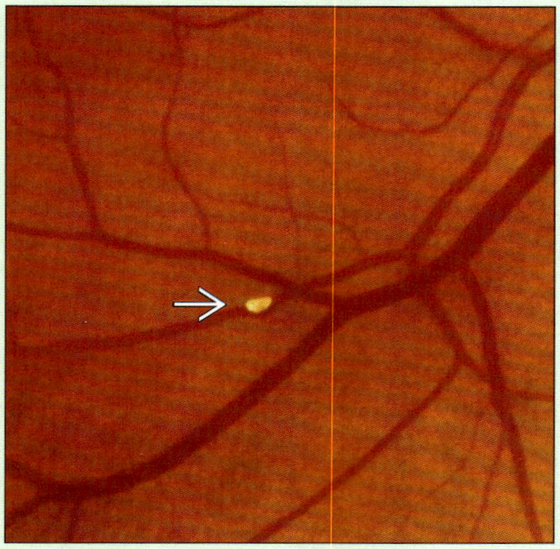

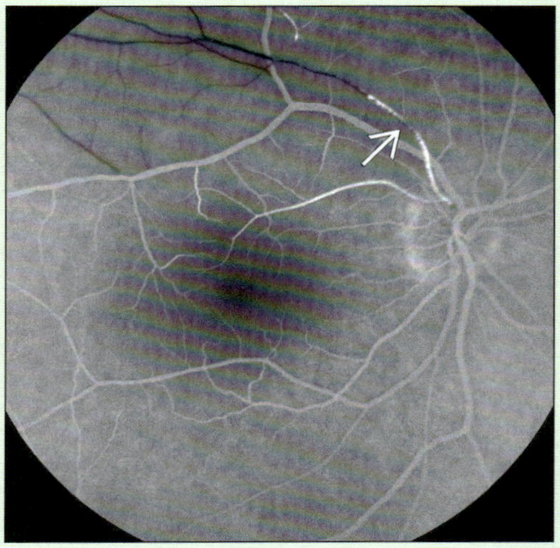

BRANCH RETINAL ARTERY OCCLUSION

INTRODUCTION

Abbreviations

- Branch retinal artery occlusion (BRAO)

Definitions

- Occurs when a branch of the central retinal artery becomes occluded, blocking blood flow to a section of retina

DEMOGRAPHICS

Etiology/Risk Factors

- Etiology
  - Embolus is most common cause
    - Cholesterol emboli from aorto-carotid atheromatous plaque
    - Platelet-fibrin emboli from thrombotic disease
    - Calcific emboli from cardiac valvular disease
      - 31% mitral valve
      - 28% aortic valve
      - 41% both valves
    - Exogenous or endogenous emboli
    - Other rare embolic causes: Leukoemboli, amniotic fluid emboli, fat emboli, air emboli, tumors, talc
  - Nonembolic causes are rare
    - Thrombosis, inflammation, vasospasm, coagulopathy, autothrombosis, compression
- Risk factors
  - Smoking
  - Hypertension, hypercholesterolemia, diabetes
  - Coronary artery disease or cerebrovascular disease
  - History of stroke or transient ischemic attack
  - Hypercoagulable state
    - Endocarditis, carotid stenosis, coagulopathies, atrial fibrillation

Epidemiology

- 2.5x more likely in men than women
- Similar incidence of BRAO between black and white patients
  - Whites were found more likely to have identifiable carotid artery disease than blacks
- Seen in 7th decade
  - Rare in patients < 30 years
- 90% of cases involve temporal retinal arteries
  - Either due to true increased incidence or undetection of nasal retinal vessel occlusions
- Occurs most commonly at arterial bifurcation site
- Makes up 38% of all retinal arterial occlusion cases
  - Central retinal artery occlusion (CRAO) (58%), cilioretinal artery occlusion (5%)

PRESENTATION

Symptoms

- Acute unilateral, painless, partial vision loss
- Patients may be asymptomatic
- History of amaurosis fugax or neurologic loss
  - Due to previous episodes of emboli that quickly dislodge, allowing retinal reperfusion

Exam Findings

- Partial visual field defect
- Segmental whitening of retina along distribution of affected artery
  - Due to intracellular edema
- Attenuation and boxcarring of blood column in occluded artery
- Narrowed branched retinal artery
- Emboli
  - Visualized in 62% of eyes with BRAO
  - Cholesterol emboli (Hollenhorst plaque)
    - Iridescent, reflective, thin yellow plate
    - Plates made up of rhomboid crystal
    - Thin size makes them translucent and allows blood to show through, giving plate its yellow color
    - Digital pressure on eye by examiner may reposition emboli within artery, allowing for better visualization
  - Platelet-fibrin emboli
    - White-gray, nonreflective, mobile
    - Often appears as multiple blockages arranged linearly within artery lumen
    - May pass through artery without causing occlusion
    - Associated with mural thrombus in carotid artery and cardiac valvular disease
  - Calcific emboli
    - Large, yellow-white, nonreflective plaque
    - Seen in larger arteries near optic disc
    - Associated with calcified cardiac valves and carotid artery atheromas

DIFFERENTIAL DIAGNOSIS

Central Retinal Artery Occlusion

- Sudden, massive loss of vision
- White, ischemic retina with cherry-red spot over macula
- Absent or poor retinal circulation on fluorescein angiography
- Caused by embolism, thrombosis, ↓ in mean arterial blood pressure below retinal perfusion pressure, ↑ in intraocular pressure > mean blood pressure, vasospasm of central retinal artery

Giant Cell Arteritis

- Systemic inflammatory vasculitis affecting temporal arteries
- Seen in patients age ≥ 50 years and associated with polymyalgia rheumatica
- Sudden, painless vision loss in 10% of cases
- ± headache, scalp pain, jaw claudication, pain with chewing, ear pain
- ↑ in C-reactive protein and erythrocyte sedimentation rate (ESR)

EVALUATION/WORK-UP

Labs

- ESR in patients > 50 years
- Test for coagulopathies in patients < 50 years
  - Antitreponemal antibody
  - Antiphospholipid antibody
  - Antinuclear antibody
  - Rheumatoid factor
  - Serum protein electrophoresis

BRANCH RETINAL ARTERY OCCLUSION

  - Hemoglobin electrophoresis
  - Prothrombin time/activated partial thromboplastin time (PT/aPTT)
  - Fibrinogen
  - Proteins C and S
  - Antithrombin III
  - Factor V Leiden
  - Homocysteine
- CBC to detect anemia, polycythemia, and platelet disorders
- Fasting blood sugar, glycosylated hemoglobin, cholesterol, triglycerides, lipid panel to asses atherosclerotic disease
- Blood cultures to evaluate for bacterial endocarditis and septic emboli

Imaging

- Fluorescein angiography
  - No or delayed filling and hypofluorescence in area of distribution of affected artery
  - Retrograde filling in arteries distal to site of obstruction
  - Late staining of artery walls at site of embolus, even if it has moved away
  - Platelet embolus may be seen
  - Artery-artery collaterals suggest old BRAO
- Red-free fundus photograph shows retinal whitening, representing ischemia in areas surrounding occluded artery
- Optical coherence tomography
  - Retinal thickening due to intracellular edema
  - ↑ reflectivity of inner retinal layers and ↓ reflectivity of photoreceptors and retinal pigment epithelium (RPE)
- Humphrey visual field testing to monitor recovery
- Electroretinogram is not helpful or recommended

Medical Work-Up

- All patients should receive a work-up to detect source of embolism
  - All patients ≥ 50 years must rule out giant cell arteritis
  - Echocardiography in elderly patients
    - Rheumatic heart disease, mitral valve prolapse, prosthetic valve, bacterial endocarditis, recent myocardial infarction/ischemia, injection drug use, valvular disease, atrial fibrillation
  - Evaluation for carotid artery disease and cerebrovascular disease
    - Carotid Doppler/angiography
      - Retinal occlusion is due to microemboli, and absence of significant carotid artery stenosis does not necessarily rule out carotid artery as a source of microembolism

TREATMENT

Medical

- Currently, there is no treatment with definitely proven benefit
- Antiplatelet therapy to prevent stroke
  - Aspirin, clopidogrel, warfarin, dipyridamole, ticlopidine
- Hyperbaric oxygen, systemic steroids, isovolumic hemodilution

Surgical

- Intraarterial thrombolysis with recombinant tissue-type plasminogen activator studied in CRAO and BRAO with varying success
- Transluminal Nd:YAG laser embolysis
  - Effective if performed within 2-3 hours of onset
  - Nd:YAG laser shatters embolus without damaging artery wall
  - Risk of retinal tear/detachment, vitreous and retinal hemorrhages, choroidal neovascularization, and epiretinal membrane formation
- Neovascularization following BRAO is rare but should be treated with sector/grid photocoagulation if it develops
  - Seen in patients with diabetes mellitus and can progress to neovascular glaucoma

Follow-Up

- Every 3-6 months to monitor progression

Prognosis

- 80-90% of patients will achieve visual acuity (VA) of 20/40 or better
  - 1 study showed that VA of 20/40 or better was seen in 74% of patients with permanent BRAO and 94% with BRAO at presentation and in 89% and 100%, respectively, at follow-up
- Vision recovery occurs over 4-6 weeks
- Nonspecific visual field defects may persist based on occlusion location
- Affected retina begins to suffer irreversible damage after 97 minutes of complete occlusion to blood flow
  - ≥ 4 hours → massive irreversible retinal damage
- Morbidity/mortality
  - 15% of patients with retinal emboli died within 1 year
    - 54% have 7-year mortality
  - ↑ risk of stroke
    - 10x ↑ in annual rate of stroke in patients with retinal emboli
    - 3x ↑ in 8-year mortality from stroke in patients with retinal emboli vs. those without emboli

SELECTED REFERENCES

1. Hayreh SS: Acute retinal arterial occlusive disorders. Prog Retin Eye Res. 30(5):359-94, 2011
2. Hayreh SS et al: Branch retinal artery occlusion: natural history of visual outcome. Ophthalmology. 116(6):1188-94, 2009
3. Hayreh SS et al: Retinal artery occlusion: associated systemic and ophthalmic abnormalities. Ophthalmology. 116(10):1928-36, 2009
4. Lim JY et al: Treatment of branch retinal artery occlusion with transluminal Nd:YAG laser embolysis. Korean J Ophthalmol. 23(4):315-7, 2009

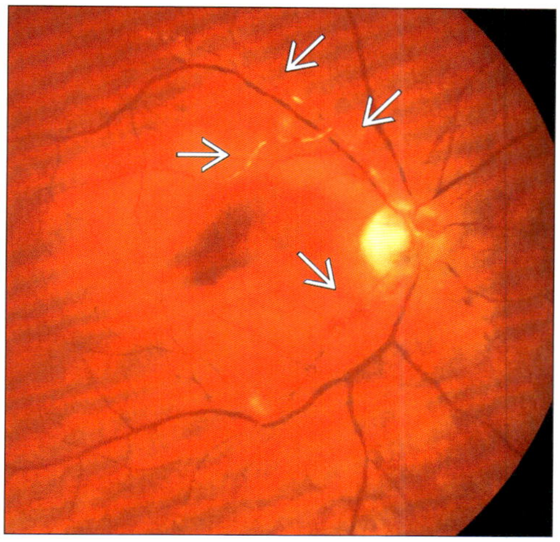

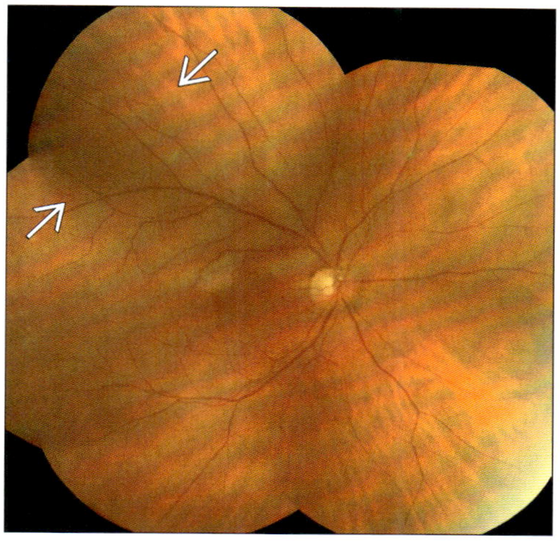

(Left) *This fundus photo shows platelet-fibrin emboli ➔ in the branches of the central retinal artery. These emboli create white-gray blockages that are mobile and often appear in "showers" that may pass through the blood vessel without causing an occlusion. They are most commonly associated with a mural thrombus in the carotid artery or cardiac valvular disease.* ***(Right)*** *This fundus photograph shows edema of the retina that results from branch retinal artery occlusion ➔.*

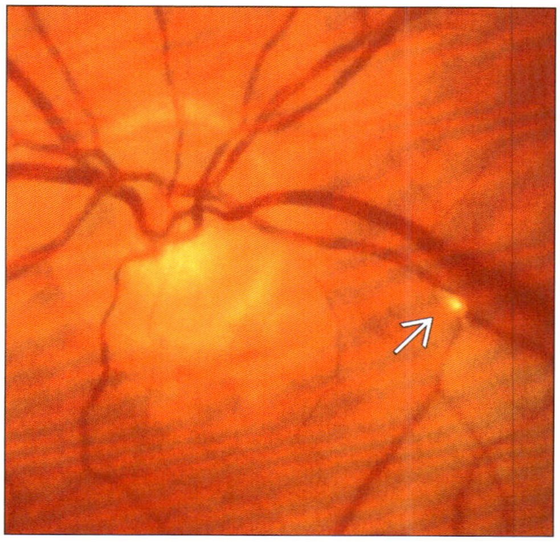

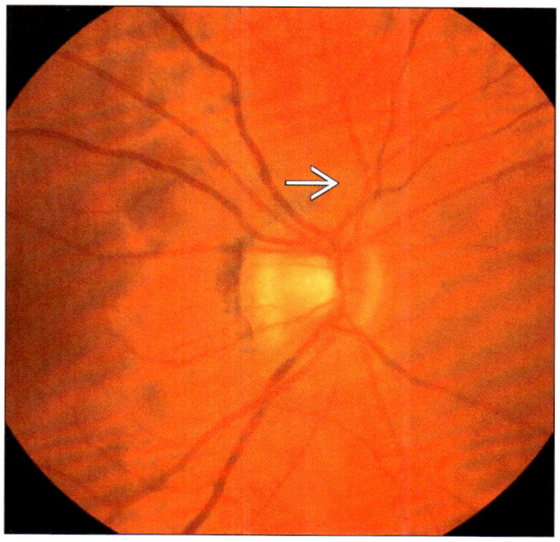

(Left) *This fundus photo shows a calcific retinal embolus ➔ in a retinal artery branch. Calcific emboli are large, yellow-white, nonreflective plaques. They are most commonly associated with calcified cardiac valves and atheromatous plaques of the carotid artery. A work-up is indicated even in asymptomatic patients; 15% of patients with retinal emboli die within 1 year.* ***(Right)*** *This fundus photograph shows a Hollenhorst plaque occluding a branch of the retinal artery ➔.*

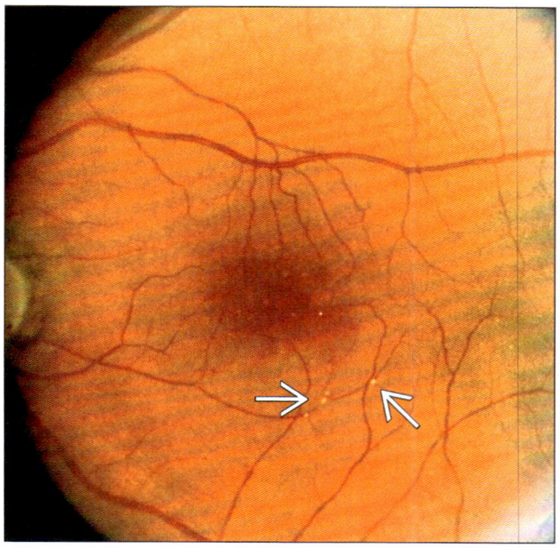

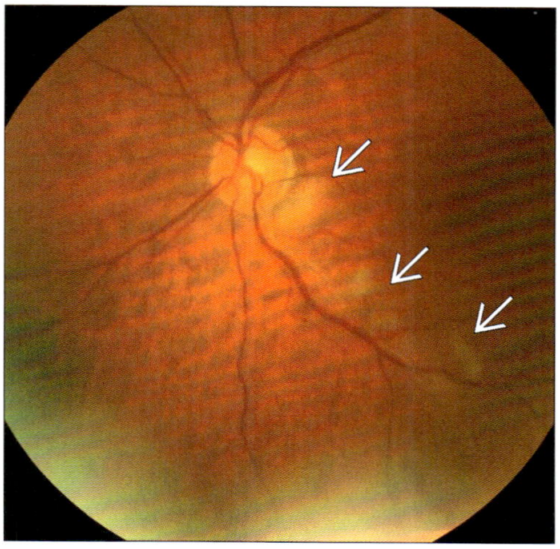

(Left) *This fundus photo demonstrates many cholesterol emboli ➔ lodged in the distal branches of the retinal artery. Small emboli in bifurcation points along the retinal artery can cause transient vision loss known as amaurosis fugax. Vision later recovers after the emboli dislodge, allowing for retinal reperfusion.* ***(Right)*** *This fundus photograph shows ischemia ➔ of the retina due to the occluded retinal artery. The ischemic retina appears pale and obscures view of the choroidal vasculature.*

BRANCH RETINAL VEIN OCCLUSION

Key Facts

Introduction

- Occlusion of either a major branch retinal vein draining a retinal quadrant, a macular branch vein draining a portion of the macula, or a peripheral branch vein draining a portion of the retinal periphery

Demographics

- Occlusions almost always occur at a site where artery crosses anteriorly over a vein
- Compression of vein creates turbulent blood flow, damage to endothelium, and subsequent thrombus formation
- Increased pressure induces leakage of blood and small molecules from the vasculature into retinal tissue, leading to edema
- Risk factors: Age, hypertension, arteriosclerosis, diabetes mellitus, dyslipidemia, high body mass index, smoking

Presentation

- Painless blurred vision corresponding to involved quadrant
- Subjects may be asymptomatic, for example, if nasal retinal quadrant is affected
- Fundus exam: Dilated tortuous veins, flame-shaped hemorrhages, cotton-wool spots, macular edema

Evaluation/Work-Up

- Fluorescein angiography (FA): Adjunct to determine if vision loss is due to macular edema or ischemia

Treatment

- Intravitreal corticosteroid
- Bevacizumab and ranibizumab
- Grid-pattern laser photocoagulation for cystoid macular edema (CME) and vision at 20/40 or worse
- Sector scatter retinal laser photocoagulation for neovascularization elsewhere (NVE)

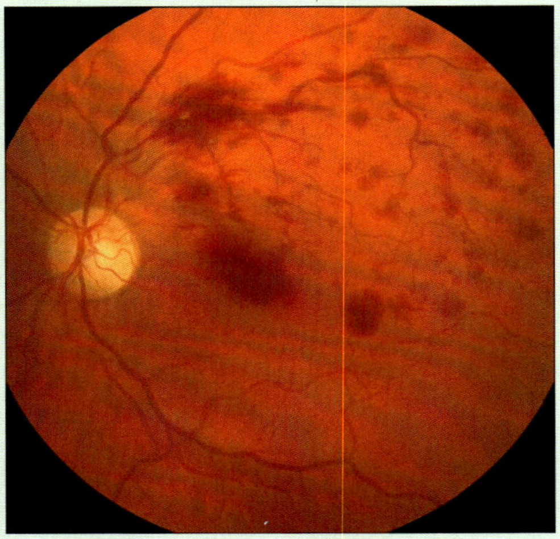

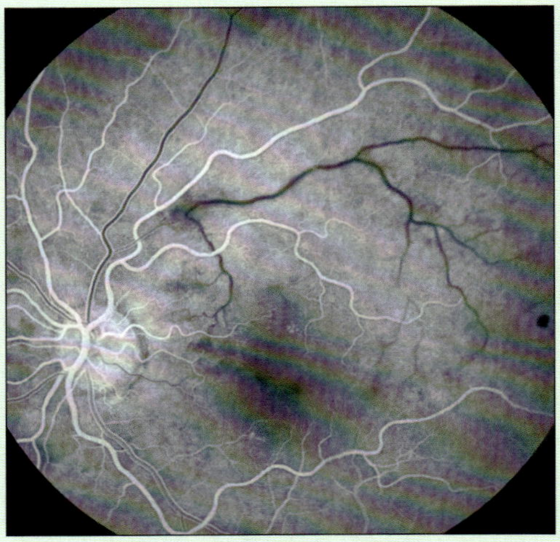

(Left) *Fundus photo shows a branch retinal vein occlusion in the superior temporal left eye. Scattered intraretinal hemorrhages are seen.* ***(Right)*** *Fluorescein angiography of the same eye shows a significant delay in draining of the superior temporal venule. Vascular tortuosity is visible.*

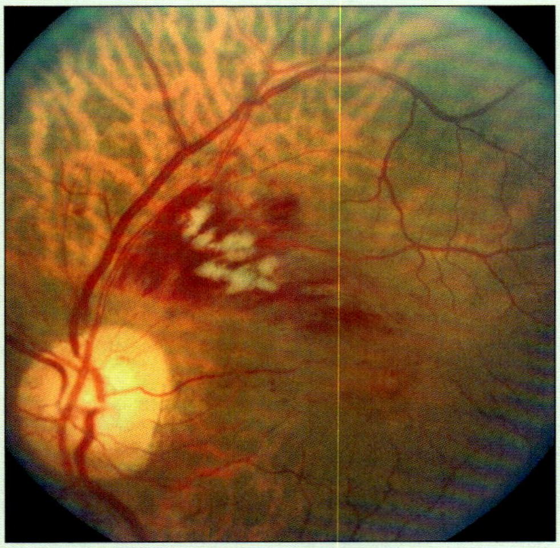

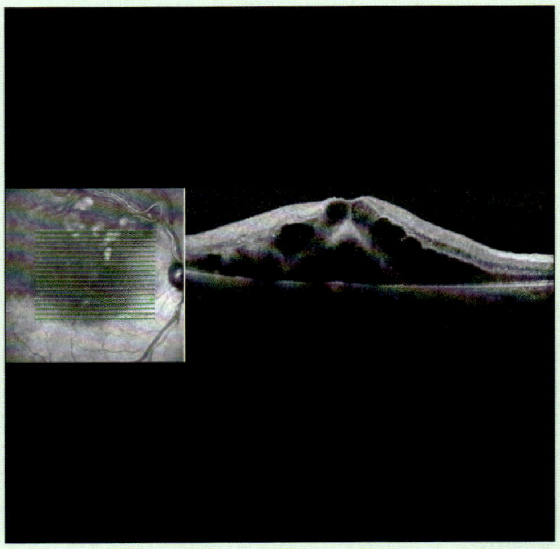

(Left) *Fundus photo shows a wedge pattern of dot-and-blot hemorrhages from a superior temporal branch retinal vein occlusion. Cotton-wool spots are present in the area of hemorrhage.* ***(Right)*** *Optical coherence tomography (OCT) shows a cystoid macular edema, suggesting that the branch retinal vein occlusion has involved vessels in the macula. If this is persistent and affects vision, consider grid laser.*

BRANCH RETINAL VEIN OCCLUSION

INTRODUCTION

Abbreviations
- Branch retinal vein occlusion (BRVO)

Definitions
- Occlusion of either a major branch retinal vein draining a retinal quadrant, a macular branch vein draining a portion of the macula, or a peripheral branch vein draining a portion of the retinal periphery

DEMOGRAPHICS

Etiology/Risk Factors
- Pathogenesis
  - Occlusions almost always occur at a site where artery crosses anteriorly over a vein
  - Arteriosclerosis in the artery causes mechanical obstruction and compression of the posterior vein
  - Compression of vein creates turbulent blood flow, damage to the endothelium, and subsequent thrombus formation
  - Increased pressure induces leakage of blood and small molecules from vasculature into retinal tissue, leading to edema
  - Vascular endothelial damage induces a release of inflammatory factors such as prostaglandins, leukotrienes, and vascular endothelial growth factor (VEGF), causing leaky vessels and neovascularization
- Risk factors
  - Age: Typical onset is > 65 years; however, may be earlier
  - Hypertension, arteriosclerosis, diabetes mellitus, dyslipidemia, high body mass index, smoking, vasculitis, polycythemia rubra vera, and multiple myeloma

Epidemiology
- ~ 0.6-1.1% prevalence in population, and 1.8% incidence
- No predilections to gender or race

PRESENTATION

Symptoms
- Painless blurred vision corresponding to involved quadrant
- Visual acuity (VA) may range from 20/20 vision to counting fingers

Exam Findings
- Fundus exam
  - Dilated tortuous veins
  - Flame-shaped hemorrhages
  - Cotton-wool spots: Caused by complete obstruction
  - Macular edema (if vessels supplying the macular are involved)
  - Retinal hemorrhages confined to distribution of occluded retinal vein
  - Late findings include cystoid macular edema (CME), atrophy of retinal pigment epithelium, and neovascularization

DIFFERENTIAL DIAGNOSIS

Central Retinal Vein Occlusion
- Involves all 4 quadrants of retina
- Occlusion occurs at level of, or posterior to, lamina cribrosa

Diabetic Retinopathy
- Progressive loss of visual acuity
- Microaneurysms, flame-shaped hemorrhages, cotton-wool spots, macular edema, and neovascularization

Hypertensive Retinopathy
- Arteriovenous nicking, retinal artery narrowing, microaneurysm, and venous tortuosity

EVALUATION/WORK-UP

Imaging
- Fluorescein angiography (FA)
  - Adjunct to determine if vision loss is due to macular edema or ischemia
- Hypervascularity work-up if young age without risk factors

TREATMENT

Medical
- Intravitreal corticosteroid
  - Triamcinolone injection or sustained-release dexamethasone
  - Side effects include increased intraocular pressure and cataract formation
- Intravitreal anti-VEGF
  - Bevacizumab and ranibizumab
  - Prevents neovascularization and development of CME

Surgical
- Grid-pattern laser photocoagulation
  - Consider in eyes with continued decreased VA at 3 months due to perfused CME
  - Not recommended for extensive intraretinal hemorrhage or in eyes with ischemic edema
- Sector scatter retinal laser photocoagulation
  - Reduces neovascularization elsewhere (NVE)
- Sheathotomy at sites of arteriovenous crossing proximal to occlusion may be useful

Prognosis
- Untreated subjects have a mean VA of ~ 20/70 after 3 years
- Subjects have a 10% risk of any RVO in the contralateral eye within 3 years following initial event

SELECTED REFERENCES

1. Ehlers JP et al: Retinal vein occlusion: beyond the acute event. Surv Ophthalmol. 56(4):281-99, 2011
2. Rehak M et al: Retinal vein thrombosis: pathogenesis and management. J Thromb Haemost. 8(9):1886-94, 2010
3. Argon laser scatter photocoagulation for prevention of neovascularization and vitreous hemorrhage in branch vein occlusion: A randomized clinical trial. Branch Vein Occlusion Study Group. Arch Ophthalmol. 104(1):34-41, 1986

CENTRAL RETINAL ARTERY OCCLUSION

Key Facts

Introduction

- Central retinal artery occlusion (CRAO): Ocular emergency caused by a sudden event in which blood supply to inner part of retina is blocked, resulting in significant vision loss
- Nonarteritic CRAO: Classic CRAO with infarction, poor retinal circulation, and no evidence of giant cell arteritis (GCA)
- Nonarteritic CRAO with cilioretinal artery sparing: Visual outcome different with collateral circulation
- Arteritic CRAO: Caused by GCA and usually associated with CRA and posterior ciliary artery (PCA) occlusion
- Transient nonarteritic CRAO: Due to transient embolus, blood pressure differences, or vasospasms

Demographics

- Most obstructions are caused by either thrombosis or embolus
- Age of occurrence: Ranges from mid 20s to 90s with mean age occurring in mid 60s

Presentation

- Sudden, painless, unilateral loss of vision
- Significant loss in visual acuity (VA), relative afferent pupillary defect (RAPD)
- Fundus exam: Retinal opacity, cherry-red spot, boxcarring of retinal vessels

Evaluation/Work-Up

- Erythrocyte sedimentation rate (ESR) and C-reactive protein; in all patients ≥ 50 years, GCA needs to be ruled out
- Fluorescein angiography (FA): Aids in diagnosis and helps distinguish between 4 subtypes of CRAO

Treatment

- Currently, there is no treatment proven to be effective

__(Left)__ This fundus photograph from a patient with central retinal artery occlusion (CRAO) demonstrates a cherry-red spot in the center of the macula ➡ due to intact retina epithelium and choroid colors in the foveola. __(Right)__ This fundus photograph from a patient with CRAO demonstrates edema of the retina as well as pallor.

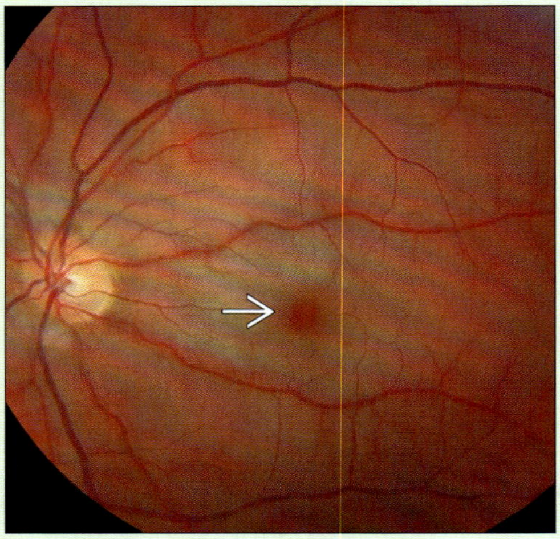

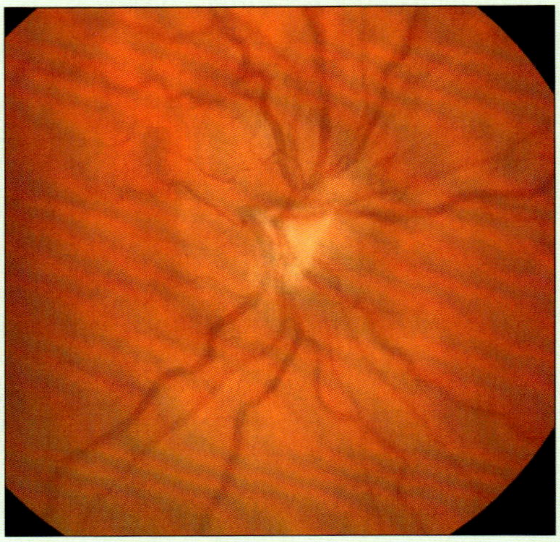

__(Left)__ This fundus photograph of another patient with CRAO shows attenuation, or narrowing, of the retinal vessels ➡. __(Right)__ This fundus photograph of a patient with central retinal artery occlusion demonstrates boxcarring, or segmentation of the blood column ➡, which can occur 4-6 weeks after the initial retinal swelling has resolved.

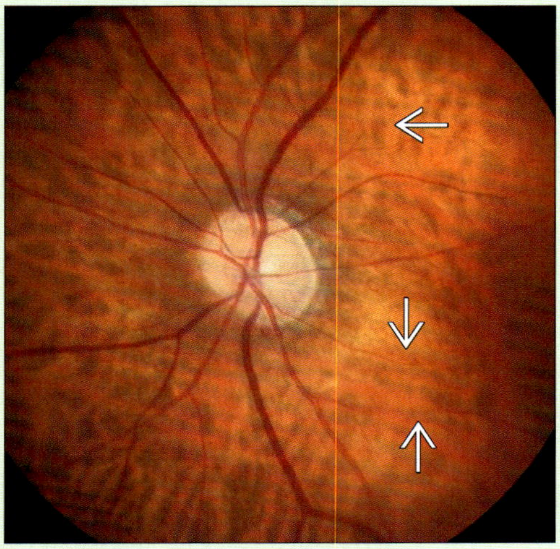

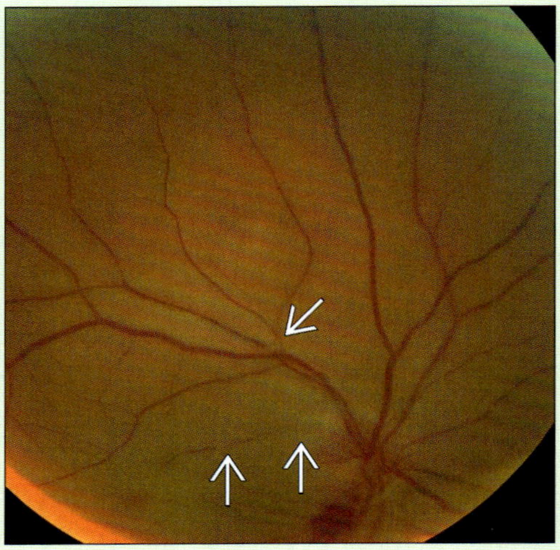

CENTRAL RETINAL ARTERY OCCLUSION

INTRODUCTION

Abbreviations

- Central retinal artery occlusion (CRAO)

Definitions

- Ocular emergency caused by a sudden event in which blood supply to inner part of retina is blocked, resulting in significant vision loss
- Cilioretinal artery: Arises from posterior ciliary artery (PCA) and provides collateral circulation to the retina in ~ 19% of the population

Subtypes

- Nonarteritic CRAO: Classic CRAO with infarction, poor retinal circulation, and no evidence of giant cell arteritis (GCA)
- Nonarteritic CRAO with cilioretinal artery sparing: Visual outcome different with collateral circulation
- Arteritic CRAO: Caused by GCA and usually associated with CRA and PCA occlusion
- Transient nonarteritic CRAO: Due to transient embolus, blood pressure differences, or vasospasms

DEMOGRAPHICS

Etiology/Risk Factors

- Etiology
  - Most obstructions are caused by either thrombosis or embolus
  - Embolic sources: Plaques in carotid arteries, carotid or coronary stenting or angiography, atrial fibrillation, mitral or aortic valve masses, bacterial endocarditis, atrial myxoma, and Takayasu arteritis
  - Other causes: Polyarteritis nodosa, granulomatosis with polyangiitis, GCA, Churg-Strauss syndrome, Behçet disease, sarcoidosis, sickle cell disease, carotid artery dissection, and oral contraceptives
- Risk factors: Atherosclerosis, valvular disease, arrhythmias, hypercoagulopathy, cancer, vasculitis, local trauma, pancreatitis, migraine, pregnancy, cocaine abuse, intravenous drug use

Epidemiology

- Age of occurrence: Ranges from mid 20s to 90s with mean age occurring in mid 60s
- Bilateral involvement in 1-2% of cases

PRESENTATION

Symptoms

- Sudden, painless loss of vision
- Usually unilateral, rarely bilateral
- Significant loss in visual acuity (VA)
- Amaurosis fugax precedes visual loss in ~ 10% of patients

Exam Findings

- Patients typically present with relative afferent pupillary defect (RAPD)
- Fundus exam
  - Early findings
    - Retinal opacity mainly in posterior pole (where ganglion cell concentration is highest)
    - Cherry-red spot
    - Boxcarring of retinal vessels
      - Segmented or interrupted columns of blood
    - Retinal arterial attenuation
    - Optic disc edema and pallor
  - Late findings
    - Optic atrophy
    - Retinal arterial attenuation
    - Macular retinal pigment epithelial changes

DIFFERENTIAL DIAGNOSIS

Branch Retinal Artery Occlusion

- Similar etiology; however, only a portion of retina affected

Commotio Retinae

- Widespread or localized whitening of retina

Purtscher Retinopathy

- Retinal white ischemic infarcts associated with traumatic angiopathy

EVALUATION/WORK-UP

Labs

- Erythrocyte sedimentation rate (ESR) and C-reactive protein; in all patients ≥ 50 years, GCA needs to be ruled out

Imaging

- Fluorescein angiography (FA)
  - Aids in diagnosis and helps distinguish between 4 subtypes of CRAO
- Carotid Doppler: Look for plaques &/or stenosis
- Echocardiogram: Detects cardiac abnormalities and sources for emboli

TREATMENT

Medical

- Currently, there is no treatment proven to be effective
- Some attempted conventional treatments include decreasing intraocular pressure by ocular massage, timolol, or acetazolamide; vasodilation with isosorbide dinitrate or rebreathing carbogen (80% oxygen and 20% CO_2); antiplatelet or heparin therapy
  - Some studies show that intraarterial thrombolytics within 3 or 6 hours may be of benefit, but other studies have found no benefit
- GCA should be treated immediately with high-dose steroids

Prognosis

- Irreversible damage to retina happens ~ 4 hours after occlusion
- VA improvement typically happens in first 7 days after occlusion
- Level of improvement or permanent vision loss depends on time of occlusion and subtype of CRAO

SELECTED REFERENCES

1. Hayreh SS: Acute retinal arterial occlusive disorders. Prog Retin Eye Res. 30(5):359-94, 2011

CENTRAL RETINAL VEIN OCCLUSION

Key Facts

Demographics

- Risk factors: Age, hypertension, diabetes, glaucoma, hypercoagulable state
- Prevalence of 0.1% in United States
- Highest prevalence in adults > age 80
- Usually associated with primary thrombus formation in central retinal vein

Presentation

- Sudden unilateral vision loss
- Painless
- Retinal hemorrhage
  - Scattered and diffuse throughout retina
  - Blood-and-thunder appearance of retina on funduscopy
- Retinal edema
- Dilated retinal veins
- May see cotton-wool spots
- May see ipsilateral relative afferent pupillary defect
- Neovascularization of iris is a very poor prognostic sign and requires urgent intervention

Evaluation/Work-Up

- Fluorescein angiogram
  - Confirms diagnosis
- Optical coherence tomography (OCT)
  - Quantifies retinal thickening due to intraretinal macular edema

Treatment

- Observation should be used in those without macular edema or neovascularization of iris
- Vascular endothelial growth factor inhibitors
- Intravitreal glucocorticoids
- Antithrombotic and thrombolytic therapy
- Isovolemic hemodilution
- Laser photocoagulation
- Prognosis depends on visual acuity at presentation

*(**Left**) This fundus photograph exhibits the characteristic blood-and-thunder appearance of retinal hemorrhage in a patient with central retinal vein occlusion (CRVO). The hemorrhage is diffuse and scattered throughout all 4 quadrants. (**Right**) This image highlights the dilated and tortuous veins that can be seen on funduscopic examination of a patient with CRVO ➡. Physical exam may also show an ipsilateral relative afferent pupillary defect.*

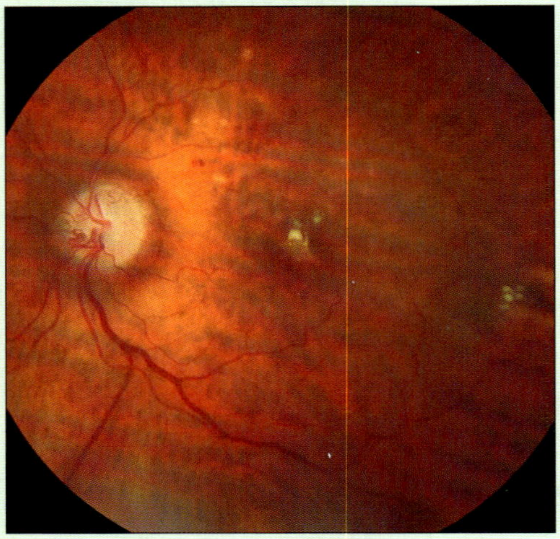

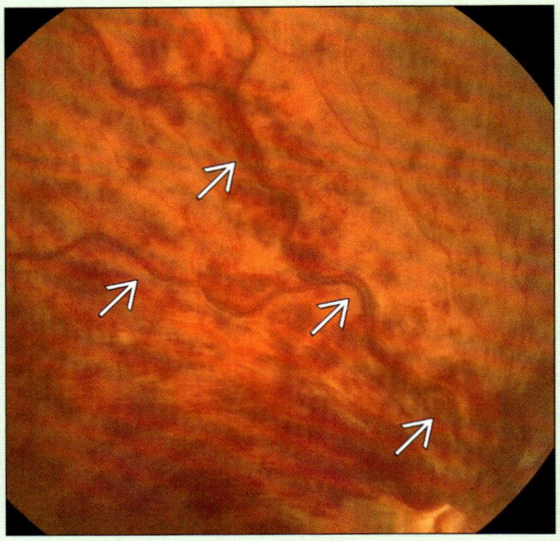

*(**Left**) Note the engorged, tortuous veins ➡ and cotton-wool spots ➡ present in this funduscopic photograph of a patient with CRVO. Cotton-wool spots indicate retinal ischemia. It is important to examine the iris of patients with CRVO because neovascularization of the iris suggests retinal ischemia. (**Right**) Note the macular edema ➡, which can be present on funduscopic examination of patients with CRVO. Macular edema is the most common cause of vision loss in these patients.*

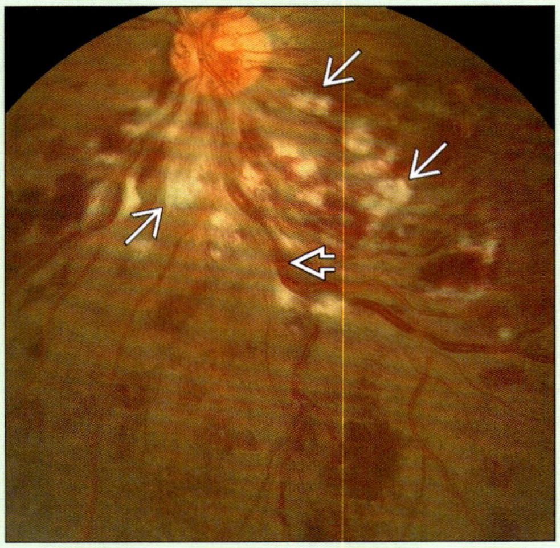

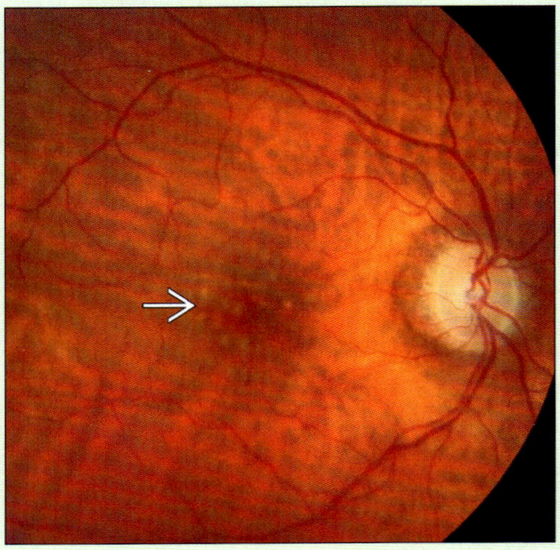

CENTRAL RETINAL VEIN OCCLUSION

INTRODUCTION

Abbreviations
- Central retinal vein occlusion (CRVO)

Definitions
- Occurs at lamina cribrosa of optic nerve
- Affects entire retina

Subtypes
- Perfused CRVO
  - < 10 disc areas (surface area of optic nerve head) of capillary nonperfusion
- Nonperfused CRVO
  - ≥ 10 disc areas of capillary nonperfusion
- Indeterminate

DEMOGRAPHICS

Etiology/Risk Factors
- Age
- Hypertension
- African American race
- Diabetes
- Smoking
- Glaucoma
- Hypercoagulable state
  - Factor V Leiden mutation
  - Deficiency in protein C or S
  - Presence of antiphospholipid antibodies
  - Antithrombin III
  - Homocysteine

Epidemiology
- Prevalence of 0.1% in United States
- Highest prevalence is in patients > age 80
- 81% of patients with CRVO have perfused CRVO

PRESENTATION

Symptoms
- Sudden unilateral vision loss, painless

Exam Findings
- Usually associated with primary thrombus formation in the central retinal vein
- Retinal hemorrhage
  - Scattered and diffuse in all 4 quadrants
  - Blood-and-thunder appearance of retina on funduscopy
    - Extensive and severe hemorrhages
- Retinal edema
- Macular edema is most frequent cause of vision loss
- Dilated retinal veins
- Cotton-wool spots in 1/2 of patients
- Ipsilateral relative afferent pupillary defect
  - Found in nonperfused CRVO
- Neovascularization of the iris mandates intervention as it indicates extensive retinal ischemia

DIFFERENTIAL DIAGNOSIS

Papillophlebitis
- Swollen optic disc
- Occurs in young, healthy adults

Diabetic Papillitis
- Swollen optic disc
- Systemic finding of diabetes

Branch Retinal Vein Occlusion
- Wedge-shaped area of retinal hemorrhages/dilations/edema
- May be asymptomatic

Ocular Ischemic Syndrome
- Ocular pain and gradual visual loss

EVALUATION/WORK-UP

Imaging
- Fluorescein angiogram
  - Confirms diagnosis
  - Distinguishes between perfused and nonperfused CRVO
  - > 10 disc areas of nonperfusion indicate ischemic or nonperfused CRVO
- Optical coherence tomography (OCT) quantifies retinal thickening due to intraretinal macular edema
- Hypercoagulability work-up in young patients without risk factors

TREATMENT

Medical
- Observation
  - Recommended if there is no macular edema or neovascularization
- Consider vascular endothelial growth factor inhibitors in setting of retinal ischemia/extensive nonperfusion (i.e., neovascularization of iris, afferent pupillary defect, > 10 disc areas of nonperfusion)
- Intravitreal glucocorticoids
- Antithrombotic and thrombolytic therapy
- Isovolemic hemodilution

Surgical
- Laser photocoagulation
  - Panretinal
  - Prophylaxis for neovascularization (in extensive nonperfusion) or treatment for neovascularization (iris, disc, retina)

Prognosis
- Depends on visual acuity at presentation
  - 65% of patient eyes maintain 20/40 vision if acuity at presentation is 20/40 or better
  - 1% of patient eyes improve to 20/40 vision if acuity at presentation is 20/200 or worse
- Worse prognosis in patients with nonperfused CRVO
- Patients with CRVO have worse prognosis than patients with branch retinal vein occlusion

SELECTED REFERENCES

1. Stem MS et al: A longitudinal analysis of risk factors associated with central retinal vein occlusion. Ophthalmology. 120(2):362-70, 2013

CENTRAL SEROUS CHORIORETINOPATHY

Key Facts

Introduction

- Serous detachment of neurosensory retina &/or retinal pigment epithelium (RPE) with monofocal or multifocal changes in RPE
- Can be acute, chronic, or recurrent

Demographics

- Associated with
  - Type A personality, stress
  - Hypertension
  - Elevated cortisol levels
  - Previous glucocorticoid treatment
- Most often occurs in mid life with peak prevalence at 45 years

Presentation

- Monocular blurred vision
- Dark spot in center of visual field
  - Fades within a few seconds
- Reduced contrast sensitivity
- RPE depigmentation with elevation of neurosensory retina on funduscopy
- May see fibrinous deposits in subretinal fluid

Evaluation/Work-Up

- Fluorescein angiography
  - Often used to make diagnosis
- 1 or 2 leakage sites usually located near fovea
  - Usually in superonasal quadrant of posterior pole

Treatment

- Usually resolves spontaneously within 3 months
- Chronic central serous chorioretinopathy (CSCR)
  - Photodynamic therapy or laser if chronic or occupational disability
  - Metoprolol and acetazolamide are alternatives
- Prognosis: Chronic CSCR may lead to subretinal neovascularization

*(**Left**) Fundus photo shows macular edema associated with central serous chorioretinopathy ➔. (**Right**) Fundus photograph shows central serous chorioretinopathy ➔, which often presents with ovoid serous retinal detachment below the macula. The patient may present with monocular blurred vision or a dark spot in the center of the visual field. Central serous chorioretinopathy (CSCR) generally resolves spontaneously within 3 months.*

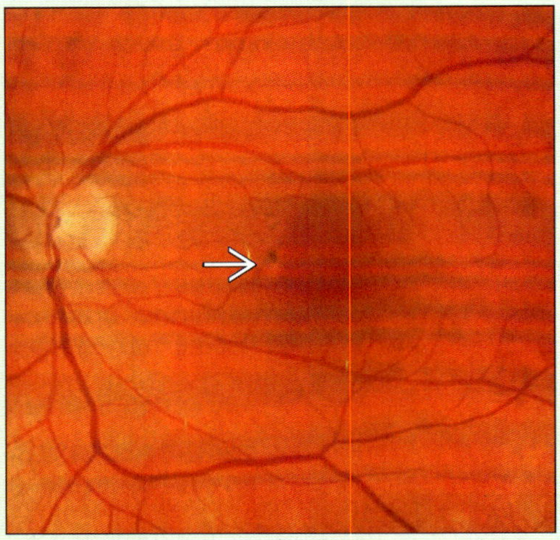

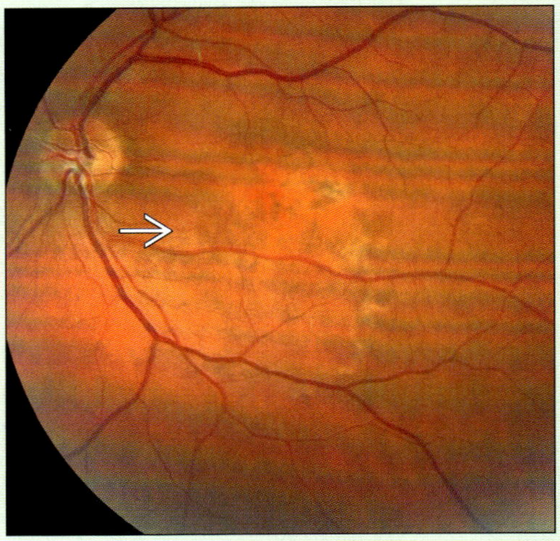

*(**Left**) Fluorescein angiogram shows central serous chorioretinopathy ➔. The fluid buildup can be localized beneath the macula under a serous detachment of the sensory retina. There are no signs of subretinal neovascularization. (**Right**) Spectral-domain OCT of the macula shows detachment of retina from retinal pigment epithelium in CSCR ➔ with a small central pigment epithelial detachment (PED), where the pigment epithelium has detached from underlying choroid ➔.*

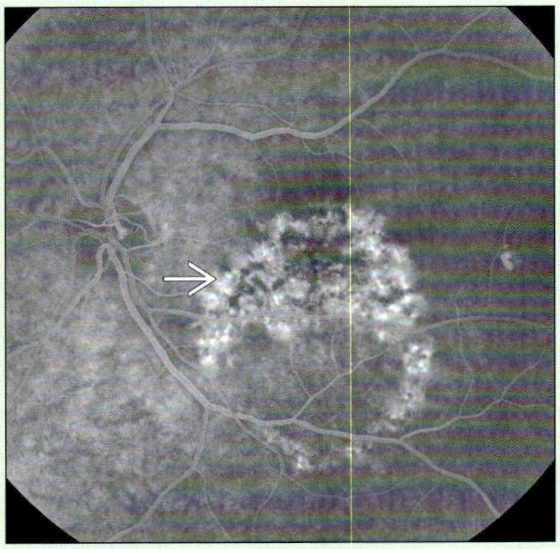

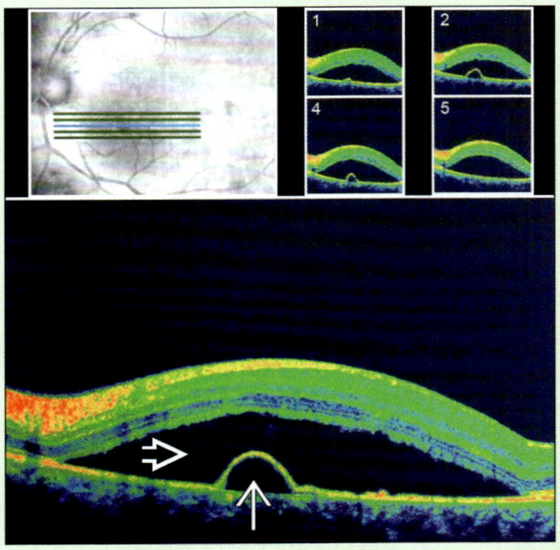

CENTRAL SEROUS CHORIORETINOPATHY

INTRODUCTION

Abbreviations
- Central serous chorioretinopathy (CSCR)

Definitions
- Serous detachment of neurosensory retina &/or retinal pigment epithelium (RPE) with monofocal or multifocal changes in RPE
- Detachment is not due to tears in retina, inflammation, neovascularization, or neoplasia

DEMOGRAPHICS

Etiology/Risk Factors
- Associations
  - Type A behavior pattern
  - Hypertension
  - Elevated cortisol levels
  - Previous glucocorticoid treatment
  - Family history of CSCR
  - Psychosocial stress and life crises

Epidemiology
- Most often occurs in mid life with peak prevalence at 45 years
- More common in men
- 1 of the 10 most common diseases of posterior segment

PRESENTATION

Symptoms
- Monocular blurred vision
- Dark spot in center of visual field
  - Worse in morning after awakening
  - Worse after blinking
  - Fades within a few seconds
- Reduced contrast sensitivity
- Metamorphopsia
- Micropsia
- Dyschromatopsia
- May have migraine headache

Exam Findings
- RPE depigmentation with elevation of neurosensory retina
- Serous detachment, usually near fovea

DIFFERENTIAL DIAGNOSIS

Rhegmatogenous Detachment
- Not usually limited to macula

Age-Related Macular Degeneration (ARMD)
- Presence of bilateral drusen and choroidal neovascularization (CNV)

Hypertensive Choroidopathy
- Elschnig spot
  - Hyperpigmentations with hypopigmented outer ring

Choroidal Tumor
- Inferior detachment of RPE may occur in choroidal hemangioma, melanoma, choroidal osteoma, or metastatic tumor

RPE Detachments
- Can be caused by CSCR, ARMD, and idiopathic polypoidal choroidal vasculopathy

EVALUATION/WORK-UP

Pathology
- Subretinal fluid is most often clear
  - May see fibrinous deposits when there is prolonged duration of symptoms

Imaging
- Fluorescein angiography (FA)
  - Often used to make diagnosis
  - Fluorescein leakage under a serous detachment of sensory retina but no CNV
  - Classic "smokestack" appearance of FA leak is seen in only 10-15% of cases
- Optical coherence tomography (OCT)
  - Shallow serous detachments
- Multifocal electroretinography (mfERG)
  - Reduced photoreceptor function of detached retina

TREATMENT

Medical
- Usually resolves spontaneously within 3 months
  - Emphasize the importance of coping with psychosocial stress
- Treatment initiated after 3 months without resolution
- Metoprolol
  - β-adrenergic inhibition may improve symptoms
- Acetazolamide
  - May improve resorption of subretinal fluid

Surgical
- Photodynamic therapy can be done in chronic cases
  - Aimed at foci of RPE leakage
  - Used when photocoagulation is not recommended due to RPE lesion located under fovea
- Photocoagulation
  - Causes earlier resolution of symptoms, but there is slightly higher risk of CNV long term
- Anti-VEGF therapy if CNV develops

Prognosis
- Acute CSCR with monofocal or paucifocal RPE changes will often resolve spontaneously
  - 90% will resolve in 1.5 months
- Chronic CSCR may lead to subretinal neovascularization
  - May result in irreversible visual acuity loss

SELECTED REFERENCES

1. Nicholson B et al: Central serous chorioretinopathy: update on pathophysiology and treatment. Surv Ophthalmol. 58(2):103-26, 2013

DIABETIC RETINOPATHY

Key Facts

Introduction

- Retinal microvascular damage caused by longstanding poorly controlled diabetes
- Divided into NPDR and PDR
- DME: Common cause of vision loss

Demographics

- Duration of diabetes is most important risk factor
- Tight glycemic control may prevent or delay development of retinopathy
- Most common cause of vision loss in patients age 25-74, higher for type 1 than type 2 diabetics

Presentation

- Microaneurysms, dot-and-blot hemorrhages, exudate, cotton-wool spots, vitreous hemorrhage, neovascularization of disc/retina/iris/angle

Differential Diagnosis

- Hypertensive retinopathy: Fewer hemorrhages that are flame-shaped, as well as arteriolar narrowing
- Sickle cell retinopathy: Shows peripheral vs. posterior neovascularization in sea fan configuration
- Central retinal vein occlusion: Usually unilateral, very dilated veins & dense nerve fiber layer hemorrhages

Treatment

- Panretinal photocoagulation for high-risk PDR or iris/angle neovascularization
- Focal or grid laser for CSME
- Intravitreal injection of anti-VEGF agents may be used alone or in combination with laser for CSME or PDR; intravitreal triamcinolone may be useful in certain select cases as well
- Strict blood glucose control with goal HbA1C ≤ 7, blood pressure control, cholesterol control; use of fenofibrate is emerging

*(**Left**) Fundus photo shows microaneurysms, dot-and-blot hemorrhages, circinate exudate, and clinically significant macular edema (delineated by the areas of exudate). (Courtesy S. Cohen, MD.) (**Right**) Red-free image depicts retinal neovascularization and small vitreous hemorrhage. Because there is > 1/2 disc diameter of neovascularization and vitreous hemorrhage, this is an example of high-risk PDR, and panretinal laser photocoagulation is indicated. (Courtesy S. Cohen, MD.)*

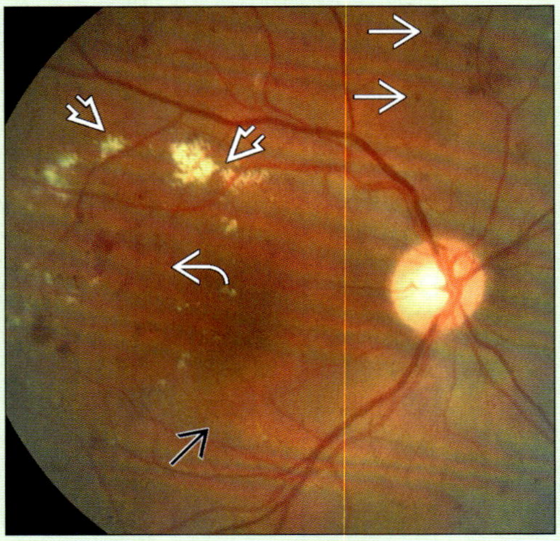

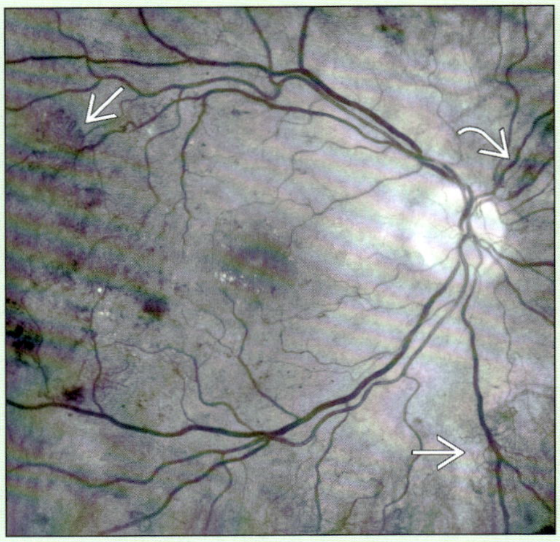

*(**Left**) Fluorescein angiogram of ischemic diabetic retinopathy demonstrates areas of capillary dropout and retinal nonperfusion. Patients with CSME and foveal ischemia are not good candidates for focal laser therapy. (Courtesy S. Cohen, MD.) (**Right**) Fundus photo shows severe proliferative diabetic retinopathy with extensive fibrovascular proliferation and tractional retinal detachments. Vitrectomy is recommended for macula-threatening tractional retinal detachments. (Courtesy S. Cohen, MD.)*

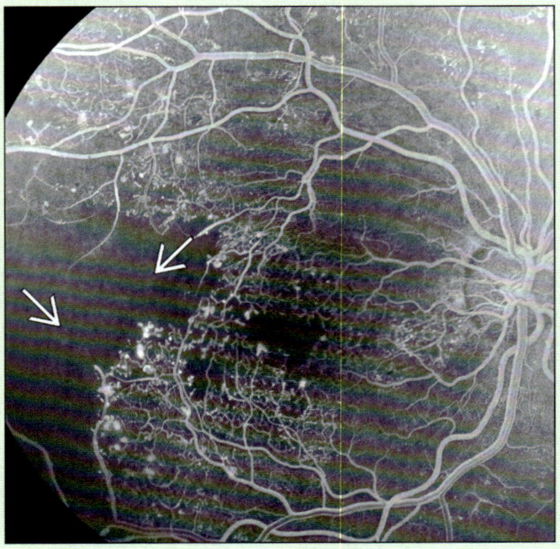

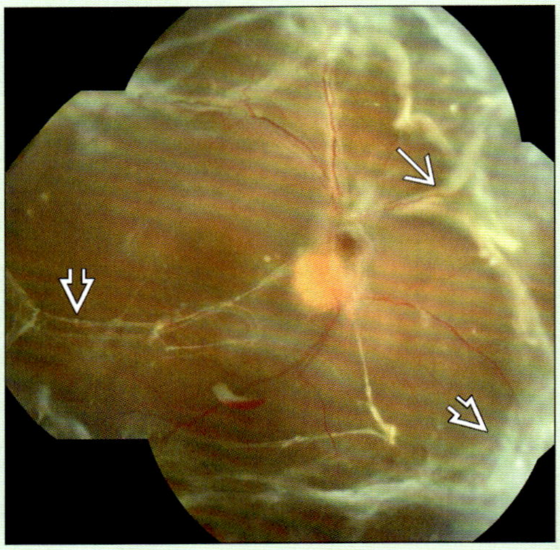

DIABETIC RETINOPATHY

INTRODUCTION

Abbreviations
- Diabetic retinopathy (DR)

Definitions
- Retinopathy secondary to diabetes mellitus

Subtypes
- Nonproliferative diabetic retinopathy (NPDR)
- Proliferative diabetic retinopathy (PDR)

DEMOGRAPHICS

Etiology/Risk Factors
- Duration of diabetes: Most important risk factor
- Glycemic control: Tight glucose control may prevent or delay development of retinopathy
- Type of diabetes: Type 1 higher risk than type 2
- Pregnancy: May accelerate progression of DR
- Hypertension: Blood pressure control decreases rate of progression and risk of vitreous hemorrhage

Epidemiology
- Among diabetes patients age 20-79, prevalence is 35% for any form of DR, 7.2% for PDR, & 7.5% for diabetic macular edema (DME)
  - Prevalence is significantly higher for type 1 diabetics over type 2, regardless of duration of disease
- Most common cause of vision loss in patients age 25-74

PRESENTATION

Symptoms
- Floaters, scotomas, decreased vision

Exam Findings
- Mild NPDR: Microaneurysms; cotton-wool spots indicate nerve fiber layer infarcts/axoplasmic stasis
- Moderate NPDR: Intermediate between mild & severe
- Severe NPDR: Any of the following in absence of PDR
  - > 20 intraretinal hemorrhages in all 4 quadrants
  - 2 quadrants of venous beading
  - 1 quadrant of intraretinal microvascular abnormality
- Early PDR: Neovascularization that does not meet criteria for high-risk PDR
- High-risk PDR: 1 or more of the following
  - Neovascularization of disc (NVD) ≥ 1/3 disc area
  - Any NVD **and** vitreous/preretinal hemorrhage
  - Neovascularization elsewhere (NVE) ≥ 1/2 disc area **and** vitreous/preretinal hemorrhage
- Clinically significant macular edema (CSME): Requires treatment and is defined by any 1 of the following
  - Retinal thickening within 500 μm of foveal center
  - Hard exudates within 500 μm of foveal center, if associated with adjacent retinal thickening
  - Retinal thickening > 1 disc area, part of which is within 1 disc diameter of foveal center

DIFFERENTIAL DIAGNOSIS

Hypertensive or Radiation Retinopathy
- Fewer hemorrhages that are flame-shaped, as well as arteriolar narrowing

Sickle Cell Retinopathy
- Shows peripheral vs. posterior neovascularization in sea fan configuration; has sickle cell disease/trait; sea fans eventually become salmon spots of focal hemorrhage and starbursts of black retinal scar tissue

Central Retinal Vein Occlusion
- Usually unilateral with very dilated veins and dense nerve-fiber layer hemorrhages

EVALUATION/WORK-UP

Labs
- Glycosylated hemoglobin (HbA1C), fasting blood sugar, glucose tolerance test

Pathology
- Basement membrane thickening, loss of vascular pericytes and endothelial cells

Imaging
- Ocular coherence tomography (OCT): Detects/quantifies macular edema
- Fluorescein angiogram (FA): Highlights microaneurysms, neovascularization, foveal ischemia

TREATMENT

Medical
- Strict blood glucose control with goal HbA1C ≤ 7, blood pressure control, cholesterol control; ruboxistaurin and aldose reductase inhibitors may be of some small benefit
  - ACCORD study shows benefit of fenofibrate in reducing diabetic retinopathy; at same time, certain glitazones (used for glycemic control) may increase macular edema over long term
- Panretinal photocoagulation (PRP) for high-risk PDR or iris/angle neovascularization
- Focal or grid laser for CSME: First-line therapy
- Intravitreal injection of anti-VEGF agents: May be used alone or in combination with laser for CSME or PDR

Surgical
- Vitrectomy surgery indicated for nonclearing vitreous hemorrhage, tractional retinal detachment, and progressive neovascularization despite PRP; endolaser, membrane peel may be necessary

Follow-Up
- Mild NPDR every 6-9 months; moderate to severe NPDR every 4 to 6 months; PDR every 2-3 months

Prognosis
- Good with good glycemic control and follow-up

SELECTED REFERENCES

1. Antonetti DA et al: Diabetic retinopathy. N Engl J Med. 366(13):1227-39, 2012
2. Cheung N et al: Diabetic retinopathy. Lancet. 376(9735):124-36, 2010
3. Wilkinson CP et al: Proposed international clinical diabetic retinopathy and diabetic macular edema disease severity scales. Ophthalmology. 110(9):1677-82, 2003

EXUDATIVE AGE-RELATED MACULAR DEGENERATION

Key Facts

Introduction
- Exudative age-related macular degeneration (EARMD)
  - Loss of central vision due to degradation and damage to photoreceptors in retinal macula

Demographics
- Risk factors
  - Age > 60
  - Cigarette smoking
  - Family history in first-degree relatives
- EARMD is most common form of irreversible visual blindness among those > age of 50

Presentation
- Acute visual distortion
- Decreased central vision
- Straight line distortion when patient views Amsler grid
- Subretinal fluid &/or hemorrhage on retinal examination

Differential Diagnosis
- Amaurosis fugax
- Dry age-related macular degeneration
- Hereditary macular dystrophies

Evaluation/Work-Up
- Optical coherence tomography
- Fluorescein dye retinal angiography

Treatment
- Intravitreal injections of anti-VEGF biologics
- Photodynamic therapy can be used as adjunct
- Patients should be strongly encouraged to stop smoking
- If not diagnosed early, damage to central photoreceptor cells can lead to irreversible loss of central vision

*(**Left**) This fundus photo shows the eye of a patient with exudative age-related macular degeneration (EARMD). Note the presence of hemorrhage → in the region of the Macula. (**Right**) Fundus changes can be further illustrated in this photo. Note the discoloration and geographic atrophy ↪ in the region of the Macula (which signifies an advanced stage of the disease) and the surrounding hemorrhaging blood vessels →.*

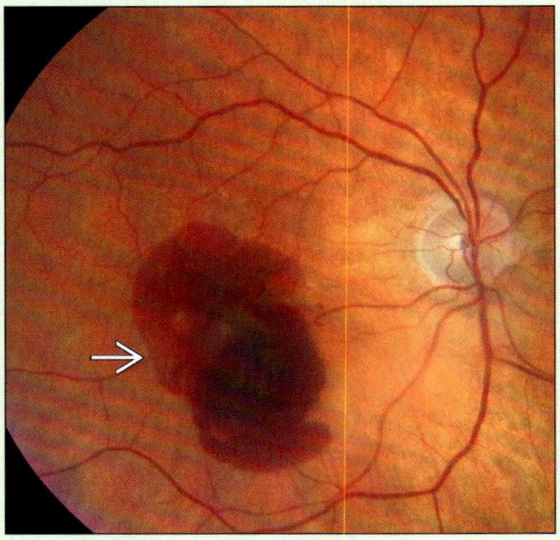

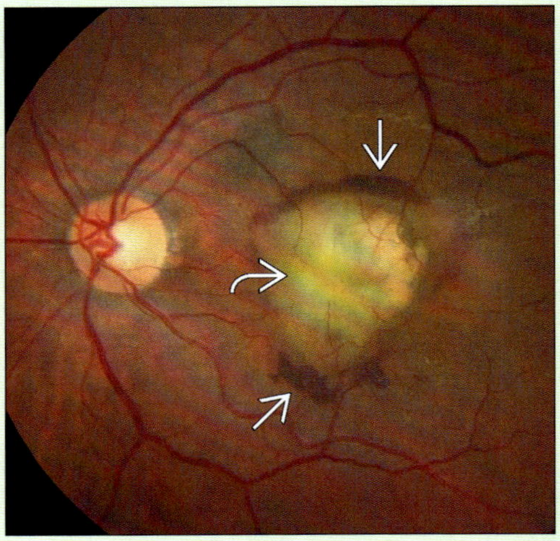

*(**Left**) Fluorescein angiography is useful in the evaluation of EARMD. This image shows the eye of a patient with a choroidal neovascular membrane →. (**Right**) Changes in the macula can be observed with optical coherence tomography. This image shows the eye of a patient with EARMD. Note the fluid → separating the retina from the choroid. The fluid layer results from hemorrhaging of the choroidal neovascularization.*

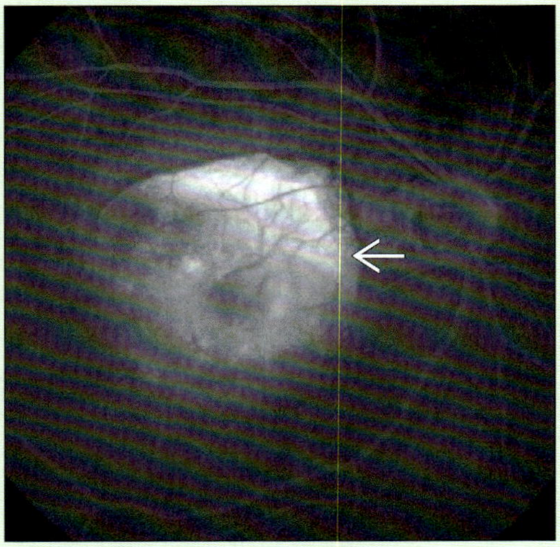

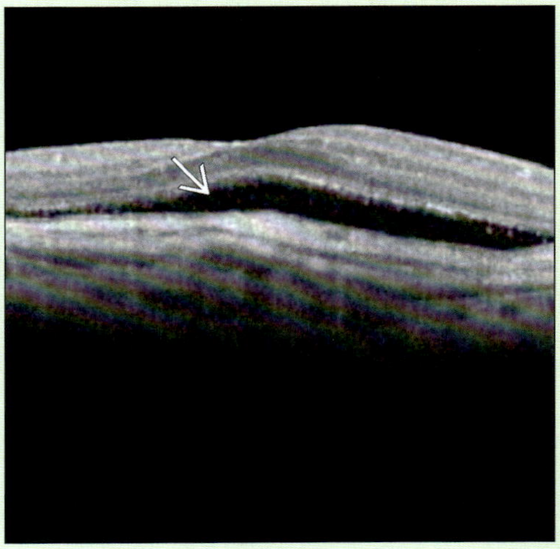

EXUDATIVE AGE-RELATED MACULAR DEGENERATION

INTRODUCTION

Abbreviations

- Exudative age-related macular degeneration (EARMD)

Definitions

- Categorized by loss of central vision due to degradation and damage to photoreceptors in retinal macula

DEMOGRAPHICS

Etiology/Risk Factors

- Inflammation and vascular endothelial growth factor (VEGF)-triggered choroidal neovascularization results in subretinal hemorrhage or fluid accumulation that then causes EARMD
- Age is strongest risk factor
  - Patients age ≥ 60 years are at most significant risk of developing EARMD
- Cigarette smoking
  - Strongest environmental risk factor for EARMD
- Family history in first-degree relatives
- Caucasians
- Hypertensive patients
- Previous diagnosis of nonneovascular (dry) macular degeneration
- HTRA1, complement factor H gene mutations have been associated

Epidemiology

- In Western world, age-related macular degeneration is most common form of irreversible visual blindness among those > age 50
- EARMD accounts for 2/3 of late-stage age-related macular degeneration and is responsible for 90% of blindness due to this disease

PRESENTATION

Symptoms

- Metamorphopsia (distortion of straight lines)
- Acute visual distortion
- Decreased central vision
- Symptoms generally present unilaterally and then spread to other eye later

Exam Findings

- Line distortion when patient views Amsler grid
- Subretinal fluid &/or hemorrhage on retinal examination
- Gray subretinal membranes

DIFFERENTIAL DIAGNOSIS

Amaurosis Fugax

- Condition also presents with acute decreased vision, but vision loss is generally characterized by darkening of entire visual field
- Patients should be evaluated for carotid artery stenosis with duplex ultrasound, as if they do, they are at increased risk of stroke

Dry Age-Related Macular Degeneration

- Gradual unilateral or bilateral vision loss
- Dilated retinal examination will reveal subretinal drusen deposits

Hereditary Macular Dystrophies

- Loss of visual acuity that progresses to blindness and affects patients of all ages
- This genetic disease affects proteins of retinal pigment epithelium and sensory retina
- Often mistaken for early-onset age-related macular degeneration

EVALUATION/WORK-UP

Labs

- Serum analysis can reveal protective or harmful biomarkers and identify those at risk of EARMD
  - Protective biomarkers include complement factors H and D
  - At-risk biomarkers: Anti-phosphodiesterase phosphatidylserine, eotaxin, IP-10

Imaging

- Optical coherence tomography
  - Will reveal subretinal fluid or retinal edema
- Fluorescein dye retinal angiography
  - Shows choroidal neovascular complexes and leaky vessels

TREATMENT

Medical

- Intravitreal injections of anti-VEGF agents including
  - Ranibuzimab, bevacizumab, aflibercept; pegaptanib (rarely used)
- Patients strongly encouraged to quit smoking

Surgical

- Laser photocoagulation
  - Uses thermal heat to coagulate patches of choroidal neovascularization
  - Best for patients with well-demarcated areas of neovascularization in extrafoveal region
  - Photodynamic therapy is an alternative and can be used in combination with anti-VEGFs
- Implantable miniature telescope is emerging

Follow-Up

- Treat and extend protocols evolving

Prognosis

- If not diagnosed early, damage to central photoreceptors can lead to irreversible central blindness
  - Most beneficial factor is early detection of EARMD

SELECTED REFERENCES

1. Renner AB et al: [Hereditary macular dystrophies in differential diagnosis of AMD.] Klin Monbl Augenheilkd. 229(9):905-9, 2012
2. Shahid H et al: Age-related macular degeneration: the importance of family history as a risk factor. Br J Ophthalmol. 96(3):427-31, 2012
3. Klein R et al: Risk assessment models for late age-related macular degeneration. Arch Ophthalmol. 129(12):1605-6, 2011

HYPERTENSIVE RETINOPATHY

Key Facts

Introduction

- Hypertensive retinopathy: Manifestation of systemic hypertension in the eye
- Retinopathy from hypertensive emergency: Retinopathy caused by acute damage from severely elevated blood pressure (BP)

Demographics

- Acute increase in BP causes arterial vasospasm causing generalized retinal-arteriolar narrowing
- Chronic elevation causes atherosclerosis and shows intimal thickening, media-wall hyperplasia, and hyaline degeneration
- Retinopathy from hypertensive emergency: Increased intracranial pressure and fibrinoid necrosis of choroidal arteries, retinal pigment epithelium (RPE) infarcts
- Risk factors: BP ≥ 140/90 mm Hg, age, family history
- 2-14% of nondiabetic population aged ≥ 40 years

Presentation

- Fundus exam: Diffuse arteriole narrowing, arteriovenous nicking, arteriolar wall opacification, flame-shaped hemorrhage, cotton-wool spots

Evaluation/Work-Up

- Assessment of BP, evaluate for other end-organ damage, evaluate for possible secondary causes of hypertension

Treatment

- BP control with lifestyle modifications and pharmacotherapy
- Malignant hypertensive retinopathy should be lowered slowly to prevent optic nerve ischemia

__(Left)__ This fundus photograph depicts cotton-wool spots ➡. These spots are a common finding in hypertensive retinopathy. Cotton-wool spots represent an area of nerve fiber layer infarct. __(Right)__ This fundus photograph shows a flame-shaped hemorrhage ➡. These hemorrhages are commonly seen in hypertensive retinopathy due to the increased pressure in vessels.

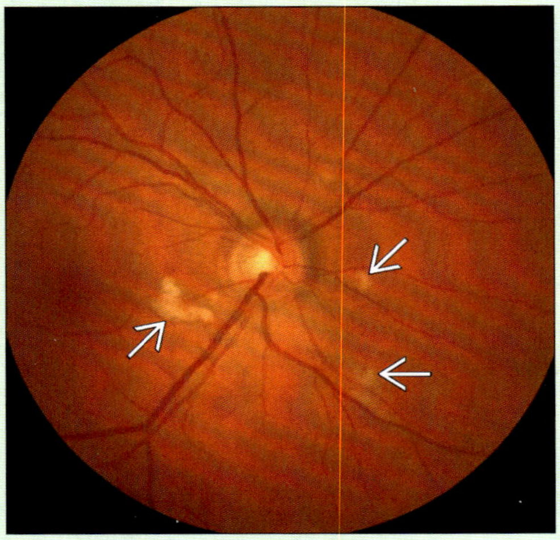

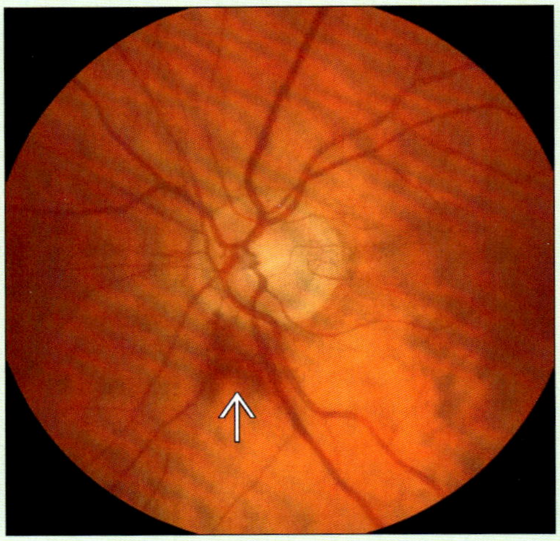

__(Left)__ This fundus photograph depicts silver wire effect of retinal vasculature ➡. Hyperplasia and thickening of the wall cause opacification in the arterial walls, giving them the classic silver wire depiction. __(Right)__ This fundus photograph shows hard exudates ➡. These white exudates are often seen in hypertensive retinopathy.

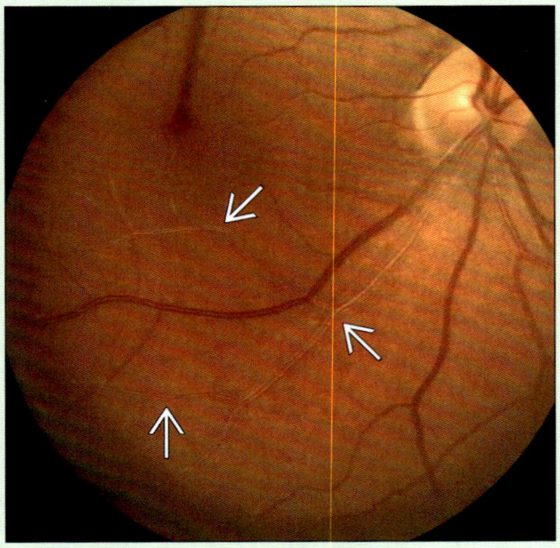

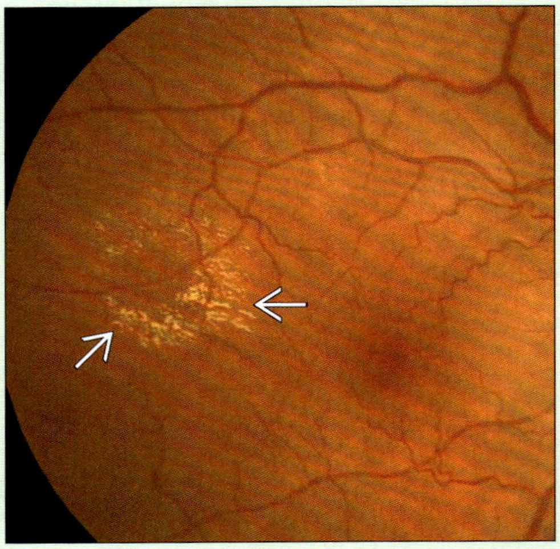

HYPERTENSIVE RETINOPATHY

INTRODUCTION

Definitions

- Hypertensive retinopathy: Manifestation of systemic hypertension in the eye
- Retinopathy from hypertensive emergency: Retinopathy caused by acute damage from severely elevated blood pressure

Subtypes

- Hypertensive retinopathy: Stepwise changes seen in chronically elevated hypertension
- Hypertensive choroidopathy: Lack of autoregulatory mechanism leads to choroidal arteriole constriction, ischemia, and subsequent choriocapillaris and retinal pigment epithelium (RPE) necrosis
- Hypertensive optic neuropathy: Vasoconstriction in prelaminar optic nerve leads to impaired axoplasmic flow and optic disc swelling

DEMOGRAPHICS

Etiology/Risk Factors

- Pathophysiology
  - Acute increase in blood pressure (BP) causes arterial vasospasm and generalized retinal-arteriolar narrowing
  - Chronic elevation causes atherosclerosis and shows intimal thickening, media-wall hyperplasia, and hyaline degeneration
    - Hyperplasia and thickening of the wall causes opacification of arterial walls, a phenomenon known as silver wire effect
    - Thickened arteriolar walls cause compression of the underlying venules, which manifest as **arteriovenous nicking**
    - More severe hypertension leads to scattered hemorrhages, lipid exudates, macular edema, and nerve ischemia (**cotton-wool spots**)
  - Retinopathy from hypertensive emergency
    - Increased intracranial pressure and fibrinoid necrosis of choroidal arteries
    - Optic nerve ischemia
    - Optic disc swelling or papilledema
    - Choriocapillaris infarction
    - RPE infarcts
    - Can cause intraretinal and preretinal hemorrhaging
- Risk factors: BP ≥ 140/90 mm Hg, age, family history

Epidemiology

- 2-14% of nondiabetic population aged ≥ 40 years

PRESENTATION

Symptoms

- Chronic hypertensive retinopathy is usually asymptomatic unless severely uncontrolled
- Malignant hypertensive retinopathy may include headache, scotoma, diplopia, and photopsia

Exam Findings

- Fundus exam
  - Diffuse arteriole narrowing
  - Arteriovenous nicking
  - Arteriolar wall opacification or copper wire effect
  - Flame-shaped hemorrhage
  - Cotton-wool spots
  - Hard exudates
  - Microaneurysms
  - Papilledema or optic disc swelling

DIFFERENTIAL DIAGNOSIS

Diabetic Retinopathy

- Hypertensive retinopathy is independent risk factor that may precipitate diabetic retinopathy

Retinal Venous Obstruction

- Backup of blood that may result in ischemic or nonischemic damage

Ocular Ischemic Syndrome

- Can present with pain around eye along with vision loss

EVALUATION/WORK-UP

Labs

- Indicated when secondary hypertension is suspected (i.e., pheochromocytoma, hyperaldosteronism)

Pathology

- Sclerosis and thickening of arteriolar walls with luminal narrowing

TREATMENT

Medical

- BP control with lifestyle modifications and pharmacotherapy
- Malignant hypertensive retinopathy should be lowered slowly to prevent optic nerve ischemia
  - Medications used include sodium nitroprusside, nitroglycerin, calcium channel blockers, β-blockers (e.g., labetalol), and angiotensin-converting enzyme inhibitors

Prognosis

- Chronic hypertensive retinopathy rarely causes visual changes
- Correlates with and is a risk factor for several other systemic and ocular diseases including retinal arterial occlusion, retinal vein occlusion, retinal macroaneurysm, diabetic retinopathy, glaucoma, age-related macular degeneration, and cardiovascular disease

SELECTED REFERENCES

1. Bhargava M et al: How does hypertension affect your eyes? J Hum Hypertens. 26(2):71-83, 2012
2. Henderson AD et al: Hypertension-related eye abnormalities and the risk of stroke. Rev Neurol Dis. 8(1-2):1-9, 2011
3. DellaCroce JT et al: Hypertension and the eye. Curr Opin Ophthalmol. 19(6):493-8, 2008

OCULAR ISCHEMIC SYNDROME

Key Facts

Introduction
- Ocular ischemic syndrome (OIS)
- Decreased vascular perfusion leads to ocular ischemia

Demographics
- Most commonly caused by atherosclerotic disease of internal carotid artery
- May also be caused by giant cell arteritis
- Occurs between 50 and 80 years of age

Presentation
- Eye pain
- Vision loss may be sudden or gradual
- Anterior segment findings
  - Cataract, asymmetric uveitis, iris neovascularization
- Posterior segment findings
  - Dilated retinal veins
  - Narrowed retinal arteries
  - Dot-and-blot retinal hemorrhage (characteristically mid peripheral)

Evaluation/Work-Up
- Obtain erythrocyte sedimentation rate (ESR) and C-reactive protein (CRP) to rule out giant cell arteritis
- Fluorescein angiography
  - Delayed and patchy choroidal filling
- Carotid duplex ultrasound (DUS)
  - Most commonly used noninvasive test
- Computed tomographic angiography (CTA) and magnetic resonance angiography (MRA)

Treatment
- Intravitreal steroids
- Topical treatments for increased intraocular pressure
- Antiplatelet therapy
- Panretinal photocoagulation
- Carotid endarterectomy

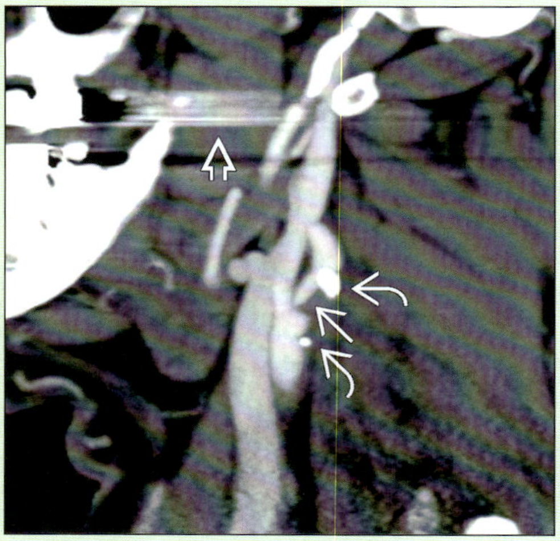

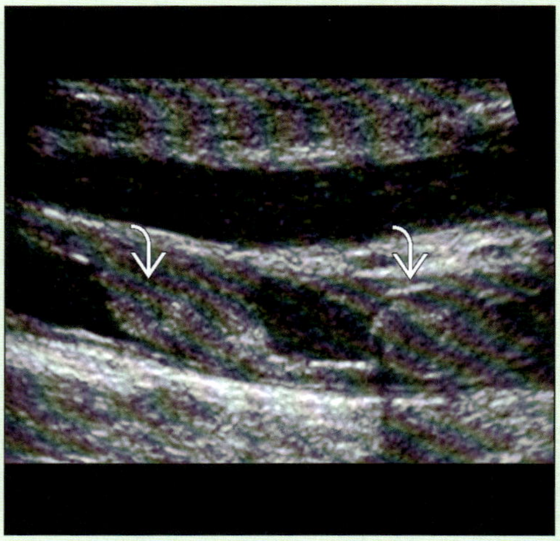

(Left) *Sagittal CTA shows a pinhole stenosis at the internal carotid artery origin ➔. Note adjacent calcifications within the atherosclerotic plaque ➔ and artifact from dental amalgam ➔. CTA is a noninvasive imaging technique that characterizes the occlusive plaque.* ***(Right)*** *Longitudinal ultrasound shows an irregular fibrous plaque ➔ in the common carotid artery, causing tight stenosis. Such a plaque is relatively stable and carries a low risk of cerebral embolism.*

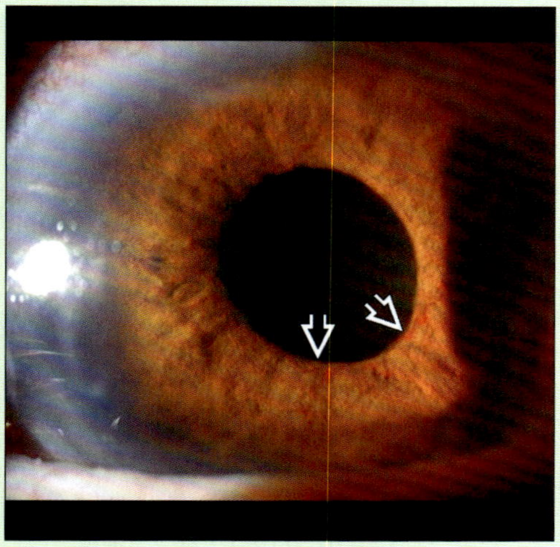

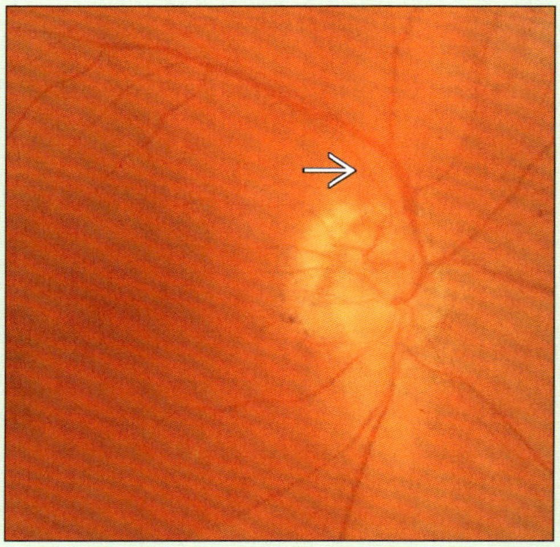

(Left) *This slit-lamp photo demonstrates neovascularization of the iris ➔. This finding is frequently found in patients with ocular ischemic syndrome. Asymmetric uveitis and cataracts may also be found in these patients. Ocular ischemic syndrome is often due to atherosclerotic disease.* ***(Right)*** *This fundus photo demonstrates the retinal arteriole narrowing ➔ or attenuation often found in association with ocular ischemic syndrome. Dilated retinal veins may also be found on funduscopy.*

OCULAR ISCHEMIC SYNDROME

INTRODUCTION

Abbreviations
- Ocular ischemic syndrome (OIS)

Definitions
- Decreased vascular perfusion leads to decreased oxygen delivery to anterior and posterior segments of eye (ocular ischemia)
  - Eventually leads to neovascularization

DEMOGRAPHICS

Etiology/Risk Factors
- Most commonly caused by atherosclerotic disease of the internal carotid artery
  - Can be secondary to disease of ophthalmic artery alone
- May also be caused by giant cell arteritis
- Risk factors
  - Hypertension
  - Diabetes mellitus
  - Age

Epidemiology
- Occurs in 5% of patients with carotid artery stenosis
- Male:female ratio is 2:1
- Occurs between 50 and 80 years of age

PRESENTATION

Symptoms
- Eye pain
  - Occurs in 40% of patients
- Vision loss may be sudden or gradual
- Amaurosis fugax
  - Transient episode of complete or partial monocular blindness

Exam Findings
- Anterior segment findings
  - Cataract
  - Asymmetric uveitis
  - Iris neovascularization
  - Neovascular glaucoma
- Posterior segment findings
  - Dilated retinal veins
  - Narrowed retinal arteries
  - Dot-and-blot retinal hemorrhage (mid peripheral)
  - Optic disc neovascularization
  - Retinal neovascularization (less common)

DIFFERENTIAL DIAGNOSIS

Diabetic Retinopathy
- Systemic findings of diabetes
- Eyes with OIS do not have hard exudates
- Disc swelling in diabetic retinopathy but not in OIS

Central Retinal Vein Occlusion
- Usually painless sudden vision loss
- Disc swelling is seen in central retinal vein occlusion, but not in OIS

Giant Cell Arteritis
- Systemic findings of fever, malaise, and weight loss
- Headache localized to temporal area

EVALUATION/WORK-UP

Labs
- Obtain erythrocyte sedimentation rate (ESR) and C-reactive protein (CRP) to rule out giant cell arteritis

Pathology
- Loss of endothelial cells in peripheral retinal vessels

Imaging
- Fluorescein angiography
  - Nonperfusion of retinal capillaries
  - Delayed and patchy choroidal filling
- Carotid duplex ultrasound (DUS)
  - Most commonly used noninvasive test
- Computed tomographic angiography (CTA) and magnetic resonance angiography (MRA)
  - Noninvasive imaging
  - Better characterization of occlusive plaque than DUS
- Carotid angiography
  - Only used if DUS and CTA/MRA are inconclusive

TREATMENT

Medical
- Intravitreal steroids
  - Suppresses anterior segment inflammation
- Topical treatments for increased intraocular pressure
- Antiplatelet therapy

Surgical
- Panretinal photocoagulation
  - Regression of iris neovascularization is usually temporary and only effective in ~ 30% of patients
- Carotid endarterectomy
  - Reduces incidence of stroke in patients with 50-99% carotid stenosis
  - May restore vision in patients with 70-99% occlusion of carotid artery
- Carotid artery stenting
- Bypass procedures
  - Superficial temporal artery to middle cerebral artery anastomoses (STA-MCA)
  - Used in 100% carotid obstruction

Follow-Up
- Counsel the patient to maintain a low-fat diet

Prognosis
- Leading cause of death is cardiac disease
- Cerebral infarction is 2nd leading cause of death
- 5-year mortality rate is 40%
- Iris neovascularization and poor initial visual acuity are associated with poor visual prognosis

SELECTED REFERENCES

1. Mendrinos E et al: Ocular ischemic syndrome. Surv Ophthalmol. 55(1):2-34, 2010
2. Foncea Beti N et al: The ocular ischemic syndrome. Clin Neurol Neurosurg. 106(1):60-2, 2003

NONEXUDATIVE AGE-RELATED MACULAR DEGENERATION

Key Facts

Introduction

- Nonexudative age-related macular degeneration (NARMD): Loss of vision in center of visual field as a result of progressive degeneration of choriocapillaris, retinal pigment epithelium (RPE), and photoreceptors

Demographics

- Common anatomical changes include loss of choriocapillaris, thickening of Bruch membrane, and loss of photoreceptors
- Geographic atrophy: Progressive atrophy of RPE, choriocapillaris, and photoreceptors associated with severe vision loss (late form of NARMD)
- Risk factors: Age (late-stage NARMD rare < 55 years), family history, white race, Asian race, obesity, smoking, and diet low in vitamin A, C, E, and zinc

Presentation

- Asymptomatic in early NARMD
- Progression over years leads to blurred vision, metamorphopsia, difficulty reading (especially in low light), glare, or difficulty with dark and light adaptation
- Fundus exam: Drusen seen as yellow excrescences and are typically found in posterior pole; may be associated with areas of hyper- and hypopigmentation of RPE
- Geographic atrophy: 1 or more large areas of depigmentation due to atrophy of RPE

Evaluation/Work-Up

- Fluorescein angiography (FA): Excludes the presence of choroidal neovascularization, identifies drusen, and locates areas of RPE atrophy

Treatment

- Patients with NARMD are advised to take a daily supplement of antioxidants plus zinc

__(Left)__ This fundus photo shows multiple soft drusen →. Drusen are an early finding in nonexudative age-related macular degeneration. Soft drusen are differentiated from hard drusen by their larger size and softer borders. __(Right)__ This fundus photo shows a fundus with multiple drusen in the region of the macula with an area of coalescence →. Increased quantity of drusen and coalescence are findings in more advanced nonexudative age-related macular degeneration.

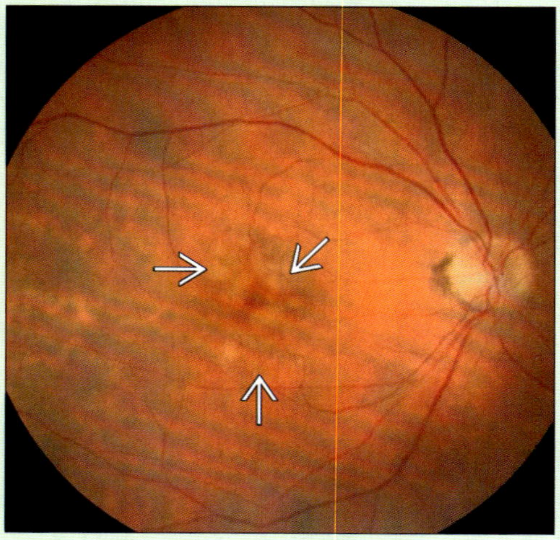

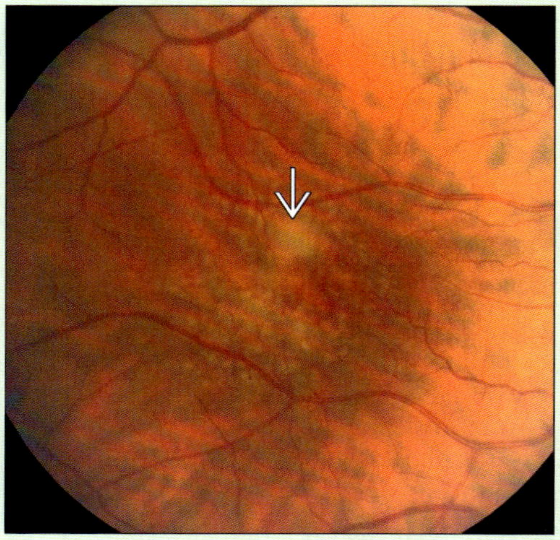

__(Left)__ This red-free image shows several drusen →. An eye such as this that is early in the course of macular degeneration may be asymptomatic. __(Right)__ This OCT image shows several drusen →. Drusen are located in between the retinal pigment epithelium → and Bruch membrane →. OCT is often necessary to further work-up and evaluate nonexudative age-related macular degeneration.

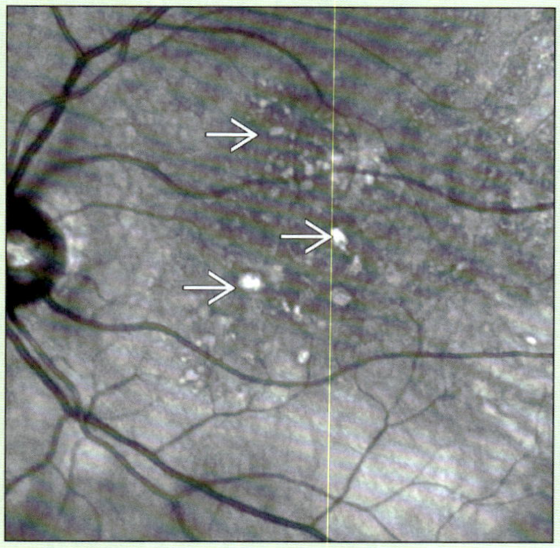

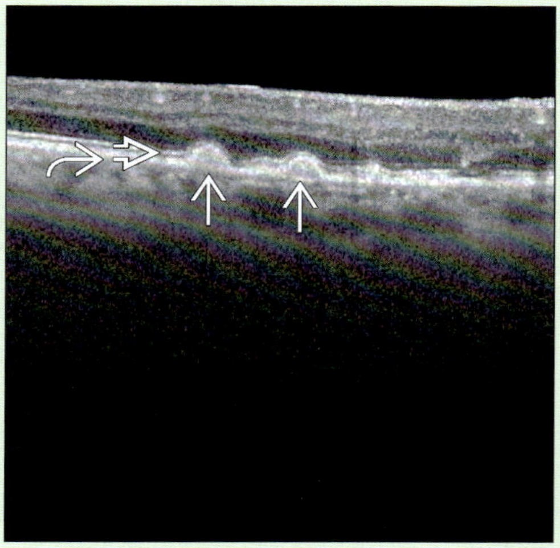

NONEXUDATIVE AGE-RELATED MACULAR DEGENERATION

INTRODUCTION

Abbreviations

- Nonexudative age-related macular degeneration (NARMD)

Synonyms

- Dry NARMD

Definitions

- Loss of vision in center of visual field as a result of progressive degeneration of choriocapillaris, retinal pigment epithelium (RPE), and photoreceptors
- Bruch membrane: Extracellular matrix that provides structural support to overlying RPE and retina

DEMOGRAPHICS

Etiology/Risk Factors

- Pathogenesis
  - Common anatomical changes seen in NARMD
    - Accumulation of deposits known as drusen under RPE is key histopathological feature of eyes with early NARMD
      - Drusen are made up of many compounds and proteins associated with RPE cell function including lipofuscin, phospholipids, cholesterol, apolipoproteins, vitronectin, immunoglobulins, amyloid, and complement
    - Loss and narrowing of choriocapillaris
    - Thickening of Bruch membrane: Thought to be effect of accumulation of phospholipid and fatty acid deposits from RPE
    - Loss of photoreceptor cells: Thought to be secondary to RPE dysfunction
  - Late-stage disease evolves into either neovascular macular degeneration or geographic atrophy (GA)
    - Neovascular macular degeneration: Choroidal neovascularization (CNV) causes a break in retina and leads to leaking of fluid and scarring
    - Geographic atrophy: Progressive atrophy of RPE, choriocapillaris, and photoreceptors associated with severe vision loss (late form of NARMD)
  - Currently, many hypotheses are being postulated about origin of degeneration
    - Genetic hypothesis
      - Single nucleotide polymorphism in complement factor H (*CFH*) is thought to lead to a dysregulation in innate complement system
      - Other genetic polymorphisms associated with NARMD include *APOE* and *FBLN5* genes, which are involved in extracellular matrix deposition
    - Choroidal hypoperfusion hypothesis: Decreased choroidal blood flow leads to impairment of waste outflow from RPE and delivery of oxygen to retina
    - Barrier hypothesis: Increased thickness of Bruch membrane impedes flow of nutrients from choroid and blocks exchange of waste from RPE
    - Lipofuscin/lysosomal failure hypothesis: Dysfunction of lysosomal enzymatic degradation of RPE byproducts causes accumulation of oxidative damaging substances
    - RPE response to injury hypothesis: Deposit formation is caused by chronic RPE damage from cellular responses to noxious stimuli
  - Risk factors: Age (late-stage NARMD rare < 55 years), family history, white race, Asian race, obesity, smoking, and diet low in vitamin A, C, E, and zinc

Epidemiology

- Incidence: ~ 14% 15-year cumulative incidence for early NARMD and 3% for late NARMD in adults aged 43-86 years
- Prevalence: > 20% of those > 60 years affected
- Predicted that by 2020 nearly 80 million people will be affected by NARMD

PRESENTATION

Symptoms

- Asymptomatic in early NARMD
- Progression over years leads to blurred vision, metamorphopsia, difficulty reading (especially in low light), glare, and difficulty with dark and light adaptation

Exam Findings

- Fundus exam
  - Drusen are seen as yellow excrescences beneath RPE
    - Typically found in posterior pole; however, may be seen in any portion of retina
  - Small: < 63 μm, round, with discrete borders (also referred to as "hard")
  - Intermediate: 63-125 μm with nondiscrete borders (when > 63 μm, referred to as "soft")
  - Large: > 125 μm
  - Diffuse: When hard and soft coalesce and lose discrete borders
  - Areas of hyperpigmentation and hypopigmentation of RPE
  - Geographic atrophy: 1 or more large areas of depigmentation due to atrophy of RPE

DIFFERENTIAL DIAGNOSIS

Angioid Streaks

- Subretinal cracks in RPE radiating from nerve showing underlying choroid; usually associated with Paget, Ehlers-Danlos, pseudoxanthoma elasticum, or sickle cell anemia

Exudative Age-Related Macular Degeneration

- CNV leads to leaking of fluid into retina and scarring

Best Disease

- Typically has an egg yolk appearance and presents early in age

Stargardt Disease

- Early onset; diffuse lipofuscin on autofluorescence imaging resulting in silent choroid on fluorescein angiography (FA)

Central Serous Chorioretinopathy

- RPE changes without drusen

Pattern Dystrophy

- Typically affects younger patients

NONEXUDATIVE AGE-RELATED MACULAR DEGENERATION

Hydrochloroquine Toxicity
- Determine any rheumatological diseases affecting patient and review medication list
- Fundus exam displays bull's-eye maculopathy

EVALUATION/WORK-UP

Labs
- No routine blood work is recommended

Pathology
- Drusen
  - Histopathologically seen as focal areas of eosinophilic material between basement membrane of RPE and Bruch membrane
  - Stain positive with periodic acid-Schiff (PAS)

Imaging
- FA
  - For the exclusion of CNV and to identify location if CNV has occurred
  - Drusen and areas of RPE atrophy display hyperfluorescence
- Optical coherence tomography (OCT)
  - May be used to visualize drusen and rule out other causes of visual acuity loss
  - May detect early signs of neovascularization
- Fundus autofluorescence
  - Identifies geographic atrophy by area of decreased autofluorescence

TREATMENT

Medical
- No current treatment exists for reversal of disease
- All persons ≥ 55 years are advised to have a dilated eye exam
- Patient who has extensive intermediate-sized drusen, at least 1 large drusen, noncentral GA in at least 1 eye, advanced NARMD, or vision loss due to NARMD in 1 eye should take a supplement of antioxidants plus zinc
- Age-related eye disease study (AREDS)
  - Design
    - Randomized clinical trial
    - 3,640 participants, aged 55-80 years, with varying degrees of NARMD were assigned to take a placebo, antioxidants (vitamin C, vitamin E, and beta carotene), zinc, or both antioxidants and zinc
    - Advancement of disease and visual acuity were determined after 5 years
  - Main outcomes
    - Statistically significant decrease (5%, 6%, 8%) in progression to advanced NARMD was observed in participants taking antioxidants, zinc, or both compared to placebo, respectively (these results were found in participants with larger drusen or noncentral GA)
    - Participants taking antioxidants, zinc, or both, compared to placebo, retained a better visual acuity
    - Higher category of NARMD, or greater pathology, was correlated with an increased chance of progression to advanced NARMD
- AREDS 2
  - Design
    - Randomized clinical trial
    - 4,203 participants, aged 50-85 years, with bilateral large drusen or large drusen in 1 eye
    - Participants were randomized to take lutein + zeaxanthin (carotenoids), omega-3 long-chain polyunsaturated fatty acids (docosahexaenoic acid [DHA] + eicosapentaenoic acid [EPA]), or both
  - Main outcomes
    - Supplemental lutein + zeaxanthin, DHA + EPA, or both did not further reduce the risk of progression to advanced NARMD

Surgical
- No laser or surgical option has been shown to break up drusen and stop progression of NARMD
- Implantable miniature telescope can be used for atrophy

Follow-Up
- Daily Amsler grid tests should be performed by patient to detect an advancement to exudative macular degeneration
- Patients should have regular follow-up to watch disease progression and assess risk for conversion to exudative macular degeneration

Prognosis
- Progression of disease is unavoidable even with daily supplement use
- Following data were seen in placebo group of the AREDS trial
  - Patients with small drusen, pigment abnormalities, or at least 1 intermediate-sized drusen (but not extensive in area) had only 1.3% probability of progression to advanced NARMD in 5 years
  - Patients with extensive intermediate drusen, large drusen, or noncentral GA had 18% probability of progression
  - Patients with large drusen in each eye or noncentral GA in at least 1 eye had a 27% probability of progression
  - Patients with advanced NARMD in 1 eye or vision loss due to nonadvanced NARMD in 1 eye had a 43% probability of progression to advanced NARMD in the other eye

SELECTED REFERENCES

1. Age-Related Eye Disease Study 2 Research Group: Lutein + zeaxanthin and omega-3 fatty acids for age-related macular degeneration: the Age-Related Eye Disease Study 2 (AREDS2) randomized clinical trial. JAMA. 309(19):2005-15, 2013
2. Lim LS et al: Age-related macular degeneration. Lancet. 379(9827):1728-38, 2012
3. Mettu PS et al: Retinal pigment epithelium response to oxidant injury in the pathogenesis of early age-related macular degeneration. Mol Aspects Med. 33(4):376-98, 2012
4. Bird AC: Therapeutic targets in age-related macular disease. J Clin Invest. 120(9):3033-41, 2010

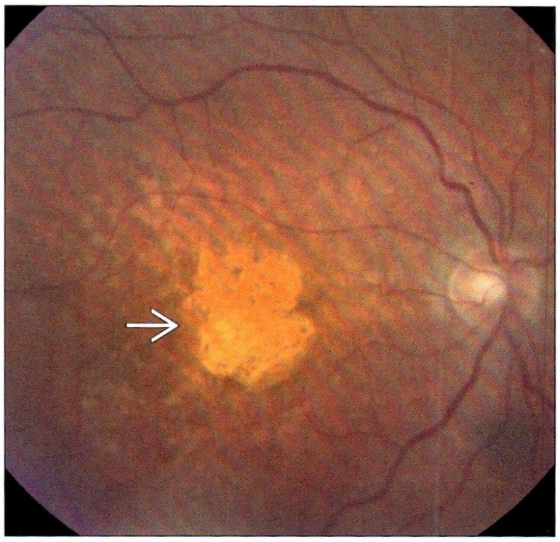

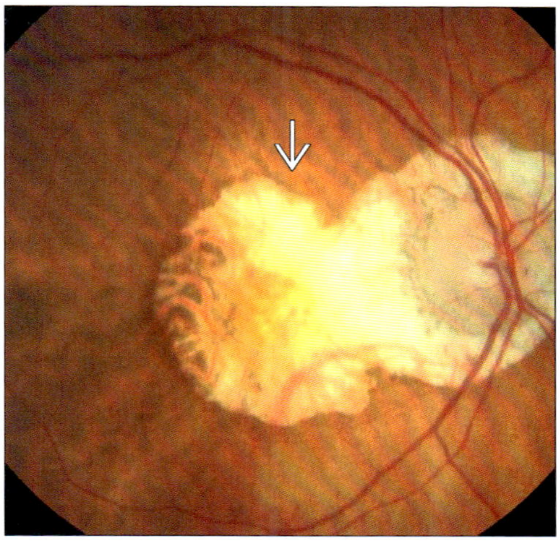

(Left) *This fundus photo shows the beginning of geographic atrophy with the disappearance of the drusen and a large area of hypopigmentation →. Geographic atrophy is the hallmark finding of advanced macular degeneration and is typically associated with poor vision.* ***(Right)*** *This fundus photo shows advanced geographic atrophy → in end-stage macular degeneration.*

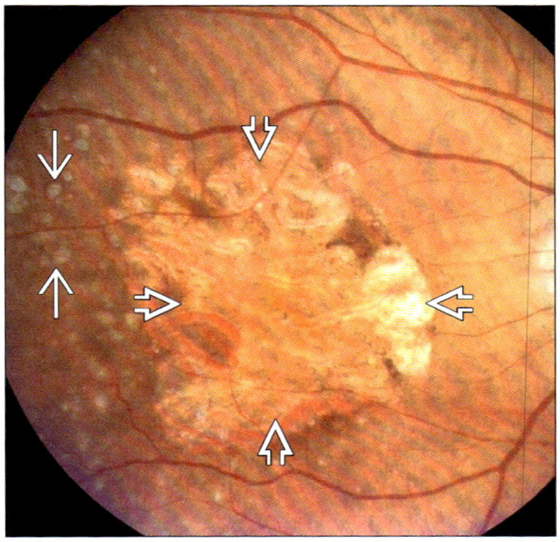

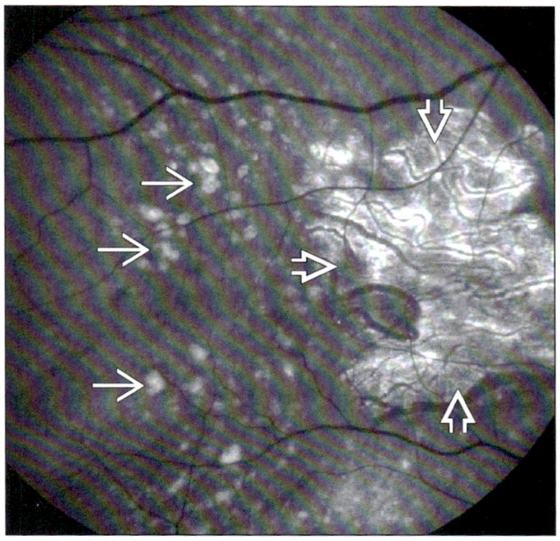

(Left) *This fundus photograph demonstrates geographic atrophy seen in advanced macular degeneration →. Multiple drusen are also present further in the periphery →.* ***(Right)*** *This fluorescein angiography image shows the same eye with geographic atrophy → and diffuse drusen → further in the periphery. The area of geographic atrophy is notable for hyperfluorescence.*

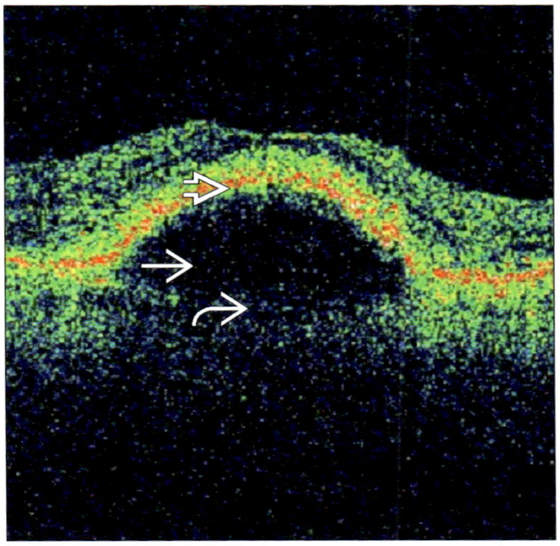

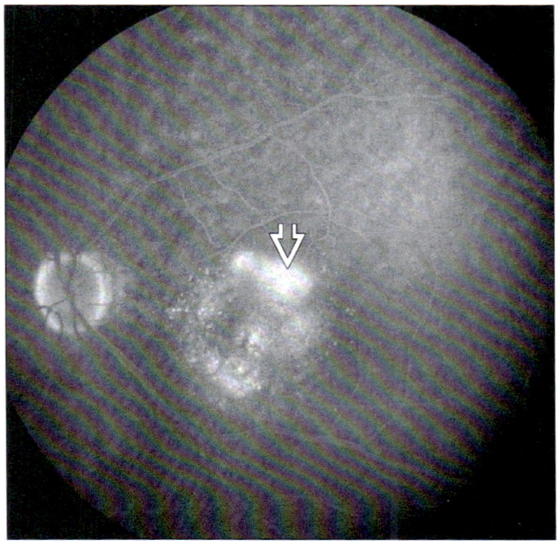

(Left) *This OCT shows an example of a retinal pigment epithelial detachment →. The retinal pigment epithelium (RPE) → is elevated and separated from the underlying Bruch membrane →. It is important to evaluate for RPE detachment in patients with macular degeneration as this is typically a sign of conversion to exudative age-related macular degeneration.* ***(Right)*** *This fluorescein angiography image shows an RPE detachment. Note the hyperfluorescence →.*

MALIGNANT MELANOMA OF THE CHOROID

Key Facts

Demographics
- Often affects those of northern European descent
- Median age of diagnosis: 55 years
- Most common primary intraocular malignant tumor
- 2nd most common site of malignant melanoma

Presentation
- Most patients are asymptomatic
- Some patients may present with visual loss
- Found on routine ophthalmic examination
- Pigmented dome-shaped or collar button-shaped tumor with exudative retinal detachment

Differential Diagnosis
- Metastasis
- Choroidal nevi
- Choroidal hemangioma
- Retinal pigment epithelium hypertrophy/hyperplasia

Evaluation/Work-Up
- Indirect ophthalmoscopy
  - Most common tool to detect melanoma of choroid

Treatment
- Medium and large choroidal melanomas
  - Enucleation
  - Sclerouvectomy
  - Plaque brachytherapy: Spares eye
  - External beam charged-particle radiation therapy (e.g., proton beam)
- Small choroidal melanoma
  - Plaque radiation therapy

Prognosis
- 5-year survival = 25%
- Liver is most common site of metastasis (90%)

__(Left)__ This fundus photograph shows a medium-sized, dark, temporally located choroidal melanoma ➔. The presence of visual loss symptoms negatively affects survival. Increased age and extrascleral extension are also associated with a negative prognosis. __(Right)__ This fundus photograph shows a dark, temporally located melanoma ➔. The large tumor size and proximity to the optic nerve is associated with a poor prognosis.

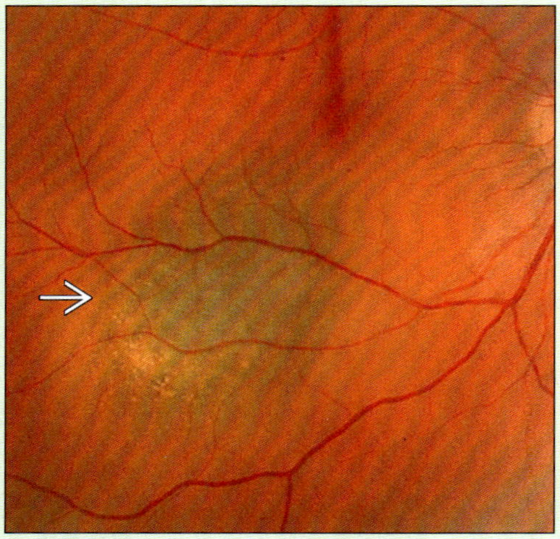

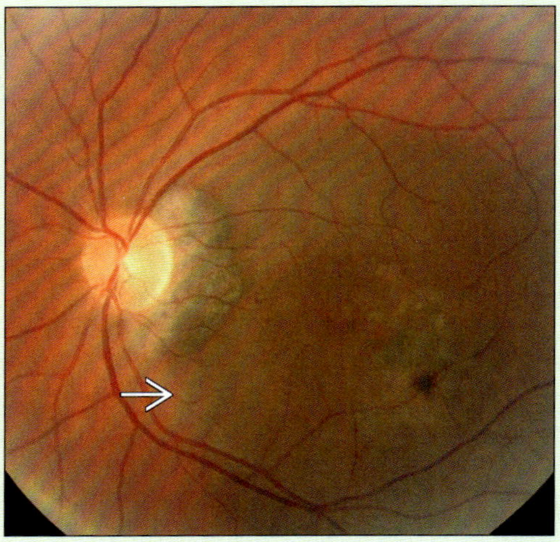

__(Left)__ This fundus photo shows an elliptical melanoma after treatment with radiation. A dark ring of RPE hypertrophy ➔ surrounds an area of radiation-induced atrophy. __(Right)__ This gross ocular cross section shows a dark-staining dome-shaped choroidal tumor located in the posterior choroid ➔. A smaller choroidal tumor is noted ➔. Retinal detachment is also present ➔.

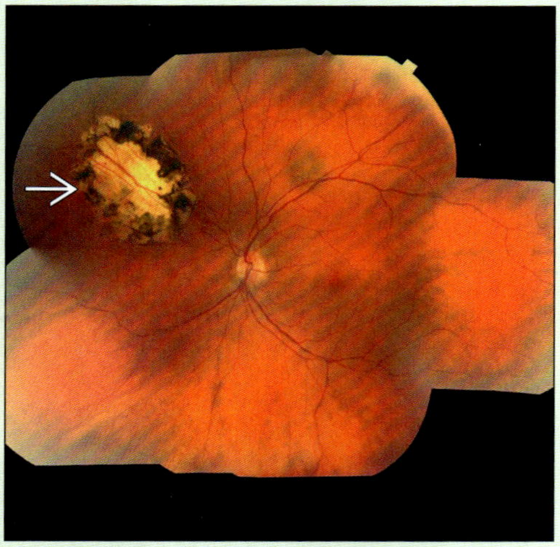

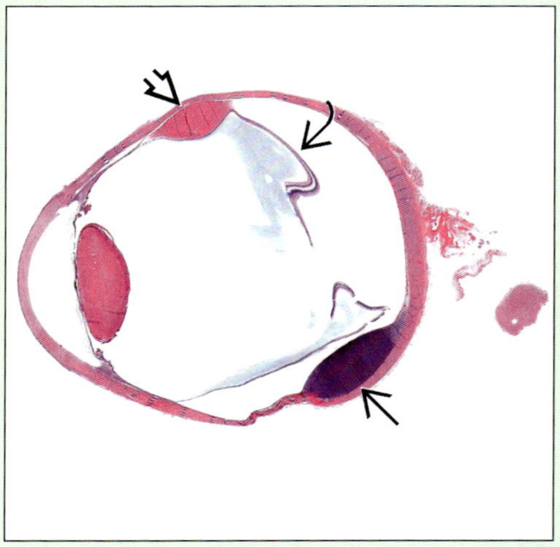

MALIGNANT MELANOMA OF THE CHOROID

DEMOGRAPHICS

Etiology/Risk Factors

- Nevi on skin
- Degree of pigmentation
- Family history of melanoma
- Important risk factors for development of choroidal nevi into melanoma
  - Tumor thickness > 2 mm
  - Subretinal fluid
  - Absence of surrounding halo
  - Tumor margin touching optic nerve
  - Symptoms of visual loss, flashes, floaters
  - Orange pigment
  - Ultrasonographic hollowness

Epidemiology

- Often affects those of northern European descent
- Median age of diagnosis: 55 years
- Most common primary intraocular malignant tumor
- 2nd most common site of malignant melanoma
- 1 in 500 choroidal nevi will evolve into a choroidal melanoma

PRESENTATION

Symptoms

- Most patients are asymptomatic
  - Found on routine ophthalmic examination
- Visual loss due to
  - Tumor moving onto fovea
  - Exudative retinal detachment
  - Tumor contact with lens
- Photopsia

Exam Findings

- Pigmented dome-shaped or collar button-shaped tumor with exudative retinal detachment
- Usually pigmented lesions
  - Lipofuscin: Orange pigment
  - However, drusen probably indicate benignity

DIFFERENTIAL DIAGNOSIS

Metastasis

- Multiple choroidal tumors

Choroidal Nevi

- Slate gray and relatively flat

Choroidal Hemangioma

- Gives fundus the typical tomato-ketchup appearance
- Usually, flat lesion
- May induce retinal detachment

Retinal Pigment Epithelium Hypertrophy/Hyperplasia

- Dark black pigmentation

EVALUATION/WORK-UP

Imaging

- A-mode ultrasonography
  - Medium to low internal echoes with smooth attenuation
  - Oscillation of height in echoes within lesions may correspond to patient's pulse
    - Indicates presence of vascularity of lesion
- B-mode ultrasonography
  - Acoustical silent zone within tumor
  - Choroidal excavation
  - Shadowing in orbit
  - Mushroom-shaped lesion
- Indirect ophthalmoscopy
  - Most common tool to detect melanoma of choroid

TREATMENT

Medical

- Choroidal nevi showing no features of disease
  - Monitored biannually
- Small choroidal melanoma in posterior fundus
  - Photocoagulation
  - Photodynamic therapy
  - Plaque radiation therapy
  - External beam charged-particle radiation therapy
- Medium and large choroidal melanomas
  - External beam charged-particle radiation therapy
    - 2x as expensive as enucleation
    - Helium ions or protons
  - Gamma knife surgery

Surgical

- Medium and large choroidal melanomas
  - Plaque brachytherapy: Spares eye
  - Enucleation
    - Prosthesis may be used after socket is rehabilitated
  - Sclerouvectomy
    - Remove entire tumor and adjacent sclera and retina
    - Scleral patch graft
  - Orbital exenteration
    - Radical treatment for cases with orbital extension

Follow-Up

- Periodic observation of choroidal nevus

Prognosis

- Melanoma size is most important factor related to prognosis
- 5-year survival = 25%
- Liver is most common site of metastasis (90%) (CT abdomen is often necessary)
  - Lung (24%)
  - Bone (16%)
- Prognosis is poor for those with chromosome 3 abnormalities (particularly monosomy 3)
  - ~ 95% metastasis by 5 years

SELECTED REFERENCES

1. Singh P et al: Choroidal melanoma. Oman J Ophthalmol. 5(1):3-9, 2012
2. Laver NV et al: Ocular melanoma. Arch Pathol Lab Med. 134(12):1778-84, 2010
3. Shields CL et al: Ocular melanoma: relatively rare but requiring respect. Clin Dermatol. 27(1):122-33, 2009

OVERVIEW OF COMMON RETINAL TOXICITIES

TERMINOLOGY

Abbreviations

- Hydroxychloroquine (HCQ)
- Chloroquine (CQ)
- Interferon (IFN)

OVERVIEW

HCQ and CQ

- Antimalarial drugs used in treatment of systemic lupus erythematosus (SLE), rheumatoid arthritis (RA), and other rheumatological diseases
- HCQ is less toxic than CQ
- Pathogenesis
  - Drugs bind to melanin in pigmented ocular structures (e.g., retinal pigment epithelium [RPE]) and can stay in body even after cessation
  - Accumulation of pigment-laden cells may cause degenerative changes to RPE and exacerbate photoreceptor destruction

Tamoxifen

- Selective estrogen-receptor modulator (SERM) used as adjuvant therapy for breast cancer
- Small crystalline deposits occur in nerve fiber and inner plexiform layers near fovea and may be accompanied by edema

Recombinant α-Interferon

- Therapy for chronic hepatitis C
- Pathogenesis is unknown

EXAM FINDINGS

HCQ and CQ

- Patients present with difficulty reading or other fine visual acuity tasks
- Central or paracentral scotomas
- Fundus exam
  - Earliest findings display irregular macular pigmentation and blunting of foveal reflex
  - Bull's-eye maculopathy: Bilateral and appears later in progression of disease
    - Hyperpigmentation of macula is surrounded by concentric depigmentation and followed by another layer of hyperpigmentation
  - Retinal arterioles show attenuation with disc pallor
- Automated threshold visual field testing with a white 10-2 pattern aids in diagnosis; multifocal electroretinopathy (MF-ERG) is alternative

Tamoxifen

- Small crystals typically do not affect VA; however, mild VA loss may occur with edema
- Foveal cystoid spaces may cause more significant visual loss
- Fundus exam
  - Small, white, refractile deposits seen in inner retina, particularly in perimacular area
  - Peripheral RPE pigmentary changes

IFN

- No visual symptoms or sequelae
- Fundus exam
  - Cotton-wool spots and retinal hemorrhages near optic disc
  - Unilateral or bilateral

IMAGING

HCQ and CQ

- Spectral-domain optical coherence tomography (SDOCT)
  - May show localized thinning of retinal layers in parafoveal region and loss of inner segment/outer segment (IS/OS) junction ("flying saucer" sign)
- Fundus autofluorescence (FAF)
  - May show subtle RPE defects with reduced autofluorescence, "bull's eye"
- Multifocal electroretinogram (mfERG)
  - May document localized paracentral ERG depression

Tamoxifen

- SDOCT
  - Cystoid spaces in fovea, loss of photoreceptors, and macular thinning

IFN

- Fluorescein angiography (FA)
  - Decreased fluorescence around area of ischemia from cotton-wool spots

TREATMENT

HCQ and CQ

- Medical
  - Stop medication (consult prescribing MD)
- Follow-up
  - Baseline examination within 1st year of use: Visual acuity (VA), dilated exam, visual field, and SDOCT
  - Annual screening exam after 5 years of use: Same as baseline

Tamoxifen

- Medical
  - Stop medication when visual impairment or macular edema is found (consult prescribing MD)
- Follow-up
  - Healthy, asymptomatic patients should be examined every 2 years and more frequently if symptomatic

IFN

- Medical
  - Retinopathy disappears spontaneously in most patients; therefore, unnecessary to stop IFN therapy
- Follow-up
  - No routine screening necessary

RELATED REFERENCES

1. Eisner A et al: Breast cancer medications and vision: effects of treatments for early-stage disease. Curr Eye Res. 36(10):867-85, 2011
2. Marmor MF et al: Revised recommendations on screening for chloroquine and hydroxychloroquine retinopathy. Ophthalmology. 118(2):415-22, 2011
3. Yam JC et al: Ocular toxicity of hydroxychloroquine. Hong Kong Med J. 12(4):294-304, 2006

ANATOMIC FEATURES

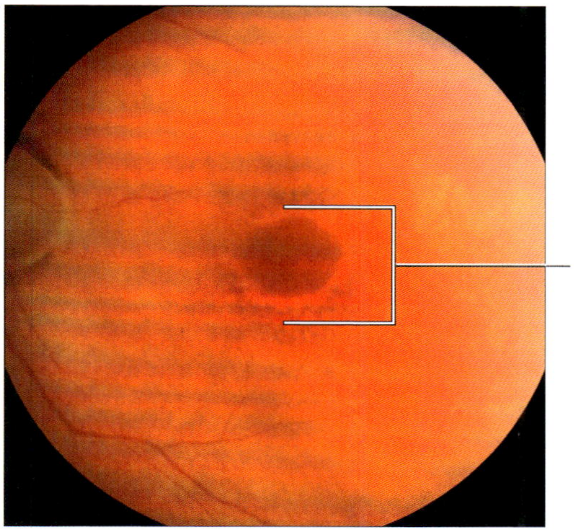

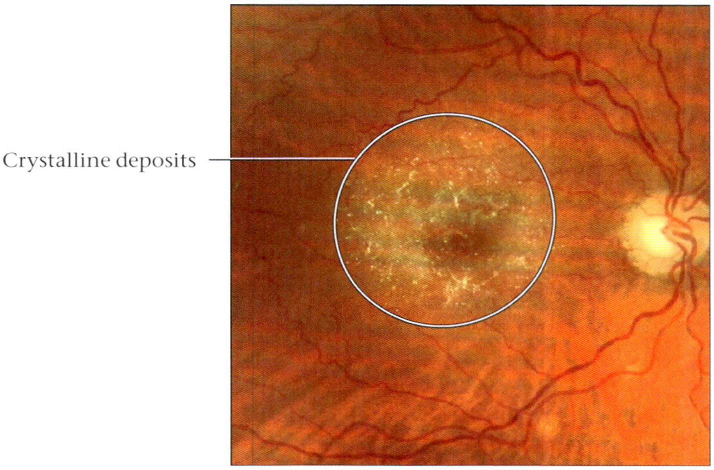

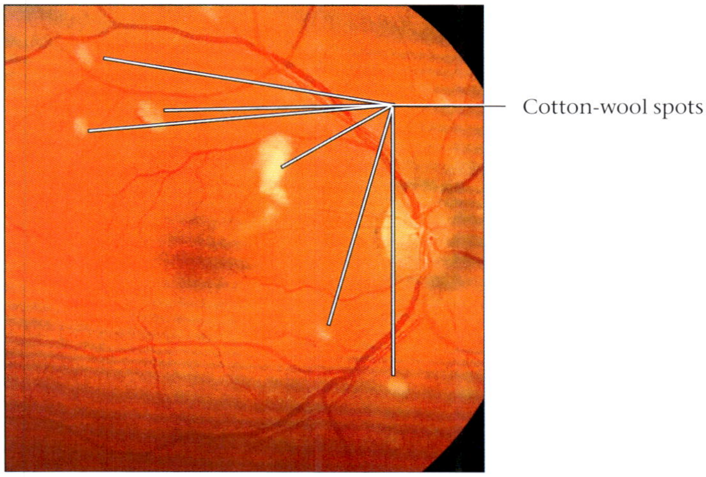

(Top) *This fundus photograph in a patient with chloroquine toxicity demonstrates a bull's-eye macular lesion, due to a zone of retinal pigment epithelium atrophy surrounded by a hyperpigmented ring.* ***(Middle)*** *This fundus photograph of a patient with crystalline maculopathy secondary to tamoxifen therapy shows many fine, yellow crystalline deposits visible in the region of the macula. Other medications that may induce this complication include canthaxanthin, methoxyflurane, or nitrofurantoin.* ***(Bottom)*** *This fundus photograph is of a patient with interferon retinopathy, characterized by cotton-wool spots due to focal areas of nonperfusion.*

CHOROIDAL DETACHMENT

Key Facts

Definitions

- Choroid
  - Meshwork of blood vessels and dense capillary beds located between retina and sclera
  - Nourishes and oxygenates outer portion of the retina and underlying structures
- Choroidal detachment
  - Separation of choroid from underlying sclera, creating a dome-shaped protrusion of the choroid and retina into center of the eye
  - Detachment of choroid from sclera is due to infiltration of fluid or blood into suprachoroidal space
  - "Kissing" choroidal detachment is caused when opposite sides of choroid are pushed inward toward center of globe
  - Can lead to major loss in visual acuity

Detachment Categorization

- Choroidal effusion (fluid)
  - Occurs when serous fluid fills suprachoroidal space, separating choroid from sclera
- Choroidal hemorrhage (blood)
  - Occurs when suprachoroidal space is filled with blood

Risk Factors

- Ocular
  - Hypotonia, uveitis, nanophthalmos, VKH, BDUMP
- Surgical
  - Intraocular/glaucoma surgery
  - Intense panretinal photocoagulation (PRP)
  - Retrobulbar anesthetic injection
- Systemic
  - Hypertension, uremia, diabetes
- General
  - Advanced age

*(**Left**) This fundus photo demonstrates a choroidal detachment. Note the course of the vessels as they travel over the detachment. This detachment is present in 360° of the fundus, which is typical for choroidal detachments. (**Right**) This fundus photo shows a choroidal detachment. The retina in the area of detachment in large part retains the coloring of normal retina. This is typical for choroidal detachment and can differentiate choroidal detachment from retinal detachment or retinoschisis.*

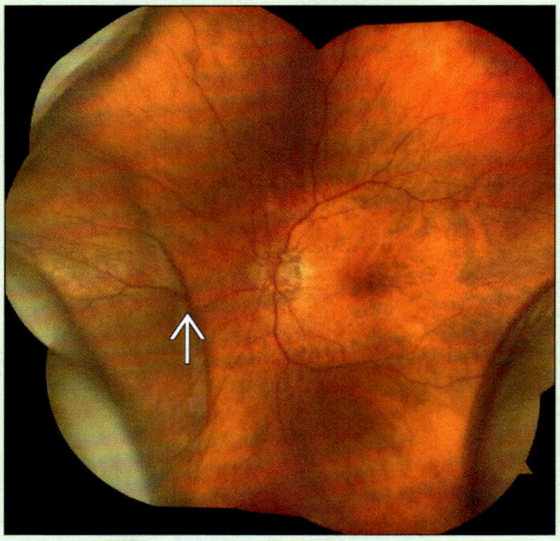

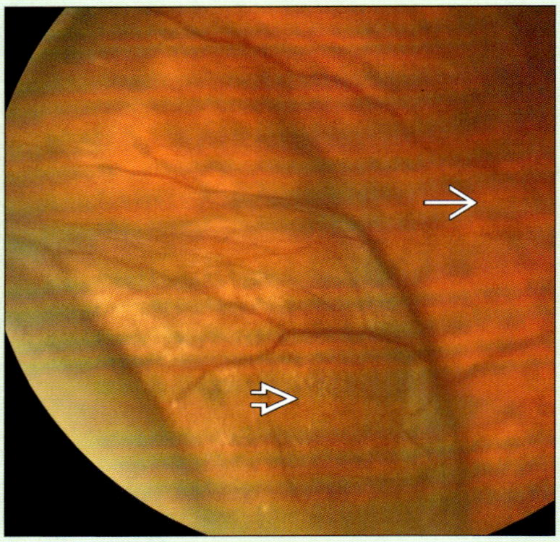

*(**Left**) This B-scan ultrasound shows an eye with a choroidal detachment. When the 2 opposite sides of choroid are further detached and in closer proximity, this gives rise to the classic finding of "kissing" choroidals. (**Right**) This fundus photo demonstrates a retinal detachment. An important finding that can help distinguish a retinal detachment from a choroidal detachment is pallor of the detached retina.*

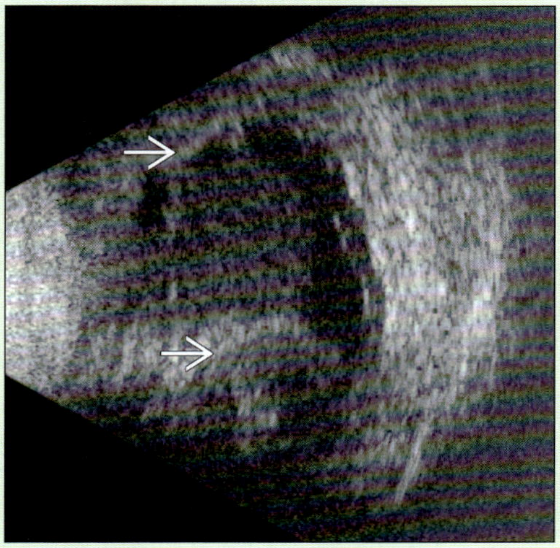

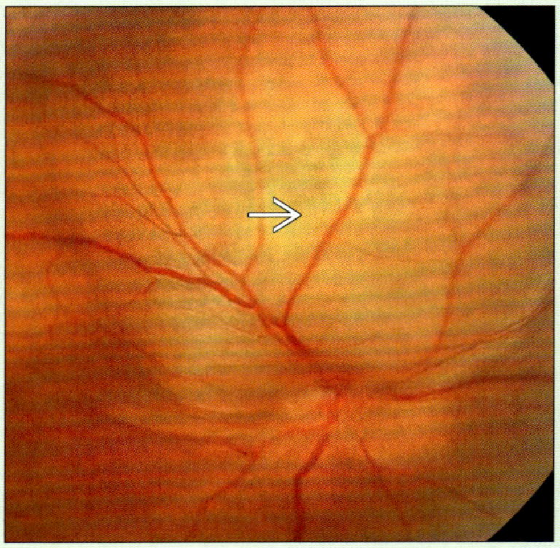

CHOROIDAL DETACHMENT

INTRODUCTION

Abbreviations

- Choroidal detachment (CD)

DEMOGRAPHICS

Etiology/Risk Factors

- Ocular
  - Hypotonia
  - Uveitis (e.g., Vogt-Koyanagi-Harada syndrome)
  - Nanophthalmos
  - Bilateral diffuse uveal melanocytic proliferation (BDUMP), a paraneoplastic syndrome
- Surgical
  - Intraocular surgery
  - Intense panretinal photocoagulation (PRP)
  - Glaucoma surgery (due to surgical induction of intraocular hypotony)
  - Retrobulbar anesthetic injection
- Systemic
  - Hypertension, uremia, diabetes

Epidemiology

- Occurs in ~ 1:10,000 people
- Limited choroidal hemorrhage occurs in ~ 2% of extracapsular cataract extractions
- Limited choroidal hemorrhage occurs in > 3% of intracapsular cataract extractions

PRESENTATION

Symptoms

- May be asymptomatic
- Loss of visual fields if severe CD
- Pain in hemorrhagic CD and severe choroidal effusions
- Occasionally, nausea and vomiting

Exam Findings

- Low IOP caused by detachment of ciliary body
- Flattening or shallowing of anterior compartment due to increased posterior pressure
- Anterior displacement of iris, lens, and vitreous humor due to increased posterior pressure
- Darkening of red reflex
- "Kissing" choroidal detachment

Complications

- Phthisis bulbi
- Retinal detachment (RD)

DIFFERENTIAL DIAGNOSIS

Retinal Detachment

- CD can be differentiated from RD by solid, even, and smooth surface, with easily visualized retinal vessels
- CD often maintains darker, more brown color

Choroidal Malignant Melanoma

- Often considered due to dark appearance of retina at CD site
- Orbital &/or ocular CT scan can differentiate between solid tumor and detached choroid/retina

EVALUATION/WORK-UP

Imaging

- B-scan ultrasound
  - Can be used to visualize fluid filling suprachoroidal space
  - CD will appear as convexing into center of globe
  - Useful to differentiate between serous (choroidal effusion) and hemorrhagic (choroidal hemorrhage) CDs
    - Serous CD will reveal a "clear" space on ultrasound between detached choroid and sclera
- Funduscopy
  - Convexing dome shape of choroid and retina
  - Often difficult to differentiate between RD
- Transillumination
  - Hemorrhagic CD will block transillumination more than a serous CD

TREATMENT

Medical

- Important to treat underlying disorder
- Topical corticosteroids
  - Prednisolone
- Cycloplegics
  - Atropine
- Mannitol IV if CD occurs during surgery

Surgical

- Drainage (sclerostomy & paracentesis)
- Can create partial thickness scleral windows
- Surgical drainage should be considered if patient is experiencing
  - Major choroidal hemorrhage coupled with extreme pain
  - Extreme IOP that causes persistent anterior chamber deformation
  - Hemorrhage extending into vitreous cavity or into suprachoroidal space directly beneath macula

Follow-Up

- Monitor
  - Visual acuity
  - Flattening of anterior chamber
  - IOP
  - Blood pressure

SELECTED REFERENCES

1. Elagouz M et al: Uveal effusion syndrome. Surv Ophthalmol. 55(2):134-45, 2010
2. Yang SS et al: Massive spontaneous choroidal hemorrhage. Retina. 23(2):139-44, 2003
3. Tabandeh H et al: Suprachoroidal hemorrhage during pars plana vitrectomy. Curr Opin Ophthalmol. 12(3):179-85, 2001
4. Mafee MF et al: Magnetic resonance imaging and computed tomography of choroidal detachment. Acta Radiol Suppl. 369:327-30. 1986
5. Bellows AR et al: Choroidal detachment. Clinical manifestation, therapy and mechanism of formation. Ophthalmology. 88(11):1107-15, 1981

CYSTOID MACULAR EDEMA

Key Facts

Introduction

- Retinal vascular hyperpermeability is causative
- Pseudophakic cystoid macular edema (PCME) (a.k.a. Irvine-Gass syndrome) subtypes
  - Angiographic: Can be diagnosed with fluorescein angiography
  - Clinical: Decreased visual acuity in addition to ophthalmic and angiographic evidence of edema
  - Acute: Occurring within 6 months post surgery
  - Chronic: Occurring after 6 months post surgery
- Nonpseudophakic CME (usually diabetic or uveitic)

Demographics

- Risks: Diabetes, age-related macular degeneration, uveitis, retinitis pigmentosa, retinal vein occlusion, prostaglandin analogue eyedrops, niacin

Presentation

- Painless edema of macula associated with blurred central vision often 4-6 weeks post surgery

Evaluation/Work-Up

- Fundus fluorescein angiography (FFA) and optical coherence tomography (OCT)

Treatment

- Topical and periocular NSAIDs and corticosteroids are first-line treatment options for PCME
- Sub-Tenon injection, retrobulbar or intravitreal corticosteroid, or anti-VEGF therapy may be beneficial in cases refractory to topical therapy
- Acetazolamide (or methazolamide) and hyperbaric oxygen are targeted treatments directed toward the disrupted blood-retinal barrier
- Pars plana vitrectomy may also be used in cases of chronic CME refractory to medical therapy

__(Left)__ This OCT image is a cross section of the central retina in a patient with cystoid macular edema. Note the cystoid formation and fluid accumulation ➔. __(Right)__ This is a fluorescein angiography image of a patient with macular edema. Note the petalloid accumulation of dye within and around the macula ➔, indicating macular edema. Fundus fluorescein angiography allows for detection of disruption to the blood-retinal barrier and is the diagnostic test of choice.

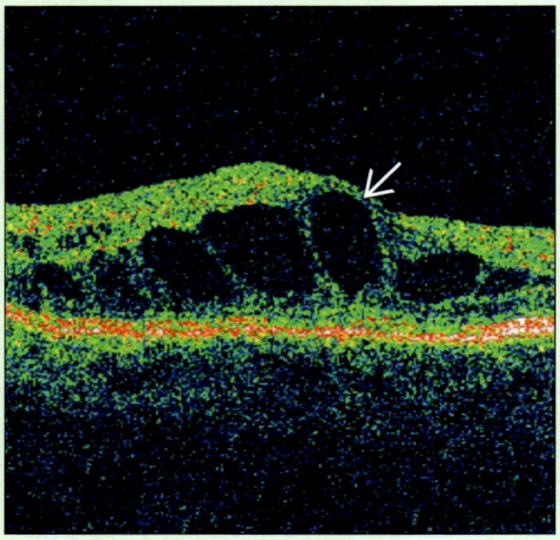

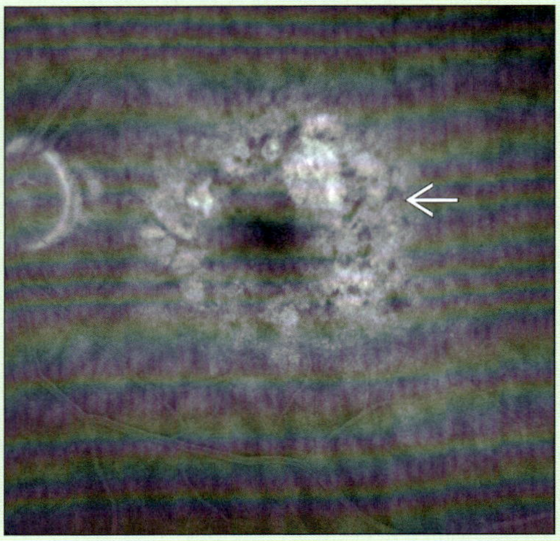

__(Left)__ This is a fluorescein angiography image of a patient with macular edema. Note the accumulation of dye ➔, indicating macular edema. __(Right)__ This fundus photo features macular edema ➔. The edema results from fluid buildup, which progresses to thickening of the layers of the retinal tissue. Macular edema is seen with many conditions, including diabetes, vein occlusion, uveitis, and as a postoperative complication of cataract surgery.

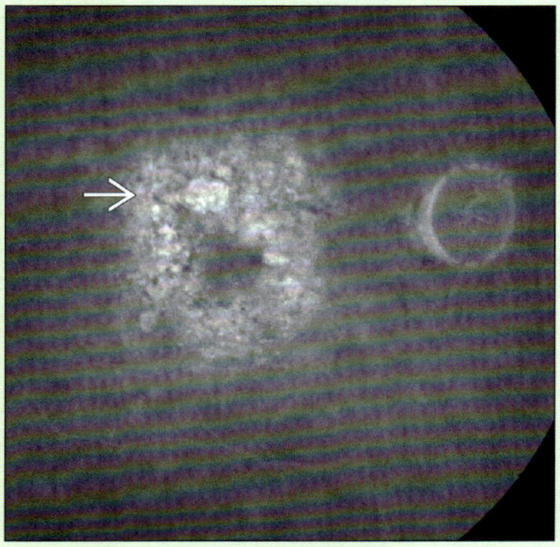

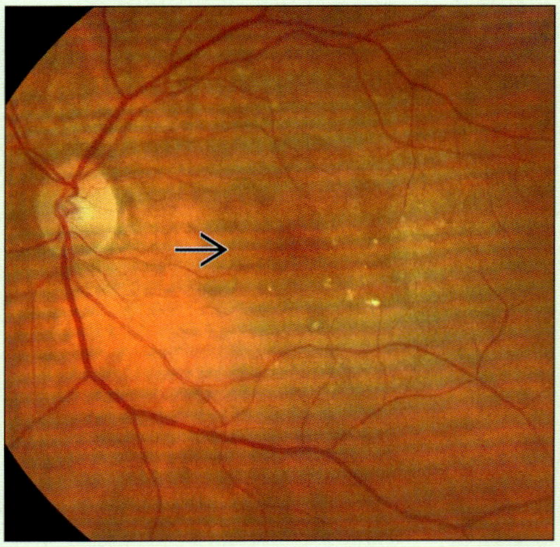

CYSTOID MACULAR EDEMA

INTRODUCTION

Abbreviations
- Cystoid macular edema (CME)

Definitions
- Accumulation of fluid in inner plexiform layer of central retina (macula) secondary to increased retinal capillary permeability
  - Cystoid describes cystic appearance of edema, though it is not truly cystic

Subtypes
- Pseudophakic cystoid macular edema (PCME) a.k.a. Irvine-Gass syndrome
  - Angiographic: Can be diagnosed with fluorescein angiography and may not be associated with visual impairment
  - Clinical: Decreased visual acuity in addition to ophthalmic and angiographic evidence of edema
  - Acute: Occurring within 6 months post surgery
  - Chronic: Occurring after 6 months post surgery
- Nonpseudophakic cystoid macular edema

DEMOGRAPHICS

Etiology/Risk Factors
- Risk factors include diabetes, age-related macular degeneration, pars planitis, retinitis pigmentosa, retinal venous occlusion, prostaglandin E2, nicotinic acid, and niacin

Epidemiology
- Incidence of clinical PCME ranges from 2-8% after cataract surgery

PRESENTATION

Symptoms
- Painless swelling and thickening of central retina associated with blurred central vision
  - Clinical PCME occurs 4-6 weeks post-cataract surgery

Exam Findings
- Biomicroscopy shows retinal thickening, loss of foveal depression, and cystic hyporeflective lesions
- Fluorescein angiography (FA) may demonstrate retinal telangiectasias, capillary dilation, and perifoveal capillary leakage in a petaloid pattern

DIFFERENTIAL DIAGNOSIS

Diabetic Macular Edema
- Macular edema due to disruption of blood-retinal barrier secondary to chronic hyperglycemia from poorly controlled diabetes
- Retinal thickening with focal macular edema associated with hard, yellow exudates

Age-Related Macular Degeneration
- Drusen, atrophy, and CNV can be distinguished from CME by OCT or FA

EVALUATION/WORK-UP

Labs
- CBC, lipid panel, and fasting blood glucose level evaluation if diabetic or retinal vein occlusion etiology is suspected

Imaging
- Fundus fluorescein angiography (FFA) is diagnostic procedure of choice
  - FFA can help rule out other causes of CME
- Optical coherence tomography visualizes fluid-filled spaces in retina and has become a more commonly used imaging technique
  - Can be used to quantify amount of edema and monitor treatment response

TREATMENT

Medical
- Topical and periocular nonsteroidal anti-inflammatory drugs (NSAIDs) and corticosteroids are first-line treatment options for PCME
  - Corticosteroids inhibit prostaglandin and leukotriene formation and reduce prostaglandin synthesis and inflammation at the macula
  - Prophylactic NSAID administration (e.g., ketorolac, bromfenac, nepafenac) may be beneficial in high-risk patients; should treat for 3 months
  - Sub-Tenon injection, retrobulbar or intravitreal corticosteroid, or anti-VEGF therapy may be beneficial in cases refractory to topical therapy
- Acetazolamide (or methazolamide) and hyperbaric oxygen are targeted treatments directed toward the disrupted blood-retinal barrier
  - Carbonic anhydrase inhibitors increase the transport of fluid across retinal pigment epithelium

Surgical
- YAG laser may be used to remove vitreous adhesions to surgical wound in cases of postoperative CME
- Pars plana vitrectomy may also be used in cases of chronic CME refractory to medical therapy

SELECTED REFERENCES

1. Yonekawa Y et al: Pseudophakic cystoid macular edema. Curr Opin Ophthalmol. 23(1):26-32, 2012
2. Moroi SE et al: Cystoid macular edema associated with latanoprost therapy in a case series of patients with glaucoma and ocular hypertension. Ophthalmology. 106(5):1024-9, 1999
3. Flach AJ: The incidence, pathogenesis and treatment of cystoid macular edema following cataract surgery. Trans Am Ophthalmol Soc. 96:557-634, 1998

EPIRETINAL MEMBRANE

Key Facts

Introduction

- Proliferations of specific cells at the vitreoretinal junction that have contractile properties and can distort the retina
- Also referred to as epimacular membrane, macular pucker, cellophane maculopathy, and epiretinal fibrosis

Demographics

- Etiologies: Idiopathic, blunt or penetrating ocular trauma, vitreous inflammatory conditions, retinal vascular diseases, or longstanding vitreous hemorrhage; postoperative complications, or retinopexy
- Risk factors: Age, hypercholesterolemia, history of smoking, arteriovenous nicking, and narrow arteriolar diameter

Presentation

- Symptoms include decreased visual acuity, metamorphopsia, central photopsia, macropsia, and micropsia
- Fundus exam: Translucent membrane, glistening light reflex, irregular wrinkling of the inner retinal surface, tortuosity of the paramacular vessels, macular pucker, and macular pseudohole

Evaluation/Work-Up

- Optical coherence tomography (OCT): Determines the presence or absence of an epiretinal membrane (ERM), which is a hyperreflective band on anterior retinal surface

Treatment

- Surgery involves 3 main steps: Pars plana subtotal vitrectomy, ERM peeling, inner limiting membrane (ILM) peeling

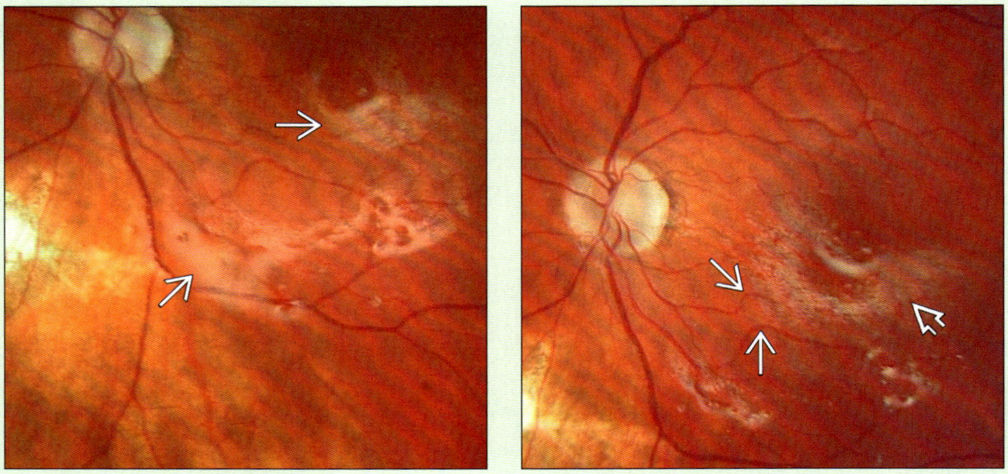

*(**Left**) This fundus photo shows the eye of a patient with epiretinal membrane. Note the translucent appearance of the epiretinal membrane ➔. (**Right**) The epiretinal membrane is displayed here ➔. Also note the tortuous path of the blood vessels ➔ due to contraction of the membrane.*

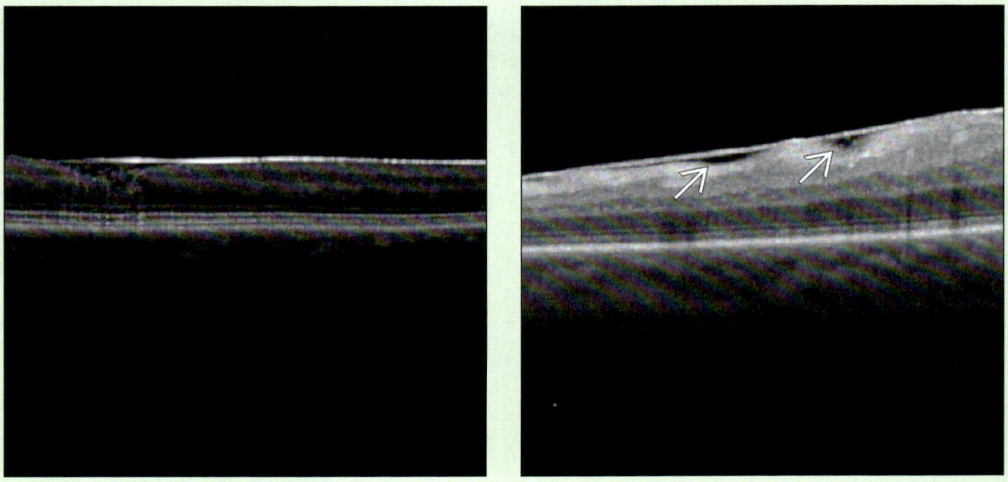

*(**Left**) This OCT image shows the eye of a patient with epiretinal membrane. The epiretinal membrane appears as a bright white layer on top of the retina. (**Right**) Seen here are 2 different areas of retinal puckering due to the epiretinal membrane contraction ➔. OCT is a good study to pinpoint the membrane and monitor preoperatively and postoperatively.*

EPIRETINAL MEMBRANE

INTRODUCTION

Abbreviations
- Epiretinal membrane (ERM)

Definitions
- Proliferations of specific cells at the vitreoretinal junction that have contractile properties and can distort retina
  - Also referred to as epimacular membrane, macular pucker, cellophane maculopathy, and epiretinal fibrosis

DEMOGRAPHICS

Etiology/Risk Factors
- Pathogenesis
  - Primary: Idiopathic
  - Secondary: Blunt or penetrating ocular trauma, vitreous inflammatory conditions, retinal vascular diseases, or longstanding vitreous hemorrhage
  - Iatrogenic: Postoperative complications or retinopexy
  - ERMs develop predominantly at sites where Müller cells proliferate; cells migrate onto inner surface of retina and extend processes into vitreous cavity
  - Growth factors in the vitreous induce a proliferation of the ERM by causing changes in glial and pigment epithelium cells
  - As membrane differentiates and grows, vitreal factors cause contraction of membrane and thus traction on adherent retina
- Risk factors: Age, hypercholesterolemia, history of smoking, arteriovenous nicking, narrow arteriolar diameter, PVD, retinal tear

Epidemiology
- Prevalence is ~ 7-11%
- 5-year incidence is ~ 5%
- Age: Prevalence peaks between 70-80 years and is rare before 60 years

PRESENTATION

Symptoms
- Patients are asymptomatic with the earliest and mildest form of ERM known as cellophane maculopathy
- With progression and contraction of retina, patients may develop decreased visual acuity, metamorphopsia, central photopsia, macropsia, or micropsia

Exam Findings
- Fundus exam
  - Early
    - Translucent membrane seen as glistening light reflex
  - Limited contraction
    - Irregular wrinkling of inner retinal surface
    - Fine, radiating folds seen as striae extend outward from contracted membrane
    - Tortuosity of paramacular vessels
  - Thicker, more contracted ERM
    - Membranes have a thick opaque/gray appearance (particularly after retinal detachment)
    - Macular pucker
    - Retinal edema
    - Small hemorrhages
    - Cotton-wool spots
    - Macular pseudohole

DIFFERENTIAL DIAGNOSIS

Tractional Retinal Detachment
- Proliferative vitreoretinopathy can pull retina away from pigment epithelium, causing a separation between layers

EVALUATION/WORK-UP

Imaging
- Fluorescein angiography (FA)
  - May help assess degree of retinal vascular distortion, differentiate pseudoholes from full-thickness macular holes, and determine leakage of perifoveal capillaries or evidence of ischemia
- Optical coherence tomography (OCT)
  - Determines presence or absence of ERM
  - ERMs appear as a hyperreflective band on anterior retinal surface
  - Identifies vitreous traction on retina, thickening of macula, and macular edema

TREATMENT

Surgical
- Mild ERM with minimal or no visual symptoms does not require surgical intervention
- Surgical intervention is reserved for more severe membranes that produce significant visual loss or metamorphopsia (20/40 or worse)
- Surgery involves 3 main steps
  - Pars plana subtotal vitrectomy
    - Eliminates any vitreal traction on retina
  - ERM peeling
    - Outer edge of membrane is identified with a vitreoretinal pick and peeled away with forceps
  - Inner limiting membrane (ILM) peeling
    - Sharp surface creates a flap in the ILM, and desired area is removed with vitreoretinal forceps with a motion similar to capsulorrhexis
- Combined ERM and ILM peeling improves recurrence rates compared with ERM alone
- Dyes like indocyanine green and brilliant blue help visualization in surgery

SELECTED REFERENCES

1. Almony A et al: Techniques, rationale, and outcomes of internal limiting membrane peeling. Retina. 32(5):877-91, 2012
2. Ng CH et al: Prevalence and risk factors for epiretinal membranes in a multi-ethnic United States population. Ophthalmology. 118(4):694-9, 2011
3. Bringmann A et al: Involvement of Müller glial cells in epiretinal membrane formation. Graefes Arch Clin Exp Ophthalmol. 247(7):865-83, 2009

RETINAL DETACHMENT

Key Facts

Subtypes

- Rhegmatogenous retinal detachment (RD): Detachment secondary to a retinal tear, which allows liquefied vitreous to pass through the retina into the subretinal space
- Exudative/serous RD: Detachment secondary to accumulation of subretinal fluid (SRF) from inflammatory, hemorrhagic, or traumatic process
- Tractional RD: Detachment secondary to vitreoretinal adhesion/traction or epiretinal membranes

Etiology

- Age-related molecular changes in collagen structure at the vitreoretinal interface, causing adhesion/traction
- Posterior migration of vitreous base
- Retinal tear, often precipitated by minor trauma
- Inflammatory or traumatic vascular leakage
- SRF accumulation between retina and retinal pigment epithelium (RPE)

Presentation

- Visual field loss
- Photopsia (rays or flashes of light) from retinal traction
- Floaters (from blood, vitreous strands, or RPE debris)

Treatment

- Rhegmatogenous RD
  - Surgical reattachment (gas + laser or cryo, vitrectomy, silicone oil, scleral buckle, or combination)
- Serous/exudative RD
  - Surgical reattachment not effective, attempt may be harmful
- Tractional RD
  - Vitrectomy with epiretinal membrane peel/ retinectomy/lysis of adhesions

Prognosis

- Macula-on RD → risk of progression to macula-off RD
- Macula-off RD → profound vision loss

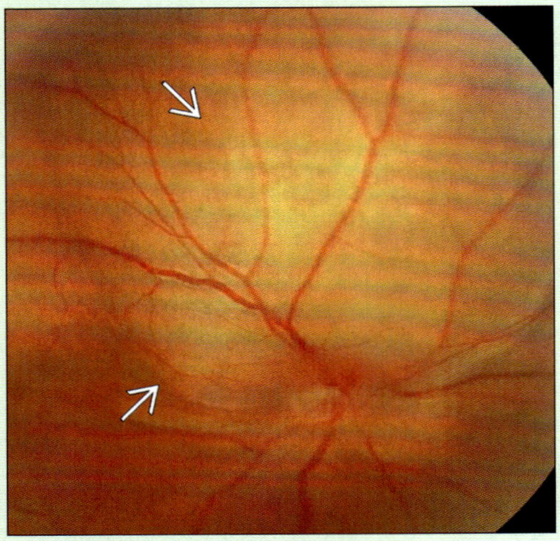
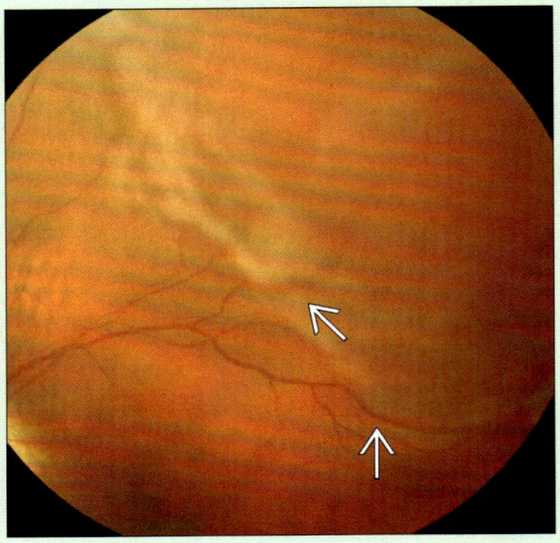

(Left) *This fundus photograph shows a retinal detachment (RD). Note the bullous serous separation of the retina ➔ from the underlying retinal pigmented epithelium. Peripheral detachments may lead to eventual macular detachment, causing serious vision impairment. Prompt diagnosis and treatment is critical to minimizing damage.* ***(Right)*** *This fundus photograph depicts a retinal detachment. Note how the retinal vessels seem to rise as they continue over the detached section of the retina ➔.*

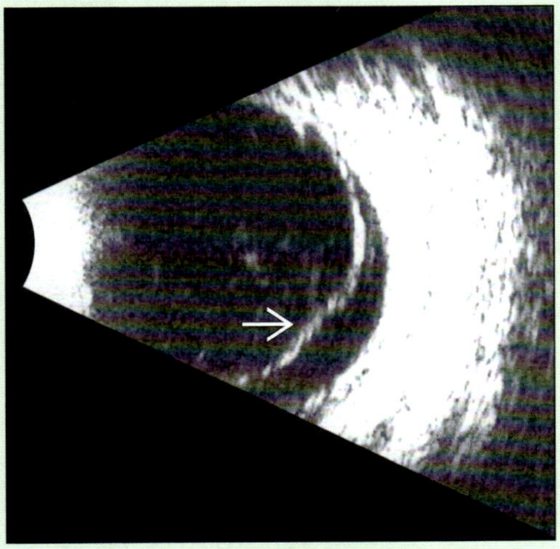
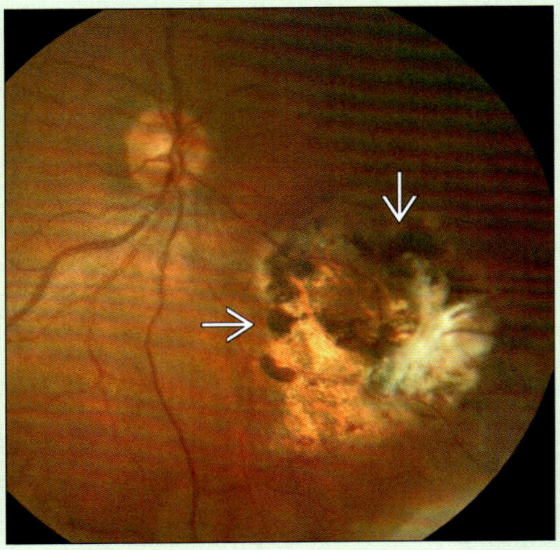

(Left) *This B-scan ultrasound image demonstrates a retinal detachment ➔, which appears as a bright signal forward of its natural anatomic position against the RPE. Often, a B-scan is necessary to rule-out retinal detachment if the view of the fundus is obscured by blood.* ***(Right)*** *This fundus photograph shows a chronic retinal detachment that resulted from trauma. Note the chorioretinal scar marked by black areas of pigment clumping ➔ resulting from surgical repair of the RD.*

RETINAL DETACHMENT

INTRODUCTION

Abbreviations
- Retinal detachment (RD)

Definitions
- RD: Detachment of the neural retina from underlying retinal pigmented epithelium (RPE)
- Retinal pigmented epithelium (RPE): Supporting cell layer underlying neural retina
- Lattice degeneration: Peripheral retina becomes atrophic in a lattice pattern and develops tears and holes, which can progress to detachment

Subtypes
- Rhegmatogenous RD: Secondary to retinal tear, which allows liquefied vitreous to pass through the retina into the subretinal space
- Exudative/serous RD: Secondary to accumulation of subretinal fluid (SRF) from inflammatory, hemorrhagic, or traumatic process
- Tractional RD: Secondary to vitreoretinal adhesion/traction or contraction of epiretinal membranes

DEMOGRAPHICS

Etiology (Rhegmatogenous)
- Age-related molecular changes in collagen structure at the vitreoretinal interface
- Posterior migration of the vitreous base
- Vitreoretinal adhesion and traction
- Retinal tear, often precipitated by minor trauma
- Passage of liquefied vitreous through a retinal break
- SRF accumulation between retina and RPE causes RD

Risk Factors
- Advanced age
- High myopia
- Retinal degenerative diseases

Epidemiology
- Annual incidence between 6.3 and 17.9 per 100,000 population
- Mean prevalence of lattice degeneration in RD patients: 45.7 ± 20.3%
- Mean prevalence of myopia in RD patients: 47.28 ± 12.59%

PRESENTATION

Symptoms
- Visual field loss, usually starting in periphery
- Vision loss spreads centrally over hours to weeks
- Photopsia (rays or flashes of light) from retinal traction
- Floaters (from blood or RPE debris)
- Frequently precipitated by traumatic deceleration/head injuries

DIFFERENTIAL DIAGNOSIS

Posterior Vitreous Detachment
- Common cause of floaters

Retinoschisis
- Commonly confused with RD
- Separation in retinoschisis is between layers of the retina itself, causes an absolute scotoma, and is usually nonprogressive
- Retinoschisis does not blanche with laser (unlike RD)

Migraine Headaches
- Common cause of photopsia/flashes

Postural Hypotension/Vasovagal Response
- Common cause of photopsia/flashes

Cerebrovascular Event
- Vision loss typically bilateral, stable, and homonymous

Retinal Vascular Occlusion
- Fixed field defects
- Generally lack flashes, floaters
- Flame-shaped hemorrhages, exudative plaques on funduscopy

Optic Neuropathy
- Typically central vision loss first
- Relative afferent pupillary defect

TREATMENT

Medical Emergency
- Prompt treatment essential for vision preservation
  - Macula-on RDs should be operated on urgently to prevent macular detachment
  - Macula-off RDs should be repaired within a few days if possible

Surgical
- Rhegmatogenous RD
  - Surgical reattachment (in clinic with combination of gas + laser or cryoretinopexy; or in OR with vitrectomy or scleral buckle ± gas/laser/cryo/silicone oil/perfluoron)
- Serous/exudative RD
  - Surgical reattachment not effective; treat cause
- Tractional RD: Vitrectomy + membrane peel/lysis of adhesions/retinectomy

Prognosis
- Macula-on detachment may progress rapidly to macula-off detachment
- Macula-off detachment leads to profound vision loss
- Prompt diagnosis and treatment essential

SELECTED REFERENCES

1. Schwartz SG et al: Update on retinal detachment surgery. Curr Opin Ophthalmol. 24(3):255-61, 2013
2. Fabian ID et al: Macular hole after vitrectomy for primary rhegmatogenous retinal detachment. Retina. 32(3):511-9, 2012
3. Mitry D et al: Pathogenesis of rhegmatogenous retinal detachment: predisposing anatomy and cell biology. Retina. 30(10):1561-72, 2010
4. Mitry D et al: The epidemiology of rhegmatogenous retinal detachment: geographical variation and clinical associations. Br J Ophthalmol. 94(6):678-84, 2010

HIGH MYOPIA

Key Facts

Introduction
- Generally considered myopia ≥ -6.0 diopters (or axial length ≥ 26.5 mm) that may be accompanied by degenerative changes of posterior segment of globe

Demographics
- Cause unknown: Likely multifactorial
- Environmental associations: May increase with more years of schooling, more near-work activity
- Genetic predispositions: Multiple genetic loci and chromosomes implicated
- Syndromes: Stickler, Marfan

Presentation
- High refractive error; > -6.0 diopters
- Long axial length
- Tigroid fundus
- Retinal pigment epithelial atrophy
- Posterior staphyloma
- Myopic crescent
- Choroidal neovascularization (CNV)
- Fuchs spot
- Rhegmatogenous retinal detachment

Evaluation/Work-Up
- Refraction, slit-lamp, and fundus exam
- Visual field exam
- OCT
- Intravenous fluorescein angiography if CNV suspected

Treatment
- Glasses or contact lenses
- Photorefractive keratectomy (PRK), LASIK, or phakic IOL for elective refractive correction
- Laser photocoagulation or anti-VEGF for CNV
- PPV with gas bubble for macular hole
- Scleral buckle, laser photocoagulation, cryotherapy, or PPV for RD

__(Left)__ This OCT image depicts a posterior vitreous detachment (PVD). The posterior hyaloid ➔ of the vitreous can be seen separated from the internal limiting membrane ➔. PVDs in myopia have an increased risk of leading to retinal detachment. __(Right)__ This fundus photo demonstrates a macular hole ➔. High myopia leads to an increased risk of macular holes as well as asymptomatic atrophic holes.

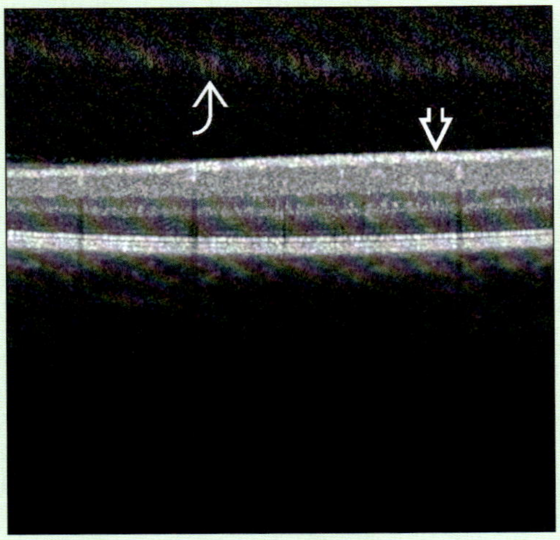

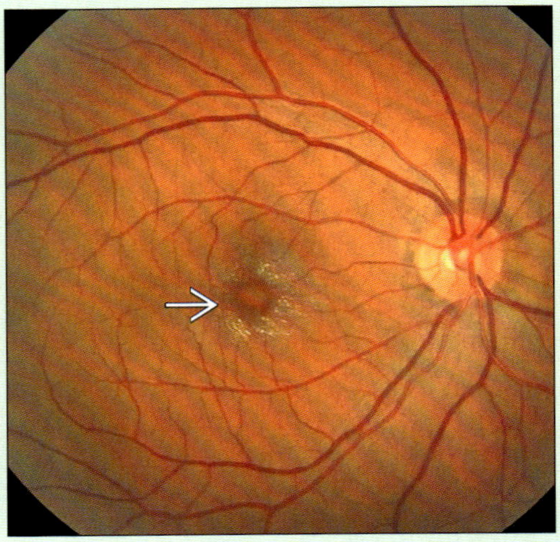

__(Left)__ This fundus photo demonstrates a retinal detachment. Note the billowing of the retinal arteries ➔ secondary to subretinal fluid accumulation. While ~10% of the general population are myopes, over 40% of all retinal detachments occur in myopic eyes. __(Right)__ This slit-lamp photo demonstrates corneal dryness ➔ after LASIK surgery. Patients with high myopia are often good candidates for refractive surgery though it is important to review risk factors with them.

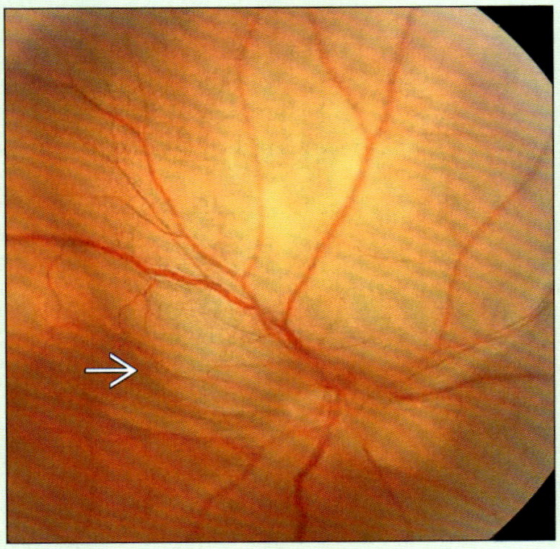

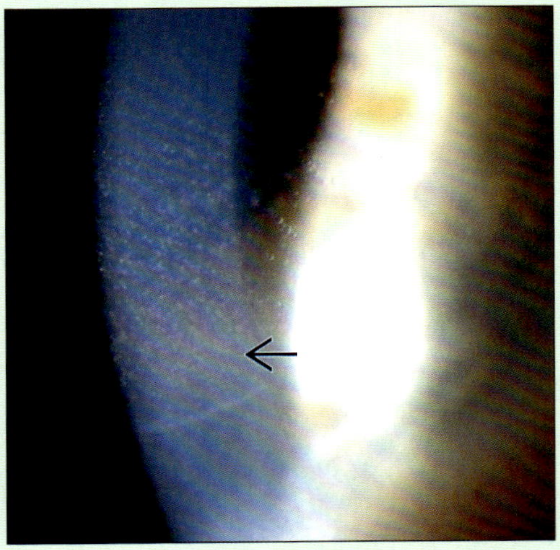

HIGH MYOPIA

INTRODUCTION

Definitions

- Myopia ≥ to -6.0 diopters (or axial length ≥ 26.5 mm) that may be accompanied by degenerative changes of posterior segment of globe
- Also called pathologic or degenerative myopia

DEMOGRAPHICS

Etiology/Risk Factors

- Cause unknown: Likely multifactorial
- Myopia generally develops in early to mid childhood
- Environmental associations: May increase with more years of schooling, more near-work activity
- Genetic predispositions: Multiple genetic loci and chromosomes implicated
- Syndromes: Stickler, Marfan
- Early insult to eye: Retinopathy of prematurity, congenital glaucoma
- Eye axial length increase causes structural changes to posterior segment of eye, increasing risk of
  - Myopic maculopathy
  - Retinal detachment (RD)
  - Myopic optic neuropathy
  - Macular holes
- Some correlation with glaucoma and cataract

Epidemiology

- 0.2-0.4% of general population in United States
- 1% of general population in Japan

PRESENTATION

Symptoms

- Decreased visual acuity

Exam Findings

- High refractive error; > -6.0 diopters
- Long axial length
- May have visual field deficits
- Fundus
  - Tigroid fundus
  - Retinal pigment epithelial atrophy
  - Tilted optic disc
  - Myopic crescent
  - Posterior staphyloma
  - Fuchs spot (not to be confused with Fuchs nodules)
  - Choroidal neovascularization (CNV)
  - Rhegmatogenous retinal detachment
  - Lacquer cracks
  - Peripheral lattice degeneration

DIFFERENTIAL DIAGNOSIS

Age-Related Macular Degeneration

- May have similar appearance to degenerative myopia, but drusen usually present

Toxoplasmosis

- Chorioretinal scar may appear similar to myopic crescent but without other features of myopic degeneration

EVALUATION/WORK-UP

Imaging

- Refraction
- Slit-lamp and fundus exam
- Intravenous fluorescein angiography if choroidal neovascularization (CNV) suspected
- Optical coherence tomography (OCT)
- Visual field exam

TREATMENT

Medical

- Refractive error correction
  - Glasses or contact lenses
- CNV
  - For subfoveal lesions consider anti-VEGF injections

Surgical

- Photorefractive keratectomy (PRK), LASIK, or phakic IOL for elective refractive correction
  - For > 6 D myopia, PRK generally needs mitomycin C to prevent haze
  - Carefully evaluate predicted residual stromal bed: should be > 270-300 μm
- Retinal breaks or RD
  - Laser photocoagulation, cryotherapy, scleral buckle surgery, PPV
- CNV
  - May consider laser photocoagulation or anti-VEGF
- Macular hole
  - Pars plana vitrectomy with gas bubble

Follow-Up

- If stable, regular follow-up to monitor for development of complications

Prognosis

- Depends on severity of disease
- For myopic CNV, there is a poor prognosis: ~ 89% of patients have marked visual impairment after 5 years

SELECTED REFERENCES

1. Morgan IG et al: Myopia. Lancet. 379(9827):1739-48, 2012
2. Alió JL et al: Ten-year follow-up of laser in situ keratomileusis for myopia of up to -10 diopters. Am J Ophthalmol. 145(1):46-54, 2008
3. Saw SM: How blinding is pathological myopia? Br J Ophthalmol. 90(5):525-6, 2006
4. Saw SM et al: Myopia and associated pathological complications. Ophthalmic Physiol Opt. 25(5):381-91, 2005
5. Saw SM: A synopsis of the prevalence rates and environmental risk factors for myopia. Clin Exp Optom. 86(5):289-94, 2003
6. Tano Y: Pathologic myopia: where are we now? Am J Ophthalmol. 134(5):645-60, 2002
7. Hersh PS et al: Photorefractive keratectomy versus laser in situ keratomileusis for moderate to high myopia. A randomized prospective study. Ophthalmology. 105(8):1512-22, discussion 1522-3, 1998

MACULAR HOLE

Key Facts

Staging
- Monitor with regular funduscopy or OCT
- Stage 1: Partial-thickness (lamellar) macular hole
- Stage 2: Small, full-thickness macular hole
- Stage 3: Full-thickness hole with surrounding SRF
- Stage 4: Full-thickness hole, surrounding SRF, and PVD

Demographics
- Usually occurs in elderly
- 3-4x more common in women

Presentation
- Minor to severe loss of visual acuity
- Distortion of visual field, central scotoma

Evaluation/Work-Up
- Funduscopy
  - Partial-thickness holes: Yellow spots or rings
  - Full-thickness holes: Darker red spots
  - SRF appears as a hazy, gray area surrounding a hole
  - Cystic edema appears as small yellow precipitates surrounding a hole
- OCT to evaluate for CME, SRF, PVD

Treatment
- Vitrectomy with membrane peel and gas or silicone oil
  - Can recover vision; strongly consider in stage 2 or 3 patients
  - Carries small risk of postoperative RD, especially in highly myopic patients
  - Earlier intervention carries a better prognosis
  - Ocriplasmin is emerging therapeutic
- Stage 1 resolves spontaneously ~ 50% of the time
- Patients with high myopia at increased risk of progressing to RD

*(**Left**) This fundus photograph demonstrates a visible macular hole ➔. Note the yellow precipitates distributed in a fanning pattern surrounding the hole ➔. (**Right**) These OCT images from 2 different patients demonstrate the variable appearance of late-stage macular holes. Note the more prominent cystic edema present in the 1st image ➔.*

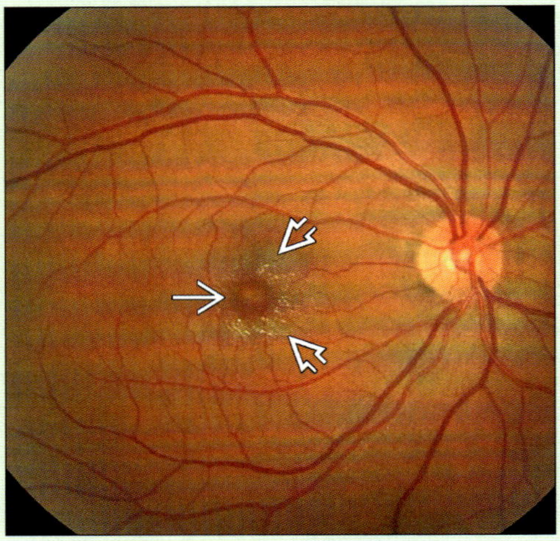

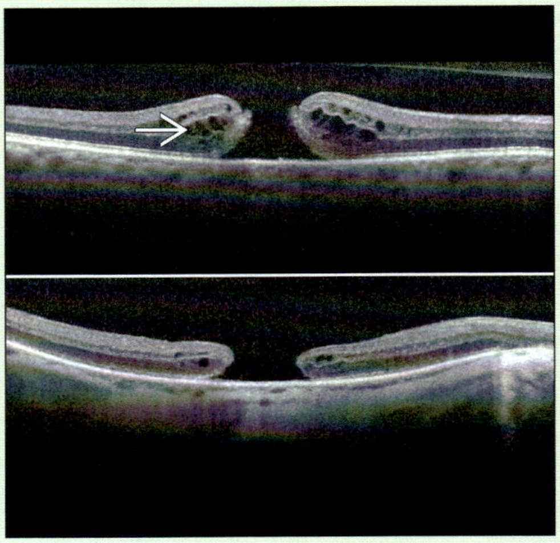

*(**Left**) This fundus photograph from a female patient demonstrates a full-thickness macular hole ➔. Women are more likely to have macular holes than men. (**Right**) Earlier stages of macular holes do not penetrate the full thickness of the retina and may appear less prominently ➔, as seen in this photo.*

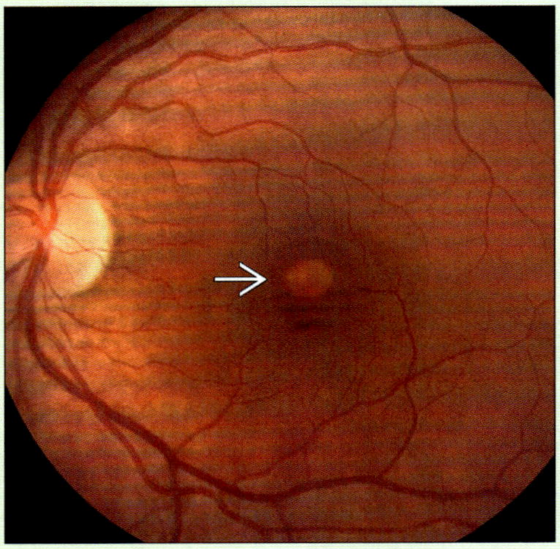

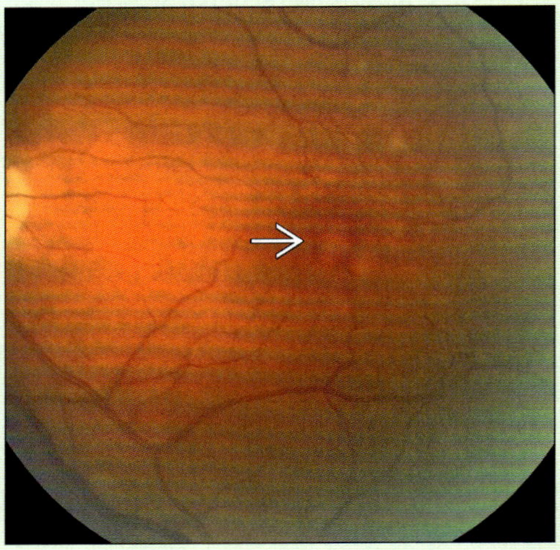

MACULAR HOLE

INTRODUCTION

Definitions

- Macular hole (MH): Round, full-thickness depletion of neural retinal tissue in the foveal center
- Scotoma: Region of compromised, nonfunctional vision surrounded by intact, functioning vision
- Amsler grid: Grid of horizontal and vertical lines used to monitor the central visual field and detect the development of physical distortions in the macula indicative of detachment, wrinkles, cystic edema, etc.

Subtypes

- Stage 1: Partial-thickness (lamellar) macular hole
- Stage 2: Small, full-thickness macular hole
- Stage 3: Full-thickness hole with surrounding subretinal fluid (SRF)
- Stage 4: Full-thickness hole, surrounding SRF, and posterior vitreous detachment (PVD)

DEMOGRAPHICS

Etiology/Risk Factors

- Typically caused by damage to retina, as opposed to intrinsic retinal diseases like age-related macular dystrophy (ARMD)
- Epiretinal membrane can cause retinal traction, leading to detachment/tear/hole
- Trauma: Microdetachment leads to loss of affected tissue, SRF accumulation, and eventual hole formation
- Cystoid macular edema (CME): Advanced cystic disease leads to loss of neural tissue, resulting in full-thickness hole
- Vitreomacular adhesion or traction (VMA/VMT)

Epidemiology

- Usually occurs in elderly patients
- 3-4x more common in women
- 10-15% chance of progression to bilateral disease

PRESENTATION

Symptoms

- Early: Blurriness or distortion of central vision
- Late: Profound central scotoma
- Distortion of visual field (Amsler grid)
- Significant loss of visual acuity

DIFFERENTIAL DIAGNOSIS

Intraretinal Cysts

- CME can cause similar funduscopic appearance
- Visible on optical coherence tomography (OCT)

Macular Pucker With Pseudohole

- Epiretinal membrane wrinkling
- Distortion on Amsler grid test

Solar Retinopathy

- Yellow spot in retina; if severe, can cause hole
- History of looking at bright light

ARMD With Geographic Atrophy

- Typically larger lesion with pigmented borders
- Profound central scotoma

EVALUATION/WORK-UP

Imaging

- Funduscopy
  - Partial-thickness holes appear as yellow spots or rings in the macula
  - Full-thickness holes appear as darker red spots in center of the macula
  - SRF appears as a hazy, gray area surrounding a hole
  - Cystic edema appears as small yellow precipitates surrounding a hole
- OCT
  - Useful for staging and tracking progression
  - Can differentiate partial thickness from full thickness
  - Evaluate for SRF and PVD
- Intravenous fluorescein angiography (IVFA)
  - Foveal hyperfluorescence indicates full-thickness hole
  - SRF accumulation visible if present

Watzke-Allen Test

- Thin slit beam placed on suspected macular hole
- Pseudohole will often result in distortion of slit beam
- True macular hole will result in disruption of slit beam

TREATMENT

Medical

- Ocriplasmin may have a role in VMT/VMA and may improve macular hole closure
- Treat CME

Surgical

- Vitrectomy with membrane peel
  - Can achieve partial visual function rescue
  - Carries small risk of postoperative retinal detachment (RD), especially in highly myopic patients
  - Earlier intervention carries a better prognosis
  - Gas with appropriate positioning or silicone oil to help tamponade

Follow-Up

- Nonmyopic: Yearly exam
- High myopia: Exam every 6 months
- Patients should be sent home with Amsler grid to monitor contralateral eye
- Patients must be instructed to return immediately with any RD symptoms (flashes, floaters, cobwebs)

Prognosis

- Stage 1 resolves spontaneously ~ 50% of the time
- High myopes at increased risk of RD
- 10% of patients will progress to bilateral disease

SELECTED REFERENCES

1. Ortisi E et al: Surgical management of retinal detachment because of macular hole in highly myopic eyes. Retina. 32(9):1704-18, 2012
2. Zheng Q et al: Vitreous surgery for macular hole-related retinal detachment after phacoemulsification cataract extraction: 10-year retrospective review. Eye (Lond). 26(8):1058-64, 2012

OPTIC PIT

Key Facts

Introduction

- Congenital excavation or regional depression of optic nerve head (ONH) from malformation during development
- Associated with posterior vitreous detachments (PVD) and retinal detachments (RD)
- Up to 50% develop RD in early adults
- Incidence: 1:11,000 people
- Usually asymptomatic and an incidental finding but may be underlying cause of PVD and RD
- 85% unilateral
- 70% found in temporal side of optic disc
- Possible autosomal dominant (check family history)

Presentation

- Blind spot or scotomas (or secondary findings from PVD or RD)
- Usually a benign incidental finding

Differential Diagnosis

- Acquired optic pits secondary to glaucoma
  - Higher frequency of hemorrhage compared to congenital form
- Other diseases of ONH (coloboma, megalopapilla, ONH hypoplasia)
  - ONH size and optic pit color may be key in differentiating optic pits

Evaluation/Work-Up

- Imaging studies, especially fundus photos and OCT
- Look carefully for CNV or retinal detachment

Treatment

- No treatment for isolated optic pits
- If CNV or RD consider
  - Photocoagulation, anti-VEGF injections, and surgery

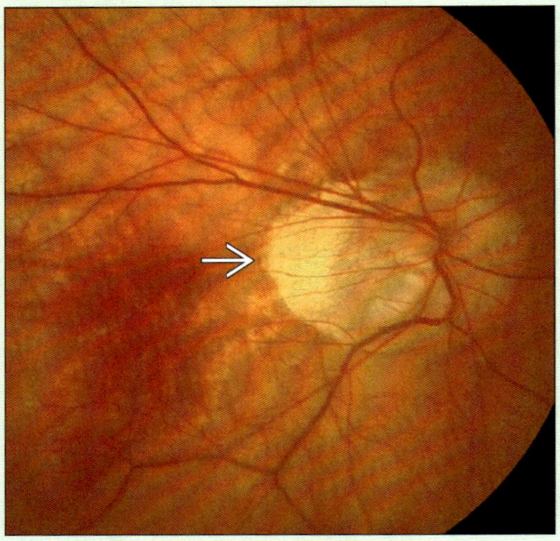
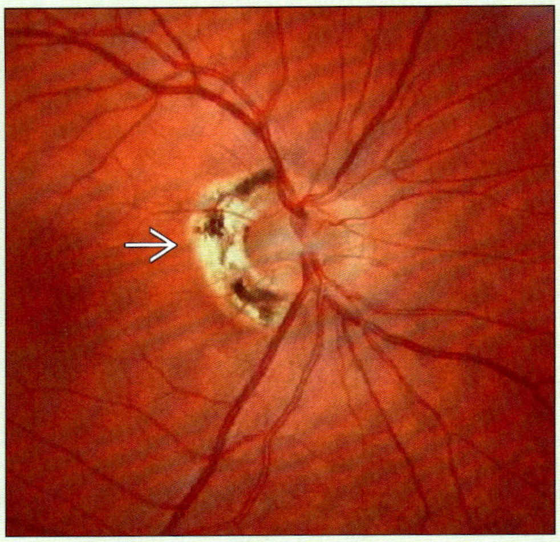

(Left) *This fundus photo shows an example of an optic pit. The oval optic pit has a more yellowish color compared with the optic disc ➔. Optic pits are often yellow, black, or gray in color.* ***(Right)*** *This fundus photo demonstrates the variability in appearance of optic pits ➔. Optic pits are thought to be predominately a congenital defect. Approximately 2/3 of optic pits are located temporally.*

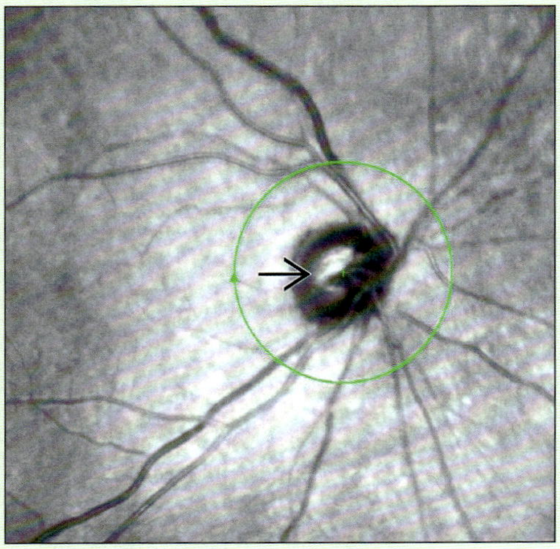
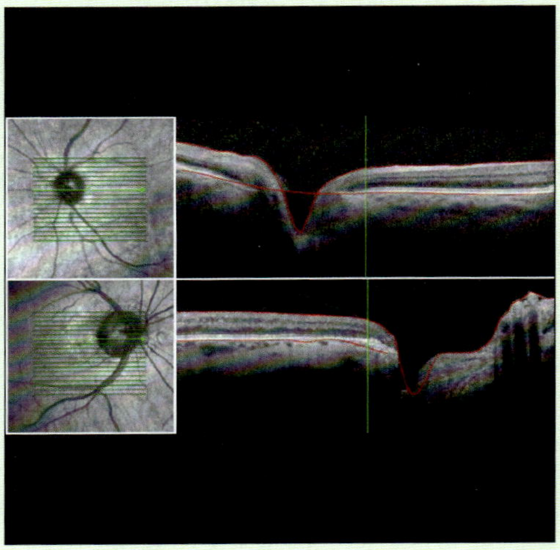

(Left) *This red-free image shows a patient with a centrally located optic pit ➔. Central optic pits are less common than temporal pits.* ***(Right)*** *These OCT images from 2 different patients demonstrate the variability possible between centrally located and temporally located optic pits.*

OPTIC PIT

INTRODUCTION

Abbreviations
- Optic disc pit (ODP)

Synonyms
- Optic nerve pits, optic holes

Definitions
- Localized oval, gray-white depression in optic disc
- Can have 1 or more pits per disc
  - 0.1-0.7 disc diameters (dd); average depth: ~ 0.3 dd
- Usually unilateral
- Usually found in inferotemporal portion of optic disc
- Usually benign (incidental finding) unless associated with macular lesions

Subtypes
- Congenital, acquired

DEMOGRAPHICS

Etiology/Risk Factors
- Thought to result from incomplete closure of fetal fissure
- Glaucoma ↑ risk for acquired optic pits (or pseudopit)

Epidemiology
- 1 in 11,000 with no gender predilection

PRESENTATION

Symptoms
- Asymptomatic (incidental finding on fundus exam)
- 25-75% develop visual deterioration in their 30s and 40s after developing macular schisis or detachment

Exam Findings
- May have visual field defects
  - Paracentral arcuate scotoma and enlarged blind spot are most common
- Normal optic nerve head (ONH) size
- Unilateral, round/oval-shaped depression with gray, white/yellowish, or black color

DIFFERENTIAL DIAGNOSIS

Congenital/Developmental
- Coloboma
  - Enlarged ONH
  - Bowl-shaped inferior excavation
- ONH hypoplasia
  - Small ONH
- Megalopapilla
  - Enlarged ONH (horizontally elongated cup)
  - Usually bilateral
- Morning glory
  - Enlarged ONH
  - Funnel-shaped excavation
  - Increased disc vessels

Macular Complications
- Idiopathic central serous retinopathy
- Subretinal neovascular membrane (CN5)

Acquired vs. Congenital Optic Pits
- Acquired
  - More common in women than men (2-3:1)
  - Located more frequently in inferior location
  - Present bilaterally 21-48% of the time
  - Higher prevalence with low-tension glaucoma (74%) than with high-tension glaucoma (15%)
  - Higher frequency of disc hemorrhage (40%) compared to congenital optic pits (8%)
  - Disease progress (visual field loss) more frequent

EVALUATION/WORK-UP

Labs
- Markers for optic pits are still unavailable; diagnosis for optic pits is clinical

Imaging
- Fundus photography
  - Round or oval depression in optic disc
  - Color of optic pit varies: 60% are gray, 30% are white/yellow, 10% are black
- Optical coherence tomography (OCT)
  - May show macular involvement: Intraretinal and subretinal fluid
- Fluorescein angiography (FA)
  - Early in disease: Optic pit hypofluorescence
  - Late in disease: Optic pit hyperfluorescent
  - Usually no fluorescein leakage
  - No fluorescein staining of macula
- Indocyanine green angiography (ICGA)
  - Hypofluorescence of optic pit

TREATMENT

Medical
- No treatment is necessary for isolated optic pits; anti-VEGF agents can be used for CNV

Surgical
- None for isolated optic pits
- Pars plana vitrectomy
  - Endolaser photocoagulation and C3F8 endotamponade for optic pits with macular involvement

Follow-Up
- Isolated optic pits from routine examination need to be monitored for possible development of macular complications
  - It is thought that development of macular lesions from isolated optic pits is a rare event

Prognosis
- Optic pits without macular involvement is benign

SELECTED REFERENCES

1. Georgalas I et al: Optic disc pit: a review. Graefes Arch Clin Exp Ophthalmol. 249(8):1113-22, 2011
2. Corbett JJ et al: Cavitary developmental defects of the optic disc. Visual loss associated with optic pits and colobomas. Arch Neurol. 37(4):210-3, 1980
3. Brockhurst RJ: Optic pits and posterior retinal detachment. Trans Am Ophthalmol Soc. 73:264-91, 1975

RETINOSCHISIS

Key Facts

Introduction
- Abnormal splitting of neurosensory layers of the retina
- Categorized as
  - Degenerative
  - Hereditary
  - Tractional
  - Exudative
- Can lead to retinal detachments

Demographics
- Prevalent in general population
- Typical degenerative retinoschisis
  - 7% of population > 40 years old

Presentation
- Commonly asymptomatic
- Acute retinal break
  - Sudden onset of dark floaters and flashes
- Examine both eyes due to high rate of bilateral retinal breaks
- Found during routine evaluation
- May use 360° scleral depression to visualize breaks

Treatment
- Retinoschisis is not treated, but retinal detachments that occur must be treated with
  - Transconjunctival cryotherapy
  - Laser photocoagulation
  - Scleral buckling

Prognosis
- Most cases of retinoschisis do not lead to retinal detachment
- Retinal detachment in 1 eye is associated with greater likelihood of retinal detachment in other eye

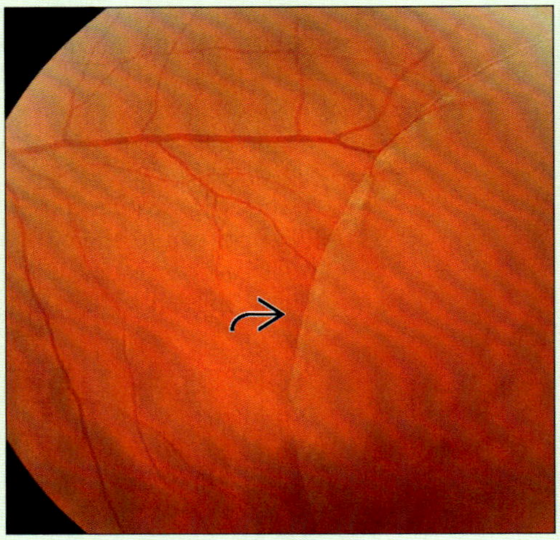
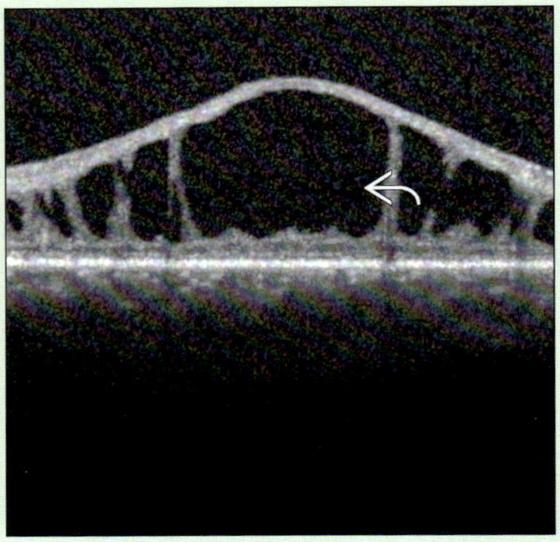

(Left) *This fundus photograph shows a clearly demarcated separation of retinal neurosensory layers typical of retinoschisis. This separation resembles a blister. Retinoschisis can be due to degeneration, hereditary disorders, traction, or exudation.* ***(Right)*** *This OCT shows separation of the retinal layers seen in retinoschisis. Retinoschisis can lead to retinal detachments and retinal breaks. These conditions require prompt treatment.*

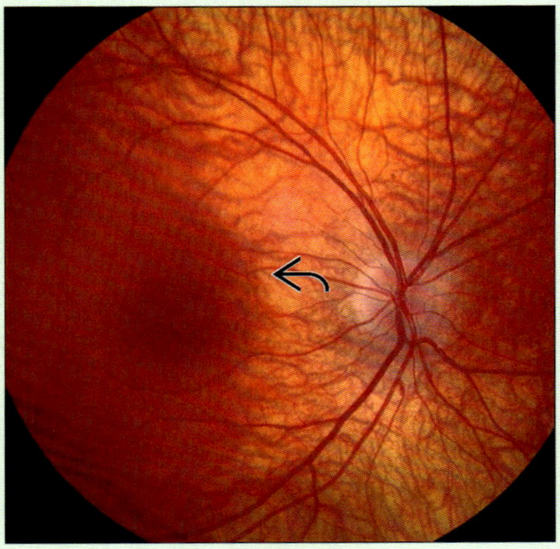
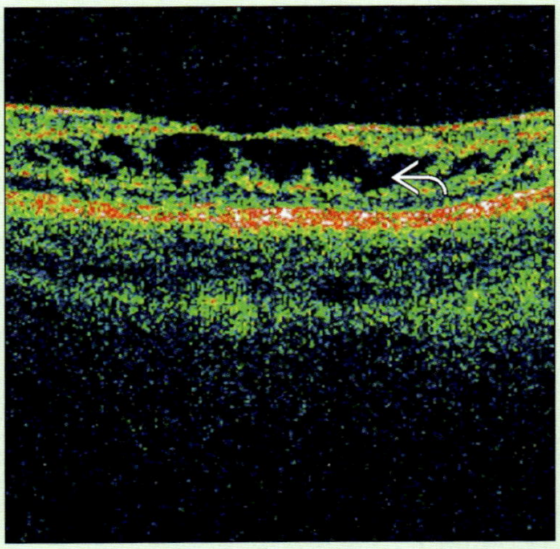

(Left) *This fundus photograph shows separation of retinal layers in X-linked juvenile retinoschisis. This condition usually presents with bilateral and symmetric retinal splitting at the nerve fiber layer. Patients present with progressive vision loss, strabismus, and nystagmus.* ***(Right)*** *This OCT shows separation of retinal layers seen in X-linked juvenile retinoschisis. Visual acuity in these patients worsens during the first 20 years of life but then remains relatively stable.*

RETINOSCHISIS

INTRODUCTION

Definitions

- Abnormal splitting of neurosensory layers of retina
  - Usually at outer plexiform and inner nuclear level in older patients in periphery
  - X-linked juvenile retinoschisis usually has a split at nerve fiber layer in macula

Subtypes

- Categorized as
  - Degenerative
    - Typical
    - Reticular
  - Hereditary
    - X-linked juvenile retinoschisis
    - Familial foveal retinoschisis
  - Tractional
  - Exudative
    - Secondary to optic disc pit

DEMOGRAPHICS

Etiology/Risk Factors

- Aging
- Vitreoretinal traction
  - Causes full-thickness breaks
- Inflammation
- Myopia
  - Major risk factor of retinal detachment
  - Associated with reticular/lattice degeneration (retinal holes)
- X-linked juvenile retinoschisis
  - Associated with mutations of *RS1* gene

Epidemiology

- Degenerative retinoschisis is prevalent in general population
- Typical degenerative retinoschisis (affects outer plexiform layer peripherally; not usually visually significant)
  - 7% of population > 40 years old
- Reticular degenerative retinoschisis
  - 6-8% of general population
  - Slowly progressive
  - 3.3x more common in females
- X-linked juvenile retinoschisis (affects nerve fiber layer centrally; can compromise vision)
  - 1 in 5,000 to 1 in 25,000 males worldwide

PRESENTATION

Symptoms

- Commonly asymptomatic
- May have absolute field defect (unlike retinal detachment, which can be relative)
- Acute retinal break
  - Sudden onset of symptoms
    - Dark floaters
    - Photopsia
- X-linked retinoschisis presents in males at around age 10 with
  - Progressive vision loss
  - Strabismus
  - Nystagmus

Exam Findings

- Found during routine evaluation
- Ballooning of inner retinal layers into vitreous
  - Resembles a blister
- May use 360° scleral depression to visualize breaks
- Examine both eyes due to high rate of bilateral retinal breaks

DIFFERENTIAL DIAGNOSIS

Rhegmatogenous Retinal Detachment

- Pigmented cells in vitreous
- Usually unilateral

Vitreous Inflammation

- Toxoplasma chorioretinitis
- Cytomegalovirus chorioretinitis

EVALUATION/WORK-UP

Labs

- Multifocal ERG can show absolute loss in areas involving retinoschisis

TREATMENT

Surgical

- Treatment generally not necessary, but retinal detachments require prompt treatment
  - Transconjunctival cryotherapy
  - Laser photocoagulation to prevent progression ("firewall")
  - Scleral buckling
  - Pneumatic retinopexy, PPV

Follow-Up

- Most retinoschisis do not lead to retinal detachment
- Combined retinoschisist retinal tear is much more serious

Prognosis

- Asymptomatic patients
  - Development of retinal detachment
    - 0.5% over 11 years
- Most retinoschisis is clinically insignificant, unless a retinal detachment occurs
- Retinal detachment in 1 eye is associated with a greater likelihood of retinal detachment in other eye
- Full recovery of visual function following surgical therapy is limited
- Juvenile retinoschisis can lead to vision loss of central and peripheral vision

SELECTED REFERENCES

1. Molday RS et al: X-linked juvenile retinoschisis: clinical diagnosis, genetic analysis, and molecular mechanisms. Prog Retin Eye Res. 31(3):195-212, 2012
2. Buch H et al: Prevalence and long-term natural course of retinoschisis among elderly individuals: the Copenhagen City Eye Study. Ophthalmology. 114(4):751-5, 2007

VITAMIN A DEFICIENCY

Key Facts

Introduction
- Vitamin A is essential for
  - Vision
  - Differentiation and proliferation of most cells

Demographics
- Due to
  - Low egg and dairy intake
  - Low dietary intake of fruits and vegetables
- Greater risk at times of growth
- Leading cause of preventable pediatric blindness
- Uncommon in industrialized countries
- Common in
  - Southern and Southeast Asia
  - Africa
  - South America

Presentation
- Night blindness
- Xerophthalmia
- Associated with increased risk of infections
- Poor growth
- Bitot spots
- Corneal ulceration and necrosis
- Keratomalacia
- Anemia

Treatment
- Vitamin A supplementation
- Supportive dietary supplementation
- Antibiotic therapy may be considered
- Prevention is key
  - Dietary diversification
  - Vitamin A fortification
  - Supplementation
- Vitamin A supplementation to children in endemic areas associated with reduction in mortality

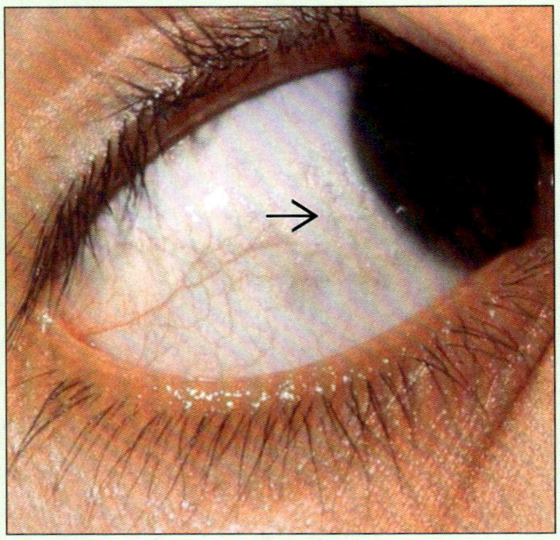

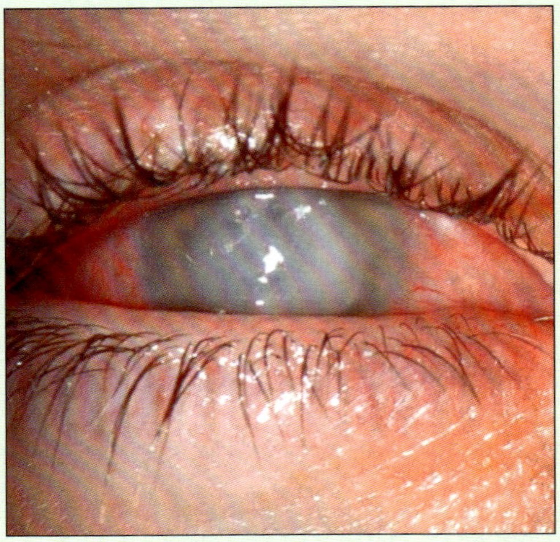

(Left) *External photo shows an example of a Bitot spot ⇨. Characteristic of vitamin A deficiency, these are triangular areas of abnormal squamous cell proliferation and keratinization of the conjunctiva.* ***(Right)*** *External photo shows keratomalacia, defined as softening and ulceration of the cornea secondary to vitamin A deficiency. Risk factors for vitamin A deficiency include poor dietary intake and age < 5 years. Low egg and dairy intake are an important predictor of vitamin A deficiency.*

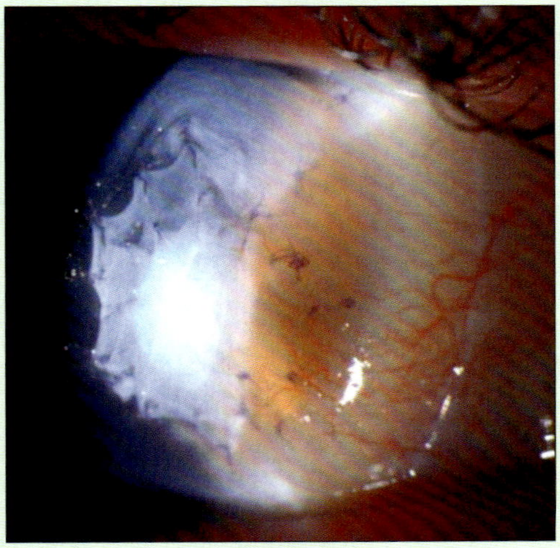

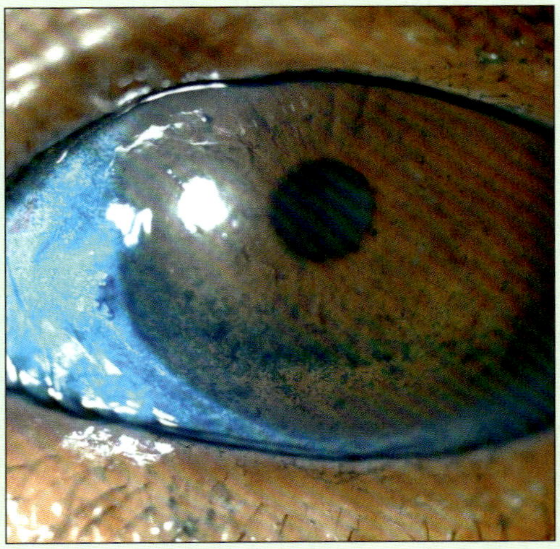

(Left) *Slit-lamp photo shows severe keratomalacia status post amniotic membrane transplant. In addition to corneal necrosis, vitamin A deficiency causes symptoms of night blindness, poor growth, and increased risk of other systemic infections.* ***(Right)*** *External photo shows significant xerophthalmia, seen in large areas of punctate corneal and conjunctival staining. Vitamin A deficiency is treated with vitamin A supplementation and treatment of corneal surface disease or inflammation, if present.*

VITAMIN A DEFICIENCY

INTRODUCTION

Abbreviations

- Vitamin A deficiency (VAD)

Definitions

- Vitamin A is essential for
  - Vision
  - Maturation
  - Differentiation and proliferation of most cells
  - Immunity
- Vitamin A is an essential fat-soluble nutrient

DEMOGRAPHICS

Etiology/Risk Factors

- Low egg and dairy intake
  - Most important predictor of vitamin A deficiency
- Low dietary intake of fruits and vegetables
  - Dark green leafy vegetables
  - Carrots
  - Mangoes
  - Papaya
- Greater risk at times of growth
  - Infancy
  - Childhood
  - Pregnancy
- Formula feeding of infants

Epidemiology

- 3rd most common nutritional deficiency in the world
- Leading cause of preventable pediatric blindness
- Uncommon in industrialized countries
- Common in
  - Southern and Southeast Asia
  - Africa
  - South America
- Low income countries
  - 125-130 million preschool-aged children
  - 7 million pregnant women

PRESENTATION

Symptoms

- Night blindness
  - Failure in rod photoreceptors in dim light
- Xerophthalmia
  - Dryness of conjunctiva and cornea
- Associated with increased risk of infections
  - Diarrhea
  - Respiratory tract infections
  - Measles
- Poor growth

Exam Findings

- Bitot spots
  - Triangular areas of abnormal squamous cell proliferation and keratinization of conjunctiva
  - Keratinizing metaplasia of mucosal surfaces
  - Best seen on oblique illumination
  - Look like "sandbanks at the receding tide"
- Keratomalacia
  - Necrosis of cornea
  - Initial opaque lesions that can expand to cover and blind cornea
- Anemia
- Keratinization
- Examine carefully to avoid further damage to cornea

DIFFERENTIAL DIAGNOSIS

Retinitis Pigmentosa

- Retinal pigmentation
- Patients also experience loss of night vision
- Dry eye syndrome

EVALUATION/WORK-UP

Labs

- Serum retinol levels
  - < 20 μg/dL
- Molar ratio of retinol:retinol binding protein (RBP)
  - < 0.8
- Vitamin A concentration in breast milk
  - < 0.70 μmol/L

Imaging

- Dark adaptometry
  - Impaired peripheral vision in dim light

TREATMENT

Medical

- Vitamin A supplementation
  - Night blindness responds within 24-48 hours
  - Dose and frequency depend on age
  - Children with severe measles should receive supplementation
- Supportive dietary supplementation
- Antibiotic therapy may be considered
- Tetracycline eye drops may be used if there is corneal inflammation

Follow-Up

- Scarring of cornea may occur

Prognosis

- Prevention is key
  - Dietary diversification
  - Vitamin A fortification
  - Supplementation
- Vitamin A supplementation to children in endemic areas associated with reduction in mortality

SELECTED REFERENCES

1. Limburg H et al: Prevalence and causes of blindness in children in Vietnam. Ophthalmology. 119(2):355-61, 2012
2. Sherwin JC et al: Epidemiology of vitamin A deficiency and xerophthalmia in at-risk populations. Trans R Soc Trop Med Hyg. 106(4):205-14, 2012
3. West KP et al: Vitamin A deficiency. In Semba RD et al: Nutrition and Health in Developing Countries. Totowa, NJ: Humana Press. 377-433, 2008
4. Humphrey JH et al: Vitamin A deficiency and attributable mortality among under-5-year-olds. Bull World Health Organ. 70(2):225-32, 1992

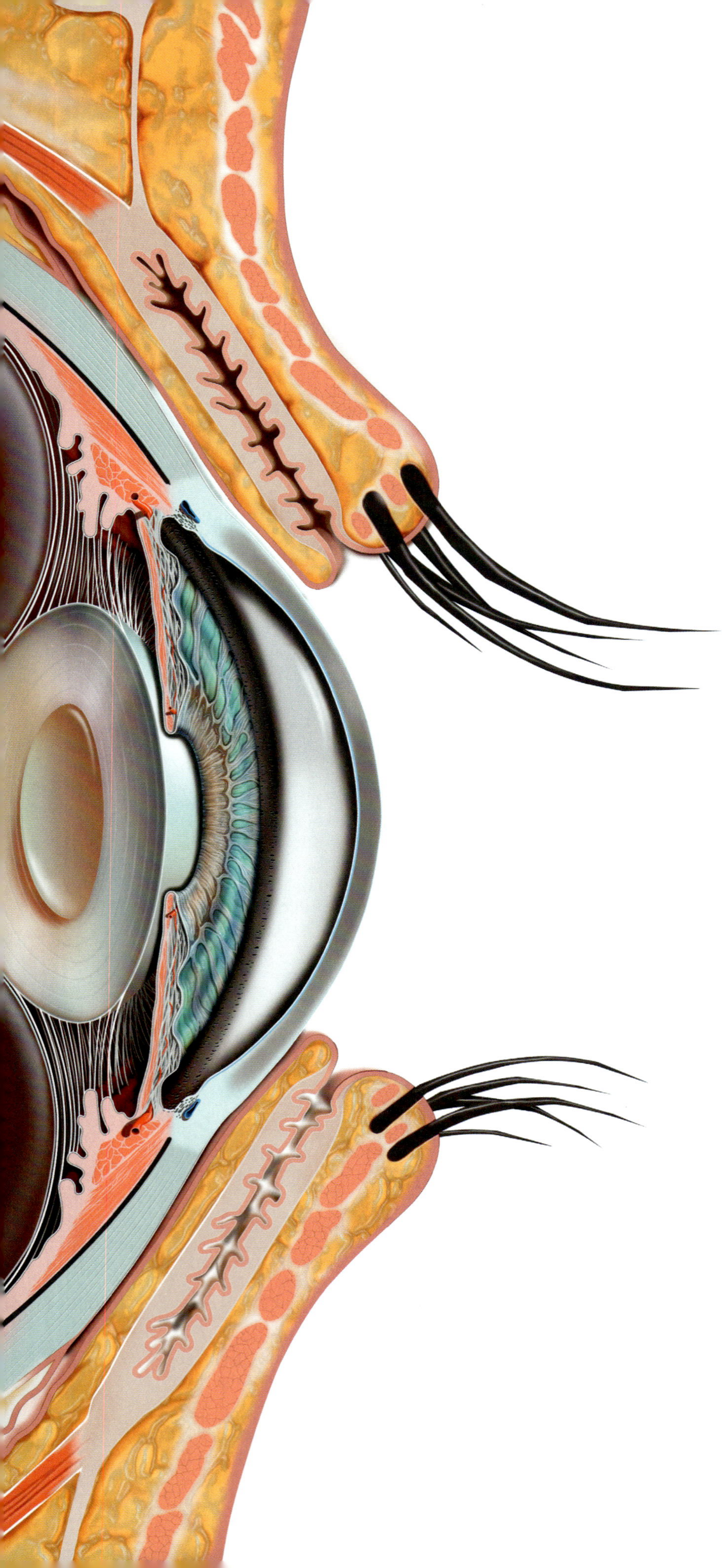

SECTION 1
Eyelids

Introduction and Overview

Autoimmune and Inflammatory Disorders

Trauma

Nonneoplastic Cysts

Malignant Neoplasms

Miscellaneous

EYELID OVERVIEW

GROSS ANATOMY

Surface Anatomy

- Upper and lower palpebrae (eyelids) are modified skin folds that close to protect the globe; consist of 5 layers
- Upper eyelid extends from the eyebrow inferiorly to the free margin that represents superior boundary of the palpebral fissure
  - Superior palpebral sulcus, or upper eyelid crease, is created by the attachment of the levator aponeurosis to the pretarsal orbicularis bundle and skin
- Lower eyelid extends from inferior boundary of the palpebral fissure inferiorly to join the cheek

Layers of Eyelid

- Skin of eyelids is among the thinnest of the body (measuring < 1 mm) and possesses few hair follicles and no subcutaneous fat
  - Nasal aspect of the skin has a higher density of fine hairs and sebaceous glands, making the skin smoother and more oily
- Orbicularis oculi muscle
  - Striated muscle innervated by the facial nerve and functions to close eyelid
  - Muscle is divided into 3 segments depending on location: Within eyelids (pretarsal), overlying orbital septum (preseptal), and outside of the lid (orbital segment)
  - Orbicularis oculi muscle and the skin together form the anterior lamella
- Areolar tissue
  - Tissue that lies deep to orbicularis oculi muscle & communicates with subaponeurotic layer of scalp
- Tarsal plates
  - Dense, fibrous layer that provides primary structural support to the eyelids
  - Attached to lateral and medial orbital margins via lateral and medial palpebral ligaments and the superior and inferior orbital margins by a thin fascia called the orbital septum
- Palpebral conjunctiva
  - Layer of mucous membrane that lines the lid posteriorly and adheres firmly to tarsal plate
  - Along with the tarsal plate, forms the posterior lamella

Lid Margin

- ~ 25-30 mm in length and 2 mm in width
- Mucocutaneous junction, or gray line, divides the lid into the anterior and posterior margins
  - Anterior margin is composed of the eyelashes, glands of Zeis, and glands of Moll
    - Eyelashes: Upper are more numerous and project upwards whereas the lower project downwards
    - Glands of Zeis: Modified sebaceous glands that open into hair follicles at base of eyelashes
    - Glands of Moll: Modified sweat glands that open in a row near base of eyelashes
  - Posterior margin
    - Meibomian glands: Modified sebaceous glands that line the posterior margin

Palpebral Fissure

- Elliptic space created when upper and lower eyelids are open
- Fissure is demarcated on either end by the lateral and medial canthi
  - Medical canthus is more elliptic, and upper and lower lids join together to form a lacrimal lake
  - Lacrimal lake is composed of 2 structures: Lacrimal caruncle and plica semilunaris
    - Lacrimal caruncle: Yellow-colored, modified skin containing large sweat and sebaceous glands that open into follicles that contain fine hair
    - Plica semilunaris: Vestigial remnant of a 3rd eyelid (nictitating membrane)
  - Lateral canthus attaches to lateral orbital wall at protuberance called Whitnall tubercle
  - Lacrimal papillae are small elevations near medial canthus of the upper and lower eyelids that contain a central opening called lacrimal punctum, which serves as the opening to the canaliculus

Lid Retractors

- Musculofascial complex composed of smooth and striated muscles that function to open eyelid
  - Smooth muscle components are innervated by sympathetic nerves
  - Levator palpebrae superioris and inferior rectus muscle are supplied by the oculomotor nerve
- Upper lid
  - Levator palpebrae superioris: Arises from apex of the orbit and divides to form an aponeurosis and a deeper smooth muscle fiber called Müller (superior tarsal) muscle
    - Aponeurosis elevates the anterior lamella of the eyelid and forms the upper lid skin crease
    - Müller muscle inserts into upper border of the tarsal plate, elevating the posterior lamella
- Lower lid
  - Capsulopalpebral fascia initiates at inferior rectus muscles and extends to inferior edge of the lower eyelid tarsal plate
  - Inferior tarsal muscle is equivalent of Muller muscle in upper eyelid

Sensory Nerve Supply

- To eyelids: Derived from 1st and 2nd divisions of the trigeminal nerve
  - Branches of ophthalmic division of the trigeminal nerve: Lacrimal, supraorbital, supratrochlear, infratrochlear, and external nasal nerves
  - Branches of maxillary division of the trigeminal nerve include: Infraorbital, zygomaticofacial, and zygomaticotemporal nerves

Blood Supply and Lymphatics

- Eyelids receive dual blood supply via the lateral and medial palpebral branches of the lacrimal and ophthalmic arteries
  - Anastomoses between lateral and medial palpebral arteries form a marginal tarsal arcade, which lies in the areolar tissue
- Venous drainage from the eyelids empties primarily into the ophthalmic vein
- Lymphatic drainage from the medial and lateral segments of the lids empties into the submandibular and preauricular/parotid nodes, respectively

EYELID

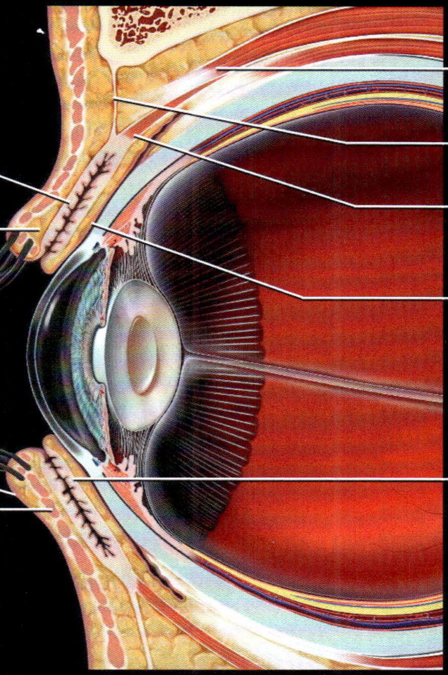

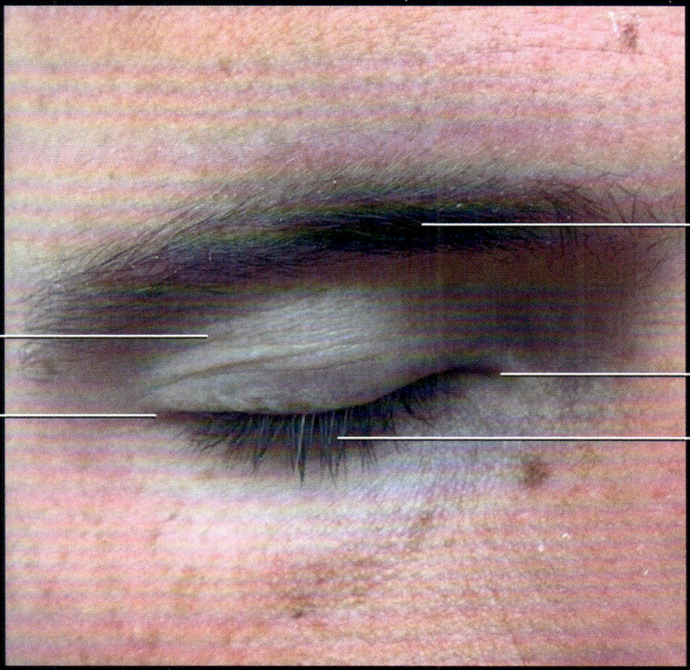

(Top) *Illustration depicts a sagittal section of the eyelid. The layers of the eyelid are easily discernible in this cross section. From superficial to deep, the layers of the eyelid include skin, orbicularis oculi muscle, areolar tissue, tarsal plate, and palpebral conjunctiva. The orbital septum separates the orbital contents from the lid contents and serves to contain the spread of infection into the orbit.* ***(Bottom)*** *This clinical photograph shows an external eyelid. The upper palpebral sulcus is created by the aponeurosis of the levator palpebrae superioris. Blood supply to the superior and inferior palpebrae is provided by the superior and inferior palpebral arteries and their branches, the superior and inferior palpebral arterial arches. The medial canthus can be covered with a skin fold (epicanthal fold) as a normal variant or in certain pathological conditions including Down syndrome, Turner syndrome, fetal alcohol syndrome, and phenylketonuria.*

BLEPHARITIS

Key Facts

Introduction

- Inflammation of eyelid typically involving skin, lashes, or meibomian glands
- Classification by location
  - Anterior blepharitis
  - Posterior blepharitis

Demographics

- Anterior blepharitis is commonly caused by bacterial infection (*Staphylococcus aureus* or *Staphylococcus epidermidis*) or seborrheic blepharitis
- Posterior blepharitis is commonly due to abnormal oil production by meibomian glands

Presentation

- Irritation, burning, or foreign body sensation in eyelids
- Red, dry, or watery eyes
- Anterior blepharitis may be associated with hard crusts around bases of cilia
- Posterior blepharitis findings
  - Oily tear film and possible frothy discharge on lid margins
  - Inspissated meibomian glands obstructed by oily secretions
  - Eyelid hyperemia and telangiectasia

Treatment

- Anterior blepharitis is treated with erythromycin, bacitracin, or fusidic acid
- Posterior blepharitis is treated with
  - Preservative-free artificial tears
  - Eyelid hygiene
  - Eyelid massage
  - Gentle eyelid scrubs
  - Warm compresses

*(**Left**) Slit-lamp photograph depicts crusting around the base of the lashes ➔, which is typical of anterior blepharitis. This appearance is common in blepharitis caused by Staphylococcus species. (**Right**) This slit-lamp photograph depicts inspissated meibomian glands ➔. This finding is indicative of meibomian gland dysfunction, which is also called posterior blepharitis. Meibomian gland dysfunction leads to an inadequate oil layer in the tear film, which can result in ocular irritation.*

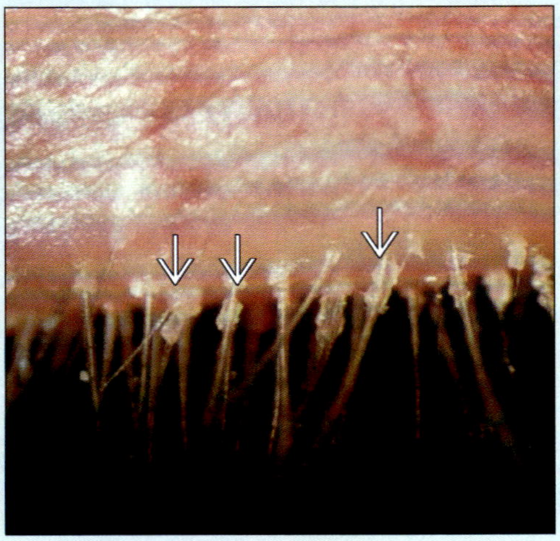

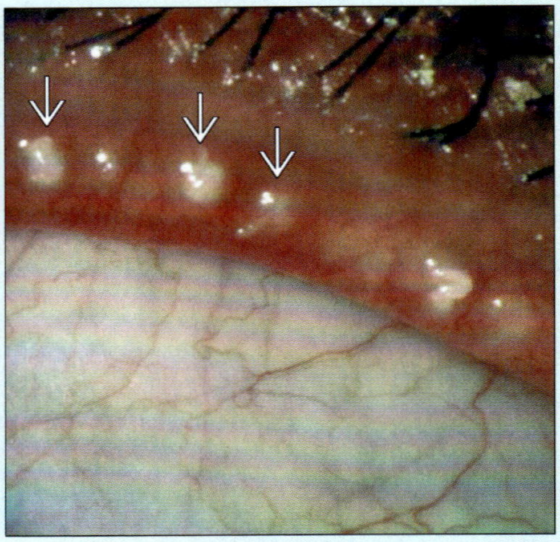

*(**Left**) Slit-lamp photograph demonstrates a thickened upper eyelid ➔, which has occurred secondary to chronic blepharitis. The thickening can inhibit eyelid functionality. (**Right**) This slit-lamp photograph demonstrates eyelash misdirection ➔, which can occur in chronic blepharitis. The misdirection of the lashes can lead to further ocular irritation and exacerbation of symptoms. The misdirection of the lashes is likely secondary to chronic inflammation.*

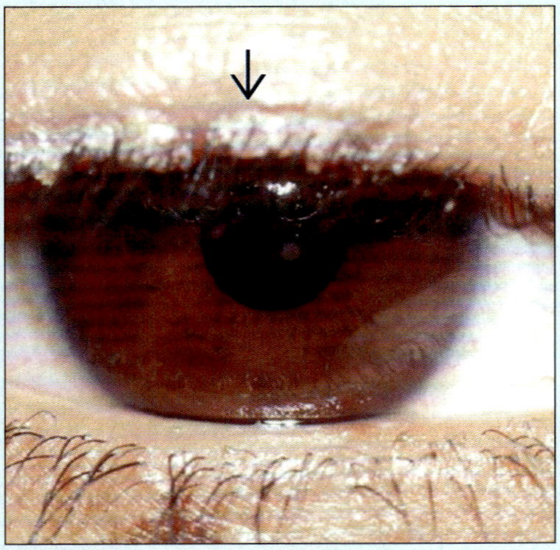

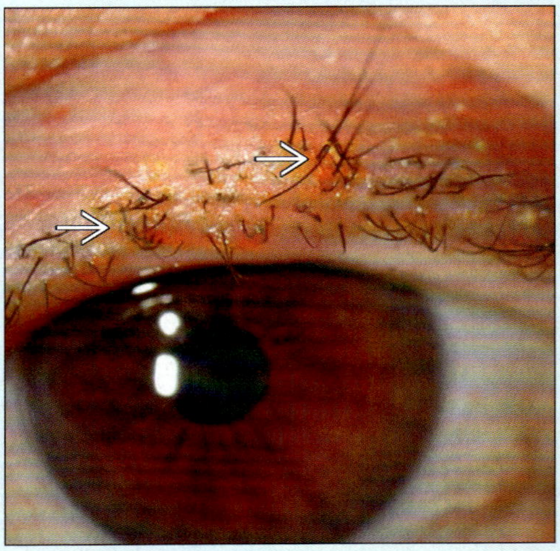

BLEPHARITIS

INTRODUCTION

Definitions
- Inflammation of eyelid typically involving skin, lashes, or meibomian glands

Subtypes
- Classification by location
  - Anterior blepharitis: Inflammation of anterior lid, eyelashes, and follicles
  - Posterior blepharitis: Inflammation of meibomian glands

DEMOGRAPHICS

Etiology/Risk Factors
- Commonly results from increased colonization of eyelid margins
- Anterior blepharitis is commonly caused by bacterial infection (*Staphylococcus aureus* or *Staphylococcus epidermidis*) or seborrheic blepharitis
  - Bacterial (*S. epidermidis, S. aureus, Propionibacterium acnes*, corynebacteria), viral (molluscum contagiosum, herpes simplex, or varicella), or parasitic (*Demodex folliculorum, Pediculosis pubis*)
- Posterior blepharitis is commonly due to abnormal oil production by meibomian glands
- May be associated with systemic diseases: Rosacea, seborrheic dermatitis, systemic lupus erythematous

PRESENTATION

Symptoms
- Photophobia; red, dry, or watery eyes typically worse in the morning
- Soreness, irritation, burning, or foreign body sensation in eyelids

Exam Findings
- Anterior blepharitis may be associated with hard crusts around bases of cilia
- Posterior blepharitis findings: Oily tear film and possible frothy discharge on lid margins, meibomian glands obstructed by oily secretions, or eyelid hyperemia and telangiectasia
- Chronic conditions may present with reddened, inspissated lid margins with scaling or crusting around lid margins

DIFFERENTIAL DIAGNOSIS

Preseptal Cellulitis
- Acute, painful, eyelid erythema and edema often accompanied with a fever
- May present with upper respiratory infection (URI) symptoms (i.e., sinus tenderness, rhinorrhea, adenopathy)

Dry Eye Syndrome
- Symptoms (i.e., excessive reflex tearing) tend to be worse at end of day
- May be a sign of systemic disease (i.e., connective tissue disease, rheumatoid arthritis, thyroid disease)

Chalazion
- Acute inflammation with firm, nontender eyelid mass
- More common in upper lid and typically follows chronic course

Keratitis
- Rapid onset of pain, photophobia, and decreased vision
- Ulceration of epithelium, folds in Descemet membrane

Basal Cell Carcinoma of Eyelid
- Slow-growing waxy papule with central depression that bleeds when traumatized
- More common in patients who sunburn

EVALUATION/WORK-UP

Labs
- Evaluate for tear insufficiency or insufficient nasolacrimal drainage
- Culture of eyelid margin for recurrent blepharitis with severe inflammation or for cases refractory to therapy
- Biopsy of eyelid to rule out carcinoma in severe cases

TREATMENT

Medical
- Posterior blepharitis is treated with preservative-free artificial tears, eyelid hygiene, eyelid massage, warm compresses, and scrubbing
  - Microwaveable eye mask is helpful
- Anterior blepharitis is treated with erythromycin, bacitracin, or fusidic acid
- Topical corticosteroids can be used for cases of severe blepharitis
  - Flaxseed oil or fish oil, 1 g p.o. t.i.d., is good for improving omega-3 fatty acid delivery (diet modifications are helpful)
    - Doxycycline 50 mg p.o. b.i.d. is helpful to modify tear film

Surgical
- Cases refractory to medical therapy should be worked up for possible squamous cell carcinoma or basal cell carcinoma
- Lipiflow or intense pulse light therapy are newer alternatives

Follow-Up
- Advise patients to return if condition worsens
- If corticosteroids are administered, follow-up should be within 2-4 weeks

Prognosis
- Typically follows chronic pattern with remissions and exacerbations
- Symptoms can improve but are rarely eliminated and may persist even after infection or inflammation resolves

SELECTED REFERENCES

1. American Academy of Ophthalmology Cornea/External Disease Panel. Blepharitis. Limited revision. San Francisco: American Academy of Ophthalmology, 2011

OCULAR ROSACEA

Key Facts

Introduction

- Chronic skin condition characterized by presence of telangiectasia, erythema, papules, pustules, and sebaceous gland hypertrophy
- Hallmark findings include bilateral chronic blepharitis, recurrent chalazia, eyelid telangiectasia, meibomian gland inspissation, and foreign body sensation

Demographics

- UV light, bacterial infection (*Staphylococcus epidermidis*, *Helicobacter pylori*), positive family history, smoking, flushing triggers (alcohol, spicy food, vasodilating medicine, emotional stress)
- ~ 10% of USA population diagnosed with rosacea, and 60% of these patients experience ocular symptoms
- Commonly found in patients 30-60 years old and up to 3x more common in women

Presentation

- Foreign body sensation, photophobia, lid margin telangiectasia, meibomian gland inflammation, inspissation, and marginal corneal ulceration and vascularization
- Bilateral chronic blepharitis, recurrent chalazia, eyelid margin telangiectasia, meibomian gland inspissation, and foreign body sensation
- May be accompanied with facial findings including facial pustules; erythema of cheek, forehead, and nose; or rhinophyma

Evaluation/Work-Up

- Resembles type IV hypersensitivity reaction

Treatment

- Tetracycline or doxycycline are usually preferred but may also use topical azithromycin eye drops

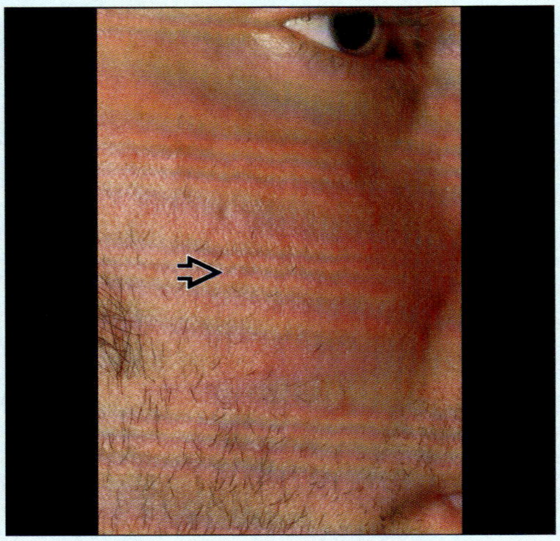

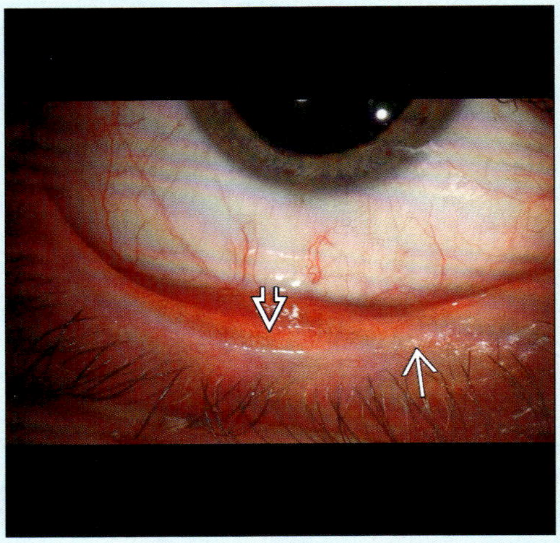

(Left) *External photo demonstrates classic skin findings of ocular rosacea, including a malar rash with increased sebum production and associated skin findings including pustules, papules, and erythema of the cheeks.* ***(Right)*** *External photo shows ocular signs of rosacea, including eyelid telangiectasias and blepharitis with inspissated meibomian glands.*

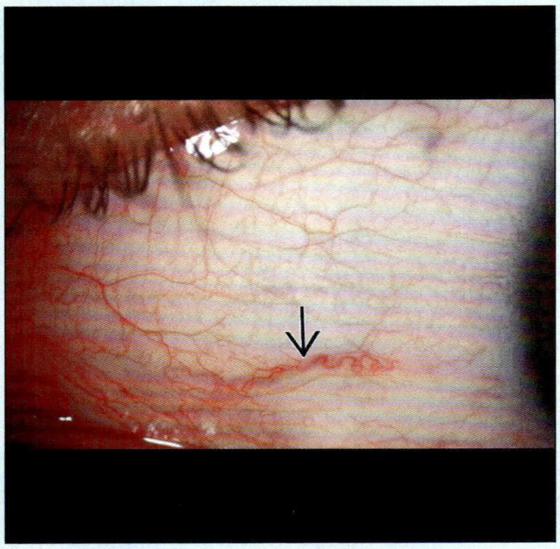

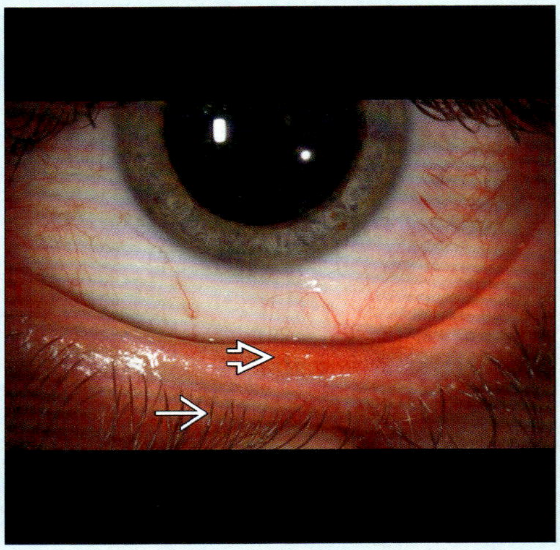

(Left) *Conjunctival hyperemia is often seen in ocular rosacea. Corneal neovascularization and thinning can develop and may lead to ulceration and opacification of the cornea if untreated.* ***(Right)*** *Diffuse conjunctival hyperemia with meibomian gland dysfunction, eyelid telangiectasias, and blepharitis are common findings with ocular rosacea.*

OCULAR ROSACEA

INTRODUCTION

Definitions

- Chronic skin condition characterized by presence of malar rash, telangiectasia, erythema, papules, pustules, and sebaceous gland hypertrophy
- Hallmark findings include bilateral chronic blepharitis, recurrent chalazia, eyelid telangiectasia, meibomian gland inspissation, and foreign body sensation

DEMOGRAPHICS

Etiology/Risk Factors

- UV light, bacterial infection (*Staphylococcus epidermidis*, *Helicobacter pylori*), positive family history, smoking, flushing triggers (alcohol, spicy food, vasodilating medicine, emotional stress)

Epidemiology

- About 10% of USA population diagnosed with rosacea, and 60% of these patients experience ocular symptoms
- Low mortality risk from rosacea, but high risk of morbidity due to symptoms and psychosocial impairment
- Commonly found in patients 30-60 years old and up to 3x more common in women

PRESENTATION

Symptoms

- Foreign body sensation, photophobia, lid margin telangiectasia, meibomian gland inflammation, inspissation, and marginal corneal ulceration and vascularization
- Recurrent eye infections or styes

Exam Findings

- Bilateral chronic blepharitis, recurrent chalazia, eyelid margin telangiectasia, meibomian gland inspissation, and foreign body sensation
- Corneal findings: Punctate epithelial keratopathy, corneal neovascularization, corneal thinning with ulceration or perforation
- May be accompanied with facial findings including facial pustules; erythema of cheek, forehead, and nose; or rhinophyma

DIFFERENTIAL DIAGNOSIS

Dry Eye Syndrome (Keratoconjunctivitis Sicca)

- Foreign body sensation, hyperemia, mucoid discharge, and photophobia exacerbated by smoke, dry environments, excessive heat, or prolonged computer use
- Symptoms tend to be worse at end of the day

Herpes Simplex Keratitis

- Pain, photophobia, blurry vision due to HSV infection of cornea
- Corneal epithelial staining in dendritic pattern

Episcleritis

- Inflammation of tissue between sclera and conjunctiva
- Mild to moderate discomfort associated with injection of bulbar conjunctiva and possibly photophobia and watery discharge
- Corneal findings are uncommon

Systemic Lupus Erythematosus (SLE)

- Most commonly presents as fever, joint pain, and a malar rash in women of child-bearing age
- Strong family history of SLE may be present

EVALUATION/WORK-UP

Pathology

- Infiltration of conjunctiva by inflammatory cells, CD4 T cells, phagocytic cells, and antigen-presenting cells
- Possible granulomatous changes with increased vascular dilation
- Resembles type IV hypersensitivity reaction

TREATMENT

Medical

- Lid hygiene with warm compresses, eye lubricant, and gentle massage provide symptomatic relief
- Antibiotics in patients with worsening disease
  - Systemic tetracyclines may decrease inflammation and are often first-line treatment for patients with moderate disease
  - Topical metronidazole can be used to treat facial lesions
  - Erythromycin ointment to eyelids if there is severe lid margin disease with suspected *Staphylococcus* infection
- Dietary modifications can reduce symptoms including
  - Flaxseed oil or fish oil (1 g p.o. t.i.d.) can help improve symptoms by giving omega-3 fatty acids
  - Reduce alcohol, caffeine, red meat; increase omega-3 fatty acids
- Consider referral to dermatology

Surgical

- Not indicated unless complications present (i.e., nonhealing epithelial defects, corneal ulceration, or limbal stem cell deficiency)
  - Can treat with amniotic membrane reconstruction, keratoplasty, or limbal cell transplant

Follow-Up

- Frequent follow-ups every 6-12 months may be required given chronic nature of this rosacea

Prognosis

- Can be managed symptomatically; however, long-term management is required to appropriately control rosacea
- Untreated ocular rosacea can lead to peripheral corneal ulceration, corneal scarring, and neovascularization

SELECTED REFERENCES

1. Wilkin J et al: Standard classification of rosacea: Report of the National Rosacea Society Expert Committee on the Classification and Staging of Rosacea. J Am Acad Dermatol. 46(4):584-7, 2002
2. Knox CM et al: Rosacea. Int Ophthalmol Clin. 37(2):29-40, 1997

EYELID LACERATION

Key Facts

Introduction
- Lacerations to eyelid and associated structures

Demographics
- Children: Most common etiologies of eyelid laceration include dog bites, biking injury, and collision with sharp objects
- Adults: Most common etiology is blunt trauma

Presentation
- Eyelid laceration where subtype may be assessed further via slit-lamp examination

Differential Diagnosis
- Trauma to orbit or globe
- Ocular burns
- Periocular hematoma

Evaluation/Work-Up
- Consider noncontrast orbit CT scan
- If lids medial to the puncta are cut, lacrimal ducts should be evaluated and reattached

Treatment
- Standard trauma evaluation to assess for life-threatening injuries
- Consider general anesthesia for lacerations in children and regional anesthesia in adults
- Surgical reconstruction methods are varied and highly dependent on the anatomy of the injury
  - Superficial lacerations: Lacerations that are horizontal and follow skin tension folds/lid lines
  - Partial thickness: Deeper lacerations that run perpendicular to skin tension folds
  - Eyelid margin: Lacerations to eyelid margin
  - Tissue loss: Lacerations with tissue loss
  - Full thickness: Lacerations involving skin, muscle, &/or tarsal plate, &/or conjunctiva

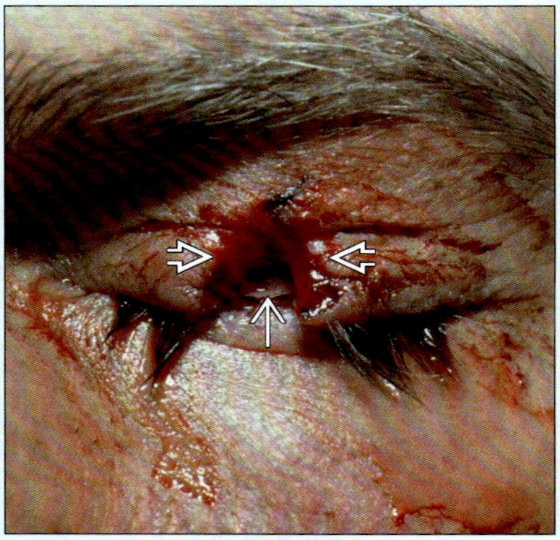
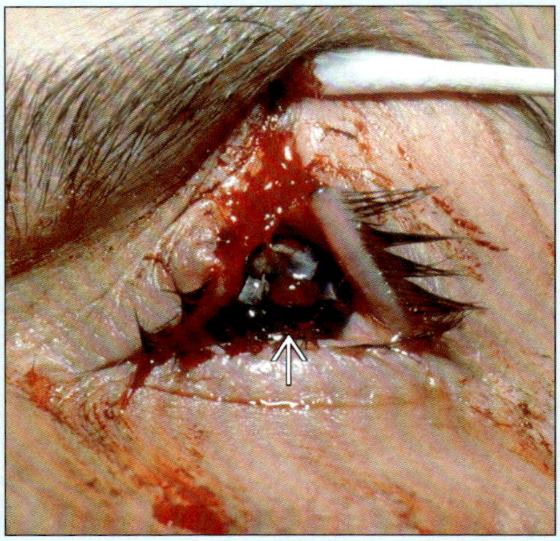

(Left) *External photograph demonstrates a full-thickness eyelid laceration of the upper eyelid ➡. Note the thickened, edematous eyelid tissue that is visible on either side of the laceration ➡.* ***(Right)*** *This external photograph depicts the same eyelid laceration with the globe exposed ➡. It is important to perform a thorough ocular exam in a patient with an eyelid laceration as the trauma can often result in injury to the intraocular structures.*

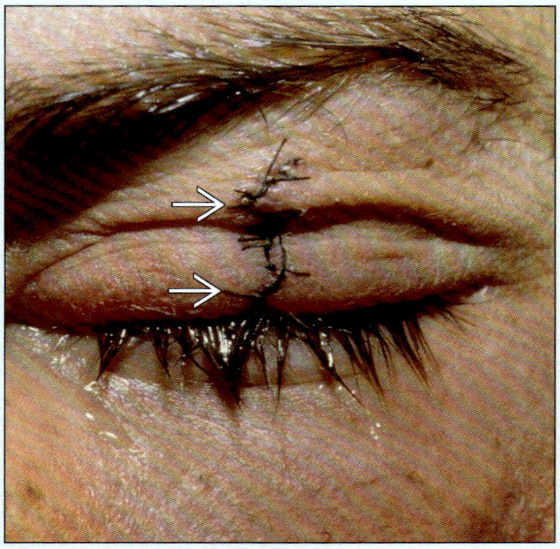
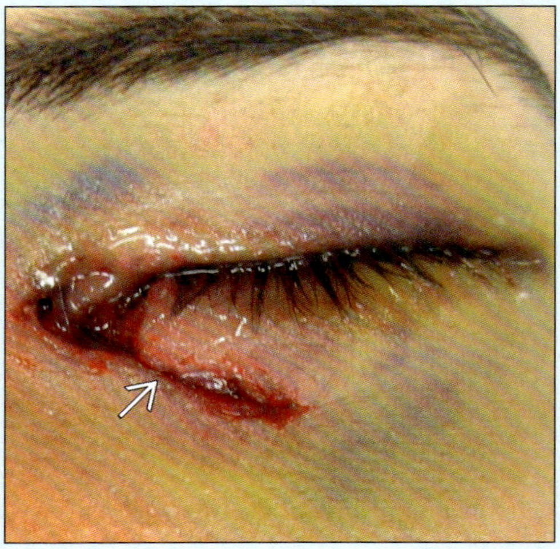

(Left) *External photograph depicts the same eyelid after repair has taken place with visible sutures ➡. The eyelids remain edematous, which can occasionally make suturing more difficult.* ***(Right)*** *This external photograph depicts an eyelid with an inferior laceration ➡. With a laceration such as the one pictured, it is important to identify the depth and extent of the lesion in addition to identifying any other structures involved, such as the inferior canaliculi.*

EYELID LACERATION

INTRODUCTION

Subtypes
- Superficial laceration
- Eyelid-margin laceration
- Partial-thickness laceration
- Tissue loss laceration
- Full-thickness laceration

DEMOGRAPHICS

Etiology/Risk Factors
- Facial trauma, including blunt or penetrating trauma
- Dog bites, biking injuries, and collision with sharp objects
- Child abuse
- Newborns delivered via cesarean section

Epidemiology
- In children, most common etiologies of eyelid laceration include dog bites, biking injury, and collision with sharp objects
- In adolescents and adults, most common etiology of eyelid laceration is blunt trauma
- Eyelid laceration is more common in men than women
- Ocular injury is seen in conjunction with eyelid laceration in up to 66% of cases

PRESENTATION

Exam Findings
- Slit-lamp examination evaluating for the following
  - Foreign body
  - Corneal or scleral laceration
  - Prolapse
  - Volume loss of eyeball
  - Pupil shape irregularities
  - Subconjunctival hemorrhage
- Assess for decrease in visual acuity and relative pupillary defect
- If lids medial to the puncta are cut, oculoplastics involvement is necessary to potentially reconstruct lacrimal ducts

DIFFERENTIAL DIAGNOSIS

Trauma to Globe or Orbit
- May present with ecchymosis and edema and a history of trauma

Ocular Burns
- Thermal or chemical exposure to eye or eyelid

Periocular Hematoma
- Collection of blood or bruising surrounding eye ("black eye")

EVALUATION/WORK-UP

Imaging
- Consider noncontrast orbit CT scan if further injury is suspected, including open globe injury (e.g., periorbital edema and significant ecchymosis)

TREATMENT

Medical
- Standard trauma evaluation to assess for life-threatening injuries
- Tetanus vaccination if needed
- Rabies protocol if animal bite suspected
- Wound should be kept moist
- Eye protection with aggressive lubrication should be used
- Consider general anesthesia for lacerations in children and regional anesthesia in adults
- For procedures requiring local anesthesia, use of lidocaine with epinephrine is preferred with injection along wound edges
  - If laceration creates skin flap, use of lidocaine only is preferred to prevent decreased blood flow to flap

Surgical
- Surgical reconstruction methods are varied and highly dependent on the anatomy of the injury
- Superficial: Lacerations that are horizontal and follow skin tension folds/lid lines
  - If laceration involves < 25% of the lid, suturing is often not required, and skin tape may be used instead
- Partial thickness: Deeper lacerations that run perpendicular to skin tension folds that need to reapproximated
  - 6-0 or 7-0 absorbable or nonabsorbable simple interrupted sutures may be placed
- Eyelid margin: Lacerations to eyelid margin that require accurate eyelid approximation to avoid eyelid notching and margin malposition
  - To align lid margin, use 6-0 absorbable or nonabsorbable suture placed 2 mm from and 2 mm deep to wound edge
  - Tarsal closure by fine, interrupted, partial thickness suture tied anteriorly
  - Skin closure by fine suture
- Tissue loss: Depending on amount and location of loss, may require skin grafts, myocutaneous flaps, advancement flaps, &/or skin grafts
- Full thickness: Lacerations involving skin, muscle, &/or tarsal plate &/or conjunctiva that may cause severe structure disruption and, therefore, necessitates careful inspection of each layer
  - To reapproximate the lash margin, use 5-0 or 6-0 absorbable or nonabsorbable suture
  - To reapproximate tarsal plate and orbicularis oculi muscle, use 5-0 absorbable suture
  - To repair eyelid skin, use 5-0 or 6-0 absorbable or nonabsorbable simple loose suture
- Postoperative care may include ice compresses, head elevation, and antibiotic ointment

Follow-Up
- Usually within 1-2 weeks, depending on surgery

Prognosis
- Occasionally, reconstructive surgery may be necessary

SELECTED REFERENCES

1. Brown DJ et al: Advanced laceration management. Emerg Med Clin North Am. 25(1):83-99, 2007

CHALAZION

Key Facts

Introduction

- Chronic obstruction of meibomian or Zeis gland resulting in chronic granulomatous inflammation

Demographics

- Associated with seborrhea, chronic blepharitis, and acne rosacea
- More common in peripubertal and adult populations due to higher androgen hormone levels and increased sebum viscosity

Presentation

- Recurrent episodes of acute-onset lid swelling, redness, and irritation
- More common on upper eyelid due to increased concentration of meibomian glands
- Firm, painless lid nodule when meibomian gland involved; superficial lid nodule if Zeis gland involved
- Applying pressure to nodule produces thick secretion instead of oily secretion

Evaluation/Work-Up

- Histology identifies numerous lipid-laden giant cells
- Mass of granulation tissue and chronic inflammation containing lymphocytes and lipid-laden macrophages

Treatment

- Conservative treatment with warm compresses and artificial tears can alleviate most acute episodes and decrease future recurrence
- Transconjunctival incision and curettage for chronic, persistent lesions (opening should be vertical, not horizontal), consider intralesional steroid injection
- Chalazion should resolve within 1 month without intervention; however, recurrence is common
- Patients undergoing incision and curettage should be seen within 1 week and then follow-up as is required

*(**Left**) In this photograph, a chalazion can be seen on the patient's upper eyelid ➔. These cysts commonly occur in this location due to the higher density of meibomian glands on the upper lid. (**Right**) Photograph demonstrates a patient with more prominent eyelid swelling and lid heaviness in association with this larger chalazion seen on the upper lid ➔.*

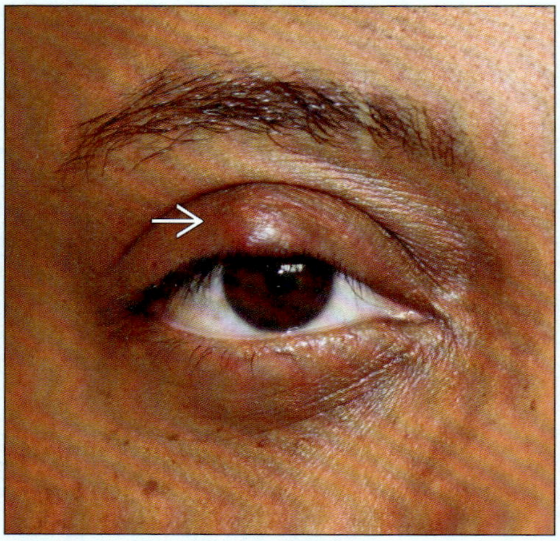

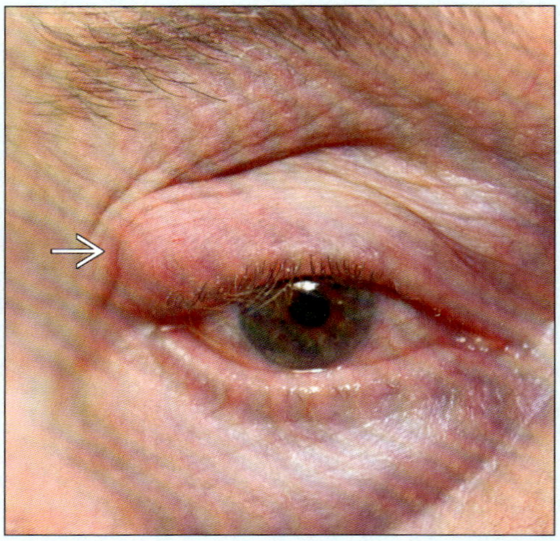

*(**Left**) Surgical removal of a chalazion usually begins with eversion of the eyelid with a special clamp, as shown in this photograph. (**Right**) The surgeon will then proceed to incision, and the contents of the chalazion will be curetted to resolve the lesion.*

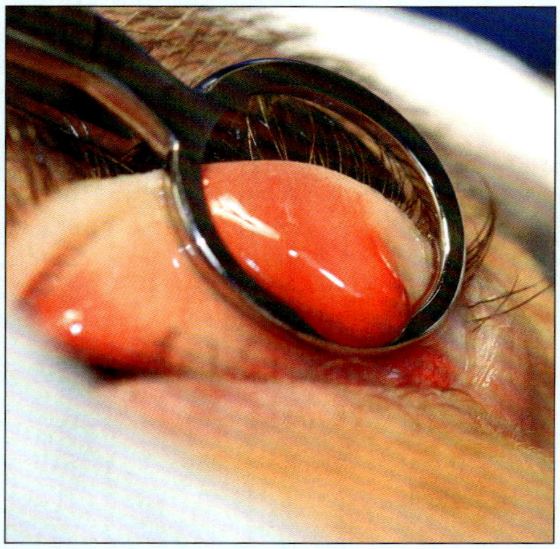

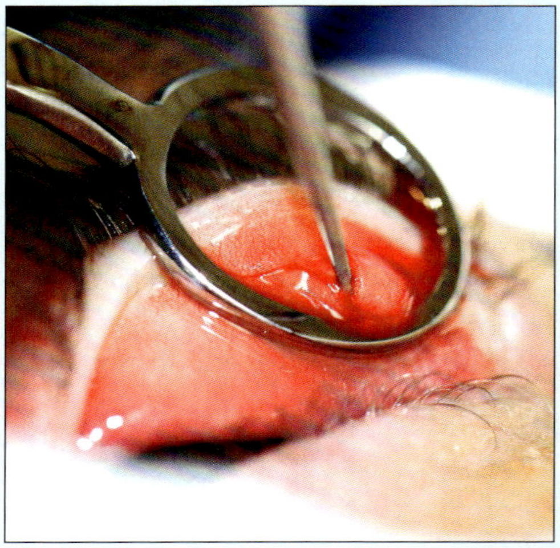

CHALAZION

INTRODUCTION

Definitions

- Noninfectious chronic obstruction of meibomian or Zeis gland resulting in chronic granulomatous inflammation

DEMOGRAPHICS

Etiology/Risk Factors

- Associated with seborrhea, chronic blepharitis, and acne rosacea

Epidemiology

- More common in peripubertal and adult populations due to higher androgen hormone levels and increased sebum viscosity

PRESENTATION

Symptoms

- Recurrent episodes of acute-onset lid swelling, redness, and irritation

Exam Findings

- More common on upper eyelid due to increased concentration of meibomian glands
- Firm, painless lid nodule when meibomian gland involved; superficial lid nodule if Zeis gland involved
- Chronic inspissation of meibomian gland
- Applying pressure to nodule produces thick secretion instead of oily secretion

DIFFERENTIAL DIAGNOSIS

Hordeolum

- Acute, painful infection of meibomian gland
- Neutrophilic inflammation associated with necrosis and pustule formation

Sebaceous Cell Carcinoma

- Insidious onset of a firm, painless mass with ulceration, associated with loss of eyelashes
- Distinguish by biopsy with lipid stain, which is characteristically positive in sebaceous cell carcinoma
- Often mimics recurrent chalazia

Trichiasis

- Prominent eyelash misdirection often secondary to posterior lamellar scarring from prior trachoma
- May be associated with distichiasis, a metaplastic change of epithelial germ cells resulting in eyelash growth from meibomian gland orifice on posterior lamella of tarsal plate

Orbital Cellulitis

- Inflammation of soft tissues of eye socket secondary to acute spread of bacterial infection from adjacent sinuses, skin, or blood
- Initially presents with increasing redness and swelling followed by proptosis and decreased extraocular motility as inflammation progresses

EVALUATION/WORK-UP

Pathology

- Histology identifies numerous lipid-laden giant cells
- Mass of granulation tissue and chronic inflammation containing lymphocytes and lipid-laden macrophages

TREATMENT

Medical

- Conservative treatment with lid massage, moist heat, and artificial tears can alleviate most acute episodes and decrease future recurrence
- Antibiotic therapy may be effective in complicated cases associated with inflammatory conditions (i.e., blepharitis) or recurrent cases
  - Treat with oral tetracycline (doxycycline 100 mg or minocycline 50 mg) once a day for 10 days to help reduce blepharitis that contributes to chalazia
  - Topical erythromycin or sulfacetamide ointment can help fight bacterial colonization of eyelids that contributes to chalazia
- Direct injection of steroids (mild, low dose, short duration) may be useful if lesions are in close proximity to the lacrimal apparatus

Surgical

- Transconjunctival incision and curettage for chronic, persistent hordeola (opening should be vertical, not horizontal, to minimize number of meibomian glands that are cut)
- Incision and curettage in combination with local intralesional corticosteroid injection
  - More effective in combination than either treatment is alone
- Extensively fibrotic chalazia may require more extensive surgical excision including a portion of tarsal plate

Follow-Up

- Patients undergoing incision and curettage should be seen within 1 week and then follow-up as is required

Prognosis

- Chalazion should resolve within 1 month without intervention; however, recurrence is common
  - Episodes that do not resolve with conservative management within 1 month should be evaluated for incision and curettage
- Persistence or multiple recurrences may be due to carcinoma and require further evaluation to rule out sebaceous cell carcinoma

SELECTED REFERENCES

1. Arbabi EM et al: Chalazion. BMJ. 341:c4044, 2010
2. Gilchrist H et al: Management of chalazia in general practice. Aust Fam Physician. 38(5):311-4, 2009
3. Carter SR: Eyelid disorders: diagnosis and management. Am Fam Physician. 57(11):2695-702, 1998

BASAL CELL CARCINOMA

Key Facts

Introduction
- Locally invasive, slowly spreading tumor that rarely metastasizes, arising in epidermis or hair follicles, and in which the peripheral cells usually simulate basal cells of epidermis
  - Nodular (most common): Rounded, pearly nodule that usually contains linear telangiectasias and can ulcerate; may contain pearly raised border
  - Morpheaform (rare): Aggressive form of BCC that resembles fibrotic scar tissue, has indeterminate margins, and may infiltrate deeply

Demographics
- Most common eyelid malignancy, accounting for 90-95% of eyelid tumors
- Vast majority of cases related to sun exposure
- Basal cell nevus syndrome (Gorlin syndrome)
  - Multiple nevoid basal cell carcinomas that appear around puberty
- Xeroderma pigmentosum
  - Present with multiple BCC and other skin malignancies at young age

Presentation
- May present as a slow-growing, plaque-like, papular, or nodular lesion around the eyelids
- May have central ulceration, bleeding, crusting

Evaluation/Work-Up
- Histology: Tumor frequently displays proliferation of small basaloid cells, peripheral palisading, and ulceration in larger tumors

Treatment
- Mohs micrographic surgery
  - Standard of care for head and neck BCC
- Surgical excision
- Radiotherapy

*(**Left**) External photo shows nodular basal cell carcinoma (BCC) of the left lower eyelid margin ➡. This small tumor has a classic pearly appearance, central ulceration, and madarosis. (**Right**) External photo depicts a larger left lower eyelid nodular BCC ➙. Tumors of this size may require more complex reconstructive surgery after full-thickness excision or MOHS micrographic surgery and are often repaired with lid-sharing techniques or flaps. (Courtesy S. Leite, MD.)*

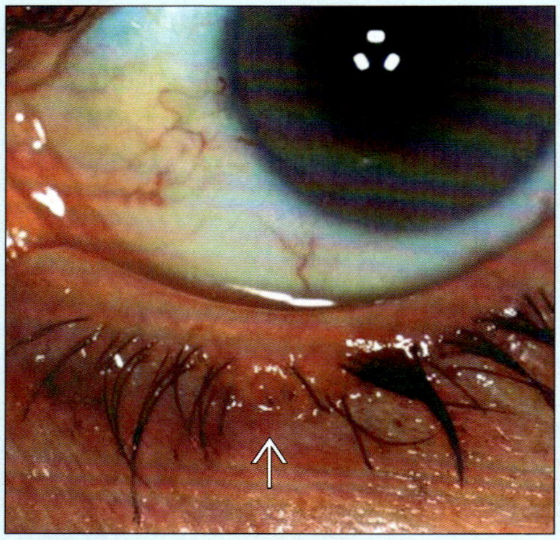

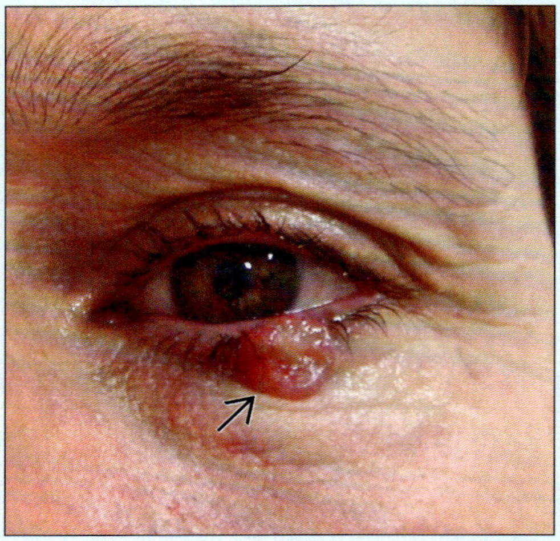

*(**Left**) Pathology slide with hematoxylin and eosin staining shows infiltrating nests and cords of basaloid cells ⇨ with peripheral palisading ➙. Cells show hyperchromatic nuclei with scant eosinophilic cytoplasm. (**Right**) External photo shows a large, advanced, morpheaform BCC. The tumor has invaded through underlying orbicularis muscle and shows extensive areas of ulceration and necrosis ➡. Smaller tumors usually resemble a flat, firm, erythematous fibrotic scar. (Courtesy B. Mack, MD.)*

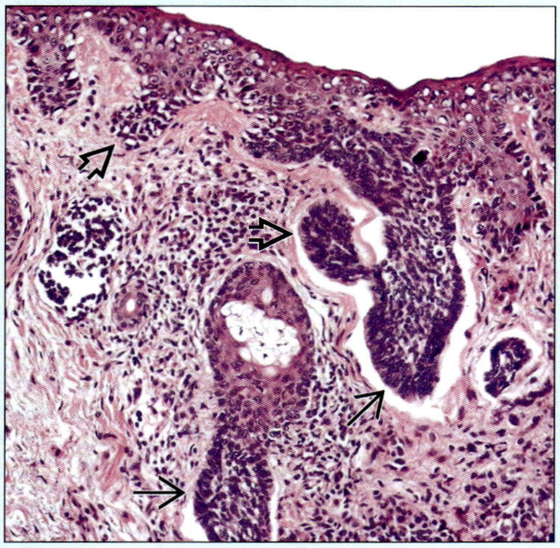

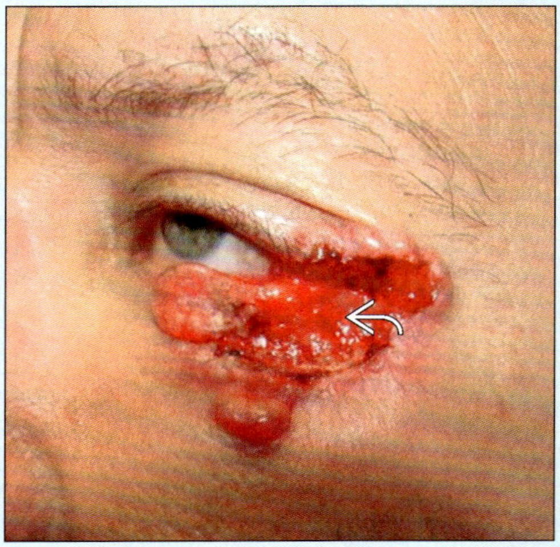

BASAL CELL CARCINOMA

INTRODUCTION

Abbreviations

- Basal cell carcinoma (BCC)

Definitions

- Locally invasive, slowly spreading tumor that rarely metastasizes, arising in epidermis or hair follicles, and in which the peripheral cells usually simulate basal cells of epidermis

Subtypes

- Nodular: Large, rounded, pearly nodule that usually contains linear telangiectasias and can ulcerate; may contain pearly raised border
  - Most common form, accounting for 75% of BCC
  - 90% found in head and neck
- Superficial: Appears as plaque or erythematous plaque
  - Most commonly found in trunk and extremities; however, 40% still found in head and neck
  - May be confused for chronic blepharitis
- Morpheaform: Rare, aggressive form of BCC that resembles fibrotic scar tissue, has indeterminate margins, and may infiltrate deeply
  - 6% of BCC cases, 95% located in head and neck
- Infiltrative: Often deeply invasive, linked to nodular or morpheaform variants
- Metatypical: Resembles both BCC and squamous cell carcinoma (SCC), has higher invasive and metastatic potential similar to SCC

DEMOGRAPHICS

Etiology/Risk Factors

- Vast majority of cases related to sun exposure
  - Risk factors: Fair-skinned patients of northern European descent, family or personal history of BCC, cigarette smoking, and advanced age
- Basal cell nevus syndrome (Gorlin syndrome)
  - Multiple nevoid BCCs that appear around puberty
  - Associated with odontogenic keratocyst, intracranial calcification, frontal bossing, hypertelorism, cleft lip or palate, and rib and skeletal malformations
- Xeroderma pigmentosum
  - Rare defect in DNA repair mechanisms to UV damage, autosomal recessive
  - Present with multiple BCCs and other skin malignancies at young age

Epidemiology

- ~ 150 cases per 100,000
- Most common cancer in humans
- Most common eyelid malignancy (90-95%)
  - Normally found in lower eyelid (50-60%) and medial canthus (25-30%)

PRESENTATION

Symptoms

- Painless, slow-growing eyelid lesion

Exam Findings

- Slow-growing, plaque-like, papular, or nodular lesion around eyelids
  - Pearly or translucent, with telangiectasias and multiple blue-gray globules visible on dermoscopy
  - May have central ulceration, bleeding, crusting, madarosis

DIFFERENTIAL DIAGNOSIS

Squamous Cell Carcinoma

- May often appear similar to BCC but less common, more aggressive, and with higher metastatic potential

Actinic Keratosis

- Premalignant lesion with scaly, erythematous macules

Sebaceous Carcinoma

- Highly malignant diffuse eyelid tumor, often confused with recurrent chalazia or blepharitis

EVALUATION/WORK-UP

Pathology

- Definitive diagnosis is obtained through incisional or excisional biopsy and histologic examination
- Tumor frequently displays proliferation of small basaloid cells, peripheral palisading, and ulceration in larger tumors
  - Nodular: Large, rounded, dermal-based nests with peripheral palisading
  - Morpheaform: Infiltrative strands and nests associated with dense sclerotic stroma, no peripheral palisading

TREATMENT

Medical

- Radiotherapy: 92-99% cure rate
  - Used either primarily or as adjunctive treatment for invasive tumors or positive margins
- Photodynamic therapy (PDT): 73-92% response rate

Surgical

- Mohs micrographic surgery: 5-year cure rate 99%
  - Standard of care for head and neck BCC
- Surgical excision: 5-year cure rate of 95.2%
  - 4 mm margins for nonmorpheaform tumors; however, depends on tumor type, size, and location
- Cryotherapy: Higher recurrence rate than surgery
  - Reserved for small tumors in patients who are otherwise unable to undergo surgery

Follow-Up

- Few weeks after surgery, then every 6-12 months

Prognosis

- Excellent with complete local excision

SELECTED REFERENCES

1. Nakayama M et al: Basal cell carcinoma of the head and neck. J Skin Cancer. 2011:496910, 2011
2. Telfer NR et al: Guidelines for the management of basal cell carcinoma. Br J Dermatol. 159(1):35-48, 2008
3. Nemet AY et al: Management of periocular basal and squamous cell carcinoma: a series of 485 cases. Am J Ophthalmol. 142(2):293-7, 2006

SEBACEOUS GLAND CARCINOMA

Key Facts

Introduction
- Neoplasm of sebaceous glands including meibomian glands, Zeis glands, or glands associated with caruncle

Demographics
- Though etiology is unknown, sebaceous gland carcinoma may be associated with *P53* mutations, HIV, and HPV
- 3rd most common eyelid malignancy after basal cell and squamous cell carcinoma
- Most cases present at mean age of 70 years
- Younger people with history of radiation exposure to the face are at increased risk

Presentation
- Insidious onset of painless, yellowish mass with associated thickening of the eyelid; often there are recurrent chalazia
- Firm, yellow-colored mass or ulceration that appears at sebaceous glands at the lid margin with possible extension to palpebral conjunctiva

Evaluation/Work-Up
- Wide excisional biopsy of all recurrent chalazia or other nonresolving lesions of the eyelid
- Hallmark feature is a Pagetoid spread: Spread of malignant cells to epithelium that is separate from primary tumor
- Foamy cytoplasm, which stains positive with fat stains, and increased mitotic figures are commonly seen in biopsy specimens
- Evaluate lymph nodes to rule out metastases

Treatment
- Wide-margin, full-thickness excision with sentinel lymph node biopsy for stage T2b or worse; also obtain map biopsies of the conjunctiva

*(**Left**) External photograph shows sebaceous gland carcinoma (SGC) involving the upper eyelid ⇒. It is more common for sebaceous gland carcinoma to involve the upper eyelid. (**Right**) This is a hematoxylin and eosin-stained slide from a lesion that is concerning for SGC. The cells form large lobules separated by small fibrous septa. These are vacuolated, epithelioid-type cells. There is a moderate degree of dysplasia with nucleoli and pleomorphism. A mitotic figure can be seen ⇒.*

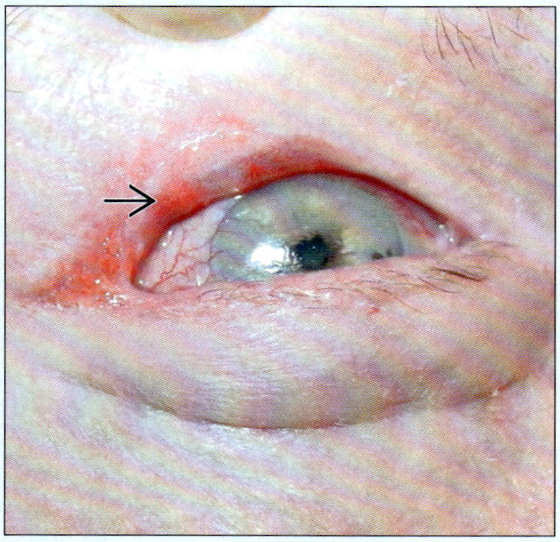

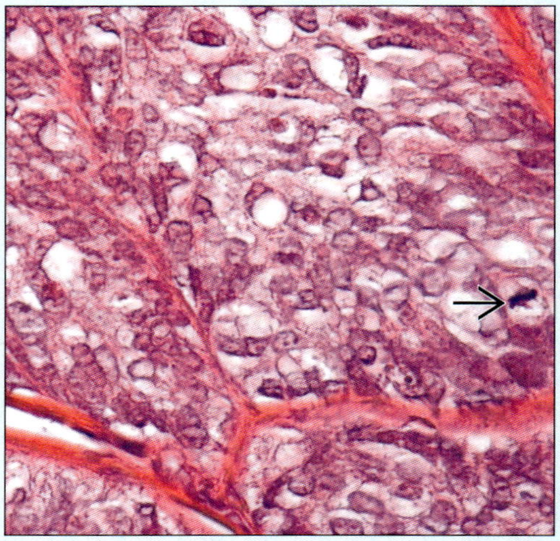

*(**Left**) External photograph shows the eye of a patient with a chalazion of the upper eyelid ⇒. SGC is often initially misdiagnosed as chalazion or blepharitis. It is important to have a degree of suspicion for SGC any time chalazion or blepharitis is diagnosed. (**Right**) This external photograph shows basal cell carcinoma of the lower eyelid ⇒. Basal cell carcinoma is an important differential diagnosis for SGC and is more typically found on the lower eyelid.*

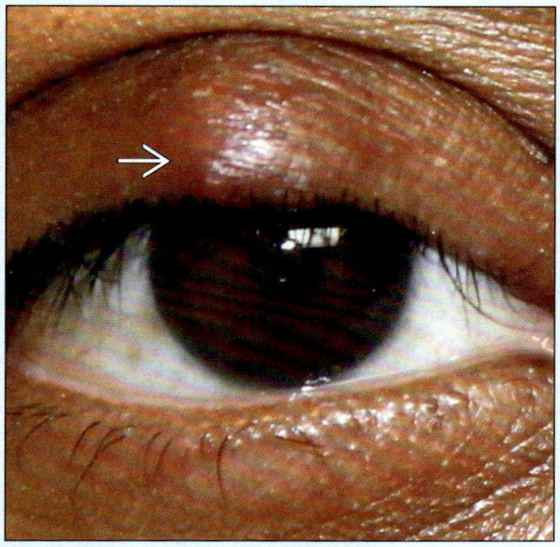

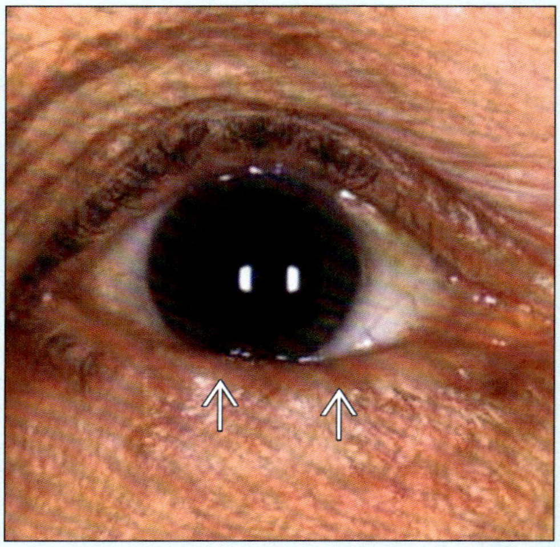

SEBACEOUS GLAND CARCINOMA

INTRODUCTION

Abbreviations
- Sebaceous gland carcinoma (SGC)

Synonyms
- Sebaceous cell carcinoma
- Meibomian gland carcinoma

Definitions
- Neoplasm of sebaceous glands including Meibomian glands, Zeis glands, glands associated with the caruncle, lacrimal gland, or skin of eyelid and eyebrow

DEMOGRAPHICS

Etiology/Risk Factors
- Though etiology is unknown, SGC may be associated with *P53* mutations, HIV, and HPV
- Younger people with a history of radiation exposure to the face are at increased risk
- Women are more commonly affected than men
- In North America, whites are more commonly affected than African Americans
- Most cases present at a mean age of 70 years

Epidemiology
- 3rd most common eyelid malignancy after basal cell and squamous cell carcinomas
- Lesions more commonly located in upper eyelid due to increased number of meibomian glands present

PRESENTATION

Symptoms
- Insidious onset of painless, yellowish mass with associated thickening of the eyelid
  - May mimic recurrent chalazia of the upper eyelid
- Keratoconjunctivitis or blepharoconjunctivitis unresponsive to treatment

Exam Findings
- Firm, yellow-colored mass or ulceration that appears at the sebaceous glands at the lid margin with possible extension to palpebral conjunctiva
  - May be associated with loss of cilia

DIFFERENTIAL DIAGNOSIS

Recurrent Chalazion
- Chronic granulomatous reaction to retained sebaceous secretions of meibomian gland; commonly found in upper eyelid
- Chalazion tends to be more painful, well circumscribed, and not associated with loss of cilia

Muir-Torre Syndrome (MTS)
- Autosomal dominant condition characterized by sebaceous tumors of the gastrointestinal, endometrial, and genitourinary organs
- Less aggressive tumor that is less likely to metastasize relative to solitary sebaceous tumors

Basal Cell Carcinoma
- Tumor of the epithelial basal cells with a predilection for lower eyelids
- Histologically distinguished by characteristic palisading of nuclei at periphery of the islands of tumor

Merkel Cell Carcinoma
- Cutaneous, neuroendocrine carcinoma that may also present as solitary subcutaneous nodule
- Unlike SGC, Merkel cell carcinoma is red or blue in color and is typically caused by polyomavirus

EVALUATION/WORK-UP

Pathology
- Wide excisional biopsy of all recurrent chalazia or other nonresolving lesions of the eyelid
  - Hallmark feature is a Pagetoid spread: Spread of malignant cells to epithelium that is separate from the primary tumor
  - Foamy cytoplasm and increased mitotic figures are commonly seen in biopsy specimens
    - Presence of foamy cytoplasm helps distinguish SGC from cutaneous squamous cell carcinoma, and positive fat staining confirms the diagnosis
- Map biopsies of the conjunctiva including bulbar and palpebral conjunctiva
- Advanced lesions may be multicentric and grow in nests with central necrosis
- Evaluate lymph nodes to rule out metastases

TREATMENT

Surgical
- Wide-margin, full-thickness excision with sentinel lymph node biopsy for stage T2b or worse; also obtain map biopsies of conjunctiva
- If bulbar conjunctiva involvement or deep invasive lesions present, then orbital exenteration is required

Follow-Up
- Monitor for metastases or additional malignancies as these patients are at increased risk of head and neck basal cell lesions and visceral malignancies

Prognosis
- Recurrence in up to 33% of cases
- 25% rate of metastasis rate in stage T2b or worse

SELECTED REFERENCES

1. Sung D et al: Early onset sebaceous carcinoma. Diagn Pathol. 6:81, 2011
2. Dasgupta T et al: A retrospective review of 1349 cases of sebaceous carcinoma. Cancer. 115(1):158-65, 2009
3. Song A et al: Sebaceous cell carcinoma of the ocular adnexa: clinical presentations, histopathology, and outcomes. Ophthal Plast Reconstr Surg. 24(3):194-200, 2008
4. Shields JA et al: Sebaceous carcinoma of the ocular region: a review. Surv Ophthalmol. 50(2):103-22, 2005

SQUAMOUS CELL CARCINOMA OF THE EYELID

Key Facts

Introduction

- Nonmelanoma skin cancer characterized by lobular proliferation of keratinocytes and intradermal invasion of keratinocytes that show prominent keratin production

Demographics

- 2nd most common malignant neoplasm of eyelid after basal cell carcinoma (BCC) but more aggressive and invasive than BCC
- Incidence: 0.09-2.42 cases/100,000 people

Presentation

- Foreign body sensation with redness or irritation of eyelids, recurrent nonhealing ulceration or bleeding
- Tender erythematous, scaly plaque or papule that enlarges over months
- Occurs more commonly on lower eyelid and interpalpebral area than upper eyelid
- Advanced cases may exhibit perineural invasion (PNI) with findings of numbness, tingling, pain, paralysis or formication

Evaluation/Work-Up

- Histologic hallmark is keratin pearls

Treatment

- Local chemotherapy with intralesional injection of 5-fluorouracil and epinephrine for metastatic SCC
- Primary excision with 4-6 mm margins if no risk for recurrence
- Mohs surgery if higher risk for recurrence
- 3-month follow-up for patients at increased risk of recurrence (i.e., transplant recipients)
- Annual follow-up for uncomplicated patients
- Daily oral 13-cis-retinoic acid plus subcutaneous interferon α-2a; imiquimod cream is emerging alternative

__(Left)__ External photograph shows hyperkeratotic SCC of the lower eyelid. SCC occurs less often on the eyelid than BCC, but is more aggressive and may arise de novo or from preexisting actinic keratosis. Differential diagnoses of keratoacanthoma and cutaneous horn may exhibit invasive SCC at deeper histologic sections. (Courtesy J. Dutton, MD, PhD.) __(Right)__ This external photograph shows a patient with a large SCC of the face with visible hyperkeratosis ➔. (Courtesy D. Cassarino, MD, PhD.)

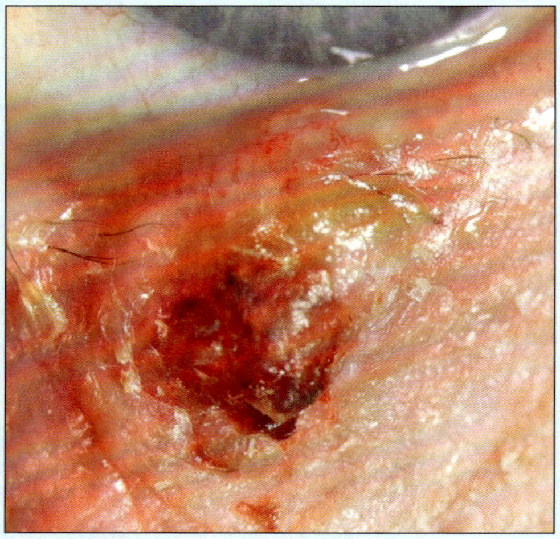

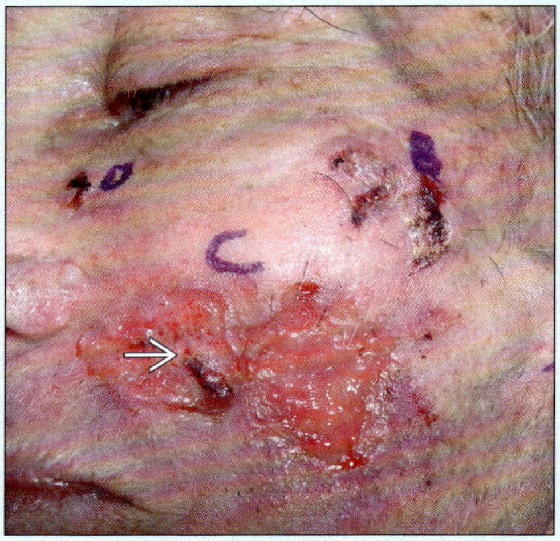

__(Left)__ This pathology slide depicts an example of SCC of the eyelid. The epithelium is moderately thickened in areas and shows focal areas of marked dysplastic changes →. There are areas of deep keratinization or dyskeratosis as well as multiple keratin pearls ➔. __(Right)__ External photo shows nodular BCC of the left lower eyelid margin ➔. This small tumor has classic pearly appearance, central ulceration, and madarosis. BCC is an important differential diagnosis for SCC.

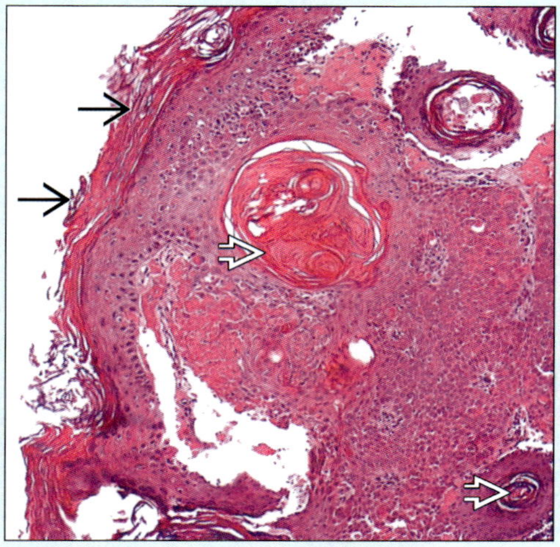

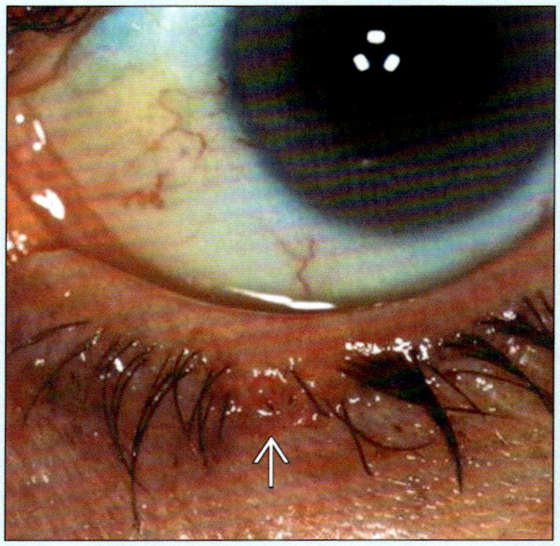

SQUAMOUS CELL CARCINOMA OF THE EYELID

INTRODUCTION

Abbreviations
- Squamous cell carcinoma (SCC)

Definitions
- Skin cancer characterized by lobular proliferation of keratinocytes and intradermal invasion of keratinocytes that show prominent keratin production

DEMOGRAPHICS

Etiology/Risk Factors
- Extrinsic risk factors
  - Family history of skin cancer, ultraviolet light exposure (UVA and UVB), toxic exposure (arsenic, hydrocarbons, radiation), HPV infection (especially types 6, 11, 16, 18), organ transplant or immunosuppressive drug therapy, smoking
- Intrinsic risk factors
  - Albinism or preexisting chronic skin lesions and genetic skin disorders (i.e., xeroderma pigmentosum and epidermodysplasia verruciformis)

Epidemiology
- 2nd most common malignant neoplasm of eyelid after basal cell carcinoma (BCC), comprising 5-10% of all eyelid malignancies (incidence: 0.09-2.42 cases per 100,000 people)

PRESENTATION

Symptoms
- Foreign body sensation with redness or irritation of eyelids, recurrent nonhealing ulceration or bleeding
- Tender erythematous, scaly plaque or papule that enlarges over months

Exam Findings
- Occurs more commonly on lower eyelid and interpalpebral area than upper eyelid
- Variable clinical presentation, including erythematous scaly patches, ulcerated lesions, or nodular or papillomatous lesions
- Advanced cases may exhibit perineural invasion (PNI) with findings of numbness, tingling, pain, paralysis, or formication

DIFFERENTIAL DIAGNOSIS

Precancerous Lesions
- Actinic keratosis
  - Scaly lesions, 2-6 mm in diameter, characterized by aggregates of atypical, pleomorphic keratinocytes at basal layer that may extend upwards to involve granular and cornified layers
- Intraepidermal SCC (Bowen disease)
  - Sharply demarcated, erythematous, and velvety plaque with follicular involvement that extends full thickness of epidermis and is commonly associated with HPV infection
- Keratoacanthoma
  - Dysplastic squamous proliferation with intradermal invasion that undergoes rapid keratinization

Basal Cell Carcinoma
- Nonmelanocytic skin cancer that arises from basal cells in lower epidermis
- Lobules of basaloid cells characterized by hyperchromatic nuclei and scant cytoplasm

EVALUATION/WORK-UP

Labs
- Consider genetic analysis for xeroderma pigmentosum, HIV status

Pathology
- Histologic hallmark of SCC: Presence of keratin pearls, desmosomal attachments, and intracytoplasmic bundles of keratin tonofilaments
- Histological grades
  - Well-differentiated SCC: Normal-appearing nuclei with abundant cytoplasm and extracellular keratin pearls
  - Poorly differentiated SCC: High degree of nuclear atypia with frequent mitoses, a greater nuclear to cytoplasmic ratio, and less keratinization

Imaging
- MR is preferred when evaluating for perineural invasion, orbital extension, or nodal staging

TREATMENT

Medical
- Local chemotherapy with intralesional injection of 5-fluorouracil and epinephrine or systemic therapy with cisplatin and doxorubicin for metastatic SCC
- Daily oral 13-cis-retinoic acid plus subcutaneous interferon α-2a for 2-3 months
  - Topical imiquimod cream can be used on skin (but not in eye)

Surgical
- Incisional, excisional, or punch biopsy depending on location and size of lesion
- Primary excision with 4-6 mm margins if no risk for recurrence or Mohs surgery if higher risk for recurrence

Follow-Up
- 3-month follow-up for patients at increased risk of recurrence (i.e., transplant recipients) or annually for low-risk patients

Prognosis
- Patients with uncomplicated, early-stage tumors have 5-year survival rate > 90%; perineural invasion (PNI) indicates poor prognosis

SELECTED REFERENCES

1. Thosani MK et al: Periocular squamous cell carcinoma. Dermatol Surg. 34(5):585-99, 2008
2. Donaldson MJ et al: Squamous cell carcinoma of the eyelids. Br J Ophthalmol. 86(10):1161-5, 2002

BLEPHAROSPASM

Key Facts

Introduction
- Uncontrollable bilateral blinking from contractions of orbicularis oculi and other lid protractors; may begin unilaterally

Demographics
- Benign essential blepharospasm: F:M ~ 2:1; typically affects individuals > 50 years of age

Presentation
- Increased blink rate
- Eyelid and additional facial spasm
- Ocular irritation &/or pain
- Photophobia
- Eye muscle spasms may be observed during exam
- Thorough slit-lamp exam may show primary signs of ocular surface irritation (dry eye syndrome, blepharitis, entropion, foreign body)

Differential Diagnosis
- Eyelid myokymia: Benign, self-resolving unilateral twitching of eyelid
- Hemifacial spasm: Twitching of upper and lower 1/2 of face, usually beginning with involuntary closure of eyelid, and is typically unilateral

Treatment
- Botulinum toxin injection is currently considered treatment of choice for benign essential blepharospasm
- For secondary blepharospasm, addressing primary cause will resolve symptoms
- In cases of benign essential blepharospasm refractory to botulinum toxin injection, partial myectomy of orbicularis oculi can be an option
- Benign essential blepharospasm is a progressive disease though most cases can be managed with botulinum toxin injection

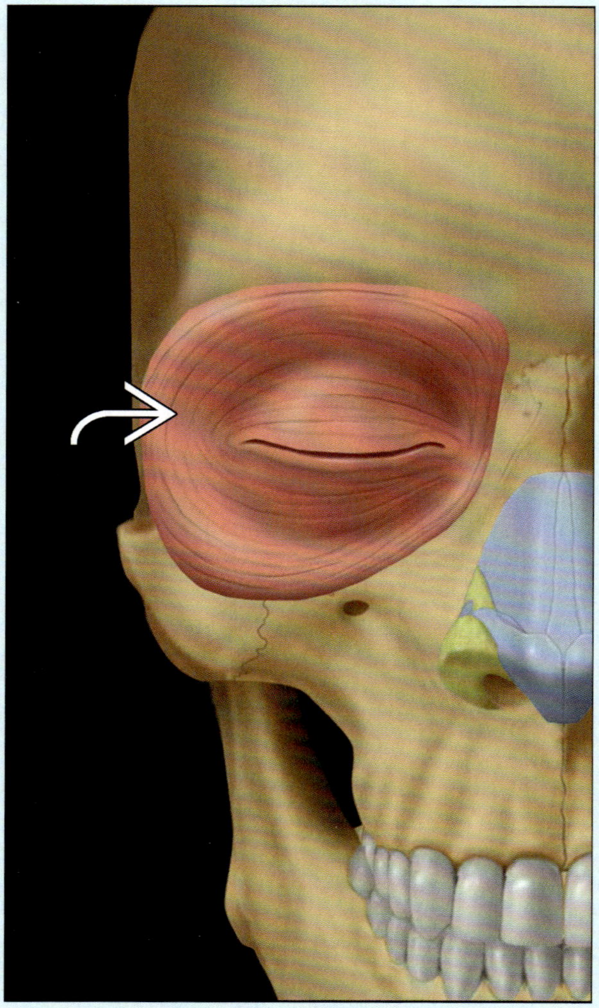

This graphic shows a frontal view of the orbicularis oculi muscle ➔, which involuntarily contracts in patients with blepharospasm.

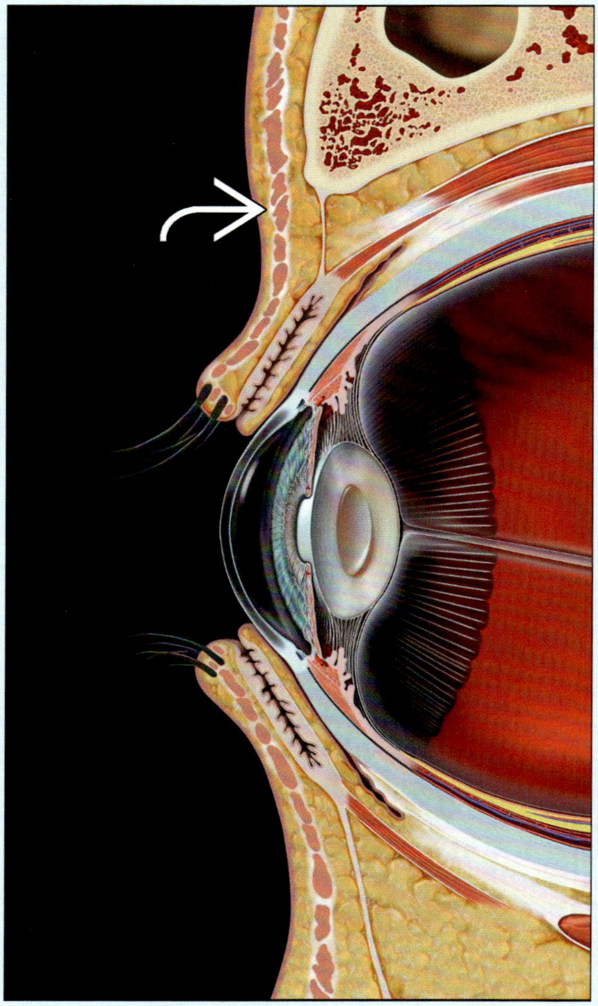

This graphic shows a cross-sectional view of the orbicularis oculi muscle ➔.

BLEPHAROSPASM

INTRODUCTION

Definitions

- Uncontrollable bilateral blinking from contractions of the orbicularis oculi and other lid protractors; may begin unilaterally

Subtypes

- Benign essential blepharospasm
- Secondary blepharospasm

DEMOGRAPHICS

Etiology/Risk Factors

- Benign essential blepharospasm
  - Exact etiology is unknown but is thought to be a multifactorial defect in the blink regulation pathway
- Secondary blepharospasm
  - Ocular irritation from blepharitis, keratoconjunctivitis sicca, foreign body, or trichiasis
  - Movement disorder secondary to medications, systemic disease, Meige syndrome

Epidemiology

- Benign essential blepharospasm
  - ~ 2x as prevalent in females
  - Patients are typically diagnosed when > 50 years of age
  - Prevalence is ~ 5 in 100,000 people with 2,000 new diagnoses per year in USA
- Secondary blepharospasm: Dependent on primary cause

PRESENTATION

Symptoms

- Increased blink rate
- Eyelid and additional facial spasm
- Ocular irritation &/or pain
- Photophobia
- Can progress to debilitating severity with spasms interrupting daily activities such as driving, reading, and watching television
- Symptoms are often relieved by sleep

Exam Findings

- Eye muscle spasms may be observed during exam
- Secondary blepharospasm
  - Thorough slit-lamp exam may show primary signs of ocular surface irritation (dry eye syndrome, blepharitis, entropion, foreign body)
  - Extraocular observation may show additional facial or bodily spasms
- Anatomical changes associated with increased spasms of eyelid may be observed and may also be clinically significant
  - Dermatochalasis, lid and brow ptosis, entropion

DIFFERENTIAL DIAGNOSIS

Eyelid Myokymia

- Benign and self-resolving, unilateral twitching of eyelid (usually induced by stress or caffeine)

Tardive Dyskinesia

- Positive history of previous use of neuroleptics
- Additional facial spasms

Hemifacial Spasm

- Twitching of 1 side of face caused by involuntary contracture of facial muscles, usually beginning with involuntary closure of eyelid
- Most often caused by compression of facial nerve by a blood vessel
- Can present bilaterally in rare cases

Apraxia of Lid Opening

- Difficulty opening the eyelid
  - No issues keeping eyes open once lids are in open position (e.g., with manual assistance)

EVALUATION/WORK-UP

Imaging

- Neuroimaging generally does not show any pathology

TREATMENT

Medical

- Botulinum toxin injection is currently considered treatment of choice for benign essential blepharospasm
  - Relief is temporary; typically needs to be repeated every 3 months
  - Often requires progressively higher doses
- Tinted sunglasses and lid hygiene can help alleviate symptoms through minimization of exacerbating factors
- For a limited number of patients, psychoactive medications may help provide transient, partial relief
- For secondary blepharospasm, addressing primary cause will resolve symptoms

Surgical

- In cases of benign essential blepharospasm refractory to botulinum toxin injection, partial myectomy of the orbicularis oculi can be an option
- Surgery to correct lid and brow ptosis and dermatochalasis secondary to blepharospasm may be warranted

Prognosis

- Benign essential blepharospasm is a progressive disease though most cases can be managed with botulinum toxin injection

SELECTED REFERENCES

1. Coscarelli JM: Essential blepharospasm. Semin Ophthalmol. 25(3):104-8, 2010
2. Hallett M et al: Update on blepharospasm: report from the BEBRF International Workshop. Neurology. 71(16):1275-82, 2008
3. Kenney C et al: Botulinum toxin in the treatment of blepharospasm and hemifacial spasm. J Neural Transm. 115(4):585-91, 2008
4. Jankovic J et al: Blinking and blepharospasm. Mechanism, diagnosis, and management. JAMA. 248(23):3160-4, 1982

ECTROPION

Key Facts

Introduction

- Eversion of eyelid margin away from the globe due to laxity of tarsoligamentous sling
- Congenital ectropion is rarely an isolated condition: Commonly seen with eyelid tumor or congenital eyelid syndromes (i.e., Kohn-Romano syndrome)
- Acquired ectropion: Involutional, paralytic, cicatricial, and mechanical

Demographics

- Age, eyelid rubbing, repeated eyelid pulling, floppy eyelid syndrome, history of periocular skin cancer or facial nerve palsy

Presentation

- Outward turning of the eyelid such that the inner, moist conjunctiva is exposed
- Abnormal positioning of the punctum
- Excessive tearing, redness, and mucoid discharge; may also complain of irritation or foreign body sensation
- Abnormal snap-back test: Lower lid does not return to resting position when pulled inferiorly

Treatment

- Aimed to minimize symptoms while awaiting surgery
  - Includes lubrication and eyelid hygiene
- Surgical treatment of involutional ectropion entails lateral tarsal strip to correct weakened lid retractors and elongated lateral tendon
- Cicatricial ectropion can be corrected surgically by lengthening the anterior lamella and tightening the lower lid
- Recurrence after surgery may occur after several years

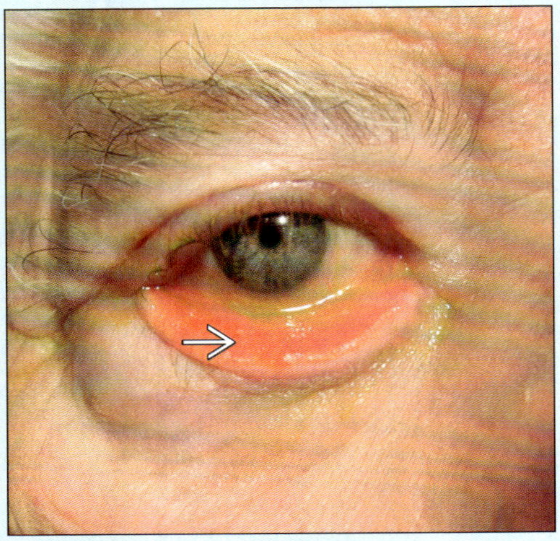

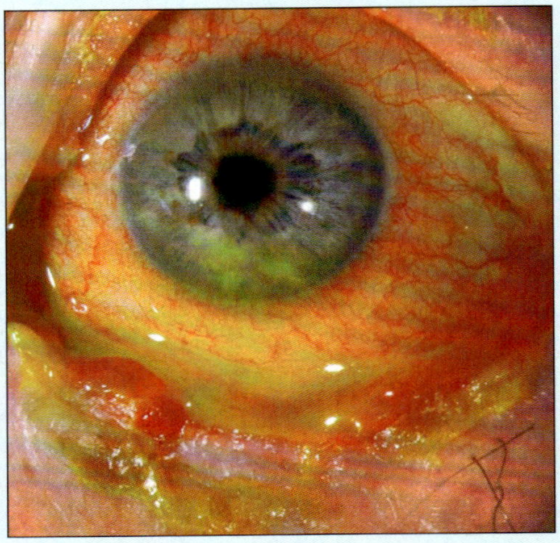

(Left) *External photograph depicts an example of classic involutional ectropion of the lower eyelid. Note how the eyelid is everted and the palpebral conjunctiva is clearly visible ➔. Ectropion often leads to poor lid closure and severe dry eye. It can be symptomatically managed with artificial tears and lubricants but often requires surgical correction.* ***(Right)*** *This external photograph shows paralytic eversion and ectropion of the lower eyelid. This may occur as a result of a CN7 palsy.*

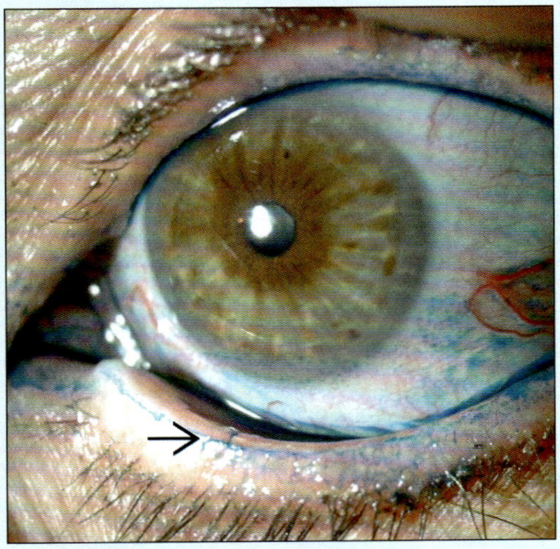

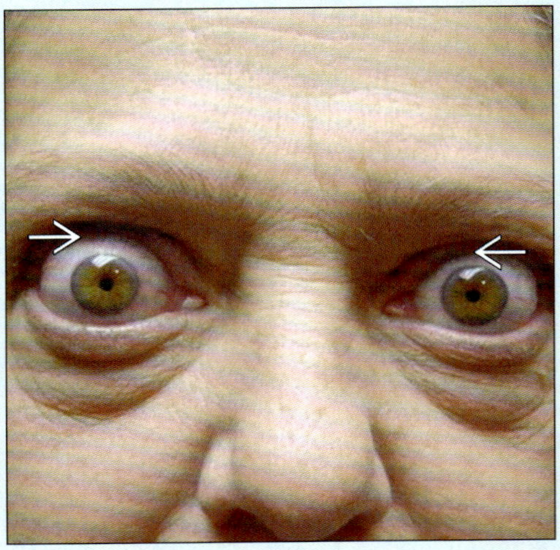

(Left) *This external photograph shows an eye with a relatively mild case of ectropion of the lower lid ➔.* ***(Right)*** *Clinical photograph shows Graves exophthalmos. Note the remarkable proptosis and retraction of the eyelids (lid lag) ➔. This is a very characteristic stare of patients with an infiltrative pathology of the extraocular muscles. The proptosis and lid retraction seen in Graves exophthalmos is occasionally confused with ectropion. (Courtesy K. B. Krantz, MD.)*

ECTROPION

INTRODUCTION

Definitions

- Eversion of eyelid margin away from the globe due to laxity of tarsoligamentous sling
- Tarsoligamentous sling attaches to orbital rim via the medial and lateral tendons and supports the eyelid

Subtypes

- Congenital ectropion is rarely an isolated condition; commonly seen with eyelid tumor or congenital eyelid syndromes (i.e., Kohn-Romano syndrome)
  - Due to either excessive horizontal lid length or vertical deficiency of the anterior lamella and primarily involves the lower eyelid
- Acquired ectropion
  - Involutional: Most common form, typically secondary to horizontal lid laxity
  - Paralytic: Secondary to CN7 palsy
  - Cicatricial: Secondary to scarring of the anterior lamella from trauma, chronic dermatitis, or excessive excision with blepharoplasty
  - Mechanical causes, including tumors (i.e., neurofibromas)

DIFFERENTIAL DIAGNOSIS

Floppy Eyelid Syndrome

- Floppy, easily everted, and rubbery eyelid that is commonly seen in obese patients
- Associated with keratoconus, decreased vision, and unilateral or bilateral chronic eye irritation

Bell Palsy

- Acute onset of unilateral upper and lower facial paralysis secondary to facial nerve paralysis
- Often associated with taste and salivation disturbances and posterior auricular pain
- Resolves over time in 80-90% of cases

Eyelid Retraction Secondary to Proptosis From Thyroid Disease

- i.e., Graves disease
- Thyroid-associated orbitopathy resulting from antibody-mediated reaction against the thyroid-stimulating hormone receptor on retroorbital fibroblast
- Symptoms include dry eyes, puffy eyelids, diplopia, vision loss, and systemic signs of hyperthyroidism (i.e., tachycardia, palpitations, heat intolerance, hair loss)

DEMOGRAPHICS

Etiology/Risk Factors

- Age, eyelid rubbing, repeated eyelid pulling, floppy eyelid syndrome, or history of periocular skin cancer or facial nerve palsy

Epidemiology

- Most commonly observed in older adults, though it can present at any age

PRESENTATION

Symptoms

- Irritated, red eyes associated with tearing, redness, and mucoid discharge
  - May also complain of irritation or foreign body sensation
  - Epiphora is commonly the 1st presenting symptom of ectropion and can exacerbate lid laxity with excessive wiping

Exam Findings

- Outward turning of the eyelid such that the inner, moist conjunctiva is exposed
- Abnormal positioning of punctum
  - Normally positioned lateral to the caruncle and inverted toward lacrimal gland
  - Abnormal positioning of the punctum leads to epiphora
- More common on lower eyelid, but upper lid can be affected, particularly with involutional ectropion
- Abnormal snap-back test: Lower lid does not return to resting position when pulled inferiorly
  - Indicates abnormal horizontal lid laxity
- Anterior lid distraction can also test for horizontal lid laxity
  - Ability to pull anterior lid > 6-8 mm from the globe is considered positive

TREATMENT

Medical

- Aimed to minimize symptoms while awaiting surgery
  - Includes lubrication and eyelid hygiene

Surgical

- Surgical treatment of involutional ectropion is directed at correcting the weakened lid retractors and elongated lateral tendon
  - Lateral tarsal strip procedure to correct horizontal eyelid laxity; medial canthal tendon resection or partial excision of the tarsus-conjunctiva may successfully correct involutional ectropions
- Cicatricial ectropion can be corrected surgically by lengthening the anterior lamella and tightening the lower lid
  - Surgical options include Z-plasty or skin replacement

Prognosis

- Complications primarily secondary to corneal and conjunctival exposure
- Recurrence after surgery may occur after several years

SELECTED REFERENCES

1. Bedran EG et al: Ectropion. Semin Ophthalmol. 25(3):59-65, 2010
2. American Academy of Ophthalmology: Eyelids and lacrimal system. In: Basic and Clinical science Course. San Francisco: The Academy. 195-201, 2006

ENTROPION

Key Facts

Introduction
- Abnormal inward rotation of lid margin and tarsus

Demographics
- Involutional entropion
  - Etiology: Associated with structural defects of the eyelid
- Cicatricial entropion
  - Etiology: Contracture secondary to scarring of the conjunctiva, rotating the margin of the lid inward
- Congenital entropion
  - Etiology: Lower eyelid retractor dysgenesis or disinsertion, structural defects in tarsal plate &/or shortening of posterior lamella
- Acute spastic entropion
  - Etiology: Excessive contracture of the orbicularis muscle secondary to ocular inflammation or irritation, forcing the tarsal plate inward

Presentation
- Ocular discomfort or foreign body sensation
- Ocular erythema and irritation
- Mucous discharge
- Visual acuity change or loss

Differential Diagnosis
- Epiblepharon; eyelid retraction
- Dermatochalasis; distichiasis; trichiasis

Treatment
- Eye lubricants, lid taping to normal position, soft bandage contact lenses, botulinum toxic injection
- Surgical treatment should be aimed to treat underlying anatomical defects
  - Quickert suture is temporary surgical maneuver; lateral tarsal strip is often long-term solution

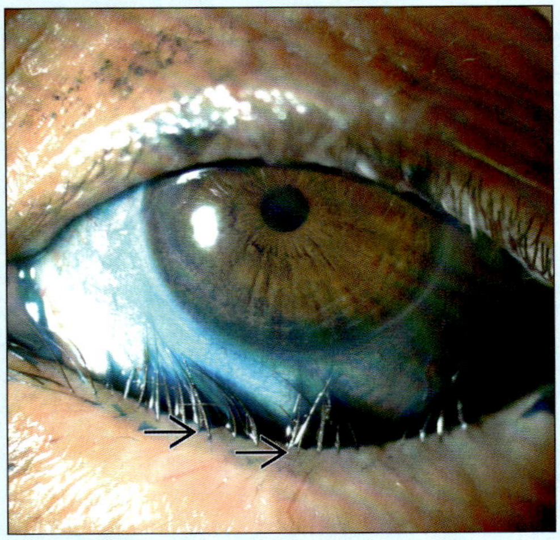
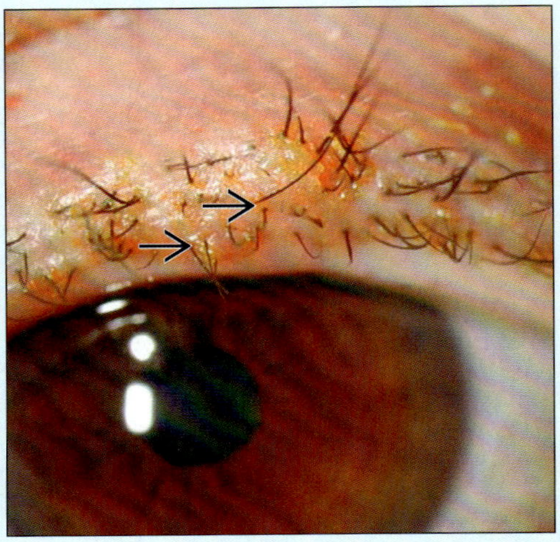

(Left) *External photograph with rose bengal stain shows an eye with involutional entropion of the lower eyelid. Note how the lashes and rim of the eyelid are oriented toward the eye →.* ***(Right)*** *This external photograph depicts an example of lash misdirection, called trichiasis →. Trichiasis is occasionally confused with entropion. Entropion is inward deviation of both the eyelid margin and lashes whereas trichiasis refers to misdirection of the lashes alone.*

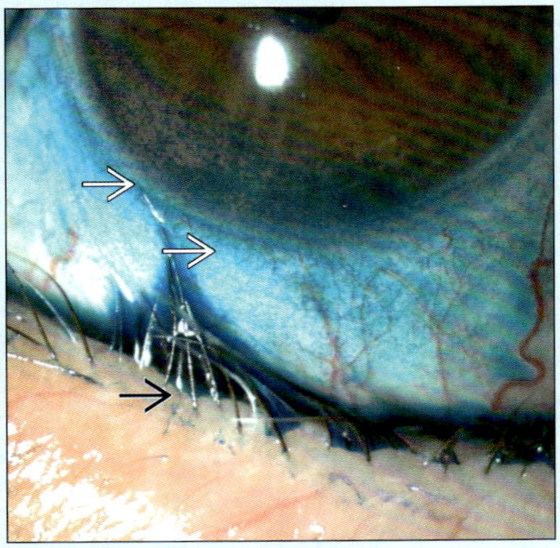
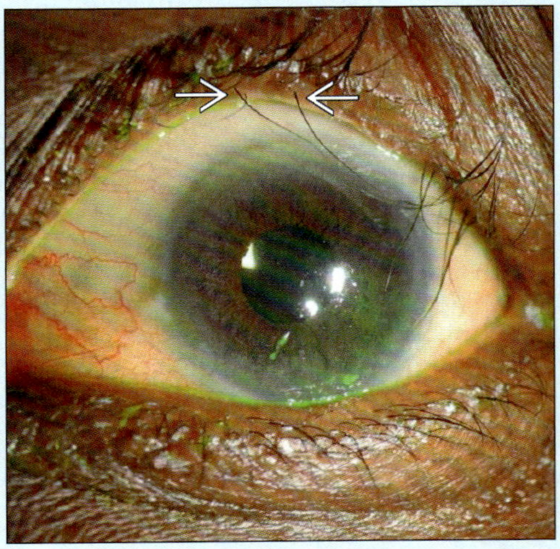

(Left) *External photograph shows an eye with involutional entropion and associated ocular surface damage. Note the inward orientation of the lashes and lid margin →. The ocular surface is covered with punctate staining →.* ***(Right)*** *This external photograph demonstrates an eye with distichiasis. Distichiasis refers to lashes that originate from the meibomian glands rather than the hair follicles →. These aberrant lashes are often misdirected toward the eye and can be confused with entropion.*

ENTROPION

INTRODUCTION

Definitions
- Abnormal inward rotation of the eyelid margin and tarsus

Subtypes
- Involutional entropion
- Cicatricial entropion
- Acute spastic entropion
- Congenital entropion

DEMOGRAPHICS

Etiology/Risk Factors
- Lower eyelid entropion is more common than upper eyelid entropion
- Involutional entropion
  - Etiology: Associated with structural defects of the eyelid
    - Preseptal orbicularis oculi muscle overriding preseptal orbicularis oculi muscle, turning the margin of the lid inward
    - Lower lid retractor complex weakening or disinsertion
    - Tarsal plate degeneration
    - Horizontal lid laxity caused by stretching of canthal tendons
  - Risk factors: Increased age
- Cicatricial entropion
  - Etiology: Contracture secondary to scarring of the conjunctiva, rotating the margin of the lid inward
  - Risk factors: Conjunctivitis, trachoma, Stevens-Johnson syndrome, trauma, or chemical injury
- Congenital entropion
  - Etiology: Lower eyelid retractor dysgenesis or disinsertion, structural defects in tarsal plate, &/or shortening of posterior lamella
    - May be associated with corneal ulceration
    - True congenital entropion not secondary to epiblepharon is rare
- Acute spastic entropion
  - Etiology: Excessive contracture of the orbicularis muscle secondary to ocular inflammation or irritation, forcing the tarsal plate inward
  - Risk factors: Recent ocular surgery, inflammatory eye disease

PRESENTATION

Symptoms
- Ocular discomfort or foreign body sensation
- Ocular erythema and irritation
- Mucous discharge
- Visual acuity change or loss

Exam Findings
- Corneal abrasion (via fluorescein cornea test)
- Conjunctival epithelial disturbance or scarring
- Lid laxity (assessed via snap-back test, medial and lateral canthal laxity test)

DIFFERENTIAL DIAGNOSIS

Epiblepharon
- Folds of skin and an overriding pretarsal orbicularis oculi push the lashes toward globe
  - Normal tarsal plate

Eyelid Retraction
- Retracted upper or lower lid hides eyelashes (can be seen in Graves disease)

Dermatochalasis
- Redundant lid skin, leading to misdirection of eyelashes

Distichiasis
- Anomalous eyelash row

Trichiasis
- Misdirection of eyelashes

TREATMENT

Medical
- Eye lubricants, lid taping to normal position, soft bandage contact lenses, botulinum toxic injection
  - Spastic entropion: Treat underlying etiology, lid taping, botulinum toxin to control spasm and thus irritation
    - May resolve without surgery

Surgical
- Surgical treatment should be aimed to treat underlying anatomical defects
  - Quickert-Rathbun method: Everting sutures to prevent inward lid rotation
    - Relatively simple procedure
    - Appealing option for correction in poor surgical candidates or temporary postponement of surgery
    - Temporary solution
  - Wies method: Transverse blepharotomy and marginal rotation including horizontal lid splitting and everting sutures
    - More permanent solution
  - Jones method: Plication of the lower lid retractors
    - More permanent solution
  - Lateral tarsal strip is generally effective in correcting lid laxity

Prognosis
- High rate of symptomatic improvement following proper treatment
- Surgical success rate > 97%

SELECTED REFERENCES

1. Boboridis K et al: Interventions for involutional lower lid entropion. Cochrane Database Syst Rev. 2002; (1):CD002221. Review. Update in: Cochrane Database Syst Rev. (12):CD002221, 2011
2. Pereira MG et al: Eyelid entropion. Semin Ophthalmol. 25(3):52-8, 2010
3. Eliasoph I: Current techniques of entropion and ectropion correction. Otolaryngol Clin North Am. 38(5):903-19, 2005
4. Vallabhanath P et al: Ectropion and entropion. Curr Opin Ophthalmol. 11(5):345-51, 2000

FLOPPY EYELID SYNDROME

Key Facts

Introduction
- Consists of the following features: Loose upper lid that readily everts by pulling it upward; a soft, rubbery tarsus that can be easily folded; and a chronic papillary conjunctival response
- Strong association with obstructive sleep apnea (OSA) and keratoconus

Demographics
- Generally seen in obese males in 40-69 age range

Presentation
- Symptoms include irritation, tearing, discharge, and sometimes visual acuity loss if cornea is involved

Differential Diagnosis
- Dermatochalasis
- Ectropion
- Blepharitis
- Conjunctivitis
- Keratoconus

Evaluation/Work-Up
- Clinical exam should focus on lid laxity, evidence of superior papillary conjunctivitis, exposure keratopathy &/or keratoconus, and signs and symptoms of OSA

Treatment
- Managed both medically and surgically with excellent outcomes
  - Medical management consists of erythromycin ointment for mild conjunctival and corneal findings, nighttime lubrication, eyelid taping, and eye shielding to prevent exposure keratopathy
  - Surgical management consists of full-thickness wedge resection, lateral tarsal strip, lateral canthal tendon plication, and lateral tarsorrhaphy

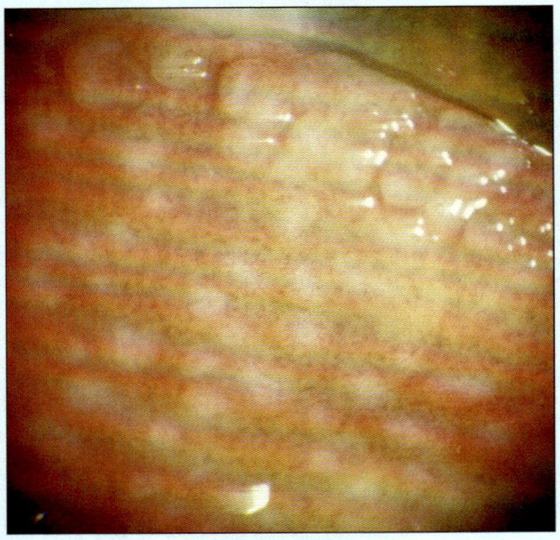

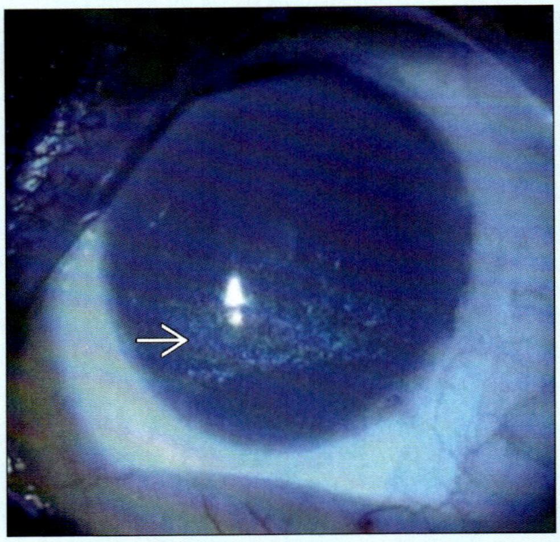

(Left) *Slit-lamp photo demonstrates papillary conjunctivitis. While not a specific sign, papillary conjunctivitis can be seen in floppy eyelid syndrome.* ***(Right)*** *This slit-lamp photo demonstrates superficial punctate keratopathy ➡. While not specific, superficial punctate keratopathy is often present in patients with floppy eyelid syndrome.*

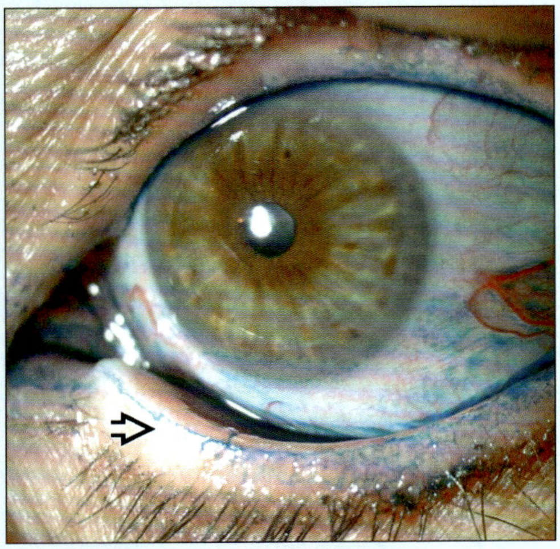

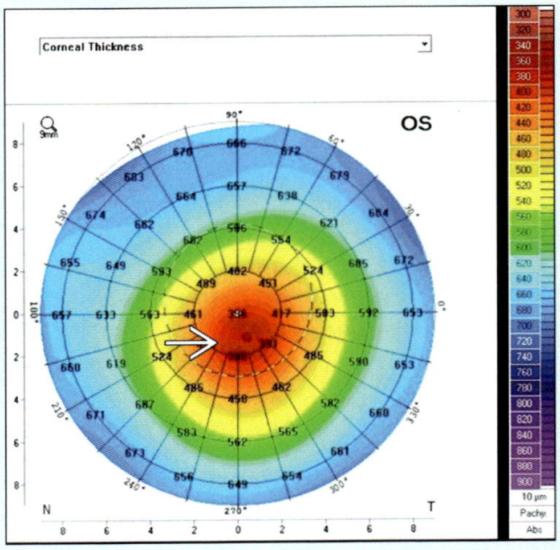

(Left) *External photo demonstrates left lower lid ectropion ⇨. While the symptoms of ectropion may be similar to that seen in floppy eyelid syndrome, the underlying etiology is different. Typically, floppy eyelid syndrome is secondary to dysfunction of the upper eyelid.* ***(Right)*** *This Pentacam image demonstrates the central corneal thinning ➡ seen in patients with keratoconus. Keratoconus is present in ~ 10% of patients with floppy eyelid syndrome.*

FLOPPY EYELID SYNDROME

INTRODUCTION

Abbreviations

- Floppy eyelid syndrome (FES)

Definitions

- Condition consisting of the following features: Loose upper lid that readily everts by pulling it upward; a soft, rubbery tarsus that can be easily folded; and a chronic papillary conjunctival response

DEMOGRAPHICS

Etiology/Risk Factors

- Male sex
- Obesity
- Obstructive sleep apnea (OSA)
- Sleep positioning (occurs more often in patients who sleep on their side or on their stomach)

Epidemiology

- Most commonly affects obese men between ages 40-69 but can also affect nonobese patients

PRESENTATION

Symptoms

- Unilateral or bilateral eye irritation, tearing, and discharge that is usually worse in morning
- Low visual acuity if cornea is involved

Exam Findings

- Eyelid and conjunctiva: Papillary conjunctivitis, blepharitis, blepharoptosis, and upper lid lash ptosis
  - Can also cause globe luxation: Herniation of the eye anteriorly through the palpebral aperture, leading to optic neuropathy
- Cornea: Superficial punctate keratopathy, scarring with neovascularization, corneal erosion, corneal endotheliopathy, and keratoconus
  - Can also cause ulcerative microbial keratitis or perforation

DIFFERENTIAL DIAGNOSIS

Dermatochalasis

- Excess of skin in upper or lower eyelid that can obstruct visual field; commonly affects elderly; associated with blepharitis, entropion, and blepharoptosis

Ectropion

- Lower eyelid turns outwards; can cause symptoms related to ocular exposure and inadequate lubrication

Blepharitis

- Chronic inflammation of eyelid

Conjunctivitis

- Inflammation of conjunctiva that is caused by allergies, viruses, bacteria, and chemicals

Keratoconus

- Condition in which cornea becomes more cone-like in shape; present in ~ 10% of FES patients

EVALUATION/WORK-UP

Pathology

- Conjunctival scrapings show predominance of neutrophils with variable amounts of eosinophils and lymphocytes

Complete Ophthalmic Exam

- External: Assess for eyelid laxity, soft or atrophic tarsal plate, eyelash ptosis with loss of lash parallelism, dermatochalasis, blepharoptosis, enophthalmos, and lagophthalmos
- Slit-lamp exam: Assess for superior tarsal conjunctival hypertrophy, conjunctival injection, corneal pannus or evidence of exposure keratopathy, abnormal fluorescein staining of cornea, and evidence of central corneal thinning consistent with keratoconus

Polysomnography

- If OSA is suspected

TREATMENT

Medical

- For mild conjunctival/corneal abnormalities: Erythromycin ointment if patient has evidence of keratitis, doxycycline if meibomian gland dysfunction is suspected, eyelid taping and lubricating drops at bedtime, nighttime eye shielding to prevent exposure keratopathy
- If OSA is suspected, referral to an internist or pulmonologist for CPAP or other airway management
- Weight loss and management for comorbidities such as diabetes and high cholesterol

Surgical

- Full-thickness wedge resection: Pentagon excision in upper lid and wound edges are reattached
- Lateral tarsal strip: Originally a lower lid technique but has been adapted to address upper lid laxity in FES; success rate > 90%
- Lateral canthal tendon plication: Involves suturing lateral end of upper tarsal plate to periosteum of lateral orbital wall
- Lateral tarsorrhaphy: Involves closing part of the palpebral aperture

Follow-Up

- Every 3-7 days if there is keratopathy keratitis, then every 2-6 weeks

Prognosis

- Medical and surgical approaches of managing symptoms caused by FES are often successful

SELECTED REFERENCES

1. Ezra DG et al: Floppy eyelid syndrome: stretching the limits. Surv Ophthalmol. 55(1):35-46, 2010
2. Ezra DG et al: Long-term outcomes of surgical approaches to the treatment of floppy eyelid syndrome. Ophthalmology. 117(4):839-46, 2010
3. Pham TT et al: Floppy eyelid syndrome. Curr Opin Ophthalmol. 18(5):430-3, 2007

TRICHIASIS

Key Facts

Introduction

- Lid margin disorder involving misdirection of eyelashes toward globe
- Major trichiasis affects ≥ 5 cilia
- Minor trichiasis involves < 5 cilia

Demographics

- Causes include epiblepharon or distichiasis, chronic inflammation of eyelid margin, skin disease (i.e., eczema, atopic disease, herpes zoster), conjunctival disease (ocular pemphigoid, chemical burns, or cicatricial trachoma), and eyelid margin scarring from surgery or trauma
- Mainly affects central portion of lower eyelid, but may involve upper eyelid if associated with trachoma
- Primary morbidity associated with trichiasis is corneal abrasion, scarring, and microbial keratitis
- Children of Asian ancestry are at increased risk of trichiasis secondary to epiblepharon

Presentation

- Foreign body sensation, photophobia, tearing, discharge, dry eye sensation, and pain
- Misdirected eyelashes, superficial keratopathy, corneal abrasion, infection, vascularization, or loss of vision

Treatment

- Eye lubricants, contact lenses, and forceps epilation provide temporary symptomatic relief
- Radiofrequency ablation has better success and fewer complications (including scarring) compared to bipolar electrolysis
- Diffuse trichiasis, complicated segmental trichiasis, and recurrent trichiasis respond well to a variety of surgical procedures including eyelash trephination, full-thickness block resection, partial excision of anterior lamella, or mucocutaneous graft

*(**Left**) Slit-lamp photograph demonstrates eyelash misdirection ➔. The misdirection of the lashes can lead to ocular irritation and is likely secondary to the chronic inflammation of the eyelid. (**Right**) This external photograph demonstrates multiple misdirected eyelashes ➔. This is known as trichiasis and will often lead to significant conjunctival and corneal irritation.*

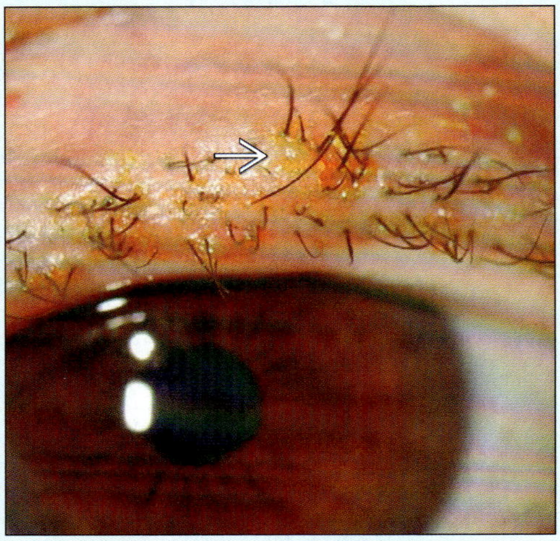

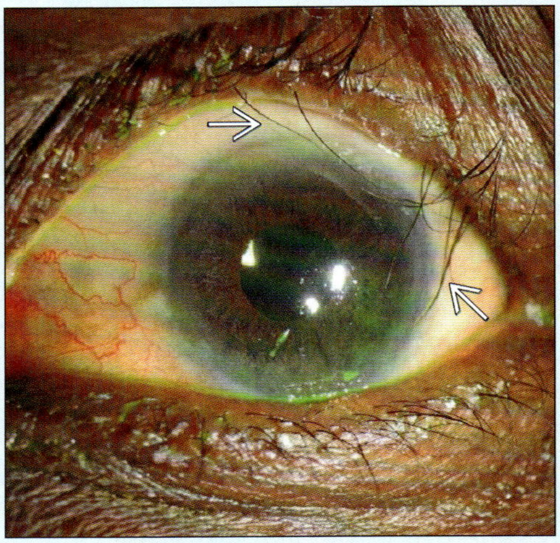

*(**Left**) Slit-lamp photograph depicts inspissated meibomian glands ➔. Chronic inflammation of these glands can lead to eyelid scarring and eyelash malposition, causing trichiasis. (**Right**) This slit-lamp photograph shows corneal neovascularization ➔, one of the possible side effects of long-term corneal irritation, which can be associated with trichiasis.*

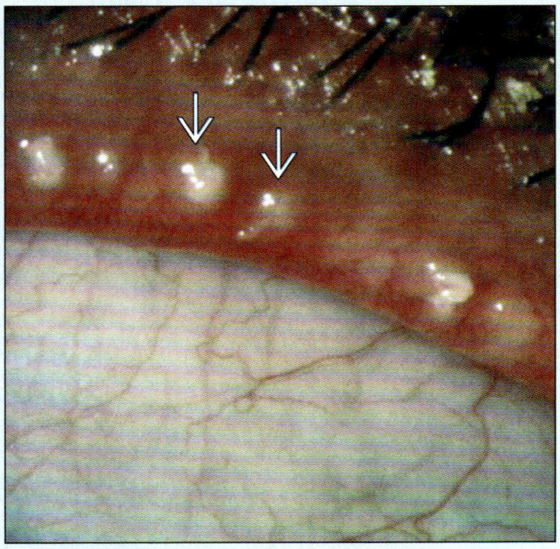

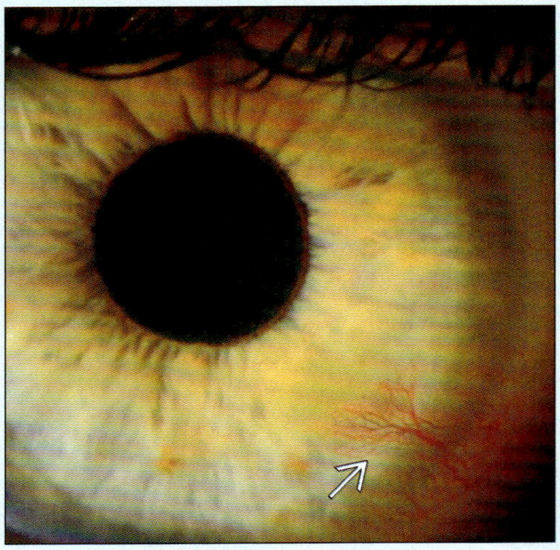

TRICHIASIS

INTRODUCTION

Definitions

- Lid margin disorder involving misdirection of eyelashes toward globe

Subtypes

- Major trichiasis affects ≥ 5 cilia
- Minor trichiasis involves < 5 cilia

DEMOGRAPHICS

Etiology/Risk Factors

- Main causes
  - Chronic inflammation of eyelids from blepharitis or meibomitis
  - Skin disease (e.g., eczema, atopic disease, herpes zoster)
  - Conjunctival disease (e.g., ocular pemphigoid, chemical burns, or cicatricial trachoma)
  - Scarring of eyelid margin from surgery or trauma
- Trachoma infection
  - Formerly the main cause of trichiasis worldwide
  - Now only prevalent in certain parts of world (i.e., sub-Saharan Africa, Middle East, Asia, and Latin America)

Epidemiology

- Location
  - Bilateral trichiasis seen in 70% of cases
  - Mainly affects central portion of lower eyelid, but may involve upper eyelid if associated with trachoma
    - Upper lid entropion is associated with trachoma infection
- Age
  - Can occur at any age
  - More commonly seen in adults, after 3rd decade of life
- Primary morbidity associated with trichiasis is corneal abrasion, scarring, and microbial keratitis
- Children of Asian ancestry are at increased risk
  - Secondary to epiblepharon
    - Congenital disorder characterized by vertical positioning of cilia due to overriding pretarsal orbicularis

PRESENTATION

Symptoms

- Foreign body sensation, photophobia, tearing, discharge, dry eye sensation, and pain

Exam Findings

- Misdirected eyelashes = main finding on examination
- Posterior lamellar scarring may be present in cases with previous herpes zoster ophthalmicus infection
- Distichiasis may be present secondary to chronic inflammation of eyelids
  - Metaplastic change resulting in eyelash growth from meibomian glands

DIFFERENTIAL DIAGNOSIS

Distichiasis

- Congenital condition associated with additional row of cilia positioned posterior to meibomian gland orifice
- Presents in young children ~ age of 5
- May also present as acquired variant characterized by metaplasia of tarsal gland

Entropion

- Involution of eyelid margin, causing eyelashes to be directed toward eye
- Cilia are directed in a normal direction

Trachoma

- Disease caused by infection with *Chlamydia trachomatis,* leading to granulation formation of middle and posterior lamella
- When left untreated, can progress to ulceration of cornea with subsequent blindness
  - A leading cause of blindness worldwide

TREATMENT

Medical

- Eye lubricants, contact lenses, and forceps epilation provide temporary symptomatic relief
- Bipolar electrolysis treats segmental and minor cases of trichiasis
- Radiofrequency ablation has better success and fewer complications (including scarring) compared to bipolar electrolysis
- Cryotherapy for segmental or diffuse trichiasis
- If trichiasis is a result of underlying disease process (Stevens-Johnson syndrome, trachoma, or ocular cicatricial pemphigoid), medical therapy should be guided toward correcting disease

Surgical

- Diffuse trichiasis, complicated segmental trichiasis, and recurrent trichiasis respond well to a variety of surgical procedures
  - Eyelash trephination to excise trichiatic eyelash bulbs
  - Full-thickness block resection
  - Partial excision of anterior lamella
  - Mucocutaneous graft
- A single, 1-gram dose of oral azithromycin after surgery reduces recurrence of severe, postsurgical trichiasis up to 1 year

SELECTED REFERENCES

1. Rajak SN et al: Trachomatous trichiasis and its management in endemic countries. Surv Ophthalmol. 57(2):105-35, 2012
2. Woreta F et al: Three-year outcomes of the surgery for trichiasis, antibiotics to prevent recurrence trial. Arch Ophthalmol. 130(4):427-31, 2012
3. Gower EW: Trichiasis: making progress toward elimination. Int Ophthalmol Clin. 47(3):77-86, 2007
4. Moosavi AH et al: Simple surgery for severe trichiasis. Ophthal Plast Reconstr Surg. 23(4):296-7, 2007
5. West ES et al: The association between epilation and corneal opacity among eyes with trachomatous trichiasis. Br J Ophthalmol. 90(2):171-4, 2006

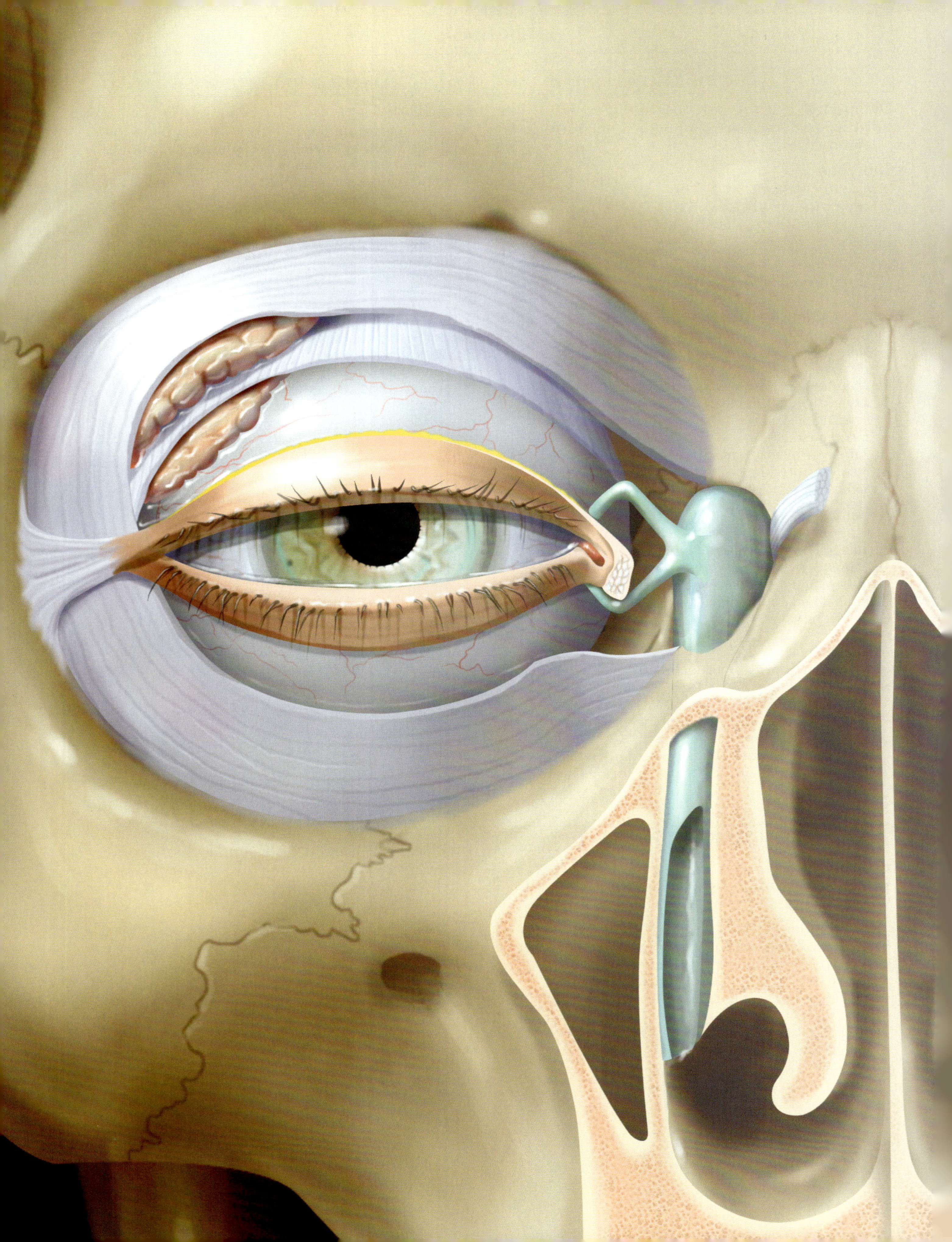

SECTION 2
Lacrimal System

Introduction and Overview

Infectious Disorders

Trauma

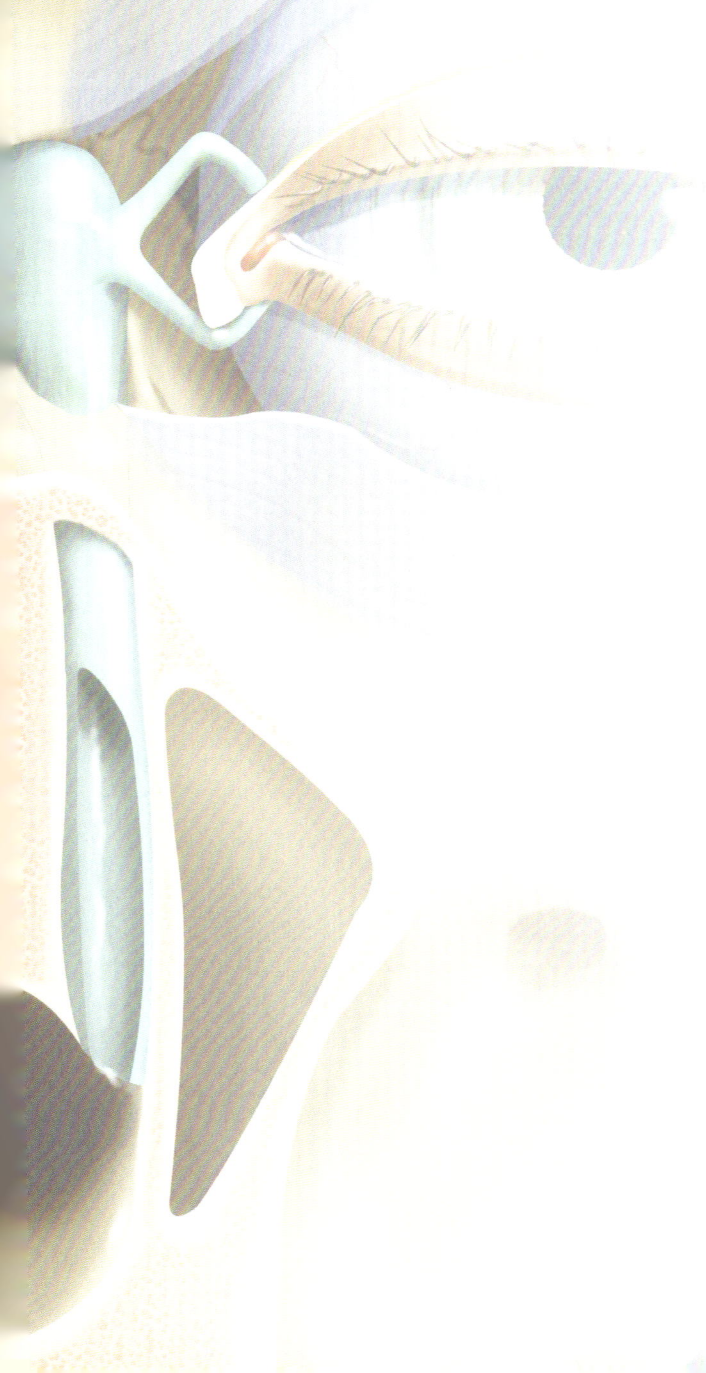

LACRIMAL SYSTEM OVERVIEW

ANATOMY

Lacrimal Gland
- Walnut-sized gland that produces lacrimal fluid
- Sits superior and lateral to eye within lacrimal fossa of frontal bone

Lacrimal Fluid
- Also known as aqueous layer of tear film
- Sits below a thin lipid layer and above a thin mucin layer, which coat the cornea and conjunctiva

Puncta
- Superior and inferior openings of lacrimal drainage system located on eyelids at medial canthus

Canaliculi
- Superior and inferior collection tubes that form the beginning of lacrimal drainage system

Lacrimal Sac
- Round sac that collects fluid from canaliculi

Nasolacrimal Duct
- Intraosseous portion of drainage system distal to lacrimal sac

Inferior Nasal Meatus
- Located on medial wall of nasal cavity
- Exit point of lacrimal system drainage

PHYSIOLOGY

Function
- Fluid production that protects against eyelid abrasion
- Part of tear film that prevents cornea and conjunctiva dryness
- Main supplier of oxygen and nutrients to cornea
- Suspends pathogens away from eye surface and removes them via drainage system

Innervation
- Parasympathetic innervation via lacrimal nerve
- Branch from CN7 (facial nerve)

PATHOLOGY

Gland Dysfunction
- Systemic inflammatory disease
  - Common symptom: Dry eyes
  - Sjögren syndrome most common
- Tumors
  - 55% benign
    - Adenomas common
  - 45% malignant
    - Adenoid cystic carcinoma common

Nerve Dysfunction
- Common symptom: Dry eyes
- Trama and surgery likely causes

Lacrimal Drainage Obstruction
- Common symptoms: Unilateral conjunctivitis, reflux of mucopurulent material, medial canthal inflammation, epiphora, and a red pouting punctum
- Infectious disease
  - Canaliculitis
    - Rare, yet often misdiagnosed as conjunctivitis
    - *Actinomyces*, *Mycobacteria*, *Nocardia*, *Staphylococcus aureus*, and *Streptococcus* are common pathogens
  - Dacryocystitis: Inflammation of lacrimal sac/ nasolacrimal duct
    - Most common in children with obstruction of drainage system
    - May lead to orbital cellulitis
- Tumors
  - Exceedingly rare, but commonly malignant when present
- Systemic inflammatory disease
  - Wegener granulomatosis or sarcoidosis
- Primary acquired nasolacrimal duct obstruction (PANDO)
  - Caused by inflammation or fibrosis with unknown etiology
  - Common in middle-aged and elderly women

Congenital Disorders
- Congenital nasolacrimal duct obstruction (CNDO)
  - Most common cause of epiphora in infants
  - Membrane over lower end of nasolacrimal duct (valve of Hasner) or embryologic tissue occluding opening
  - Commonly resolves spontaneously in 1st year of life
    - If problem continues past 1st year, massage or probing techniques may be indicated
- Other defects
  - Often due to failure of drainage system to fully canalize during embryonic development
  - Agenesis or imperforation of openings or tubing along any point of drainage pathway

IMAGING

Dacryocystography (DCG)
- Contrast medium injected into puncta to visualize blockage of drainage system
- Available in many modalities (MRI, CT, simple x-ray)

Radioscintillography
- Technetium-99 delivered to lacrimal drainage system
- Continuous photo sequence

RELATED REFERENCES

1. Cher I: Fluids of the ocular surface: concepts, functions and physics. Clin Experiment Ophthalmol. 40(6):634-43, 2012
2. Lefebvre DR et al: Update on imaging of the lacrimal drainage system. Semin Ophthalmol. 27(5-6):175-86, 2012
3. Dantas RR: Lacrimal drainage system obstruction. Semin Ophthalmol. 25(3):98-103, 2010
4. Heindl LM et al: Tumors of the lacrimal drainage system. Orbit. 29(5):298-306, 2010
5. Levy J et al: Lesions of the caruncle: a description of 42 cases and a review of the literature. Eye (Lond). 23(5):1004-18, 2009
6. Bernardini FP et al: Epithelial tumors of the lacrimal gland: an update. Curr Opin Ophthalmol. 19(5):409-13, 2008
7. Schmitt NJ et al: Superior ophthalmic vein thrombosis in a patient with dacryocystitis-induced orbital cellulitis. Ophthal Plast Reconstr Surg. 21(5):387-9, 2005
8. Bartley GB. Acquired lacrimal drainage obstruction: an etiologic classification system et al: Part 1. Ophthal Plast Reconstr Surg. 8(4):237-42, 1992

GRAPHICS

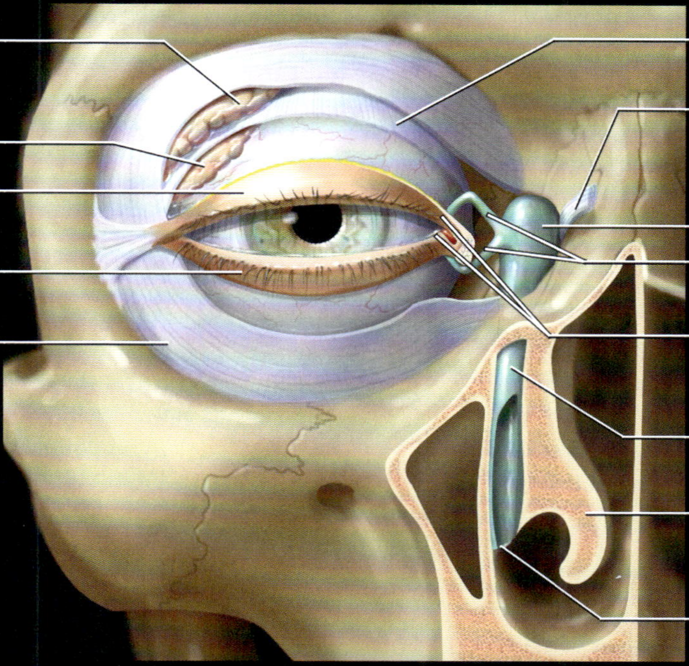

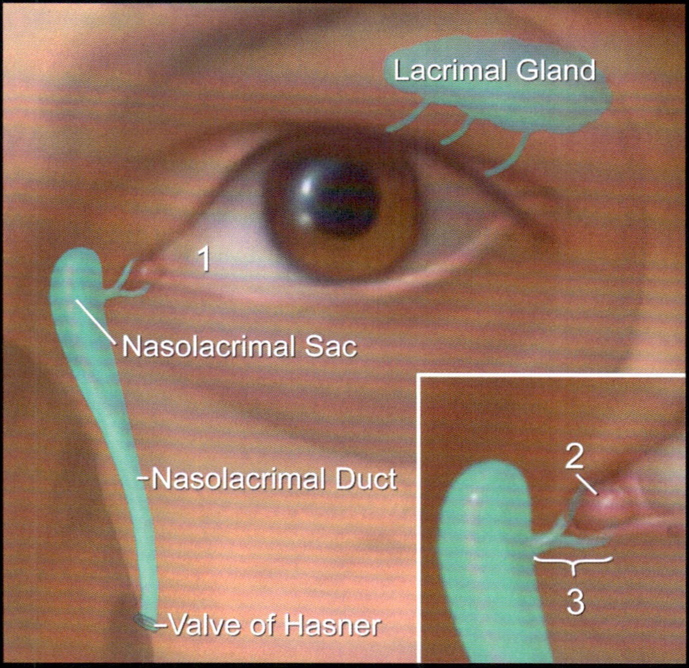

(Top) *Illustration depicts lacrimal fluid pathway. Lacrimal fluid is produced by the lacrimal gland, which is located in the superior-lateral region of the orbit. The orbicularis oculi then uses peristalsis-like movements to move the tear film toward the nasal bulbar direction, where it is drained by the superior and inferior puncta. The inferior puncta is responsible for draining the majority of the lacrimal fluid. The fluid then moves through the canaliculi into the lacrimal sac, the nasolacrimal duct, and finally exits into the inferior nasal meatus.* ***(Bottom)*** *(1) Illustration depicts basic overview of the lacrimal system in relation to surface anatomy. (2) Lacrimal caruncle: This wart-like structure is made of skin covering sudoriferous and sebaceous glands. (3) Canaliculi of the lacrimal apparatus: These tubes are responsible for draining lacrimal fluid. Fluid moves from the puncta into the vertical portion (2 mm) and into the horizontal portion (8 mm). Then, the inferior and superior canaliculi join to form the common canaliculus (2 mm).*

DACRYOADENITIS

Key Facts

Introduction
- Inflammation of the lacrimal gland; may be subdivided into acute and chronic
  - Acute: Usually secondary to infectious causes including viral, bacterial, and fungal organisms
  - Chronic: Commonly secondary to inflammatory and systemic causes such as sarcoidosis, Sjögren syndrome, reactive arthritis, Wegener disease, and inflammatory orbital pseudotumor

Presentation
- Acute: Painful, swollen, and erythematous lacrimal gland; commonly unilateral
- Chronic: Normally painless; enlarged but freely mobile lacrimal gland; frequently bilateral

Differential Diagnosis
- Malignancy: Lacrimal gland neoplasms may cause similar presentation and must be ruled out
- Preseptal or orbital cellulitis: Also presents with erythema, edema, and tenderness of eyelid
- Chalazion: Usually more well defined and located closer to eyelid margin by tarsal plate

Evaluation/Work-Up
- Gram stain and culture of discharge
- Complete blood count with differential if febrile or infectious cause suspected; systemic work-up for autoimmune or infectious etiologies
- CT scan of orbit and brain with contrast including axial and coronal views
- Chest x-ray or CT scan for suspected sarcoidosis

Treatment
- Appropriate antibiotics for infectious etiologies; may require admission and IV antibiotics for severe cases
- Treat underlying cause: Oral steroids are the mainstay of therapy for inflammatory etiologies

*(**Left**) Graphic demonstrates position of the lacrimal gland in the orbit. Palpebral lobe ⇨ is more often involved than orbital lobe → in acute dacryoadenitis. The palpebral lobe's direct connection with the conjunctiva through the lacrimal ductules allows easier access for pathogens. (**Right**) External photo depicts dacryoadenitis in a child. Note the superotemporal edema ➔, erythema, and apparent ptosis. The palpebral lobe of the lacrimal gland was visibly enlarged and prolapsed on eyelid eversion.*

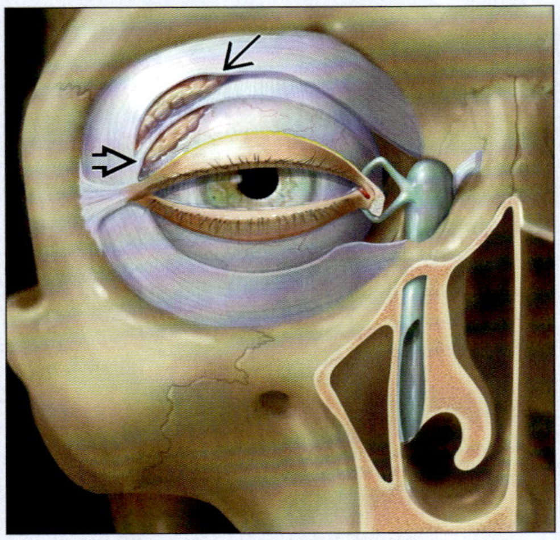

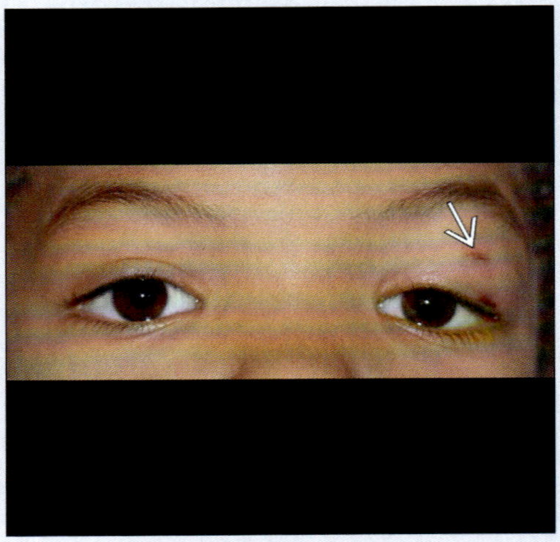

*(**Left**) This CT shows lacrimal gland enhancement → seen in dacryoadenitis. Dacryoadenitis can be infectious or inflammatory and must be distinguished from malignant lacrimal gland masses. (**Right**) Axial contrast-enhanced CT shows an infiltrative tumor centered in the right lacrimal gland ➔ with evidence of bony erosion that is visible even on soft tissue windows ➔. Malignancy is an important differential for dacryoadenitis.*

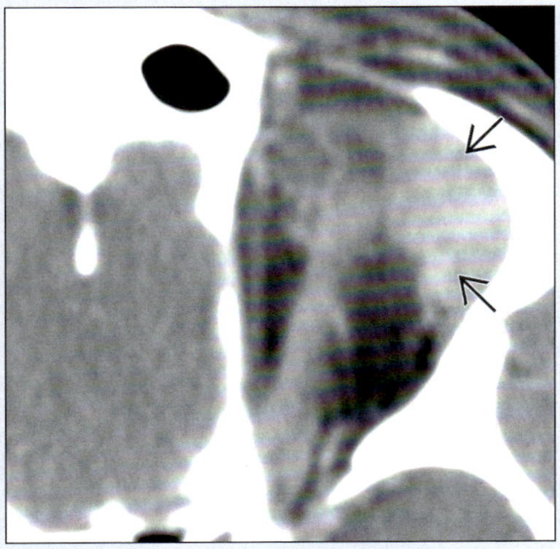

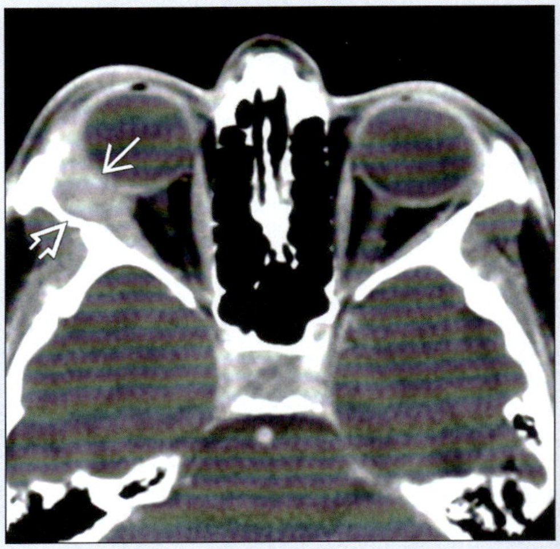

DACRYOADENITIS

INTRODUCTION

Definitions
- Inflammation of the lacrimal gland

Subtypes
- Acute: Usually secondary to infectious causes
- Chronic: Commonly secondary to inflammatory and systemic causes

DEMOGRAPHICS

Etiology/Risk Factors
- Infectious dacryoadenitis is likely secondary to ascension of microorganisms from the ocular surface into the lacrimal gland through lacrimal ductules
  - Viral: Mumps, Epstein-Barr, herpes simplex, varicella zoster, Cytomegalovirus
  - Bacterial: *Staphylococcus*, *Streptococcus*, *Neisseria gonorrhoeae*, *Chlamydia trachomatis*, *Pseudomonas*, *Mycobacterium tuberculosis*, syphilis, Lyme disease
  - Fungal: *Acanthamoeba*, histoplasmosis, blastomycosis
- Inflammatory dacryoadenitis may be caused by multiple conditions including
  - Sarcoidosis: May have lymphadenopathy, skin, and lung involvement
  - Sjögren syndrome: Autoimmune disease affecting lacrimal and salivary glands
  - Mikulicz disease: Consists of self-limited and benign symmetric enlargement of the lacrimal, submandibular, and parotid glands
  - Reactive arthritis: 1 case described secondary to *C. trachomatis* urethritis
  - Orbital inflammatory pseudotumor: Diagnosis of exclusion

Epidemiology
- Rare, ~ 1 in 10,000 ophthalmic patients
- No age, sex, or race predilection

PRESENTATION

Symptoms
- Acute: Rapid onset of pain, pressure, tenderness, and redness over superotemporal orbit
- Chronic: Slow enlargement of lacrimal gland over superotemporal orbit, usually painless, frequently bilateral

Exam Findings
- Acute: Painful, swollen, and erythematous lacrimal gland, prolapsed and enlarged on eyelid eversion; may accompany ocular discharge, conjunctivitis, chemosis, or globe displacement
- Chronic: Normally painless; enlarged but freely mobile lacrimal gland

DIFFERENTIAL DIAGNOSIS

Lacrimal Gland Neoplasm
- Important to rule out malignancy; lacrimal gland neoplasms (e.g., pleomorphic adenoma, adenoid cystic carcinoma) may cause proptosis
  - CT scan or MRI facilitates differentiation

Preseptal/Orbital Cellulitis
- Also presents with erythema, edema, and tenderness of eyelid; orbital cellulitis will frequently cause proptosis and extraocular movement limitation

Chalazion
- Occurs lower in the eyelid in the tarsal plate

EVALUATION/WORK-UP

Labs
- Gram stain and culture of discharge
- Complete blood count with differential if febrile or infectious cause suspected
- ACE for suspected sarcoidosis; rapid plasma reagin and fluorescent treponemal antibody for suspected syphilis; ESR, CRP, ANA for suspected autoimmune cases; C-ANCA for suspected Wegener granulomatosis; PPD for suspected tuberculosis; Lyme titers

Pathology
- Orbital biopsy with pathologic review should be performed for suspected malignancy or cases unresponsive to medical treatment

Imaging
- CT scan of the orbit and brain with contrast including axial and coronal views
- MRI may be considered if CT not diagnostic
- Chest x-ray or CT scan for suspected sarcoidosis or TB

TREATMENT

Medical
- Appropriate antibiotics for infectious causes
  - May be managed as outpatient if mild; may require admission and IV antibiotics for more severe cases
- Oral steroids are the mainstay of therapy for inflammatory causes

Surgical
- Intralesional steroids have been used successfully for a few inflammatory cases

Follow-Up
- Daily for acute cases until improvement documented

Prognosis
- Depends on underlying etiology, but generally good

SELECTED REFERENCES

1. Madge SN et al: Bilateral dacryoadenitis: a new addition to the spectrum of reactive arthritis? Ophthal Plast Reconstr Surg. 25(2):152-3, 2009
2. Mohammad Ael-N: Intralesional steroid injection for management of acute idiopathic dacryoadenitis: a preliminary result. Ophthal Plast Reconstr Surg. 21(2):138-41, 2005
3. Soheilian M et al: Dacryoadenitis as the earliest presenting manifestation of systemic Wegener's granulomatosis. Eur J Ophthalmol. 12(3):241-3, 2002
4. Rhem MN et al: Epstein-Barr virus dacryoadenitis. Am J Ophthalmol. 129(3):372-5, 2000

CANALICULITIS

Key Facts

Introduction
- Inflammation of the canaliculus typically secondary to a bacterial infection
- Can be seen secondary to plug insertion or intubation

Demographics
- Most common organisms involved are *Actinomyces* spp., *Nocardia asteroides,* and *Staphylococcus* spp.
- Adults are more commonly affected
- More common in women
- Often misdiagnosed, which leads to delay in diagnosis and treatment

Presentation
- Mucopurulent discharge
- Epiphora
- Red eyes
- Slit-lamp examination to evaluate puncta

Differential Diagnosis
- Dacryocystitis
- Conjunctivitis
- Chalazion/hordeolum

Evaluation/Work-Up
- Cultures of samples from tears, discharge, conjunctiva, etc.
- Histopathology is most commonly performed to diagnosis canaliculitis

Treatment
- Medical management alone is rarely effective
- Consider canaliculostomy as it is a definitive treatment

__(Left)__ This illustration depicts normal anatomy of the lacrimal system. The superior ⇒ and inferior ➡ canaliculi are noted. Inflammation of these canaliculi presents clinically as canaliculitis. __(Right)__ This external photograph shows mucopurulent discharge from the superior puncta ⇒.

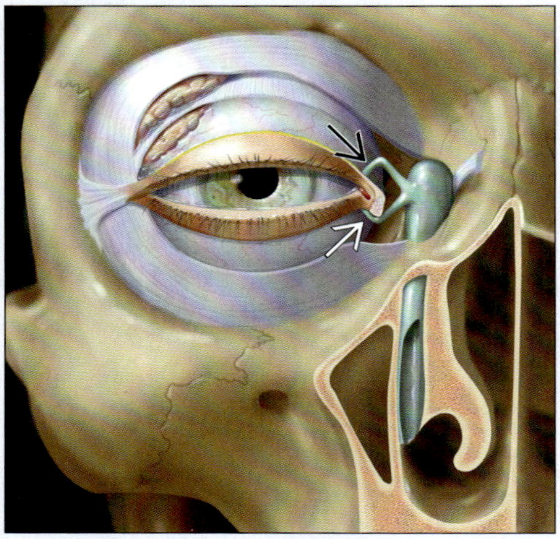

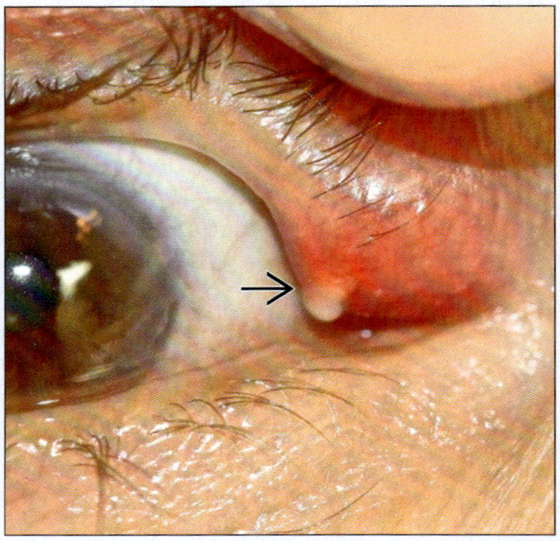

__(Left)__ This external photograph shows inflammation in the medial canthus ⇒, likely indicative of dacryocystitis. The location of inflammation is important in distinguishing from canaliculitis. __(Right)__ This external photo shows purulent discharge protruding from the inferior puncta ⇒. This discharge likely indicates drainage from an abscess due to dacryocystitis.

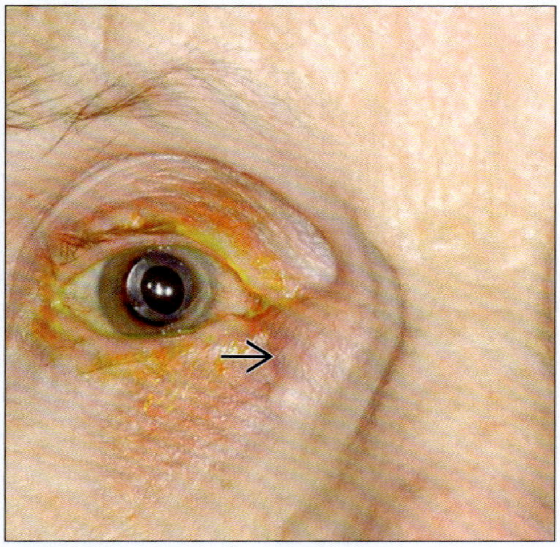

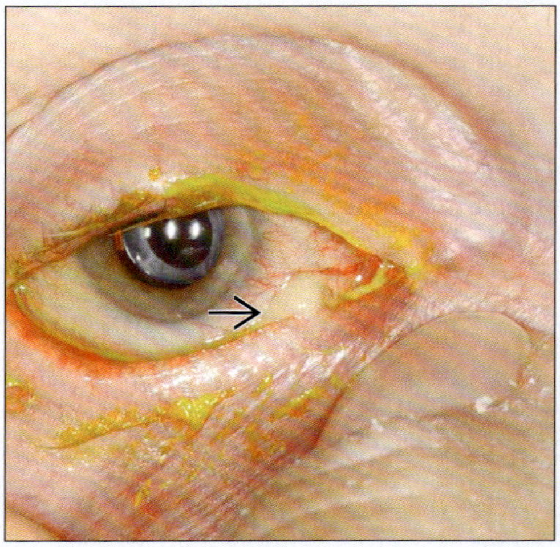

CANALICULITIS

INTRODUCTION

Definitions

- Inflammation of the canaliculus, typically secondary to bacterial infection
  - Canaliculi originate at lacrimal puncta
  - In upper eyelid, horizontal canaliculi ~ 6 mm; in lower eyelid, horizontal canaliculi are ~ 8 mm in length
  - In most people, canaliculi meet to form the common canaliculus, which then empties into the lacrimal sac
- May be seen secondary to plug insertion or intubation

DEMOGRAPHICS

Etiology/Risk Factors

- Most common organisms involved are *Actinomyces* spp., *Nocardia asteroides,* and *Staphylococcus* spp.
  - Other organisms include: *Arcanobacterium haemolyticum, Eikenella corrodens, Haemophilus aphrophilus, Lactococcus lactis cremoris, Molluscum contagiosum, Mycobacterium chelonae, Propionibacterium propionicus*
  - Viral infections are seen in younger populations, often primary herpetic infections
  - *Actinomyces* spp. may form stones known as canaliculiths
- No obvious predisposing conditions have been identified, although obstruction or deformities of lacrimal tract may promote stasis and bacterial growth

Epidemiology

- Adults are more commonly affected (≥ 50 years)
- More common in women
  - Thought to be secondary to changes during menopause including decreased tear production and decreased immunity
  - May be partially attributed to cosmetics usage
- Typically unilateral with lower eyelid canaliculus more often affected
- Makes up ~ 2% of lacrimal disease
- Often misdiagnosed, which leads to delay in diagnosis and treatment (by ~ 10 months)

PRESENTATION

Symptoms

- Mucopurulent discharge
- Epiphora
- Red eyes
- Tenderness
- Can be chronic in nature, leading to months of painless discharge

Exam Findings

- Slit-lamp examination evaluating puncta
  - "Pouting" puncta, erythema, and regurgitation
  - Thickening of eyelid margin
  - Medial canthal swelling
- Attempts to express material from puncta
  - "Granules" of pus may sometimes be expressed
- Palpation of lacrimal sac
  - Important to distinguish between dacryocystitis and canaliculitis
- Lacrimal syringing to assess for stenosis

DIFFERENTIAL DIAGNOSIS

Dacryocystitis

- Infection or inflammation of lacrimal drainage system may be secondary to nasolacrimal duct obstruction

Conjunctivitis

- Inflammation of conjunctiva

Chalazion/Hordeolum

- Infection or obstruction of meibomian or Zeis glands

EVALUATION/WORK-UP

Labs

- Cultures tears, discharge, conjunctiva etc.
  - Samples sent for aerobic and anaerobic cultures, may culture for bacteria, fungus, and mycobacteria
  - Often polymicrobial in nature
  - *Actinomyces israelii* is a gram-positive rod anaerobe bacteria that is difficult to isolate

Pathology

- Histopathology is most commonly performed to diagnosis canaliculitis
  - Concretions may be seen
  - Sulfur granules are pathological for *Actinomyces* spp.
- Secondary canaliculitis will show signs of inflammation and infiltrates

Imaging

- Consider dacryocystography or ultrasound biomicroscopy
  - Typically a clinical diagnosis as these diagnostic methods may further inflame canaliculi

TREATMENT

Medical

- Medical management alone is rarely effective
  - Warm compresses
  - Punctal dilation and canalicular expression
  - Topical antibiotic ointment and steroids
  - Oral penicillin/amoxicillin

Surgical

- In more severe cases, consider canaliculostomy as it is a definitive treatment
  - 6 mm incision along canaliculus and expression of all affected contents including canaliculiths
  - May lead to narrowing or scarring and lacrimal pump dysfunction
- Punctoplasty with canalicular curettage

Prognosis

- Good prognosis and low recurrence rate with surgical intervention

SELECTED REFERENCES

1. Freedman JR et al: Primary and secondary lacrimal canaliculitis: a review of literature. Surv Ophthalmol. 56(4):336-47, 2011

DACRYOCYSTITIS

Key Facts

Introduction
- Infection or inflammation of lacrimal drainage system

Demographics
- Majority of disease is caused by blockage of drainage system and subsequent stagnation of tears
- Bimodal distribution affecting infants and elderly

Presentation
- Acute: Sudden onset of pain, swelling, and erythema in area below medial canthal tendon
- Chronic: Insidious onset of epiphora that may be accompanied by mattering and irritation and inflammation of conjunctiva
- Congenital: Can easily progress to orbital cellulitis, abscess formation, meningitis, and death due to incompletely developed orbital septum

Evaluation/Work-Up
- Diagnosis is clinical, based on history and symptoms
- Complete blood count, culture of discharge may assist in treatment decision
- Antineutrophil cytoplasmic antibody and antinuclear antibody testing to rule out systemic disease (Wegener granulomatosis, lupus)

Treatment
- Acute
  - Surgical treatment should be delayed until after initial infection is controlled
- Chronic
  - Dacryocystorhinostomy or balloon dacryoplasty
- Congenital
  - Probing or placement of silicone tube; rarely, dacryocystorhinostomy may be required
- Recurrence is not uncommon; surgery is a definitive treatment

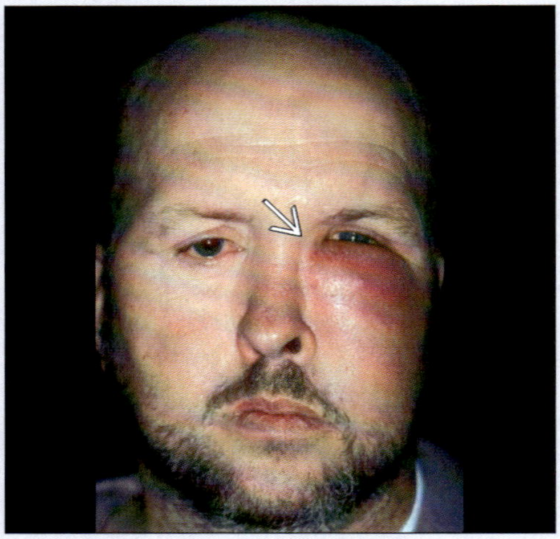
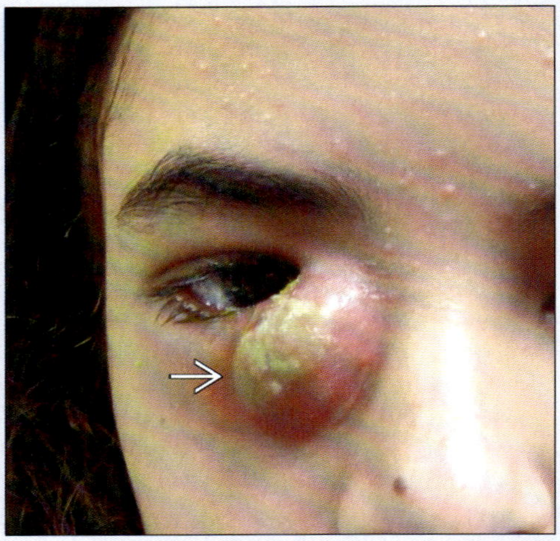

(Left) *This external photo demonstrates left-sided dacryocystitis. Notice the significant swelling and erythema below the level of the medial canthal tendon* ➔. ***(Right)*** *This external photo demonstrates severe dacryocystitis with significant swelling, erythema, and evidence of purulent discharge* ➔, *concerning for fistula formation. (Courtesy R. Nosé, MD.)*

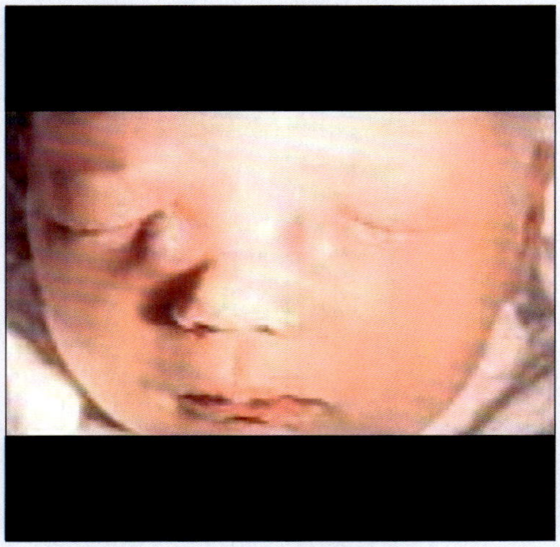
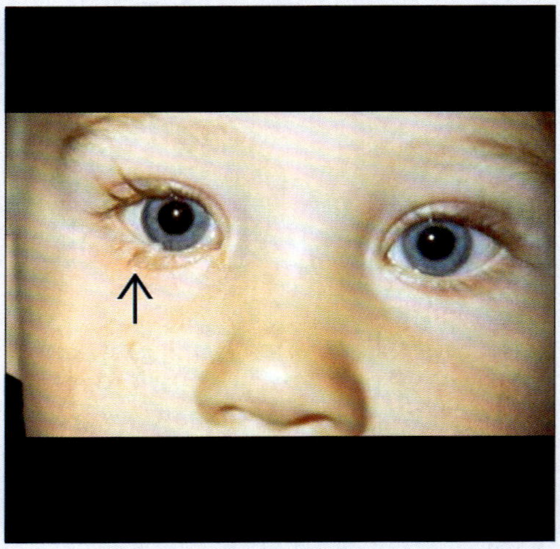

(Left) *This external photo shows a child with bilateral bilateral dacryocystocele. Note the lack of inflammation or signs of infection. This is likely secondary to incomplete canalization of the lacrimal system, most commonly at the valve of Hasner.* ***(Right)*** *This external photo demonstrates increased tear meniscus and mucoid discharge along the lid margin* ➔. *This patient has congenital nasolacrimal duct obstruction, which predisposes to the development of dacryocystitis.*

DACRYOCYSTITIS

INTRODUCTION

Definitions
- Infection or inflammation of lacrimal drainage system

Subtypes
- Acute, chronic, congenital

DEMOGRAPHICS

Etiology/Risk Factors
- Majority of disease is caused by blockage of drainage system and subsequent stagnation of tears, resulting in infection
- Congenital: Most often due to incomplete canalization, particularly at valve of Hasner

Epidemiology
- More prevalent in females
- Bimodal distribution affecting infants and elderly between 60-70 years

PRESENTATION

Symptoms
- Acute
  - Sudden onset of pain, swelling, and erythema in area below medial canthal tendon
  - Additional symptoms include epiphora, mattering, purulent discharge from lacrimal punctum, and fever
  - Often, there will be associated conjunctival injection and inflammation and cellulitis that can progress to orbital cellulitis due to buildup of bacterial debris
  - Fistula formation to superficial skin surface can occur
  - Decreased visual acuity from altered tear film and inflammatory changes to corneal surface
- Chronic
  - Insidious onset of epiphora that may be accompanied by mattering and irritation and inflammation of conjunctiva
  - Lacrimal sac cyst or mucocele may form
- Congenital
  - Can easily progress to orbital cellulitis, abscess formation, meningitis, and death due to incompletely developed orbital septum

DIFFERENTIAL DIAGNOSIS

Nasolacrimal Duct Obstruction
- Most common cause; does not have redness/pain

Canaliculitis
- Presents similarly to dacryocystitis, but symptoms are more focal and mild, surrounding medial canthus

Preseptal Cellulitis
- More diffuse, periorbital involvement without discharge from or blockage of punctum

EVALUATION/WORK-UP

Clinical
- Diagnosis is typically made clinically, based on history and symptoms
- Manual expression of purulent material from punctum
- Schirmer test: Helps rule out epiphora due to lid malposition

Labs
- Complete blood count may show leukocytosis
- Culture of discharge may assist in treatment decision
- Antineutrophil cytoplasmic antibody and antinuclear antibody testing to rule out systemic disease (Wegener granulomatosis, lupus)

Pathology
- Dependent on etiology of blockage but typically shows inflammatory changes and fibrosis

Imaging
- Plain films are useful to identify skeletal anomalies, foreign bodies, or mass lesions
- Computed tomography of orbit and paranasal cavities in atypical cases

TREATMENT

Medical
- Acute: Topical and oral antibiotics (cover skin and upper respiratory flora [e.g., cefuroxime/Augmentin])
- Chronic: Topical steroid drops
- Congenital: In majority of cases, oral or intravenous antibiotics, warm compresses, and massage are sufficient
  - Lacrimal syringing if previous fails to result in improvement

Surgical
- Acute: Surgical treatment should be delayed until after initial infection is controlled
  - Current preferred treatment is external dacryocystorhinostomy
- Chronic: Dacryocystorhinostomy or balloon dacryoplasty
- Congenital: Probing or placement of silicone tube; rarely, dacryocystorhinostomy may be required

Follow-Up
- Daily to track improvement with hospital admission for intravenous antibiotics if necessary

Prognosis
- Surgery is a definitive and effective treatment

SELECTED REFERENCES

1. Mueller JB et al: Ocular infection and inflammation. Emerg Med Clin North Am. 26(1):57-72, vi, 2008
2. Brook I et al: Aerobic and anaerobic microbiology of dacryocystitis. Am J Ophthalmol. 125(4):552-4, 1998
3. Cahill KV et al: Management of acute dacryocystitis in adults. Ophthal Plast Reconstr Surg. 9(1):38-41; discussion 42, 1993
4. Boruchoff SA et al: Infections of the lacrimal system. Infect Dis Clin North Am. 6(4):925-32, 1992

PRESEPTAL CELLULITIS

Key Facts

Introduction

- Infection or inflammation of soft tissue of periorbital area anterior to orbital septum

Demographics

- Most often associated with upper respiratory infections, sinusitis, dacryocystitis, and recent eyelid lesions
- Presents predominantly in pediatric population

Presentation

- Unilateral swelling, redness, and tenderness of periocular area
- It is imperative to rule out orbital cellulitis, which can quickly threaten vision

Differential Diagnosis

- Orbital cellulitis: Proptosis, ophthalmoplegia; requires prompt admission for intravenous antibiotics

Evaluation/Work-Up

- Gram stain and culture of discharge should be obtained prior to starting antibiotics
- Systemic manifestations are uncommon and indicate that orbital cellulitis is more likely
- Computed tomography can be used for cases in which orbital cellulitis cannot be ruled out

Treatment

- Empiric treatment of common upper respiratory infection agents is recommended
- In severe cases, consider hospital admission for intravenous antibiotics and monitoring
- Moderate cases and cases that show marked improvement after intravenous antibiotics can be treated with oral antibiotics
- Excellent outcome if identified and treated early

*(**Left**) This external photograph shows a patient with preseptal cellulitis with erythema of the eyelid ➲. The distinction between preseptal cellulitis and orbital cellulitis is important. Proptosis is typically not present in preseptal cellulitis. (**Right**) Axial contrast-enhanced CT in an older patient with facial impetigo shows typical findings of preseptal cellulitis. The preseptal soft tissues show edema and enhancement ➔ with a normal appearance of the intraorbital fat ➲.*

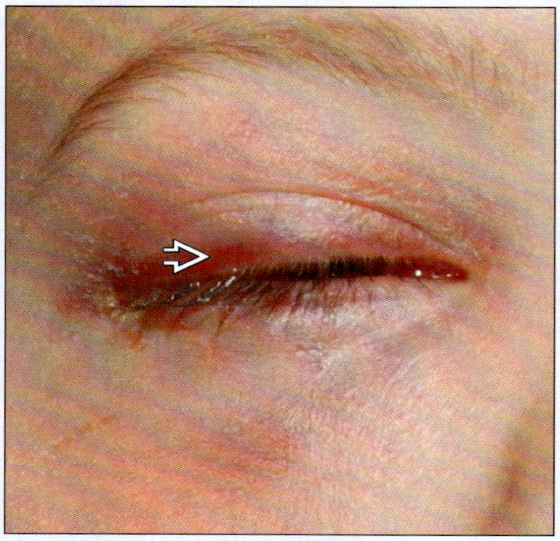

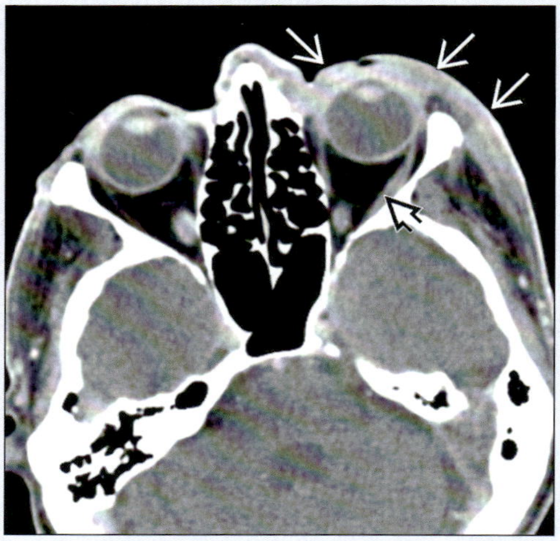

*(**Left**) This external photograph shows a patient with orbital cellulitis. Orbital cellulitis is an important differential diagnosis for preseptal cellulitis since orbital cellulitis is more likely to be visually threatening. Symptoms and findings concerning for orbital cellulitis include proptosis, vision changes, and impaired ocular motility. (**Right**) Axial contrast-enhanced CT in a patient with orbital cellulitis shows preseptal ➔ and postseptal ➲ cellulitis, as well as mild proptosis without focal abscess.*

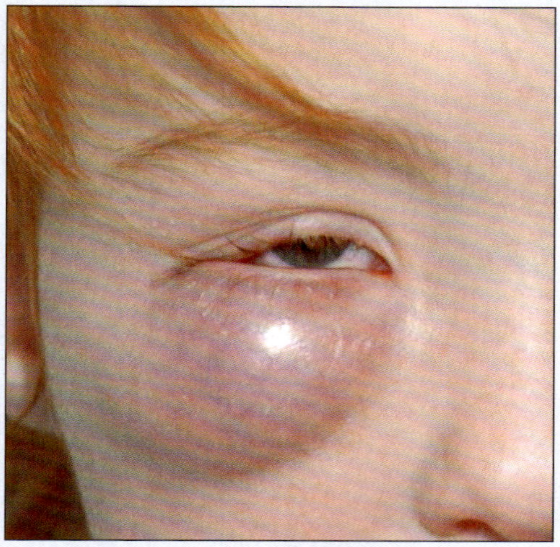

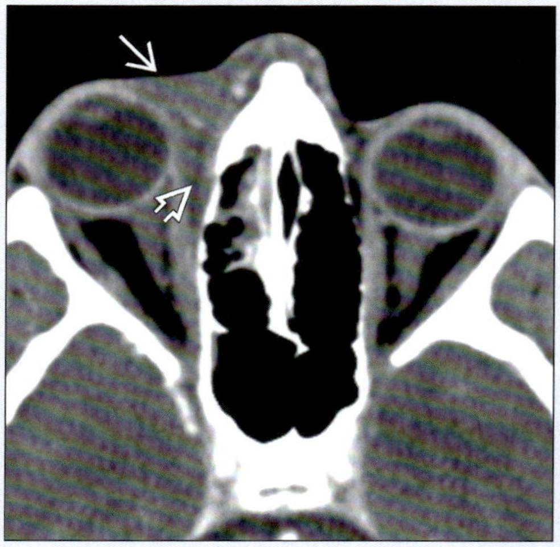

PRESEPTAL CELLULITIS

INTRODUCTION

Synonyms
- Periorbital cellulitis

Definitions
- Infection or inflammation of soft tissue of periorbital area anterior to orbital septum

DEMOGRAPHICS

Etiology/Risk Factors
- Most often associated with upper respiratory infections, sinusitis and dacryocystitis
- Recent eyelid lesions are also predisposing factors
  - Hordeolum
  - Chalazion
  - Insect bites
  - Trauma
  - Recent ocular surgery
- Most common responsible organisms
  - *Staphylococcus aureus* or *Staphylococcus epidermidis*, *Pneumococcus*, *Moraxella*, *Streptococcus* species

Epidemiology
- Presents predominantly in pediatric population

PRESENTATION

Symptoms
- Unilateral swelling, redness, and tenderness of periocular area
- May be associated with mild conjunctivitis, epiphora, chemosis, and visual acuity changes (from changes in tear film)
- In severe cases, voluntary opening of eyelids may be prevented by edema

Exam Findings
- It is imperative to rule out orbital cellulitis, which can quickly threaten vision
- Signs of orbital cellulitis
  - Resistance to retropulsion
  - Extraocular muscle restriction and diplopia
  - Afferent pupillary defect
  - Extensive involvement of the globe itself
  - Reduced vision or color vision

DIFFERENTIAL DIAGNOSIS

Orbital Cellulitis
- Proptosis, restriction of eye movement; requires admission for intravenous antibiotics

Idiopathic Orbital Inflammatory Disease
- More frequently occurs in adult population; unknown etiology

Allergies
- Usually bilateral, nontender, and has pruritus

Chalazion
- Localized hard nodule from clogged meibomian glands

Cavernous Sinus Thrombosis
- Cranial nerve and systemic manifestations

EVALUATION/WORK-UP

Labs
- Gram stain and culture of discharge should be obtained prior to starting antibiotics
- Leukocytosis is less likely to be elevated in preseptal cellulitis vs. orbital cellulitis
- Blood cultures rarely reveal infectious organisms and are not recommended

Imaging
- Not typically indicated in clear cases of preseptal cellulitis
- Computed tomography can be used for cases in which orbital cellulitis cannot be ruled out
- Magnetic resonance imaging is increasingly preferred in pediatric population due to concerns with radiation exposure

TREATMENT

Medical
- Empiric treatment of common skin and upper respiratory flora recommended (e.g., cefuroxime, amoxicillin + clavulanate)
- In severe cases, consider hospital admission for intravenous antibiotics and monitoring
  - Ampicillin + sulbactam
  - Ceftriaxone
  - Vancomycin if methicillin-resistant *S. aureus* is suspected
- Moderate cases and cases that show marked improvement after intravenous antibiotics can be treated with oral antibiotics
  - Amoxicillin + clavulanate
  - Cefaclor, cefuroxime, ceftriaxone
  - Trimethoprim + sulfamethoxazole

Surgical
- Preseptal cellulitis typically does not warrant surgical management unless complicated by orbital abscesses

Prognosis
- Excellent outcome if identified and treated early
- Treatment delay can result in multiple complications: Orbital cellulitis, abscess, meningitis, cavernous sinus thrombosis

SELECTED REFERENCES

1. Hauser A et al: Periorbital and orbital cellulitis. Pediatr Rev. 31(6):242-9, 2010
2. Liu IT et al: Preseptal and orbital cellulitis: a 10-year review of hospitalized patients. J Chin Med Assoc. 69(9):415-22, 2006
3. Howe L et al: Guidelines for the management of periorbital cellulitis/abscess. Clin Otolaryngol Allied Sci. 29(6):725-8, 2004
4. Tovilla-Canales JL et al: Orbital and periorbital infections. Curr Opin Ophthalmol. 12(5):335-41, 2001
5. Lessner A et al: Preseptal and orbital cellulitis. Infect Dis Clin North Am. 6(4):933-52, 1992

LACRIMAL TRACT TRAUMA

Key Facts

Introduction
- Trauma to any structures of the lacrimal tract: Puncta, canaliculi, lacrimal sac, and nasolacrimal duct

Demographics
- Seen secondary to trauma, motor vehicle accidents, biking injuries, falls, and animal bites
- More common in children and young adults
- Canalicular lacerations are the most common lacrimal tract injury

Presentation
- Typically associated with history of trauma
- Warrants full ophthalmic evaluation (including Bowman probe and irrigation of tract)

Differential Diagnosis
- Epiphora
- Eyelid laceration
- Lacrimal outflow obstruction

Evaluation/Work-Up
- Consider CT orbit

Treatment
- Standard trauma evaluation to assess for life-threatening conditions
- Wide variety of surgical techniques for repair
  - Bicanalicular injuries require immediate stenting (Crawford tubes) and repair
  - Monocanalicular injury may be managed conservatively, with bicanalicular stenting or monocanalicular intubation
- Good surgical prognosis
- Late repair is difficult given distortion and scarring of anatomical features

__(Left)__ Notice the damage to the medial aspect of the inferior lid. A careful search of the periorbital tissue is necessary to identify the canaliculus ➡. __(Right)__ This external photograph clearly demonstrates involvement of the lacrimal system in this lid laceration. Notice the probe entering the punctum ➡ and exiting in the lid laceration ➡. Identification of the remainder of the canaliculus and lacrimal system is critical in this situation.

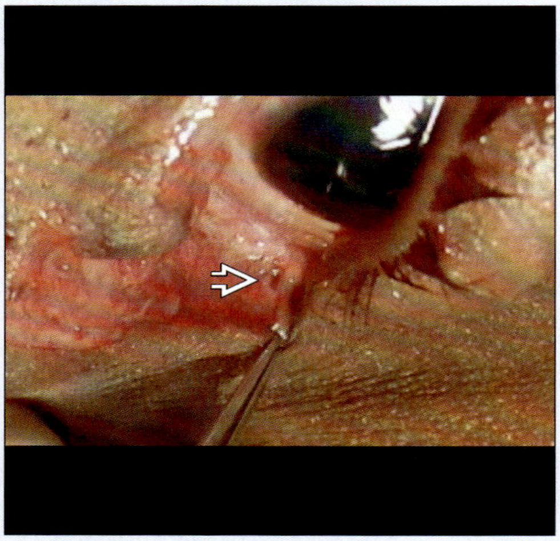

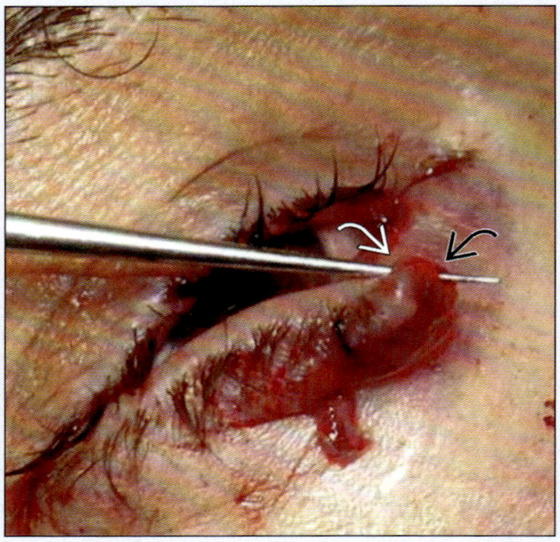

__(Left)__ This external photograph demonstrates a lacrimal stent ➡ in place in the lower punctum. Notice that this stent has an endplate and does not extend into the superior punctum, features that identify it as monocanalicular. These stents help reduce long-term complications of lacrimal trauma. __(Right)__ After sufficient healing has occurred, the canalicular stents can be removed. If monocanalicular, they are typically removed from the eyelid, and if bicanalicular, they are removed through the nose.

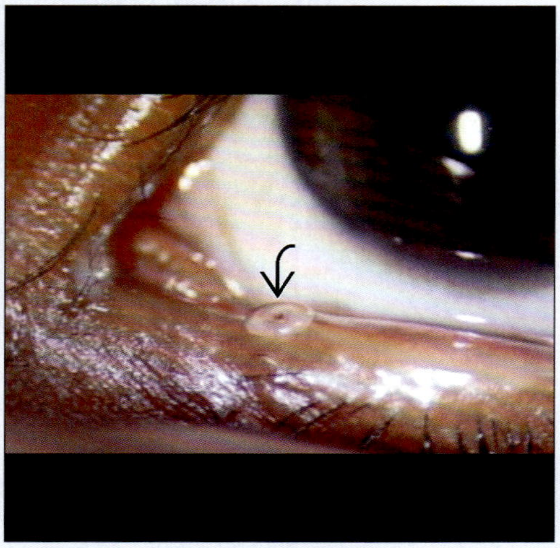

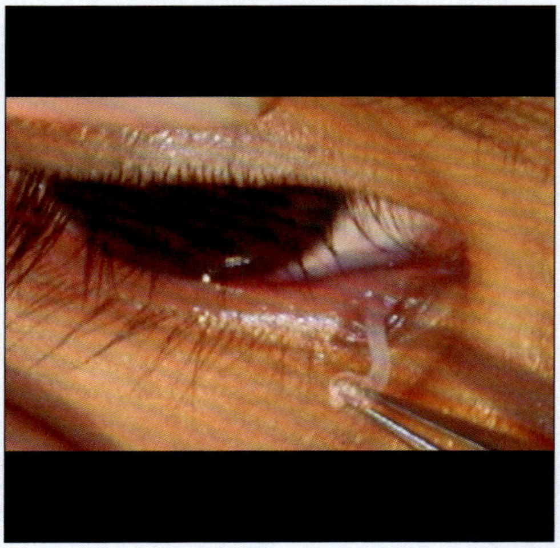

LACRIMAL TRACT TRAUMA

INTRODUCTION

Definitions

- Trauma to tear drainage system of eye
- Trauma to any structures of the lacrimal tract: Puncta, canaliculi, lacrimal sac, and nasolacrimal duct

DEMOGRAPHICS

Etiology/Risk Factors

- Seen secondary to blunt trauma, sharp trauma, motor vehicle accidents, biking injuries, falls, and animal bites
  - May be due to direct or indirect trauma
- Tends to occur in conjunction with orbit or eyelid injury
- More common in children and young adults
- Seen more often in men

Epidemiology

- Canalicular lacerations are the most common lacrimal tract injury
  - Canalicular involvement is estimated in 16-30% of **all** eye trauma
  - Injury most often involves lower canaliculus

PRESENTATION

Symptoms

- Typically associated with history of trauma
- Orbit pain (although presentation may be asymptomatic)

Exam Findings

- Full ophthalmic evaluation with special attention to the following
  - Slit-lamp examination
  - Retained foreign bodies
  - Bowman probe insertion following dilation of puncta to assess for disruption of lacrimal tract
    - Injury should be suspected if a hard stop at the nose is not felt
  - Irrigation of system by methylene blue or fluorescein stain through the puncta to assess for disruption of lacrimal tract
    - Injury to the system may not be readily visualized
  - Lacerations medial to the punctum often accompany canalicular injury

DIFFERENTIAL DIAGNOSIS

Epiphora

- May be preexisting and due to prior ocular inflammation or irritation

Eyelid Laceration

- Assess for any coexisting lacerations, especially to eyelid

Lacrimal Outflow Obstruction

- Loss of compliance or stenosis of lacrimal outflow tract

EVALUATION/WORK-UP

Imaging

- Consider CT of orbit in axial and coronal planes for suspected orbit or facial fracture

TREATMENT

Medical

- Standard trauma evaluation to assess for life-threatening conditions
- Tetanus vaccination if needed and rabies protocol if animal bite suspected
- Consider general anesthesia for children
- Depending on extent of injury, local anesthesia may be used in adults
  - 1% lidocaine in 1:100,000 epinephrine

Surgical

- Wide variety of surgical techniques for repair
  - Most surgeons tend to agree that if repair is to be performed, it should occur as soon as possible; 48-72 hours is ideal
  - Common goals include restoring anatomy of eyelid, reapproximating the disrupted canaliculus and providing support to this structure (usually via stenting of canaliculi to prevent obstruction)
- Bicanalicular injuries require immediate stenting (Crawford tubes) and repair
- Monocanalicular injury may be managed in the following ways
  - Bicanalicular annual stenting via round-tipped pigtail probe
    - Possibility of unintentional injury to intact canaliculi
  - Monocanalicular intubation of canaliculi to prevent restenosis
    - May be done with or without surgical repair
    - Insufficient studies on timing of stent removal (range: 3-12 months)
  - Conservative treatment as monocanalicular injury may not directly cause epiphora
    - Note that other symptoms may persist, including intermittent watery eye and mild blurred vision
- Evaluation for medial canthal ligament injury
  - Crucial to be repaired in its anatomical position
  - Influences lid function and appearance

Follow-Up

- Continued use of broad-spectrum systemic antibiotics and topical ophthalmic antibiotics

Prognosis

- Good surgical prognosis if repaired before scarring &/or epiphora occurs
- Late repair is difficult given distortion and scarring of anatomical features

SELECTED REFERENCES

1. Naik MN et al: Management of canalicular lacerations: epidemiological aspects and experience with Mini-Monoka monocanalicular stent. Am J Ophthalmol. 145(2):375-380, 2008

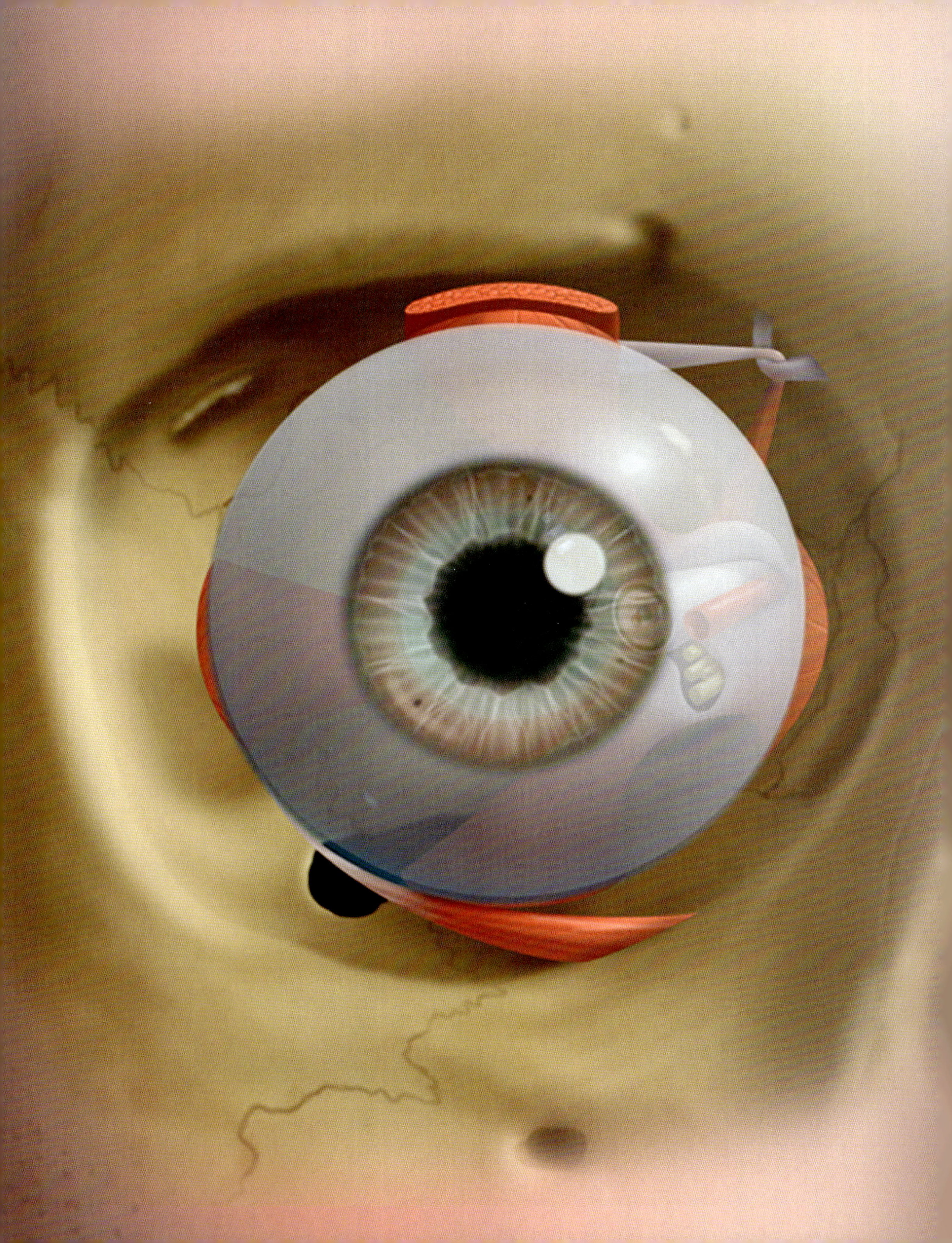

SECTION 3
Orbit

Introduction and Overview

Congenital Disorders

Infectious Disorders

Autoimmune Disorders

Trauma

Nonneoplastic Cysts

Benign Neoplasms

Malignant Neoplasms

ORBIT OVERVIEW

GROSS ANATOMY

Bony Structures

- Cone-shaped cavity with the apex toward the back of the head and boundaries formed by 7 bones
- Orbital roof
  - Frontal bone and lesser wing of sphenoid
  - Landmarks: Lacrimal gland fossa, trochlea, supraorbital notch/foramen
- Orbital floor: Typically 1st to break from trauma
  - Maxillary bone, orbital processes of the palatine and zygomatic bones
  - Landmarks: Infraorbital groove, infraorbital canal
- Lateral wall: Strongest and thickest wall of orbit
  - Zygomatic bone
  - Lesser and greater wings of the sphenoid
  - Landmarks: Lateral orbital tubercle of Whitnall 10 mm inferior to the zygomaticofrontal suture
- Medial wall
  - Lacrimal bone
  - Ethmoid bone
    - Thinnest portion of orbit and susceptible to erosion from sinus infections
  - Palatine bone
  - Landmark: Lacrimal fossa inferior to the frontoethmoidal suture
- Orbital apex
  - Sphenoid bone
    - Forms superior orbital fissure and optic canal
    - Superior border of inferior orbital fissure
- Optic canal
  - 8-19 mm long in lesser wing of the sphenoid
  - Path for optic nerve, ophthalmic artery, central retinal vein, and sympathetic nerves
- Superior orbital fissure
  - Formed by greater and lesser wings of the sphenoid
  - Path for CN3, CN4, CN5 (ophthalmic division), CN4, sympathetic nerve fibers and venous drainage (via superior orbital vein and superior ophthalmic vein)
- Inferior orbital fissure
  - Formed by the sphenoid, maxillary, and palatine bones
  - Path for CN5 (maxillary division, includes infraorbital nerve and zygomatic nerve), infraorbital artery and vein, parasympathetics to lacrimal gland, and branches of inferior ophthalmic vein
- Ethmoidal foramina
  - Anterior and posterior apertures located along frontoethmoidal suture
  - Important surgical landmarks that transmit the anterior and posterior ethmoidal arteries
  - Provides a potential conduit for infections and neoplasm to enter orbit

ORBITAL CONTENTS

Periorbital Fat

- Separated into intraconal and extraconal areas by intermuscular septum

Connective Tissue

- Multiple septa exist in the orbit to provide barriers and stability to extraocular muscles, optic nerve, and the globe itself

Muscles

- 4 recti muscles: Originate at annulus of Zinn and attach to the sclera
  - Intermuscular septum: Membrane that connects recti muscles anteriorly
  - Superior: Elevation, adduction, intorsion
  - Inferior: Depression, adduction, extorsion
  - Medial rectus: Adduction
  - Lateral rectus: Abduction
- 2 oblique muscles
  - Superior oblique: Originates at the apex of the orbit, hooks through the trochlea to attach to the sclera and performs intorsion, depression, abduction
  - Inferior oblique: Originates on the posterior orbital floor, inserts inferolateral to the macula and performs extorsion, elevation, abduction
  - May hypertrophy due to various medical conditions (i.e., Graves disease, pseudotumor, orbital tumor) and cause proptosis or diplopia
- Nerves
  - Sensory
    - CN5 is the afferent sensory nerve of the periorbital region with 3 main branches
    - CN5 splits into its ophthalmic division (lacrimal, frontal, nasociliary), maxillary division, and mandibular division
    - Ophthalmic division innervates medial canthus, upper eyelid, forehead, and eye itself
  - Motor
    - CN3 (oculomotor nerve) innervates the levator muscles; inferior, medial, and superior recti; and inferior oblique
    - CN4 (trochlear nerve) innervates the superior oblique muscle
    - CN6 (abducens nerve) innervates the lateral rectus
    - CN7 (facial nerve) innervates the muscles of facial expression including the orbicularis oculi and frontalis
  - Sympathetic
    - Controls pupil dilation, vasoconstriction, and smooth muscles of orbit and lids
  - Parasympathetic
    - Controls pupil constriction, accommodations, and lacrimation
- Vasculature
  - Supply is primarily from the ophthalmic artery that branches into the central retinal artery and posterior ciliary arteries and feeds extraocular muscles
  - High density of anastomoses with facial and periorbital branches of the external carotid artery
  - Drainage is performed by the superior ophthalmic vein into the cavernous sinus and inferior ophthalmic vein into the pterygoid venous plexus
- Lacrimal gland
  - Located in the superotemporal orbit in the lacrimal fossa of the frontal bone
  - Divided into an orbital lobe and palpebral lobe

RELATED REFERENCES

1. Lemke BN et al: Anatomy of the ocular adnexa, orbit, and related facial structures. Smith and Nesi's Ophthalmic Plastic and Reconstructive Surgery. New York: Springer. 3-58, 2012

ORBIT ANATOMY

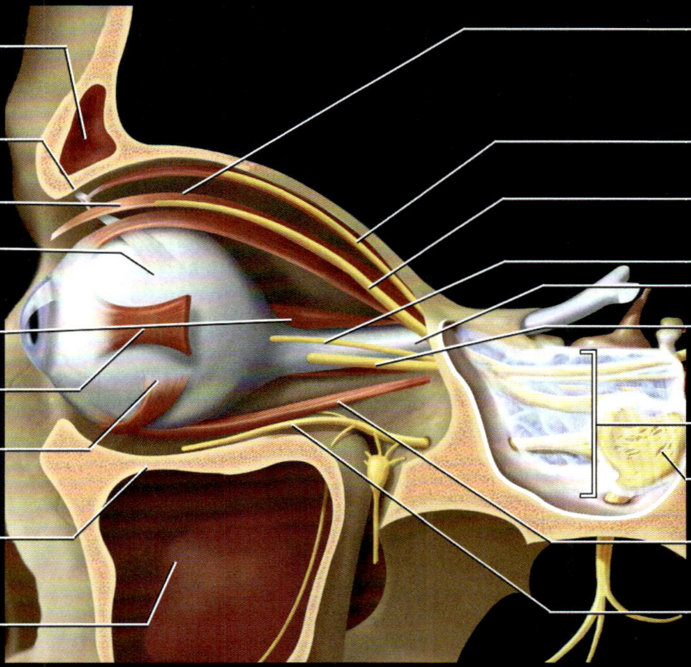

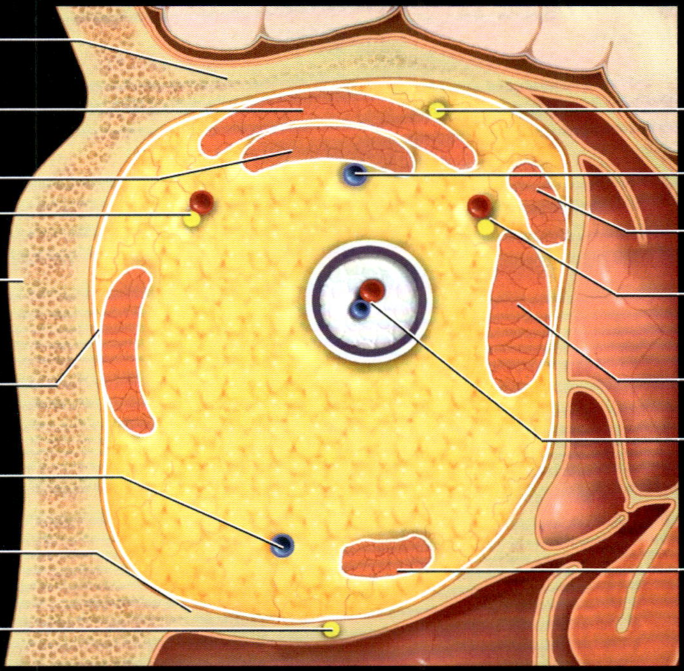

(Top) *This is an illustration of the left orbit in cross sectional view. The average human orbit is cone shaped with the apex pointing medial and posterior and occupying 30 mL of space. The fibrous orbital septum (not pictured) acts as a barrier between superficial, preorbital infections and much more dangerous orbital infections that can spread to the surrounding sinuses and brain. Infectious, inflammatory, autoimmune, and neoplastic processes can occur in this space and cause varying degrees of proptosis. Severe cases can threaten vision by compression of nerves and vasculature. The medial wall is the thinnest and most often compromised by infiltrative processes. It is, however, well buttressed by surrounding structures such that the floor of the orbit is the 1st to break in direct ocular trauma.* ***(Bottom)*** *This is an illustration of the orbit in coronal view. The orbit contains intraocular fat, multiple muscles, nerves, and vessels serving the globe itself and surrounding structures.*

Key Facts

Introduction

- Rare condition involving premature closure and fusion of fontanels and sutures during embryogenesis or early childhood
- Occurs in ~ 1 per 2,000 live births
- Can be syndromic or nonsyndromic
- Many craniosynostosis syndromes are sporadic, although often follow autosomal dominance inheritance
- Results in many facial and ocular malformations

Bone Fusion Syndromes

- Crouzon syndrome
  - Premature fusion of coronal &/or sagittal sutures (coronal suture fusion occurs more often)
- Apert syndrome
  - Premature fusion of coronal sutures (often both) &/or skull base
- Saethre-Chotzen syndrome
  - Usually involves premature fusion of only 1 coronal suture
- Pfeiffer syndrome
  - Premature fusion of coronal &/or lambdoidal sutures and occasionally sagittal sutures
- Carpenter syndrome
  - Premature fusion of sagittal, lambdoidal, &/or coronal sutures

Facial Malformation Syndromes

- Treacher Collins syndrome (TCS)
  - Mandibulofacial dysostosis
  - Malformation of 1st and 2nd pharyngeal arches
- Goldenhar syndrome
  - Oculoauriculovertebral dysplasia
  - Malformation of 1st and 2nd pharyngeal arches; more severe than TCS

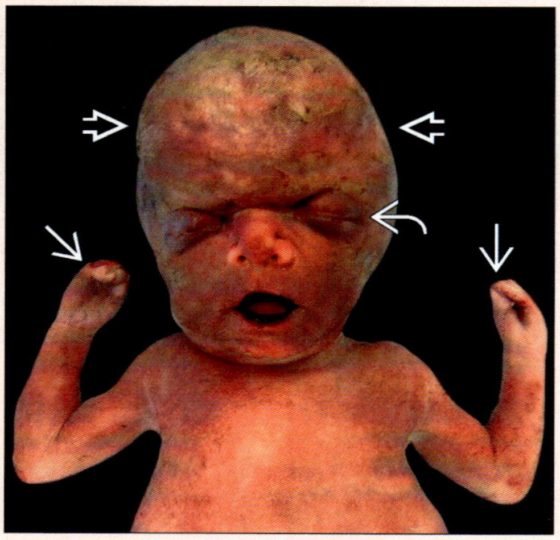

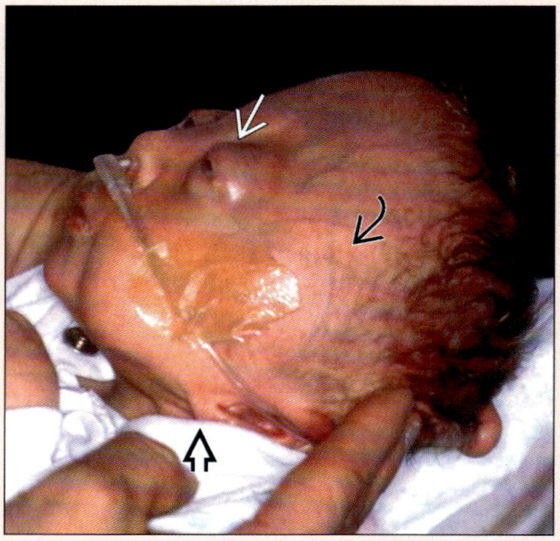

(Left) *Clinical photograph of a stillborn fetus shows the typical facial phenotype of Apert syndrome. Bilateral severe "mitten" syndactyly of the hands is seen ➔. There is a "tower" shape to the calvaria due to the craniosynostosis ➔. Note also the proptosis due to shallow orbits ➔.* ***(Right)*** *Clinical photograph shows a preterm infant with Carpenter syndrome. Note the severe proptosis ➔, the parietal bulge ➔, and low-set ear ➔ due to craniosynostosis.*

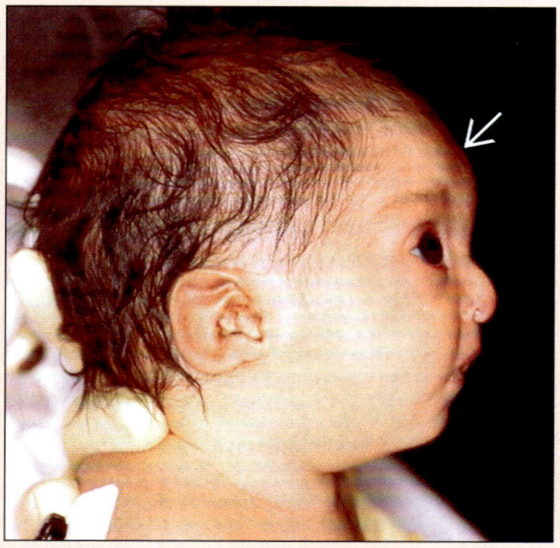

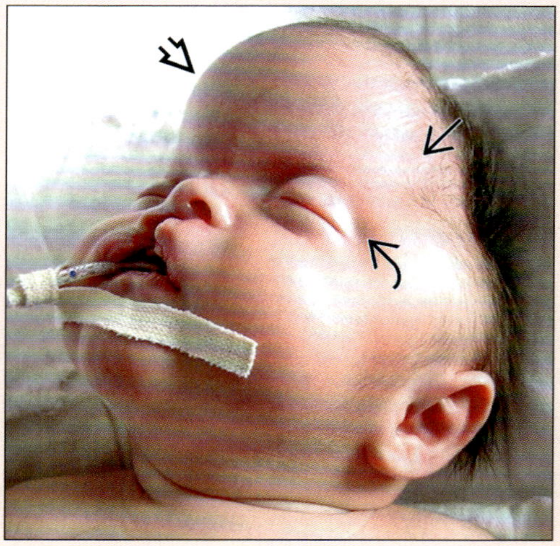

(Left) *Profile of an infant with trigonocephaly shows a very prominent metopic ridge ➔.* ***(Right)*** *Clinical photograph shows the abnormal calvarial shape due to complex craniosynostosis associated with Pfeiffer syndrome. Note the very prominent frontal bossing ➔ due to coronal synostosis ➔. The eyes are proptotic ➔ due to shallow orbits. The cleft lip is also seen.*

CRANIOSYNOSTOSIS

DEMOGRAPHICS

Etiology/Risk Factors

- Crouzon syndrome
  - Autosomal dominant inheritance, although 25% result from de novo mutation
  - > 30 mutations in fibroblast growth factor receptor 2 (*FGFR2*) gene on chromosome 10 have been implicated in syndrome
  - Most common autosomal dominant craniosynostosis syndrome: ~ 1 per 62,500 live births
- Apert syndrome
  - Most cases are sporadic and associated with increased parental age, although also follows autosomal dominant inheritance pattern
  - 2 mutations in *FGFR2* gene are responsible for majority of cases
  - Often associated with cardiovascular and genitourinary malformations and mental deficiency
- Saethre-Chotzen syndrome
  - Autosomal dominant inheritance with mutations often found in *TWIST* gene on chromosome 7
- Pfeiffer syndrome
  - Autosomal dominant with genetic heterogeneity
  - Occurs in ~ 1 per 100,000 live births
- Carpenter syndrome
  - Autosomal recessive inheritance
  - Occurs in < 1 per 1,000,000 live births
- Treacher Collins syndrome
  - Autosomal dominant inheritance, although 60% result from de novo mutation
  - Most mutations occur in *TCOF1* gene on chromosome 5q, affecting the "treacle" protein
  - Occurs in 1 per 50,000 live births
- Goldenhar syndrome
  - Usually sporadic
  - Prevalence estimates vastly vary; range: 1 per 3,500 to 1 per 26,600 live births

PRESENTATION

Exam Findings

- Many craniosynostosis syndromes result in elevated intracranial pressure, leading to papilledema
  - Can lead to a spectrum of vision-threatening complications
- Crouzon syndrome
  - Proptosis as a result of shallow orbits
  - "V" pattern exotropia (eyes naturally rest up and out)
  - Ametropia and amblyopia
  - Hypertelorism
  - Elevated intracranial pressure
  - Inverted V-shape palate
- Apert syndrome
  - Tower-shaped head (turri- or oxycephaly)
  - "Beak nose" with midfacial hypoplasia
  - Proptosis
  - Shallow orbits
  - Exotropia
  - Extreme syndactyly: Key finding to differentiate from Crouzon syndrome
    - Complete fusion of most or all digits on hands and feet ("mitten" syndactyly)
- Saethre-Chotzen syndrome
  - Features are generally more mild than other craniosynostosis syndromes
  - Plagiocephaly
    - Causes face to become asymmetrical
  - Ptosis
  - Small, unusually shaped ears
  - Low hairline
  - Brachydactyly (shortened digits) on hands and feet with mild syndactyly
- Pfeiffer syndrome
  - Disproportionately wide head with flat occiput
  - Frontal bossing of forehead
  - Shallow orbits
  - Hypertelorisms
  - Downslanting palpebral fissures
  - Abnormally broad thumbs and great toes
  - Ankylosis of elbow
  - Most patients with Pfeiffer syndrome do not suffer any mental deficiencies
- Carpenter syndrome
  - Often severe mental retardation
  - Proptosis
  - Polydactyly
  - Brittle bones, often resembling osteogenesis imperfecta
  - Congenital heart disease
  - Hypogenitalism
  - Mild soft tissue syndactyly
- Treacher Collins syndrome
  - Lower lid coloboma
  - Often thin or absent orbicularis oculi muscles &/or meibomian glands
  - Downslanting palpebral fissures
  - Bilateral malar hypoplasia (abnormally small cheek bones)
    - Underdevelopment or agenesis of zygomatic bone
  - Malformed, low-set ears
    - Hearing loss common
  - Mandibular micrognathia (abnormally small jaw) with macrostomia (abnormally wide mouth)
- Goldenhar syndrome
  - Dermoids
    - Epibulbar (lipodermoid)
      - Usually occur in lower lateral portion of upper and lower eyelids
      - Often covered by conjunctiva
    - Limbal
      - Occur more frequently than epibulbar dermoids
  - Lower and upper lid coloboma
  - Dermolipomas
  - Bilateral or unilateral hemifacial microsomia
  - Associated with Duane syndrome

SELECTED REFERENCES

1. Forrest CR et al: Craniofacial syndromes and surgery. Plast Reconstr Surg. 131(1):86e-109e, 2013
2. Chang CC et al: Treacher collins syndrome. Semin Plast Surg. 26(2):83-90, 2012
3. Newman SA: Ophthalmic features of craniosynostosis. Neurosurg Clin N Am. 2(3):587-610, 1991

ORBITAL CELLULITIS

Key Facts

Introduction
- Infection of soft tissue posterior to orbital septum of frontal bone

Demographics
- Sinus disease (including acute sinusitis)
- Eyelid or facial infection
- Foreign body or trauma to orbit
- Most common pathogens are *Staphylococcus* sp. and *Streptococcus* sp.
- Most common in children and young adults

Presentation
- Orbital pain ± movement
- Lid edema and erythema
- Visual disturbances/loss
- Systemic symptoms including malaise, fevers, and chills

Differential Diagnosis
- Preseptal (periorbital) cellulitis
- Mucormycosis
- Cavernous sinus thrombosis
- Herpes simplex or herpes zoster ophthalmicus
- Tumors (i.e., lymphoproliferative, neuroblastoma, rhabdomyosarcoma)

Treatment
- If orbital cellulitis is suspected, patient should be admitted to hospital for prompt treatment with IV antibiotics
- If unresponsive to medical treatment or worsening of symptoms, consider sinus &/or abscess drainage
- If treatment is not delayed, prognosis is excellent

*(**Left**) This external photograph shows proptosis and severe unilateral inflammation associated with orbital cellulitis, an infection of the soft tissues posterior to the orbital septum. (**Right**) This external photo shows mild orbital cellulitis. Note that this patient exhibited minimal external findings, but the diagnosis of orbital cellulitis was confirmed by radiologic imaging.*

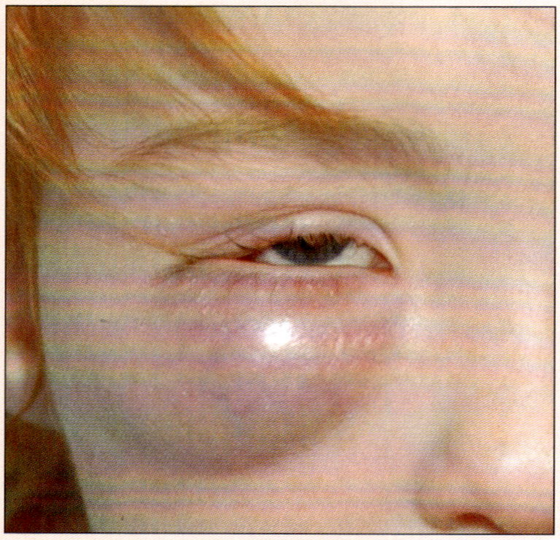

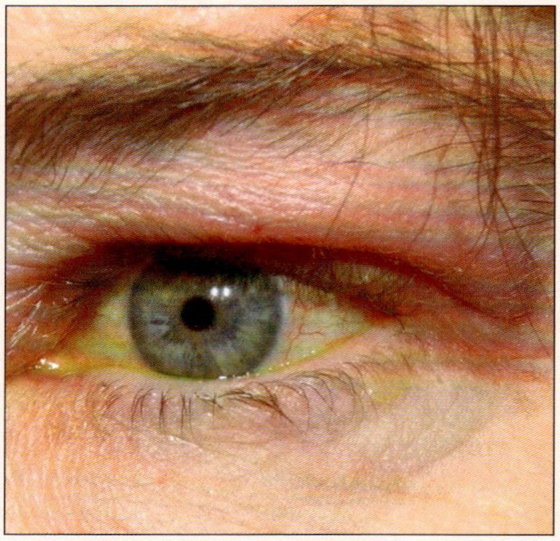

*(**Left**) This external photograph shows periorbital edema typical of preseptal cellulitis, an infection of the subcutaneous tissue anterior to the orbital septum. For proper treatment, it is important to distinguish preseptal from orbital cellulitis. (**Right**) Axial CT in a patient with aggressive cellulitis shows periorbital swelling and enhancement ➔. There is also postseptal infiltration of the intraconal fat ➔. The infection was polymicrobial with resistant organisms.*

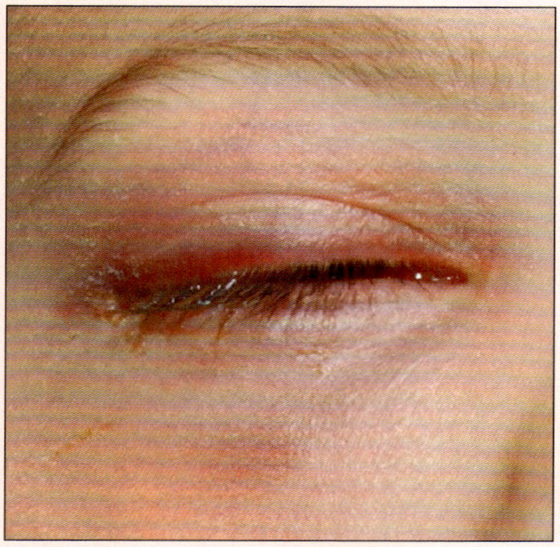

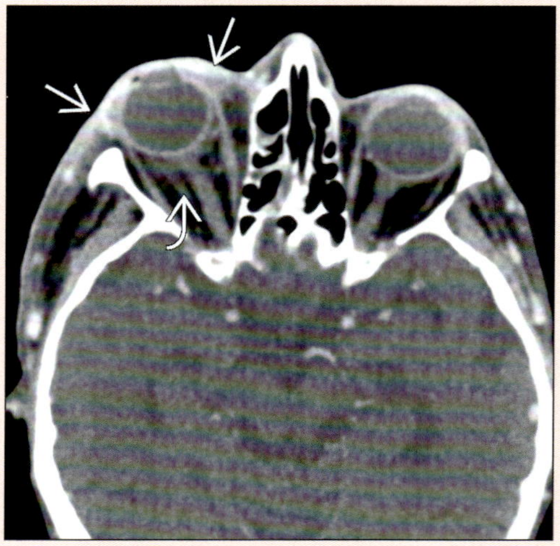

ORBITAL CELLULITIS

INTRODUCTION

Definitions
- Infection of soft tissue posterior to orbital septum of frontal bone

DEMOGRAPHICS

Etiology/Risk Factors
- Sinus disease (including acute sinusitis) extension via the ethmoid or maxillary sinuses
- Eyelid or facial infection
- Foreign body or trauma to orbit
- Hematogenous spread
- Post surgical
- Most common pathogens are *Staphylococcus* sp. and *Streptococcus* sp.
  - Pathogens include *Streptococcus pneumoniae, Haemophilus influenzae, Moraxella catarrhalis, Staphylococcus pyogenes, Staphylococcus aureus*, α- and nonhemolytic streptococci, and anaerobic bacteria associated with upper respiratory tract
  - *H. influenzae* orbital cellulitis is less likely since the advent of the Hib vaccination, but it should always be considered, especially in unvaccinated individuals

Epidemiology
- Most common in children and young adults

PRESENTATION

Symptoms
- Orbital pain ± movement
- Lid edema and erythema
- Visual disturbances/loss; diplopia
- Systemic symptoms including malaise, fevers, and chills

Exam Findings
- Unilateral lid &/or periorbital edema and erythema
- Ophthalmoplegia or resistance to ocular motility
- Proptosis, most frequently seen as eye displacement lateral and downward
- Afferent pupillary defect signifying involvement of optic nerve
- Papilledema secondary to increase in intraocular pressure
- Violaceous eyelids (may or may not be present)

DIFFERENTIAL DIAGNOSIS

Preseptal (Periorbital) Cellulitis
- Infection of soft tissues **anterior** to orbital septum of frontal bone

Mucormycosis
- Opportunistic infection caused by fungi of the order Mucorales (high risk in patients with diabetes or acidosis)

Cavernous Sinus Thrombosis
- Thrombosis in the cavernous sinus formed secondary to facial infection

Viral Infection
- Infection of the ocular region with *herpesvirdae* virus (i.e., herpes simplex, herpes zoster ophthalmicus)

Ocular Tumors
- Lymphoproliferative, neuroblastoma, and rhabdomyosarcoma

EVALUATION/WORK-UP

Labs
- Complete blood count with differential (for leukocytosis)
- Blood culture (if positive, can be helpful for narrowing antibiotics)
- Erythrocyte sedimentation rate (ESR) and C-reactive protein (CRP) for baseline analysis and response tracking
- Consider lumbar puncture if meningitic signs present or suspicion for intracranial involvement

Imaging
- Orbital and sinus CT or MRI with contrast: Often shows diffuse edema and infiltrate of orbital soft tissues
  - May show opacification of sinuses or intraorbital abscess

TREATMENT

Medical
- If orbital cellulitis is suspected, patient should be admitted to hospital for prompt treatment with IV antibiotics
  - Obtain ophthalmology and otolaryngology consult
- Broad-spectrum antibiotics, narrow if organisms are identified on blood culture or for known pathogenesis
  - Ampicillin/sulbactam
  - **Or** piperacillin/tazobactam
  - **Or** vancomycin **and** 3rd generation cephalosporin (i.e., ceftriaxone, cefotaxime) if concerned for methicillin-resistant *S. aureus* (MRSA)
  - **Or** clindamycin if concerned for MRSA
  - If signs of intracranial involvement, treatment should cover anaerobes
  - IV antibiotics may be transitioned to oral therapy as patient begins to show signs of clinical improvement (i.e., afebrile for 4 or more days) for a total treatment course of 21 days

Surgical
- If unresponsive to medical treatment or worsening of symptoms, consider sinus &/or abscess drainage
  - Depending on location, can be performed endoscopically; otherwise, open procedure is required
  - Consider biopsy if suspicious for alternative etiology

Prognosis
- If treatment is not delayed, prognosis is excellent

SELECTED REFERENCES

1. Papier A et al: Differential diagnosis of the swollen red eyelid. Am Fam Physician. 76(12):1815-24, 2007

ORBITAL INFLAMMATORY PSEUDOTUMOR

Key Facts

Introduction
- Also known as idiopathic orbital inflammation, nonspecific orbital inflammation, and orbital inflammatory syndrome
- Localized or diffuse benign, noninfectious idiopathic swelling of any or all orbital soft tissue

Demographics
- Idiopathic nature but has been associated with immune processes and infections
- Most common cause of painful orbital swelling in adults

Presentation
- Sudden, painful onset of swelling, erythema, and proptosis; typically unilateral
- In severe cases, there may be extraocular muscle restriction and loss in visual acuity, color, and contrast sensitivity

Differential Diagnosis
- Thyroid eye disease, lymphoma, orbital cellulitis, sarcoidosis

Evaluation/Work-Up
- Diagnosis of exclusion, complete systemic work-up is recommended
- Classic histopathologic characteristics: Cellular polymorphism, lymphoid follicles with granulomas, lack of atypia, ancillary evidence of inflammation

Treatment
- Steroids are the mainstay of treatment and aid in diagnosis
- Radiation can be used in elderly patients or steroid nonresponder
- Surgical resection of focal lesions that are refractory to medical treatment can be effective
- Highly variable outcome depending on subtype

__(Left)__ This external photograph demonstrates proptosis, which is a common finding in orbital inflammatory pseudotumor. __(Right)__ Coronal T1WI C+ FS MRI demonstrates extensive orbital inflammation with ill-defined enlargement and enhancement of the rectus muscles ➔, extraconal infiltration extending to the lacrimal gland ➔, and intraconal enhancement partially surrounding the optic nerve ➔.

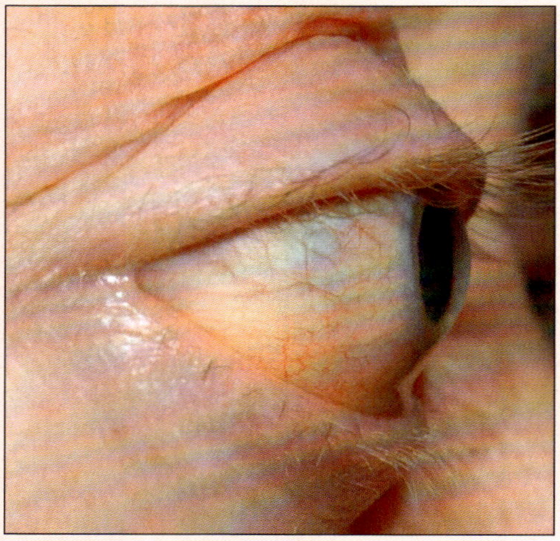

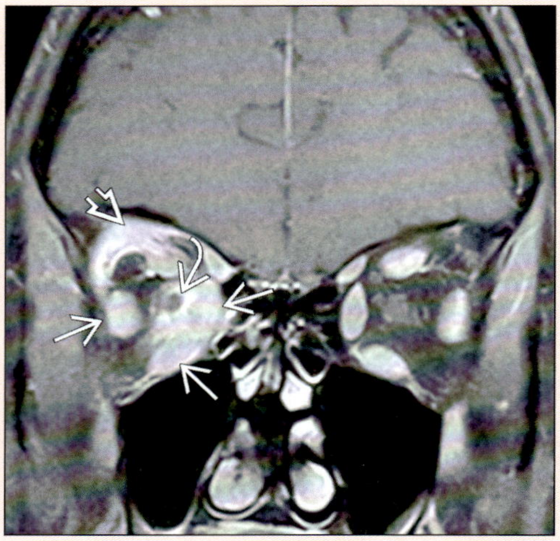

__(Left)__ Axial CECT in a patient with acute-onset orbital pseudotumor shows bilateral marked enlargement and enhancement of the lacrimal glands ➔. __(Right)__ Micropathology in the same patient shows a mixed inflammatory cell infiltrate with little fibrosis. Lacrimal glandular elements ➔ are visible.

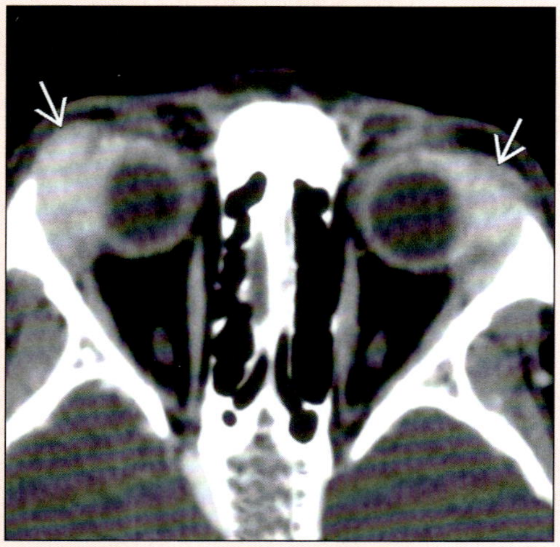

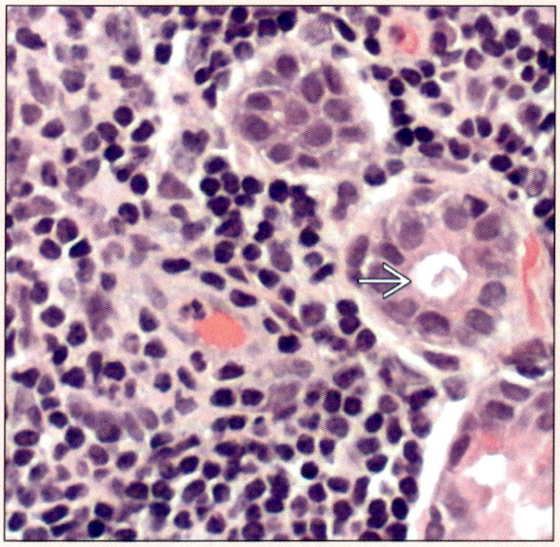

ORBITAL INFLAMMATORY PSEUDOTUMOR

INTRODUCTION

Synonyms

- Idiopathic orbital inflammation, nonspecific orbital inflammation, orbital inflammatory syndrome

Definitions

- Localized or diffuse benign, noninfectious idiopathic swelling of extraocular contents and adnexa affecting muscles, lacrimal gland, optic nerve, and orbital fat
- Related condition is ophthalmoplegia + cavernous sinus inflammation (Tolosa-Hunt syndrome)
  - Both are responsive to steroids

Subtypes

- Granulomatous
  - Rare, noncaseating granulomas with histiocytic infiltrate and giant cells on histology
- Vasculitic
  - Swelling of endothelial cells, white cells destroy muscularis and elastic lamina of arteries
- Sclerosing
  - Associated with IgG4 inflammation; may be end stage of the disease process
    - Dearth of inflammatory infiltrate; abundant fibrosis
- Eosinophilic
  - Comprise 50% of cases in children, eosinophils form cuffs around small vessels and invade

DEMOGRAPHICS

Etiology/Risk Factors

- Idiopathic but has been associated with immune processes and infections

Epidemiology

- Most common cause of painful orbital edema in adults

PRESENTATION

Symptoms

- Sudden, painful onset of swelling, erythema, and proptosis
  - Typically unilateral
- Can progress to ophthalmoplegia with subsequent diplopia and vision loss from optic neuropathy

Exam Findings

- Conjunctival injection and chemosis may be present
- In severe cases, there may be motility restriction and loss in vision, color, and contrast sensitivity

DIFFERENTIAL DIAGNOSIS

Thyroid Eye Disease

- Typical bilateral presentation; may have thyroid dysfunction

Lymphoma

- Gradual, painless course (often with mass lesion)

Orbital Cellulitis

- Occurs with fever and leukocytosis (often there is sinusitis or orbital abscess)

Sarcoidosis

- Systemic involvement, particularly shortness of breath and hilar lymphadenopathy

EVALUATION/WORK-UP

Labs

- Complete systemic work-up is recommended due to possibility of systemic rheumatologic involvement

Pathology

- Biopsy is indicated only in the following situations
  - Acute lesion that does not respond to medical treatment, atypical or recurrent presentation, bilateral presentation in adults, positive history of cancer
- Malignancy process must be excluded
  - Immunohistochemical staining may be necessary
- Classic histopathologic characteristics
  - Cellular polymorphism, lymphoid follicles with granulomas, lack of atypia, inflammation

Imaging

- Radiographic findings are highly variable
- Magnetic resonance imaging with fat suppression is the preferred method for diagnosis
- CT is useful in differentiating bony structures, air, and fat and delineating the mass or infiltrate
- Ultrasound will show a reduced signal from the mass

TREATMENT

Medical

- Observation in cases that are not worsening (can sometimes resolve on their own)
- NSAIDs can be used in mild cases
- Steroids are the mainstay and can aid in diagnosis
- Radiation is option in elderly patients or patients who do not respond to steroids
- Immunosuppressants
  - Methotrexate, cyclophosphamide, mycophenolate mofetil
- Inflammatory modulators
  - Infliximab, etanercept

Surgical

- Surgical resection of focal lesions that are refractory to medical treatment can be effective

Prognosis

- Highly variable depending on subtype although the majority of patients do improve

SELECTED REFERENCES

1. Berry-Brincat A et al: Idiopathic orbital inflammation: a new dimension with the discovery of immunoglobulin G4-related disease. Curr Opin Ophthalmol. 23(5):415-9, 2012
2. Jacobs D et al: Diagnosis and management of orbital pseudotumor. Curr Opin Ophthalmol. 13(6):347-51, 2002
3. Mombaerts I et al: What is orbital pseudotumor? Surv Ophthalmol. 41(1):66-78, 1996

THYROID EYE DISEASE

Key Facts

Introduction
- Autoimmune inflammatory disease that causes upper eyelid retraction, proptosis, and conjunctivitis due to swelling of extraocular muscles and fat in association with hyperthyroidism

Demographics
- Women: 16 per 100,000
- Men: 3 per 100,000
- Smoking: Major risk factor in patients with Graves disease; 4x increased risk of thyroid eye disease
- Occurs in 25-50% of Graves disease patients

Presentation
- Pain
- Photophobia
- Diplopia
- Systemic symptoms of hyperthyroidism
- Proptosis
- Eyelid retraction
- Dry eye syndrome
- Impaired eye movement
- Afferent pupillary defect

Evaluation/Work-Up
- TSH, T3/T4
- Thyroid autoantibody panel
- Orbital CT or MRI

Treatment
- Comanagement with endocrinologist to achieve euthyroid state
- Steroid, orbital irradiation, symptom managements with lubricating drops
- Surgery: Orbital decompression, strabismus surgery, eyelid surgery

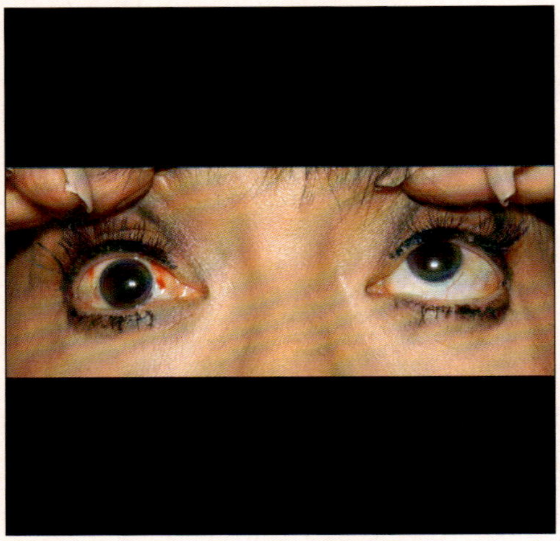
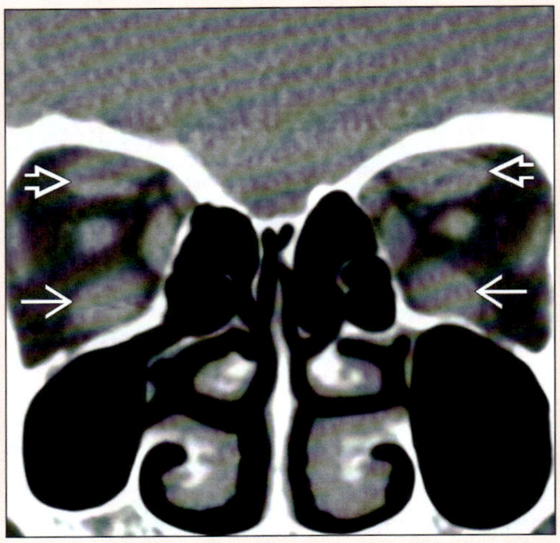

(Left) *This patient is attempting to gaze upward. Due to restrictive thyroid myopathy, she is unable to elevate the right eye.* ***(Right)*** *Coronal NECT in a patient with Graves disease with thyroid-associated ophthalmopathy shows inferior and superior recti, uniformly enlarged bilaterally.*

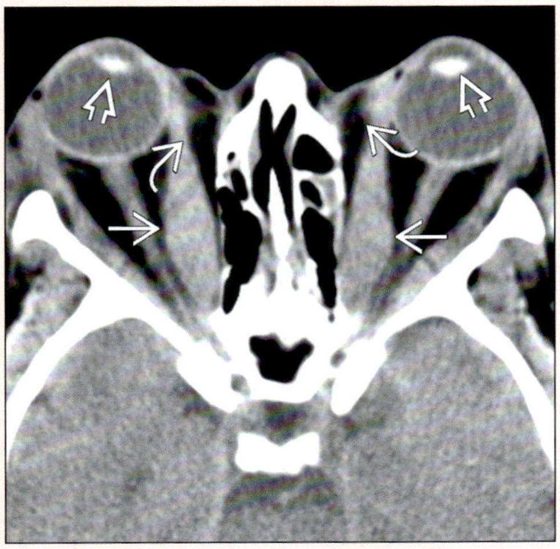
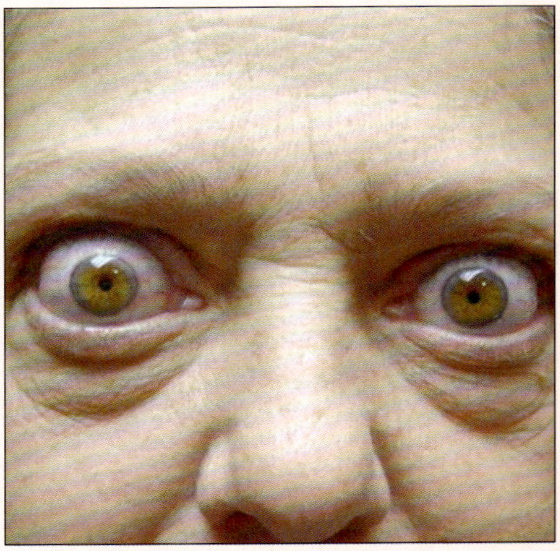

(Left) *Axial contrast-enhanced CT shows marked thickening of the medial rectus bellies, with relative sparing of the tendinous insertions. The disconjugate orientation of the lenses is evidence of impaired muscle movement.* ***(Right)*** *Clinical photograph shows Graves exophthalmos. Note the remarkable proptosis and retraction of the eyelids (lid lag). This is a very characteristic stare of patients with an infiltrative pathology of the extraocular muscles. (Courtesy K. B. Krantz, MD.)*

THYROID EYE DISEASE

INTRODUCTION

Abbreviations
- Thyroid eye disease (TED)

Synonyms
- Graves ophthalmopathy (GO)

Definitions
- Autoimmune inflammatory disease that causes upper eyelid retraction, proptosis, and conjunctivitis due to swelling of extraocular muscles and fat in association with hyperthyroidism
  - Swelling is caused by accumulation of glycosaminoglycans in orbital muscles and increase in orbital fat
  - Accompanied by fibroblast proliferation
  - May be the 1st symptom of hyperthyroidism

DEMOGRAPHICS

Etiology/Risk Factors
- Etiology
  - T cells induce B cells to produce IgG antibodies against TSH receptor: Type II hypersensitivity reaction
  - Causes stimulation of thyroid gland
  - Infiltrative ophthalmopathy is due to fat and glycosaminoglycan deposits in extraocular muscles and orbit
- Risk factors
  - Smoking: Major risk factor in patients with Graves disease; 4x increased risk of TED
  - Women: 5x more likely
  - Genetic predisposition

Epidemiology
- Women: 16 per 100,000
- Men: 3 per 100,000
- Occurs in 25-50% of Graves disease patients but can occur in those with hypothyroidism or euthyroidism

PRESENTATION

Symptoms
- Pain, pressure behind eyes, diplopia, photophobia
- Systemic symptoms of hyperthyroidism
  - Heat/cold intolerance, rapid heart rate, weight loss, anxiety, tremor

Exam Findings
- Proptosis, eyelid retraction (scleral show), chemosis, corneal dryness, afferent pupillary defect, optic nerve pallor
- Decreased vision, decreased color vision
- Diplopia: Muscle enlargement most likely in inferior > medial > superior > lateral rectus

DIFFERENTIAL DIAGNOSIS

Orbital Tumors
- Melanoma, lymphoma, leukemia, metastasis, rhabdomyosarcoma

Myasthenia Gravis & Lambert-Eaton Myasthenic Syndrome
- Diplopia may be present

Allergic Conjunctivitis
- May have swollen eyelids that appear proptotic

Orbital Cellulitis
- Frequently causes swelling of eyelid and periorbital area

EVALUATION/WORK-UP

Labs
- TSH, T3/T4, thyroid autoantibody panel

Pathology
- Infiltrate of glycosaminoglycans and fat into orbit
- Can see fibroblast proliferation

Imaging
- Orbital CT/MRI shows muscle enlargement with tendon sparing (unlike orbital pseudotumor)

TREATMENT

Medical
- Comanage thyroid with endocrinology
- Steroid: Pulse therapy with IV steroids shown to be more effective than oral steroids
- Orbital irradiation
- Lubrication with protective eyewear and artificial tears
- Encourage smoking cessation

Surgical
- Surgical decompression
- Strabismus surgery to relieve diplopia
- Eyelid surgery
- Sequence surgery if multiple procedures required: Decompress first, then muscle surgery, and eyelid surgery last

Follow-Up
- Continue comanagement with endocrinologist to achieve euthyroid state
- Frequent exams to monitor for sight-threatening conditions, such as optic neuropathy or corneal ulceration

Prognosis
- Initial phase of TED lasts a few months and reaches a peak in severity
- Symptoms then gradually begin to improve over a longer period of time

SELECTED REFERENCES

1. Perros P et al: Thyroid eye disease. BMJ. 338:b560, 2009
2. Garrity JA et al: Pathogenesis of graves ophthalmopathy: implications for prediction, prevention, and treatment. Am J Ophthalmol. 142(1):147-153, 2006
3. Cawood T et al: Recent developments in thyroid eye disease. BMJ. 329(7462):385-90, 2004

ORBITAL FOREIGN BODY

Key Facts

Introduction
- Orbital foreign body is defined as material that penetrates the orbit but remains outside the globe

Demographics
- Incidence is highest in males between ages 10 and 30 years

Presentation
- Patients may be asymptomatic or present with changes in vision such as
  - Decreased visual acuity, diplopia

Differential Diagnosis
- Orbital cellulitis
- Intraocular foreign body
- Orbital granuloma

Evaluation/Work-Up
- 1st imaging study should always be CT or x-ray
  - Orbital CT scan is gold standard
- MRI is indicated if suspected particle is wood or other organic material; avoid if metallic

Treatment
- Broad-spectrum antibiotics are recommended to prevent secondary infection
- Patients who are not current on tetanus vaccination should be immunized
- Early evaluation and intervention is key to prevent vision compromise
- Surgical removal of orbital foreign bodies is dependent on location, nature, and material of the particle
- Surgery is indicated for all organic materials and anteriorly accessible foreign bodies
  - Nonorganic foreign bodies that are not easily accessible can usually be left in place

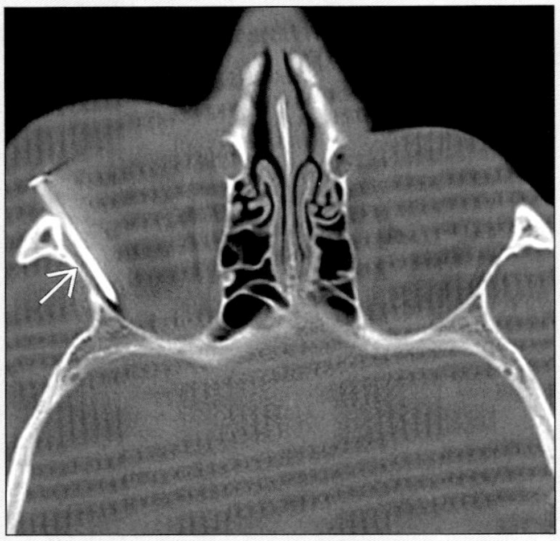
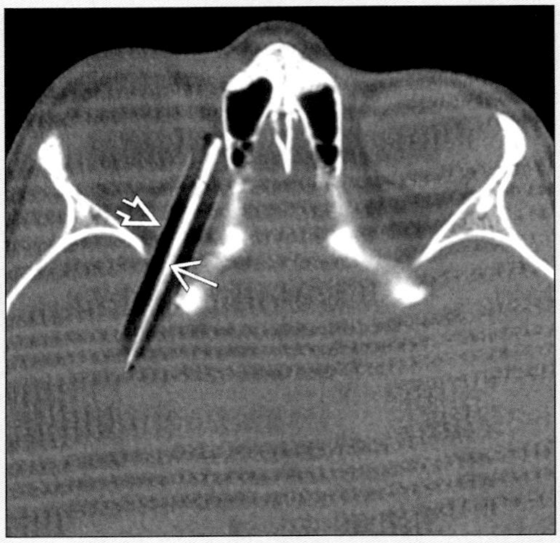

(Left) *Axial bone CT in a patient who had been using a nail gun demonstrates a foreign body ➔ (nail) within the extraconal fat of the right orbit. Fortunately, the patient's globe was not ruptured in this case.* ***(Right)*** *Axial bone CT shows a piece of a broken pencil within the right orbit. The center dense core represents the pencil "lead" ➔ and the outer casing of wood is low density ➔.*

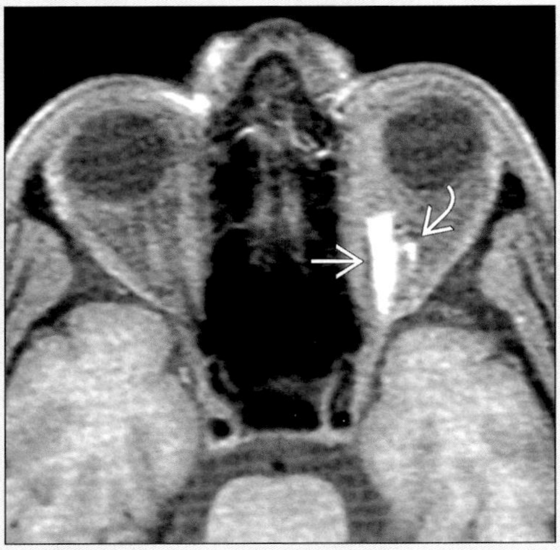
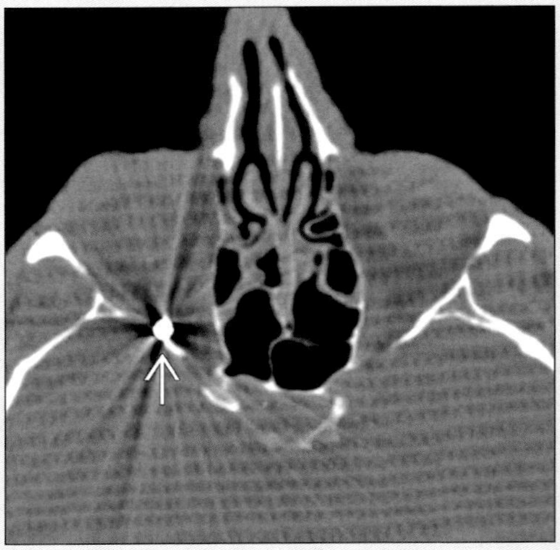

(Left) *This Axial T1 C+ FS MRI shows a retained orbital foreign body (OFB). The patient presented with a foreign body granuloma. The granuloma ➔ shows increased T1 signal and is medial to the optic nerve ➔. The OFB was determined to be organic plant material from a hiking injury 2 years prior.* ***(Right)*** *Axial bone CT confirms the location of 1 foreign body lateral to the right orbital apex ➔. The posterior position of object is a relative contraindication to surgical removal. Note the metallic streak artifact.*

ORBITAL FOREIGN BODY

INTRODUCTION

Abbreviations
- Orbital foreign body (OFB)

Definitions
- Material that penetrates the orbit but remains outside globe

DEMOGRAPHICS

Etiology/Risk Factors
- Incidence of penetrating injuries resulting in OFB is highest in males between ages 10 and 30 years

PRESENTATION

Symptoms
- Patients may be asymptomatic or present with changes in vision such as
  - Decreased visual acuity, diplopia
- Pain, redness, and swelling are also common, depending on nature of trauma

Exam Findings
- Some OFBs may be easily visualized protruding from orbit
  - Surgical removal of the foreign body is preferred over in-office removal
  - It is always important to image foreign bodies to rule out fragmentation within orbit

DIFFERENTIAL DIAGNOSIS

Orbital Cellulitis
- Possible complication of OFB and should be considered when patients present with fever, purulence, decreased ocular motion, and diplopia

Intraocular Foreign Body
- Differs from OFB in that foreign body penetrates globe
- Surgical emergency and must be treated promptly to best preserve vision in affected eye

Orbital Granuloma
- Granuloma formation can occur months to years after introduction of organic material (such as wood) into orbit
- To decrease the chances of granuloma formation, MRI should be used if wood or other organic material causes initial injury

EVALUATION/WORK-UP

Imaging
- 1st imaging study should always be CT or x-ray as these are nonmagnetic and will not disrupt positioning of metallic foreign bodies
  - Orbital CT scan is gold standard to determine exact location, consequential injury to surrounding tissue, and material of the particle
    - Axial and coronal scans of 1-1.5 mm of tissues ideal for detection of small particles
- MRI is indicated for full investigation if suspected particle is wood
  - MRI contraindicated if suspected particle is metallic
- Orbital ultrasonography can also be employed as an adjunct to CT when trying to identify wood in orbit

TREATMENT

Medical
- Broad-spectrum antibiotics are recommended to prevent secondary infection
- Patients who have not received a tetanus vaccination or booster in the past 10 years should be given one during initial evaluation
  - In cases where the wound is visibly contaminated with dirt and debris, consider a dose of tetanus immunoglobulin

Surgical
- Surgical removal of orbital foreign bodies is dependent on location, nature, and material of particle
  - Surgery is indicated for all organic materials and anteriorly accessible foreign bodies and in cases of
    - Large particle with sharp edges
    - Signs of inflammation, infection, or abscess
    - Evidence of optic nerve compression
    - Restricted ocular mobility
  - Certain materials are more important to remove than others
    - Materials that are better tolerated if left in orbit include inorganic materials such as
      - Glass, rock, and some metals
    - Materials that can be immunogenic and should be removed include
      - Copper, nickel, and organic materials

Follow-Up
- Whether the foreign body is retained or surgically removed, patients should return for any changes in vision or increased pain

Prognosis
- Depends upon the nature of penetration and management
- Surgery is ideal treatment for OFB, but in the case of foreign bodies that are not easily accessible, often they can be left in place
  - Complications of retained foreign bodies can include
    - Globe rupture, optic neuropathy, intraocular infection, and loss of vision

SELECTED REFERENCES

1. Al-Mujaini A et al: Intraorbital foreign body: clinical presentation, radiological appearance and management. Sultan Qaboos Univ Med J. 8(1):69-74, 2008
2. Fulcher TP et al: Clinical features and management of intraorbital foreign bodies. Ophthalmology. 109(3):494-500, 2002
3. Finkelstein M et al: Projectile metallic foreign bodies in the orbit: a retrospective study of epidemiologic factors, management, and outcomes. Ophthalmology. 104(1):96-103, 1997

ORBITAL BLOWOUT FRACTURE

Key Facts

Introduction
- "Pure" blowout fracture is an internal fracture (does not involve orbital rim or surrounding bones)

Demographics
- Motor vehicle accidents (MVA), blunt trauma, sports-related injury, and falls
- Force of blow to orbit is dissipated to surrounding bony structures (hydraulic vs. buckling mechanism)
- Orbit floor &/or medial orbital wall are structures most commonly involved
- More common in young adults and men

Presentation
- Pain &/or restriction with extraocular movements (especially with upward gaze)
- Loss of sensation over superior cheek
- Eyelid swelling
- Warrants a full ophthalmic examination including thorough slit-lamp and fundus examination

Differential Diagnosis
- Periorbital hematoma
- Cranial nerve palsy
- Skull fracture

Evaluation/Work-Up
- CT of orbit is preferred imaging modality

Treatment
- Most fractures heal without surgical intervention
- For surgical intervention (merited if diplopia, entrapment, or enophthalmos)
  - Transconjunctival or subciliary approach or
  - Endoscopic repair via endonasal or transmaxillary approach
  - Waiting till edema subsides

*(**Left**) This coronal bone CT demonstrates a mildly depressed left orbital floor blowout fracture ➔ just medial to the infraorbital canal ➔. The inferior rectus muscle ➔ is grossly normal in position and configuration. (**Right**) This coronal CT reveals a chronic right orbital floor fracture with herniation of a small volume of fat ➔ and a portion of the inferior rectus muscle ➔ through the fracture defect. The muscle also demonstrates an abnormal vertical orientation.*

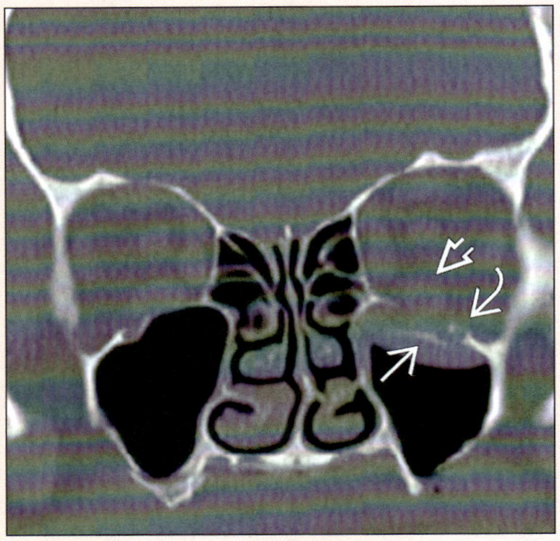

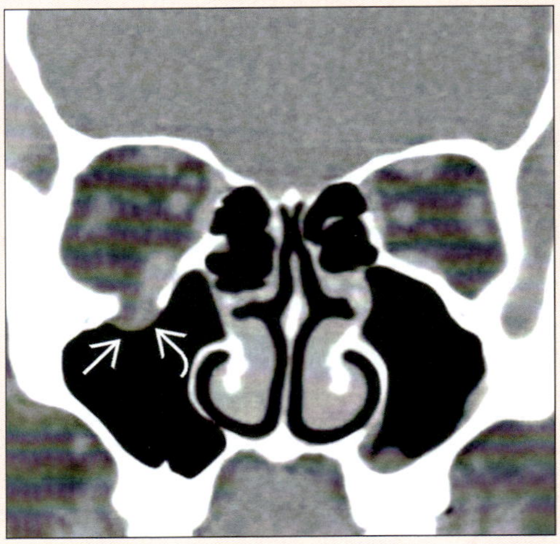

*(**Left**) This axial bone CT reveals a large medial wall fracture ➔. The medial rectus muscle ➔ can be seen herniating through the bony defect. The medial wall is the thinnest wall of the orbit. (**Right**) 3D reformation demonstrates the classic features of a zygomatic fracture. Fractures involve the walls of the left maxillary sinus ➔, the left zygomatic arch ➔, and the lateral orbital wall ➔. This patient also sustained trauma to the nasal dorsum ➔. The lateral wall of the orbit is the least frequent fracture of the orbit.*

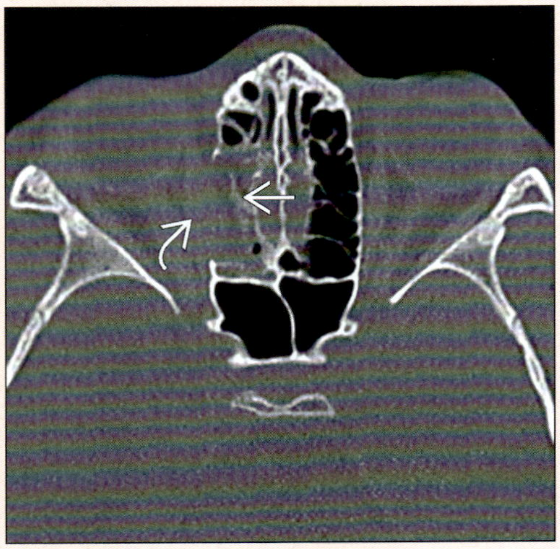

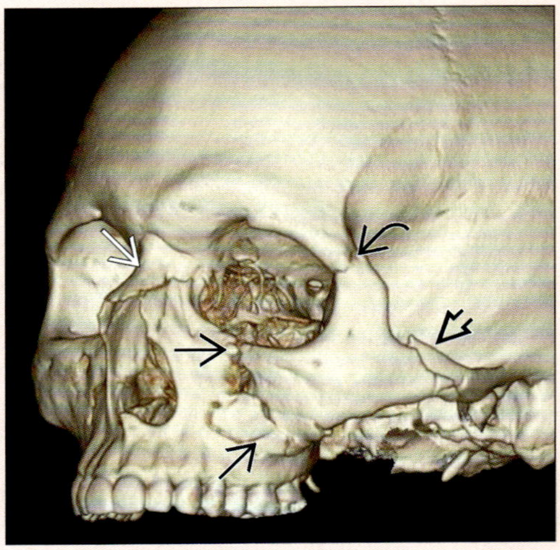

ORBITAL BLOWOUT FRACTURE

INTRODUCTION

Definitions

- Orbit is composed of frontal, zygomatic, maxilla, lacrimal, ethmoid, palatine, and sphenoid bones
- "Pure" blowout fracture does not involve orbital rim or other bones besides floor of orbit (internal fractures)

DEMOGRAPHICS

Etiology/Risk Factors

- Motor vehicle accidents (MVA), blunt trauma, sports-related injury, and falls
  - Some reports suggest MVA to be most common etiology
- Force of blow to orbit is dissipated to surrounding bony structures
  - Hydraulic mechanism: Retropulsion and compression of orbital contents leads to increased intraocular pressure and subsequent fracturing of bones
  - Buckling mechanism: Direct trauma to orbital rim causes fracturing of bones
- Orbit floor &/or medial orbital wall are structures most commonly involved
- Associated intracranial and intraocular injury is common (i.e., retroorbital and vitreous hemorrhage, ruptured globe, etc.)

Epidemiology

- More common in young adult males

PRESENTATION

Symptoms

- Pain &/or restriction with extraocular movements (especially with upward gaze)
- Eyelid swelling
- Loss of sensation over superior cheek (CNV2 distribution)
- Binocular diplopia
- Subconjunctival hemorrhage
- Periorbital ecchymosis
- May be asymptomatic depending on etiology

Exam Findings

- Warrants a full ophthalmic examination including thorough slit-lamp and fundus examination
- Hess test to evaluate for diplopia

DIFFERENTIAL DIAGNOSIS

Periorbital Hematoma

- Collection of blood or bruising surrounding the eye ("black eye")

Cranial Nerve Palsy

- Loss of function or dysfunction of nerve

Skull Fracture

- Any break of a cranial bone (skull)

EVALUATION/WORK-UP

Imaging

- CT is preferred imaging modality given most surgeons order preoperative CTs
  - Coronal CT of orbit
  - High-resolution axial CT of orbit
- MRI does not provide adequate information of bony structures of orbit
- Transantral exploration of orbit floor
- May initially be clinical diagnosis

TREATMENT

Medical

- Most fractures heal without surgical intervention
- Icing of affected area for 1st 48 hours following fracture
- Consider steroids, broad-spectrum antibiotics, nasal decongestants
- Avoidance of blowing of nose
- Avoidance of anticoagulation

Surgical

- If the following are present, surgery is indicated
  - Double vision on primary or downward gaze not improving over 2 weeks
    - Seen secondary to entrapment of extraocular muscles
  - Enophthalmos > 2 mm
    - Typically corresponds to a fracture > 50% of orbital floor
- Consider orbital floor exploration depending on extent of injury
- Immediate surgery is typically not needed (typically performed within 14 days but can be delayed up to 6 weeks)
- Transconjunctival or subciliary approach
  - Elevation of periosteum to expose orbital floor
  - Removal of affected orbital contents
  - Repair of floor by synthetic materials including Supramid, Teflon, or porous polyethylene to overlap defect
  - Suturing of periosteum and incision
  - Complications included hematoma, ectropion, entropion, conjunctival granuloma
- Endoscopic repair via endonasal or transmaxillary approach

Follow-Up

- Depends on extent of injury and interventions performed

Prognosis

- If evaluated and treated properly, prognosis tends to be favorable with relatively few postoperative complications

SELECTED REFERENCES

1. Chang EL et al: Update on orbital trauma. Curr Opin Ophthalmol. 15(5):411-5, 2004
2. Brady SM et al: The diagnosis and management of orbital blowout fractures: update 2001. Am J Emerg Med. 19(2):147-54, 2001

RETROBULBAR HEMORRHAGE

Key Facts

Introduction
- Hemorrhagic space-occupying lesion in the orbit with potential for compartment syndrome, potentially leading to optic neuropathy if untreated

Demographics
- Numerous causes including spontaneous (orbital lymphangiomas, arteriovenous malformations, or orbital varices), post-traumatic, postanesthesia (retrobulbar, peribulbar), postsurgical
- Majority of cases occur within hours of surgery

Presentation
- Pain, pressure, proptosis, and vision loss in affected eye are most common symptoms
- Relative afferent pupillary defect is most common abnormality of the pupil
- Eyelid ecchymosis or hematoma is most common presenting sign postoperatively

Evaluation/Work-Up
- CBC, PT/INR, PTT, and factor Xa assay can help provide information on coagulation status of an individual

Treatment
- Aimed toward reducing intraorbital and intraocular pressure and protecting optic nerve from damage
- If vision loss is present or IOP is very high, surgical intervention should be emergently performed
- Most common initial surgical treatment is lateral canthotomy and cantholysis
- Vision should improve within a short period of time after surgical intervention
  - If vision and IOP do not immediately improve, then further orbital decompression should be considered

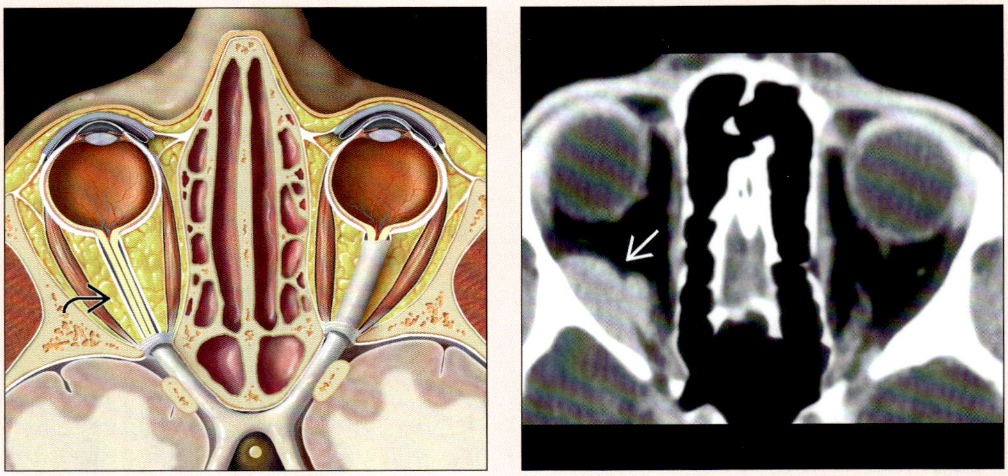

(Left) *Graphic representation shows the potential retrobulbar space ↷. Retrobulbar hemorrhages increase in size in the restricted intraorbital space, leading to compartment syndrome that may lead to irreversible damage to the optic nerve.* ***(Right)*** *Axial CT was taken of a patient holding his breath in Valsalva maneuver and shows distention of a large extraconal varix posteriorly and laterally in the right orbit ➡. The right globe is slightly proptotic. Varices such as these can lead to spontaneous retrobulbar hemorrhage.*

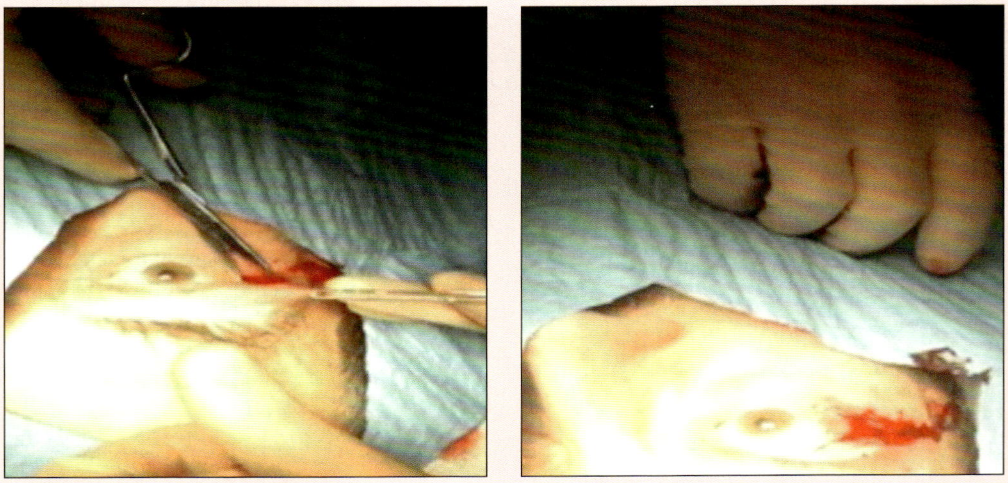

(Left) *External photo shows a patient undergoing lateral canthotomy and cantholysis. This procedure may be necessary in patients with retrobulbar hemorrhages with increased intraocular pressures and vision changes.* ***(Right)*** *External photo shows a patient after lateral canthotomy and cantholysis. Note the patient's ability to adduct his eye after release of the tendon.*

RETROBULBAR HEMORRHAGE

INTRODUCTION

Definitions

- Hemorrhagic space-occupying lesion in the orbit with potential for compartment syndrome and eventual optic neuropathy
  - Retrobulbar hemorrhage occurs posterior to orbital septum, while a preseptal hemorrhage would be confined to area anterior to orbital septum
  - Considered a medical emergency

DEMOGRAPHICS

Etiology/Risk Factors

- Numerous causes including
  - Spontaneous (orbital lymphangiomas, arteriovenous malformations, or orbital varices)
  - Post-traumatic
  - Postanesthesia (retrobulbar, peribulbar)
  - Postsurgical (such as with blepharoplasty)
- Risk factors include
  - Hypertension
  - Anticoagulant medication
  - Valsalva maneuvers
  - Vascular diseases
  - Coagulopathies
- Majority of cases occur within hours of surgery

PRESENTATION

Symptoms

- Pain, pressure, and vision loss in affected eye are most common symptoms
  - Pain is typically severe and described as lancinating in quality
  - Vision loss may include
    - Visual flashes
    - Hemianopsia
    - Amaurosis fugax
- May also complain of diplopia, nausea, and vomiting

Exam Findings

- Proptosis (possibly expanding), ophthalmoplegia, increased intraocular pressure, loss of pupillary reflexes, or pallor of optic disc or retina
- Relative afferent pupillary defect is the most common abnormality of the pupil
- Eyelid ecchymosis or hematoma is the most common presenting sign postoperatively
- Decreased vision &/or color vision

EVALUATION/WORK-UP

Labs

- CBC, PT/INR, PTT, and factor Xa assay can help provide information on coagulation status of an individual

Imaging

- Given the urgent nature of retrobulbar hemorrhage, imaging is not always necessary
- In cases of spontaneous retrobulbar hemorrhage, imaging can aid in diagnosing underlying pathology
  - Orbital CT scan without contrast is the preferred imaging choice given its ability to quickly detect hemorrhage

TREATMENT

Medical

- Small retrobulbar hemorrhages without significant IOP spike or evidence of optic nerve damage may be observed closely
- Medical therapy is aimed at reducing intraorbital and intraocular pressure and protecting optic nerve from damage
- Supplemental oxygen therapy, IV mannitol, IV acetazolamide, IV methylprednisolone, and topical β-blockers may be used to reduce ischemia, lower intraocular pressure, and reduce inflammation
  - Medical intervention is only sufficient in mild cases of retrobulbar hemorrhage without any signs of vision loss or significant IOP spike

Surgical

- If any signs of vision loss or orbital compartment syndrome are present, then surgical intervention is necessary immediately
  - Frequently the case with postseptal hemorrhages
- Treatment depends on the nature of the inciting event, but the overall aim is to reduce intraorbital pressure
- Lateral canthotomy with inferior cantholysis relieves orbital compression better than lateral canthotomy alone
  - Superior cantholysis can be used to further decrease intraorbital pressure if above procedure is insufficient
- Orbital exploration, drainage, and cautery of bleeding vessels may be necessary

Follow-Up

- Vision should be improved within a short period of time after surgical intervention
  - If patient does not notice any improved vision, then further orbital decompression should be considered

Prognosis

- Central retinal artery occlusion > 105 minutes results in irreversible optic nerve damage
  - Occlusion > 240 minutes results in complete optic nerve atrophy

SELECTED REFERENCES

1. Jamal BT et al: Orbital hemorrhage and compressive optic neuropathy in patients with midfacial fractures receiving low-molecular weight heparin therapy. J Oral Maxillofac Surg. 67(7):1416-9, 2009
2. Hass AN et al: Incidence of postblepharoplasty orbital hemorrhage and associated visual loss. Ophthal Plast Reconstr Surg. 20(6):426-32, 2004
3. Sullivan TJ et al: Non-traumatic orbital haemorrhage. Clin Experiment Ophthalmol. 28(1):26-31, 2000

DERMOID/EPIDERMOID CYSTS

Key Facts

Introduction
- Embryologic remnants of ectodermal elements that have been sequestered between orbital bones and slowly develop into choristomas
- Anterior lesions: Superficial to orbital septum and present in early childhood
- Deep lesions: Deep to orbital septum and present in young adulthood

Demographics
- Most common noninflammatory orbital mass in children and young adults

Presentation
- Unilateral, painless, slow growth
- Well-circumscribed, smooth mass superior to either the medial or lateral canthus (more common)
- Motility restriction and diplopia
- Proptosis and globe displacement

Differential Diagnosis
- Orbital cellulitis: Most common cause of proptosis in children, more acute and painful onset
- Rhabdomyosarcoma: Acute presentation with rapid growth

Evaluation/Work-Up
- Histopathologic findings: Cyst lined with keratinized stratified squamous epithelium and containing keratin, sebaceous fluid, calcium, and possible skin adnexal elements
- Computed tomography to evaluate deeper lesions, or magnetic resonance imaging used to avoid high radiation doses in children

Treatment
- Surgical excision is desired and definitive treatment

*(**Left**) This coronal graphic depicts a superotemporal dermoid cyst ➔ located adjacent to the frontozygomatic suture of the right orbit ➔. Notice resultant mass effect on the globe, with remodeling of the bony orbit ➔. (**Right**) This external photo demonstrates the appearance of a dermoid cyst located superotemporal to the eye itself.*

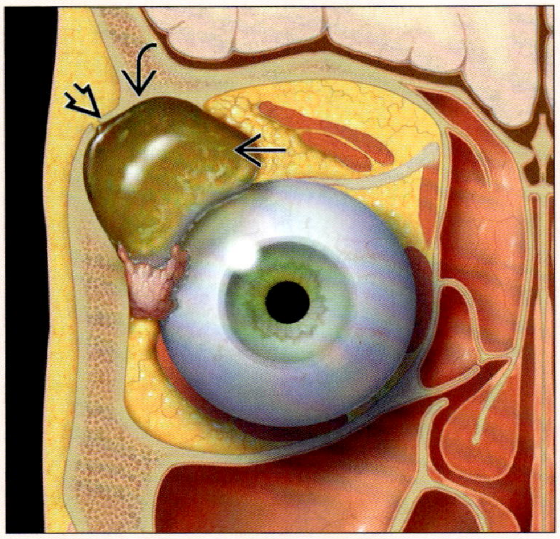

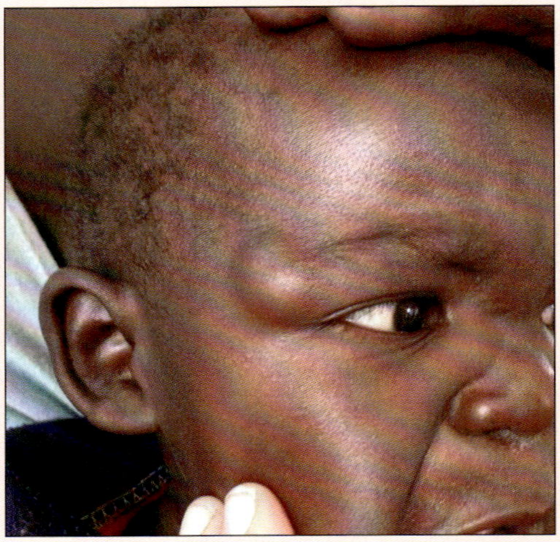

*(**Left**) Gross pathology of an orbital dermoid cyst shows a white-yellow mass with a relatively thick fibrous capsule. During surgery, care was taken not to rupture the cyst, as releasing contents may lead to significant inflammation. (**Right**) Coronal CT demonstrates an ovoid, well-marginated cystic mass in the superotemporal quadrant of the right orbit ➔. Even on bone windows, the lipid density within the mass can be readily appreciated. Smooth remodeling of the adjacent bony orbit is evident ➔.*

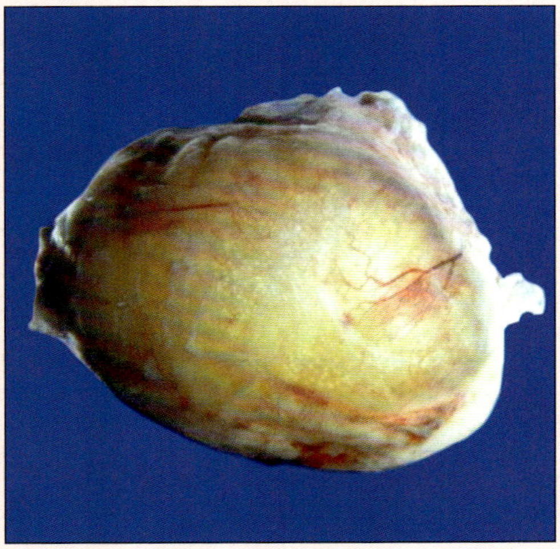

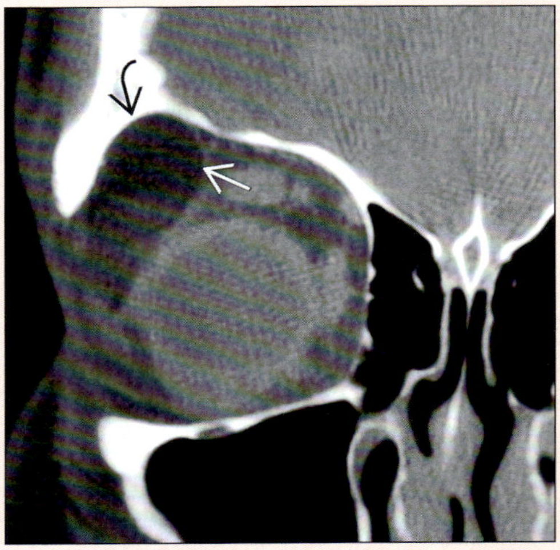

DERMOID/EPIDERMOID CYSTS

INTRODUCTION

Definitions
- Embryologic remnants of ectodermal elements that have been sequestered between orbital bones and slowly develop into choristomas

Subtypes
- Epidermoid cysts: Contain keratin, sebaceous fluid, and calcium
- Dermoid cysts: In addition to elements in epidermoid cysts, contain adnexal structures such as hair and sweat and sebaceous glands
- Anterior lesions: Superficial to orbital septum and present in early childhood
- Deep lesions: Deep to orbital septum and present in young adulthood
- Dumbbell: Bilobed lesion occupying both anterior and posterior orbit

DEMOGRAPHICS

Etiology/Risk Factors
- No known predilection for race or gender

Epidemiology
- Most common noninflammatory orbital mass in children and young adults
- Anterior lesions
  - Typically present in infancy or early childhood
- Posterior lesions
  - Typically present later, in adolescence or early adulthood

PRESENTATION

Symptoms
- Unilateral
- Anterior lesions
  - Painless, slow growth can cause ptosis
  - Well-circumscribed, smooth mass superior to either the medial or lateral canthus (thus superonasal or superotemporal)
  - Limbal dermoids are associated with Goldenhar syndrome
- Posterior lesions
  - Painless progression
  - Motility restriction and diplopia
  - Proptosis and globe displacement
- If dermoid/epidermoid cyst leaks or ruptures, severe inflammation and orbital cellulitis can occur

DIFFERENTIAL DIAGNOSIS

Orbital Cellulitis
- Most common cause of proptosis in children, more acute and painful onset

Plexiform Neurofibroma
- Occurs with neurofibromatosis type 1, S-shaped deformity

Mucocele
- Typically presents in older population, rule out with imaging

Encephalocele
- Associated with developmental, neurological delays, rule out with imaging

Rhabdomyosarcoma
- Acute presentation with rapid growth

EVALUATION/WORK-UP

Pathology
- Histopathologic findings
  - Cyst walls are lined with keratinized stratified squamous epithelium
  - Contents of the cyst can contain any or all of the following
    - Sebaceous fluid
    - Keratin
    - Calcium
    - Cholesterol crystals
    - Skin adnexa (hair and follicles, sebaceous glands, sweat glands)

Imaging
- Fully palpable masses do not need imaging
- Computed tomography to evaluate deeper lesions and rule out mucocele and encephalocele
  - Bony changes are often seen
- Magnetic resonance imaging used to avoid high radiation doses in children

TREATMENT

Surgical
- Surgical excision is desired and definitive treatment
- Anterior lesions
  - Can be approached through eyelid crease
- Posterior lesions
  - Should be approached through orbit
  - Extension intracranially requires collaboration with other surgical specialties for excision

Prognosis
- Cysts that are surgically removed in entirety rarely recur
- There have been rare case reports of squamous cell carcinoma and melanoma arising from dermoid/epidermoid cysts

SELECTED REFERENCES

1. Golden BA et al: Craniofacial and orbital dermoids in children. Oral Maxillofac Surg Clin North Am. 24(3):417-25, 2012
2. Veselinović D et al: Orbital dermoid and epidermoid cysts: case study. Srp Arh Celok Lek. 138(11-12):755-9, 2010
3. Ahuja R et al: Orbital dermoids in children. Semin Ophthalmol. 21(3):207-11, 2006
4. Chawda SJ et al: Computed tomography of orbital dermoids: a 20-year review. Clin Radiol. 54(12):821-5, 1999
5. Forbes G: Radiologic evaluation of orbital tumors. Clin Neurosurg. 32:474-513, 1985

CAPILLARY HEMANGIOMA

Key Facts

Introduction
- Vascular tumor composed of abnormal proliferations of endothelial cells

Demographics
- More common in females and premature infants
- Most common orbital tumor of childhood
- Hypoxia-inducible factor 1-α may contribute

Presentation
- Superficial lesions have a strawberry-like appearance
- Subcutaneous lesions are darker with "bluish" discoloration
- Deeper lesions typically do not correspond with skin changes

Differential Diagnosis
- Nevus flammeus, lymphangioma, encephalocele, rhabdomyosarcoma, neuroblastoma, capillary malformation
- Phacomatoses/neurocutaneous syndromes

Evaluation/Work-Up
- Biopsy is typically not necessary for diagnosis
- Doppler ultrasonography
- Orbital CT or MRI with gadolinium contrast

Treatment
- Typical care involves close monitoring;
  - However, may require further treatment if amblyopia, anisometropia, proptosis, or optic neuropathy are present
- Ongoing ophthalmic examinations to assess for visual development

__(Left)__ Clinical photograph shows a superficial vascular mass involving the medial orbit and nose, with typical violaceous discoloration seen in infantile hemangioma. __(Right)__ Axial CT without contrast demonstrates the most common location for orbital infantile hemangioma, within the superior medial preseptal soft tissues ➔. There is no evidence of postseptal extension.

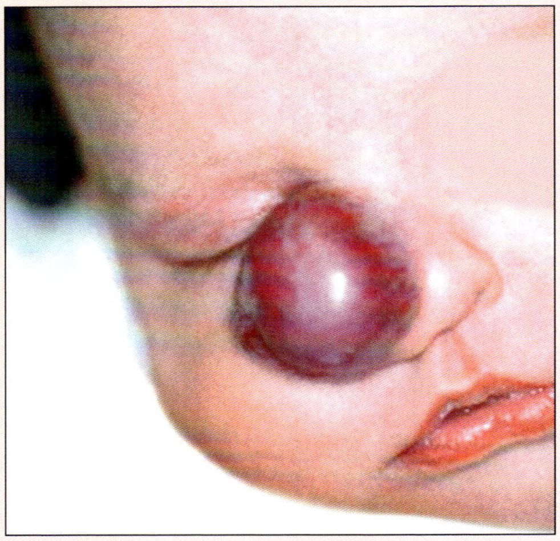

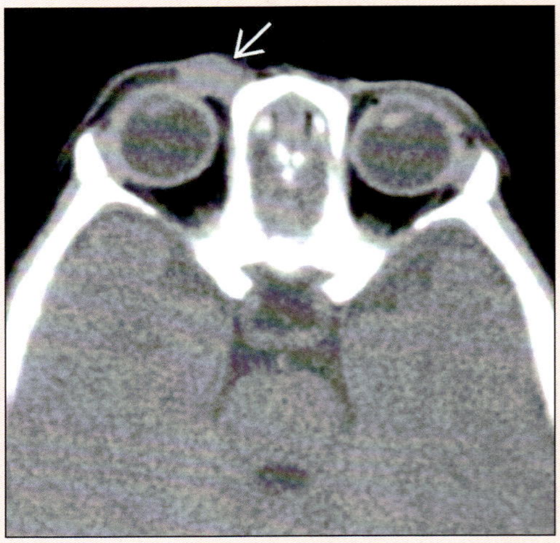

__(Left)__ Axial contrast-enhanced CT demonstrates an intensely enhancing, lobular, primarily retrobulbar hemangioma. The mass is multicompartmental, with intraconal ➔ and extraconal ⇨ components, as well as a small superficial preseptal component laterally ➔. The globe is markedly proptotic. __(Right)__ Clinical photograph shows a raised superficial hemangioma near the inferior orbital rim. Hemangioma is the most common tumor of the orbit and periorbital area in children.

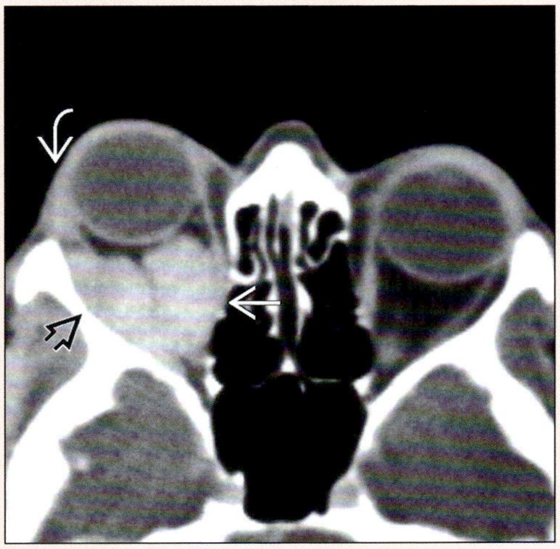

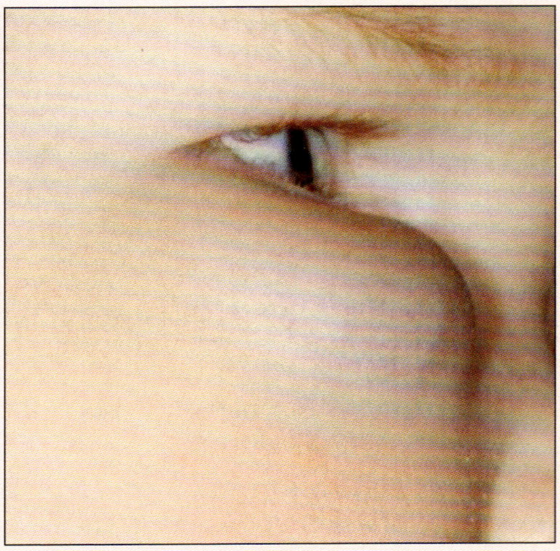

CAPILLARY HEMANGIOMA

INTRODUCTION

Definitions

- Vascular tumor composed of abnormal proliferations of endothelial cells (also known as infantile hemangioma or benign hemangioendothelioma)

Subtypes

- Superficial/cutaneous
- Subcutaneous
- Deep orbit/retrobulbar

DEMOGRAPHICS

Etiology/Risk Factors

- Characterized by 3 stages
  - Nascent phase
  - Proliferative phase (days to ~ 9 months)
  - Involutional phase (5-12 years)
  - Complete involution present in most cases by 7-9 years of age
- Unknown etiology but likely due to defects of angiogenesis with placental origins
  - Evidence of increased placental cells in circulation
  - Hypoxia-inducible factor 1-α may contribute
- More common in females (1.5x) and premature infants

Epidemiology

- Common benign tumor of childhood
  - Seen in 1-2% of infants
- Most common orbital tumor of childhood

PRESENTATION

Symptoms

- 30-50% of neonates will have markings at birth
  - Most infants will manifest markings by 6 months

Exam Findings

- Superficial lesions typically have a strawberry-like appearance
  - Red, raised, nodular, blanching lesion
- Subcutaneous lesions are darker or "bluish"
  - May be palpated as a spongy mass
- Deeper lesions typically do not correspond with superficial skin changes
  - Can cause proptosis and orbital derangement
- On each ophthalmic examination, assess for visual acuity, lid movement, ocular alignment, extraocular movements, and refraction with cycloplegia and track photographs of lesion
  - Mass can cause
    - Astigmatism
    - Ptosis
    - Amblyopia

DIFFERENTIAL DIAGNOSIS

Tumors

- Nevus flammeus, lymphangioma, encephalocele, rhabdomyosarcoma, neuroblastoma, capillary malformation

Phacomatoses/Neurocutaneous Syndromes

- Congenital or hereditary syndromes with characteristic skin and eye lesions (e.g., Sturge-Weber, tuberous sclerosis)

EVALUATION/WORK-UP

Pathology

- Biopsy is typically not necessary for diagnosis
- Proliferative-phase histology demonstrates plump lobules of endothelial cells and mitotic figures
- Involutional-phase histology demonstrates fibrofatty tissue and decreased endothelial lobules

Imaging

- Doppler ultrasonography will show high vessel density and high Doppler shift
- Orbital CT or MRI with gadolinium contrast may be necessary for deeper lesions

TREATMENT

Medical

- Most lesions resolve spontaneously (40% by age 4, 80% by age 8)
- Most common associated ocular complications include amblyopia and anisometropia
  - Amblyopia is thought to occur secondary to occlusion of pupil or visual axis
    - Early amblyopia can be corrected with occlusion of nonaffected eye
    - May further result in strabismus
  - Anisometropia results from induced astigmatism
    - Early anisometropia can be corrected with prescription glasses
  - Typical care involves close monitoring; however, may require further treatment if amblyopia, anisometropia, proptosis, or optic neuropathy are present
    - Topical high-potency steroids have been shown to shrink or stabilize small lesions
    - Intralesional steroids are effective (but can cause depigmentation in dark patients)
      - 1-2 mL of triamcinolone acetonide 40 mg or betamethasone 4 mg into lesion, which may be repeated after 2 months
    - Systemic steroids may be used for lesions with large orbital component
    - β-blocker use is a new and promising treatment

Surgical

- Consider surgery if failure to respond to medical therapy or for small localized lesions

Follow-Up

- Ongoing ophthalmic examinations to assess for visual development (initially every 3-6 weeks)

SELECTED REFERENCES

1. Bang GM et al: Periocular capillary hemangiomas: indications and options for treatment. Middle East Afr J Ophthalmol. 17(2):121-8, 2010

LYMPHANGIOMA

Key Facts

Introduction
- Benign abnormal proliferation of lymphatic vessels
  - Can occur anywhere in the body
  - Orbital lymphangiomas may be found in conjunctiva, eyelid, or orbit
  - Can fill with venous blood or experience an intralesional hemorrhage, producing a "chocolate" cyst
  - Spontaneous involution is rare
- Complications
  - Anisometropia, amblyopia, strabismus
- Lesion subtypes
  - No flow, arterial flow, venous flow

Presentation
- Acute orbital pain
- Bluish coloration in involved eyelid
- Proptosis, ptosis, chemosis
- Diplopia, hypotropia, esotropia
- Cystic mass on conjunctiva, orbit, or eyelid = "chocolate" cyst
  - "Chocolate" cysts may resolve on their own over time
- Lesion may appear as an edematous patch of vesicles
- Characteristically worsens with illness such as URI
- Cellulitis

Evaluation/Work-Up
- MRI, CT, ultrasound

Classification
- Superficial lymphangioma
  - Usually presents as multilobulated cystic mass in bulbar conjunctiva or eyelid
  - Little effect on visual acuity
- Orbital lymphangioma
  - Found behind orbital septum
  - Occupies intraconal &/or extraconal space

(Left) Axial graphic shows typical features of orbital lymphangioma. Note multilocular, transcompartmental nature of this lesion involving extraconal, conal, & intraconal orbit. Also notice the fluid-fluid levels →, characteristic of this lesion. (Right) Axial T2 fat-saturated MRI in an older child with acute worsening of longstanding right proptosis shows a large retrobulbar mass with characteristic fluid-fluid levels →. Differing heights of the levels are indicative of the multilocular nature of a lymphangioma.

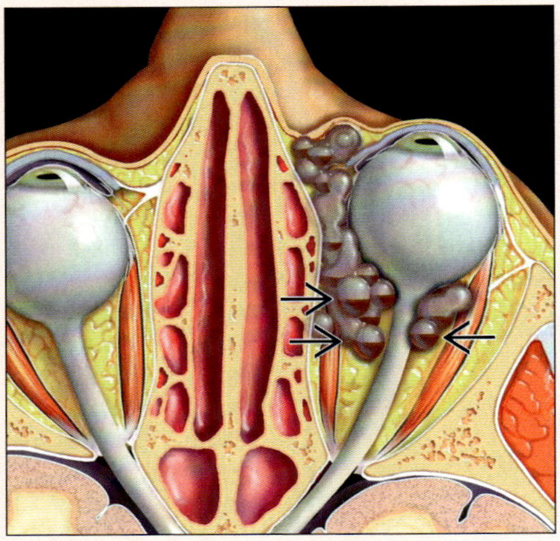

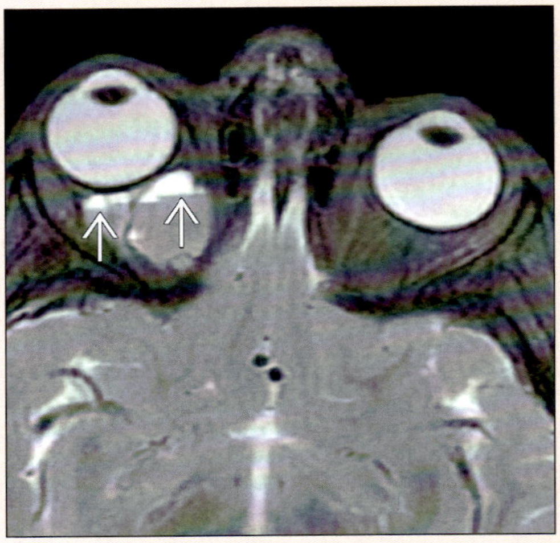

(Left) Axial T2-weighted fat-saturated MRI shows a massive, complex left orbital malformation → with proptosis. Striking signal variability with fluid-fluid levels → represents sequelae of multiple bouts of hemorrhage. Additional preseptal component is also evident →. (Right) Micropathology of lymphangioma shows channels resembling lymphatics, lined by attenuated endothelium →, containing blood and eosinophilic fluid →, and surrounded by loose connective tissue → with lymphocytes.

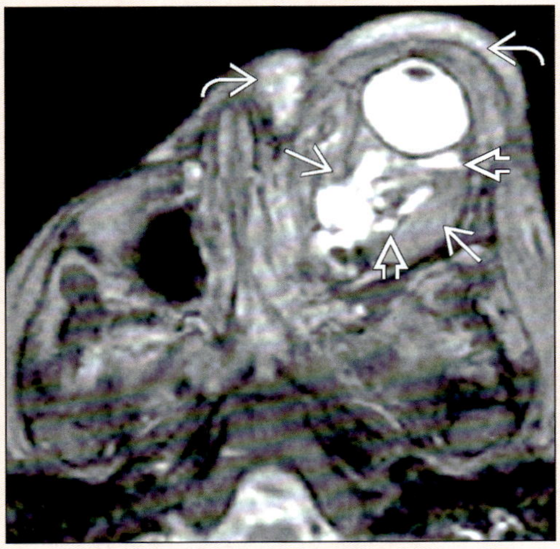

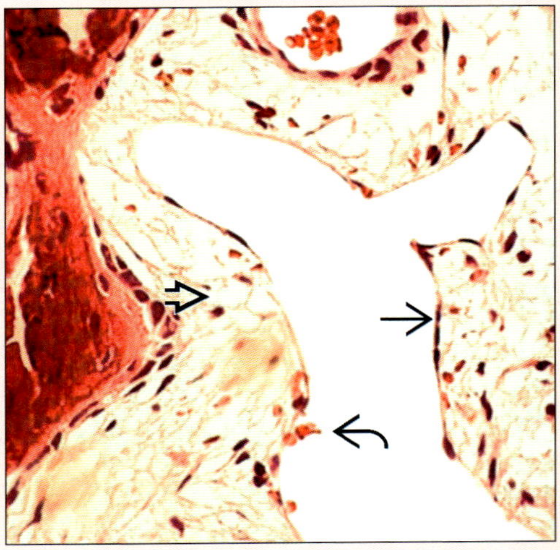

LYMPHANGIOMA

DEMOGRAPHICS

Etiology/Risk Factors

- Etiology unknown but thought to be caused by obstruction of conjunctival lymphatic vessels in the orbit, eyelids, or conjunctiva
  - Often occurs in bulbar conjunctiva
  - Can cause thickening and distortion of eyelid and surrounding areas
- Conjunctival lymphangiomas can be exacerbated by upper respiratory infections
- Usually unilateral unless associated with Turner Syndrome or Nonne-Milroy-Meige disease
- Often diagnosed during 1st or 2nd decade of life

Epidemiology

- Rare condition, only representing 1-3% of all orbital masses
- Usually appears at birth or shortly after
  - Rarely appears in adulthood
- Seen slightly more often in females than males (1.4:1)

PRESENTATION

Symptoms

- Acute orbital pain
- Bluish coloration in involved eyelid
  - Often seen in upper nasal quadrant

Exam Findings

- Ptosis, chemosis, esotropia, and proptosis (which increases upon Valsalva maneuver)
- Cystic mass on conjunctiva, orbit, or eye lid = "chocolate" cyst
- Lesion may appear as an edematous patch of vesicles

DIFFERENTIAL DIAGNOSIS

Hemangioma

- More often presents as an encapsulated lesion
- Often grows very quickly during infancy
- More likely to regress spontaneously
- Superficial lesions have a bright red color
- Less likely to bleed upon excision
- Focal calcifications (cavernous hemangioma)
- Less invasive and often follows anatomical boundaries
- Deeper orbital lesions often lack skin discoloration

Orbital Venous Varix

- Of venous origin
- Often involves the superior ophthalmic vein (can be visualized on MRI)
- Spontaneous orbital hemorrhage less likely to occur
- Histopathology will show a dilated vein with thickened vessel walls
- Ultrasonography reveals a lesion with a single cystic space
- Presents with pseudoenophthalmis

EVALUATION/WORK-UP

Labs

- Biopsy useful to confirm diagnosis

Pathology

- Dilated, unencapsulated lymphatic vessels lined by endothelium
- Cysts often have a well-defined endothelium

Imaging

- MRI
  - Ideal diagnostic imaging technique
  - Often identified as multilobulated intraorbital mass
  - Internal hyperintense areas can signify bleeding
  - Often indistinct margins
  - Lesions often do not show gadolinium enhancement, indicating that tumors are isolated from systemic circulation
- CT
  - May show infiltrating, lobular, cystic mass
- Ultrasound
  - B-scan ultrasonography is particularly useful
  - Should provide good sound transmission
  - Will show large, multiple, irregular cystic spaces
  - Limited efficacy when lesion expands beyond orbit

TREATMENT

Medical

- "Chocolate" cysts
  - Will sometimes regress on their own
  - Drainage
  - Vaporization by carbon dioxide laser
- Intralesional injections of OK432 (picibanil)

Surgical

- Resection
  - Often difficult because cysts are friable, not encapsulated, bleed easily, and may infiltrate normal orbital tissues
  - Recurrence is often common with surgery
- Surgery is recommended if lymphangioma is impinging optic nerve, causing facial disfiguration, or displacing eyelid

SELECTED REFERENCES

1. Sekhar LN et al: Orbital lymphangiomas: surgical treatment and clinical outcome. World Neurosurg. Epub ahead of print, 2013
2. Seca M et al: Conjunctival lymphangioma: a case report and brief review of the literature. Case Rep Ophthalmol Med. 2012:836573, 2012
3. Wiegand S et al: Pathogenesis of lymphangiomas. Virchows Arch. 453(1):1-8, 2008
4. Kalisa P et al: Orbital lymphangioma: clinical features and management. Bull Soc Belge Ophtalmol. (282):59-68, 2001
5. Suzuki Y et al: Management of orbital lymphangioma using intralesional injection of OK-432. Br J Ophthalmol. 84(6):614-7, 2000
6. Goble RR et al: Lymphangioma circumscriptum of the eyelids and conjunctiva. Br J Ophthalmol. 74(9):574-5, 1990
7. Graeb DA et al: Orbital lymphangiomas: clinical, radiologic, and pathologic characteristics. Radiology. 175(2):417-21, 1990

MALIGNANT ORBITAL TUMORS

Key Facts

Introduction
- Tumor that develops within orbit or adnexal structures including the globe, extraocular muscles, fat, vascular, nerve, glandular, or connective tissue structures
  - May be primary or metastatic
- Pediatric malignant tumors
  - Rhabdomyosarcoma: Most common primary malignancy of orbit in children
  - Retinoblastoma: Malignant neoplasm of retina arising from immature retinal cells
  - Granulocytic sarcoma
- Adult malignant tumors
  - Lacrimal gland tumor
  - Ocular adnexal lymphoma (OAL) is a localized lymphoproliferative tumor affecting the orbit, lacrimal gland, lids, &/or conjunctiva

Presentation
- Proptosis with or without pain
- Weakness, weight loss, or fever may indicate systemic malignancy with secondary involvement of orbit

Evaluation/Work-Up
- Fine-needle aspiration biopsy (FNAB) is used primarily to diagnose orbital tumors
- Orbital ultrasound, PET/CT, CAT scan, or MRI with and without contrast can aid in evaluating intraorbital masses

Treatment
- Surgical intervention is mainstay of therapy for majority of orbital tumors
- Local disease may be treated with radiotherapy
- Systemic disease is primarily treated with chemotherapy

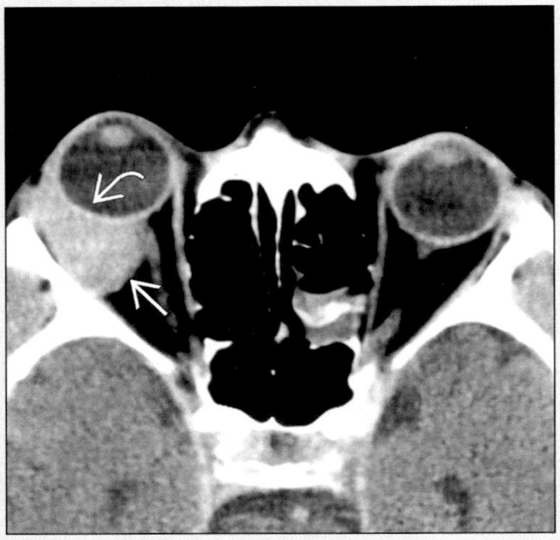
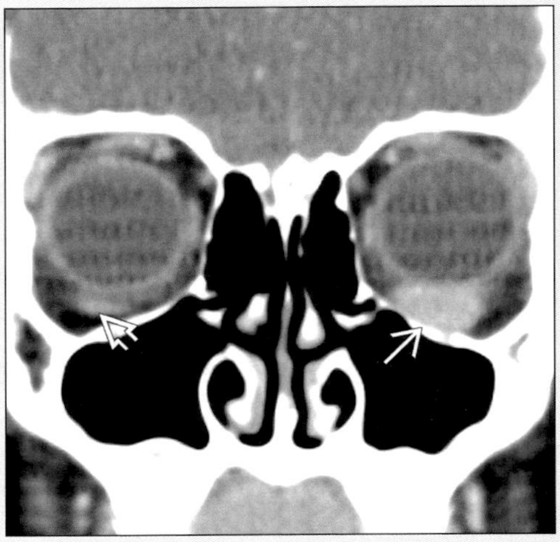

(Left) *Axial contrast-enhanced CT demonstrates a lobular retrobulbar mass ➔ conforming to the shape of the posterior aspect of the right globe ➔. Only minimal flattening of the scleral margin is present. This tumor was found to be mucosa-associated lymphoid tissue lymphoma.* ***(Right)*** *Coronal contrast-enhanced CT in a 5 year old shows a well-defined, mildly enhancing left orbital rhabdomyosarcoma ➔, inseparable from the left inferior rectus muscle. Notice contralateral normal inferior rectus muscle ➔.*

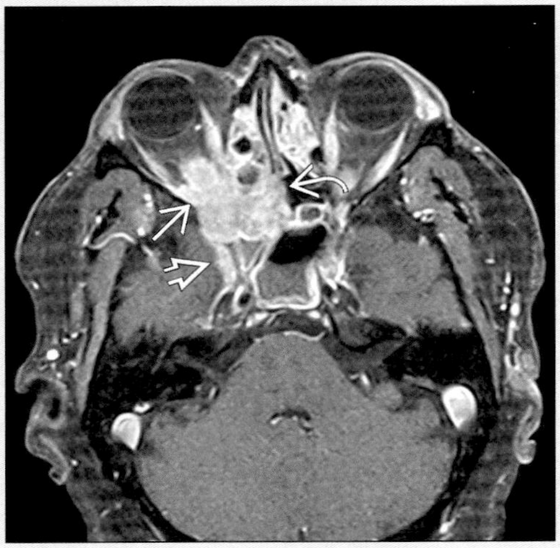
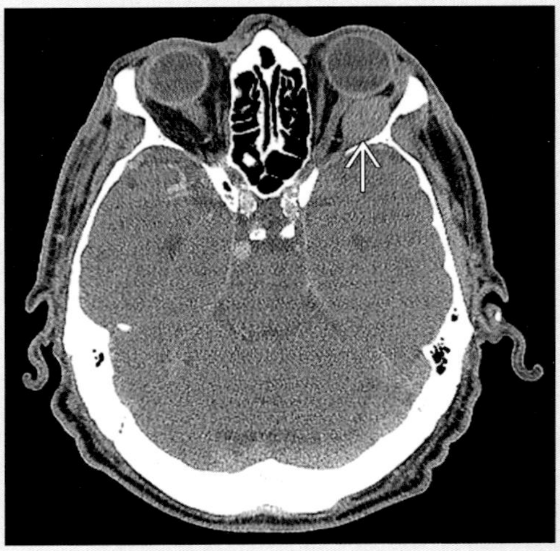

(Left) *Axial T1-weighted MRI shows extensive infiltrating idiopathic inflammatory pseudotumor involving the orbital apex ➔, ethmoid sinus ➔, and foramen rotundum ➔. Pseudotumor is an important differential consideration of orbital masses.* ***(Right)*** *Axial CT shows a discrete mass of the left lateral rectus muscle belly ➔ in a patient who presented with diplopia and proptosis. Further imaging demonstrated a renal mass, and biopsy of the orbital mass was consistent with metastatic renal cell carcinoma.*

MALIGNANT ORBITAL TUMORS

INTRODUCTION

Definitions

- Tumor that develops within orbit or adnexal structures including globe, extraocular muscles, fat, vascular, nerve, glandular, or connective tissue structures
  - May be primary or metastatic

Subtypes

- Pediatric malignant tumors
  - Rhabdomyosarcoma: Most common primary malignancy of orbit in children
    - Soft tissue sarcoma with findings on CT demonstrating homogeneous, well-circumscribed, round mass, which is isodense to muscle
    - Embryonal histological subtype is the most common, occurring in ~ 2 out of every 3 cases
  - Retinoblastoma: Malignant neoplasm of retina that may have extraocular extension
    - Leukocoria, white discoloration of the pupil, is a common finding
  - Granulocytic sarcoma
    - Rapidly developing localized form of myeloblastic leukemia
    - Biopsy demonstrates green discoloration of the surface secondary to myeloperoxidase within the tumor, giving rise to its alternate name, chloroma
- Adult malignant tumors
  - Lacrimal gland tumor
    - Epithelial neoplasms account for 1/2 of lacrimal gland tumors
      - Adenoid cystic carcinoma is the most common primary, malignant, epithelial neoplasm of the lacrimal gland
    - Lymphoproliferative disorders account for the other 1/2 and include malignant lymphoma and leukemia
  - Ocular adnexal lymphoma (OAL) is a localized lymphoproliferative tumor affecting the orbit, lacrimal gland, lids, &/or the conjunctiva
    - Most OALs are non-Hodgkin low-grade B-cell tumors, and mucosa-associated lymphoid tissue (MALT) is the most common primary form of OAL
  - Metastatic disease (prostate, lung, breast, melanoma)

DEMOGRAPHICS

Etiology/Risk Factors

- Most childhood tumors are a result of developmental abnormalities

Epidemiology

- Rhabdomyosarcoma presents with a bimodal distribution, presenting in children < 2 years or > 6 years
- Epithelial lacrimal gland tumor occurs primarily in adults ages 20-50 years
- Orbital lymphoma primarily presents in adults between ages of 50-70 years

PRESENTATION

Symptoms

- Proptosis (secondary to mass effect) is the most common presenting symptom and may also present with pain, ptosis, excessive tearing, headache, vision changes, and nosebleeds
  - Displacement of the globe may elucidate underlying pathological process and can be measured via Hertel exophthalmometry
- Weakness, weight loss, or fever may indicate systemic malignancy with secondary involvement of the orbit

Exam Findings

- Hyperemic conjunctiva, ptosis, lid retraction, or ophthalmoplegia may be present on exam
- Lymphoid neoplasms classically have a smooth, pink-orange subconjunctival mass ("salmon patch")

DIFFERENTIAL DIAGNOSIS

Graves Disease

- Thyroid-associated orbitopathy associated with increased production of glycosaminoglycans by orbital fibroblasts, resulting in characteristic exophthalmos

Orbital Inflammatory Pseudotumor

- Most common cause of painful orbital mass in adults
- Characterized by the acute onset of benign inflammation of the orbit, lymphoid infiltrate, fibrosis, and associated with increased ESR and CRP

EVALUATION/WORK-UP

Labs

- Complete blood count, erythrocyte sedimentation rate, and thyroid function tests can help elucidate infectious, autoimmune, or thyroid disease

Pathology

- Fine-needle aspiration biopsy (FNAB) is used primarily to diagnose orbital tumors
  - If FNAB is unsuccessful in obtaining adequate tissue for pathological assessment, open biopsy is reliable

Imaging

- Orbital ultrasound, PET/CT, CAT scan or MRI with and without contrast

TREATMENT

Medical

- Treatment is oriented against the primary disease
- Radiation + chemotherapy; immunotherapy with chimeric antigen-receptor altered T cells is emerging

Surgical

- Debulking or removal

SELECTED REFERENCES

1. Gündüz K et al: Optic nerve biopsy via a medial transconjunctival orbitotomy approach in the diagnosis of optic nerve and sheath tumors. Orbit. 29(4):190-3, 2010

Key Facts

Introduction

- Optic nerve gliomas are astrocytomas found in the optic nerve, optic chiasm, or both
- Also referred to as optic pathway glioma (OPG)
- Derived from astroglia, oligoglia, and interstitial cells
- Usually does not metastasize
- Most common intracranial tumor of childhood

Demographics

- Often affects children
  - 75% of tumors are diagnosed in 1st decade of life
  - Over 90% of tumors are diagnosed by age 20
- Neurofibromatosis type 1 (NF1)
  - Affects up to 11-30% of children with NF1
  - Tumor often lacks chiasm involvement in patients with NF1
- Accounts for 1% of all intracranial tumors
- Accounts for 66% of primary optic nerve tumors
- Represents 3-5% of intracranial childhood tumors

Presentation

- Depends on which portion of optic pathway or brain structures are affected by tumor
- Symptoms
  - Proptosis: Often unilateral, common in patients with gliomas affecting optic nerve
  - Nystagmus: Seen in 25% of cases
  - Loss of vision
  - Strabismus
  - Endocrine disturbances
- Exam findings
  - Optic disc pallor
  - Optic disc edema
  - Papilledema
- Orbital optic nerve gliomas may cause
  - Optic disc swelling
  - Chorioretinal folds

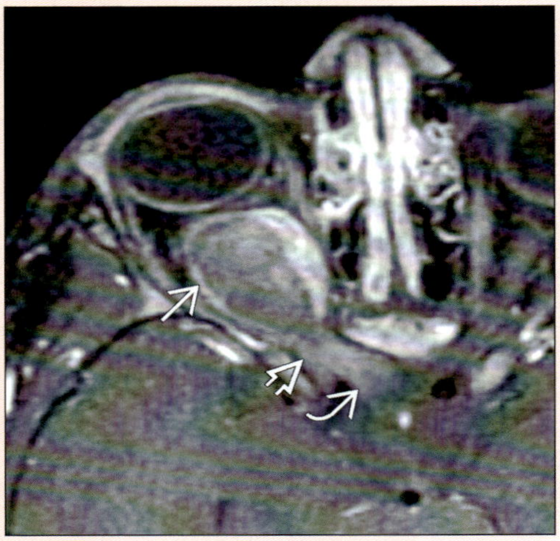
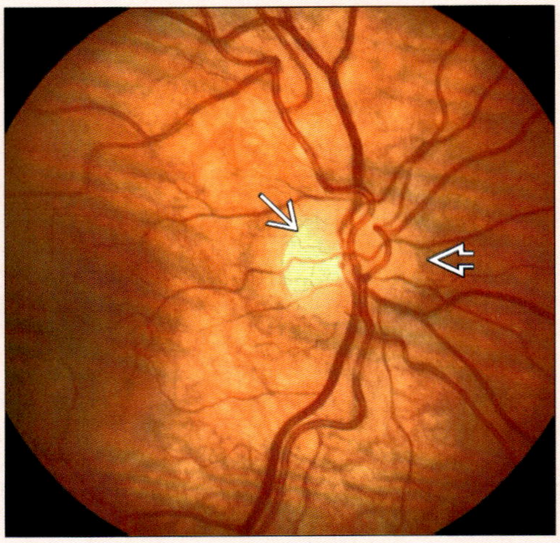

(Left) *Axial T1-weighted MRI with contrast shows mild patchy enhancement and marked fusiform enlargement of the intraorbital ➔, intracanalicular ➔, and prechiasmatic ➔ segments of the right optic nerve.* ***(Right)*** *As seen in this fundus photograph, optic nerve tumors can cause fundus changes such as optic disc edema ➔ and formation of enlarged opticociliary collaterals ➔, both due to compression of the intraorbital optic nerve and central retinal veins.*

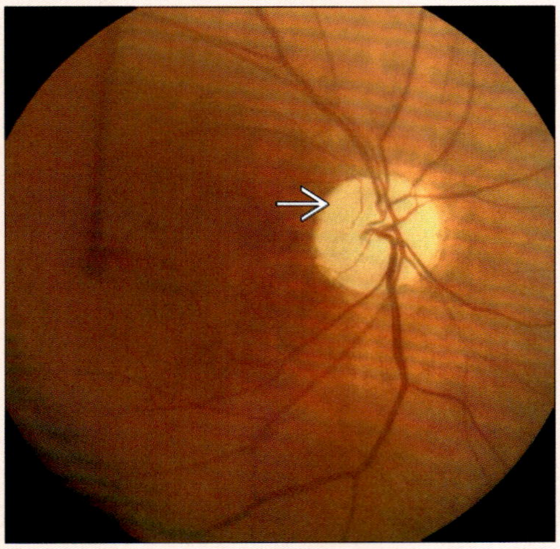
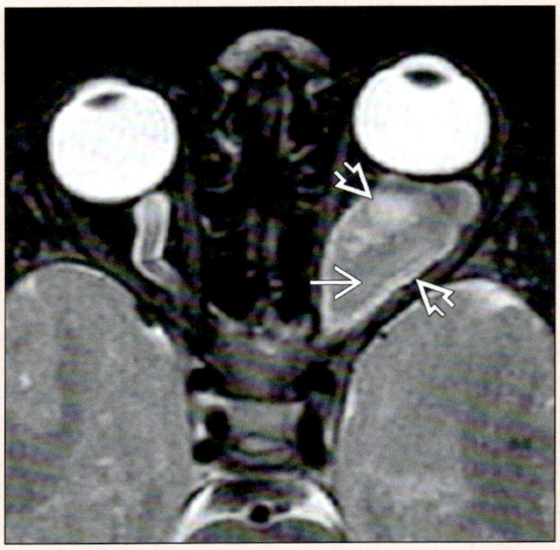

(Left) *This fundus photograph shows optic atrophy in a patient with optic nerve glioma ➔. Atrophy is another common feature of compressive optic nerve tumors and may be preceded by disc swelling.* ***(Right)*** *This axial STIR MRI shows an optic pathway glioma affecting the left optic nerve ➔, with heterogeneous peripheral hyperintensity indicating gliomatosis ➔. Proptosis of the left eye is also evident. Proptosis and painful vision loss often accompany these tumors.*

OPTIC NERVE GLIOMA

INTRODUCTION

Abbreviations
- Optic nerve glioma (ONG)

Synonyms
- Optic pathway glioma (OPG)
- Visual pathway glioma (VPG)

PRESENTATION

Tumor Location Involvement
- 24% confined solely to optic nerve
- 46% invade into 3rd ventricle or midbrain
- 40-76% occupy optic chiasm
- Symptoms and exam findings can help to locate area of tumor involvement

DIFFERENTIAL DIAGNOSIS

Optic Nerve Sheath Meningioma
- Usually occurs in adults; often affects middle-aged women
- Tumor involves nerve sheath and only encircles nerve rather than invading into nerve itself
- Originates from meningothelial cap cells of arachnoid villi
- Classic triad of optic atrophy, decrease in vision, and presence of optocilliary shunt vessels

Optic Neuritis
- Can be of autoimmune origin (multiple sclerosis or lupus)
- May also be due to infection such as bacterial meningitis or Lyme disease
- Can be associated with pain or discomfort if due to infectious origin
- MRI will show white matter abnormalities (especially with optic neuritis secondary to multiple sclerosis)

EVALUATION/WORK-UP

Labs
- Biopsy

Pathology
- Categorized by World Health Organization (WHO) as grade I pilocytic astrocytoma
  - Often called juvenile pilocytic astrocytoma (JPA)
- Appears as spindle-shaped pilocytic astrocytes and glial filaments on histology
- Can visualize astrocytic and oligodendroglial proliferation
- Rosenthal fibers common

Imaging
- MRI
  - Should be performed every 6-12 months
  - Spindle-like or globular enlargement of optic nerve
  - Optic nerve or chiasm thickening
  - Kinking or buckling of optic nerve
  - Isointense or mildly hypointense to brain on T1-weighted MRI scan
  - Hyperintense on T2-weighted MRI scan
- CT
  - Calcification of nerve sheath
  - Adjacent bony hyperostosis
  - Enlargement of optic foramen
- Cerebral angiography

TREATMENT

Medical
- Chemotherapy
  - First-line treatment for symptomatic cases
  - Involves various combinations of chemotherapeutics such as
    - Vincristine, actinomycin D, carboplatin, cisplatin, procarbazine, etoposide, cyclophosphamide
- Radiotherapy
  - Often only given if chemotherapy fails
  - Metastatic tumors
  - Corticosteroids often prescribed during radiotherapy to reduce swelling and inflammation
- No treatment for malignant gliomas of visual pathway

Surgical
- Complete surgical excision is recommended if patient experiences severe vision loss or disfiguring proptosis
- Partial resection

Follow-Up
- Regular MRI follow-up screenings

Prognosis
- Highly variable
  - > 90% survival at 15 years after resection for optic gliomas confined to optic nerve
  - NF1 patients as well as children often have a more favorable prognosis
  - Malignant gliomas in adults are often fatal within 1 year
  - Some patients may suffer from loss of peripheral vision
  - Combination of globular hypothalamic/chiasmatic glioma and electrolyte abnormalities in a child without NF1 are related to a poor prognosis

SELECTED REFERENCES

1. Yeung JT et al: Optic pathway glioma as part of a constitutional mismatch-repair deficiency syndrome in a patient meeting the criteria for neurofibromatosis type 1. Pediatr Blood Cancer. 60(1):137-9, 2013
2. Avery RA et al: Optic pathway gliomas. J Neuroophthalmol. 31(3):269-78, 2011
3. Shapey J et al: Diagnosis and management of optic nerve glioma. J Clin Neurosci. 18(12):1585-91, 2011
4. Moreno L et al: Does chemotherapy affect the visual outcome in children with optic pathway glioma? A systematic review of the evidence. Eur J Cancer. 46(12):2253-9, 2010
5. Binning MJ et al: Optic pathway gliomas: a review. Neurosurg Focus. 23(5):E2, 2007
6. Cnossen MH et al: Endocrinologic disorders and optic pathway gliomas in children with neurofibromatosis type 1. Pediatrics. 100(4):667-70, 1997

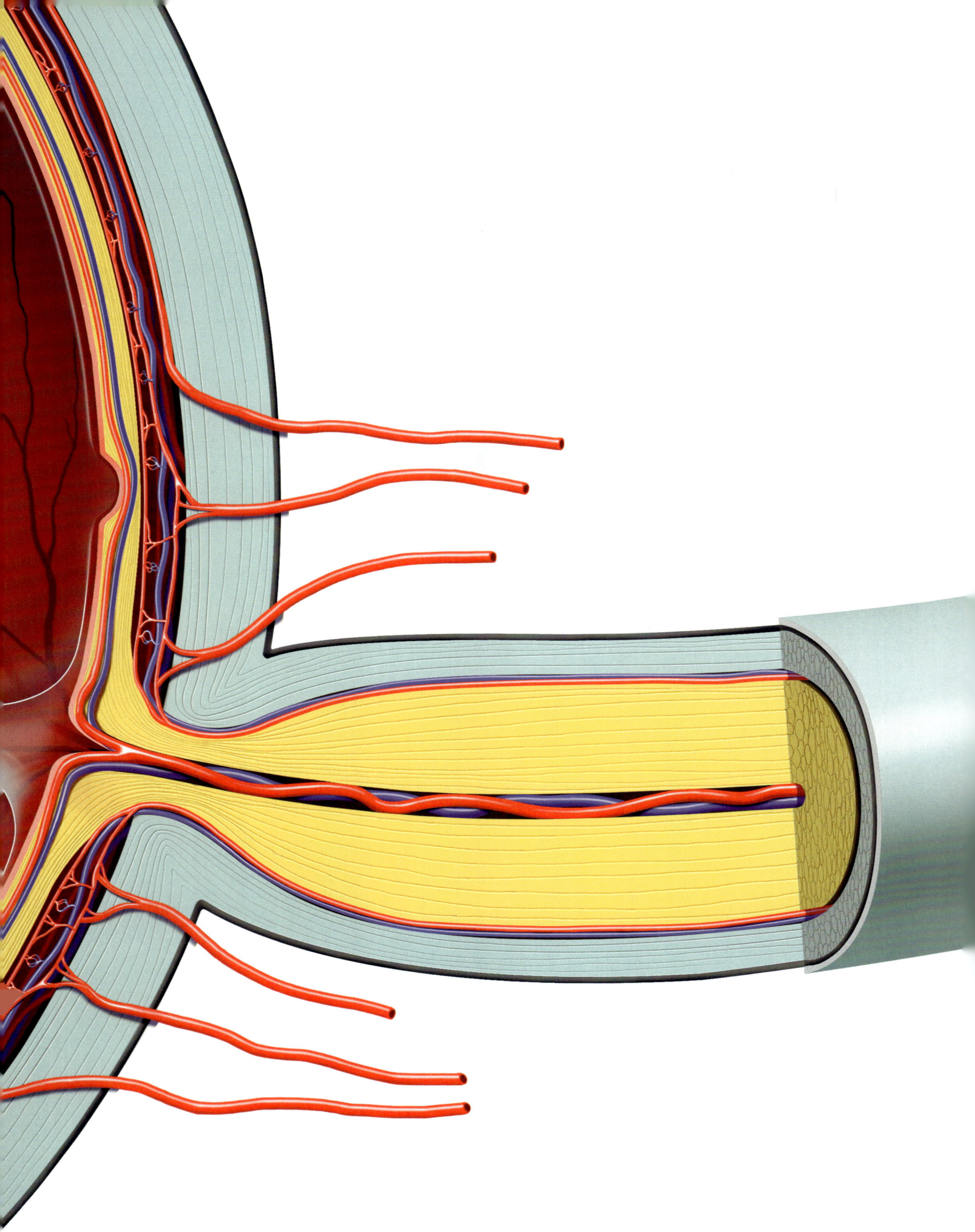

SECTION 1
Optic Nerve

MAJOR CLINICAL STUDIES: OPTIC NERVE

OPTIC NEURITIS TREATMENT TRIAL (ONTT)

Objectives
- Determine benefit of optic neuritis (ON) corticosteroids
- Describe clinical course of ON
- Determine risk factors for developing multiple sclerosis (MS) in patients with ON

Inclusion Criteria
- Age 18-46 years
- Active unilateral ON with visual symptoms for ≤ 8 days
- Relative afferent pupillary defect (RAPD) with visual field defect
- No previous history of ON in study eye
- No previous history of steroid treatment for MS
- No systemic disease that could be causing ON, other than MS

Randomization Method
- Patients were randomized to 3 groups
  - Oral prednisone 1 mg/kg/day for 14 days
  - IV methylprednisolone 250 mg every 6 hr for 3 days followed by oral prednisone 1 mg/kg/day for 11 days
  - Placebo for 14 days

Results
- Treatment with oral prednisone should be avoided
- Consider IV methylprednisolone if patient requires rapid improvement in vision or brain MRI suggests MS
- Reasonable to consider no pharmacologic intervention in treating ON
- Brain MRI should be done to assess risk of MS; however, chest x-ray, blood tests, and lumbar puncture are not necessary in evaluating a patient with clinical features of acute onset ON

LONGITUDINAL OPTIC NEURITIS STUDY (LONS)

Objective and Principal Conclusion
- Determine risks and benefits of corticosteroids for ON and risk of developing MS in patients with ON
- Treatment with oral prednisone in standard doses should be avoided, but treatment with intravenous methylprednisolone should be considered, especially if brain MRI shows lesions consistent with MS or if patient must recover vision rapidly

Inclusion Criteria
- Age 18-46 years
- Active unilateral ON with visual symptoms for ≤ 8 days
- Relative afferent pupillary defect (RAPD) with visual field defect
- No previous history of ON in study eye
- No previous history of steroid treatment for MS
- No systemic disease that could be causing ON, other than MS

Randomization Method
- Long-term follow-up phase of ONTT with same randomization

Results
- Routine blood tests, chest x-ray, brain MRI, and lumbar puncture are of limited value in diagnosing ON in a patient with classic clinical features of ON
  - Classic ON presents as a young adult with sudden vision loss, symptoms progressing over 1 week with pain on eye movement, and visual improvement beginning within 1 month
- Brain MRI predicts early risk of MS following ON
- In a patient with ON and no lesions on brain MRI, 5 features are associated with a low 5-year risk of developing MS
  - Lack of pain, optic disc edema, peripapillary hemorrhage, retinal exudates, mild vision loss
- Treatment
  - High-dose, intravenous corticosteroids followed by oral corticosteroids accelerated vision recovery, but did not improve long-term visual outcome
  - Standard-dose oral prednisone alone did not improve visual outcome and was associated with an increased rate of recurrent ON
  - Intravenous corticosteroids followed by oral corticosteroids ↓ rate of developing MS, but by 3 years this risk reduction was no longer observed
  - Treatments are generally well tolerated and adverse effects during treatment are mild
- Visual recovery begins within 2 weeks in most ON cases without any intervention and improvement continues for 1st year
  - Most patients recover to 20/20 visual acuity (VA), although possible symptomatic deficits in vision
- Probability of recurrent ON in either eye within 5 years is 28%; visual recovery after 2nd episode of ON in same eye is generally good

ISCHEMIC OPTIC NEUROPATHY DECOMPRESSION TRIAL (IONDT) AND IONDT FOLLOW-UP

Objective
- Determine if optic canal decompression is useful for nonarteritic ischemic optic neuropathy (NAION)

Inclusion Criteria
- Age ≥ 50 years
- Acute NAION + visual symptoms for ≤ 14 days
- VA of 20/64 or worse

Randomization Method
- Patients were randomized to receive either decompression surgery or observation

Results
- Neither surgery nor steroids useful in traumatic optic neuropathy
  - Patients undergoing surgery had 25% less chance of visual recovery & 2x risk of visual loss vs. observed patients
    - 33% of patients undergoing surgery recovered 3 or more lines of vision after 6 months vs. 43% of patients undergoing observation
    - 24% of patients undergoing surgery lost 3 or more lines of vision after 6 months vs. 12% undergoing observation
  - No benefit to decompression surgery for ischemic optic neuropathy; may actually be harmful
- Decompression should be avoided unless patient clearly has bone fragment impinging on optic nerve

MAJOR CLINICAL STUDIES: OPTIC NERVE

INTRAVENOUS IMMUNOGLOBULIN THERAPY IN OPTIC NEURITIS

Objective
- Assess risk and benefits of high-dose intravenous immunoglobulin (IVIg) in restoring vision in ON

Inclusion Criteria
- History of ≥ 1 episode of previous demyelinating optic neuritis in setting of classic, adult-onset MS
- Age < 50 years
- Irreversible loss of VA
  - Worse than 20/40 for at least 6 months
  - Must read at least 1 letter on 1-meter eye chart
  - Visual function unchanged from screening visit & enrollment visit separated by 1 month
  - Optic disc pallor on funduscopic exam
  - Visual field mean deviation of -4.00
- Must not have received ACTH or corticosteroids within preceding 2 months

Randomization Method
- 60 patients assigned to receive either IVIg or a placebo over 3 months
  - IVIg group: 0.4 g/kg Gamimune N intravenously q.i.d. for 5 days, then 1x month for 3 months
  - Placebo group: 0.1% human serum albumin in 10% maltose q.i.d. for 5 days, then 1x month for 3 months

Results
- IVIg does not reverse persistent visual loss from ON to a degree that merits general use
- Trial was terminated after interim analysis showed that treatment was not effective at improving VA

TREATMENT OF TRAUMATIC OPTIC NEUROPATHY: INTERNATIONAL OPTIC NERVE TRAUMA STUDY

Objective and Principal Conclusion
- Compare observation, optic canal decompression, and steroids for treating indirect traumatic optic neuropathy (TON)
- No difference in final VA with steroids or surgery

Inclusion Criteria
- Diagnosis of traumatic optic neuropathy
- Initial visual assessment ≤ 3 days after injury
- Excluded for penetrating optic nerve injuries

Randomization Method
- Comparative nonrandomized interventional study
- Patients were treated based on usual clinical routine of each investigator
- Untreated: No corticosteroids and no optic canal decompression surgery
- Steroid: Corticosteroids given within 7 days of injury, no surgery
- Surgery: Optic canal decompression surgery was performed ± corticosteroid within 7 days of injury

Results
- Vision improved ≥ 3 lines in 57% of observed patients, 52% in steroid group, and 32% in surgery group

HIGH-DOSE INTRAVENOUS METHYLPREDNISOLONE IN RECENT TRAUMATIC OPTIC NEUROPATHY

Objective and Principal Conclusions
- Compare high-dose intravenous corticosteroid therapy with placebo in TON
- No difference in VA improvement between high-dose corticosteroids and placebo in treatment of TON

Inclusion Criteria
- Diagnosis of indirect TON based on ↓ vision and RAPD
- ≤ 7 days between injury and treatment
- Normal fundus on examination
- Exclusion criteria: Unconscious patients, penetrating trauma, candidates for decompression surgery, other lesions that may cause low vision, hazy ocular media, optic nerve avulsion, TON with blowout fracture

Randomization Method
- Double-masked placebo-controlled trial
- Intravenous methylprednisolone 250 mg every 6 hours for 3 days, then oral prednisolone 1 mg/kg for 14 days
- Intravenous 50 mL normal saline (placebo) every 6 hours for 3 days, then placebo for 14 days

Results
- Mean BCVA in treated group was 1.11 ± 1.14 vs. 1.78 ± 1.23 in placebo group ($P = .13$)
- VA improved in 68.8% of treated group and 53.3% of placebo group ($P = .38$)

RELATED REFERENCES

1. National Institutes of Health, National Eye Institute: Intravenous Immunoglobulin Therapy in Optic Neuritis (NEI Clinical Studies). http://www.nei.nih.gov/neitrials/static/study13.asp. Updated September 21, 2001. Accessed September 6, 2013
2. National Institutes of Health, National Eye Institute: Ischemic Optic Neuropathy Decompression Trial (IONDT). http://www.nei.nih.gov/neitrials/static/study26.asp. Updated October 21, 1999. Accessed September 6, 2013
3. National Institutes of Health, National Eye Institute: Ischemic Optic Neuropathy Decompression Trial Followup (IONDT Followup). http://www.nei.nih.gov/neitrials/static/study25.asp. Updated October 21, 1999. Accessed September 6, 2013
4. National Institutes of Health, National Eye Institute: Longitudinal Optic Neuritis Study (LONS). http://www.nei.nih.gov/neitrials/static/study48.asp. Updated February 4, 2003. Accessed September 6, 2013
5. National Institutes of Health, National Eye Institute: Optic Neuritis Treatment Trial (ONTT). http://www.nei.nih.gov/neitrials/static/study47.asp. Updated February 4, 2003. Accessed September 6, 2013
6. Levin LA et al: The treatment of traumatic optic neuropathy: the International Optic Nerve Trauma Study. Ophthalmology. 106(7):1268-77, 1999

OPTIC NERVE OVERVIEW

TERMINOLOGY

Synonyms

- Cranial nerve 2, CN2

Definitions

- Optic nerve relays visual information from retina to brain
- Optic neuropathy is a common cause of vision loss
  - Signs include visual field defects and abnormal pupillary response
  - Imaging of optic nerve may be important for disease diagnosis

ANATOMY

Structure

- Retinal ganglion cell axons converge to form optic nerve
- Optic nerve exits the globe posteriorly through the optic disc, also called physiological blind spot
  - Absence of photoreceptor cells in optic disc
- Retro-bulbar optic nerve is covered by CNS meninges (dura, arachnoid, and pia mater)
- Myelinated by oligodendrocytes
- Incapable of regeneration after damage, leading to irreversible loss of vision

Anatomical Course

- Exits eye through optic canal
- Optic nerve fibers decussate in optic chiasm (temporal visual field fibers)
- Axons synapse in lateral geniculate nucleus (LGN)
- Fibers of optic radiation from the LGN terminate to visual cortex in occipital lobe

OPTIC NERVE AND DISEASE

Optic Neuropathies

- Hereditary optic neuropathy
  - Leber hereditary optic neuropathy (LHON)
  - Dominant optic neuropathy (Kjer type)
  - Recessive optic neuropathy (Wolfram syndrome)
  - Spinocerebellar degeneration
  - Friedreich ataxia
  - Olivopontocerebellar atrophy
  - Charcot-Marie-Tooth disease
  - Hereditary spastic paraplegias (Strumpell-Lorrain disease)
- Glaucoma
  - Most common cause of optic nerve dysfunction
  - Loss of ganglion cells
  - Increased intraocular pressure (IOP) is a major risk for optic nerve damage
  - Initial peripheral vision loss with central vision sparing
  - Increased cup to disc ratio
- Acute demyelinating optic neuritis
  - Inflammation of optic nerve myelin sheath most commonly associated with multiple sclerosis
  - MRI of brain to detect white matter lesions
- Nonarteritic ischemic optic neuropathy (NAION)
  - Severe disc edema with hemorrhages early
  - Altitudinal scotomas are characteristic visual field change
- Arteritic anterior or posterior ischemic optic neuropathy
  - Caused by giant cell arteritis (GCA)
- Inflammatory (nondemyelinating) optic neuropathy
  - Ocular inflammation
    - Posterior uveitis, retinitis, optic perineuritis
  - Systemic inflammation
    - Sarcoidosis, systemic lupus erythematosus, Behçet disease, inflammatory bowel disease, Sjögren syndrome, Wegener granulomatosis, syphilis, Lyme disease, cat scratch disease
- Neuromyelitis optica (NMO) (or Devic disease)
  - Optic neuritis with myelopathy
- Optic nerve hypoplasia
  - Most common congenital optic nerve disease
  - Fewer nerve fibers resulting in smaller than normal optic disc
- Toxic-nutritional optic neuropathies
  - Typically cecocentral scotomas
  - Ethambutol, amiodarone, methanol, ethanol, tobacco, vitamin B12 deficiency
- Compressive optic neuropathy
  - Intracranial meningioma
  - Pituitary adenoma
  - Intracranial aneurysms
  - Craniopharyngiomas/gliomas of anterior visual pathway
  - Thyroid eye disease
  - Retrobulbar hemorrhage
- Traumatic optic neuropathy
- Radiation optic neuropathy (RON)
- Infiltrative optic neuropathy (malignancies)
- Paraneoplastic optic neuropathy
- Myotonic dystrophy

Visual Field Loss From Disease

- Optic nerve damage
  - Loss of all visual fields in 1 eye
- Optic nerve damage in optic chiasm
  - Loss of temporal vision in both vision fields (bitemporal hemianopsia)
  - Pituitary adenoma may compress optic nerve in optic chiasm
- Optic tract damage
  - Loss of contralateral hemifield

Optic Nerve Imaging

- Fundus photography
- Confocal scanning laser ophthalmoscopy (CSLO)
  - Heidelberg retinal tonograph (HRTII and III)
  - 3D reconstruction of the optic nerve head
- Scanning laser polarimetry (SLP)
  - GDx nerve fiber analyzer, Carl Zeiss Meditec
  - Measures retinal nerve fiber layer thickness
- Optical coherence tomography
  - Measures retinal nerve fiber layer thickness

RELATED REFERENCES

1. Behbehani R: Clinical approach to optic neuropathies. Clin Ophthalmol. 1(3):233-46, 2007
2. Newman NJ et al: Hereditary optic neuropathies. Eye (Lond). 18(11):1144-60, 2004
3. Jonas JB et al: Ophthalmoscopic evaluation of the optic nerve head. Surv Ophthalmol. 43(4):293-320, 1999

OPTIC NERVE

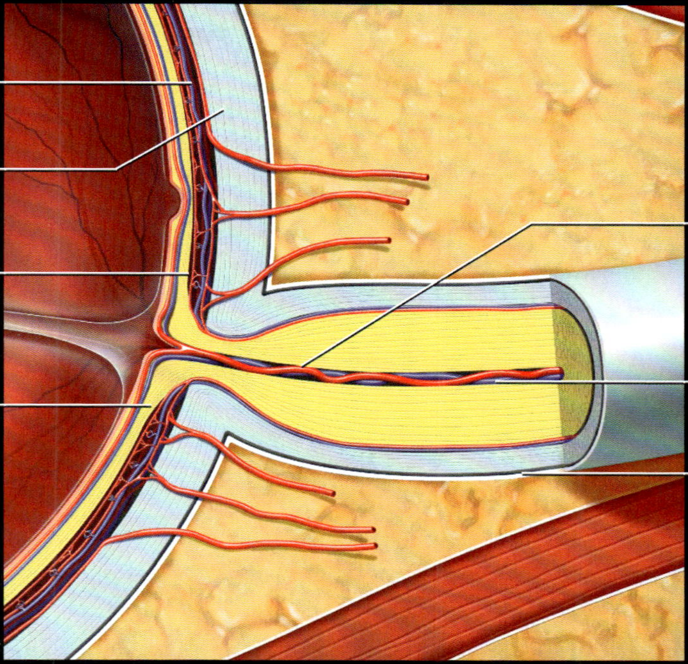

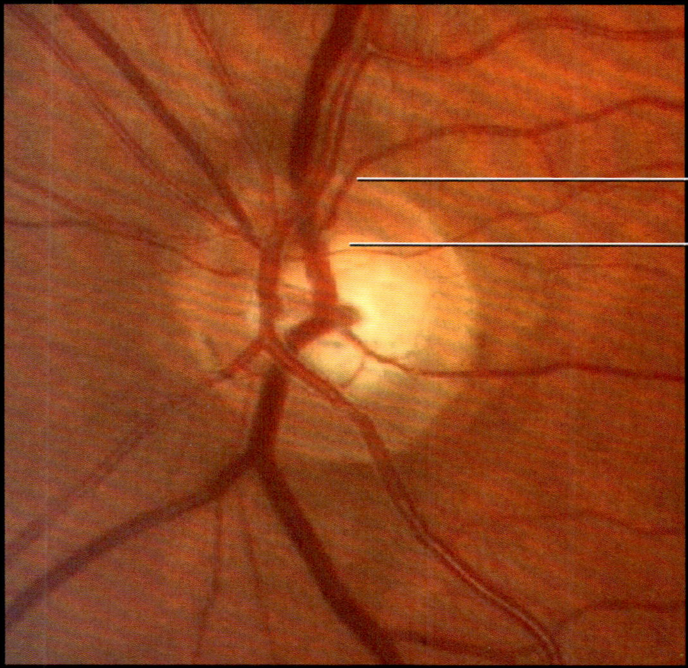

(Top) *Retinal ganglion cell axons converge to form the optic nerve (yellow). The optic disc, or physiologic blind spot, is the area where the optic nerve exits the eye. The optic nerve is ensheathed by the CNS meninges (dura, arachnoid, and pia mater) and is myelinated after exiting the eye.* ***(Bottom)*** *This image shows a normal optic disc. The optic disc consists of a smaller white cup in the center and an outer rim. The optic disc is the location where the optic nerve and blood vessels exit the eye. The ratio between the cup to the entire optic disc is called the cup to disc ratio. This image shows a cup to disc ratio of ~ 0.5. An enlarged cup to disc ratio may suggest underlying pathology such as glaucoma.*

DOMINANT OPTIC NEUROPATHY

Key Facts

Introduction

- Autosomal dominant disorder resulting in bilateral degeneration of optic nerve
- Defects have been identified in 2 genes (*OPA1*, *OPA3*), 3 loci (*OPA4*, *OPA5*, *OPA8*)

Presentation

- Insidious vision loss
- Optic atrophy
  - Isolated, translucent optic disc pallor
  - Commonly, a temporal crescent/wedge
  - Temporal excavation (triangular)
  - Neuroretinal rim atrophy
  - Peripapillary atrophy

Evaluation/Work-Up

- *OPA1* gene mutation in 75% of DON patients
- *OPA3* gene mutation in 1% of DON patients
- Optical coherence tomography
  - Nonspecific thinning of peripapillary RNFL
  - Normal photoreceptors layers
- Visual evoked potentials
  - Diminished amplitude
  - Prolonged latency
- Electroretinography
  - Reduced N95 component
- Perimetry
  - Central, cecocentral, paracentral scotomas
  - Normal peripheral fields

Treatment

- No current treatment for DON
- Low vision aids
- Genetic counseling
- Gene therapies are under investigation
- Prognosis
  - Very slow, mild progression in some patients
  - Spontaneous recovery does not occur

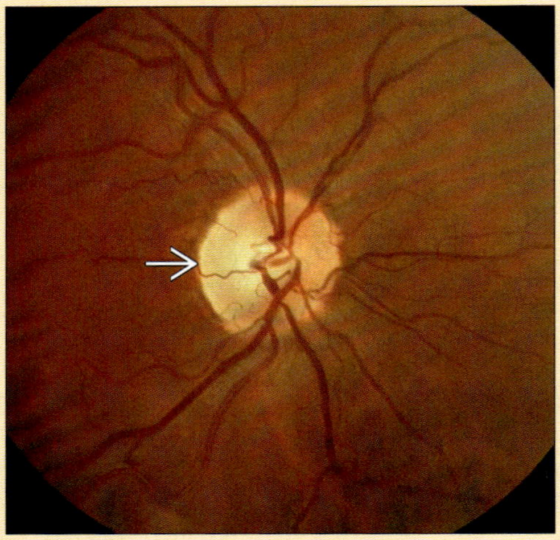

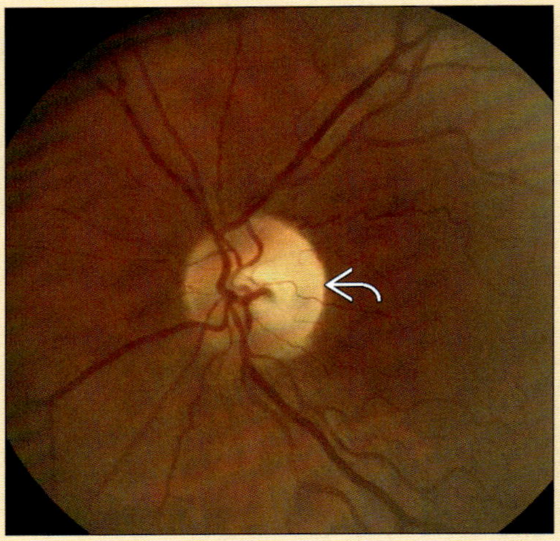

(Left) *This fundus photo shows the right eye of a patient with dominant optic neuropathy. Note the temporal pallor ➔.* ***(Right)*** *This fundus photo shows the left eye of the same patient revealing bilateral temporal pallor ↩, a finding commonly seen in dominant optic neuropathy.*

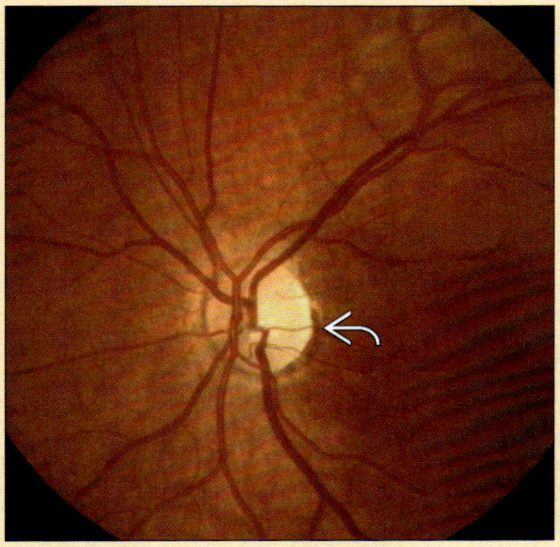

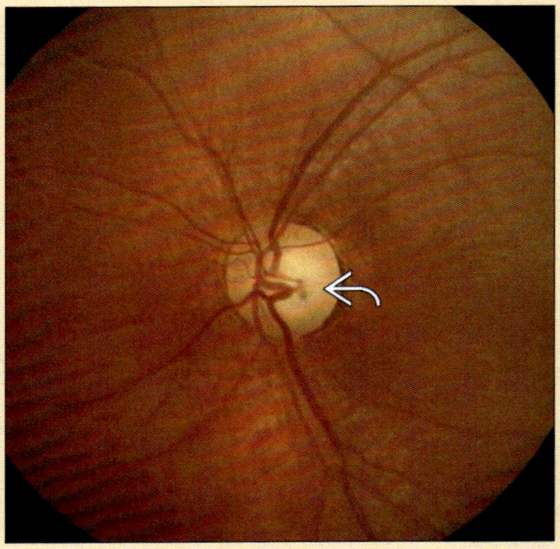

(Left) *This fundus photo shows the left eye of a patient with dominant optic neuropathy. Note the contour of blood vessels suggesting optic disc excavation ➔. Temporal pallor is also evident.* ***(Right)*** *This fundus photo shows the left eye of a patient with dominant optic neuropathy. Less intense temporal pallor ↩ suggests that the disease is at its early stage in this patient.*

DOMINANT OPTIC NEUROPATHY

INTRODUCTION

Abbreviations
- Dominant optic neuropathy (DON)

Synonyms
- Kjer disease

Definitions
- Autosomal dominant disorder resulting in bilateral degeneration of optic nerve
  - Defect in 2 genes (*OPA1*, *OPA3*)
    - 3 loci (*OPA4*, *OPA5*, *OPA8*)
    - Product is a mitochondrial dynamin-related GTPase
      - Likely role is mitochondrial membrane stability
  - Primary effect is on retinal ganglion cells (RGCs) and axons

DEMOGRAPHICS

Etiology/Risk Factors
- Family history of DON
  - Autosomal dominant, ~ 70% penetrance
  - Severity is highly variable

Epidemiology
- Prevalence ~ 1 per 10,000 in Denmark (founder effect)
- Prevalence ~ 1 per 50,000 outside of Denmark
- Most common hereditary optic neuropathy

PRESENTATION

Symptoms
- Insidious vision loss
  - Bilateral, central, symmetric
  - Color blindness
    - Generalized dyschromatopsia > isolated tritanopia
  - Onset in first 2 decades, often early childhood

Exam Findings
- Visual field deficits vary
  - Normal peripheral fields
- Optic atrophy
  - Isolated, translucent optic disc pallor
    - Commonly, a temporal crescent/wedge
    - May be diffuse, subtle
  - Temporal excavation (triangular cupping)
  - Neuroretinal rim atrophy
  - Peripapillary atrophy
  - Saucerization of optic cup
- Absent foveal reflex
- Mild macular pigmentary changes
- Arterial attenuation
- Color vision defects
- Cataracts
- Chronic external ophthalmoplegia
- Nystagmus
  - Suggests early visual impairment
  - Not correlated with central involvement
- Systemic/neurologic findings
  - Sensorineural hearing loss
  - Peripheral neuropathy
  - Myopathy
  - Multiple sclerosis-like illness
  - Spastic paraplegia
  - Diabetes insipidus or mellitus

DIFFERENTIAL DIAGNOSIS

Normal Pressure Glaucoma
- No family history of unexplained optic atrophy
- Later age of onset
- No pallor of remaining neuroretinal rim
- No sparing of peripheral fields

EVALUATION/WORK-UP

Labs
- Molecular genetic testing
  - *OPA1* gene mutation in 75% of DON patients
  - *OPA3* gene mutation in 1% of DON patients

Pathology
- Diffuse atrophy of RGC layer
- Loss of myelin within optic nerves

Imaging
- Optical coherence tomography
  - Nonspecific thinning of peripapillary retinal nerve fiber layer (RNFL)
  - Normal photoreceptor layers
- Visual evoked potentials
  - Diminished amplitude, prolonged latency
- Electroretinography
  - Reduced N95 component → RGC dysfunction
- Perimetry
  - Central, cecocentral, paracentral scotomas
  - Normal peripheral fields

TREATMENT

Medical
- No current treatment
- Low vision aids
- Genetic counseling
- Avoid alcohol, tobacco, and medications interfering with mitochondrial metabolism
- Gene therapies are under investigation

Prognosis
- Very slow, mild progression in some patients
- Systemic involvement is a poor prognostic indicator
- Spontaneous recovery does not occur (unlike Leber)

SELECTED REFERENCES

1. Newman NJ et al: Hereditary optic neuropathies. Eye (Lond). 18(11):1144-60, 2004
2. Eliott D et al: Visual prognosis in autosomal dominant optic atrophy (Kjer type). Am J Ophthalmol. 115(3):360-7, 1993
3. Kline LB et al: Dominant optic atrophy. The clinical profile. Arch Ophthalmol. 97(9):1680-6, 1979
4. Smith DP: Diagnostic criteria in cominantly inherited juvenile optic atrophy. A report of three new families. Am J Optom Arch Am Acad Optom. 49(3):183-200, 1972
5. KJER P: Hereditary infantile optic atrophy with dominant transmission. Acta Genet Stat Med. 7(2):290-1, 1957

Key Facts

Introduction
- Hereditary loss of central vision

Demographics
- Mitochondrially inherited
  - Caused by replacement mutation in mitochondrial DNA
- Males more commonly affected (81.9%)
- Diagnostic key is maternal family history of vision loss

Presentation
- Ocular symptoms
  - Vision blurring
  - Painless loss of central vision; vision might return, even years later
  - RNFL swelling in 80%
- Systemic symptoms
  - Muscular tremors
  - Cardiac arrhythmia

Evaluation/Work-Up
- Test for mitochondrial DNA point mutations
- Muscle biopsy looking for mitochondrial abnormalities
- MRI shows increased optic nerve signal in affected eye(s)
- Perimetry analysis
- Visual acuity testing
- Referral for EKG for associated cardiac abnormalities

Treatment
- Preventative: Incomplete penetrance of LHON indicates that there are environmental factors associated with presentation of disease
  - Patients with LHON should not smoke and should drink alcohol only in moderation
- Genetic counseling for known carriers
- Result in affected individuals is significant visual impairment

*(**Left**) The disease process causes degeneration of the axons in the central portion of the optic nerve ⇨ and degeneration of retinal ganglion cells and axons ➡. (**Right**) Fundus photo illustrates changes to the optic disc. Note the telangiectasia of the peripapillary vessels ➡ and disc swelling. (Courtesy P. Bernstein, MD.)*

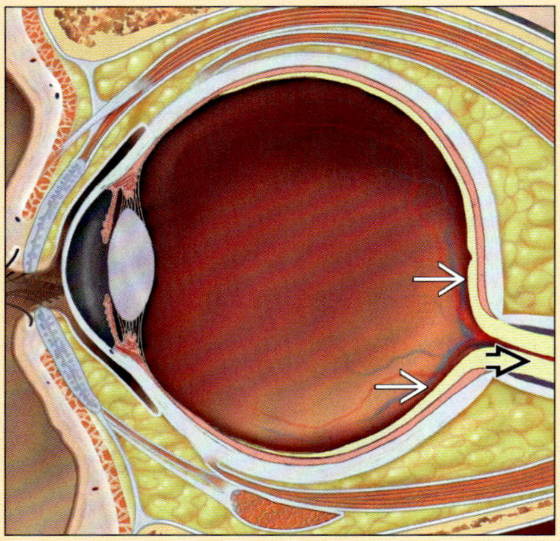

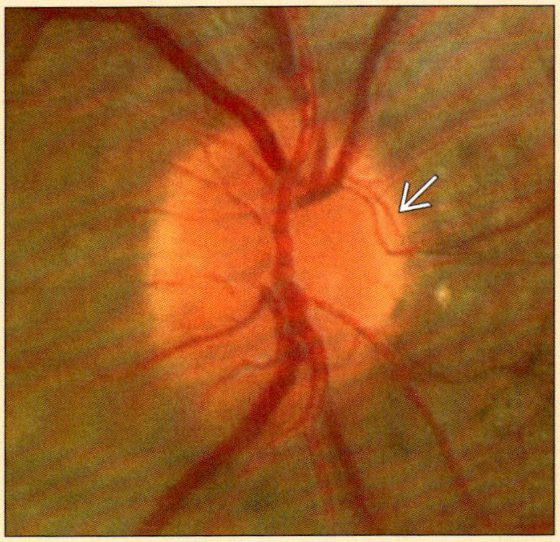

*(**Left**) Fundus photo illustrates enlarged peripapillary vessels ➡ and slight optic disc pallor ⇨. (Courtesy P. Bernstein, MD.) (**Right**) This graphic illustrates a pedigree chart for Leber hereditary optic neuropathy (LHON). Only females can pass mitochondrial DNA (mDNA) to offspring. There is variable penetration of LHON. Consequently, unaffected carrier mothers can pass the disease on to male or female children, but males do not pass mDNA on to their children. Blue indicates carrier; black indicates noncarrier.*

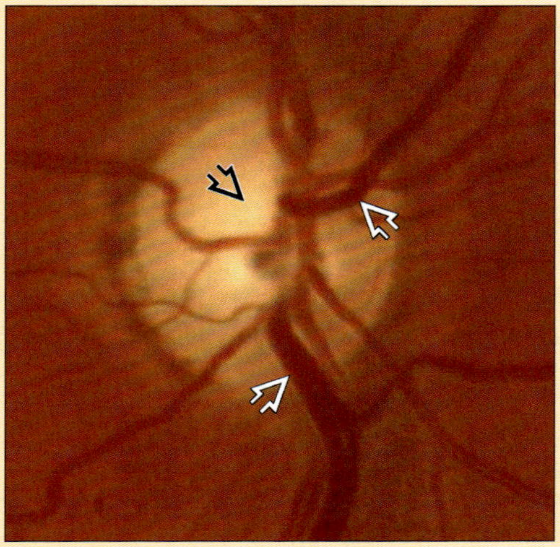

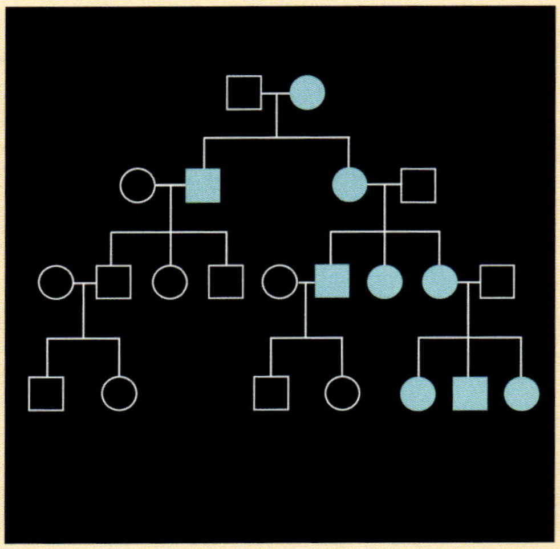

LEBER HEREDITARY OPTIC NEUROPATHY

INTRODUCTION

Abbreviations

- Leber hereditary optic neuropathy (LHON)

Definitions

- Hereditary loss of central vision

Subtypes

- Based on location of mitochondrial DNA (mDNA) mutation
  - M14484T = least severe
  - M3460G = moderately severity
  - M11778G = most severe

DEMOGRAPHICS

Etiology/Risk Factors

- Mitochondrially inherited
  - Caused by replacement mutation in mDNA that leads to
    - Degeneration of geniculate bodies via cell loss and gliosis
    - Damage/degeneration of axons in central portion of optic nerve
    - Decreased number of ganglionic cells in retina

Epidemiology

- Males more commonly affected (81.9%)
- Onset of vision loss is typically between 1st and 6th decades
- Mean time from onset of vision loss to complete vision loss is 3.7 months
- Diagnostic key is maternal family history of vision loss

PRESENTATION

Symptoms

- Ocular symptoms
  - Vision blurring
  - Painless loss of central vision
- Systemic symptoms
  - Muscular tremors
  - Cardiac arrhythmia

Exam Findings

- Ophthalmoscopic findings
  - Telangiectatic microangiopathy
  - Retinal nerve fiber layer swelling in 80%
  - Vascular tortuosity
- Cecocentral scotoma
- Loss of color vision

DIFFERENTIAL DIAGNOSIS

Other Optic Neuropathies

- Compressive
- Infiltrative
- Inflammatory
- Thyroid related

Neuromyelitis Optica

- Most commonly arises in early childhood but is not a hereditary disease

Multiple Sclerosis

- Average age of onset in women is 23.5 and men 30
- Symptoms/findings include vision loss, optic neuritis (unilateral eye pain), nystagmus, and internuclear ophthalmoplegia

EVALUATION/WORK-UP

Labs

- Test for mDNA point mutations

Pathology

- Muscle biopsy looking for mitochondrial abnormalities
- Electron microscopy looking for groupings in subsarcolemma of enlarged mitochondria along with myofilament disorganization

Imaging

- MRI showing ↑ optic nerve signal in affected eye(s)
- Optical coherence tomography to measure thickness of retinal nerve fiber layer

Medical

- Referral for EKG and cardiological work-up due to associated cardiac abnormalities

TREATMENT

Medical

- Preventative: Incomplete penetrance of LHON indicates that there are environmental factors associated with presentation of disease
  - Patients with LHON should not smoke and should drink alcohol in moderation
- Some evidence for effectiveness of idebenone

Follow-Up

- Genetic counseling for known carriers
- Visual acuity testing, perimetry analysis

Prognosis

- Significant visual impairment is common; in some patients, vision may recover even years later

SELECTED REFERENCES

1. Hashemi N et al: Leber hereditary optic neuropathy mimicking thyroid-related optic neuropathy. J Neuroophthalmol. 32(1):95-6, 2012
2. Sabet-Peyman EJ et al: Is leber hereditary optic neuropathy treatable? Encouraging results with idebenone in both prospective and retrospective trials and an illustrative case. J Neuroophthalmol. 32(1):54-7, 2012
3. Yu H et al: Gene delivery to mitochondria by targeting modified adenoassociated virus suppresses Leber's hereditary optic neuropathy in a mouse model. Proc Natl Acad Sci U S A. 109(20):E1238-47, 2012
4. Maguire AM et al: Age-dependent effects of RPE65 gene therapy for Leber's congenital amaurosis: a phase 1 dose-escalation trial. Lancet. 374(9701):1597-605, 2009
5. Barboni P et al: Retinal nerve fiber layer evaluation by optical coherence tomography in Leber's hereditary optic neuropathy. Ophthalmology. 112(1):120-6, 2005
6. Sorajja P et al: Cardiac abnormalities in patients with Leber's hereditary optic neuropathy. Heart. 89(7):791-2, 2003

OPTIC NEURITIS

Key Facts

Introduction

- Temporary inflammation of the optic nerve, commonly resulting in pain and loss of vision
- Subtypes
  - Retrobulbar neuritis (accounts for 66% of cases)
  - Papillitis
  - Perineuritis
  - Neuroretinitis

Demographics

- Etiology
  - Demyelinating disease (may be isolated event, but most often secondary to multiple sclerosis)
  - Infectious
  - Parainfectious
  - Noninfectious
  - Idiopathic
- Females most often affected (> 2:1)

Presentation

- Visual loss that occurs over hours to days
- Most often monocular but may be binocular
- Periorbital pain associated with eye movement
- Dyschromatopsia (loss of color vision), particularly red

Treatment

- MRI can help predict risk of MS
- Corticosteroid therapy has been shown to increase only rate of visual return, not final visual outcome
- Referral to neurologist when suspicious of underlying multiple sclerosis
- Prognosis
  - Typical optic neuritis shows improvement within 1-3 months
  - Recurrence rate is 1/3

__(Left)__ Axial T1 MRI in an adult woman with left eye pain and decreased color vision shows intense segmental enhancement of the left intraorbital optic nerve ➔. A component of peripheral nerve sheath enhancement is seen extending posteriorly ➔. __(Right)__ Fundus photo shows the normal-appearing optic nerve of a patient with retrobulbar neuritis.

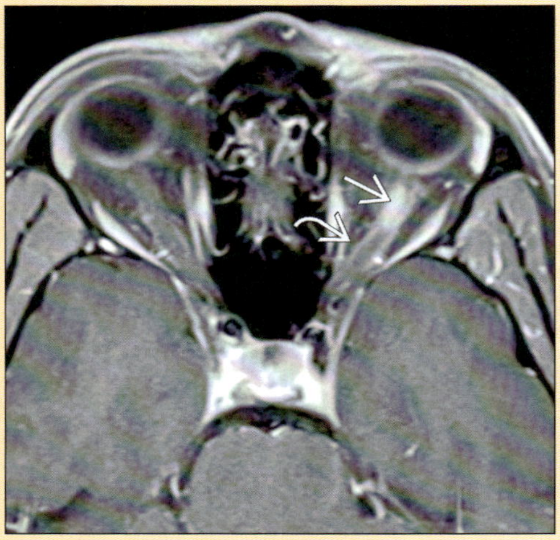

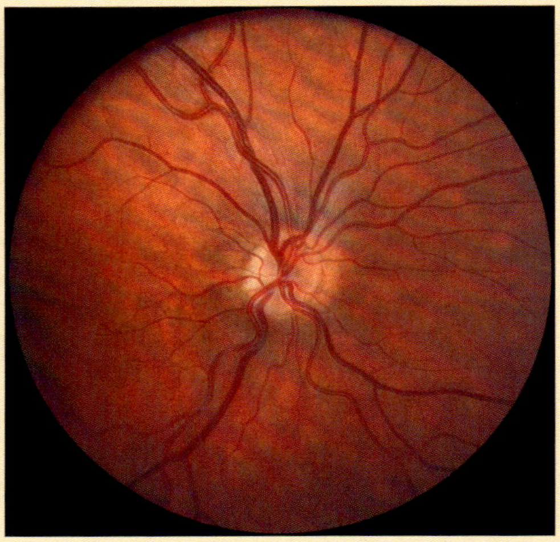

__(Left)__ Funduscopic image in a child with postviral optic neuritis shows typical appearance of papillitis. The fundus returned to normal after corticosteroid therapy. __(Right)__ Funduscopic image demonstrates the characteristic exudative macular star pattern of neuroretinitis. Papillitis is also present.

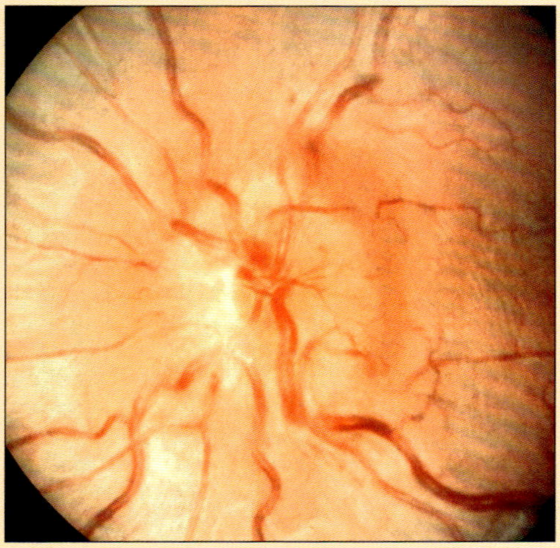

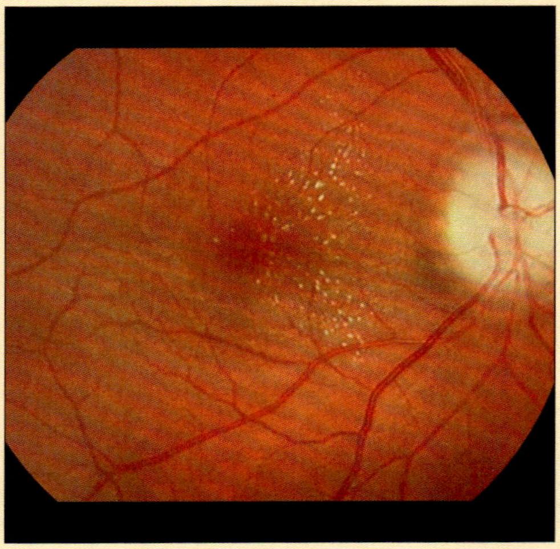

OPTIC NEURITIS

INTRODUCTION

Abbreviations
- Optic neuritis (ON)

Definitions
- Temporary inflammation of optic nerve, commonly resulting in pain and loss of vision

Subtypes
- **Retrobulbar neuritis**
  - Accounts for 2/3 of adult cases
  - Affected portion of optic nerve is posterior to optic nerve head
    - Funduscopy appears normal
  - Associated with multiple sclerosis (MS)
- **Papillitis**
  - Most common form of optic neuritis in children
  - Edematous optic disc
  - Flame-shaped hemorrhages often present peripheral to optic disc
  - Vitreous cell may be present
- **Perineuritis**
  - Inflammation of nerve sheath
  - Less likely to be associated with MS
- **Neuroretinitis**
  - Least common form
  - Papillitis and inflammation of retinal nerve fiber layer
  - 1-2 weeks following acute onset of neuritis, a macular star may appear

DEMOGRAPHICS

Etiology/Risk Factors
- **Demyelinating disease**
  - May present as isolated demyelinating optic neuritis but most often secondary to MS, a demyelinating disease involving white matter of CNS
  - 15-20% of MS patients present with optic neuritis
  - 50% of MS patients will suffer from at least 1 episode of optic neuritis
- **Infectious**
  - Associated with herpes zoster, tuberculosis, syphilis, mononucleosis, cat scratch disease, Lyme disease, and infectious encephalitis
- **Parainfectious**
  - May follow a childhood viral infection (measles, mumps, rubella, chickenpox)
  - May occur following vaccination
- **Noninfectious**
  - Causes include sarcoidosis, lupus, and various forms of vasculitis
- **Idiopathic**

Epidemiology
- Occurs in young patients (mean age of onset = 32 years)
- Females most often affected (> 2:1)
- Incidence: 4-6 per 100,000 in USA and Europe
- Highest incidence among whites of Northern European ancestry
  - 8:1 ratio of Northern Europeans to Africans and Asians
- Several HLA alleles are associated with increased risk of ON and MS
  - DR2, DW2, DRB1, others

PRESENTATION

Symptoms
- Visual loss that occurs over hours to days
- Most commonly monocular but may be binocular
- Periorbital pain associated with eye movement
  - Present in 92% of cases
- Dyschromatopsia (loss of color vision), particularly red
  - Present in > 90% of cases
- Flashes of light
- Uhthoff phenomenon
  - Worsening of symptoms with exercise, fever, or hot weather

Exam Findings
- In unilateral or asymmetric cases, a relative afferent pupillary defect (RAPD) will be present
- Visual field defects
  - Scotoma
    - Most commonly, diffuse visual loss within central 30° of vision
    - 2nd most common type of defect is altitudinal or arcuate defects
    - Focal, cecocentral, and paracentral scotomas are also associated with ON
- Funduscopy may reveal swollen disc, but most often the disc appears normal (retrobulbar neuritis)
  - Papillitis occurs in only 35% of cases; flame-shaped hemorrhages can occur
- Concomitant neurologic findings such as focal weakness, tingling, and numbness are often present

DIFFERENTIAL DIAGNOSIS

Acute Papilledema
- Secondary to increased intracranial pressure
- Typically present with bilateral disc edema

Severe Hypertensive Disease
- Bilateral findings including flame-shaped hemorrhages, cotton-wool spots, and disc edema
- Elevated blood pressure

Acute Angle-Closure Glaucoma
- Acute onset of severe eye pain and sudden loss of vision
- Associated with nausea, vomiting, and headache
- Increased intraocular pressure

Anterior Ischemic Optic Neuropathy
- Onset of visual loss is rapid
- Nonarteritic anterior ischemic optic neuropathy
  - Induced by cardiovascular risk factors such as diabetes, hypertension, and high cholesterol
- Arteritic anterior ischemic optic neuropathy
  - Caused by giant cell arteritis

Compressive Optic Neuropathy
- Slowly progressive visual loss
- Loss of color vision and RAPD
- CN2, CN4, or CN6 palsy may be present
- Compressive mass on orbital/brain CT or MRI

OPTIC NEURITIS

- Etiologies include orbital mass, intracranial mass, pseudotumor cerebri, thyroid ophthalmopathy, and carotid-ophthalmic artery aneurysm

Toxic and Nutritional Optic Neuropathies

- Visual loss may be acute or insidious in onset
- Detailed history should be obtained regarding the following
  - Diet (B1, B6, B12, folate)
  - Past alcohol and tobacco use
  - Medication list
  - Chemical exposures (heavy metals, solvents, aerosols)
  - Toxin (methanol, carbon monoxide)

EVALUATION/WORK-UP

Labs

- Consider CBC, ESR, CRP, TSH, ANA, ACE, lysozyme, RPR, FTA-ABS, PPD, Lyme serology, *Bartonella* serology, and monospot
  - In absence of associated clinical signs and symptoms of systemic disease, yield of these tests is very low
- CSF analysis is often noncontributory
  - However, leukocytosis, increased IgG index, myelin basic protein, and oligoclonal banding are suggestive of a diagnosis of MS

Pathology

- Nerve edema acutely, with atrophy resulting from chronic inflammation
- Microscopic features
  - Acute
    - Macrophage and lymphocytic infiltrate resulting in myelin loss, cholesterol droplets, and axonal damage
  - Chronic
    - Atrophy, gliosis, astrocytic scar

Imaging

- MRI of brain, spine, and orbits with gadolinium and fat suppression
  - Acute demyelinating plaques will be visible with gadolinium and T1-weighted scans; 2 or more enhancing lesions indicate high probability of evolving to MS
  - Periventricular and spinal cord plaques are characteristic of associated MS
- Humphrey visual field test

TREATMENT

Medical

- Treatment varies based on etiology
  - Demyelinating
    - Potential benefits of corticosteroid therapy must be carefully weighed against risks of steroid
    - Optic Neuritis Treatment Trial recommended the following for ON accompanied by 2 enhancing lesions on MRI
      - 1 g IV methylprednisolone for 3 days, then 1 mg/kg oral prednisone for the next 11 days
      - Discontinue therapy with 3-day taper
    - Corticosteroid therapy has been shown to increase only rate of visual return, not final visual outcome
    - For patients with possible MS, treatment with immunomodulators (interferon-β, glatiramer acetate) has been shown to be beneficial
  - Infectious
    - Pathogen-specific antimicrobial agents as appropriate
  - Parainfectious
    - Prognosis is excellent without treatment
  - Noninfectious
    - Sarcoid
      - Typically demonstrates rapid response to corticosteroid therapy
      - Methotrexate may be used as adjunct therapy or alone in steroid-intolerant patients
    - Autoimmune
      - Corticosteroid therapy or immunomodulators as appropriate for specific autoimmune etiology

Surgical

- Extracranial venous angioplasty is being explored in clinical trials for patients with MS who have chronic cerebrospinal venous insufficiency

Follow-Up

- Return to clinic in 1-2 months initially
- Surveillance every 3-6 months thereafter
- Referral to neurologist when suspicious of underlying MS

Prognosis

- Typical optic neuritis shows improvement within 1-3 months independent of treatment
- Optic Neuritis Treatment Trial: 15-year follow-up
  - 72% of patients recovered best corrected visual acuity of at least 20/20
  - > 90% of patients had visual acuity 20/40 or better
  - 3% of patients never improved to better than 20/200 vision
- Longer optic nerve lesions as demonstrated on MRI are associated with worse visual outcome
- African Americans typically have poorer visual outcomes when compared to whites
- Recurrence rate affecting either eye is 1/3
  - Patients with recurrent optic neuritis are more likely to develop MS

SELECTED REFERENCES

1. Optic Neuritis Study Group: Multiple sclerosis risk after optic neuritis: final optic neuritis treatment trial follow-up. Arch Neurol. 65(6):727-32, 2008
2. Optic Neuritis Study Group: Visual function 15 years after optic neuritis: a final follow-up report from the Optic Neuritis Treatment Trial. Ophthalmology. 115(6):1079-1082, 2008
3. The 5-year risk of MS after optic neuritis: Experience of the optic neuritis treatment trial. Optic Neuritis Study Group. Neurology. 49(5):1404-13, 1997
4. Beck RW et al: The effect of corticosteroids for acute optic neuritis on the subsequent development of multiple sclerosis. The Optic Neuritis Study Group. N Engl J Med. 329(24):1764-9, 1993
5. Beck RW et al: A randomized, controlled trial of corticosteroids in the treatment of acute optic neuritis. The Optic Neuritis Study Group. N Engl J Med. 326(9):581-8, 1992

OPTIC NEURITIS

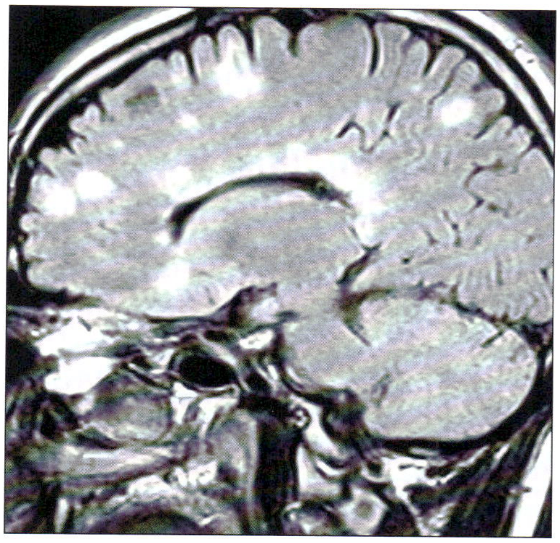

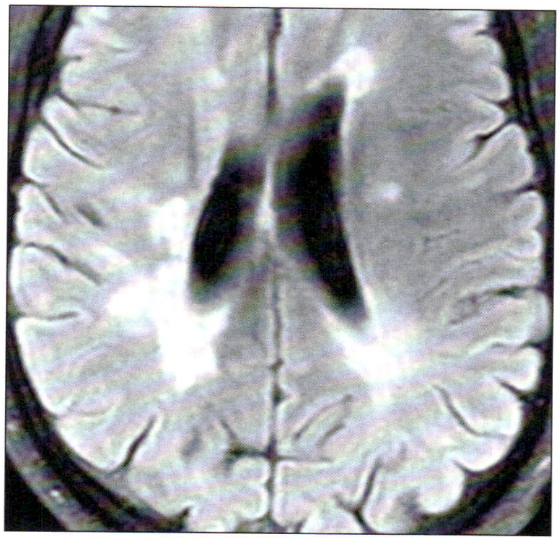

(Left) *Sagittal FLAIR MRI shows multiple sclerosis plaques with typical perpendicular orientation at the callososeptal interface along penetrating venules ("Dawson fingers"), as well as involving subcortical white matter.* ***(Right)*** *Axial FLAIR MRI at 3.0 tesla shows confluent multiple sclerosis plaques in commonly seen periventricular locations.*

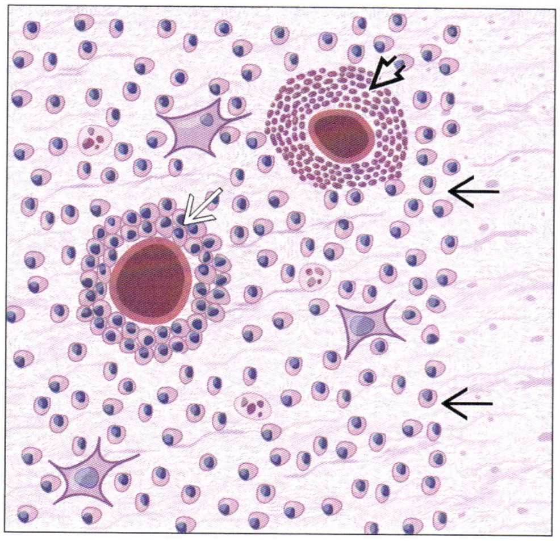

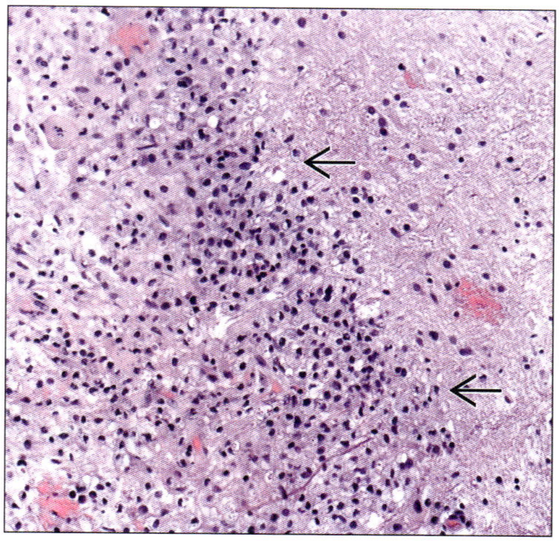

(Left) *This illustration demonstrates that in H&E sections, demyelinating plaques typically have (1) sharp borders →, (2) macrophages, both interstitial and perivascular ➡, and (3) perivascular chronic inflammation ⇨. Scattered large stellate reactive astrocytes complete the picture.* ***(Right)*** *Macrophages crowding along the edge of plaque → emphasize the lesion's typically sharp border and are seen in chronic active (smoldering) lesions. (Courtesy B. DeMasters, MD.)*

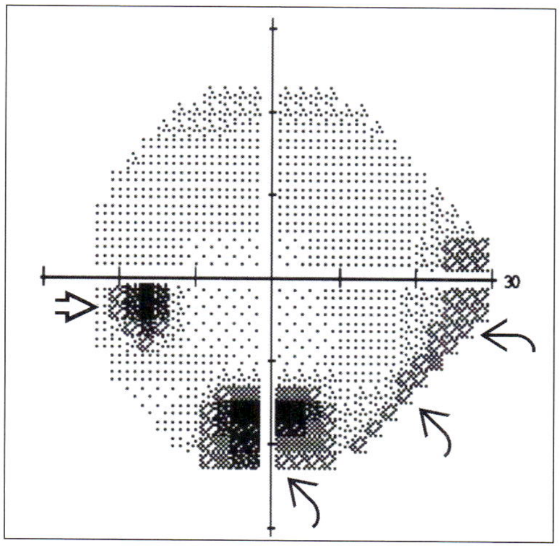

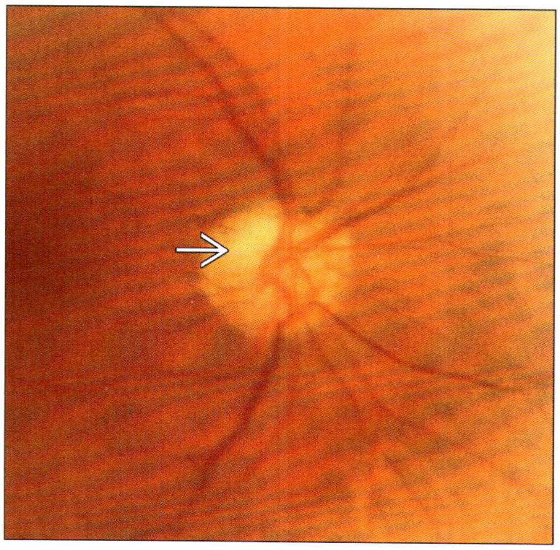

(Left) *Humphrey visual field central 24-2 threshold testing most commonly reveals a central scotoma in patients with active optic neuritis. Here, testing of the left eye reveals an arcuate scotoma located over the inferonasal field ↶. The physiologic or normal blind spot ⇨ is also present.* ***(Right)*** *Funduscopy of a patient suffering from ocular sarcoid shows a sarcoid granuloma of the optic nerve head ➡. Characteristic vitreous haze is also present, obscuring the image slightly.*

RADIATION OPTIC NEUROPATHY

Key Facts

Introduction
- Radiation injury to optic nerves and chiasm

Demographics
- Rare complication in patients irradiated for tumors near optic nerves
  - Incidence is dose dependent

Presentation
- Reported onset ranges from 3 months to 8 years after irradiation
- Decreased visual acuity
  - Sudden
  - Painless
  - Irreversible
  - Unilateral or bilateral
- Retina exam
  - Sparse vascularity
  - Flame-shaped hemorrhages
  - Optic nerve atrophy, pallor
- Visual field defect
  - Any optic nerve or chiasmal pattern may be seen

Evaluation/Work-Up
- T1-weighted MRI with gadolinium-DTPA enhancement
  - Segmental enhancement of the optic nerve, optic chiasm, or optic tracts
  - Abnormalities may be visible prior to visual loss
- Fluorescein angiography may show coexisting radiation retinopathy
  - Segmental narrowing of retinal arteries, scattered hemorrhages, retinal microaneurysms, capillary nonperfusion or leakage, macular edema, stained disc

Treatment
- Hyperbaric oxygen therapy
  - Best if started within 48-72 hours of vision loss

__(Left)__ This fundus photo is of the eye of a patient with radiation optic neuropathy. Note the optic nerve pallor → as well as the generalized sparse vascularity. __(Right)__ This axial T1WI C+ FS MRI shows marked enhancement of the right optic nerve, involving the cisternal segment and extending from the optic canal to the chiasm →. These MRI findings in a patient with a history of radiotherapy to the head suggest radiation optic neuropathy.

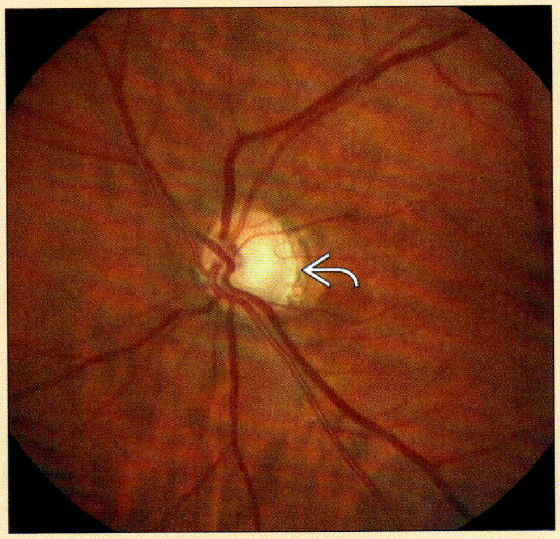

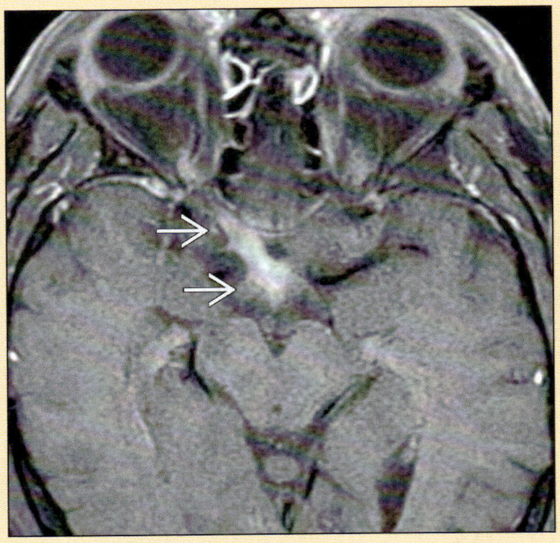

__(Left)__ This fundus photo features peripapillary flame-shaped hemorrhages →, which is a characteristic finding of radiation optic neuropathy. __(Right)__ This fundus photo demonstrates cotton-wool spots →, which are associated with radiation optic neuropathy.

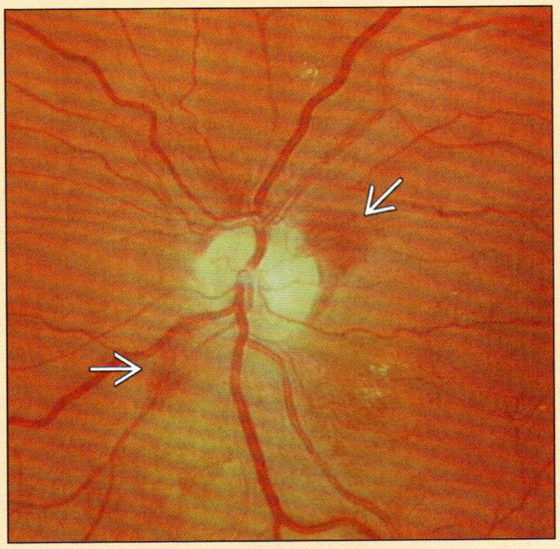

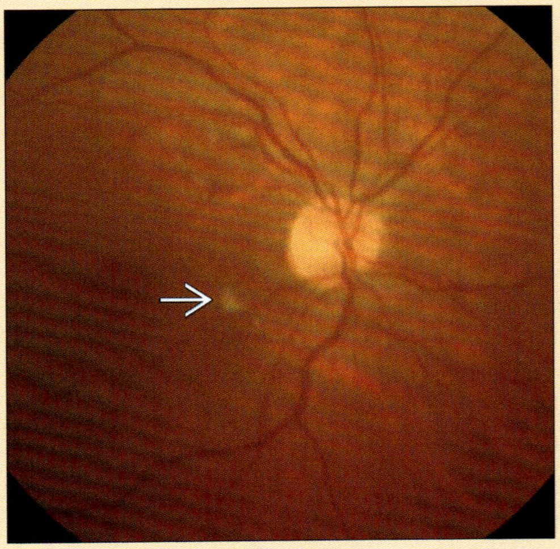

RADIATION OPTIC NEUROPATHY

INTRODUCTION

Abbreviations
- Radiation optic neuropathy (RON)

Definitions
- Radiation injury to optic nerves and chiasm
  - Inability of vasculature to respond to metabolic demands of damaged glial cells

DEMOGRAPHICS

Etiology/Risk Factors
- Radiotherapy to head and neck
  - Incidence is dose dependent
    - Total dose ≥ 50-55 Gy
    - Single dose ≥ 10 Gy
    - Radiation fraction size ≥ 2 Gy
- Factors increasing risk at lower radiation doses
  - Concomitant radiotherapy and chemotherapy
  - Diabetes mellitus
  - Visual impairment
  - Advanced age
  - Compression of optic nerve by tumor

Epidemiology
- Rare complication in patients irradiated for tumors near optic nerves

PRESENTATION

Symptoms
- Onset ranges from 3 months to 8 years after irradiation
  - Average presentation is 18 months after irradiation
  - Majority present within 3 years of radiation therapy
- Decreased visual acuity
  - Sudden
  - Painless
  - Irreversible
  - Unilateral or bilateral
    - Bilateral may be simultaneous or sequential
  - May progress to total blindness

Exam Findings
- Retina exam
  - Sparse vascularity
  - Flame-shaped hemorrhages
  - Optic nerve atrophy, pallor
  - Cotton-wool spots
- Visual field defect
  - Any optic nerve or chiasmal pattern may be seen

DIFFERENTIAL DIAGNOSIS

Tumor Recurrence With Optic Nerve Compression
- Slower course of visual loss; rule out with MRI

Arachnoidal Adhesions Around Chiasm
- History of intrathecal infection or trauma

Radiation Retinopathy
- Fluorescein angiogram → vessel occlusion

Giant Cell Arteritis
- Jaw/tongue claudication, headache

EVALUATION/WORK-UP

Imaging
- T1-weighted MRI with gadolinium-diethylenetriamine pentaacetic acid (DTPA) enhancement
  - Segmental enhancement of the optic nerve, optic chiasm, or optic tracts
  - Abnormalities may be visible prior to visual loss
- Fundus fluorescein angiography may show coexisting radiation retinopathy
  - Early phase
    - Segmental narrowing of retinal arteries
    - Scattered punctuate hemorrhages
    - Retinal microaneurysms
  - Late phase
    - Capillary nonperfusion
    - Telangiectasia
    - Leakage from abnormal perifoveal capillaries
    - Macular edema
    - Stained disc

TREATMENT

Medical
- Hyperbaric oxygen (HBO) therapy
  - 100% oxygen at 2-3 atmospheres for 30-60 minutes
  - Most effective if started within 48-72 hours of vision loss
  - Reverses radiation-induced ischemic injury
    - Promotes angiogenesis in areas of hypoxia
- Glucocorticoid and anticoagulant use controversial

Follow-Up
- Serial MRIs of unaffected eye if unilateral

Prognosis
- Progression to complete blindness is common
- Rare cases of spontaneous recovery
- Early HBO associated with significant improvement and, rarely, complete recovery

Prevention
- Stereotactic radiosurgery with focused irradiation
- Consider radiation effects in treatment plans
- Frequent screening MRIs in high-risk patients

SELECTED REFERENCES

1. Zhao Z et al: Late-onset radiation-induced optic neuropathy after radiotherapy for nasopharyngeal carcinoma. J Clin Neurosci. 20(5):702-6, 2013
2. Danesh-Meyer HV: Radiation-induced optic neuropathy. J Clin Neurosci. 15(2):95-100, 2008
3. Borruat FX et al: Visual recovery from radiation-induced optic neuropathy. The role of hyperbaric oxygen therapy. J Clin Neuroophthalmol. 13(2):98-101, 1993
4. Zimmerman CF et al: Magnetic resonance imaging of radiation optic neuropathy. Am J Ophthalmol. 110(4):389-94, 1990
5. Kline LB et al: Radiation optic neuropathy. Ophthalmology. 92(8):1118-26, 1985

TRAUMATIC OPTIC NEUROPATHY

Key Facts

Introduction
- Acute injury to optic nerve caused by traumatic force
- Direct
  - Caused by actual anatomic disruption of optic nerve fibers
- Indirect
  - Results from transmission of forces (shear or compressive) to optic canal
  - Often compromises blood flow, resulting in ischemic event to nerve

Demographics
- Motor vehicle accidents are the leading cause of traumatic optic neuropathy (TON)
- Bicycle accidents
- Falls
- Assault
- Recreational and action sports

Presentation
- Funduscopy may reveal a normal-appearing optic nerve acutely
- Nerve atrophy and pallor develop by 6-8 weeks following traumatic event
- Relative afferent pupillary defect
- Visual field defects

Evaluation/Work-Up
- CT
  - Imaging test of choice for suspected TON
- MRI
  - Superior for detecting changes in soft tissue (e.g., hematoma)

Treatment
- Observation alone is current standard of care

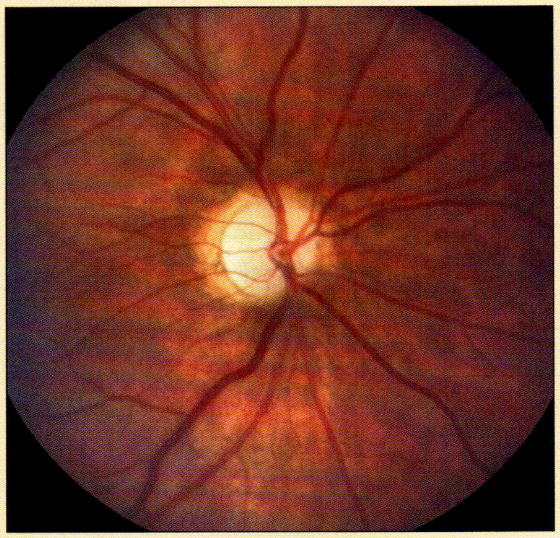

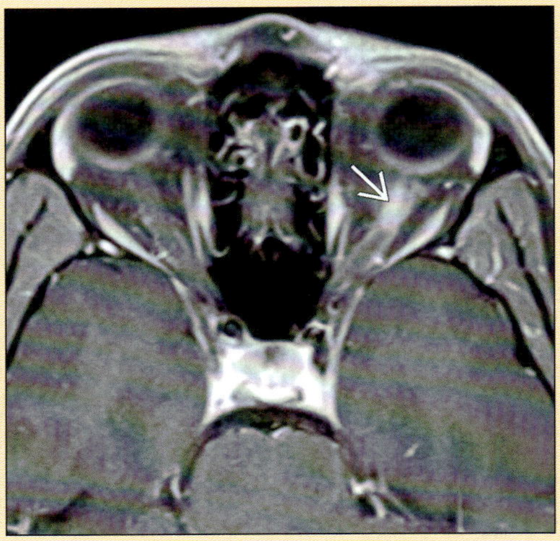

(Left) *Optic nerve pallor, as seen in this fundus photo, is a subacute finding in traumatic optic neuropathy (TON), developing roughly 6-8 weeks after the initial traumatic injury.* ***(Right)*** *Optic neuritis, which may be included in the differential diagnosis of TON, is seen in this axial T1-weighted MRI of an adult woman with left eye pain and decreased color vision. Note enhancement of the left optic nerve →. Lack of a trauma history and pain with eye movement may point toward the diagnosis of optic neuritis rather than TON.*

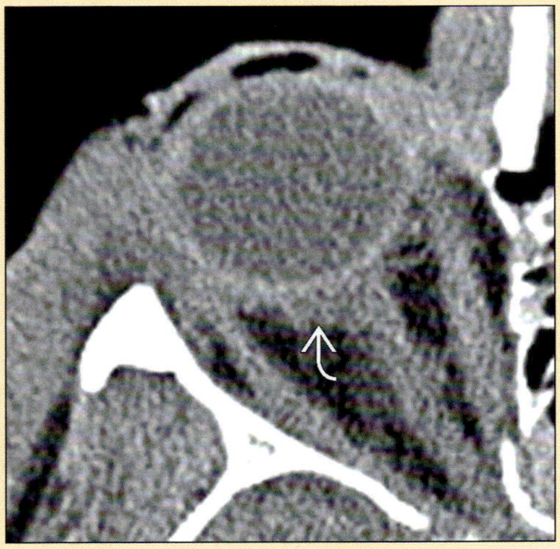

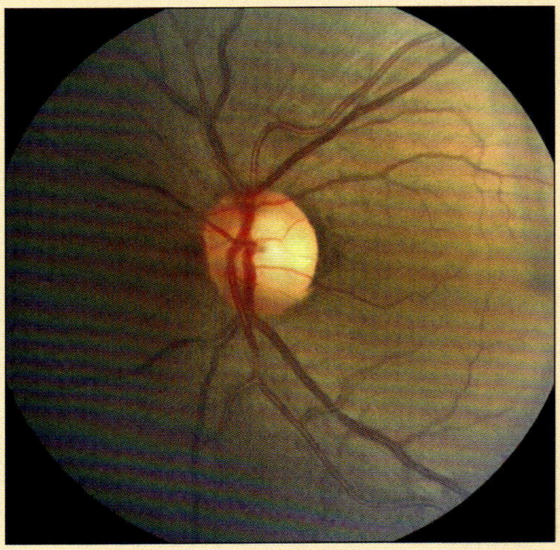

(Left) *Axial NECT shows a retrobulbar hematoma in a patient following a motor vehicle crash, indicated by abnormal density in retrobulbar fat at the optic nerve head →. If large enough, a retrobulbar hematoma can cause orbital compartment syndrome with optic nerve compression, which may clinically imitate TON and often requires urgent surgical intervention.* ***(Right)*** *This fundus photo shows optic nerve pallor in a patient with traumatic optic neuropathy.*

TRAUMATIC OPTIC NEUROPATHY

INTRODUCTION

Abbreviations
- Traumatic optic neuropathy (TON)

Definitions
- Acute injury to optic nerve caused by traumatic force

Subtypes
- Direct
  - Caused by actual anatomic disruption of optic nerve fibers
    - Penetrating orbital trauma (foreign bodies, knife and gunshot wounds)
    - Bone fragments created by blunt trauma may also result in direct injury
- Indirect
  - Results from transmission of forces (shear or compressive) to optic canal
    - Blunt trauma
  - Often compromises blood flow, resulting in ischemic event to nerve

DEMOGRAPHICS

Etiology/Risk Factors
- Motor vehicle accidents are leading cause of TON
- Bicycle accidents
- Falls
- Assault
- Recreational and action sports

Epidemiology
- Males most commonly affected (up to 85%)
- More common among young adults (mean age of onset: 34)
- Incidence of TON in closed head injuries is 0.5-5%

PRESENTATION

Symptoms
- Partial to complete vision loss
- Visual field defects
- Dyschromatopsia

Exam Findings
- Funduscopy may reveal a normal-appearing optic nerve acutely
  - Nerve atrophy and pallor develop by 6-8 weeks following traumatic event
- Relative afferent pupillary defect
- Visual field defects
- Poor visual acuity
  - Up to 60% of cases have visual acuity of light perception only, or worse

DIFFERENTIAL DIAGNOSIS

Compressive Orbital Hemorrhage
- Potentially reversible cause of traumatic visual loss
- May result in irreversible vision loss secondary to optic nerve compression without prompt surgical intervention

Optic Neuritis
- Sudden loss of vision in absence of orbital trauma
- Strong female predilection
- Often associated with multiple sclerosis

Orbital Inflammatory Conditions
- Variety of etiologies including infectious, sarcoid, thyroid eye disease, Wegener granulomatosis, or orbital pseudotumor

Compressive Neoplasm
- Often lymphoma or metastatic disease
- Evident on imaging

EVALUATION/WORK-UP

Imaging
- CT
  - Imaging test of choice for suspected TON
  - Superior for detection of optic canal fractures
- MRI
  - Superior for detecting changes in soft tissue (e.g., hematoma)

TREATMENT

Medical
- Historically, IV steroids have been used for those with severe or progressive visual loss
- The International Optic Nerve Trauma Study demonstrated no clear benefit for corticosteroid therapy in the setting of TON
  - Observation alone is current standard of care

Surgical
- Optic nerve decompression has also been performed in treatment of TON
- The International Optic Nerve Trauma Study demonstrated no clear benefit for optic nerve decompression or steroids

Prognosis
- Spontaneous visual improvement occurs in ~ 50% of indirect TON cases
- No light perception at presentation carries a very poor visual prognosis
- Visual loss is irreversible if axons are sheared or otherwise damaged

SELECTED REFERENCES

1. Yu-Wai-Man P et al: Steroids for traumatic optic neuropathy. Cochrane Database Syst Rev. (1):CD006032, 2011
2. Warner N et al: Traumatic optic neuropathy: a review of the current literature. Curr Opin Ophthalmol. 21(6):459-62, 2010
3. Levin LA et al: The treatment of traumatic optic neuropathy: the International Optic Nerve Trauma Study. Ophthalmology. 106(7):1268-77, 1999
4. Warner JE et al: Traumatic optic neuropathy. Int Ophthalmol Clin. 35(1):57-62, 1995
5. Joseph MP et al: Extracranial optic nerve decompression for traumatic optic neuropathy. Arch Ophthalmol. 108(8):1091-3, 1990

AMAUROSIS FUGAX

Key Facts

Introduction
- Transient monocular or binocular vision loss from any origin

Demographics
- Carotid artery stenosis
- Hypercoagulability disorders
- Can occur at any age
  - > age 40: Most likely secondary to atherosclerosis of the internal carotid artery
  - In children and young adults with transient vision loss, migraines must be considered

Presentation
- Due to the transient nature of the vision loss, most patients do not present for examination while experiencing vision loss
- Positive symptoms such as zig-zagging patterns, flashing lights, or visual patterns
- Negative symptoms such as blurring, dimming, fogging, blacking out of vision, shades dropping over eyes
- Painful or painless loss of vision

Treatment
- No treatment/observation if labs and examination are normal
- Treatments to decrease risk of stroke (anticoagulation)
- Treatment of migraines and autoimmune diseases (if indicated by labs)
- Carotid endarterectomy: Open or endoscopic for > 50% stenosis with symptoms
- Generally resolves spontaneously; most episodes of transient vision loss do not reoccur
- May be a warning sign of impending stroke &/or ischemic heart disease

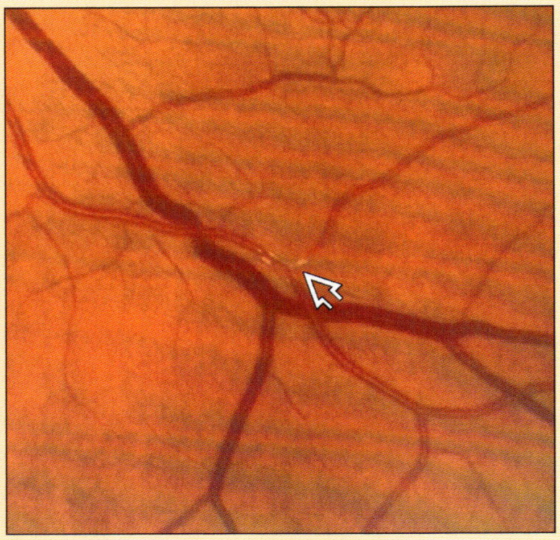
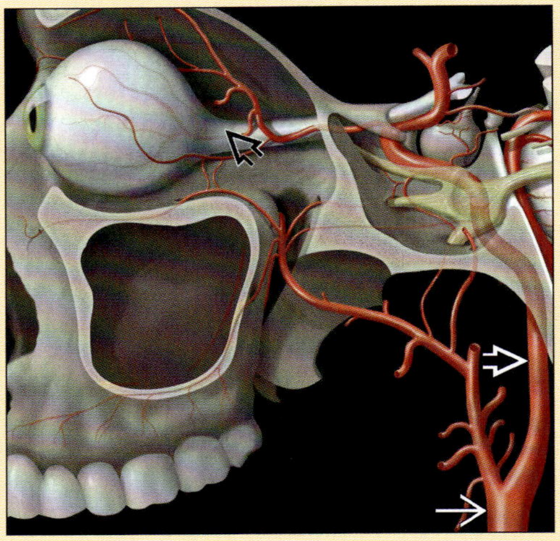

(Left) *This cholesterol Hollenhorst plaque is lodged in a bifurcation of a retinal arteriole. Most plaques originate from carotid artery (CA). Plaques lead to ischemia, which can cause visual disruption, characteristic of amaurosis fugax. (Courtesy P. Morris, MD.)* ***(Right)*** *Common locations of pathology that can lead to amaurosis fugax include the optic nerve, common CA, & internal CA. Emboli to optic nerve can cause ischemic optic neuropathy, which can be a sequela of amaurosis fugax.*

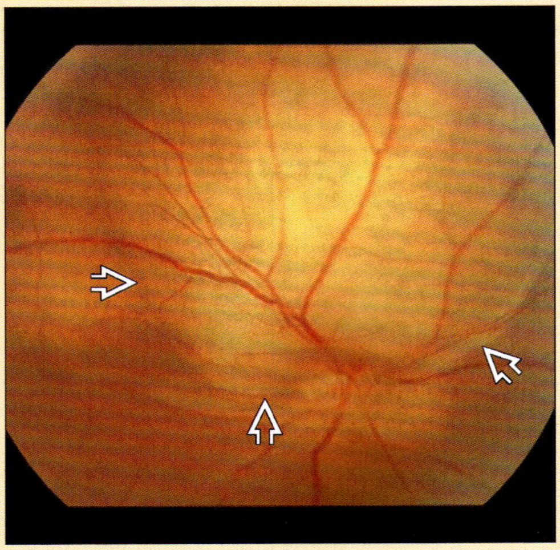
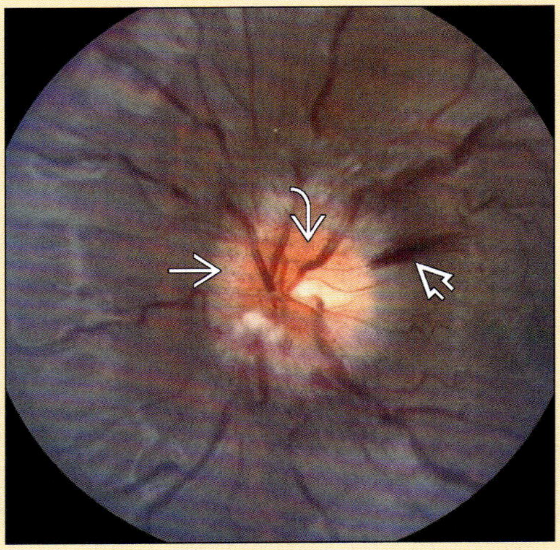

(Left) *Fundus photo shows a retinal detachment (RD), which causes distortion & loss of vision. Patients may describe RD in a way similar to amaurosis fugax. RDs can present like amaurosis fugax but are distinguished by physical examination. (Courtesy A. Vitale, MD.)* ***(Right)*** *Fundus photo shows optic disc edema. Characteristics include blurring of the optic disc margins, optic nerve hyperemia, and papillary hemorrhages. The symptoms of optic disc edema may be confused with amaurosis fugax.*

AMAUROSIS FUGAX

INTRODUCTION

Definitions
- Transient monocular or binocular vision loss from any origin

Subtypes
- Circulatory
- Ocular
- Neurologic

DEMOGRAPHICS

Etiology/Risk Factors
- Carotid artery stenosis
- Family history of stroke
- Hypercoagulability disorders
- Epilepsy

Epidemiology
- Can occur at any age
- > age 40: Most likely secondary to atherosclerosis of internal carotid artery
- In children and young adults with transient vision loss, migraines must be considered

PRESENTATION

Symptoms
- Due to transient nature of the vision loss, most patients do not present for examination while experiencing vision loss
  - Most valuable information will be gained from patient description of visual loss, including duration of episode, vision loss description, and monocular or binocular pattern
- Positive visual symptoms such as zig-zagging patterns and flashing lights
  - Gradual onset of these symptoms is indicative of migraine
  - Rapid symptom onset can indicate seizure
- Negative symptoms such as blurring, dimming, fogging, blacking out of vision, and shades dropping over eyes are more characteristic of ischemia
- Painless loss of vision
- Pain with disturbance of vision
  - Migraines, vasospasm, and hypoperfusion

Exam Findings
- Funduscopic exam
  - May show optic disc pallor, vascular abnormalities, optic nerve distortion, or embolic plaques
- Possible visual field scotomas
- ↑ IOP may indicate angle-closure glaucoma
- Carotid bruits
- Hypertension
- Hollenhorst plaque

DIFFERENTIAL DIAGNOSIS

Neurologic
- Migraine, optic neuropathies, papilledema, psychogenic, autoimmune (MS and lupus), and intracranial tumors

Circulatory
- Carotid stenosis, IV drug use, cardiac failure, hypoperfusion, coagulopathies, embolic event, inflammatory arteritis, ophthalmic artery stenosis, malignant hypertension, and choroidal or retinal artery damage

Ocular
- Retinal detachment/break, angiospasm, vasospasm, dry eyes, glaucoma, and orbital tumor

EVALUATION/WORK-UP

Labs
- ESR and CRP to rule in/out giant cell arteritis
- Consider clotting studies including
  - Factor V Leiden, antithrombin-3, partial thromboplastin time, prothrombin time, protein C and S levels

Pathology
- Temporal artery biopsy

Imaging
- Carotid duplex ultrasound and echocardiogram looking for embolic sources
- Brain MRI looking for evidence of stroke, demyelination, or intracranial tumor
- B-scan ultrasound for media opacity

TREATMENT

Medical
- No treatment/observation if labs and examination are normal
- Treatment directed to decrease risk of stroke
  - Diet, exercise, and cholesterol-lowering medications
  - Warfarin &/or other blood thinners (aspirin; ticlopidine; clopidogrel bisulfate; aspirin/extended-release dipyridamole)
- Treatment of migraines and autoimmune diseases
- Corticosteroids if inflammatory causes (e.g., temporal arteritis) are suspected

Surgical
- Carotid endarterectomy: Open or endoscopic; ACAS and NASCET trials show benefit if > 50% stenosis is present with symptoms

Follow-Up
- After initial loss of vision has been addressed, follow-up examination should focus on finding primary cause of disease

Prognosis
- Generally resolves spontaneously; most episodes of transient vision loss do not reoccur
  - May be a warning sign of impending stroke &/or ischemic heart disease

SELECTED REFERENCES

1. Hooshmand H et al: Amaurosis fugax: diagnostic and therapeutic aspects. Stroke. 5(5):643-7, 1974

ARTERITIC ISCHEMIC OPTIC NEUROPATHY

Key Facts

Introduction

- Ischemic damage to optic nerve caused by vasculitis
  - Most commonly giant cell arteritis (GCA)
- Arteritic anterior ischemic optic neuropathy (AION)
  - Most common form of AION
- Arteritic posterior ischemic optic neuropathy (A-PION)
  - Rare, a diagnosis of exclusion

Demographics

- Most common cause of blindness in GCA
- A-AION is far more common than A-PION
- Elderly; Caucasian > other races; female > male

Presentation

- Amaurosis fugax without inciting event
- Sudden, unilateral vision loss
- Eye pain, diplopia
- Systemic symptoms of GCA may **not** be present
- Exam findings depend on vascular involvement
  - Chalky white optic disc edema
  - Optic disc cupping with pale rim
  - Cotton-wool spots
  - Central retinal/cilioretinal artery occlusions

Evaluation/Work-Up

- Fluorescein fundus angiography → PCA occlusion
- Acute phase reactants: Combination ESR/CRP

Treatment

- Emergent treatment if AION is suspected
  - Immediate, high-dose systemic corticosteroids
  - Treatment should **not** be withheld for TAB
  - Continue steroids until ESR and CRP normalize
- Lifelong steroid therapy to prevent further vision loss
- Prognosis
  - Early, adequate treatment prevents vision loss
  - Vision loss in GCA is permanent

__(Left)__ This fundus photograph shows the optic nerve of a patient with arteritic anterior ischemic optic neuropathy. Note the optic nerve swelling, evidenced by obscuration of the disc margin ➔. Optic disc swelling suggests anterior rather than posterior ischemic optic neuropathy. __(Right)__ This fundus photograph of a patient with temporal arteritis demonstrates significant optic nerve swelling, evidenced by vessel obscuration ➔. Significant nerve pallor is also present.

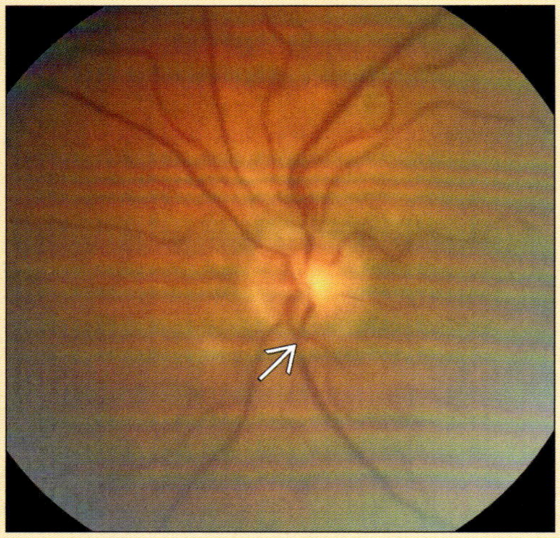

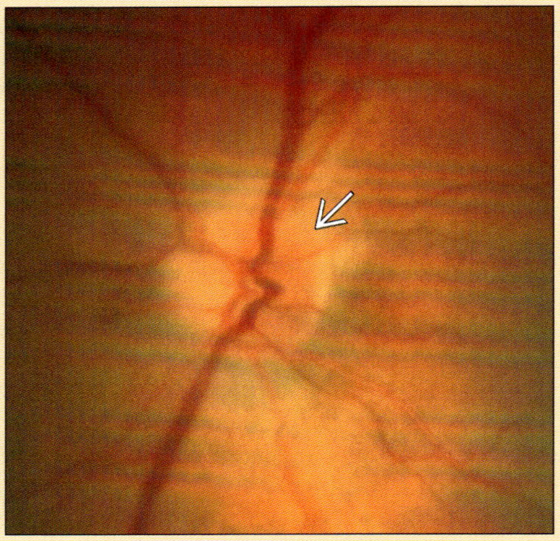

__(Left)__ This histopathologic image shows a temporal artery biopsy in giant cell arteritis. Note the presence of inflammatory cells ➔, giant cells ➔, and loss of the elastic lamina ➔, which contribute to arterial occlusion and ischemic damage. __(Right)__ This coronal CE-MRA shows an irregular long-segment stenosis of the left common carotid artery ➔ and a moderate right subclavian artery stenosis ➔ due to mural thickening. These findings are typical of giant cell arteritis involving the great vessels.

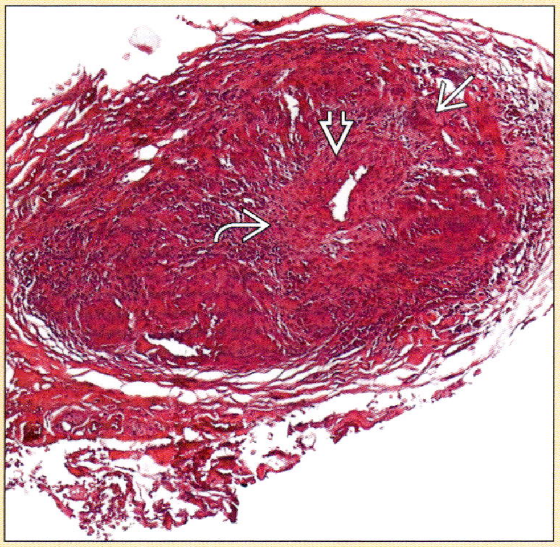

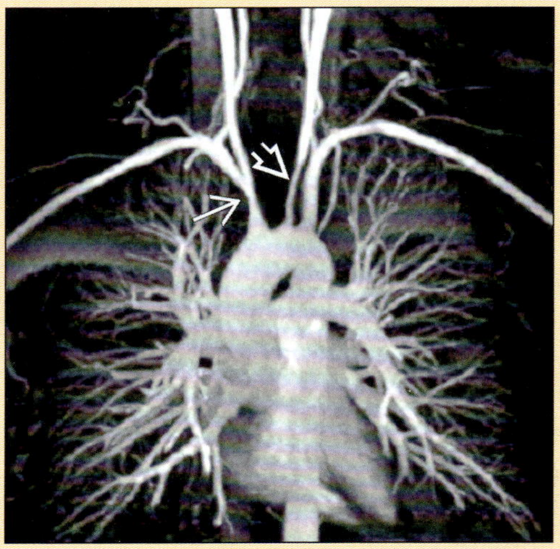

ARTERITIC ISCHEMIC OPTIC NEUROPATHY

INTRODUCTION

Abbreviations

- Arteritic anterior ischemic optic neuropathy (A-AION)
- Arteritic posterior ischemic optic neuropathy (A-PION)

Definitions

- Ischemic damage to optic nerve caused by vasculitis
  - Most commonly giant cell arteritis (GCA)

Subtypes

- A-AION: Ischemia of optic nerve head
  - Most common form of AION
  - Occlusion of posterior ciliary artery (PCA)
- A-PION: Ischemia of posterior optic nerve
  - Rare, diagnosis of exclusion
  - Several arteries involved but **not** PCA

DEMOGRAPHICS

Etiology/Risk Factors

- Elderly
- Caucasian > other races
- Female > male

Epidemiology

- Most common cause of blindness in GCA

PRESENTATION

Symptoms

- A-AION
  - Amaurosis fugax without inciting event
  - Sudden, unilateral vision loss
  - Eye pain, diplopia
  - Systemic symptoms of GCA may or may not be present
    - Jaw claudication, neck pain, headache, scalp tenderness, polymyalgia rheumatica
- A-PION
  - Sudden, painless vision loss; may be progressive

Exam Findings

- Findings depend on vascular territory involved
  - Chalky white optic disc edema
  - Optic disc cupping with pale rim
    - Appears after edema resolves
  - Cotton-wool spots
  - Central retinal artery occlusion
  - Cilioretinal artery occlusion
  - Choroidal lesions (triangle-shaped, midperiphery)
  - Visual acuity/visual field abnormalities vary
  - Afferent pupillary defect (if unilateral)
  - Anterior chamber exudate (if involved)
  - Extraocular motility dysfunction (if involved)
  - Temporal artery abnormalities
    - Tender, decreased pulse, unable to flatten

DIFFERENTIAL DIAGNOSIS

Nonarteritic Anterior Ischemic Optic Neuropathy

- No GCA, no amaurosis fugax, less severe vision loss
- No chalky white disc edema or artery occlusion
- Fluorescein fundus angiography is definitive

Nonarteritic Posterior Ischemic Optic Neuropathy

- No clinical or laboratory evidence of GCA
- Meets other criteria for A-PION

EVALUATION/WORK-UP

Labs

- Acute phase reactants
  - Erythrocyte sedimentation rate (ESR) may be markedly high to low/normal
  - Elevated C-reactive protein (CRP) is more sensitive
  - Combination ESR/CRP is most sensitive
- Complete blood count
  - Leukocytosis, thrombocytosis, anemia

Pathology

- Temporal artery biopsy (TAB)
  - ≥ 2.5 cm, ipsilateral to vision loss

Imaging

- A-AION
  - Fluorescein fundus angiography → PCA occlusion
    - Obtain early
    - Defects resolve by collateral flow
- A-PION
  - Normal fluorescein fundus angiography

TREATMENT

Medical

- Emergent treatment if AION is suspected
  - Immediate, high-dose systemic corticosteroids
  - Treatment should **not** be withheld for TAB
    - TAB should occur within ~ 7 days of steroids
  - Continue steroids until ESR and CRP stabilize, then taper steroids over 2-4 weeks
  - Lifelong steroid therapy to prevent further vision loss
    - Immunosuppressants are an alternative
  - Antiplatelet therapy with aspirin

Prognosis

- Vision loss in GCA is permanent
  - Very rarely, immediate steroids improve vision slightly
- Early, adequate treatment prevents vision loss
- Lifelong steroid therapy prevents further vision loss

SELECTED REFERENCES

1. Hayreh SS: Ischemic optic neuropathy. Prog Retin Eye Res. 28(1):34-62, 2009
2. Fontal MR et al: Ischemic optic neuropathy. Semin Neurol. 27(3):221-32, 2007
3. Hayreh SS: Posterior ischaemic optic neuropathy: clinical features, pathogenesis, and management. Eye (Lond). 18(11):1188-206, 2004
4. Arnold AC et al: Treatment of ischemic optic neuropathy. Semin Ophthalmol. 17(1):39-46, 2002

NONARTERITIC ISCHEMIC OPTIC NEUROPATHY

Key Facts

Introduction

- Vision loss resulting from infarction of optic nerve due to compromise in circulation to anterior optic nerve
- Subtypes
  - Nonprogressive NAION
  - Progressive NAION

Demographics

- Associated risk factors
  - Atherosclerosis, hyperlipidemia, diabetes, hypertension
  - Nocturnal hypotension
  - Obstructive sleep apnea
  - Smoking
  - Typically, age > 50 years

Presentation

- Sudden decrease in visual acuity, often upon awakening
- Visual field defects, classically altitudinal
- Segmental or diffuse disc edema
- Flame-shaped hemorrhages
- "Crowded" discs

Evaluation/Work-Up

- Consider lipid profile, glucose tolerance, and blood pressure; echocardiogram; carotid ultrasound

Treatment

- No proven treatment for NAION
- Carotid endarterectomy may prevent future episodes if there is stenosis
- Aspirin has not been shown to decrease risk
- Visual function usually remains stable after initial decrease in vision
- 5-year risk of contralateral involvement is 15%

(Left) *Funduscopic image demonstrates classic appearance of nonarteritic anterior ischemic optic neuropathy (NAION). Optic disc blurring along inferior margin reveals segmental edema. A characteristic flame-shaped hemorrhage is also present. Note the small cup indicative of a crowded disc.* ***(Right)*** *This fundus photo of stage V papilledema and multiple hemorrhages demonstrates the extent of optic disc involvement possible with NAION.*

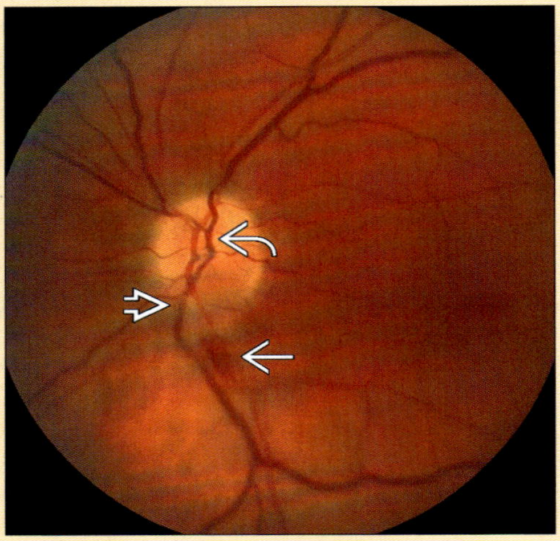

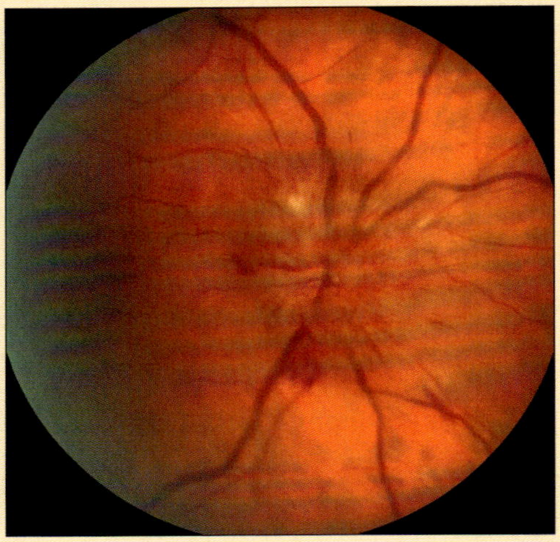

(Left) *Fundus photo shows the right eye of a 58-year-old man following a diagnosis of NAION. The photo reveals segmental pallor of the optic nerve, which typically develops 6-8 weeks after the initial onset of NAION.* ***(Right)*** *Central 24-2 Humphrey visual field threshold testing was subsequently performed on the same eye. Testing revealed a corresponding inferior visual field defect.*

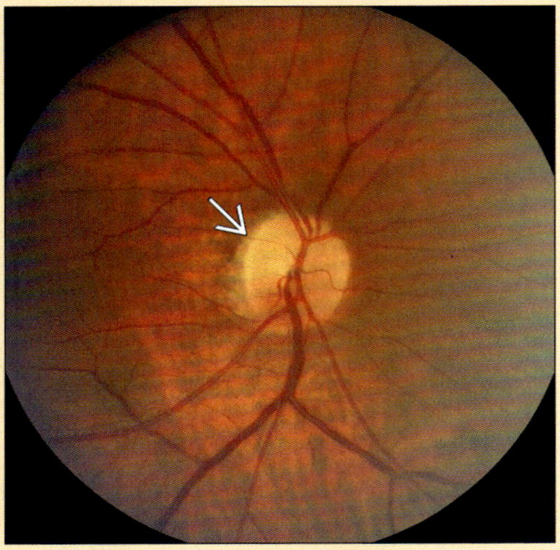

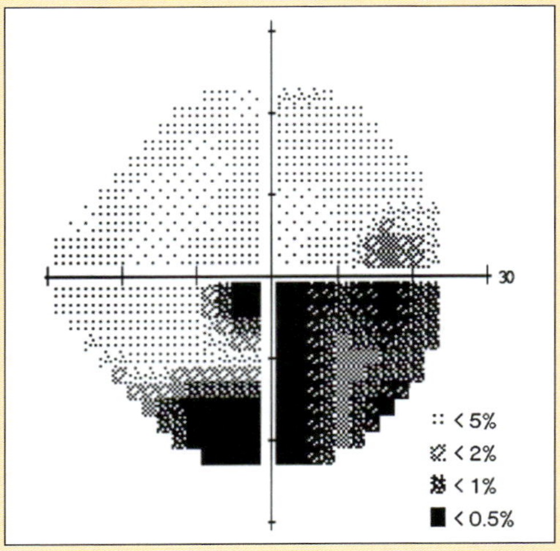

NONARTERITIC ISCHEMIC OPTIC NEUROPATHY

INTRODUCTION

Abbreviations
- Nonarteritic anterior ischemic optic neuropathy (NAION)

Definitions
- Vision loss resulting from infarction of optic nerve due to compromise of short posterior ciliary arteries

Subtypes
- Nonprogressive NAION
- Progressive NAION
  - Progressive decrease in visual acuity or field for 3-4 weeks following initial insult
  - As many as 30% of cases

DEMOGRAPHICS

Etiology/Risk Factors
- Associated risk factors
  - "Crowded" discs
  - Atherosclerosis, hyperlipidemia, diabetes, hypertension
  - Obstructive sleep apnea
  - Nocturnal hypotension
  - Smoking

Epidemiology
- Typically age > 50 years

PRESENTATION

Symptoms
- Sudden decrease in visual acuity, often upon awakening
- Visual field defects (altitudinal more common than central)
- Dyschromatopsia

Exam Findings
- Segmental or diffuse disc edema
- Hyperemic disc, which later becomes pale
- Flame-shaped hemorrhages
- Focal narrowing of retinal arterioles in peripapillary region
- Contralateral optic disc is usually small with accompanying small or absent physiologic cup ("disc at risk")
- Atrophy of optic disc in 4-8 weeks

DIFFERENTIAL DIAGNOSIS

Arteritic Ischemic Optic Neuropathy
- Associated headache, jaw claudication, and scalp tenderness
- Elevated ESR, CRP secondary to temporal arteritis

Optic Neuritis
- Typically age < 40 years
- Pain with eye movement

Orbital Mass
- May compress optic nerve

Diabetic Papillopathy
- Diabetic retinopathy often present

EVALUATION/WORK-UP

Labs
- Normal ESR (in contrast to elevated value found in arteritic ischemic optic neuropathy)
  - Always check ESR to exclude temporal arteritis
- Consider lipid profile, glucose tolerance, and blood pressure

Imaging
- Fluorescein angiography
  - May be helpful in unclear cases
  - 75% of NAION cases demonstrate delayed optic disc filling
- Contrast-enhanced MRI
  - Normal in NAION
- Echocardiogram and carotid ultrasound

TREATMENT

Medical
- No proven treatment for NAION
- Aspirin has not been shown to decrease risk
- Neuroprotective agents (e.g., brimonidine)
- Avoid BP medications at night (nocturnal hypotension)

Surgical
- Ischemic Optic Neuropathy Decompression Trial showed no benefit to surgery
- North American Symptomatic Carotid Endarterectomy Trial (NASCET) and Asymptomatic Carotid Atherosclerosis Study (ACAS)
  - Showed no benefit to carotid endarterectomy (if < 50% stenosis) for preventing future embolic events

Follow-Up
- Optic nerve edema resolves in 6-8 weeks
- 1/3 of patients may show mild improvement in vision

Prognosis
- Visual function usually remains stable after initial decrease in vision
- 5-year risk of contralateral involvement is 15%
- Recurrent visual loss in affected eye after 3 months is uncommon (6%)

SELECTED REFERENCES

1. Wilhelm B et al: Efficacy and tolerability of 0.2% brimonidine tartrate for the treatment of acute non-arteritic anterior ischemic optic neuropathy (NAION): a 3-month, double-masked, randomised, placebo-controlled trial. Graefes Arch Clin Exp Ophthalmol. 244(5):551-8, 2006
2. Newman NJ et al: The fellow eye in NAION: report from the ischemic optic neuropathy decompression trial follow-up study. Am J Ophthalmol. 134(3):317-28, 2002
3. Hayreh SS et al: Ipsilateral recurrence of nonarteritic anterior ischemic optic neuropathy. Am J Ophthalmol. 132(5):734-42, 2001
4. Optic nerve decompression surgery for nonarteritic anterior ischemic optic neuropathy (NAION) is not effective and may be harmful: The Ischemic Optic Neuropathy Decompression Trial Research Group. JAMA. 273(8):625-32, 1995

COMPRESSIVE OPTIC NEUROPATHY

Key Facts

Introduction

- Consider glioma, meningioma, arteriovenous malformations, infections, granulomas, leukemia, hemorrhage, trauma
- Decreased vision due to compression of optic nerve
  - Compression of nerve leads to ischemia and mechanical damage, ultimately resulting in decreased vision

Demographics

- Patients with intracranial/intraorbital tumors or Graves disease

Presentation

- Gradual or acute onset of vision loss
  - Can be binocular or monocular
- Headaches and eye pain
- Constriction/decrease of visual fields in affected eye(s)
- Funduscopic examination revealing
  - Optic nerve atrophy
  - Optic disc edema

Evaluation/Work-Up

- Lumbar puncture with CNS fluid cytology and culture after MRI to rule out mass effect
- TSH and T4 blood analysis for thyroid disease
- Optic nerve biopsy if malignant lesion is suspected
- Optic nerve MRI
- Head CT with and without contrast

Treatment

- Systemic corticosteroids to decrease inflammation around optic nerve
- Optic nerve decompression
- Removal of tumor
- Systemic antibiotics if cause is infectious

*(**Left**) This axial T2-weighted MRI of the left orbit shows a cavernous hemangioma ➡. The mass is impinging on the lateral side of the optic nerve sheath ➡. (**Right**) Two of the funduscopic findings characteristic of compressive optic neuropathy (CON) are pallor and edema ➡ of the optic disc.*

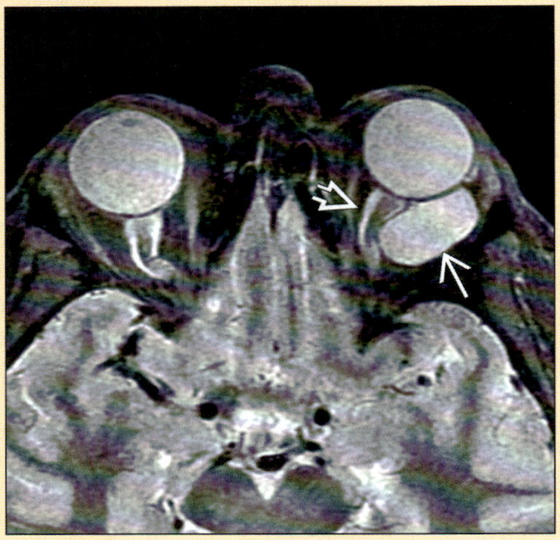

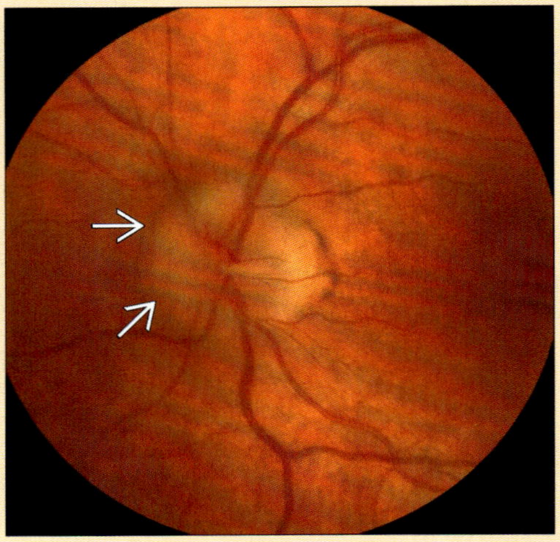

*(**Left**) There are several visual field defects that can occur in CON. In this graphic, black illustrates an area of lost/decreased vision. Visual field "A" represents bitemporal hemianopsia, while "B" illustrates right monocular blindness, and left homonymous hemianopsia is shown in "C". (**Right**) This is an axial T1WI MRI of a patient with thyroid orbitopathy. This MRI reveals increased orbital fat ➡, which causes proptosis, and compression of the optic nerve ➡.*

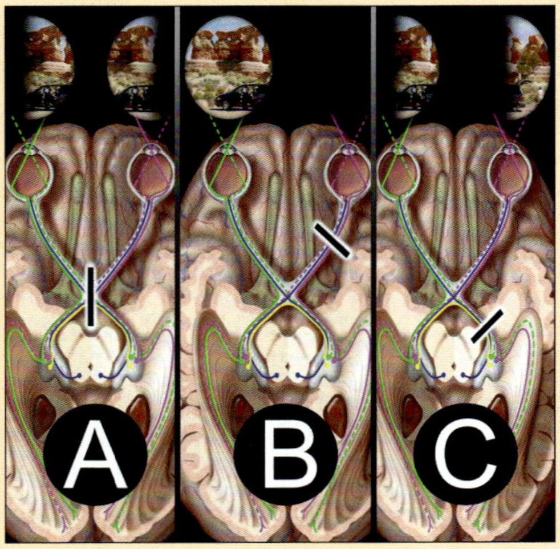

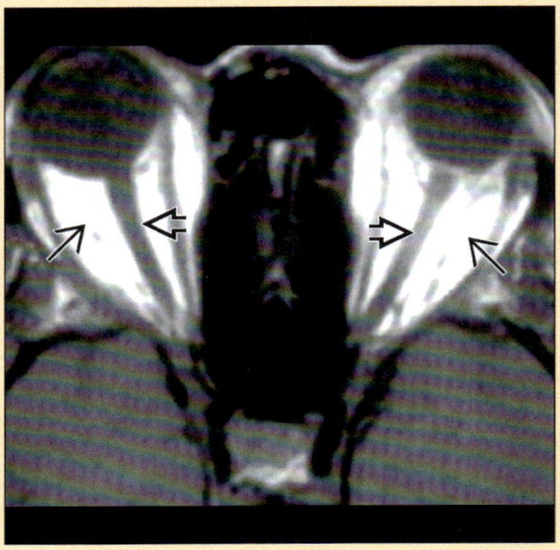

COMPRESSIVE OPTIC NEUROPATHY

INTRODUCTION

Abbreviations
- Compressive optic neuropathy (CON)

Definitions
- Decreased vision due to compression of optic nerve

Subtypes
- Traumatic
- Neoplastic
- Infectious
- Autoimmune

DEMOGRAPHICS

Etiology/Risk Factors
- Caused by anything that impinges on optic nerve
  - Can include inflammation or space-occupying mass in intraorbital or intracranial space that compresses optic nerve
    - Compression of nerve leads to ischemia and mechanical damage, ultimately resulting in decreased vision
- Risk factors include
  - Graves thyroiditis
  - Eye infection leading to orbital cellulitis
  - Orbital trauma resulting in swelling of tissues around optic nerve
  - Intracranial/intraorbital tumors

PRESENTATION

Symptoms
- Gradual or acute onset of vision loss
  - Can be binocular or monocular
- Headaches and eye pain
- Decreased vision that changes with eye movement

Exam Findings
- Afferent pupillary defect in affected eye
- Funduscopic examination reveals
  - Optociliary shunt vessels
  - Choroidal folds
  - Foster-Kennedy syndrome, which occurs when a frontal lobe tumor causes
    - Optic nerve edema in the contralateral eye caused by acutely elevated intracranial pressure
    - Optic nerve atrophy in ipsilateral eye due to chronic pressure of tumor on nerve
      - Pseudo-Foster-Kennedy syndrome is due to sequential ischemic optic neuropathy
- Visual fields testing
  - Constriction/decrease of visual fields in affected eye(s)
- Exophthalmos, ↓ extraocular motility, ↓ color vision

DIFFERENTIAL DIAGNOSIS

Glaucoma
- Can also present with gradual onset vision loss
  - Orbital MRI/CT will be negative for presence of mass/inflammation compressing optic nerve
- Patients will often have family history of glaucoma

Pseudotumor Cerebri
- Gradual vision loss due to increased intracranial pressure
  - Cerebrospinal fluid pressure is increased
  - Normal CNS imaging
  - Papilledema present on funduscopic exam
- Most common in overweight females

Leber Hereditary Optic Neuropathy
- Male patients with positive family history of vision loss
  - Vision loss is very gradual, often occurring over several months

EVALUATION/WORK-UP

Labs
- Lumbar puncture with CNS fluid cytology and culture
- TSH and T4 blood analysis for thyroid disease

Pathology
- Optic nerve biopsy
  - Can be performed if vision is declining rapidly, eye is blind, or there is suspicion of a malignant lesion (e.g., glioma, neurofibroma, or lymphoma)

Imaging
- Orbital MRI
- Head CT with and without contrast
  - Contrast is useful if carotid or ophthalmic artery aneurysm is suspected

TREATMENT

Medical
- Systemic corticosteroids to decrease inflammation around optic nerve
- Graves treatment with methimazole (Tapazole) and propylthiouracil
- Systemic antibiotics if cause of CON is infectious

Surgical
- Optic nerve decompression
- Removal of intracranial or intraorbital tumor
- Removal of thyroid gland in Graves disease

Follow-Up
- Depends on etiology and clinical course

Prognosis
- Good if identified early
- Vision generally returns with prompt treatment
  - May lead to blindness if left untreated
- Rapid onset of vision loss holds worse prognosis than gradual onset

SELECTED REFERENCES

1. Tourbah A: Contribution of imaging to the diagnosis of optic neuropathies. Rev Neurol (Paris). 168(10):702-5, 2012
2. Bulters DO et al: Visual recovery following optic nerve decompression for chronic compressive neuropathy. Acta Neurochir (Wien). 151(4):325-34, 2009
3. Behbehani R: Clinical approach to optic neuropathies. Clin Ophthalmol. 1(3):233-46, 2007

DIABETIC PAPILLOPATHY

Key Facts

Introduction
- Diagnosis of exclusion
- Occurs in patients with diabetes and is characterized by transient unilateral or bilateral hyperemic disc edema with minimal or no visual loss
- Normal intracranial pressure
- Absence of infection or infiltration

Demographics
- Pathogenesis of diabetic papillopathy (DP) is uncertain
- Associated with small cup to disc ratio
- Unclear relationship between DP and metabolic control
- < 150 cases of DP have been described in literature
- Some believe this disease to be on spectrum of nonarteritic anterior ischemic optic neuropathy (NAION) and, therefore, progression to NAION may occur

Presentation
- Commonly asymptomatic
- Blurry vision or distortion may occur
- 70-100% of patients with acuity deficits have comorbid pathology (e.g., diabetic retinopathy &/or macular edema)
- Optic disc edema may be unilateral or bilateral
- Dilation of optic disc vasculature
- Optic nerve vessels have a radiating pattern in contrast to neovascularization of the optic disc

Evaluation/Work-Up
- Fluorescein angiogram

Treatment
- Condition is most often considered benign with minimal long-term vision changes
- Vision changes are usually transient

*(**Left**) This fundus photograph shows diabetic papillopathy (DP). Note the blurring edge of the optic disc ➔, suggesting edema of the optic cup. (**Right**) This fundus photograph shows papilledema and bulging of the optic disc. Note the dilation of the inner optic disc vasculature ➔. This is a common finding in diabetic papillopathy.*

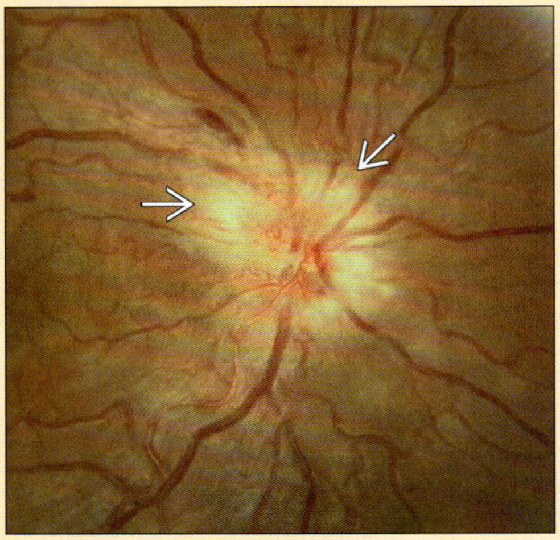

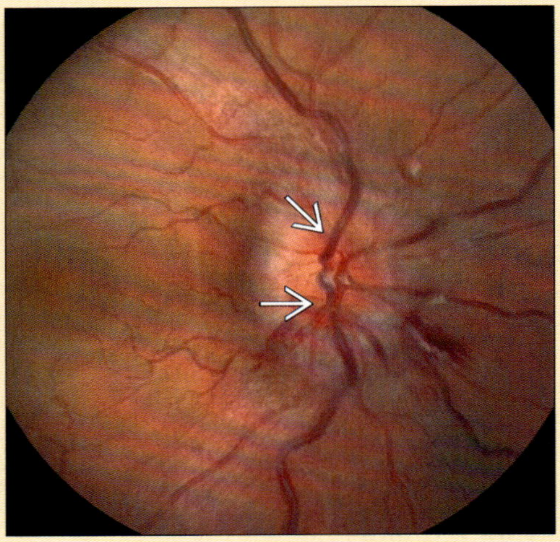

*(**Left**) This fundus photography shows diabetic papillopathy. Note how the vessels appear to rise as they protrude from the optic disc ➔, suggesting optic disc swelling. (**Right**) This fundus photograph shows optic disc swelling ➔. Note the bulging appearance of the optic cup. Optic disc edema is always present in diabetic papillopathy.*

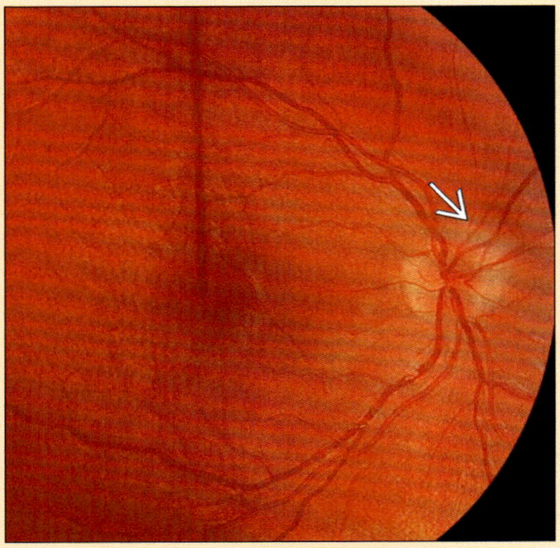

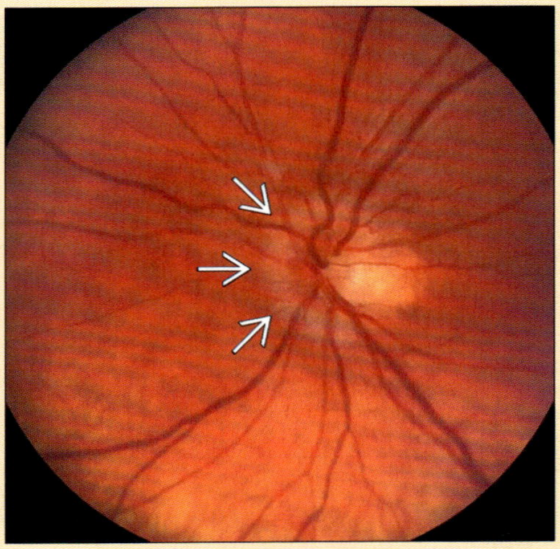

DIABETIC PAPILLOPATHY

INTRODUCTION

Abbreviations
- Diabetic papillopathy (DP)

Definitions
- Diagnosis of exclusion
- Occurs in patients with diabetes and is characterized by transient unilateral or bilateral hyperemic disc edema with minimal or no visual loss

DEMOGRAPHICS

Etiology/Risk Factors
- Pathogenesis of DP is uncertain
- Associated with small cup to disc ratio
- Unclear relationship between DP and metabolic control
  - Recent study shows potential association between drastic recent reduction in glycemia and development of DP
- Occurs in patients with normal intracranial pressure in absence of infection or infiltration
- Some authors believe DP represents a mild form of nonarteritic anterior ischemic optic neuropathy (NAION)

Epidemiology
- < 150 cases of DP have been described in literature

PRESENTATION

Symptoms
- Commonly asymptomatic
- Blurry vision

Exam Findings
- Visual acuity normal or mildly abnormal
  - 70-100% of patients with acuity deficits have comorbid pathology (e.g., diabetic retinopathy &/or macular edema)
- Fundus exam
  - Optic disc swelling
  - Dilation of optic disc vasculature
  - Optic nerve vessels have a radiating pattern in contrast to neovascularization of the optic disc

DIFFERENTIAL DIAGNOSIS

Nonarteritic Anterior Ischemic Optic Neuropathy (NAION)
- Sudden onset and permanent vision loss
- Vision changes include scotomas and dyschromatopsia
- Afferent pupil defect
- Delayed filling of optic disc common with late leakage of the optic nerve in fluorescein angiography

Increased Intracranial Pressure
- Neuroimaging and lumbar puncture should rule out suspected etiologies

Optic Disc Neovascularization
- Abnormal vasculature will be superior to plane of optic disc and vessels are usually randomly oriented

Malignant Hypertension
- Severely elevated blood pressure
- Hemorrhages, exudates, cotton-wool spots visualized in posterior pole

Papillitis
- Loss of vision and abnormal pupillary reflex
- Pain with eye movement is common
- Vasculitis, viral syndromes, syphilis, toxoplasmosis, sarcoidosis, and Lyme disease possible

Central Retinal Vein Occlusion
- Occlusion of central retinal vein may be related to chronic glaucoma, atherosclerotic risk factors, or coagulopathy
- Disc is enlarged and hemorrhages are evident

Papillophlebitis
- Central retinal vein occlusion occurring in young healthy adults
- Spontaneous improvement is common

Iatrogenic
- Disc swelling after eye surgery

EVALUATION/WORK-UP

Labs
- CBC and lumbar puncture to rule out infection
- ESR and ANA testing to rule out autoimmune causes

Imaging
- Fluorescein angiogram
- MRI or lumbar puncture if there is concern for ↑ intracranial pressure or optic neuritis

TREATMENT

Medical
- Condition is usually benign with minimal long-term vision loss
- Occasionally, periocular or intravitreal injections of corticosteroids are used to prevent associated macular edema and prevent progression to NAION
- Treat diabetes and diabetic retinopathy as indicated

Follow-Up
- Monitoring is recommended to evaluate for resolution of disc swelling and changes in vision

Prognosis
- Vision changes are often transient
- Some believe this disease to be on spectrum of NAION and, therefore, progression to NAION may occur

SELECTED REFERENCES

1. Ostri C et al: Bilateral diabetic papillopathy and metabolic control. Ophthalmology. 117(11):2214-7, 2010
2. Slagle WS et al: Diabetic papillopathy and its relation to optic nerve ischemia. Optom Vis Sci. 86(4):e395-403, 2009
3. Bayraktar Z et al: Diabetic papillopathy in type II diabetic patients. Retina. 22(6):752-8, 2002
4. Regillo CD et al: Diabetic papillopathy. Patient characteristics and fundus findings. Arch Ophthalmol. 113(7):889-95, 1995

PAPILLEDEMA

Key Facts

Introduction

- Swelling of optic nerve head secondary to increased intracranial pressure (ICP)
- Optic nerve swelling secondary to causes other than increased ICP is referred to as "optic nerve edema" and is **not** papilledema

Demographics

- Increased ICP may be caused by
  - Idiopathic intracranial hypertension (IIH)
  - Mass effect
  - CSF abnormalities
  - Medications
  - Cerebral edema secondary to blunt head trauma
  - Severe systemic hypertension
  - Craniosynostosis

Presentation

- Visual obscurations, double vision, field defects (often enlarged blind spot)
- Headaches, worse in recumbent position
- Nausea and vomiting
- Pulsatile tinnitus or vascular "whooshing" sounds
- Bilateral swelling of optic nerves (may be asymmetric)
- Disc hyperemia and hemorrhages
- Absent venous pulsations
- Paton lines (retinochoroidal folds) may develop

Evaluation/Work-Up

- Lumbar puncture (performed to confirm elevated ICP and rule out a meningeal process)
- All patients with papilledema need to rule out an intracranial space-occupying lesion
  - CNS imaging (CT or MRI)

__(Left)__ Slit-lamp photo demonstrates very early (stage 1) papilledema with obscuration of the nasal disc border but preservation of the temporal disc border. Differential diagnosis for optic nerve edema is broad but includes optic nerve head drusen, anterior optic neuropathy, optic neuritis, and diabetic papillopathy. __(Right)__ Slit-lamp photo shows early (stage 2) papilledema, with obscuration of all disc margins and mild elevation nasally. Optic nerve edema may be asymmetric early in disease course.

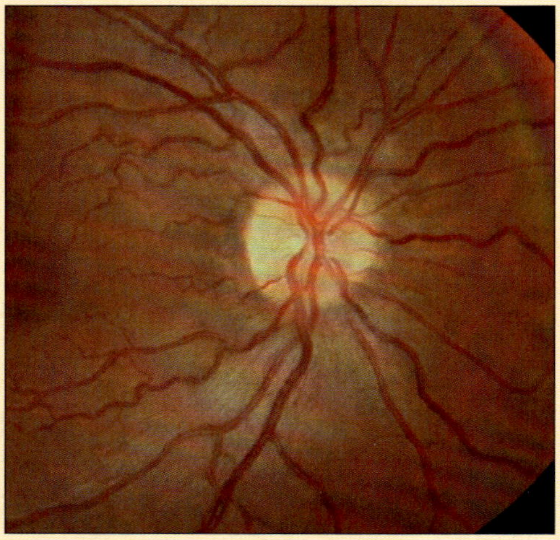

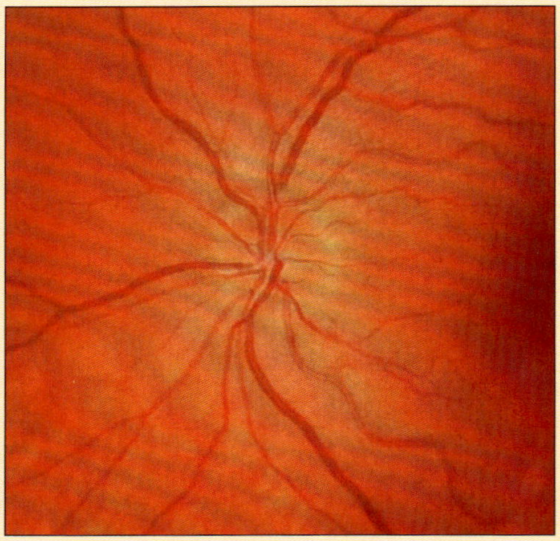

__(Left)__ Slit-lamp photo shows papilledema in a 34-year-old woman with idiopathic intracranial hypertension. This photo demonstrates stage 3 papilledema, with obscuration of all disc borders and increased optic nerve head diameter. __(Right)__ Slit-lamp photo shows marked (stage 4) papilledema, characterized by elevation of the entire optic nerve head. Note obliteration of blood vessels ➔. Symptoms of papilledema include transient visual obscurations, often brought on by standing or bending over.

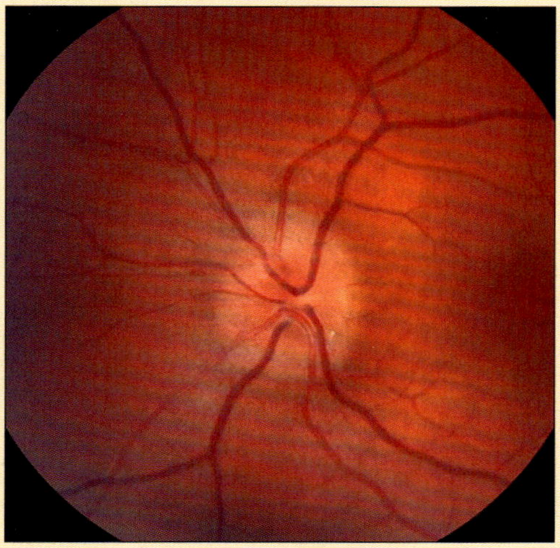

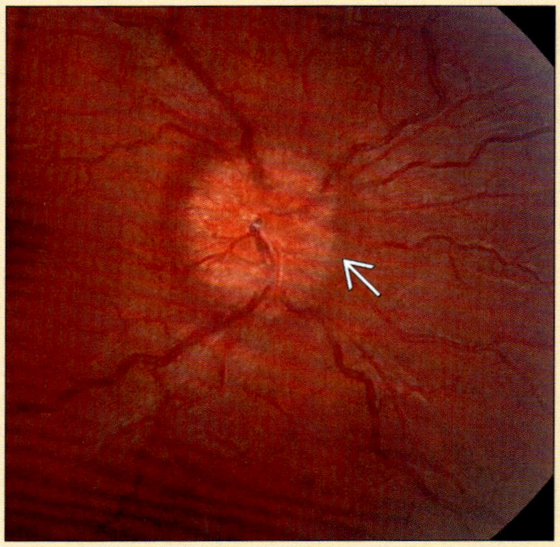

PAPILLEDEMA

INTRODUCTION

Definitions

- Swelling of optic nerve head secondary to increased intracranial pressure (ICP)
  - Optic nerve swelling secondary to causes other than increased ICP is referred to as "optic nerve edema" and is **not** papilledema
- Normal ICP < 250 mm water

Subtypes

- Papilledema grading system (Frisen scale)
  - Stage 1: Very early papilledema
    - Obscuration of nasal disc border without elevation
    - Concentric or radial retrochoroidal folds
  - Stage 2: Early papilledema
    - Obscuration of all disc borders with elevation nasally
  - Stage 3: Moderate papilledema
    - Obscuration of all borders with increased diameter of optic nerve head
  - Stage 4: Marked papilledema
    - Elevation of entire nerve head
  - Stage 5: Severe papilledema
    - Dome-shaped protrusions representing anterior expansion of optic nerve head
    - Obliteration of optic cup
- Papilledema may be further classified as acute (days-weeks) or chronic (month-years)

DEMOGRAPHICS

Etiology/Risk Factors

- Increased ICP may be caused by
  - Idiopathic intracranial hypertension (IIH)
    - Strong female predilection
    - Most patients with IIH are overweight or obese
  - Mass effect
    - Intracranial tumor
    - Hemorrhage
      - Subdural and epidural hematomas
    - Cerebral venous sinus thrombosis
    - Brain abscess
  - CSF abnormalities
    - Obstructive hydrocephalus
      - Congenital
      - Acquired
    - Decreased CSF absorption due to arachnoid villi impairment
      - Meningitis
      - Trauma
      - Subarachnoid hemorrhage
      - Venous sinus thrombosis
    - CSF hypersecretion by choroid plexus tumor
  - Medications
    - Tetracyclines
    - Vitamin A
    - Steroids
    - Cyclosporine
    - Oral contraceptives
    - Nalidixic acid
  - Cerebral edema secondary to blunt head trauma
  - Severe systemic hypertension
  - Craniosynostosis

PRESENTATION

Symptoms

- Visual obscurations, diplopia, field defects
- Headaches, worst in recumbent position
- Nausea and vomiting
- Pulsatile tinnitus or vascular "whooshing" sounds

Exam Findings

- Bilateral swelling of optic nerves
  - May be asymmetric (especially early in process)
  - Absent venous pulsations
- Disc hyperemia or hemorrhages
- Splinter hemorrhages, cotton-wool spots, or hard exudates may be present
- Severe disc leakage
  - May result in formation of macular star
- Paton lines (retinochoroidal folds) may develop
- Horizontal diplopia
  - Unilateral or bilateral 6th nerve palsy may result from increased ICP
- Field defects
- Longstanding papilledema may result in
  - Disc losing hyperemic appearance and instead becomes pale from chronic axonal loss
  - Gliosis of peripapillary nerve fiber layer (NFL)
    - Grayish appearance
    - Gliosis frequently follows vascular distribution, resulting in vascular sheathing
  - Development of optociliary shunt vessels
  - Refractile bodies may develop on disc surface
    - Formed by lipid-rich exudates
    - Similar in appearance to optic nerve drusen
  - Permanent vision loss

DIFFERENTIAL DIAGNOSIS

Anterior Optic Neuropathy

- Most often monocular (resulting in relative afferent pupillary defect [RAPD])
- Etiology may include
  - Ischemic
  - Inflammatory
  - Infiltrative
  - Compressive

Pseudopapilledema

- Optic nerve drusen
  - Optic nerves appear elevated
  - Result from refractile and often calcified nodules within optic nerve head
  - Most patients are asymptomatic, but visual obscurations have been reported
  - B-scan ultrasonography or fluorescein angiography may be used to help distinguish calcified drusen from true papilledema
- Tilted or hypoplastic discs
- Leber hereditary optic neuropathy
  - Typically affects males age 10-30 years
  - Fluorescein angiography reveals no leakage or staining of disc

- Related to mitochondrial DNA mutation
- Family history

Central Retinal Vein Occlusion
- Painless and sudden vision loss
- Usually unilateral with very dilated veins
- Dense nerve-fiber layer hemorrhages
- Fluorescein angiogram confirms diagnosis

Optic Neuritis
- Temporary inflammation of optic nerve
- Most often unilateral, but may present with bilateral inflammation
- Periorbital pain associated with eye movement
- Commonly associated with multiple sclerosis
- F:M = 2:1

Hypertensive Optic Neuropathy
- Bilateral flame-shaped hemorrhages, arteriolar narrowing, disc edema, and cotton-wool spots
- Elevated blood pressure

Diabetic Papillopathy
- Vision may be normal or decreased
- Associated retinopathy is present in > 2/3 of patients with diabetic papillopathy
  - Diabetic retinopathy is manifest by presence of microaneurysms, dot-and-blot hemorrhages, exudate, cotton-wool spots, and possible vitreous hemorrhage
  - Neovascularization of disc/retina/iris/angle may ensue
- Systemic findings of diabetes

Papillophlebitis
- Unilateral retinal venous congestion with associated optic disc edema
- Occurs in healthy, young patients
- Typically resolves spontaneously within a year
  - Little to no visual impairment retained following resolution

EVALUATION/WORK-UP

Labs
- Lumbar puncture with opening pressure (performed to confirm elevated ICP and rule out meningeal process)
  - Labs to include
    - Glucose
    - Protein
    - Cell count and differential
  - Culture

Imaging
- All patients with papilledema require imaging to rule out intracranial space-occupying lesion
  - CNS imaging (CT or MRI)
    - Used to rule out CNS mass lesion
    - Consider MRI venography for venous sinus thrombosis
- B-scan ultrasonography
  - May be used to confirm enlarged optic nerve diameter
  - Used to identify drusen
- Fluorescein angiography
  - Preformed to detect disc leakage
- Fundus photos

TREATMENT

Medical
- Underlying cause should be addressed
  - If medications (e.g., tetracyclines, steroids) are implicated, discontinue
- Acetalzolaminde and Lasix
  - In addition to weight loss, mainstay of treatment for IIH
- Emergent causes must be considered, assessed, and ruled out with urgency

Surgical
- Surgery may be considered depending on underlying etiology
- Intracranial mass lesion may require
  - Ventriculoperitoneal or lumboperitoneal shunts
  - Optic nerve sheath fenestration
    - Will decompress optic nerve but typically does not resolve headaches

Prognosis
- Varies widely with underlying etiology

SELECTED REFERENCES

1. Thurtell MJ et al: Idiopathic intracranial hypertension (pseudotumor cerebri): recognition, treatment, and ongoing management. Curr Treat Options Neurol. 15(1):1-12, 2013
2. Wall M: Idiopathic intracranial hypertension and the idiopathic intracranial hypertension treatment trial. J Neuroophthalmol. 33(1):1-3, 2013
3. Abubaker K et al: Idiopathic intracranial hypertension: lumboperitoneal shunts versus ventriculoperitoneal shunts--case series and literature review. Br J Neurosurg. 25(1):94-9, 2011
4. Lam BL et al: Drusen of the optic disc. Curr Neurol Neurosci Rep. 8(5):404-8, 2008
5. Trick GL et al: Quantitative evaluation of papilledema in pseudotumor cerebri. Invest Ophthalmol Vis Sci. 39(10):1964-71, 1998

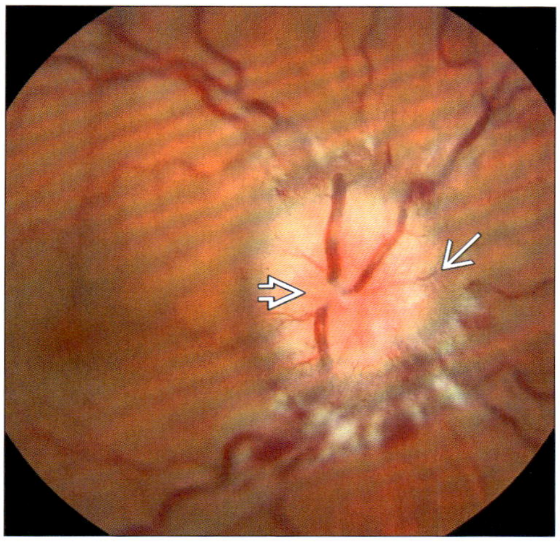

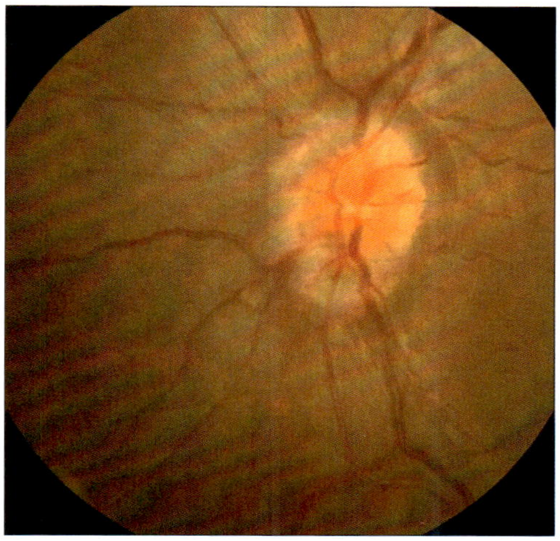

(Left) *Slit-lamp photo shows severe (stage 5) papilledema. Note complete obliteration of the optic cup* → *and significant anterior protrusion of the optic nerve head. There is also complete obscuration of the vessels* →. ***(Right)*** *Fundus photo shows hypertensive papillitis, which is 1 differential consideration when papilledema is suspected. It is important to note that papilledema refers only to optic nerve edema secondary to elevated intracranial pressure (ICP).*

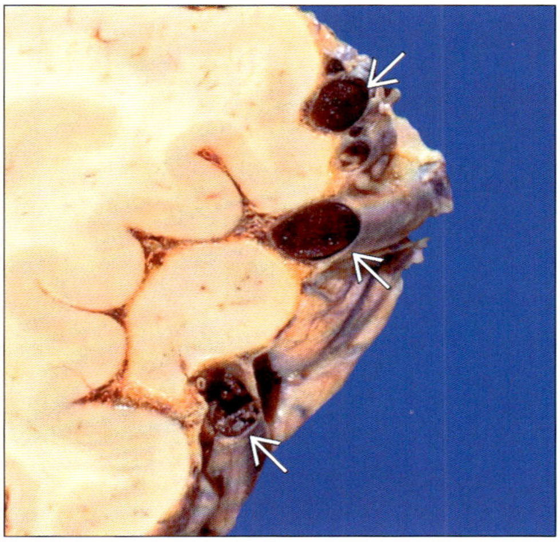

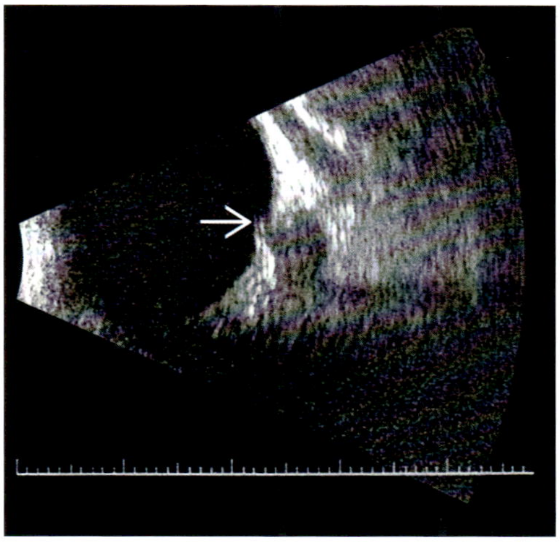

(Left) *Autopsy photo of superior sagittal sinus thrombosis (not shown) reveals clots extending into multiple superficial cortical veins* →. *Elevated ICP leading to papilledema may be caused by venous sinus thrombosis.* ***(Right)*** *B-scan ultrasound shows optic nerve head swelling in papilledema* →. *All patients with papilledema must undergo imaging of the central nervous system to rule out a mass lesion. CT or MRI venography can be used to rule out venous sinus thrombosis.*

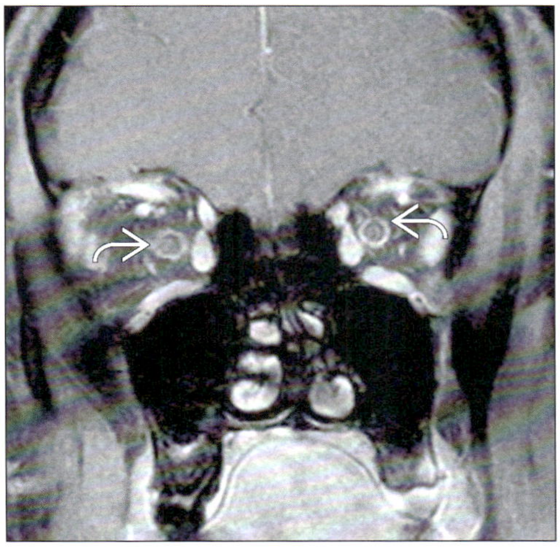

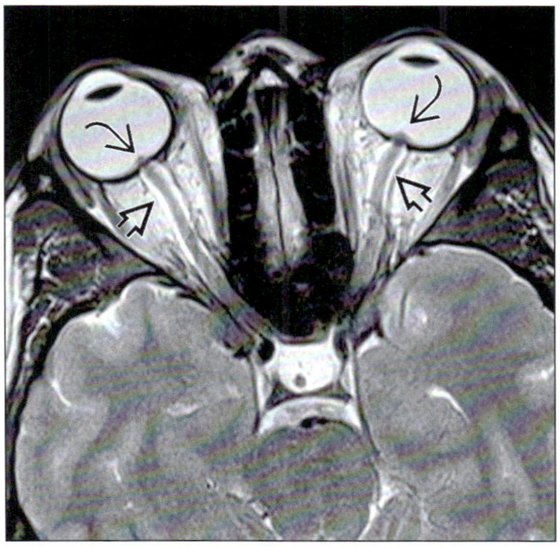

(Left) *Coronal T1WI MRI shows diffuse enhancement of the optic nerve sheaths* → *associated with prominent subarachnoid spaces along the optic nerves, consistent with idiopathic intracranial hypertension (IIH).* ***(Right)*** *Axial T2WI MRI shows dilated CSF spaces around the optic nerves* → *and protrusion of the optic nerve papilla into the posterior globes* →. *These findings are consistent with IIH, a common cause of papilledema in younger obese females.*

PSEUDOTUMOR CEREBRI

Key Facts

Introduction
- Process that mimics intracranial tumor but is usually reversible

Demographics
- Female predominance
- Obesity
- Can occur at any age

Presentation
- Bilateral decrease in vision
- Headaches
- Diplopia
- Pulse-synchrous tinnitus
- Papilledema on funduscopy
- Decreased light sensitivity

Differential Diagnosis
- Intracranial mass
  - Tumor or abscess
- Hydrocephalus
- Intracranial arteriovenous fistulas/malformations

Evaluation/Work-Up
- CSF analysis: Looking for cytogenic abnormalities
- Brain imaging: CT, MRI, MRV to look for venous sinus thrombosis
- Confocal scanning laser tomography of optic nerve
- Visual field testing often shows enlarged blind spot

Treatment
- Acetazolamide or methazolamide
- Weight reduction
- Corticosteroids (be cautious)
- Optic nerve sheath fenestration
- Lumboperitoneal or ventriculoperitoneal shunt to relieve CSF pressure
- Vision loss due to pseudotumor cerebri is often reversible

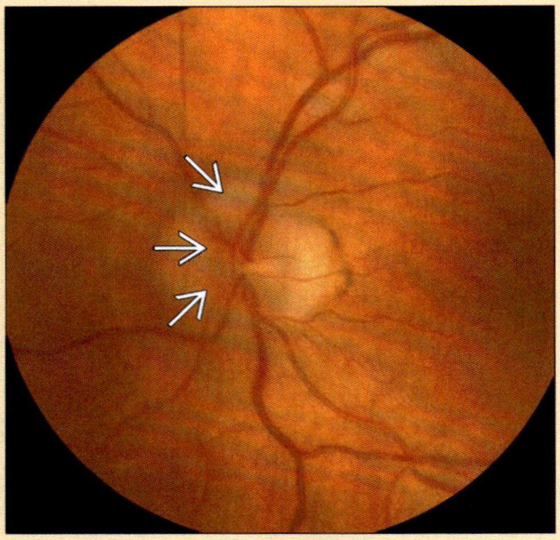
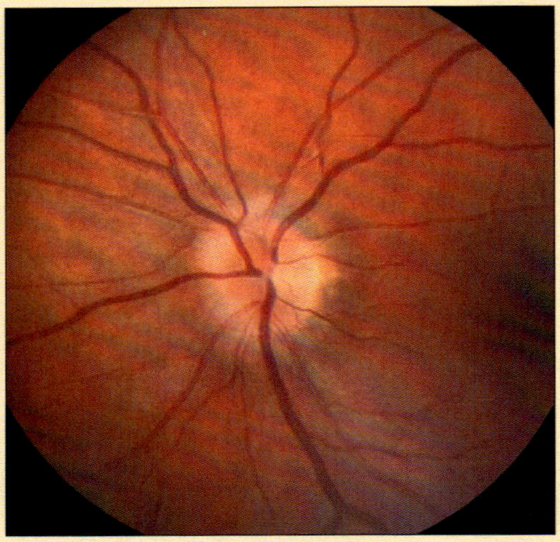

(Left) *Papilledema is key in the diagnosis/prognosis of pseudotumor cerebri and can also help determine the response to treatment. The Frisen scale is used to gauge the level of papilledema. Frisen stage 1 is the earliest stage of papilledema and is characterized by a C-shaped halo* ➔ *of blurred optic disc. (Courtesy J. Warner, MD.)* ***(Right)*** *In Frisen stage 2, the halo of peripapillary edema around the optic disc becomes circumferential. (Courtesy B. Katz, MD.)*

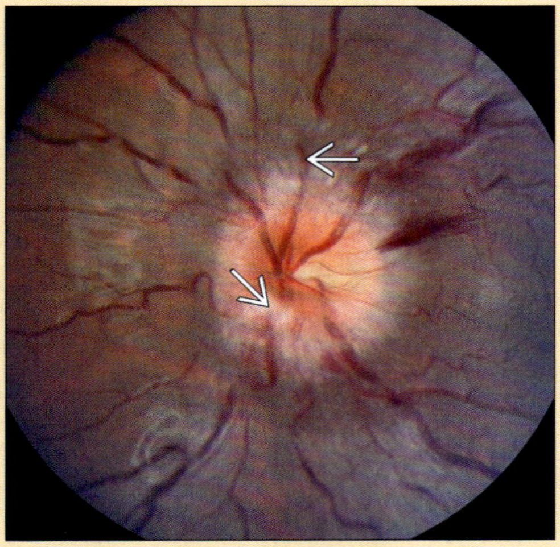
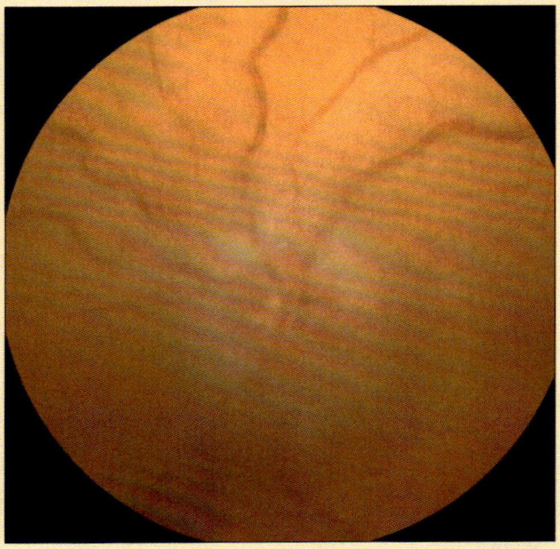

(Left) *This photo illustrates Frisen stage 3. In this stage, the peripapillary edema has progressed to the point of obscuring 1 or more of the blood vessels that exit the optic disc* ➔. ***(Right)*** *The worst stage is Frisen stage 4/5. This is characterized by an obscuration of all of the vessels exiting the optic disc, caused by the high level of edema. Stage 5 carries the worst prognosis of vision recovery from pseudotumor cerebri. (Courtesy A. Vitale, MD.)*

PSEUDOTUMOR CEREBRI

INTRODUCTION

Abbreviations

- Pseudotumor cerebri (PC)
- Also known as idiopathic intracranial hypertension (IIH)

Definitions

- Process that mimics intracranial tumor but is usually reversible

DEMOGRAPHICS

Etiology/Risk Factors

- Caused by increased intracranial pressure
  - Diagnosis of exclusion when space-occupying lesion and hydrocephalus have been ruled out
- Risk factors include obesity and female gender
  - Pregnancy can contribute to exacerbation

Epidemiology

- Can occur at any age
  - In adults, there is a direct correlation between recent weight gain and onset of vision loss
  - PC in children and adolescents is usually not directly associated with obesity

PRESENTATION

Symptoms

- Typically presents as bilateral decrease in vision but can be unilateral
  - In late stages, there may be complete loss of vision
- Headache
- Diplopia
- Pulse synchronous tinnitus
- Photopsia

Exam Findings

- Funduscopic examination
  - Bilateral papilledema (optic disc edema) is 1 of the most diagnostic features
- Visual field defects (enlarged blind spot, peripheral constriction)
- Abducens nerve (CN6) palsy
- Lumbar puncture with high CSF pressure and normal CSF studies
- Decreased light sensitivity on perimetry

DIFFERENTIAL DIAGNOSIS

Intracranial Mass

- Usually has similar presentation to PC
- CT and MRI will reveal a space-occupying lesion

Hydrocephalus

- Caused by increased production/decreased absorption of CSF
  - Imaging will illustrate enlargement of ventricles, which is not found in PC
    - Distinction between communicating and noncommunicating hydrocephalus must be made
      - In communicating, patient may have history of meningitis
      - In noncommunicating, cause of CSF obstruction is usually an intracranial mass

Intracranial Arteriovenous Fistulas/ Malformations

- Can be ruled in or out by CT or MRI with contrast

EVALUATION/WORK-UP

Pathology

- CSF analysis without cytogenic abnormalities
- No evidence of cerebral edema on histology

Imaging

- Brain MRI and CT to look for enlargement of ventricles indicating hydrocephalus, rule in or out presence of tumor or abscess
- MRI may show empty sella
- Optical coherence tomography of optic nerve for quantitative measurement of papilledema

TREATMENT

Medical

- Acetazolamide or methazolamide
- Corticosteroids (be cautious as this can sometimes worsen symptoms, or reducing steroids can worsen symptoms; also, steroids increase weight)
- Weight reduction
- Repeated lumbar punctures to decrease CSF pressure by small decreases in CSF volume

Surgical

- If medical management and weight loss are not effective
  - Optic nerve sheath fenestration
  - Lumboperitoneal or ventriculoperitoneal shunt to relieve CSF pressure

Follow-Up

- Both lumbar puncture and funduscopy (to assess the grade of papilledema) should be used on follow-up to monitor level of intracranial pressure and treatment response

Prognosis

- Vision loss due to PC is often reversible
  - High-grade papilledema is associated with greater risk of blindness

SELECTED REFERENCES

1. Abubaker K et al: Idiopathic intracranial hypertension: lumboperitoneal shunts versus ventriculoperitoneal shunts--case series and literature review. Br J Neurosurg. 25(1):94-9, 2011
2. Spennato P et al: Pseudotumor cerebri. Childs Nerv Syst. 27(2):215-35, 2011
3. Friedman DI et al: Diagnostic criteria for idiopathic intracranial hypertension. Neurology. 59(10):1492-5, 2002
4. Trick GL et al: Quantitative evaluation of papilledema in pseudotumor cerebri. Invest Ophthalmol Vis Sci. 39(10):1964-71, 1998
5. Frisén L: Swelling of the optic nerve head: a staging scheme. J Neurol Neurosurg Psychiatry. 45(1):13-8, 1982

TOXIC/NUTRITIONAL OPTIC NEUROPATHY

Key Facts

Introduction

- Toxin-induced vision loss resulting from damage to optic nerve, chiasm, or optic tracts
- Nutritional; drug induced

Presentation

- Typically bilateral, symmetric, insidious, painless vision loss
- Color blindness
- Methanol ingestion → nausea/vomiting, abdominal pain
- Optic disc
  - Swelling, hyperemia, hemorrhage, temporal pallor
- Pupils
  - Normal size early, dilated if severe
  - Normal light response early, weak or absent if severe
- Visual field examination
  - Symmetric, central or cecocentral scotoma
  - Soft margins with colored targets
- Dyschromatopsia out of proportion to vision loss

Evaluation/Work-Up

- Screening for specific toxins or metabolites
- CBC with differential, urinalysis
- Heavy metal screening if exposure is suspected
- Serum B-12, folate if bilateral central/cecocentral scotomas
- Magnetic resonance imaging
- Electrophysiologic testing

Treatment

- Remove offending agent
- Vitamin supplementation if there is deficiency
- Antidote for specific toxins
- Reversal of vision loss over weeks-months is possible
  - Both toxin- and severity-dependent
  - Visual recovery may be dramatic, even in severe cases
- Total blindness is uncommon (except with methanol)

__(Left)__ This funduscopic photograph of a patient with amiodarone-induced toxic optic neuropathy demonstrates swelling of the optic disc ➡. __(Right)__ This funduscopic photograph of the same patient with amiodarone-induced toxic optic neuropathy demonstrates more severe swelling and edema of the optic disc ➡.

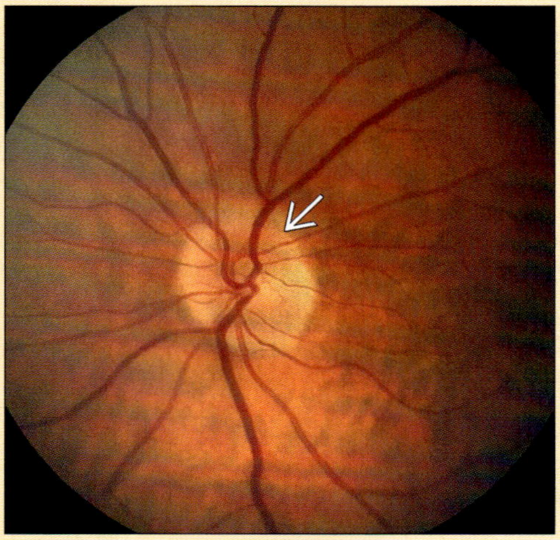

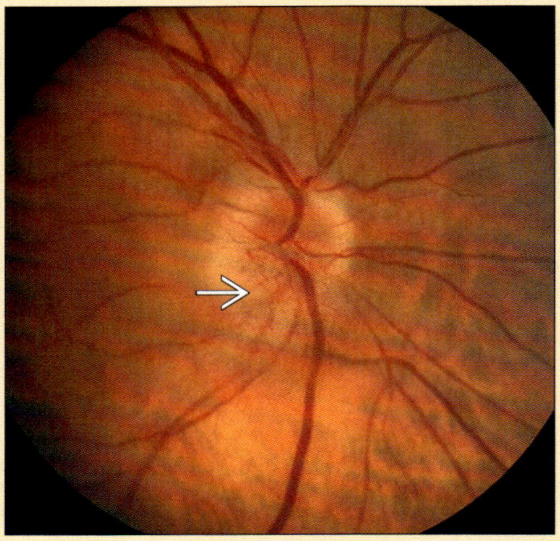

__(Left)__ This fundus photograph depicts nonarteritic anterior ischemic optic neuropathy (NAION) with characteristic optic disc edema ➡. NAION is an important differential diagnosis for toxic optic neuropathy. One of the key differences is the rate of onset. NAION typically has very sudden onset of symptoms. __(Right)__ This fundus photograph demonstrated optic nerve pallor and atrophy ➡, which may develop as long-term sequelae after toxic optic neuropathy.

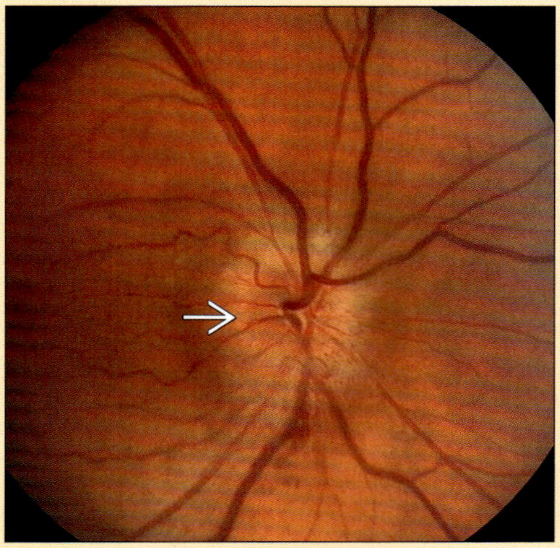

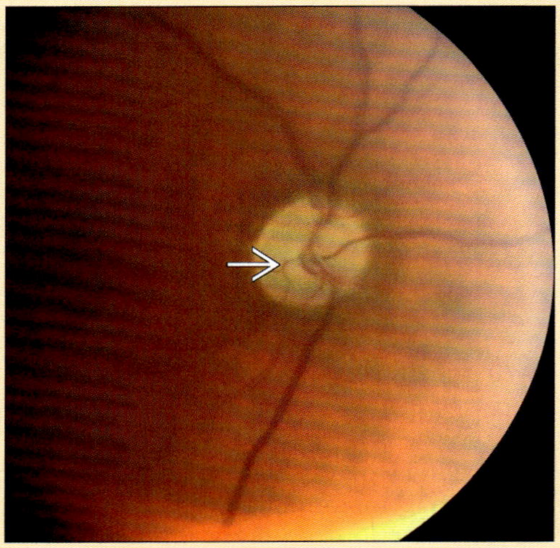

TOXIC/NUTRITIONAL OPTIC NEUROPATHY

INTRODUCTION

Abbreviations
- Toxic optic neuropathy (ToxON)

Definitions
- Toxin-induced vision loss resulting from damage to optic nerve, chiasm, or optic tracts
  - Toxins alter mitochondrial oxidative phosphorylation

Subtypes
- Nutritional
  - B-complex vitamin deficiency
    - B1-thiamine
    - B12-cyanocobalamin
- Drug induced
  - Alcohol (chronic use → malnutrition, acute use → metabolic deficiency), tobacco, amiodarone, chloramphenicol, cimetidine, cyclosporine, dapsone, disulfiram, ethambutol, halogenated hydroquinolones, isoniazid, linezolid, methanol (wood alcohol), sildenafil citrate, vincristine

DEMOGRAPHICS

Etiology/Risk Factors
- Exposure to neurotoxins
  - Ingestion, environmental, ↑ serum drug level
- Systemic diseases resulting in toxin buildup
  - Renal failure, diabetes, thyroid/metabolic disorders
- Toxic and nutritional factors may play a synergistic role

Epidemiology
- Nutritional optic neuropathy
  - Developing countries, chronic alcoholics
- Drug-induced optic neuropathy
  - Developed countries
- No gender, race, or age predilection

PRESENTATION

Symptoms
- Insidious, painless vision loss or color blindness
  - Progressive, bilateral, symmetric, central
- Methanol → nausea/vomiting, abdominal pain

Exam Findings
- Optic disc
  - Swelling, hyperemia, hemorrhage, temporal pallor
- Pupils
  - Normal size early, dilated if severe
  - Normal light response early, weak or absent if severe
- Visual field examination
  - Symmetric, central or cecocentral scotoma
  - Soft margins with colored targets
- Dyschromatopsia out of proportion to vision loss
- Isoniazid-induced ToxON
  - Swollen discs, bitemporal hemianopic scotomas
- Amiodarone-induced ToxON
  - Disc swelling (reverses after amiodarone is withheld)
- Ethambutol-induced ToxON
  - Dyschromatopsia then vision loss, bitemporal or central scotoma, contrast sensitivity may detect subclinical ToxON

DIFFERENTIAL DIAGNOSIS

Anterior Ischemic Optic Neuropathy
- Typically has a sudden onset

EVALUATION/WORK-UP

Labs
- Screening for specific toxins or metabolites
  - Guided by history
- CBC with differential, urinalysis, B-12, folate
- Heavy metal screening if exposure is suspected

Imaging
- Magnetic resonance imaging
  - ± gadolinium enhancement
  - Normal in ToxON, indicated to confirm diagnosis
- Optical coherence tomography
  - Can detect preclinical ethambutol-induced ToxON
- Electrophysiologic testing
  - P100 wave amplitude markedly reduced, normal latency

TREATMENT

Medical
- Remove offending agent
- Vitamin supplementation
- Isoniazid-induced ToxON
  - Pyridoxine 25-100 mg/day may be beneficial
- Methanol-induced ToxON
  - Sodium bicarbonate, IV ethanol/fomepizole, pulse steroids, hemodialysis if indicated

Follow-Up
- Examine every 4-6 weeks initially
- Every 6-12 months thereafter until recovery

Prognosis
- Reversal of vision loss over weeks to months is possible
  - Both toxin- and severity-dependent
  - Visual recovery may be dramatic, even in severe cases
- Visual acuity recovers first, then color vision
- Total blindness is uncommon (except with methanol)

SELECTED REFERENCES

1. Lee E et al: Toxic optic neuropathy. Indian J Ophthalmol. 60(2):159, 2012
2. Sharma P et al: Toxic optic neuropathy. Indian J Ophthalmol. 59(2):137-41, 2011
3. Lloyd MJ et al: Drug-induced optic neuropathies. Drugs Today (Barc). 43(11):827-36, 2007
4. Kesler A et al: Toxic optic neuropathy. Curr Neurol Neurosci Rep. 3(5):410-4, 2003
5. Melamud A et al: Ocular ethambutol toxicity. Mayo Clin Proc. 78(11):1409-11, 2003
6. Van Stavern GP et al: Optic neuropathies. An overview. Ophthalmol Clin North Am. 14(1):61-71, viii, 2001

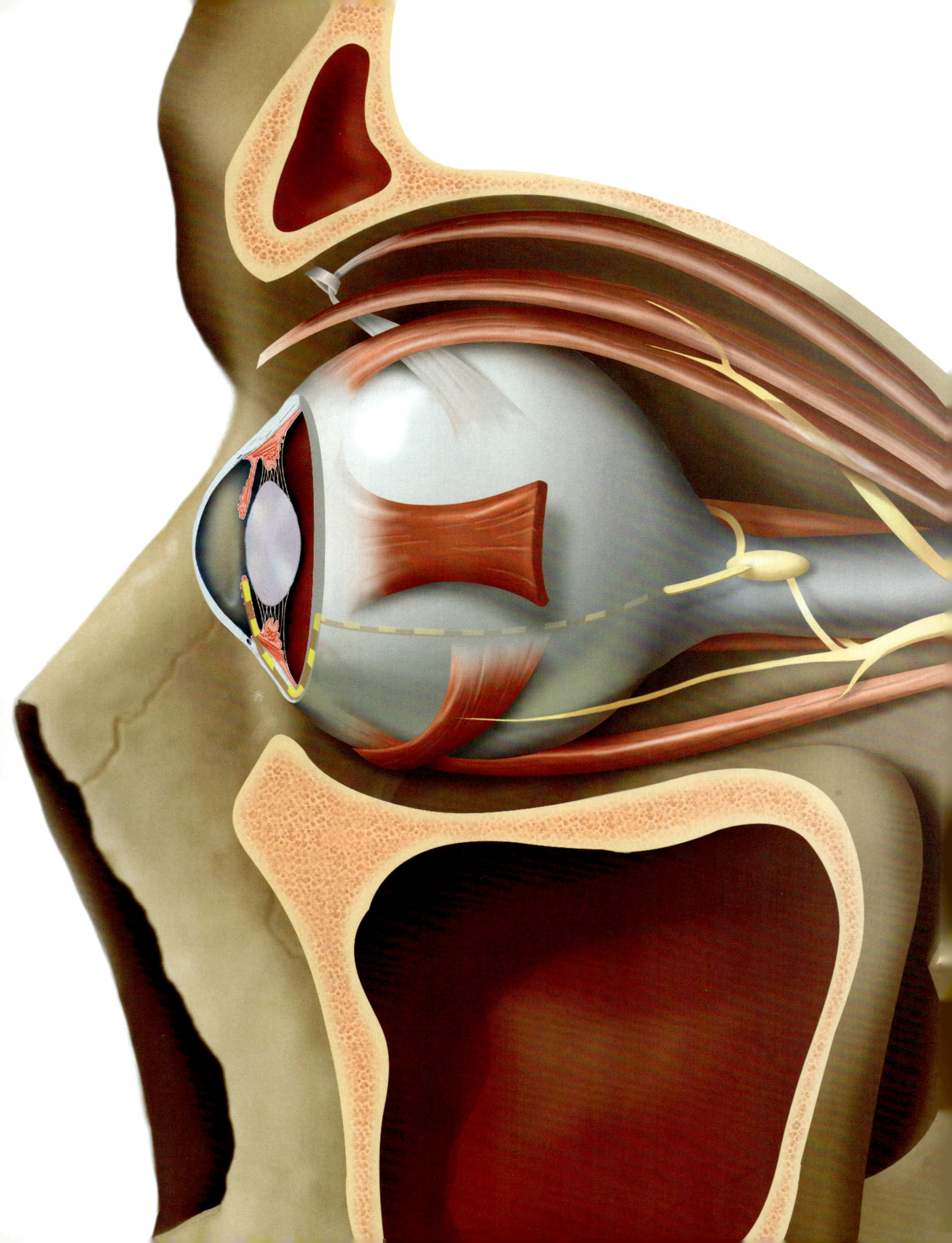

SECTION 2
Ocular Motility and Cranial Nerves

Introduction and Overview

Congenital Disorders

Autoimmune Disorders

Vascular Disorders

Degenerations

Malignant Neoplasms

Miscellaneous

CRANIAL NERVES OVERVIEW

TERMINOLOGY

Abbreviations

- Cranial nerve (CN)
  - Optic nerve (CN2)
  - Oculomotor nerve (CN3)
  - Trochlear nerve (CN4)
  - Trigeminal nerve (CN5)
  - Abducens nerve (CN6)
  - Facial nerve (CN7)

Definitions

- Group of nerves that arise directly from brain or brainstem
  - Can control motor function, sensory function, or a mixture of both (depending on individual nerve)
- CN nucleus
  - Collection of neurons within central nervous system where cranial nerves originate

EMBRYOLOGY

CN Origins

- Forebrain: CN1
- Thalamus: CN2
- Midbrain: CN3 and CN4
- Pons: CN5-CN8
- Medulla: CN9-CN12

ANATOMY AND PHYSIOLOGY

CN Actions

- CN reflexes involving eye
  - Corneal reflex
    - Afferent branch: CN5
    - Efferent branch: CN7
  - Pupillary light reflex
    - Afferent branch: CN2
    - Efferent branch: CN3
- Vision
  - CN2: Afferent nerve that transmits visual stimuli from retina to visual cortex
- Action of nerve is helpful in diagnosis of CN pathology on physical examination
  - Purely sensory: 1, 2, 8
  - Motor: 3, 4, 6, 11, 12
  - Sensory and motor: 5, 7, 9, 10

CN Anatomy Special Considerations

- CN4 is the longest intracranial nerve
  - Only CN that emerges dorsally from brainstem
  - Based on long length, this nerve is more susceptible to damage than other intracranial CNs

IMAGING

Recommendations

- Best modality: Magnetic resonance imaging (MRI)
  - In general, cranial MRI combined with MRI brain sequences augmented by 3D gradient echo steady-state sequence is appropriate
  - Gadolinium contrast can aid in detection and diagnosis
    - Sometimes only indication of underlying CN disease on MRI is abnormal CN enhancement
- CT is useful if pathology is suspected to originate from bony portions of skull or sinuses
- Most accurate imaging takes into account
  - Focused physical examination
  - Precise CN symptoms
- CNs and CN symptoms must be considered in context of
  - Bony structures of skull and relationship to CN
  - Dural structures
  - Vascular anatomy
  - Changes in contrast enhancement
- When imaging CN2, CN3, CN4, and CN6 for suspected pathology, always order orbital sequences

Pitfalls

- Cisternal segments of CNs are very small and difficult to visualize on imaging, yet are very important in diagnosis origin of CN deficit
  - Steady-state free precession imaging best for inspecting CN cisterns and nerve segments
- Neglecting to image pathway of CN from nuclei (origin) to endpoint
  - CNs have very long and complex pathways, often traveling through soft tissue and bony structures before reaching their target
    - May require additional imaging of extracranial structures such as head/neck and mandible

CN DYSFUNCTION

Clinical Implications

- Some CN disorders can be isolated with no other neurological abnormalities
  - Full neurologic examination must be performed every time patient presents with CN deficits
- Ocular symptoms of CN pathology can be manifested by deficits in
  - Ocular motility
  - Visual function
  - Pupillary defects
  - Loss of sensation of eye and periocular tissue
- Neoplasms can also affect function of CNs by
  - Mass effect: Compressing nerve
  - Directly affecting CN nuclei
- CNs supply nerves to side of body ipsilateral to origin of nerve
  - Only exception is CN4, which innervates contralateral side
  - CN3 levator subnucleus supplies both 3rd nerves

RELATED REFERENCES

1. Liang C et al: Anatomical features of the cisternal segment of the oculomotor nerve: neurovascular relationships and abnormal compression on magnetic resonance imaging. J Neurosurg. 111(6):1193-200, 2009
2. Sheth S et al: Appearance of normal cranial nerves on steady-state free precession MR images. Radiographics. 29(4):1045-55, 2009

CN PATHWAYS AND THE OPTIC TRACT

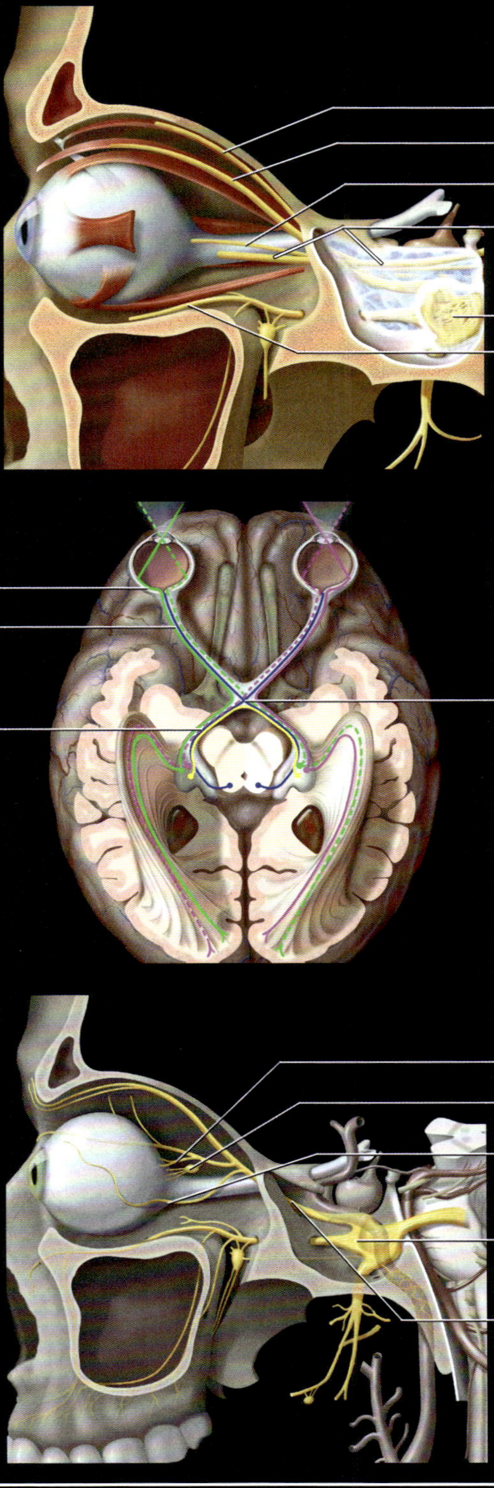

(Top) *The optic nerve (CN2) enters the orbit via the optic canal, and the oculomotor nerve (CN3), trochlear nerve (CN4), ophthalmic nerve (division of CN5), and abducens nerve (CN6) enter the orbit via the superior orbital fissure.* ***(Middle)*** *This illustration of the optic chiasm shows medial retinal fibers crossing the optic chiasm so that fibers from the left halves of both retinas course in the left optic tract (purple), and fibers in the right halves of both retinas course in the right optic tract (green). The medial fibers of the optic tracts cross in the chiasm to connect the lateral geniculate bodies of both sides (yellow).* ***(Bottom)*** *The ophthalmic division of CN5 enters into the orbit via the superior orbital fissure, where it divides into frontal, ciliary, and lacrimal branches.*

GROSS ANATOMY FEATURES

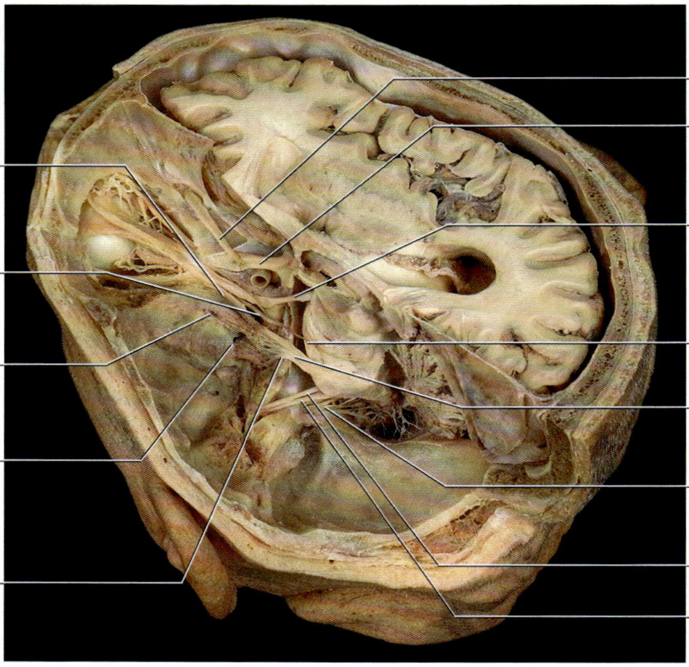

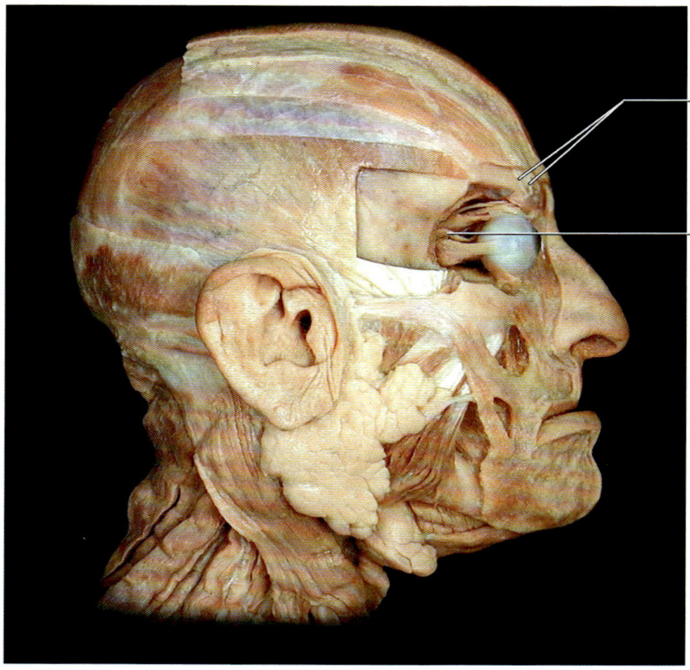

(Top) *The cranial nerves are visible in this transected brain (superolateral view). (Courtesy M. Nielsen, MS.)* ***(Bottom)*** *Step dissection of head exposes scalp, muscles of orbit, and parotid gland. (Courtesy M. Nielsen, MS.)*

CRANIAL NERVES AND OCULAR MOTIONS

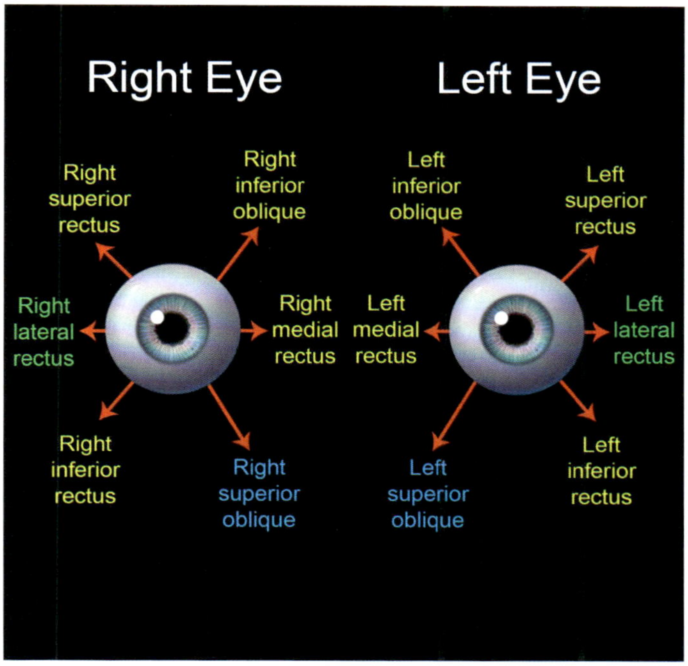

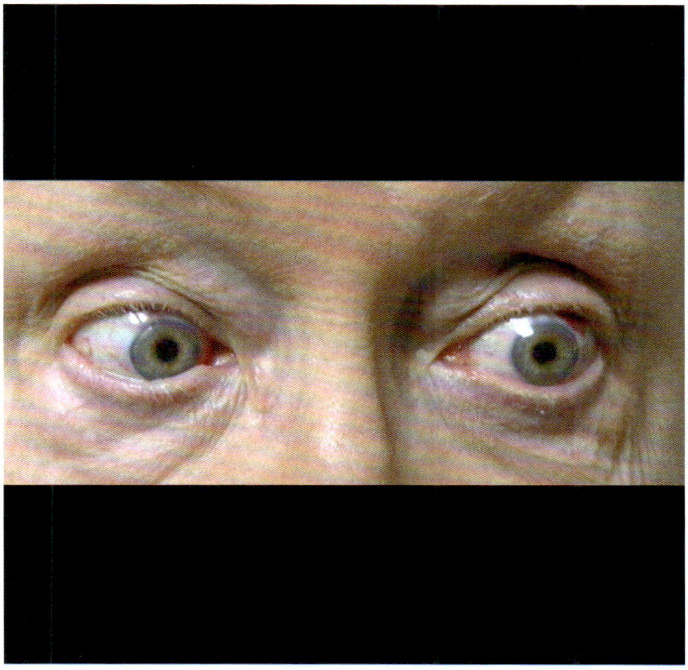

(Top) *The movements of the eyes and the muscles that correspond to each movement are illustrated in this figure. Cranial nerves 3, 4, and 6 control all of the extraocular muscles. The muscle labeled in blue is innervated by the trochlear nerve (CN4), those in yellow are controlled by the oculomotor nerve (CN3), and the green labeled muscle corresponds to the abducens nerve (CN6).* ***(Bottom)*** *This clinical photo shows a patient attempting left gaze. Note that the patient is unable to abduct the left eye, a finding suggestive of a left CN6 palsy.*

OPSOCLONUS

Key Facts

Introduction
- Acute neurologic process causing involuntary, chaotic, conjugate, large-amplitude saccades in vertical, horizontal, and torsional planes
  - Neonatal
  - Paraneoplastic
  - Toxic/metabolic
  - Encephalopathic/infectious
  - Idiopathic

Presentation
- Persistent chaotic involuntary saccades
- Blurred vision
- Opsoclonus/myoclonus syndrome includes motor symptoms
  - Myoclonus
  - Ataxia
  - Dysarthria

Evaluation/Work-Up
- Neoplastic work-up (look for neuroblastoma)
- Toxicology studies
- Infectious work-up
- Head MRI
- Chest, abdomen, pelvis CT to rule out other malignancies

Treatment
- Treat underlying etiology when possible
- Immunosuppression
  - Adrenocorticotrophic hormone, steroids, intravenous immunoglobin, cyclophosphamide, rituximab
- Paraneoplastic: Treat underlying neoplasm in addition to immunosuppression
- Symptom management
  - Propranolol, clonazepam, thiamine, baclofen

*(**Left**) Graphic shows anatomic extent of sympathetic chain ➔ in an infant. Neuroblastoma can arise anywhere in the chain and is a common cause of paraneoplastic opsoclonus in children. (**Right**) External photo shows classic bilateral ecchymosis ➔ and proptosis ➔ caused by bilateral orbital neuroblastomas in a patient with metastatic neuroblastoma. Neuroblastoma should always be ruled-out in children with opsoclonus.*

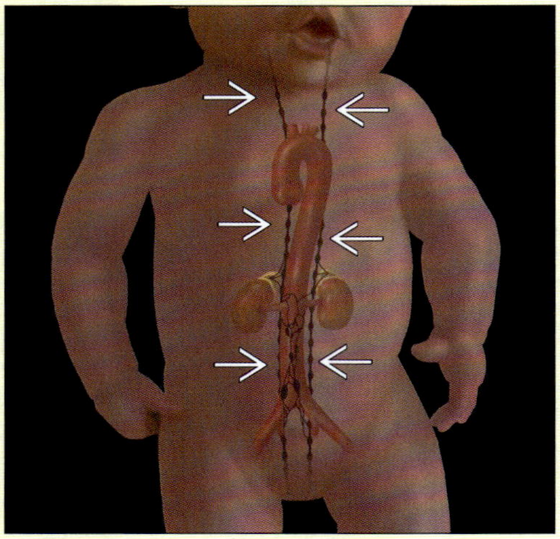

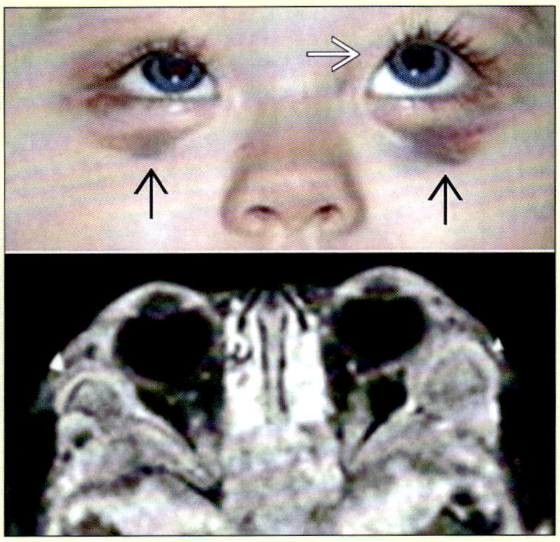

*(**Left**) Graphic depicts intracranial hemorrhage ➔, another possible cause of opsoclonus. MRI or CT scan are helpful in ruling out intracranial hemorrhage. (**Right**) Graphic shows fine-needle aspiration of breast mass. Breast cancer with anti-Ri antibodies is the most frequent cause of paraneoplastic opsoclonus in adult females. Small cell lung cancer with onconeural antibodies is another leading cause of paraneoplastic opsoclonus in adults.*

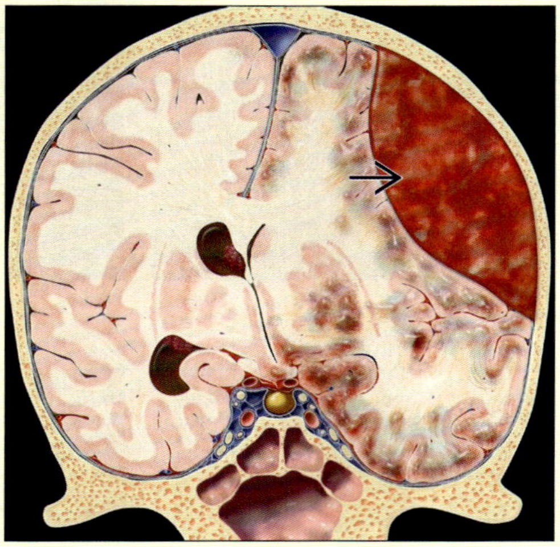

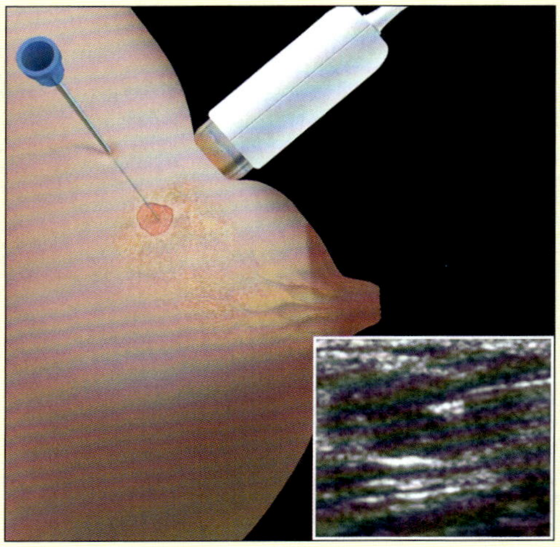

OPSOCLONUS

INTRODUCTION

Definitions

- Acute neurologic process causing involuntary, chaotic, conjugate, fast, large-amplitude saccades in vertical and horizontal planes, as well as torsional

Subtypes

- Neonatal: Idiopathic, intrauterine anoxia, intracranial hemorrhage, benign transient phenomenon in normal infants
- Paraneoplastic: Neuroblastoma, ganglioneuroma, small cell lung carcinoma, medullary thyroid carcinoma, breast carcinoma, renal cell carcinoma, malignant melanoma
- Drugs: Cocaine, chlorthalidone, lithium, amitriptyline
- Parainfectious: Meningitis, HIV, coxsackie virus, mumps, mycoplasma
- Idiopathic

DEMOGRAPHICS

Etiology/Risk Factors

- Cause unknown: Thought to be immune-mediated
- Several associations with antineuronal antibodies, but most patients are seronegative for any antineuronal antibodies

Epidemiology

- Rare disorder
- 3-5% of children with neuroblastoma

PRESENTATION

Symptoms

- Persistent chaotic involuntary saccades
- Blurred vision
- Opsoclonus/myoclonus syndrome includes motor symptoms: Myoclonus, ataxia, dysarthria

Exam Findings

- Persistent chaotic involuntary saccades in all directions
- Conjugate eye movements
- Large amplitude and high frequency of saccades
- No slow component
- Present during sleep
- May have myoclonic limb jerking
- Ataxia
- Children may have developmental delay

DIFFERENTIAL DIAGNOSIS

Ocular Flutter

- Transient rapid nystagmus only in horizontal direction

Ocular Dysmetria

- Characterized by object overshoot and rapid correction

Ocular Nystagmus

- Usually has a slow component and is only in 1 direction

EVALUATION/WORK-UP

Labs

- Neoplasm work-up
  - Children: Look for neuroendocrine tumor markers
    - 24-hour urine homovanillic acid and vanillylmandelic acid
- Toxicology studies
- Infectious studies
  - Evaluate CSF
  - Viral serologies
- Although thought to be immune-mediated, most seronegative for antineuronal antibodies
  - May evaluate for antineuroleukin, antigliadin, anti-Ri

Imaging

- Head MRI
- Chest, abdomen, pelvis CT or MRI with contrast
- Consider EEG testing
- Consider PET scan

TREATMENT

Medical

- Treat underlying etiology
- Immunosuppression
  - Adrenocorticotrophic hormone, steroids, intravenous immunoglobin, cyclophosphamide, rituximab
- Paraneoplastic
  - Treat underlying neoplasm in addition to immunosuppression
- Symptom management
  - Propranolol, clonazepam, thiamine, baclofen

Surgical

- In paraneoplastic opsoclonus, consider removing underlying tumor
  - Children: Neuroblastoma and other neural crest tumors
  - Adults: Small cell lung cancer, breast cancer, ovarian cancer

Prognosis

- Depends on underlying cause
- Children
  - Idiopathic: Relapsing and may cause developmental delay
  - Paraneoplastic: More severe course, 70-80% have persistent developmental deficits
- Adults
  - Idiopathic: May recover with immunosuppression therapy
  - Paraneoplastic: Often more severe progressive course
  - Toxic and metabolic: Improves with treatment of underlying cause

SELECTED REFERENCES

1. Sahu JK et al: The opsoclonus-myoclonus syndrome. Pract Neurol. 11(3):160-6, 2011
2. Straube A et al: Neuro-ophthalmology, neuronal control of eye movements. In Behrens-Baumann W: Developments in Ophthalmology. Vol 40. Switzerland: Karger. 185, 2007
3. Wong A: An update on opsoclonus. Curr Opin Neurol. 20(1):25-31, 2007

MYASTHENIA GRAVIS

Key Facts

Introduction

- Antibody-mediated, T-cell-dependent immunological attack on postsynaptic ACh receptors resulting in fatigable weakness of ocular, bulbar, extremity, and respiratory muscles

Demographics

- Females affected 2x as often as males
- Ocular involvement
  - Occurs in 90% of cases
  - Presenting symptom in 2/3 of cases
  - Ophthalmologists play a crucial role in detecting cases of myasthenia gravis

Presentation

- Ptosis or diplopia
- Orbicularis oculi weakness
- Limb weakness
- Dysphagia, dysarthria, or hoarseness
- Symptoms are worse at end of day or following prolonged exercise
- Sensation is always preserved
  - If sensation is reduced, consider other diagnoses

Evaluation/Work-Up

- Acetylcholine receptor antibodies (AchR-Ab)
  - Binding, blocking, and modulating
- Muscle specific receptor tyrosine kinase (MuSK) antibodies
- Edrophonium (Tensilon) test
- Sleep test
- Ice pack test
- Chest CT to rule out thymoma

Treatment

- Cholinesterase inhibition, immunosuppression, thymectomy are options to consider

*(**Left**) This external photo demonstrates left-sided ptosis in a patient with myasthenia gravis prior to an ice pack test. (**Right**) This external photo demonstrates mild improvement in the same patient's left-sided ptosis after a 2-minute ice pack test.*

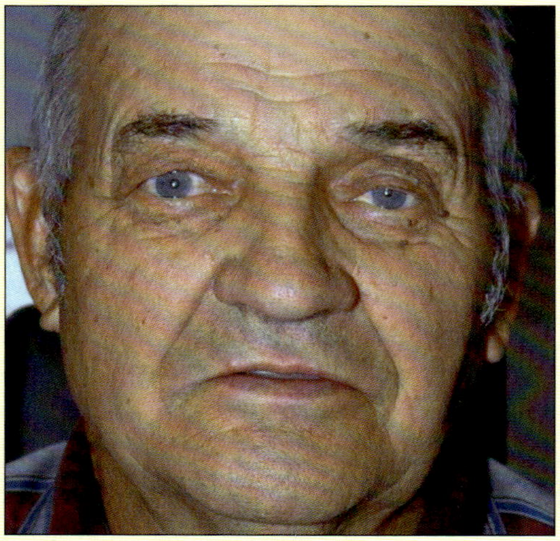

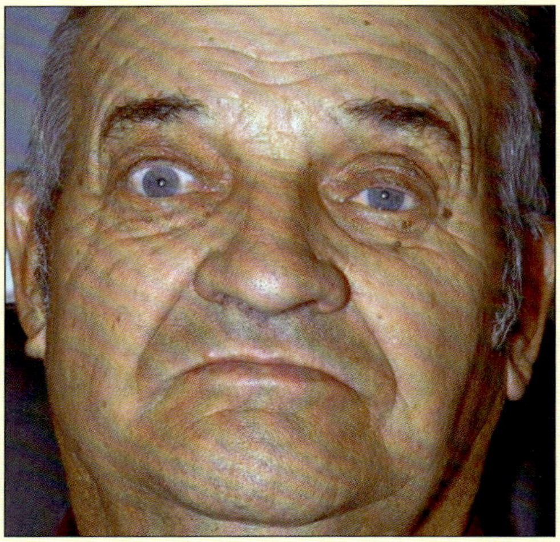

*(**Left**) Thymomas are epithelial neoplasms of the anterior mediastinum, which often project to one side. They are the most common anterior mediastinal mass, especially in patients > 40 years old. Of patients with myasthenia gravis, 10-15% have a thymoma ⇨. (**Right**) Axial CECT shows an encapsulated thymoma ➡ manifesting as a well-marginated, roughly spherical, right anterior mediastinal mass of homogeneous attenuation.*

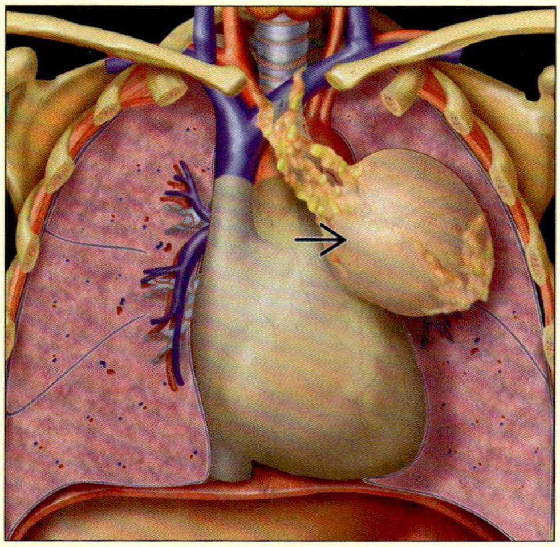

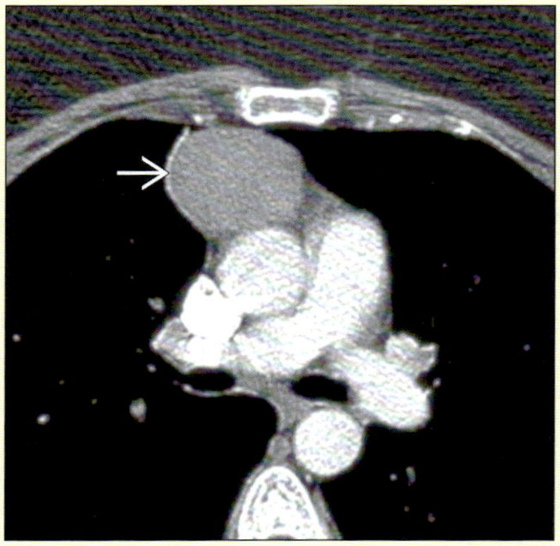

MYASTHENIA GRAVIS

INTRODUCTION

Abbreviations

- Myasthenia gravis (MG)

Definitions

- Antibody-mediated, T-cell-dependent immunological attack on postsynaptic acetylcholine (ACh) receptors resulting in fatigable weakness of ocular, bulbar, extremity, and respiratory muscles

Subtypes

- Generalized
- Ocular
- Bulbar

DEMOGRAPHICS

Etiology/Risk Factors

- Autoimmune disease (antibodies vs. postsynaptic junction)
  - MG is frequently associated with other autoimmune disorders
- No known exposure risk factors for acquiring MG
  - Increased stress, infection, excessive UV exposure, and extremes of temperature may worsen symptoms and precipitate myasthenic crisis

Epidemiology

- Females affected 2x as often as males
- Most commonly occurs in 3rd decade
- Ocular involvement
  - Occurs in 90% of cases
  - Presenting symptom in 2/3 of cases
  - Ophthalmologists play a crucial role in detecting cases of MG

PRESENTATION

Symptoms

- Ocular weakness
  - Manifest by diplopia or ptosis
  - Original presenting symptom in 50% of patients with MG
- Limb weakness
- Dysphagia, dysarthria, or hoarseness
- Symptoms are worse at end of day or following prolonged exercise

Exam Findings

- Ocular
  - Most common sign is ptosis
    - May be unilateral or bilateral
    - Worse in evening and least severe upon awakening
    - Worse after exertion or following sustained upward gaze (fatigable ptosis)
  - Diplopia
    - Variable and fatigable
    - Frequently, vertical diplopia, though any of the extraocular muscles may be affected
    - May manifest as intranuclear ophthalmoplegia, isolated gaze palsy, or simulate an oculomotor cranial nerve paresis
      - Total ophthalmoplegia may occur
  - Orbicularis oculi weakness
  - Cogan eyelid twitch
    - Brief overelevation of upper eyelid when patient moves from downgaze to upgaze
  - Enhancement of ptosis
    - If the more ptotic eyelid is manually elevated, other eyelid will lower (Herring law)
  - Pupillary abnormalities are notably absent
- Bulbar
  - Dysphagia, hoarseness, dysarthria, and hypernasality
- Generalized
  - Proximal > distal muscle weakness
  - Dyspnea
- Sensation is always preserved
  - If sensory deficits are present, consider another diagnosis

DIFFERENTIAL DIAGNOSIS

Lambert-Eaton Myasthenic Syndrome

- Spares optic and bulbar muscles
- Diminished deep tendon reflexes
- Post exercise facilitation
  - Strength improves with continued muscle contraction (unlike MG)
- Nearly 50% of patients have small cell lung cancer (need chest CT)
- Antibodies against presynaptic junction

Amyotrophic Lateral Sclerosis

- Bulbar involvement leading to dysphagia and dysarthria
- Spares optic muscles
  - Ptosis and diplopia are notably absent

Botulism

- Affects both bulbar and ocular muscles
- Commonly produces pupillary paralysis
- Distinguished from MG by its rapid progression

Thyroid Ophthalmopathy

- Associated with hyperthyroidism; may produce diplopia secondary to compressive ophthalmopathy
- Proptosis, lid retraction, lid lag, and periorbital edema
- Ptosis is notably absent
- 5% of patients with thyroid ophthalmopathy will also have MG

Chronic Progressive External Ophthalmoplegia

- Mitochondrial disorder resulting in progressive ptosis and ophthalmoparesis
- Slowed saccades (saccades are normal in MG)

Muscular Dystrophies

- Myotonic dystrophy
  - Ptosis accompanied by weakness of face, neck, and extremities
  - Associated with cataracts, characteristic facies, frontal balding, and cognitive impairment
- Oculopharyngeal dystrophy
  - Slowly progressive ptosis and dysphagia
  - Ophthalmoparesis typically develops late in disease
  - Onset in 4th or 5th decade

MYASTHENIA GRAVIS

EVALUATION/WORK-UP

Labs

- Acetylcholine receptor antibodies (AchR-Ab)
  - Binding, blocking, and modulating
    - Binding antibody is most sensitive
      - Positive in 80-90% of those with systemic disease
      - Sensitivity decreases to 40-55% for those with ocular myasthenia only
    - Blocking antibodies have high specificity
- Muscle specific receptor tyrosine kinase (MuSK) antibodies
  - Present in 38-50% of those with MG who are AchR-Ab negative
- Consider thyroid panel and pernicious anemia work-up
  - MG is frequently associated with other autoimmune disease

Clinical Tests

- Edrophonium (Tensilon) test
  - Objective baseline measurements of ptosis and diplopia are recorded
  - Short-acting acetylcholinesterase inhibitor, edrophonium is given IV at a dose of 2 mg
    - Patient is observed for 60 seconds; if ptosis or motility improve, then test is considered positive
    - If no response is elicited, up to 2 more doses of edrophonium are given at a dose of 4 mg
      - If there is no improvement in ptosis or motility compared to baseline, test is considered negative
  - Prior to edrophonium testing, the clinician must consider the potential but uncommon possibility of a cholinergic crisis with bradycardia, syncope, and possible cardiorespiratory arrest
    - Vitals should be monitored throughout
    - Atropine (0.4-0.6 mg) should be available prior to dosing of edrophonium
    - Resuscitation cart should be available
- Sleep test
  - Alternative to edrophonium testing
  - Document baseline ptosis and motility deficits
  - Have patient rest with eyes closed for at least 30 minutes
  - Repeat measurements and compare to baseline
    - Improvement in symptoms suggests a diagnosis of MG
- Ice pack test
  - Only relevant in patients with ptosis
  - Place ice pack over closed eyelids for at least 2 minutes
  - Cooling effect results in improvement of ptosis in most patients with MG
    - Cold temperature improves neuromuscular junction transmission
- Repetitive nerve stimulation testing
  - Nerve is electrically stimulated 6-10 times
  - Muscle surface electrodes record compound muscle action potentials
  - Test is considered positive when recorded action potential amplitudes decrease with each subsequent stimuli
- Single-fiber electromyography
  - Most sensitive (88-99%) test for MG

Imaging

- Chest CT
  - All MG patients need to have thymoma ruled out by imaging
  - Evaluate for thymic hyperplasia (85%) or thymoma (10-15%)
- CT and ultrasonography of orbits
  - Helpful in differential for MG and thyroid ophthalmopathy

TREATMENT

Medical

- Mainstay is corticosteroids to temporize followed by bridge to other immunosuppressant agents or acetylcholinesterase inhibitors
  - Common anticholinesterase
    - Pyridostigmine or neostigmine
  - Common immunosuppressants
    - Azathioprine or cyclosporin
- Intravenous immunoglobulin or plasmapheresis
  - Reserved for myasthenic crisis or emergent situation

Surgical

- Thymectomy
  - Treatment of choice for patients with generalized disease and concomitant thymic enlargement
  - Useful in cases with associated thymoma
  - Not typically required in patients with pure ocular MG

Follow-Up

- All patients with MG should be managed in cooperation with a neurologist
  - Respiratory and other life-threatening manifestations of MG may develop

Prognosis

- 85% of patients who present with pure ocular MG will develop systemic MG within 2 years
- Symptoms are typically well controlled under tightly controlled medical management
- Respiratory and oropharyngeal muscle involvement may be fatal

SELECTED REFERENCES

1. Keesey JC: Clinical evaluation and management of myasthenia gravis. Muscle Nerve. 29(4):484-505, 2004
2. Richman DP et al: Treatment of autoimmune myasthenia gravis. Neurology. 61(12):1652-61, 2003
3. Smith KH: Myasthenia gravis. In American Academy of Ophthalmology: Focal Points: Clinical Modules for Ophthalmologists. Module 4. San Francisco: American Academy of Ophthalmology, 2003
4. Sommer N et al: Ocular myasthenia gravis. A critical review of clinical and pathophysiological aspects. Doc Ophthalmol. 84(4):309-33, 1993
5. Perlo VP et al: The role of thymectomy in the treatment of myasthenia gravis. Ann N Y Acad Sci. 183:308-15, 1971

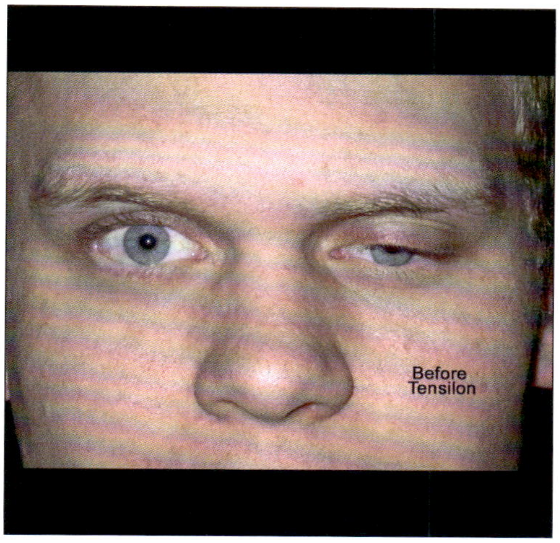

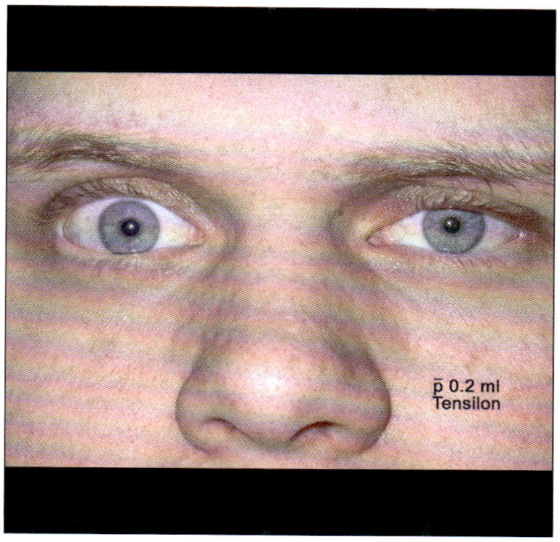

(Left) *This external photo demonstrates severe left-sided ptosis in a patient with myasthenia gravis prior to edrophonium chloride (Tensilon) administration.* ***(Right)*** *This external photo of the same patient demonstrates significant improvement in patient's ptosis after administration of 0.2 mL of edrophonium.*

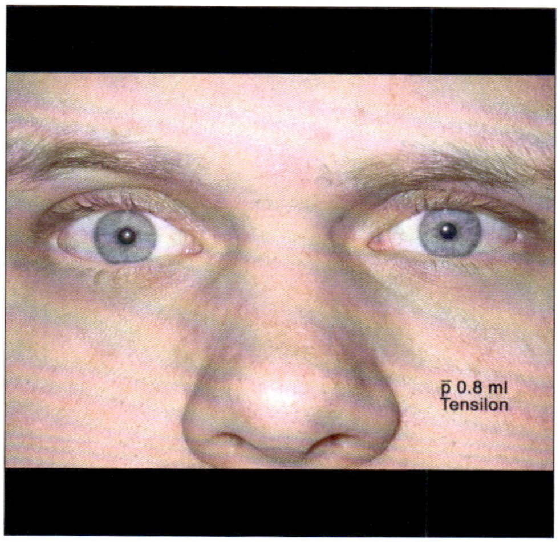

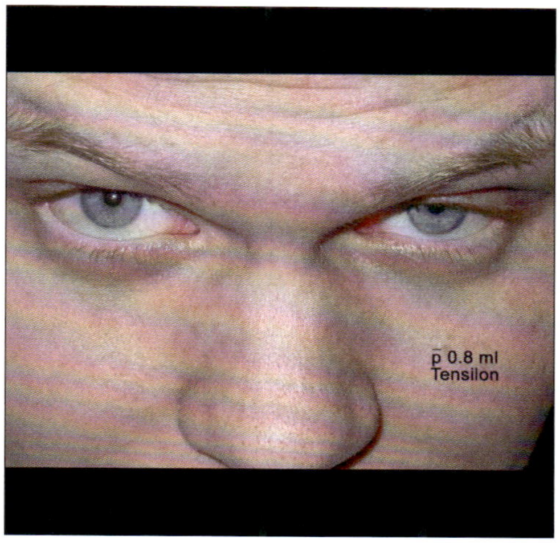

(Left) *This external photo of the same patient demonstrates continued improvement in left-sided ptosis after 0.8 mL administration of edrophonium.* ***(Right)*** *This external photo of the same patient demonstrates patient in upgaze after administration of 0.8 mL edrophonium with evidence of mild left-sided ptosis.*

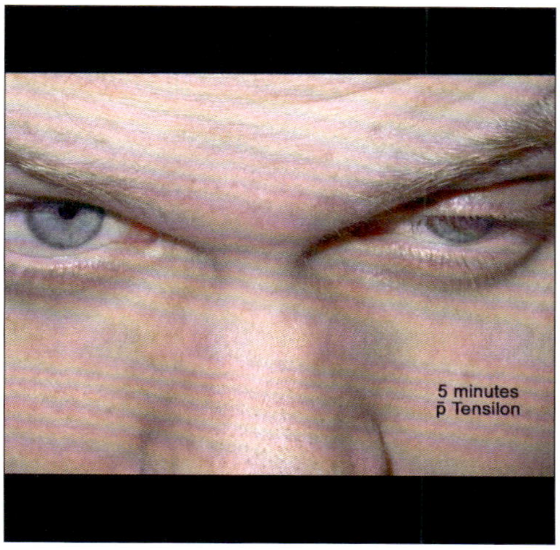

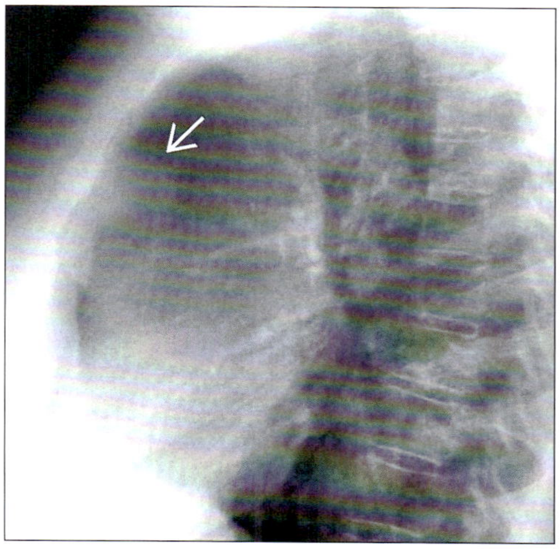

(Left) *This external photo of the same patient demonstrates return of significant left-sided ptosis 5 minutes after administration of edrophonium.* ***(Right)*** *Lateral chest radiograph shows a retrosternal anterior mediastinal mass ➔. Some thymomas are best visualized on lateral chest radiographs.*

Key Facts

Introduction
- Midbrain, also known as the mesencephalon, acts as the relay center for motor function and sensory information from the eyes and ears

Demographics
- Common locations of midbrain stroke are the posterior cerebral artery and middle cerebral artery
- Risk factors
  - Chronic hypertension
  - Smoking
  - Diabetes
  - Family history of stroke
- 15% of strokes are hemorrhagic; 85% are ischemic

Presentation
- Vertical or horizontal gaze palsy (e.g., skew deviation)
- Hearing impairment
- Dysconjugate gaze
- Dysfunction of cranial nerves 3 &/or 4
- Focal motor deficits

Differential Diagnosis
- Isolated cranial nerve palsy
- Neoplastic metastasis to brain
- Demyelinating disease

Evaluation/Work-Up
- CT and MRI ± contrast

Treatment
- Recombinant tissue plasminogen activator
- Endovascular treatments such as intraarterial thrombolytic therapy, or catheter embolectomy for ischemic strokes
- Time is key factor in diagnosis and treatment of strokes
  - Earlier therapy improves prognosis

*(**Left**) This external photograph shows the eye of a patient with an oculomotor nerve lesion. Note the ptosis ➡ and blown pupil ➡. Cranial nerve 3 lesions are a common finding in midbrain strokes. (**Right**) Axial FLAIR MRI shows hyperintensity in the occipital lobes and left pons ➡ in this patient with visual changes and confusion. Top-of-the basilar syndrome is most commonly caused by embolic disease, as in this case.*

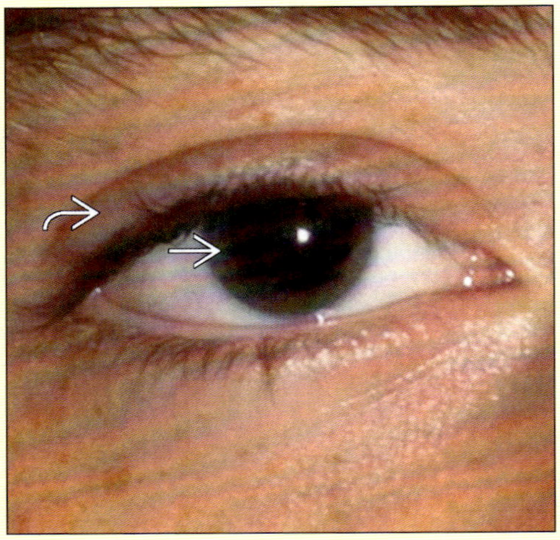

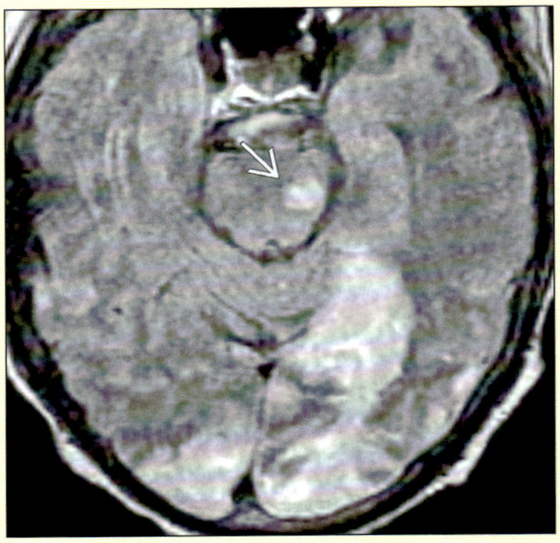

*(**Left**) Axial DTI trace shows bilateral rostral midbrain ischemia ➡, which extended into the cerebral peduncles (not shown). This patient presented with oculomotor symptoms. Note the dorsal extension of ischemia ➡ involving the medial longitudinal fasciculus. (**Right**) This external photograph demonstrates severe ocular surface damage and punctate fluorescein staining ➡. Patients with midbrain strokes affecting the facial nerve can develop exposure keratopathy.*

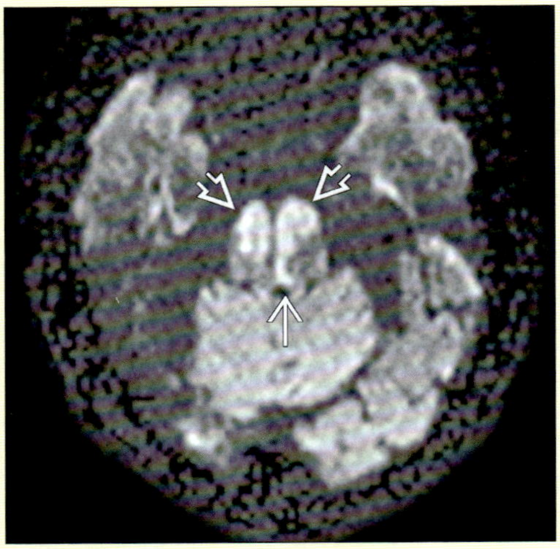

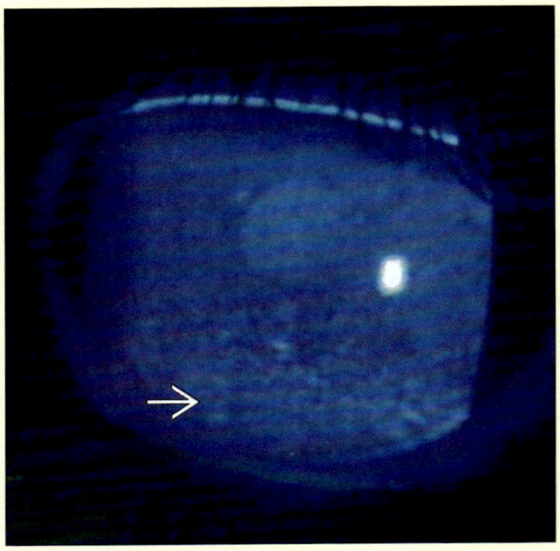

MIDBRAIN STROKES

INTRODUCTION

Definitions
- Midbrain, also known as the mesencephalon, acts as the relay center for motor function and sensory information from the eyes and ears

Subtypes
- Ischemic stroke: Hypoperfusion of the brain due to embolism, thrombosis, or systemic hypoperfusion
- Hemorrhagic stroke: Caused by rupture of a blood vessel within the brain, which leads to bleeding within intracerebral space

DEMOGRAPHICS

Etiology/Risk Factors
- Common locations of midbrain stroke are the posterior cerebral artery and middle cerebral artery
- Risk factors
  - Advanced age
  - Hypercoagulability states
  - Chronic hypertension
  - Smoking
  - Diabetes
  - Family history of stroke

Epidemiology
- 15% of strokes are hemorrhagic; 85% are ischemic
- Gender: Males > Females

PRESENTATION

Symptoms
- Hemiparesis
- Headache
- Vertical or horizontal gaze palsy (e.g., skew deviation)
- Diplopia
- Dysconjugate gaze; can involve internuclear ophthalmoplegia
- Ptosis
- Hearing impairment

Exam Findings
- Oculomotor nerve (cranial nerve 3) dysfunction
  - Decreased range of motion of extraocular muscles
  - Sluggish or absent pupillary light reflex
  - Blown pupil on affected side
- Trochlear nerve dysfunction
  - Incomplete depression of eye when looking down in adduction
- Focal motor deficits

DIFFERENTIAL DIAGNOSIS

Isolated Cranial Nerve Palsy
- Loss/decreased cranial nerve 3 or 4 function without damage to midbrain
- MRI &/or CT of midbrain will show intact cranial nerve origins and no signs of ischemia or hemorrhage
  - Along with ruling out midbrain stroke, MRI can help to locate site of cranial nerve damage

Neoplastic Metastasis to Brain
- Metastases may infiltrate into the midbrain or compress the structures, mimicking stroke
- Typically enhance on MRI
- May have signs of vasogenic edema

Demyelinating Disease
- May present with limb weakness and visual symptoms similar to midbrain stroke
- Diagnosed by presence of white matter lesions on MRI

EVALUATION/WORK-UP

Labs
- Hematocrit and platelet count
- Partial thromboplastin time and prothrombin time
- Total cholesterol, HDL, LDL, and triglycerides

Imaging
- CT and MRI ± contrast are used
  - CT has high sensitivity for hemorrhage and should be initial imaging study
    - CT perfusion imaging and CT angiography increase image quality
  - Diffusion and perfusion MRI to detect areas of ischemia

TREATMENT

Medical
- Strokes can be treated with recombinant tissue plasminogen activator (TPA) if
  - Imaging confirms that stroke is ischemic
  - TPA treatment can be started < 4.5 hours after onset of symptoms
- Risk factors such as diabetes, hypertension, and coagulopathies should be treated to prevent future strokes

Surgical
- Endovascular treatments, such as intraarterial thrombolytic therapy for ischemic strokes, or catheter embolectomy
- Decompressive craniotomy if stroke is causing cerebral swelling that could lead to further damage
- Hemorrhagic strokes may require neurosurgery to repair vessels and stop bleeding
- If present, carotid stenosis, cardiac arrhythmias, or cardiac valve issues should be dealt with once patient is stable to prevent future events

Follow-Up
- If there are residual neurologic deficits, patient should follow-up with physical/occupational therapy

Prognosis
- Time is the key factor in strokes; the earlier the midbrain stroke is caught, the better the prognosis

SELECTED REFERENCES

1. Rosamond WD et al: Stroke incidence and survival among middle-aged adults: 9-year follow-up of the Atherosclerosis Risk in Communities (ARIC) cohort. Stroke. 30(4):736-43, 1999

CHRONIC PROGRESSIVE EXTERNAL OPHTHALMOPLEGIA

Key Facts

Introduction
- Genetic disease characterized by weakness of extraocular muscles and eyelid muscles

Demographics
- Caused by mutations in skeletal muscle cells, which over time leads to decreased muscle function
- Commonly affects adults between ages 18 and 40
- Mitochondrial, autosomal dominant, and autosomal recessive inheritance patterns

Presentation
- Ptosis
- Dysconjugate gaze
- Symmetric ophthalmoplegia with decreased horizontal and vertical range of motion

Differential Diagnosis
- Kearns-Sayre syndrome
- Miller-Fisher syndrome
  - Variant of Guillain-Barré syndrome
- Myasthenia gravis

Evaluation/Work-Up
- Skeletal muscle biopsy with trichrome stain may show ragged-red fibers
- Head MRI showing
  - Slight reduction of extraocular muscle volume
  - Cerebral atrophy
- Acetylcholine receptor antibody test
- Anti-ganglioside antibody test

Treatment
- Tetracycline treatment
- Surgical ptosis correction
- Monitoring of ocular motility range and degree of proptosis
- A cure has not been identified, but treatments are effective in decreasing symptoms

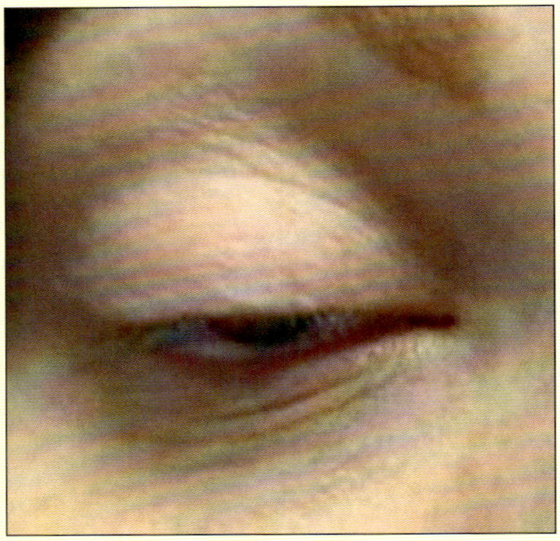
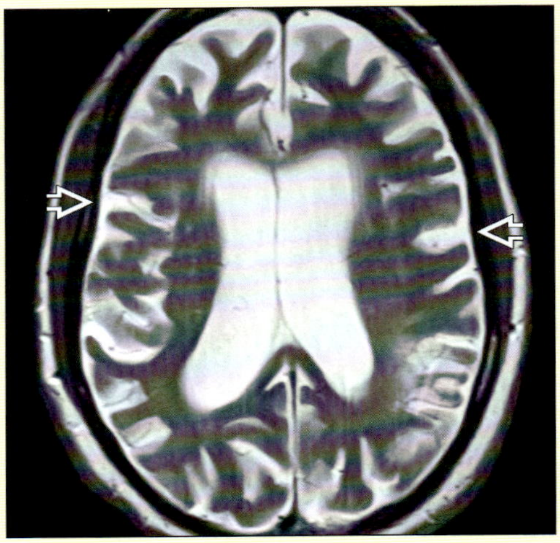

(Left) *This external photograph is an example of the severe ptosis associated with chronic progressive external ophthalmoplegia (CPEO). Ptosis is often the 1st sign noticed in the disease process. While this finding is most commonly bilateral, the degree of ptosis between the 2 eyes may be asymmetric. Orbicularis dysfunction in CPEO can lead to exposure keratopathy.* ***(Right)*** *This MRI depicts cerebral atrophy and enlarged sulci ⇨, findings consistent with a diagnosis of CPEO.*

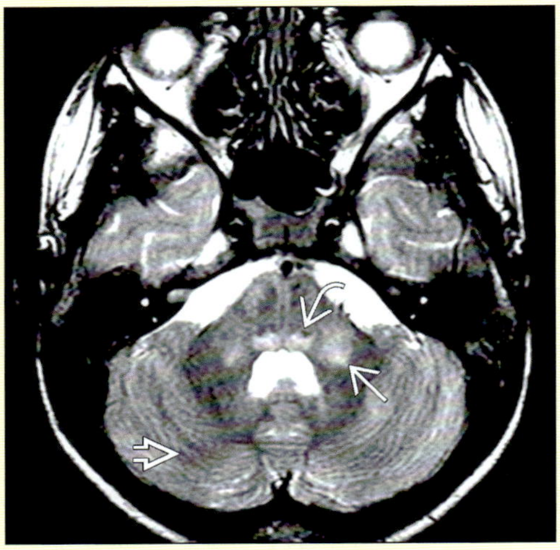
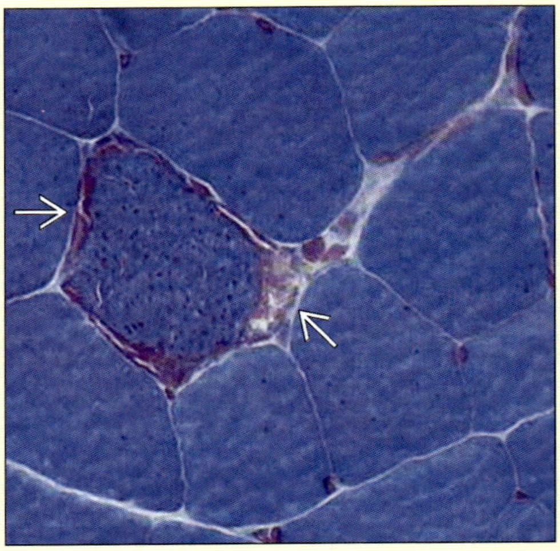

(Left) *Axial T2-weighted MRI in a teenager with symptomatic Kearns-Sayre syndrome demonstrates abnormal increased signal intensity bilaterally in the brachium pontis ➔ and the dorsal pons ↪. Widening of the interfoliate sulci ⇨ results from mild cerebellar atrophy.* ***(Right)*** *This skeletal muscle biopsy depicts ragged-red fibers ➔. Ragged-red fibers are a finding typical of diseases with mitochondrial inheritance, such as Kearns-Sayre syndrome. (Courtesy E. Rushing, MD.)*

CHRONIC PROGRESSIVE EXTERNAL OPHTHALMOPLEGIA

INTRODUCTION

Abbreviations

- Chronic progressive external ophthalmoplegia (CPEO)

Definitions

- Genetic disease characterized by weakness of extraocular muscles and eyelid muscles

Subtypes

- Isolated CPEO
- CPEO in conjunction with Kearns-Sayre syndrome

DEMOGRAPHICS

Etiology/Risk Factors

- Caused by mutations in skeletal muscle cells, which leads to decreased muscle function over time
- Can be caused by sporadic mutations
- Risk factors
  - Maternal family members with CPEO
  - Mutations in *POLG* or *PEO1* genes

Epidemiology

- Commonly affects adults between ages 18 and 40

PRESENTATION

Symptoms

- Drooping eyelids
- Impaired eye movement
- Patients rarely complain of diplopia
- Skeletal muscle myopathies
  - Systemic muscular weakness and exercise intolerance
- Other neuropathies
  - Sensorineural hearing loss
  - Ataxia
  - Dysphagia

Exam Findings

- Ptosis
- Dysconjugate gaze
- Ocular motility examination/measurement
  - Symmetric ophthalmoplegia with decreased horizontal and vertical range of motion
- Funduscopic examination looking for salt-and-pepper retinopathy

Kearns-Sayre Syndrome

- Syndrome may include
  - Progressive external ophthalmoplegia
  - Pigmentary retinopathy
  - Cardiac conduction block
  - Cerebellar ataxia
- Mitochondrial inheritance
- Histology of muscle cells shows ragged-red fibers; can be associated with myoclonic epilepsy with ragged-red fibers (MERRF)
- Generally presents before age 20

DIFFERENTIAL DIAGNOSIS

Miller-Fisher Syndrome

- Variant of Guillain-Barré syndrome
- Presents with external ophthalmoplegia, loss of deep tendon reflexes, and ataxia
- Positive anti-ganglioside antibody test

Myasthenia Gravis

- Autoimmune disorder caused by dysfunction of neuromuscular junction that lead to weakness and fatigability of skeletal muscles
- Symptoms include
  - Ptosis
  - Skeletal muscles fatigability and weakness
    - Fatigability is a key difference from CPEO
  - Isolated ophthalmoparesis
  - Acetylcholine receptor antibodies

EVALUATION/WORK-UP

Labs

- Acetylcholine receptor antibody test
- Anti-ganglioside antibody test

Pathology

- May have ragged-red fibers on muscle biopsy using trichrome stain
- EKG: Looking for cardiac conduction block

Imaging

- Head MRI showing
  - Cerebral atrophy
  - Findings characteristic of Kearns-Sayre syndrome
    - Increased signal intensity bilaterally in brachium pontis and dorsal pons

TREATMENT

Medical

- Ptosis props mounted on frame of glasses
- Prism lenses for diplopia, if present
- Tetracycline treatment
  - Case-based evidence of improved ocular motility
- Lubrication for exposure keratopathy

Surgical

- Surgical ptosis correction
  - Levator advancement surgery
  - Brow suspension surgery

Follow-Up

- Monitor ocular motility and exposure keratopathy

Prognosis

- Cure has not been identified, but treatments are effective in decreasing symptoms

SELECTED REFERENCES

1. Omar A et al: Tetracycline delays ocular motility decline in chronic progressive external ophthalmoplegia. Neurology. 68(14):1159-60, 2007
2. Laforêt P et al: Chronic progressive external ophthalmoplegia with ragged-red fibers: clinical, morphological and genetic investigations in 43 patients. Neuromuscul Disord. 5(5):399-413, 1995
3. Lane CM et al: Treatment of ptosis in chronic progressive external ophthalmoplegia. Br J Ophthalmol. 71(4):290-4, 1987

PINEALOMA

Key Facts

Introduction
- Tumor of the pineal gland
- Subtypes
  - Germinoma
  - Teratoma
  - Pineocytoma
  - Pineoblastoma
  - Retinoblastoma (trilateral)
  - Germ cell neoplasms, not otherwise specified
  - Diffuse astrocytoma

Presentation
- Headache, nausea, vomiting, and lethargy secondary to increased intracranial pressure
- Mental status changes
- Parinaud (dorsal midbrain) syndrome
  - Bilateral mid-dilated pupils
  - Pupils react poorly to light but constrict normally to convergence (light-near dissociation)
  - Eyelid retraction (Collier sign)
  - Supranuclear upgaze paralysis
  - Convergence retraction nystagmus

Evaluation/Work-Up
- High-resolution brain MRI with gadolinium
  - Sagittal images are ideal for pineal region anatomy
- CT helpful in identifying areas of calcium deposition
- Visual field testing

Treatment
- Guided by tumor type and histology
- Lifelong follow-up of children with pineal region tumors is requisite

(Left) This graphic demonstrates normal anatomy of the pineal region. Note the close proximity of the pineal gland ⇨ to the superior colliculi →. Compression of the superior colliculi and other structures of the dorsal midbrain by an enlarged pineal gland leads to Parinaud syndrome. (Right) Sagittal T1 C+ MRI shows a heterogeneously enhancing pineal mass consistent with pineoblastoma (PB). Proximity of the lesion to the cerebral aqueduct causes hydrocephalus, seen in nearly all cases of PB.

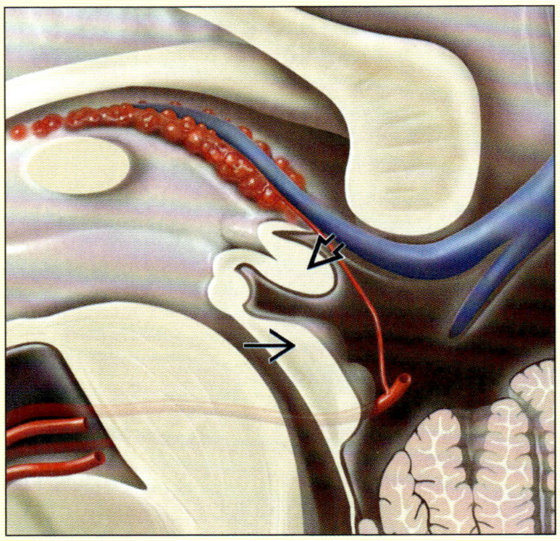

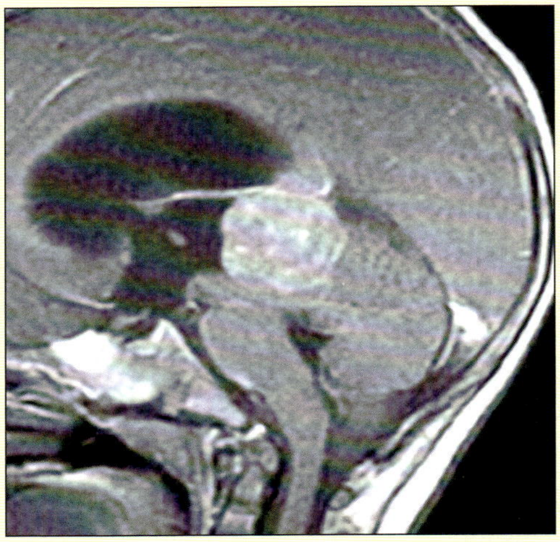

(Left) Sagittal T1 C+ MRI shows a classic benign pineal cyst ➔ with rim enhancement and mild mass effect. Note the slight compression and displacement of the tectal plate. (Courtesy L. Rudolf, MD.) (Right) Axial T1 C+ MRI shows an inhomogeneously enhancing midline mass of the pineal region ➔ in a boy who presented with double vision, nausea, vomiting, & headache in the frontal region. After surgical removal, histological analysis revealed a pineal germinoma.

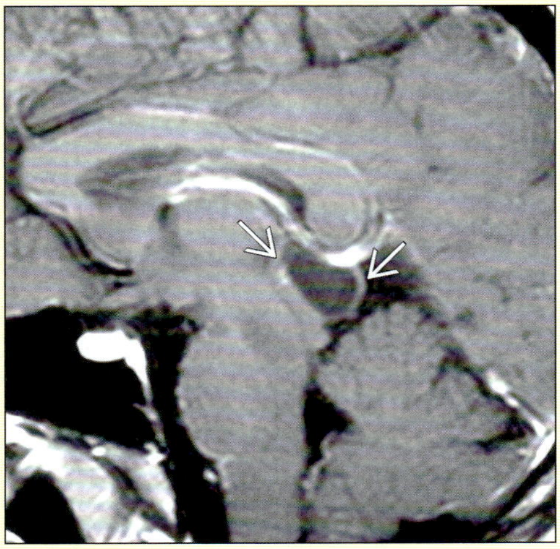

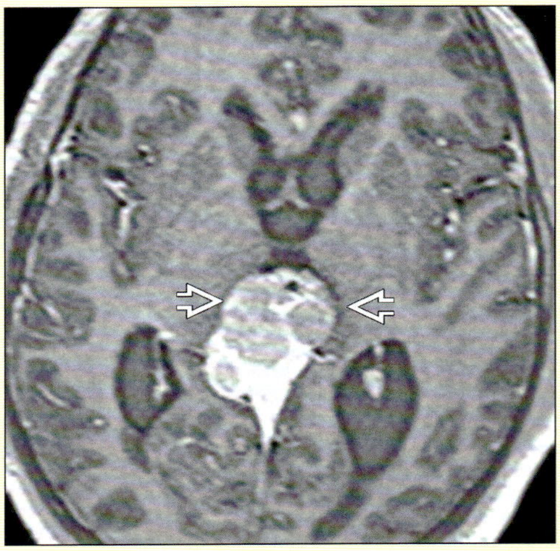

PINEALOMA

INTRODUCTION

Definitions
- Tumor of the pineal gland

Subtypes
- Germinoma
  - Most common pineal tumor
  - Classically occurs in young males
    - 90% are < 20 years old
    - Male:female = 10:1
- Teratoma
  - 2nd most common pineal tumor
  - Multicystic mass with calcium and fat deposition
- Pineocytoma
  - Differentiated tumor arising from pineal gland parenchymal cell
  - Rarely invasive
- Pinealoblastoma
  - Highly malignant, primitive embryonal tumor
  - 45% present with spinal dissemination
  - Mean age of diagnosis in children = 3 years
- Retinoblastoma (trilateral)
  - Bilateral retinoblastomas accompanied by midline intracranial tumor
    - 80% are pineal tumors (especially pinealoblastoma): Very poor prognosis
- Germ cell neoplasms, not otherwise specified
  - Uncommon, highly malignant
- Diffuse astrocytoma
  - May rarely arise from pineal gland
  - Typically do not present with Parinaud syndrome

PRESENTATION

Symptoms
- Headache, nausea, vomiting, and lethargy secondary to increased intracranial pressure (ICP)
- Mental status changes
- Paralysis of upward gaze (Parinaud)

Exam Findings
- Parinaud (dorsal midbrain) syndrome
  - Bilateral mid-dilated pupils
    - Pupils react poorly to light but constrict normally to convergence
  - Eyelid retraction (Collier sign)
  - Supranuclear upgaze paralysis
  - Convergence retraction nystagmus
- Signs consistent with increased ICP
  - Papilledema
  - Possible abducens nerve palsy
  - Ataxia
  - Decrease in cognitive function
- Concomitant endocrine abnormalities may be present
  - Diabetes insipidus, secondary amenorrhea, growth arrest

DIFFERENTIAL DIAGNOSIS

Pineal Cyst
- Found in 1-5% of normal MRI studies
- Most commonly asymptomatic
  - Large cysts may become symptomatic, resulting in Parinaud syndrome or hydrocephalus

Cerebrovascular Accident
- Parinaud syndrome may result from stroke to the midbrain
- More common in elderly patients

Mass Lesion Near Dorsal Midbrain
- Possible causes include hemorrhage, hydrocephalus, arteriovenous malformation, trauma, histiocytosis, sarcoid, neoplastic and infectious etiologies

EVALUATION/WORK-UP

Labs
- Germ cell tumors often have positive CSF or serum tumor markers
  - α-fetoprotein (AFP)
  - β-human chorionic gonadotropin (β-HCG)

Imaging
- High-resolution brain MRI with gadolinium
  - Sagittal images are ideal for pineal region anatomy
- CT helpful in identifying areas of calcium deposition
- Visual field testing

TREATMENT

Medical
- Treatment guided by tumor type and histology
  - Possible radiation and chemotherapy
    - Germinomas are among the most radiosensitive tumors

Surgical
- Dependent upon tumor type and histology
  - Surgical excision or stereotactic biopsy
  - CSF shunt may be necessary

Follow-Up
- Lifelong follow-up of children with pineal region tumors is requisite
  - May recur locally or distally

Prognosis
- Varies widely with differing tumor subtypes
  - Patients with nongerminomatous germ cell tumors have significantly worse prognosis than do those with germinomas

SELECTED REFERENCES

1. Goldenberg-Cohen N et al: Long-term ophthalmological follow-up of children with Parinaud syndrome. Ophthalmic Surg Lasers Imaging. 41(4):467-71, 2010
2. Cho BK et al: Pineal tumors: experience with 48 cases over 10 years. Childs Nerv Syst. 14(1-2):53-8, 1998
3. Keane JR: The pretectal syndrome: 206 patients. Neurology. 40(4):684-90, 1990

ACCOMMODATIVE SPASM

Key Facts

Introduction
- Difficulty viewing distant objects due to tonic contraction of ciliary muscle

Demographics
- Caused by overstimulation of parasympathetic nervous system
  - Leads to loss of ability to change shape of the lens
- Organic causes include alcohol, cholinergic drugs, and morphine
- Risk factors include
  - Head trauma
  - Brain tumors
  - Systemic or topical cholinergic drugs (e.g., pilocarpine)

Presentation
- Blurred vision when viewing distant objects
- Macropsia
- Normal near point of convergence
- Low accommodative amplitude relative to age

Differential Diagnosis
- Myasthenia gravis
- Myopia
- Spasm of the near reflex

Evaluation/Work-Up
- MRI of the dorsal midbrain and quadrigeminal plate

Treatment
- Topical antimuscarinic drops
- Cycloplegic agents
- Optometric vision therapy
- Follow-up for increased frequency/duration of spasms
- Visual symptoms improve in most patients with medical treatment
  - Few have complete disappearance of spasm

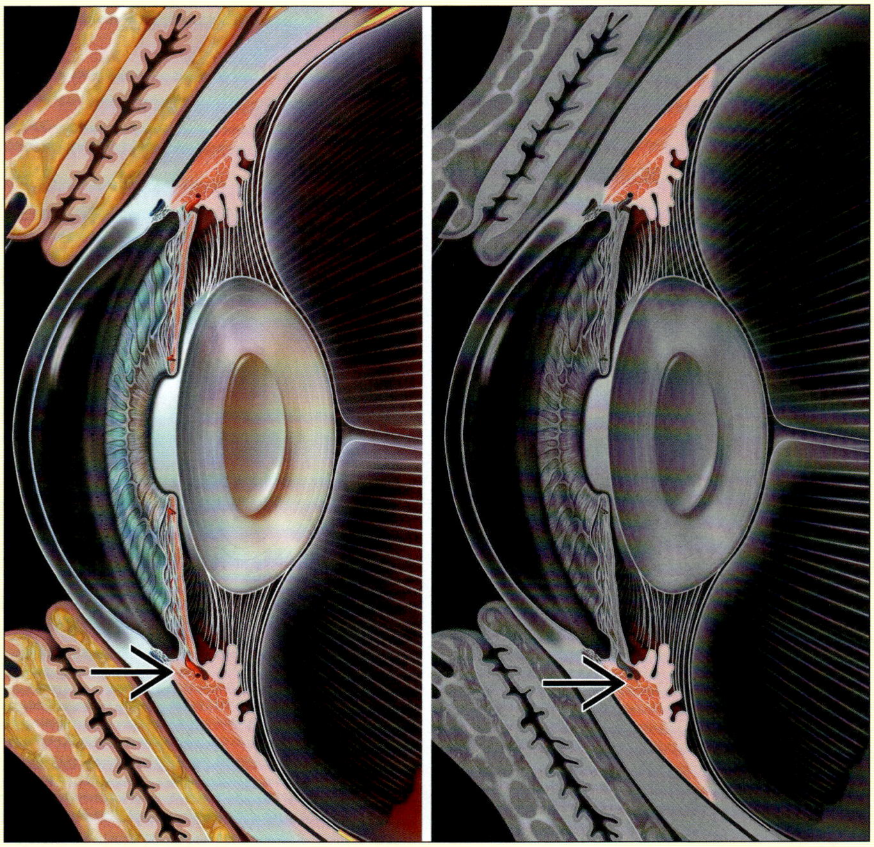

Graphic illustrates the location of the ciliary muscle ⇒. Contraction of the ciliary muscle results in relaxation of the zonules and a resulting thickening of the lens and accommodation. The ciliary muscle receives excess parasympathetic stimulation in patients with accommodative spasm. Overstimulation results in a loss of ability to properly shape the lens to focus on distant objects.

ACCOMMODATIVE SPASM

INTRODUCTION

Abbreviations
- Accommodative spasm (AS)

Definitions
- Difficulty viewing distant objects due to tonic contraction of ciliary muscle

DEMOGRAPHICS

Etiology/Risk Factors
- Caused by overstimulation of parasympathetic nervous system
  - Results in ciliary muscle of the eye remaining in a constant state of contraction
    - Leads to loss of ability to change shape of the lens to view distant objects
- Organic causes include alcohol, cholinergic drugs, and morphine
- Risk factors include
  - Head trauma
  - Brain tumors
  - Systemic or topical cholinergic drugs (e.g., pilocarpine)

Epidemiology
- In general population, 16.8% of people have an accommodative disorder
  - Of these, ~ 3% have accommodative spasm

PRESENTATION

Symptoms
- Blurred vision when viewing distant objects
- Macropsia
- Eye strain
- Headache
- Diplopia
- Symptom duration and frequency may increase with eye fatigue

Exam Findings
- Rapid worsening of existing myopia
- Normal near point of convergence
- Decreased negative relative accommodation
- Full range of eye movement in the doll's head maneuver
- Abnormal lag of accommodation
- Low accommodative amplitude relative to age (can evaluate accommodative convergence:accommodation [AC:A] ratio)
- Cycloplegic refraction
  - If AS is suspected, cycloplegic refraction using muscarinic antagonist can be used as a confirmatory test
    - If vision returns to baseline after cycloplegic agent administration, then diagnosis is confirmed

DIFFERENTIAL DIAGNOSIS

Myasthenia Gravis
- Autoimmune neuromuscular disorder
- Symptoms can include double vision and difficulty maintaining gaze
  - Systemic muscular weakness sets this apart from AS
- Diagnostic tests include acetylcholine receptor antibody assays and nerve conduction testing

Myopia
- Sudden worsening of existing myopia is a red flag for AS but can simply be part of a natural deterioration of vision
- Cycloplegic refraction will not show a difference in vision before vs. after antimuscarinic administration
- Macropsia and diplopia are not factors

Spasm of the Near Reflex
- Features include
  - Transient episodes of variable esotropia
  - Accommodative spasm
  - Pseudomyopia
  - Miosis

EVALUATION/WORK-UP

Imaging
- MRI of dorsal midbrain and quadrigeminal plate
  - There have been associations between pathology of these anatomical portions of the brain and accommodative disorders

TREATMENT

Medical
- If cause of spasm is organic (alcohol, cholinergic drugs, or morphine), remove the offending substance
- Topical antimuscarinic drops: To relax the ciliary muscles
  - Side effects include
    - Overrelaxation of the ciliary muscles resulting in difficulty with near vision
    - Excessive dilation of the pupil
- Cycloplegic agents (atropine)
  - Daily atropine treatments until spasm has fully relaxed
    - This treatment must be combined with reading glasses for near vision
- Optometric vision therapy
  - Pencil push-ups can teach the patient how to control the accommodative system (useful especially if patient has poor AC:A ratio)

Follow-Up
- If frequency or duration of spasm increases after initiation of treatment

Prognosis
- Visual symptoms improve in most patients with medical treatment, but few have complete disappearance of spasm

SELECTED REFERENCES

1. Rutstein RP et al: Accommodative spasm: a study of 17 cases. J Am Optom Assoc. 59(7):527-38, 1988

Key Facts

Introduction
- Unequal pupil sizes ≥ 0.4 mm

Demographics
- 20% of people have physiological anisocoria

Presentation
- Acute onset anisocoria is an emergency
- In anisocoria, presume pathologic eye (whether constricted or dilated) is same side as that of ptosis
  - Ptosis is associated with both Horner syndrome and oculomotor nerve palsy

Differential Diagnosis
- Potentially life-threatening causes of anisocoria
  - Horner syndrome (carotid dissection)
  - Oculomotor nerve palsy (brain aneurysm, uncal herniation, head trauma)
- Anisocoria greater in dim light: Horner syndrome, mechanical anisocoria
- Greater in bright light: Adie tonic, oculomotor nerve palsy, pharmacologic dilation

Evaluation/Work-Up
- Old photographs of patients (e.g., driver's license) may help determine whether anisocoria is physiologic
- Anisocoria accompanied by confusion, decreased mental status, and severe headache may point to a neurosurgical emergency (hemorrhage, tumor)
- Adie tonic pupil will constrict with low-dose (0.1%) pilocarpine; a normal pupil will not
- Normal pupil will dilate > Horner syndrome pupil after 4-10% cocaine challenge, increasing difference of anisocoria

Treatment
- Medical treatment depends on underlying cause of anisocoria

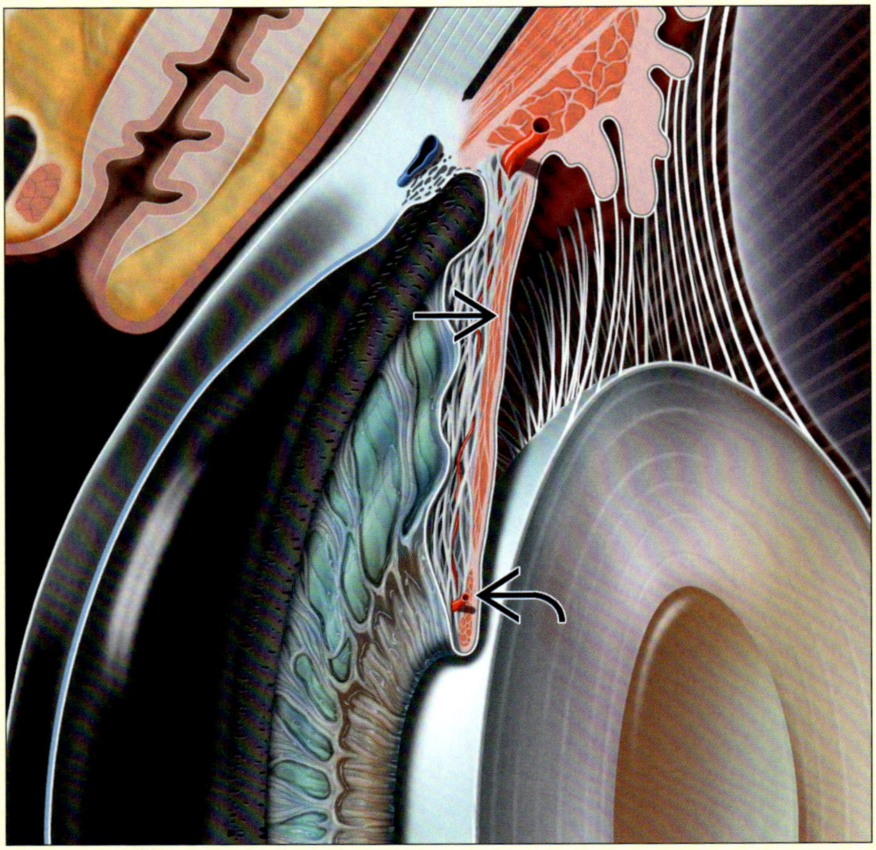

Anisocoria describes the condition of 1 pupil being larger than the other. If the anisocoria increases in darkness, the cause is likely physiologic anisocoria or Horner syndrome. Horner syndrome can be central, preganglionic, or postganglionic. Denervation of the iris dilator muscle ➡ leads to the affected eye having a smaller pupillary aperture in the dark. If the anisocoria increases in light, then the likely cause is a CN3 palsy, pharmacologic mydriasis, or Adie tonic pupil. A CN3 palsy may manifest with associated abnormal ocular motility and affect the parasympathetic-controlled iris sphincter muscle ↱.

ANISOCORIA

INTRODUCTION

Definitions

- Anisocoria: Unequal pupil size

PRESENTATION

Symptoms

- Noted pupil difference
- Photosensitivity, decreased near vision, diplopia, ptosis
- Acute onset anisocoria with confusion, severe headache, and decreased mental status is a neurosurgical emergency

Exam Findings

- Pupillary diameter difference of ≥ 0.4 mm (either in bright light or dim light)
- Anisocoria greater in dim light
  - Small pupil is abnormal: Pupil cannot dilate
- Anisocoria greater in bright light
  - Larger pupil is abnormal: Pupil cannot constrict

DIFFERENTIAL DIAGNOSIS

Physiologic Anisocoria

- Anisocoria is same in light and dark
- < 1 mm pupillary difference without underlying cause, present in 20% of people
- May have been present for a long time (check old photos of patient)

Horner Syndrome

- Anisocoria greater in dim light than bright light (affected pupil is miotic)
- Unilateral ptosis of upper and lower lids
- Anhidrosis of affected side of face if lesion is proximal to bifurcation of carotid artery (affect sudomotor nerves that travel with external carotid)
- Lesion in sympathetic pathway causing denervation of iris dilator muscle
  - 1st order = brainstem and spinal cord (synapse at ciliospinal center of bundle at about C8-T2 vertebrae)
  - 2nd order = preganglionic: Neck, pulmonary apex, and upper chest lesions
  - 3rd order = postganglionic: Superior cervical ganglion, internal carotid artery, sellar and parasellar lesions (pituitary), and cavernous sinus lesions
- Pharmacologic testing
  - Cocaine test (4-10%): Dilate normal pupil, but do not dilate Horner pupil
  - Hydroxyamphetamine (Paredrine) 1%: Will dilate normal pupil **and** Horner pupil if 1st- or 2nd-order lesion; increases anisocoria if 3rd-order Horner lesion
  - Apraclonidine: Reverses anisocoria by dilating Horner pupil, without change in normal pupil size
- Congenital Horner syndrome: Requires work-up
  - Present at birth
  - Is usually benign; may be associated with birth trauma to brachial plexus
  - Intrauterine trauma is a possible but rare cause
  - Lighter iris on Horner side
- Acquired Horner: Requires work-up
  - In children, may represent neuroblastoma of sympathetic chain in upper chest or neck

Mechanical Anisocoria

- Trauma: May cause miosis (spasm of pupil sphincter) or mydriasis (damage to sphincter muscle)
- Previous surgery affecting iris
- Inflammation/iritis causing posterior synechiae

Pharmacologic Constriction

- Pilocarpine or organophosphates including fertilizers, chemical weapons (e.g., sarin)

Pharmacologic Dilation

- Cycloplegics (e.g., atropine, homatropine, tropicamide)
- Oral anticholinergics (e.g., diphenhydramine)

Adie Tonic Pupil

- Greater in bright light than dark
- Mydriasis in affected pupil with poor or absent constriction in response to light
- Constricts slowly with near effort, then dilates slowly
- Segmental palsy of constriction
- Caused by viral or bacterial infection or idiopathic
- Pupil dilates with dilute pilocarpine (0.125% or 0.1%)

Hutchinson Pupil

- Unilateral dilated pupil ("blown pupil") in a patient with mental status changes or coma
- Uncal herniation entrapping CN3 along tentorial edge
- Pupillomotor nerves travel at peripheral nerve and are affected early in compressive lesions of CN3

Oculomotor Nerve Palsy (CN3 Palsy)

- Usually associated with muscle palsy, diplopia, and ptosis
- Intracranial aneurysm, head trauma, or tumor
- Diabetic and vascular CN3 palsies often spare the pupil

Glaucoma

- Acute angle closure may produce a fixed, mid-dilated pupil
  - Associated with cloudy cornea, pain, nausea, and high IOP
- Pilocarpine is sometimes used to treat glaucoma and results in pupil constriction

Meningitis or Encephalitis

- Argyll Robertson pupil: Better response to near than light
- Classically neurosyphilis, but other causes are possible

Benign Episodic Pupillary Dilation

- 1 pupil dilated, may last for minutes to hours
- May have discomfort or accommodative symptoms
- May have associated migraine
- Benign; occurs in young and healthy adults

SELECTED REFERENCES

1. Ettinger ER et al: Anisocoria. Variation and clinical observation with different conditions of illumination and accommodation. Invest Ophthalmol Vis Sci. 32(3):501-9, 1991
2. Lam BL et al: The prevalence of simple anisocoria. Am J Ophthalmol. 104(1):69-73, 1987

CAVERNOUS SINUS LESIONS

Key Facts

Introduction

- Insult to the cavernous sinus resulting in ophthalmoplegia, proptosis, Horner syndrome, ocular and conjunctival congestion, or trigeminal sensory loss

Demographics

- Aneurysm, thrombosis
- Trauma
- Carotid cavernous fistulas (CCF)
- Tumors
- Inflammatory disorders

Presentation

- Horner syndrome, along with 6th nerve palsy, helps localize lesion to cavernous sinus
- Painful and isolated CN3, CN4, or CN6 palsy
- Decreased or absent corneal reflex (CNV1)
- Funduscopic exam: Retinal hemorrhages and possible optic nerve edema

Evaluation/Work-Up

- Infectious or inflammatory causes: CBC, CMP, ESR, ANA, ANCA labs and serum protein electrophoresis
- Infection, malignancy: Cerebrospinal fluid (CSF) with cytology
- Mass lesions: MRI
- Vascular lesions: CT &/or DSA

Treatment

- Tumors: Radiation vs. expectant observation
- Infection: High-dose antibiotic therapy should be directed against most common pathogens
- Aneurysm: Endovascular balloon occlusion may be indicated if symptomatic
- Fistula: Endovascular obliteration of the fistula with coils if indicated

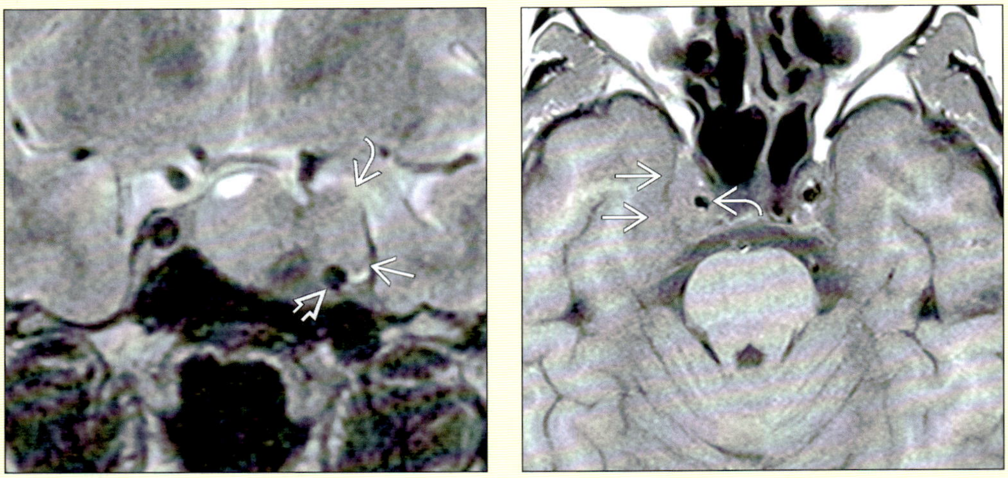

(Left) *Coronal T2 MRI shows macroadenoma that extends into the left cavernous sinus →, displacing and encasing the cavernous internal carotid artery (ICA) →. The tumor lateral to the ICA → confirms cavernous sinus invasion.* ***(Right)*** *Axial T1 MRI shows enlargement of the right cavernous sinus →. There is mild narrowing of the cavernous internal carotid artery →. The patient presented with sphenoethmoidal sinusitis, headache, right 6th nerve palsy, and mild right proptosis.*

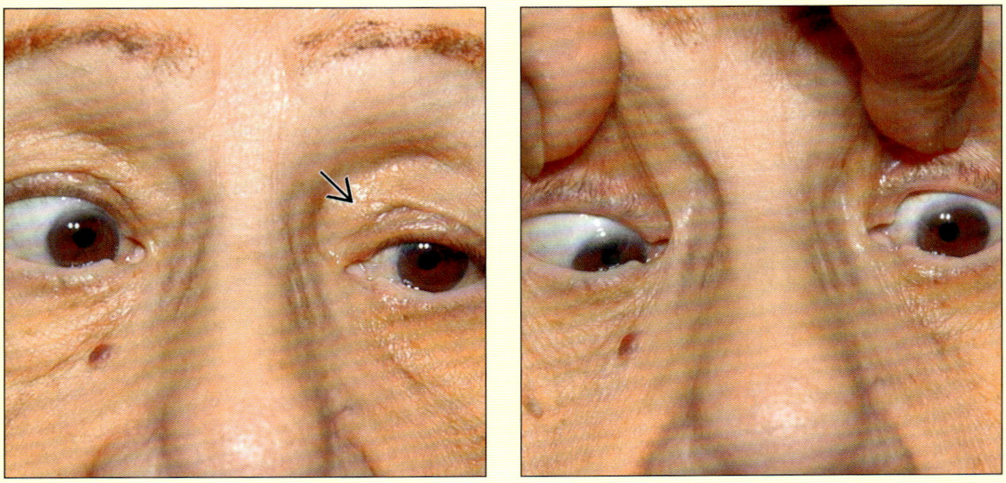

(Left) *This external photograph demonstrates a patient with ptosis and paralysis of the left eye → resulting from a cavernous sinus lesion.* ***(Right)*** *When eyelids of the same patient are retracted, the paralysis of the left eye becomes more prominent. In this image, the patient demonstrates paralysis of the left eye upon attempt to gaze down and out, due to involvement of the cranial nerves passing through the cavernous sinus.*

CAVERNOUS SINUS LESIONS

INTRODUCTION

Definitions
- Insult to the cavernous sinus resulting in possible ophthalmoplegia, proptosis, Horner syndrome, ocular and conjunctival congestion, or trigeminal sensory loss

Anatomy of Cavernous Sinus
- Contains sympathetic plexus; internal carotid artery; CN3, CN4, and CN6; and ophthalmic (V1) and sometimes maxillary (V2) branch of trigeminal nerve

DEMOGRAPHICS

Etiology/Risk Factors
- Vascular
  - Aneurysm
    - Slow-growing aneurysm that may compress various structures, causing painful ophthalmoplegia
  - Carotid cavernous fistulas (CCF)
    - Direct: Subacute presentation after trauma or rupture of aneurysm, causing carotid artery and cavernous sinus to connect
    - Indirect: Indolent presentation as a result of smaller meningeal branches from carotid system connecting with cavernous sinus
  - Thrombosis
    - Infectious spread from paranasal sinus, orbital cellulitis, facial furuncle, or dental origin, causing a prothrombotic environment
- Tumors
  - Local spread: Nasopharyngeal, pituitary, meningioma, neurofibroma, others
  - Metastatic spread: Lung, breast, prostate, lymphoma, multiple myeloma
- Inflammatory disorders
  - Wegener granulomatosis, sarcoidosis, polyarteritis nodosa, or Tolosa-Hunt syndrome

Epidemiology
- In USA, ~ 5% of ophthalmoplegias are secondary to damage of cranial nerves in the cavernous sinuses

PRESENTATION

Symptoms
- Orbital fullness or pain, double vision, proptosis, sensory loss, miosis, ptosis

Exam Findings
- Varies with cause, but may include
  - Horner syndrome, along with 6th nerve palsy, helps localize lesion to cavernous sinus
  - Painful and isolated CN3, CN4, or CN6 palsy
  - Fixed pupil due to palsies of sympathetic and parasympathetic nerves
  - Decreased or absent sensation in ophthalmic branch (V1) of trigeminal nerve and sometimes maxillary branch (V2)
  - Funduscopic exam: Possible retinal hemorrhages or optic nerve edema
- CCF: Classic triad of chemosis, pulsatile exophthalmos, and bruit over eye
- Pituitary tumors: May have endocrine signs

DIFFERENTIAL DIAGNOSIS

Orbital Tumors
- Imaging will localize

Meningitis or Subarachnoid Hemorrhage
- Isolated 6th nerve palsy

Vasculopathic CN3 Palsy
- Isolated CN3 with presence of major risk factors such as diabetes, hypertension, and hyperlipidemia

EVALUATION/WORK-UP

Labs
- Infectious or inflammatory causes: CBC, CMP, ESR, ANA, ANCA labs and serum protein electrophoresis

Pathology
- Infection, malignancy: Cerebrospinal fluid (CSF) with cytology
- Inflammatory disease, malignancy: Biopsy if etiology unknown

Imaging
- Mass lesions: MRI
- Vascular lesions: CT &/or digital subtraction angiography (DSA)

TREATMENT

Medical
- Tumors: Radiation vs. expectant observation
- Cavernous sinus thrombosis
  - High-dose antibiotic therapy should be directed against most common pathogens
- Inflammatory cavernous sinus syndromes
  - Response to usual treatment for the specific etiology
  - Tolosa-Hunt syndrome responds to high-dose steroid therapy

Surgical
- Aneurysm: Endovascular balloon occlusion may be indicated if symptomatic
- Fistula: Endovascular obliteration of fistula with coils if indicated
- Tumor: Resections are rarely done due to sensitive nature of area of interest

SELECTED REFERENCES

1. Altay T et al: Sellar and parasellar metastatic tumors. Int J Surg Oncol. 2012:647256, 2012
2. Bone I et al: Syndromes of the orbital fissure, cavernous sinus, cerebello- pontine angle, and skull base. J Neurol Neurosurg Psychiatry. 76 Suppl 3:iii29-iii38, 2005
3. Bhatia K et al: Septic cavernous sinus thrombosis secondary to sinusitis: are anticoagulants indicated? A review of the literature. J Laryngol Otol. 116(9):667-76, 2002
4. Keane JR: Cavernous sinus syndrome. Analysis of 151 cases. Arch Neurol. 53(10):967-71, 1996

CONVERGENCE INSUFFICIENCY

Key Facts

Introduction
- Inability to maintain binocular vision, due to decreased ability to converge the eyes
  - Causes difficulty focusing on near images

Demographics
- Caused by pathology to portions of the brain responsible for ocular convergence
- General population incidence of 0.1-0.2%
- Children and young adults are most commonly affected

Presentation
- Eye discomfort after reading (most common symptom); headaches; diplopia
- Decreased convergence amplitude with near vision
- Normal distance vision

Differential Diagnosis
- Exotropia
- Oculomotor nerve palsy
- Myasthenia gravis

Evaluation/Work-Up
- MR imaging of the head in adults with new onset, looking for pathology to oculomotor nerve/nucleus or extraocular muscles
- Assess AC:A ratio

Treatment
- Orthoptic therapy (pencil push-ups)
- Base-in prism glasses
- Resection of medial rectus muscle in 1 or both eyes
- Patients generally have successful treatment with ocular exercises alone and rarely need further treatment

__(Left)__ External photo depicts intact convergence when fixing at a near object. Increased accommodative demand is usually accompanied by convergence to allow for binocular fixation at near targets. __(Right)__ With convergence insufficiency, increased accommodative demand caused by near fixation does not lead to accommodative convergence, thus preventing binocular fusion with near targets. Patients with convergence insufficiency usually present with diplopia with near fixation and asthenopia.

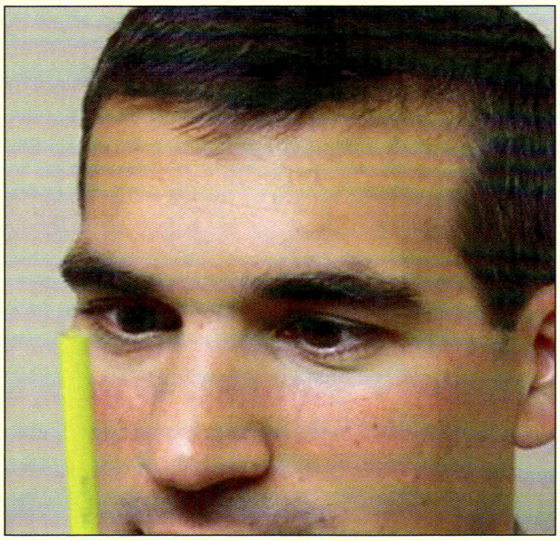

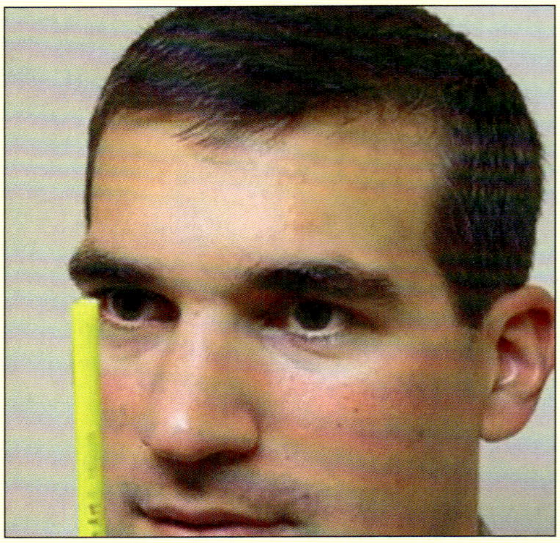

__(Left)__ The oculomotor nerve ➔ (cranial nerve 3) innervates the extraocular muscles that control ocular convergence. Pathology of this nerve can lead to a clinical picture similar to convergence insufficiency due to adductor muscle dysfunction. __(Right)__ This external photograph shows a patient with left-sided ptosis ➔ and extraocular muscle weakness due to myasthenia gravis. Myasthenia may also cause a clinical picture similar to convergence insufficiency due to adductor (medial rectus) weakness/fatigability.

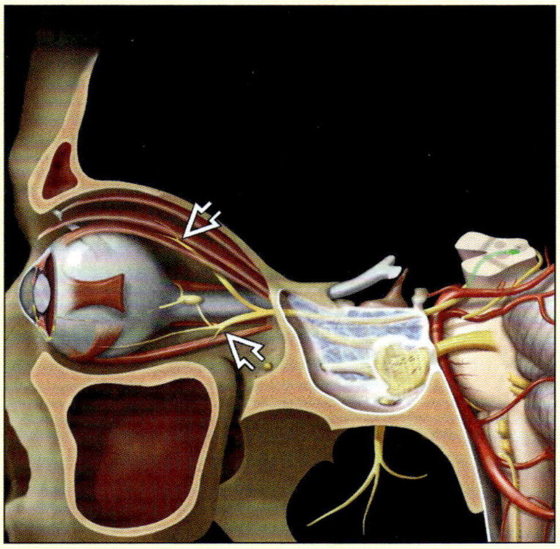

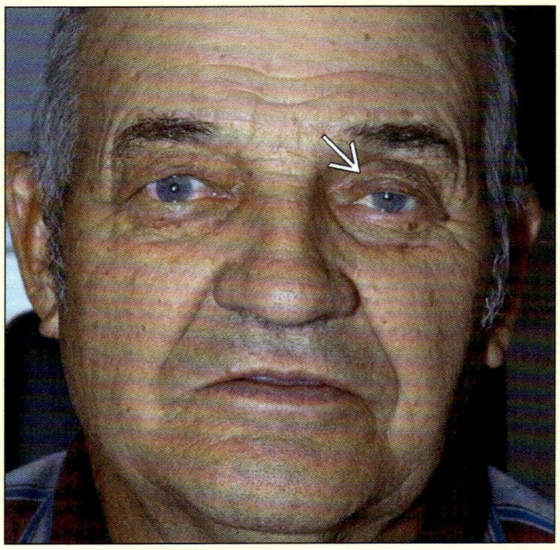

CONVERGENCE INSUFFICIENCY

INTRODUCTION

Abbreviations

- Convergence insufficiency (CI)

Definitions

- Inability to maintain binocular vision, due to decreased ability to converge the eyes
  - Causes difficulty focusing on near images

DEMOGRAPHICS

Etiology/Risk Factors

- Risk factors include
  - Damage/lesions to portions of the brain responsible for convergence movements of the eyes including
    - Midbrain reticular formation
    - Nucleus raphe interpositus
    - Reticularis tegmenti pontis
- Can be caused by trauma, neurologic disease, or congenital abnormalities affecting cranial nerve 3, which controls the action of convergence

Epidemiology

- General population incidence of 0.1-0.2%
- Children and young adults are most commonly affected

PRESENTATION

Symptoms

- Eye discomfort after reading (most common symptom)
- Frontal headaches
- Asthenopia
- Increased fatigue
- Diplopia
- Decreased ability to concentrate

Exam Findings

- Remote near point of convergence
- Decreased convergence amplitude with near vision
- Exophoria and or exotropia on alternate prism cover testing
- Normal distance vision

DIFFERENTIAL DIAGNOSIS

Exophoria/Exotropia/Intermittent Exotropia

- Patients usually present with chief complaint of diplopia
- Examination will reveal exodeviation both at near and distance
- In children, this condition must be identified early as it can lead to amblyopia

Oculomotor Nerve Palsy

- CN3 palsy can lead to convergence insufficiency
- Patients commonly complain of diplopia
- Exam will often reveal ptosis on affected side &/or loss of pupillary light reflex

Myasthenia Gravis

- Can present with convergence and accommodation insufficiency
  - Also commonly features fluctuating weakness of skeletal muscles
- Test for antibodies to acetylcholine receptor

EVALUATION/WORK-UP

Imaging

- MR imaging of the head looking for pathology to the oculomotor nerve/nucleus or extraocular muscles

TREATMENT

Medical

- Orthoptic therapy
  - Should be first-line treatment
  - "Pencil push-up" exercises improve fusional convergence
  - Ocular exercises can be performed either in office or at home and include
    - Stereograms
    - Vergence facility exercises
    - Computer-based programs
- Base-in prism glasses for reading and near vision
  - Good alternative if exercises are not successful

Surgical

- Resection of medial rectus muscle on 1 or both eyes
  - Carries a risk of diplopia

Follow-Up

- For in-office orthoptic therapy
- If medical/surgical treatment does not alleviate symptoms

Prognosis

- Patients generally have successful treatment with ocular exercises alone and rarely need further treatment

SELECTED REFERENCES

1. Cooper J et al: Convergence insufficiency-a major review. Optometry. 83(4):137-58, 2012
2. Arnoldi K et al: A review of convergence insufficiency: what are we really accomplishing with exercises? Am Orthopt J. 57:123-30, 2007
3. Colavito J et al: Non-ptotic ocular myasthenia gravis: a common presentation of an uncommon disease. Optometry. 76(7):363-75, 2005
4. Scheiman M et al: A randomized clinical trial of treatments for convergence insufficiency in children. Arch Ophthalmol. 123(1):14-24, 2005
5. Scheiman M et al: A randomized clinical trial of vision therapy/orthoptics versus pencil pushups for the treatment of convergence insufficiency in young adults. Optom Vis Sci. 82(7):583-95, 2005
6. Demer JL et al: Magnetic resonance imaging of human extraocular muscles in convergence. J Neurophysiol. 89(4):2072-85, 2003

HORNER SYNDROME

Key Facts

Introduction

- Neurological syndrome caused by interruption of sympathetic nerve pathways to the eye resulting in classic triad of ptosis, miosis, and anhidrosis
- Classified by location of lesion (1 of 3 neurons)
  - Central (1st-order neuron)
  - Preganglionic (2nd-order neuron)
  - Postganglionic (3rd-order neuron)

Presentation

- Mild ptosis (2 mm)
- Slight elevation of inferior eyelid (reverse ptosis)
- Miosis
- Anhidrosis is present in central or preganglionic lesions
- Depending on underlying etiology, may present with additional neurological deficits
- Iris heterochromia occurs in congenital cases where affected iris is lighter in color

Evaluation/Work-Up

- Confirmation of Horner syndrome
  - Cocaine testing
  - Apraclonidine testing
- Localization of Horner syndrome
  - Hydroxyamphetamine testing
- Possibility of underlying life-threatening condition (especially if there is pain after neck injury or surgery) often necessitates emergent imaging
- Associated neurological findings and hydroxyamphetamine testing should dictate selection of imaging modalities

Treatment

- Treat underlying condition
- If benign, no further treatment is necessary
- Prognosis varies with etiology of disease

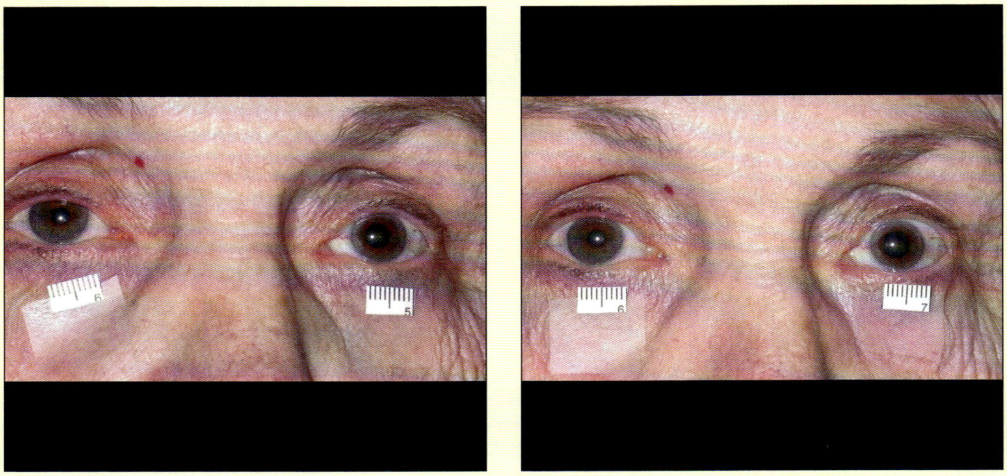

(Left) *This photo shows a 72-year-old woman who presented to the clinic with complaints of mild ptosis and miosis of the right side.* ***(Right)*** *This photo of the same patient was taken after administration of topical 4% cocaine to each eye. Greater than 1 mm of anisocoria remained after 45 minutes, confirming the diagnosis of Horner syndrome.*

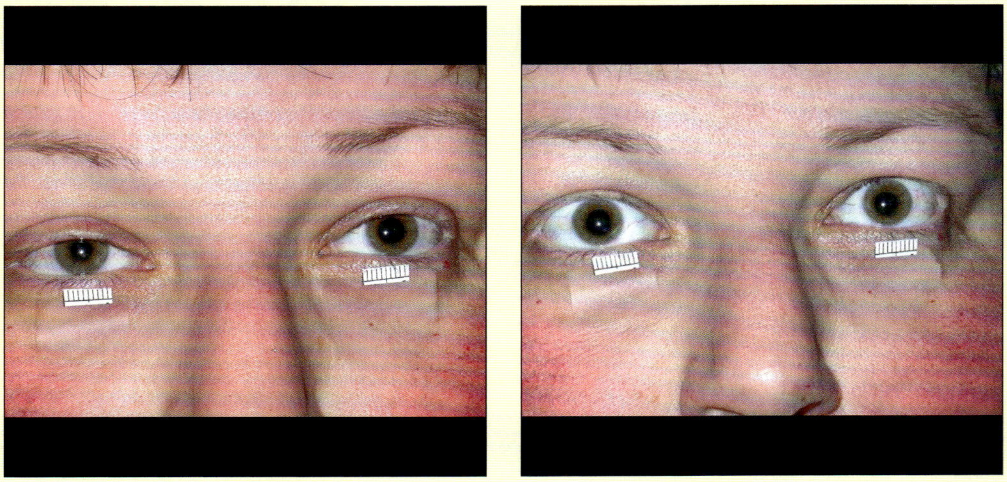

(Left) *This clinical photo demonstrates right-sided Horner syndrome present in a 41-year-old woman. The classic features of mild ptosis, lower eyelid elevation (reverse ptosis), and miosis of the affected eye are readily apparent.* ***(Right)*** *This photo was taken after administration of 1% hydroxyamphetamine to each eye. This resulted in bilateral mydriasis, indicating that the lesion causing the right-sided Horner syndrome was preganglionic.*

HORNER SYNDROME

INTRODUCTION

Synonyms
- Oculosympathetic paresis

Definitions
- Neurological syndrome caused by an interruption of sympathetic nerve pathways to the eye resulting in classic triad of ptosis, miosis, and anhidrosis

Subtypes
- Classified by location of lesion (1 of 3 neurons)
  - Central (1st-order neuron)
    - Originates in posterior hypothalamus and descends uncrossed to cervical spinal cord (C8-T2)
  - Preganglionic (2nd-order neuron)
    - Travels from sympathetic trunk, through brachial plexus, over lung apex, and synapses at superior cervical ganglion near angle of mandible at bifurcation of carotid artery
  - Postganglionic (3rd-order neuron)
    - Ascends within adventitia of internal carotid artery, through cavernous sinus, where it then joins the V1 branch of trigeminal nerve and terminates at iris dilator muscle

DEMOGRAPHICS

Etiology/Risk Factors
- Up to 40% of cases are of unknown etiology
- Classified by location of underlying lesion
  - Central
    - Vascular occlusion (frequently associated with lateral medullary syndrome [Wallenberg syndrome])
    - CNS tumor
    - Demyelinating disease
    - Cervical disc disease
    - Syringomyelia
    - Diabetic autonomic neuropathy
    - Arteriovenous malformation
  - Preganglionic
    - Pancoast (superior sulcus of lung or mediastinal tumor)
    - Thoracic aortic aneurysm
    - Subclavian artery aneurysm
    - Thyroid mass
    - Iatrogenic (jugular cannulation, thoracic surgery)
  - Postganglionic
    - Internal carotid dissection (can occur with sudden deceleration injury), aneurysm, thrombosis, or arteritis
    - Cavernous sinus lesion
    - Lymphoma
    - Tolosa-Hunt syndrome
    - Jugular venous ectasia
    - Nasopharyngeal tumor
    - Otitis media
    - Cluster headache
    - Iatrogenic (carotid endarterectomy, neck surgery, chiropractic manipulation, or stenting)
  - Congenital (frequently accompanied by iris heterochromia)
    - Birth trauma to brachial plexus
    - Neuroblastoma
    - Congenital infections
    - Idiopathic

Epidemiology
- Congenital cases occur with a prevalence of 1 per 6,250 births
- In a pediatric population (< 19 years), incidence was estimated to be 1.42 per 100,000 patients

PRESENTATION

Symptoms
- Ipsilateral classic quartet
  - Ptosis
  - Miosis
  - Anhidrosis
  - Pseudoenophthalmos can be present as upper lid comes down and lower lid comes up
- Ocular redness
- Nasal congestion
- Headache
- Depending on underlying etiology, may present with additional neurological deficits
- Vast majority of cases are unilateral
- Pediatric populations may have a difference in eye color or impaired facial flushing

Exam Findings
- Anisocoria is more apparent in dim illumination
- Dilation lag of affected pupil
- Mild ptosis (2 mm)
  - Weakness of the Müller muscle
- Slight elevation of inferior eyelid (reverse ptosis)
  - Weakness of inferior tarsal muscle
- Anhidrosis is present in central or preganglionic lesions
  - In children, impaired facial flushing (harlequin sign) is more apparent than anhidrosis
- Light and near pupillary reactions remain intact
- Iris heterochromia occurs in congenital cases where the affected iris is lighter in color

DIFFERENTIAL DIAGNOSIS

Mechanical Anisocoria
- Distinguished easily by applying topical phenylephrine
  - Mechanically restricted pupil remains miotic while a Horner pupil dilates
- Slit-lamp examination reveals adhesions and synechiae

Physiologic Anisocoria
- Most common cause of anisocoria
- Usually, difference in pupil diameter is < 1.0 mm
- Degree of anisocoria may vary from day to day
- Cocaine testing will demonstrate symmetric mydriasis

Pharmacologic Anisocoria
- Unilateral use of pilocarpine may result in poorly reactive pupil
- Patient will often have history of glaucoma
- Less common due to wide array of alternatives for glaucoma treatment

HORNER SYNDROME

Raeder Paratrigeminal Syndrome
- Horner syndrome associated with daily unilateral headaches not consistent with cluster
- Typically, middle-aged males
- Diagnosis of exclusion

EVALUATION/WORK-UP

Labs
- If a child presents with Horner syndrome, consider urine catecholamine analysis
  - Possibility of underlying neuroblastoma
- Consider CBC

Pharmacology
- Confirmation of Horner syndrome
  - Cocaine testing
    - Cocaine acts as a norepinephrine, reuptake inhibitor causing mydriasis of a normal pupil
      - Instill 2 drops of 4% or 10% cocaine in each eye, and measure the amount of anisocoria present after 45 minutes
      - In Horner syndrome, affected pupil will dilate poorly because little or no norepinephrine is being released into synaptic cleft
      - Post-cocaine testing is diagnostic of Horner syndrome if at least 1 mm of anisocoria is present
  - Apraclonidine testing
    - Apraclonidine is a weak α-1 agonist that produces no significant effect on iris dilator muscle of a normal pupil
    - Horner pupil develops adrenergic supersensitivity, resulting in mydriasis of the affected eye
      - Application of either 0.5% or 1.0% apraclonidine results in dilation of only the Horner pupil
      - Subsequent paradoxical reversal of anisocoria occurs
- Localization of Horner syndrome
  - Hydroxyamphetamine acts by releasing norepinephrine from axon terminal
    - Central or preganglionic lesion
      - 3rd-order neuron remains intact, and the drop will dilate the Horner pupil equal to that of normal pupil
    - Postganglionic lesion
      - 3rd-order neuron has degenerated, and poor dilation of Horner pupil will result following hydroxyamphetamine application

Imaging
- Possibility of underlying life-threatening condition often necessitates imaging
- Associated neurological findings and hydroxyamphetamine testing should dictate selection of imaging modalities
  - Suspected cerebrovascular disease
    - Diffusion-weighted brain MRI
  - Suspected CNS tumor
    - Brain MRI with gadolinium enhancement
  - Suspected demyelinating disease
    - FLAIR sequence
  - Acute Horner syndrome with associated neck or face pain (carotid dissection until proven otherwise)
    - MRI/MRA neck
    - CTA neck
    - Carotid ultrasonography
    - Conventional angiography remains gold standard
  - Horner syndrome with accompanying ophthalmoparesis
    - Brain MRI focused on cavernous sinuses
  - 2nd-order Horner syndrome without localizing symptoms to CNS
    - CT chest

TREATMENT

Medical
- Treat underlying condition
  - If benign, no further treatment is necessary

Surgical
- If life-threatening conditions have been excluded and ptosis is persistent and stable, blepharoplasty may be considered

Follow-Up
- Varies widely depending on underlying cause
  - If benign, no follow-up is needed

Prognosis
- Varies with etiology of disease

SELECTED REFERENCES

1. Adamec I et al: Beware of "old" Horner syndrome. Optom Vis Sci. 89(10):e12-5, 2012
2. Wang FM et al: Unilateral straight hair and congenital horner syndrome. J Neuroophthalmol. 32(2):132-4, 2012
3. Smith SJ et al: Incidence of pediatric Horner syndrome and the risk of neuroblastoma: a population-based study. Arch Ophthalmol. 128(3):324-9, 2010
4. Koc F et al: The sensitivity and specificity of 0.5% apraclonidine in the diagnosis of oculosympathetic paresis. Br J Ophthalmol. 89(11):1442-4, 2005
5. Morales J et al: Ocular effects of apraclonidine in Horner syndrome. Arch Ophthalmol. 118(7):951-4, 2000
6. Digre KB et al: Selective MR imaging approach for evaluation of patients with Horner's syndrome. AJNR Am J Neuroradiol. 13(1):223-7, 1992
7. Cremer SA et al: Hydroxyamphetamine mydriasis in Horner's syndrome. Am J Ophthalmol. 110(1):71-6, 1990
8. Kardon RH et al: Critical evaluation of the cocaine test in the diagnosis of Horner's syndrome. Arch Ophthalmol. 108(3):384-7, 1990
9. Maloney WF et al: Evaluation of the causes and accuracy of pharmacologic localization in Horner's syndrome. Am J Ophthalmol. 90(3):394-402, 1980

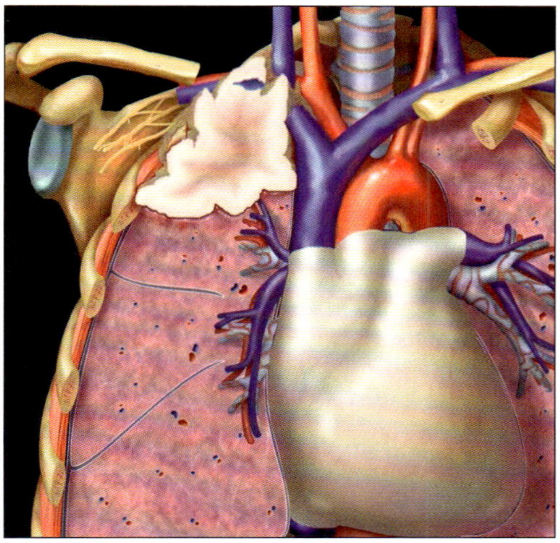

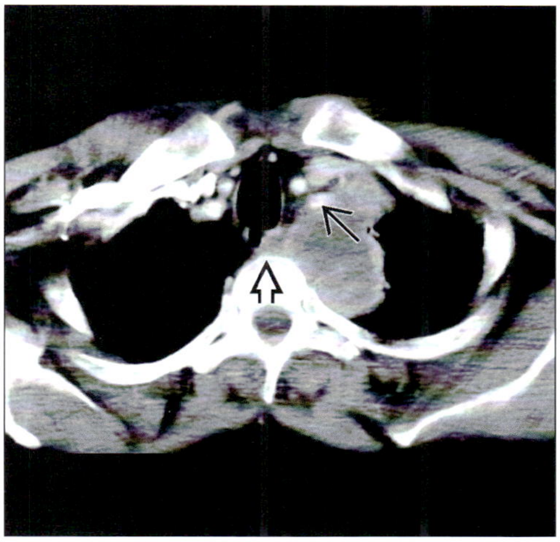

(Left) *Graphic shows the characteristic features of a Pancoast tumor. From the lung apex, the tumor usually extends through the chest wall and into the brachial plexus. A 2nd-order Horner syndrome is often caused by a Pancoast tumor.* ***(Right)*** *Axial contrast-enhanced CT shows an unresectable Pancoast tumor surrounding the left subclavian artery ⇨ and extending into the mediastinum ⇨.*

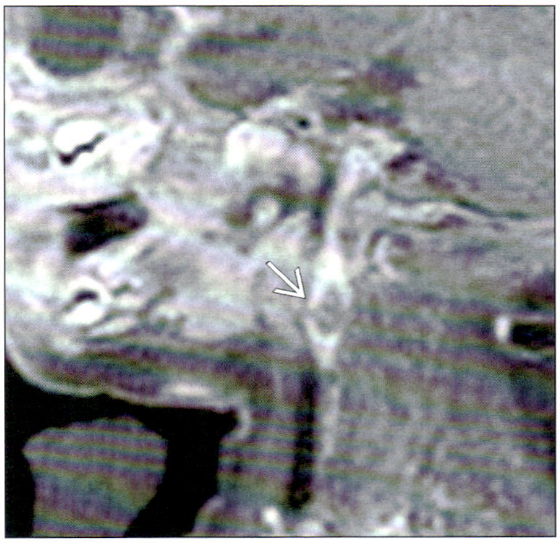

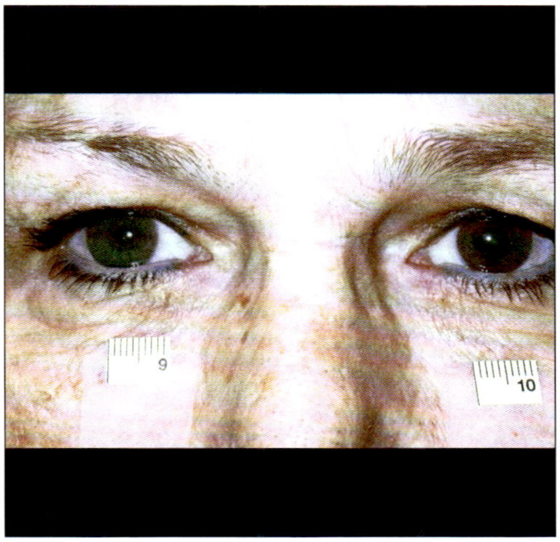

(Left) *Sagittal MRI in a 9-month-old child with Horner syndrome shows a small, rim-enhancing cervical neuroblastoma ➡ in the oropharyngeal carotid space.* ***(Right)*** *In addition to the ptosis and miosis of the right side, note that the affected iris is much lighter in color than the one on the left. This hypochromic heterochromia is indicative of a congenital Horner syndrome.*

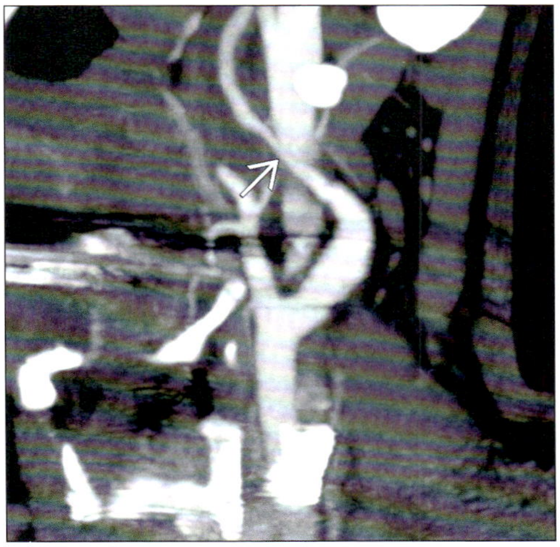

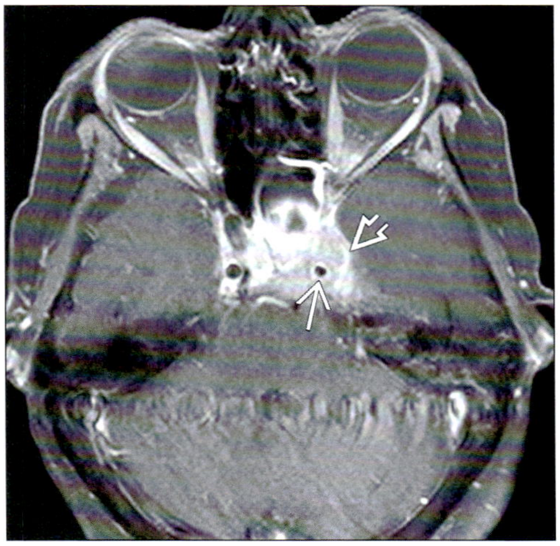

(Left) *Sagittal oblique CTA demonstrates tapered narrowing ➡ of the internal carotid artery (ICA) above the carotid bifurcation, secondary to dissection. Acute-onset Horner syndrome associated with ipsilateral face or neck pain is an ICA dissection until proven otherwise.* ***(Right)*** *Axial MRI shows a nasopharyngeal carcinoma spreading cephalad through the nasopharynx roof into the cavernous sinus ➡ with encasement of the left cavernous internal carotid artery ➡ resulting in Horner syndrome.*

INTERNUCLEAR OPHTHALMOPLEGIA

Key Facts

Introduction

- Gaze abnormality characterized by paresis of adduction in one eye combined with abduction nystagmus of other eye
- May be unilateral or bilateral
- Caused by lesions of medial longitudinal fasciculus
  - Multiple sclerosis, ischemia, infection, trauma, tumor

Presentation

- Ipsilateral paresis/paralysis of adduction with horizontal jerk nystagmus of contralateral, abducting eye
- Possible horizontal diplopia, transient oscillopsia, reading fatigue, loss of stereopsis, adduction slowing
- Normal convergence
- Diminished vertical-gaze holding
- Inadequate vertical vestibuloocular reflex
- Abnormal opticokinetic and pursuant responses
- Vertical gaze evoked nystagmus
- Skew deviation

Evaluation/Work-Up

- Infrared oculography (rarely used)
- Magnetic resonance imaging
  - Rule out multiple sclerosis, stroke
- Diagnosis
  - Based on history and clinical presentation

Treatment

- Treat underlying condition (e.g., multiple sclerosis, stroke)
- Patching 1 eye may relieve diplopia
- Botulinum toxin injection may reduce diplopia
- Prognosis
  - Partial-complete recovery occurs in in 78% of patients over weeks to months

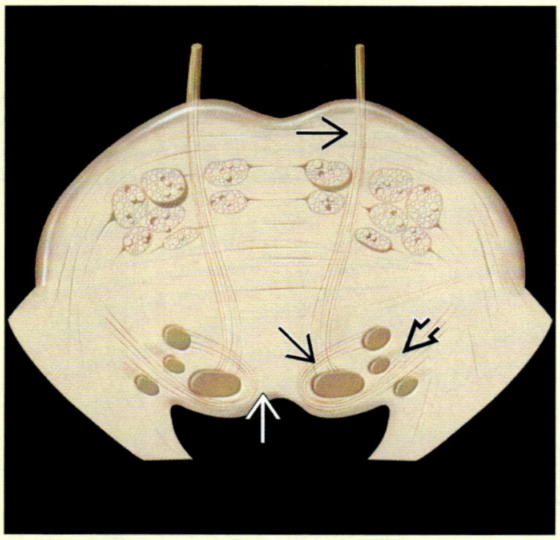
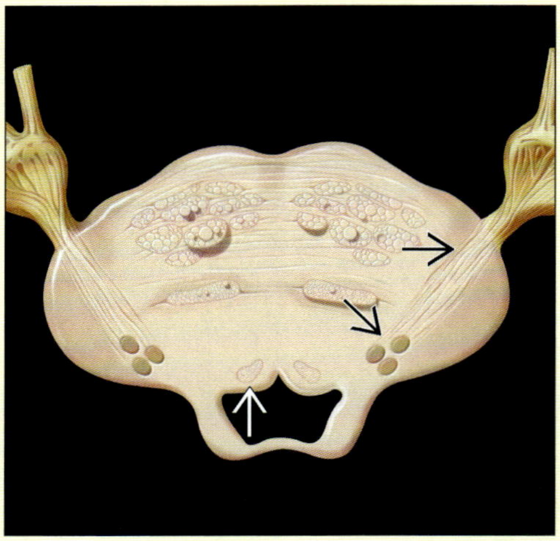

(Left) *This illustration shows an axial view of the mid pons. Note the CN6 nucleus with fibers extending anteriorly ➔. Several CN7 nuclei ➔ are located lateral to CN6. The medial longitudinal fasciculus ➔ travels through the posteromedial pons.* ***(Right)*** *This illustration shows an axial view of the superior pons. Note the CN5 nucleus located posteriorly with fibers ➔ extending anteriorly. The paired medial longitudinal fasciculi ➔ can again be seen posteromedially.*

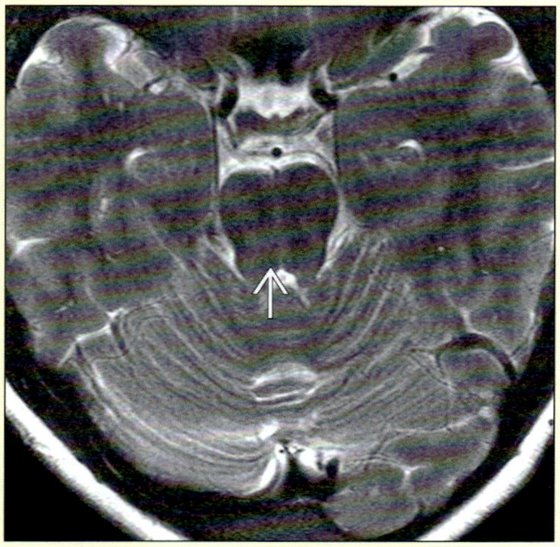
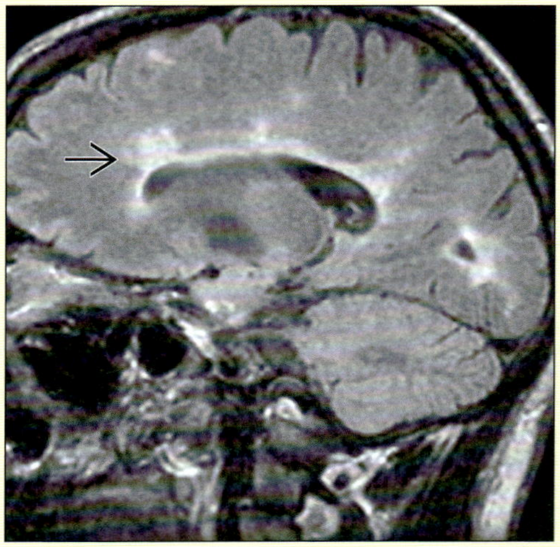

(Left) *This axial T2-weighted MRI shows structures at the junction of the pons and midbrain. Major white matter tracts, including the corticospinal tracts and medial longitudinal fasciculus ➔, cannot be seen directly and are identified by typical location.* ***(Right)*** *This sagittal FLAIR MRI shows callososeptal hyperintensities radiating from the lateral ventricles with a perpendicular orientation ➔, characteristic of multiple sclerosis (MS), the most common cause of internuclear ophthalmoplegia.*

INTERNUCLEAR OPHTHALMOPLEGIA

INTRODUCTION

Abbreviations
- Internuclear ophthalmoplegia (INO)

Definitions
- Gaze abnormality characterized by paresis of adduction in one eye combined with abduction nystagmus of other eye
  - May be unilateral or bilateral
- Caused by lesions of medial longitudinal fasciculus (MLF); signals from 6th nerve to opposite 3rd nerve are impaired
  - Located in dorsomedial brainstem tegmentum of either pons or midbrain
  - Carries interneurons from contralateral abducens nerve nucleus to medial rectus subnucleus of oculomotor nerve complex of affected eye

DEMOGRAPHICS

Etiology/Risk Factors
- Unilateral INO commonly caused by
  - Multiple sclerosis (MS) in young adults
  - Infarction in elderly
- Bilateral INO commonly caused by
  - Brainstem glioma in children
  - MS in adults
- Other causes
  - Infection, tumor, trauma, vasculitis, drug overdose

Epidemiology
- Up to 70% caused by MS

PRESENTATION

Symptoms
- Horizontal diplopia
- Transient oscillopsia
- Reading fatigue
- Loss of stereopsis
- Difficulty tracking fast objects (such as tennis balls)

Exam Findings
- Ipsilateral paresis/paralysis of adduction with horizontal jerk nystagmus of contralateral, abducting eye
- Adduction slowing
- Normal convergence, except in anterior midbrain lesion
- Diminished vertical-gaze holding
- Inadequate vertical vestibuloocular reflex
- Abnormal opticokinetic and pursuant responses
- Vertical gaze evoked nystagmus

DIFFERENTIAL DIAGNOSIS

Myasthenia Gravis
- Pseudo-INO on exam
- Ptosis, lid lag

Guillain-Barré Syndrome
- Areflexia, limb weakness, ataxia

Partial Cranial Nerve 3 (CN3) Palsy
- Additional CN3 defects (ptosis, pupil dilation)
- Impaired convergence, absence of contralateral abduction nystagmus

Associated Syndromes
- 1-and-a-half syndrome
  - Lesion of paramedian reticular formation (PPRF) &/or abducens nucleus and MLF
  - Gaze palsy in 1 direction with INO on horizontal gaze in opposite direction, normal convergence
- 8-and-a-half syndrome
  - 1-and-a-half syndrome + 7th nerve palsy
- Wall-eyed bilateral INO
  - Midbrain lesion involving both medial rectus subnuclei and MLF
  - Bilateral INO with exotropia and loss of convergence (a.k.a. wall-eyed)

EVALUATION/WORK-UP

Imaging
- Infrared oculography
- Magnetic resonance imaging
  - Rule out MS, stroke

Diagnosis
- Based on history and clinical presentation

TREATMENT

Medical
- Treat underlying condition (e.g., MS, stroke, tumor)
- Patching 1 eye may relieve diplopia
  - Inexpensive
- Botulinum toxin injection may reduce diplopia

Follow-Up
- Regular ophthalmologic examinations
- Referral to neurologist or neuroophthalmologist

Prognosis
- Partial-complete recovery is very common in MLF ischemia within weeks to months

SELECTED REFERENCES

1. Keane JR: Internuclear ophthalmoplegia: unusual causes in 114 of 410 patients. Arch Neurol. 62(5):714-7, 2005
2. Bolaños I et al: Internuclear ophthalmoplegia: causes and long-term follow-up in 65 patients. Acta Neurol Scand. 110(3):161-5, 2004
3. Kim JS: Internuclear ophthalmoplegia as an isolated or predominant symptom of brainstem infarction. Neurology. 62(9):1491-6, 2004
4. Atlas SW et al: Internuclear ophthalmoplegia: MR-anatomic correlation. AJNR Am J Neuroradiol. 8(2):243-7, 1987
5. Müri RM et al: The clinical spectrum of internuclear ophthalmoplegia in multiple sclerosis. Arch Neurol. 42(9):851-5, 1985

ISOLATED 3RD NERVE PALSY

Key Facts

Introduction

- Palsy of CN3 causing range of symptoms including ophthalmoplegia, ptosis, and mydriasis
  - Pupil sparing: No pupillary involvement
  - Relative pupil sparing: Sluggishly reactive and partially dilated pupil
  - Pupil involving: Poorly reactive, fixed, dilated pupil (more risk for compressive lesions)
- Aberrant regeneration: Frequently seen with trauma and compressive lesions, rare with microvascular etiology
  - Requires imaging when present

Demographics

- Causes include trauma, tumor, diabetes, aneurysm, surgery, stroke, infection

Presentation

- Generalized ophthalmoplegia with exotropia and hypotropia due to unopposed abducens and superior oblique action
- Ptosis due to levator paralysis
- Fixed, dilated pupil if pupillomotor fibers affected

Evaluation/Work-Up

- Urgent MRI and MRA of central nervous system
  - Critical for for patients with pupil involvement, children, patients < 50 years without vasculopathic risk factors, patients with evidence of aberrant regeneration, and for pupil-sparing palsy lasting > 3 months
  - Must rule out aneurysm

Treatment

- Treat underlying cause

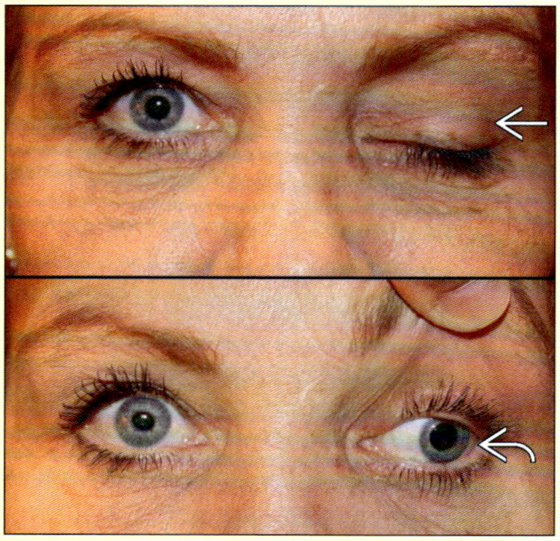

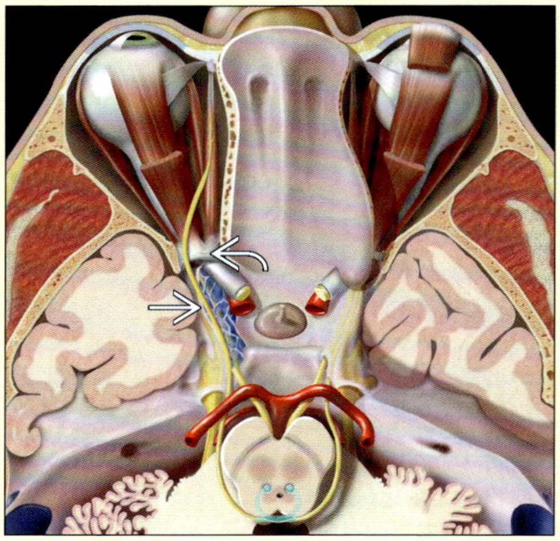

(Left) *External photo shows an acute pupil-involving CN3 palsy on the left secondary to a posterior communicating aneurysm. Note the pronounced ptosis →, adduction deficit with pronounced left exotropia, and blown left pupil → with consequent anisocoria.* ***(Right)*** *Axial graphic depicts CN3 originating from the oculomotor nucleus complex, traversing the cavernous sinus →, and entering the orbit through the superior orbital fissure via the annulus of Zinn →, before dividing into superior and inferior divisions.*

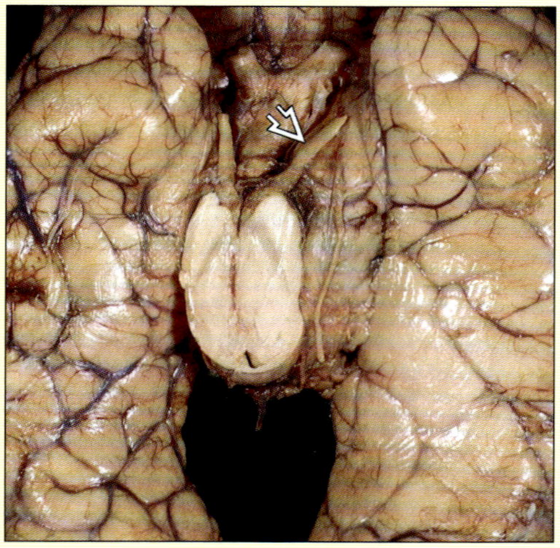

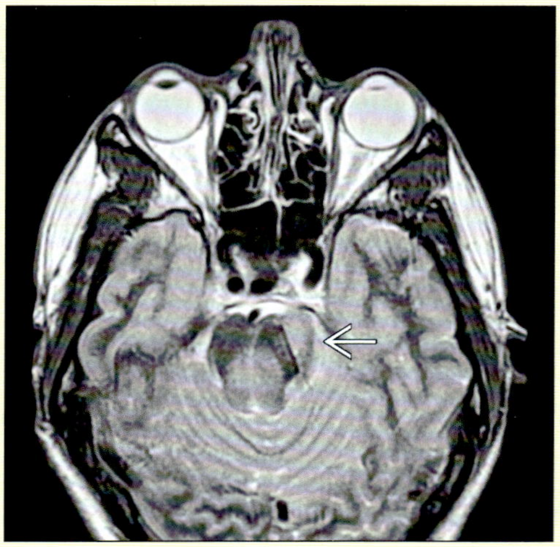

(Left) *Gross pathology shows findings of transtentorial herniation, which has led to compression of CN3 →. As parasympathetic fibers run superficially in this nerve, any pupil-involving CN3 palsy requires urgent imaging to rule out compressive pathology.* ***(Right)*** *Axial T2 MRI shows the temporal lobe herniated into the posterior fossa →, where it may potentially cause compression of CN3. Other differential considerations for CN3 palsy include vascular disease, trauma, or aneurysm.*

ISOLATED 3RD NERVE PALSY

INTRODUCTION

Synonyms
- Oculomotor nerve (CN3)

Definitions
- Palsy-causing deficits in CN3 function including ocular motility restriction, decreased levator palpebrae function, and diminished pupillary constriction

Subtypes
- Pupil sparing: No pupillary involvement (generally due to vasculopathies [e.g., diabetes, hypertension])
- Relative pupil sparing: Sluggishly reactive and partially dilated pupil
- Pupil involving: Poorly reactive, fixed, dilated pupil
  - Pupillomotor fibers compose outermost nerve fibers of CN3; more susceptible to compressive lesions such as aneurysms (posterior communicating artery most common), uncal herniation, and masses
  - Require immediate brain MRI and MRA to rule out aneurysm
- May present with complete (full gaze limitation other than abduction) or partial ophthalmoplegia; if lesion after annulus of Zinn, may only affect 1 division
  - Superior-division palsy: Deficits in supraduction and ptosis
  - Inferior-division palsy: Deficits in infraduction and adduction, with possible pupillary involvement
- Aberrant regeneration: Findings may include pupil-gaze or eyelid-gaze dyskinesis
  - Frequently seen following CN3 palsy secondary to trauma and compressive lesions
  - Rare with microvascular etiology; requires imaging

DEMOGRAPHICS

Etiology/Risk Factors
- In analysis of 1,400 patients, causes included trauma (26%), tumor (12%), diabetes (11%), aneurysm (10%), surgery (10%), stroke (8%), infection (5%), Guillain-Barré and Fisher syndromes (5%), idiopathic cavernous sinusitis (3%), benign self-limited (2%), miscellaneous (4%), and unknown (3%)

PRESENTATION

Symptoms
- Diplopia, visual obscuration secondary to ptosis, pain (affects 94% of aneurysms and 69% of diabetic cases)

Exam Findings
- Exotropia due to unopposed abducens action
- Ptosis due to levator paralysis
- Enlarged and poorly reactive pupil if pupillomotor fibers affected

DIFFERENTIAL DIAGNOSIS

Myasthenia Gravis
- No pupil involvement; symptoms tend to worsen toward end of day
- Positive Tensilon, ice pack, fatigue, or rest test

Cavernous Sinus Syndrome
- May present with ophthalmoplegia and proptosis; frequently involves more than 1 cranial nerve

Orbital Inflammatory Pseudotumor
- Inflammation usually accompanied by pain; eyelid may be edematous and conjunctiva injected

Chronic Progressive External Ophthalmoplegia
- No pupil involvement; slowly progressive and bilateral

Giant Cell Arteritis (GCA)
- No pupil involvement; has associated systemic symptoms; age frequently > 50-60 years

EVALUATION/WORK-UP

Labs
- Urgent erythrocyte sedimentation rate, C-reactive protein, and platelets for suspicion of GCA
- Lumbar puncture for pupil-involving palsy with negative imaging and angiography

Imaging
- Gadolinium-enhanced MRI and MRA of central nervous system
  - Urgently performed for patients with pupil involvement, children, patients < 50 years without vasculopathic risk factors, patients with evidence of aberrant regeneration, and for pupil-sparing palsy lasting > 3 months
- Angiography of cerebral circulation should be performed for suspected aneurysm or inconclusive imaging

TREATMENT

Medical
- Treat underlying cause
- Blood pressure and diabetes control for ischemic disease

Surgical
- Patients with persistent strabismus or ptosis may require surgical correction

Follow-Up
- Daily initially; coordinate with other departments depending on etiology

Prognosis
- Varies with underlying etiology
- Most patients with ischemic CN3 palsy have improvement in symptoms within 3 months

SELECTED REFERENCES

1. Keane JR: Third nerve palsy: analysis of 1400 personally-examined inpatients. Can J Neurol Sci. 37(5):662-70, 2010
2. Santillan A et al: Early endovascular management of oculomotor nerve palsy associated with posterior communicating artery aneurysms. Interv Neuroradiol. 16(1):17-21, 2010
3. Bruce BB et al: Third nerve palsies. Semin Neurol. 27(3):257-68, 2007

ISOLATED 4TH NERVE PALSY

Key Facts

Introduction
- Dysfunction of CN4
  - Without evidence of pathology to other cranial nerves
- Causes include
  - Idiopathic, traumatic, congenital, ischemic, compressive

Demographics
- CN4 has longest intracranial length of any cranial nerve, increasing risk of injury
- Hypertension and vasculopathies
- Diabetes

Presentation
- Torsional, horizontal, and vertical diplopia
- Head tilting in old photos and large vertical fusional amplitude (indicates longstanding palsy)
- Inability to look down and inward
- Excyclotorsion
- Otherwise normal cranial nerve exam

Differential Diagnosis
- Non-isolated CN4 palsy
- Idiopathic inflammatory pseudotumor of orbit
- Orbital cellulitis

Evaluation/Work-Up
- If 4th nerve palsy is isolated, imaging not needed
  - MRI/CT if other cranial nerve deficits are found or if other neurologic signs are present
- Ischemic should resolve in < 3 months

Treatment
- Prism lenses
  - Be wary of doing refractive surgery or refractive cataract surgery as these patients are used to wearing prisms in their glasses
- Harada-Ito surgical procedure

__(Left)__ Graphic shows a frontal view of the superior oblique muscle and tendon ➔ and trochlea ➔ in the right orbit. CN4 palsies cause deficits in eye depression (especially in adduction) and incyclotorsion. __(Right)__ Graphic shows side view of cavernous sinus ➔. If the etiology of the CN4 palsy is secondary to pathology within the cavernous sinus, there will often be involvement of other CNs (CN3, CN5, and CN6). Isolated CN4 palsies are more likely due to trauma or small vessel disease.

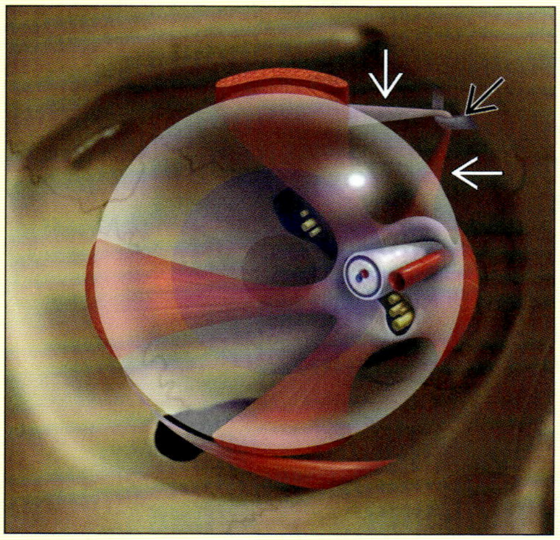

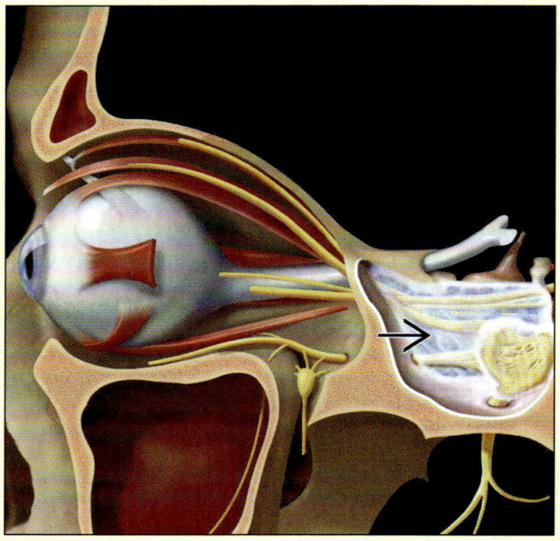

__(Left)__ This graphic demonstrates the pathway of CN4 ➔. Notice the immediate decussation of fibers ➔ and that the nerve exits on the posterior surface of the brainstem ➔. CN4 has the longest intracranial length of any nerve, increasing the risk of injury. __(Right)__ External photo shows a patient with a left superior oblique palsy and left hypertropia in adduction. Patients present with diplopia, an inability to look down and in, and may have a head tilt to the opposite side of the involved eye.

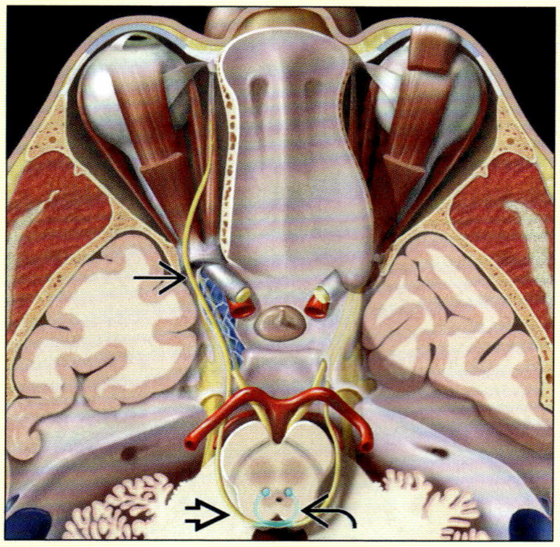

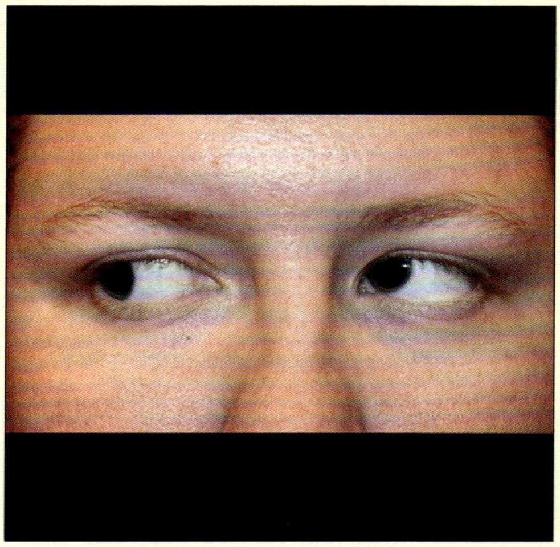

ISOLATED 4TH NERVE PALSY

INTRODUCTION

Definitions
- Dysfunction of cranial nerve 4 (CN4), a.k.a. trochlear nerve, without evidence of pathology to other cranial nerves
  - CN4 innervates superior oblique muscle

Subtypes
- Congenital, ischemic, idiopathic, traumatic, compressive

DEMOGRAPHICS

Etiology/Risk Factors
- Can occur from lesions anywhere along CN4
  - Pathway of CN4 is from trochlear nucleus, located in tegmentum of midbrain, to the orbit
- CN4 has longest intracranial length of any cranial nerve, increasing risk of injury due to trauma
- Clinical risk factors include
  - Hypertension and vasculopathies
  - Diabetes
  - Head trauma

PRESENTATION

Symptoms
- Torsional diplopia
- Horizontal diplopia
- Vertical diplopia
  - Causes difficulty reading
- Head tilting in old photos (indicates longstanding palsy)
- Inability to look down and inward

Exam Findings
- Excyclotorsion: When relaxed, eye is rotated outward
- Positive Bielschowsky test (3-step test)
  - Tilting head to side of CN4 palsy increases diplopia
  - Hypertropic in primary gaze
  - Worse with gaze away from the affected side
- Large vertical fusional amplitude with congenital cases (10-15 diopters)
- Full cranial nerve and neurological examination should be performed
  - If a truly isolated palsy, there should not be any other abnormal neurological findings

DIFFERENTIAL DIAGNOSIS

Non-Isolated 4th Nerve Palsy
- Will have other neurological or neuroophthalmologic signs in addition to trochlear nerve palsy
- Causes of non-isolated palsy can include
  - Myasthenia gravis (including ptosis)
  - Systemic inflammatory disease (e.g., giant cell arteritis)

Decompensation of Congenital 4th Nerve Palsy
- Usually accompanied by large fusional amplitudes

Idiopathic Inflammatory Pseudotumor of Orbit
- Inflammation that restricts eye movement and causes diplopia and eye pain
- Work-up includes orbital CT and MRI looking for inflammation

Orbital Cellulitis
- Generally unilateral, causes swelling and inflammation within orbit, leading to eye pain, diplopia, and decreased movement
- Ophthalmological emergency requiring orbital CT, antibiotics, and possible surgical intervention

EVALUATION/WORK-UP

Labs
- Anti-acetylcholine receptor antibodies for myasthenia gravis
- Fasting blood sugar &/or hemoglobin A1C
  - Especially in adult patients with new onset CN4 isolated palsy

Imaging
- Isolated 4th nerve palsy without other neurologic deficits, and lasting < 3 months, may be observed without imaging
- Head MRI/CT
  - If signs of additional neurologic findings on physical examination

TREATMENT

Medical
- Prism lenses

Surgical
- Harada-Ito procedure (anterolateral superior oblique transposition)
  - Best results in patients with symptoms of torsional diplopia
- Be wary of doing refractive surgery or refractive cataract surgery as these patients are used to wearing prisms in their glasses

Follow-Up
- If patient or their primary care doctor notice development of other cranial nerve palsies

Prognosis
- Varies with underlying cause; many cases are benign; however, must use caution
  - 10% due to aneurysm/neoplasm
  - 20% ischemic
  - 30% other
  - 40% trauma

SELECTED REFERENCES

1. Bradfield YS et al: Outcomes of Harada-Ito surgery for acquired torsional diplopia. J AAPOS. 16(5):453-7, 2012
2. Raghavendra S et al: Isolated trochlear nerve palsy with midbrain hemorrhage. Indian J Ophthalmol. 58(1):66-7, 2010
3. Brazis PW: Isolated palsies of cranial nerves III, IV, and VI. Semin Neurol. 29(1):14-28, 2009

ISOLATED 6TH NERVE PALSY

Key Facts

Introduction
- Dysfunction of CN6 (abducens nerve)
  - Lateral rectus muscle paralysis → unable to abduct eye
  - Horizontal gaze paralysis toward side of lesion

Demographics
- Annual incidence ~ 11 per 100,000 people
- Most common ocular motor cranial nerve palsy

Presentation
- Binocular, horizontal diplopia
  - Worse with gaze toward affected muscle
- Abduction deficit
  - Esotropia increasing toward affected muscle
- Small vertical deviation may be present

Evaluation/Work-Up
- ESR, CRP, evaluate blood pressure, CBC, diabetes work-up, VDRL, FTA-ABS, and ANA as appropriate
- Lumbar puncture
  - Consider in adults < 50 years, or if clinically indicated
- Brain MRI
  - Imaging should be obtained in children with persistent CN6 palsy and all patients < age 50
  - Consider imaging patients > 50 years if vascular risk factors are not present

Treatment
- Patching
  - Relieves diplopia, inexpensive
- Prism therapy
  - May be effective for small deviations
  - Ineffective if deviation is incomitant
- Botulinum toxin injection
- Strabismus surgery after recovery is complete
  - Lateral rectus resection possibly combined with medial rectus recession depending on size of deficit

*(**Left**) This graphic shows a frontal view of the brainstem with exiting cranial nerves (CN). CN6 exits at the pontomedullary junction ➔, medial to CN7 and CN8. CN6 palsy may be caused by ischemia, compression, trauma, or infection. (**Right**) This graphic shows a coronal section through the cavernous sinus (CS). CN6 is central ➔ along with CN3 ➔, CN4 ➔, CNV1 ➔, and CNV2 ➔ peripherally. Pathology of the cavernous sinus very rarely presents as isolated CN6 palsy since multiple CNs are affected.*

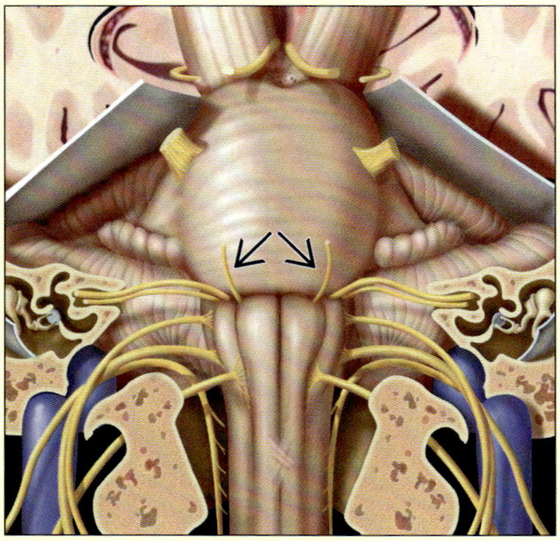

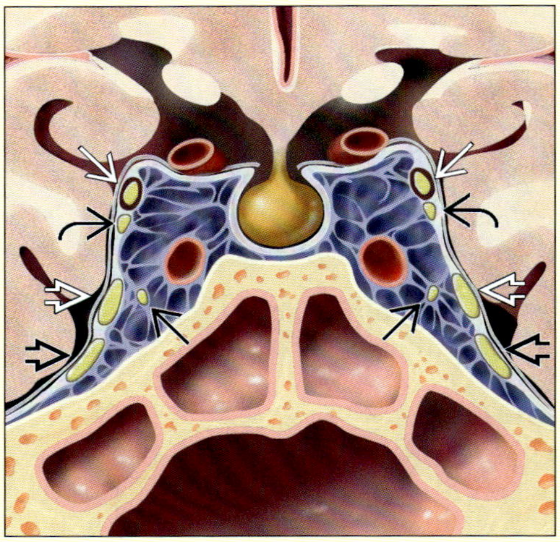

*(**Left**) External photo depicts extraocular motility of a patient with a left-sided CN6 palsy. Patient has intact right gaze; however, he is unable to abduct his left eye past the midline on attempted left gaze. (**Right**) Axial T2-weighted MRI shows hyperintensity and enlargement of the pons ➔ associated with acute ischemia. CN6 palsy can result from ischemia to the abducens nucleus (mid-pons). Nuclear damage would cause bilateral gaze palsy toward affected side, unlike fascicular or nerve lesions.*

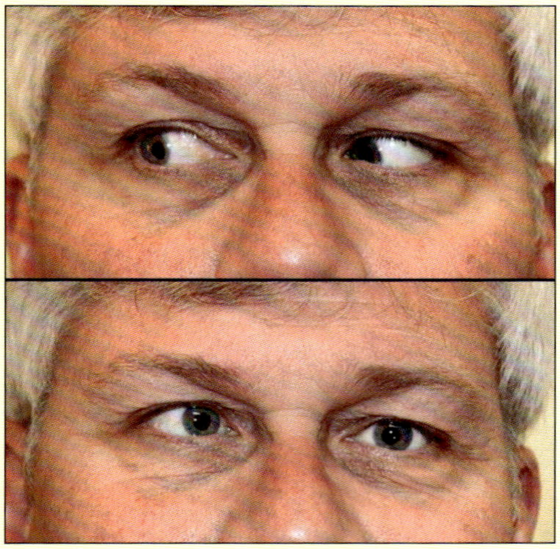

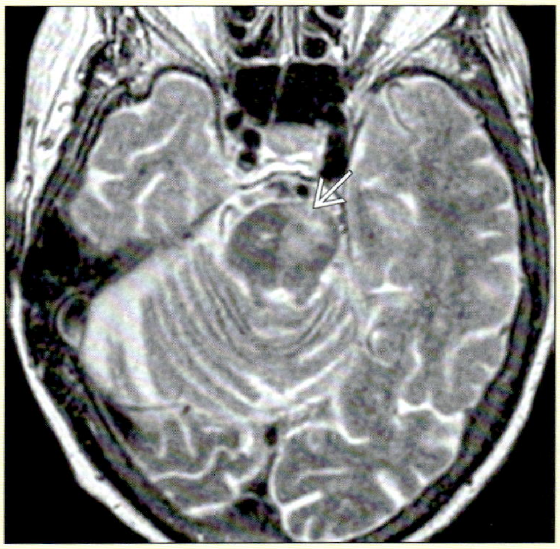

ISOLATED 6TH NERVE PALSY

INTRODUCTION

Definitions

- Dysfunction of CN6 (abducens nerve)
  - Lateral rectus muscle paralysis → inability to abduct affected eye
  - Bilateral horizontal gaze paralysis toward side of lesion if nucleus involved

Subtypes

- By anatomic location of lesion
  - Nucleus (rare) + fasciculus (rare)
    - Concomitant facial nerve palsy, internuclear ophthalmoplegia (INO) are possible
  - Subarachnoid (common): Longest subarachnoid course of all CNs, more susceptible to damage
    - Hearing loss, facial pain/numbness possible
    - Associated with pseudotumor cerebri, hemorrhage, meningitis, inflammation, tumor
  - Intracavernous/superior orbital fissure
    - Usually, a multiple cranial neuropathy/Horner syndrome, rarely, isolated CN6 palsy
  - Orbit
    - Proptosis, conjunctival inflammation are possible
    - Rarely, isolated CN6 involvement

DEMOGRAPHICS

Etiology/Risk Factors

- Adult
  - Ischemia, compression (aneurysm, neoplasm, ↑ or ↓ intracranial pressure [ICP]), trauma (neurosurgery, closed-head trauma), infection, inflammation
  - Vasculopathic risk factors: Diabetes, hypertension
- Pediatric
  - Post-viral illness, congenital, trauma, infection, inflammation, compression (neoplasm, ↑ or ↓ ICP)

Epidemiology

- Annual incidence ~ 11 per 100,000 people
- Most common ocular motor cranial nerve palsy

PRESENTATION

Symptoms

- Binocular, horizontal diplopia
  - Worse with gaze toward affected muscle
  - Worse with distance

Exam Findings

- Abduction deficit
- Esotropia
  - Increases with gaze toward affected muscle
- Small vertical deviation may be present
  - If > 4 prism diopters, consider additional causes

DIFFERENTIAL DIAGNOSIS

Myasthenia Gravis

- Fatigable ptosis, transient diplopia, weakness of orbicularis oculi

Thyroid Orbitopathy

- Proptosis, lid retraction, lid lag

Duane Syndrome (Type 1)

- Globe retraction and narrowing of palpebral fissure on abduction

Spasm of Near Reflex

- Pupillary constriction, excessive convergence on attempted lateral gaze, variable esotropia, normal abducting saccades, intact abduction with oculocephalic maneuvers, full ocular motility when testing individual eyes

EVALUATION/WORK-UP

Labs

- Lumbar puncture
  - Consider in adults < 50 years, or if clinically indicated
- Erythrocyte sedimentation rate (ESR), C-reactive protein (CRP), evaluate blood pressure, CBC, diabetes work-up, VDRL, FTA-ABS, and ANA as appropriate

Imaging

- Brain MRI
  - Clinical judgment should be used when utilizing neuroimaging
  - Imaging should be obtained in children with persistent CN6 palsy and all patients < age 50
  - Consider imaging patients > 50 years if vascular risk factors are not present or if there are other focal neurologic deficits, chronic pain/headache, loss of consciousness, or other worrisome signs

TREATMENT

Medical

- Treat underlying medical cause if any
- Patching
  - Relieves diplopia; inexpensive
- Prism therapy
  - May be effective for small deviations
  - Ineffective if deviation is incomitant
- Botulinum toxin injection
  - Inject opposing medial rectus muscle
  - Temporarily reduces tonic opposition, diplopia

Surgical

- Strabismus surgery after recovery is complete
  - Lateral rectus resection combined with medial rectus recession

Follow-Up

- Regular follow-up is necessary until recovery is complete

Prognosis

- Partial to complete recovery is very common
  - Bilateral involvement has worse prognosis
  - Median recovery time is 3-6 months

SELECTED REFERENCES

1. Brazis PW: Isolated palsies of cranial nerves III, IV, and VI. Semin Neurol. 29(1):14-28, 2009
2. Bennett JL et al: Palsies of the third, fourth, and sixth cranial nerves. Ophthalmol Clin North Am. 14(1):169-85, ix, 2001

ISOLATED 7TH NERVE PALSY

Key Facts

Introduction
- Results in ipsilateral paralysis of facial muscles
- Idiopathic Bell palsy
  - Most common type of facial palsy
- Infections
  - Lyme disease
  - Herpes simplex
  - Otitis media
- Pontine lesion (infarct or hemorrhage)
- Neoplasm
- Trauma
- Sarcoid
- Diabetes mellitus
- Guillain-Barré syndrome
- Melkersson-Rosenthal syndrome

Presentation
- Orbicularis oculi weakness
  - Corneal exposure keratopathy may ensue
- Absent corneal blink reflex
- Synkinetic movements
- Taste, lacrimation, and salivation can be altered

Treatment
- Eyelid weakness may necessitate treatment of corneal exposure
- Corticosteroids (and antivirals) may be used to treat Bell palsy
- Tarsorrhaphy, bandage contact lens may be indicated to ensure adequate eyelid closure
- Implantable gold eyelid weights
- Prognosis
  - 85% of patients with Bell palsy experience spontaneous recovery within 6 months

__(Left)__ Axial T2 MRI through the cerebellopontine angle cistern and internal auditory canal shows the facial nerve root → exit anterior to the vestibulocochlear nerve ↷ bilaterally. CN7 supplies motor innervation to facial muscles, taste input from the anterior tongue, and autonomic innervation to lacrimal, submandibular, and sublingual glands. __(Right)__ Axial T1 MRI shows classic findings of Bell palsy with ➔ facial nerve enhancement. Bell palsy is the most common cause of CN7 palsy.

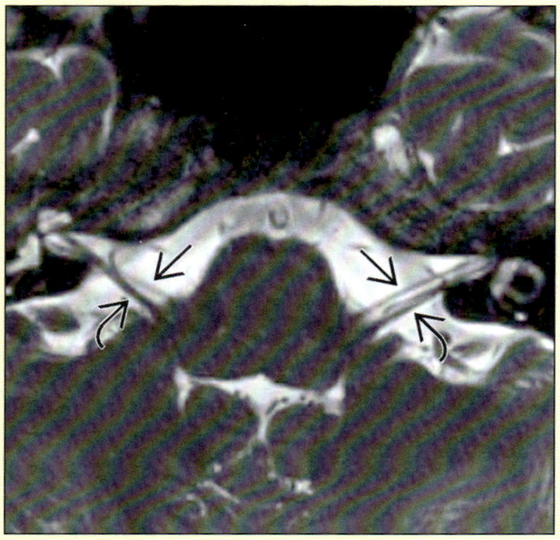

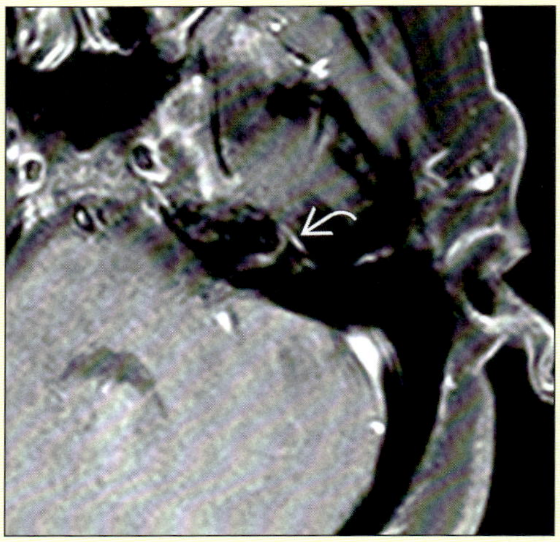

__(Left)__ Slit-lamp photo shows fluorescein staining inferiorly involving the cornea and conjunctiva. Such a pattern may be seen in exposure keratopathy, a frequent finding in patients with CN7 palsy. __(Right)__ Axial T1 MRI shows a mass in the right cerebellopontine angle ➔. Mass in this area, such as an acoustic neuroma, is 1 potential cause of 7th nerve palsy. Other differential considerations include Bell palsy, infection, infarction, trauma, or other neoplasms.

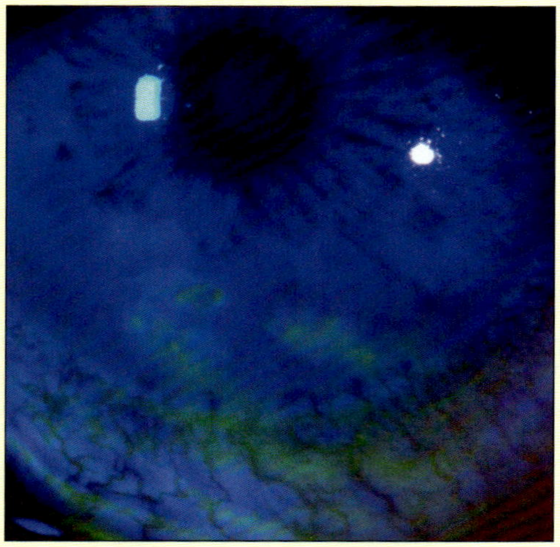

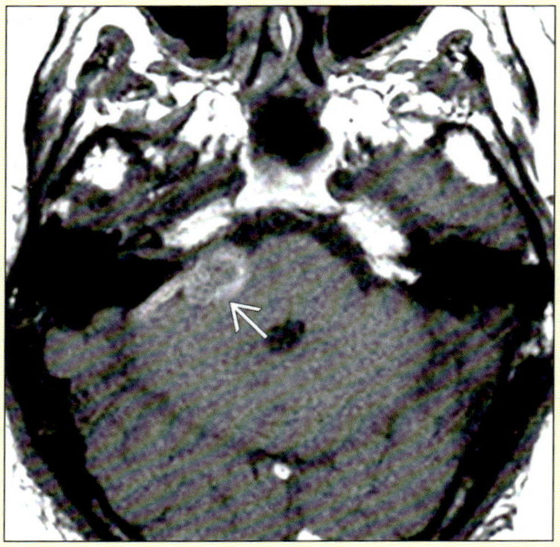

ISOLATED 7TH NERVE PALSY

INTRODUCTION

Definitions

- Ipsilateral paralysis of facial muscles
  - May be accompanied by
    - Loss of taste over anterior portion of tongue
    - Altered secretion of lacrimal and salivary glands

Anatomy

- Functions of CN7 (facial nerve)
  - Motor: Innervates facial muscles
  - Sensory
    - Taste for anterior 2/3 of tongue
    - Sensation for external auditory canal and pinna
  - Autonomic
    - Parasympathetic innervation to lacrimal, submandibular, and sublingual glands

Subtypes

- Central: Classically spares forehead
- Peripheral: Involves forehead

DEMOGRAPHICS

Etiology

- Idiopathic Bell palsy
  - Most common type of facial palsy
  - Diagnosis of exclusion
  - Autoimmune or postviral inflammation
- Infectious
  - Lyme disease
    - Caused by spirochete *Borrelia burgdorferi*
      - Transmitted by *Ixodes* tick
    - Associated rash, arthritis, and heart block
  - Herpes simplex
    - Associated vesicle formation over pinna, external auditory canal, and tympanic membrane
  - Otitis media
- Pontine lesion (infarct or hemorrhage)
- Neoplastic
  - Intracranial mass
    - Cerebellopontine angle masses may also cause associated CN5, CN6, or CN8 palsy
  - Parotid tumor
  - Leukemia or lymphoma
- Traumatic (e.g., postsurgical, temporal bone fracture)
- Other
  - Sarcoid
  - Diabetes mellitus
  - Guillain-Barré syndrome
  - Melkersson-Rosenthal syndrome
    - Recurrent unilateral or bilateral facial palsy associated with facial swelling and lingua plicata

PRESENTATION

Symptoms

- Facial weakness: Difficulty with eye closure, smiling, and facial movements

Exam Findings

- Orbicularis oculi weakness
  - Corneal exposure keratopathy may ensue
- Absent corneal blink reflex
- Synkinetic movements
  - Aberrant movements that occur when regenerating axons innervate inappropriate musculature (e.g., eyelid closes when smiling)
- Absent taste over anterior 2/3 of tongue

EVALUATION/WORK-UP

Clinical Tests

- Corneal blink reflex
- Testing salivation, lacrimation, and sensation can help to localize 7th nerve lesions
- Testing CN5, CN6, and CN8 may also aid localization

TREATMENT

Medical

- Eyelid weakness may necessitate treatment of corneal exposure
  - Preservative-free artificial tears and lubricants
  - Taping eyelid shut or temporary tarsorrhaphy
  - Moisture chambers
  - Punctal plugs
  - Botox injection
  - Bandage contact lens
  - Albumin drops can promote reepithelialization
  - Oral vitamin C, doxycycline, or medroxyprogesterone drops prevent corneal melting
- Corticosteroids may be used to treat Bell palsy
  - 7-10 day course
  - Antiviral (acyclovir or famciclovir) agents may be added to steroid regimen

Surgical

- Tarsorrhaphy may be used to ensure adequate eyelid closure
- Gold eyelid weights
  - Select heaviest weight that does not block visual axis
- Nerve reanimation surgery is emerging

Prognosis

- Varies with underlying etiology of palsy
- 85% of patients with Bell palsy experience spontaneous recovery
  - Recovery is gradual and typically takes 2-3 months

SELECTED REFERENCES

1. Lee HY et al: Steroid-antiviral treatment improves the recovery rate in patients with severe Bell's palsy. Am J Med. 126(4):336-41, 2013
2. Bhatti MT et al: Neuro-ophthalmologic complications and manifestations of upper and lower motor neuron facial paresis. Curr Neurol Neurosci Rep. 10(6):448-58, 2010
3. Rahman I et al: Ophthalmic management of facial nerve palsy: a review. Surv Ophthalmol. 52(2):121-44, 2007
4. Grogan PM et al: Practice parameter: Steroids, acyclovir, and surgery for Bell's palsy (an evidence-based review): report of the Quality Standards Subcommittee of the American Academy of Neurology. Neurology. 56(7):830-6, 2001

Key Facts

Introduction

- Rhythmic, involuntary oscillation of eyes including jerk and pendular subtypes
  - Congenital (infantile) nystagmus
  - Acquired nystagmus
- Causes of nystagmus
  - Vision loss (e.g., cataracts, cone dystrophy, macular hypoplasia, Leber congenital amaurosis)
  - Toxic: Caused by alcohol or drugs (e.g., lithium, dextromethorphan, barbiturates, MDMA, phencyclidine, benzodiazepines, anticonvulsants)
  - Metabolic (e.g., thiamine deficiency)
  - CNS disorders (e.g., stroke, thalamic hemorrhage, tumor, Chiari malformation, MS)

Differential Diagnosis

- Convergence-retraction nystagmus
  - Co-contraction of extraocular muscles on upgaze, most prominently medial recti
- Opsoclonus
  - Unpredictable, rapid, involuntary, high-frequency, multidirectional eye movements
- Superior-oblique myokymia
  - Monocular, paroxysmal bursts of superior-oblique muscle contraction

Evaluation/Work-Up

- Head MRI

Treatment

- Treat underlying etiology, amblyopia, or any uncorrected refractive errors
- Baclofen, gabapentin, and clonazepam may alleviate symptoms in some forms of nystagmus
- Botulinum toxin A injections and prism lenses may also help
- Symmetric recession or resection of horizontal rectus muscles to bring null point into primary position

*(**Left**) This graphic demonstrates the external ➪, middle ➦, and inner ear →. Nystagmus of vestibular origin may be either secondary to pathology of the otolithic organs or the semicircular canals of the inner ear (peripheral vestibular nystagmus) or to central vestibular nystagmus. (**Right**) This close-up graphic shows the semicircular canals and otolithic organs → that are often responsible for peripheral vestibular nystagmus. Central vestibular nystagmus is usually due to alcohol, medications, or brainstem disease.*

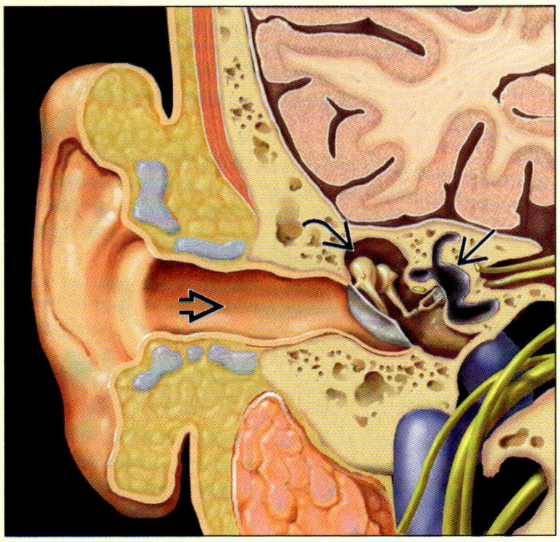

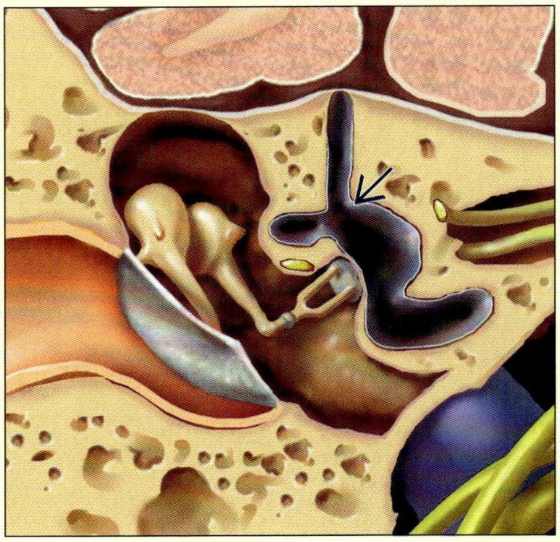

*(**Left**) This graphic depicts a low nucleus gracilis → and compressed, pointed cerebellar tonsils ➦ protruding through foramen magnum. These findings are consistent with Arnold-Chiari 1 malformation and are typically associated with Downbeat Nystagmus. (**Right**) Sagittal T1WI MRI shows a Chiari 1 malformation with the fastigium ➡ in normal position, helping to distinguish from Chiari 2 malformation. There is inferior displacement of the ectopic cerebellar tonsils ➡ through the foramen magnum.*

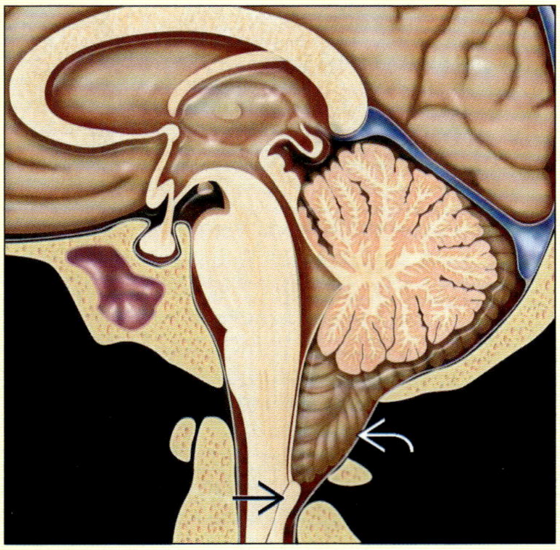

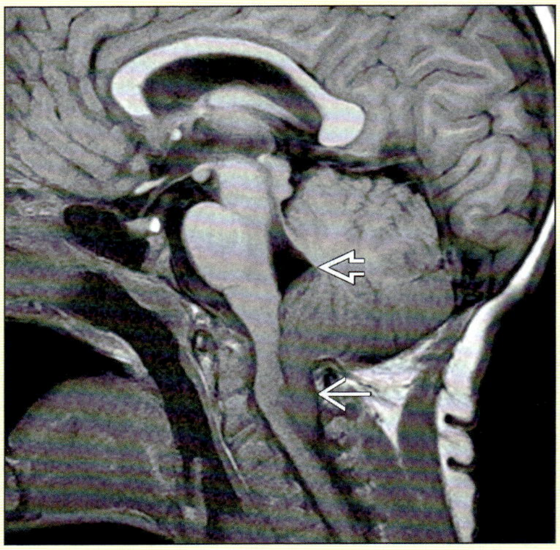

NYSTAGMUS

INTRODUCTION

Definitions

- Rhythmic, involuntary oscillation of eyes in horizontal, vertical, or torsional planes
  - Jerk nystagmus (most common)
    - Made up of slow (defoveating drift away from target) and fast (saccade realigning eye with target) phases
  - Pendular nystagmus
    - Sinusoidal eye movements where both directions are equal in amplitude and velocity

Subtypes

- Congenital (Infantile) nystagmus
  - Onset between 6 weeks and 3 months of age
  - Patients usually do not have oscillopsia
  - Typically pendular or jerk horizontal nystagmus present in all gaze positions
  - Presence of null point with possible anomalous head position
  - Dampened by convergence, worsened with distance fixation
  - Not present during sleep
- Acquired nystagmus
  - Many types and causes
  - Patients typically experience oscillopsia

DEMOGRAPHICS

Etiology/Risk Factors

- Main causes of nystagmus
  - Vision loss
    - e.g., cataracts, cone dystrophy, macular hypoplasia, Leber congenital amaurosis
    - Typically horizontal and conjugate
  - Toxic
    - Caused by alcohol or drugs (e.g., lithium, dextromethorphan, barbiturates, MDMA, phencyclidine, benzodiazepines, anticonvulsants)
  - Metabolic
    - e.g., thiamine deficiency
  - CNS disorders
    - e.g., stroke, thalamic hemorrhage, tumor, Chiari malformation, MS
- Risk factors
  - Trauma, CNS disorders, medications/drug use
  - Family history (e.g., nystagmus, albinism, aniridia)
    - Congenital nystagmus is inheritable in recessive, dominant, and x-linked patterns

Epidemiology

- Most common in patients of European descent
- Prevalence estimated at 24 per 10,000 people

PRESENTATION

Symptoms

- Vision difficulty
- Nausea
- Vertigo
- Oscillopsia
  - Depends on age of onset
- Head turn

Exam Findings

- Decreased visual acuity
  - By tilting or turning head, patient may be able to find a position that decreases the nystagmus enough (null point) to see the eye chart
- **Latent nystagmus**
  - Only apparent in monocular viewing conditions with 1 eye occluded
  - Fast phase toward viewing eye
  - Usually associated with esotropia, benign
- **Manifest latent nystagmus**
  - Similar to latent nystagmus, except that both eyes are open
  - Found in esotropia (suppression of deviating eye vs. occlusion in latent nystagmus)
- **Spasmus nutans**
  - Intermittent horizontal small-amplitude, high-frequency, pendular nystagmus
  - Associated with head nodding
  - May be idiopathic and benign, which resolves by age 3
- **Monocular nystagmus of childhood**
  - Small vertical eye movements occurring only in 1 eye
  - Associated with optic nerve or chiasmal gliomas
  - May also be seen with amblyopia
  - Patients should be imaged
- **Vestibular nystagmus**
  - Peripheral
    - Pathology of otolithic organs or semicircular canals of inner ear, deafness/tinnitus may be present; fast phase opposite side of lesion
  - Central
    - Characterized by jerk nystagmus; most commonly caused by medications or CNS disease, frequently in brainstem
    - Bruns nystagmus
      - Combination of peripheral and central vestibular nystagmus, associated with cerebellar pontine angle tumors
  - Alexander law
    - Central nystagmus has fast component in direction of gaze position; peripheral nystagmus increases with gaze toward side of fast component
- **Downbeat nystagmus**
  - Present in primary but worse in downgaze
  - Must rule out Arnold-Chiari type 1
- **Upbeat nystagmus**
  - Fast-phase up; worse in upgaze
  - Caused by posterior fossa tumors, stroke, MS, drugs
- **See-saw nystagmus**
  - Pendular; 1 eye elevates and intorts while other depresses and extorts
  - Rule out craniopharyngioma
- **Periodic alternating nystagmus (PAN)**
  - Horizontal jerk nystagmus that frequently reverses direction
  - Starts in 1 direction, increases in frequency and amplitude, and eventually subsides into nystagmus-free period, followed by a reinitiation of pattern in opposite direction
  - Associated with posterior fossa disease
- **Torsional nystagmus**

NYSTAGMUS

- Rhythmic rotation of eyes (incyclotorsion or excyclotorsion)
- May be associated with medullary lesion

DIFFERENTIAL DIAGNOSIS

Convergence-Retraction Nystagmus
- Co-contraction of extraocular muscles on upgaze, most prominently the medial recti
- Differs from most nystagmus because lacks slow and fast phases
- May be caused by pinealoma or dorsal midbrain syndrome

Opsoclonus
- Unpredictable, rapid, involuntary, high-frequency, multidirectional eye movements
- No intersaccadic interval
- Associated with
  - Neuroblastoma
  - Encephalitis
  - Breast cancer
  - Small cell lung cancer

Superior Oblique Myokymia
- Monocular, paroxysmal bursts of superior oblique muscle contraction
- Unknown etiology

EVALUATION/WORK-UP

Labs
- ERG or VEP may prove useful, especially with congenital nystagmus
- Urine vanillylmandelic acid may be ordered if opsoclonus cannot be ruled out
- Blood and urine testing for suspected toxic causes

Imaging
- Head MRI looking for
  - Intracranial mass, hemorrhage, stroke, or demyelinating disease
  - Cerebellar pathology
  - Evidence of Arnold-Chiari malformation

TREATMENT

Medical
- Treat underlying etiology
- Treat amblyopia or any uncorrected refractive errors
- PAN: Use baclofen
- Acquired pendular nystagmus: Use gabapentin
- Downbeat nystagmus: Use gabapentin, clonazepam, or baclofen
- In toxic nystagmus: Stop causative drug
- Botulinum toxin A injections
  - Injected into retrobulbar space of affected eye(s)
    - Decreases symptoms of nystagmus temporarily
      - Effects lasts for ~ 8 weeks
- Prism lenses

Surgical
- Symmetric recession or resection of horizontal rectus muscles (Anderson/Kestenbaum procedure)
  - Moves null zone toward primary position to minimize nystagmus
  - Postoperatively, patients have had increased visual acuity and decreased symptoms of nystagmus

Follow-Up
- Depends on etiology and symptoms
- Work-up for CNS disease ASAP

Prognosis
- Varies with underlying etiology
- Congenital nystagmus often improves with age
- Surgery is very effective in congenital nystagmus, less so in acquired cases
- Symptoms usually decrease or cease with medical management

SELECTED REFERENCES

1. Ehrhardt D et al: Medical treatment of acquired nystagmus. Curr Opin Ophthalmol. 23(6):510-6, 2012
2. Tränkner D et al: Molecular basis of an inherited form of incomplete achromatopsia. J Neurosci. 24(1):138-47, 2004
3. Lee J: Surgical management of nystagmus. J R Soc Med. 95(5):238-41, 2002
4. Pieh C et al: Arnold-Chiari malformation and nystagmus of skew. J Neurol Neurosurg Psychiatry. 69(1):124-6, 2000
5. Atilla H et al: Surgical treatment in nystagmus. Eye (Lond). 13 (Pt 1):11-5, 1999
6. Repka MX et al: Treatment of acquired nystagmus with botulinum neurotoxin A. Arch Ophthalmol. 112(10):1320-4, 1994
7. Helveston EM et al: Treatment of acquired nystagmus with botulinum A toxin. Am J Ophthalmol. 106(5):584-6, 1988
8. Halmagyi GM et al: Treatment of periodic alternating nystagmus. Ann Neurol. 8(6):609-11, 1980

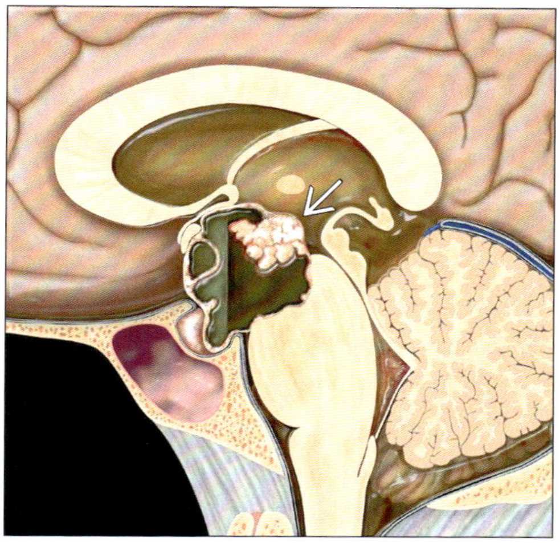

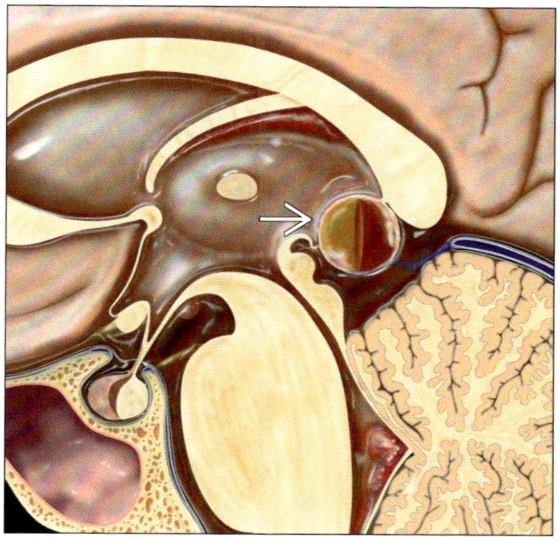

(Left) *Graphic shows a craniopharyngioma ➔. Craniopharyngiomas are the most frequent cause of see-saw nystagmus. Optic chiasm compression from the tumor may also lead to bitemporal hemianopia.* ***(Right)*** *Graphic depicts a pinealocytoma ➔ of the pineal gland. This tumor is benign and slowly growing. Pineal tumors are frequently associated with convergence-retraction nystagmus, where there is co-contraction of extraocular muscles on upgaze (especially the medial recti).*

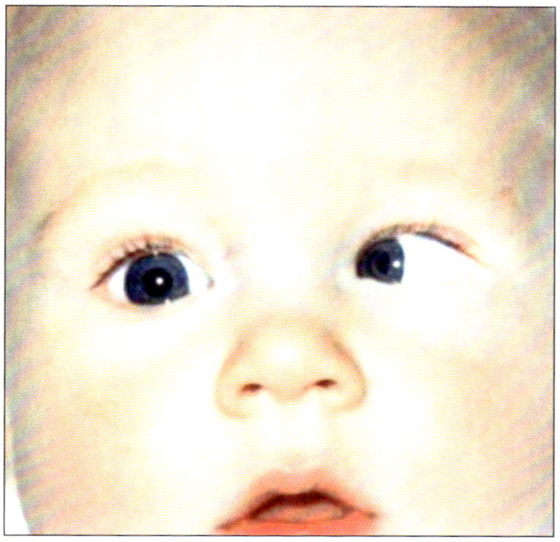

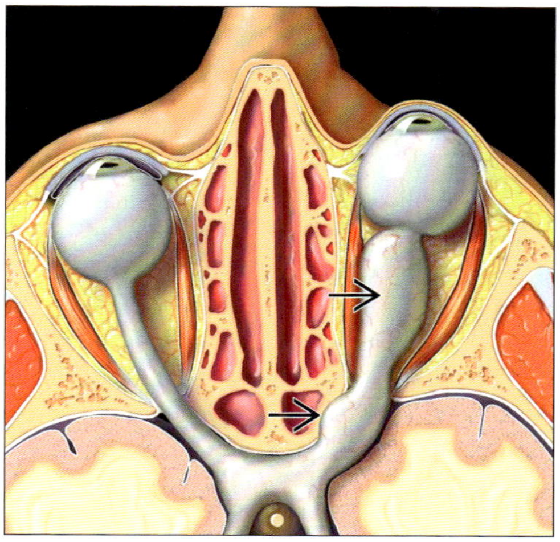

(Left) *This external photo shows congenital esotropia in an infant. Congenital esotropia is associated with latent nystagmus, which usually goes along with cross-fixation, dissociated vertical deviation, and inferior oblique overaction.* ***(Right)*** *Graphic shows optic nerve glioma ➔ extending from the chiasm to the globe. Optic nerve gliomas have been implicated in monocular nystagmus of childhood, and patients presenting with monocular nystagmus of childhood should be imaged to rule-out tumors.*

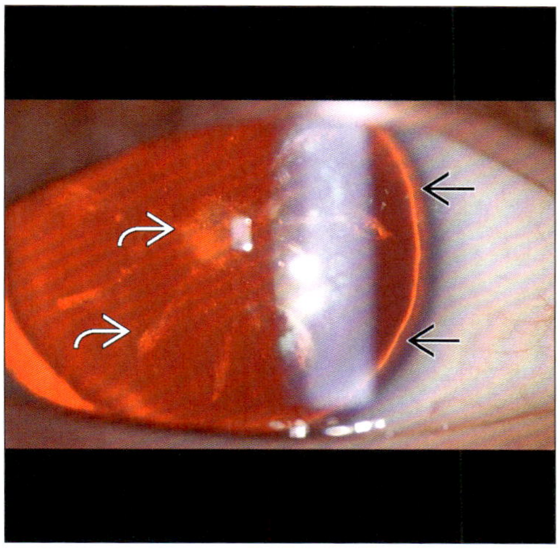

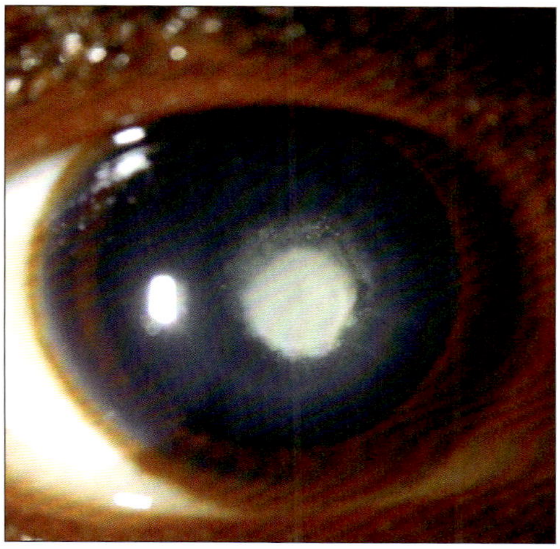

(Left) *This slit-lamp photo demonstrates aniridia ➔ as well as a cortical cataract ➔. Aniridia as well as macular hypoplasia are a possible cause of sensory deprivation nystagmus due to decreased visual acuity.* ***(Right)*** *Slit-lamp photo shows a congenital posterior cataract. Dense cataracts are another cause of visual loss responsible for nystagmus. Nystagmus in these cases tends to be vertically-oriented and monocular. Other causes include cone dystrophy and trauma.*

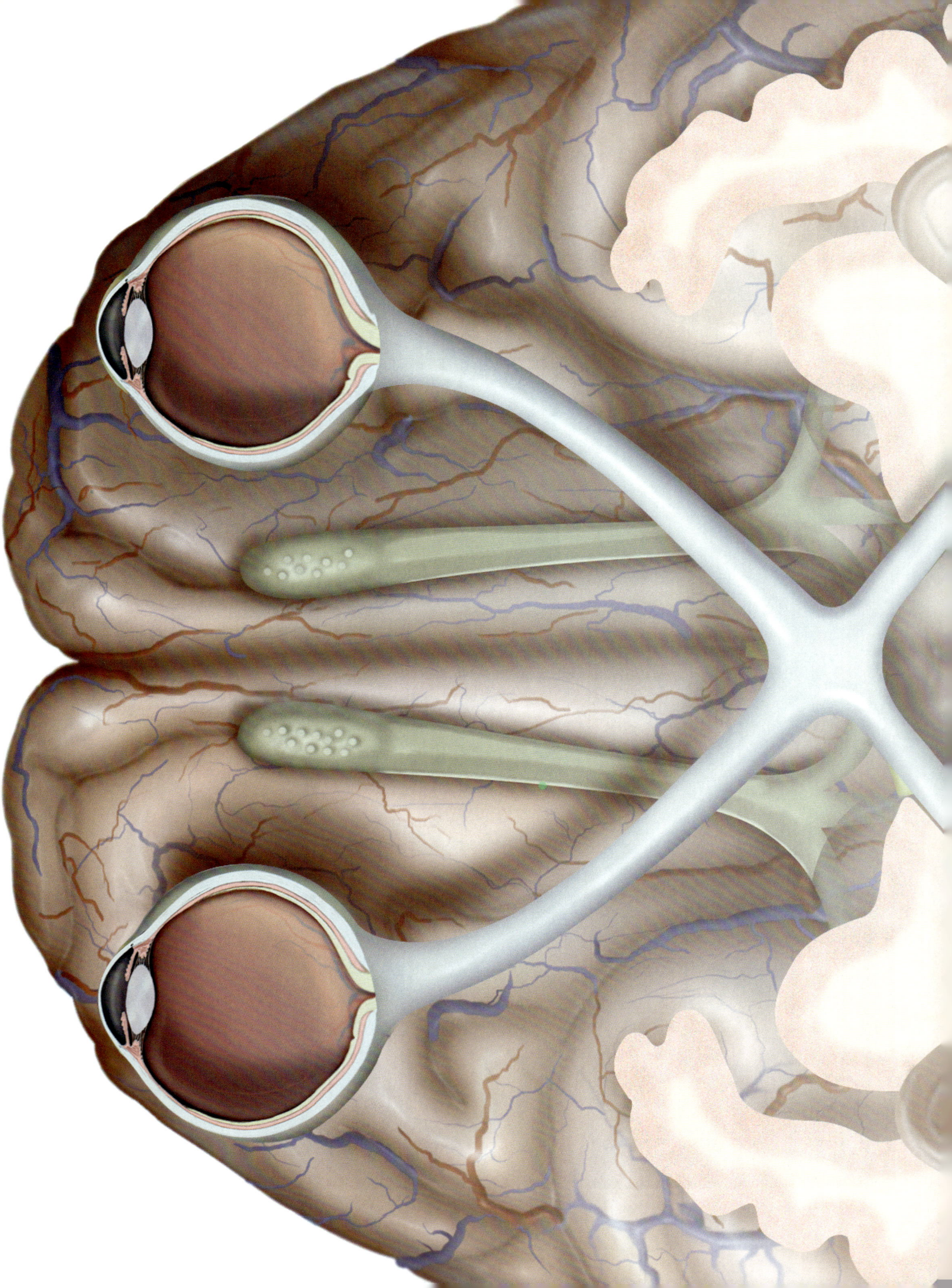

SECTION 3
Central Nervous System Visual Disorders

Introduction and Overview

Vascular Disorders

Miscellaneous

CENTRAL NERVOUS SYSTEM OVERVIEW

TERMINOLOGY

Definitions

- Central nervous system (CNS) consists of brain, spinal cord, cranial nerves, and retina

GROSS ANATOMY

Retina

- Ganglion cells of retina and their axons are part of CNS and thus will not regenerate

Optic Nerve

- Axons arise from retinal ganglion cells and emerge from globe via posterior scleral foramen
- Myelination begins outside of globe
- Anatomical segments
  - Prelaminar, laminar, retrolaminar segments
    - Associated with lamina cribrosa
  - Intraorbital (IO) segment: Within optic muscle cone
  - Intracanalicular (ICL) segment: In bony optic canal
  - Intracranial (IC) segment: Ends at optic chiasm
- Blood supply
  - Retinal arterioles → optic disc surface
  - Short posterior ciliary arteries → prelaminar, laminar, retrolaminar segments
  - Central retinal artery → anterior intraorbital segment
  - Pial network of vessels (ophthalmic artery) → posterior intraorbital, ICL, IC segments

Optic Chiasm

- Junction of the 2 optic nerves
- Allows decussation of optic fibers to contralateral tracts
- Located ~ 1 cm superior to diaphragm of sella turcica at junction of floor and anterior wall of 3rd ventricle; internal carotid arteries and cavernous sinuses lie laterally
- Blood supply via circle of Willis

Retrochiasmatic Visual Pathways

- Optic tracts
  - Begin at optic chiasm, curve around peduncles
  - Terminate in lateral geniculate nucleus
  - A few retinal nerve fibers involved in optic reflexes bypass lateral geniculate to pretectal nuclei
- Geniculocalcarine tract
  - Arises from afferent visual fibers in lateral geniculate nucleus, courses through posterior limb of internal capsule, and then fans out to become optic radiations
- Optic radiations
  - Curve around anterior temporal horn of lateral ventricle, and then course medially and terminate in calcarine cortex of occipital lobe
- Afferent pupillary fibers
  - Exit tracts anterior to geniculate nucleus, travel via brachium of superior colliculus to midbrain
- Primary visual cortex
  - Calcarine fissure on medial occipital lobe
  - Receives fibers from each ipsilateral half-retina
    - Making up contralateral visual field
  - Visual field is organized on visual cortex in retinotopic pattern

Cranial Nerves

- Oculomotor nerve (CN3)
  - Passes lateral to posterior communicating artery, lateral to pituitary gland near optic tract, and through lateral wall of cavernous sinus before dividing into superior and inferior divisions and entering orbit via superior orbital fissure (SOF)
  - Superior division supplies superior rectus and levator palpebrae superioris muscles
  - Inferior division supplies medial rectus, inferior rectus, and inferior oblique muscles as well as sending parasympathetic fibers to ciliary ganglion
- Trochlear nerve (CN4)
  - Emerges just below inferior colliculus on dorsal surface, courses around crus cerebri, beneath free edge of tentorium, through lateral wall of cavernous sinus, and through SOF to superior oblique muscle
- Trigeminal nerve (CN5)
  - Ophthalmic division courses through wall of cavernous sinus and divides into 3 nerves
    - Lacrimal nerve enters orbit via SOF and supplies sensation to lacrimal gland
    - Facial nerve enters orbit via SOF and divides into supraorbital and supratrochlear nerves, which supply sensation to forehead and brow
    - Nasociliary nerve (sensory nerve of eye) enters orbit via SOF, supplies sensory fibers to ciliary ganglion and ciliary nerves (cornea, iris, and ciliary body), and then branches into infratrochlear nerve (medial conjunctiva and eyelids) and anterior ethmoidal nerve (nose tip)
  - Maxillary division passes through foramen rotundum, enters orbit via inferior orbital fissure, enters infraorbital canal (where it becomes infraorbital nerve), exits infraorbital foramen, and supplies sensation to lower eyelid/cheek
- Abducens nerve (CN6)
  - Emerges at pontomedullary junction, courses up clivus to posterior clinoid, travels through cavernous sinus, enters orbit via SOF, and innervates lateral rectus muscle
- Facial nerve (CN7)
  - Emerges from pons, passes through internal acoustic meatus and facial canal, exits stylomastoid foramen, passes through parotid gland, and branches across face to muscles of facial expression including orbicularis oculi
  - Parasympathetic fibers extend to lacrimal gland through pterygopalatine ganglion via geniculate ganglion from nerve of pterygoid canal (Vidian nerve), made up of greater and lesser petrosal nerves

RELATED REFERENCES

1. Sheth S et al: Appearance of normal cranial nerves on steady-state free precession MR images. Radiographics. 29(4):1045-55, 2009
2. Grill-Spector K et al: The human visual cortex. Annu Rev Neurosci. 27:649-77, 2004
3. Tamraz JC et al: MR imaging anatomy of the optic pathways. Radiol Clin North Am. 37(1):1-36, ix, 1999

ANATOMIC FEATURES

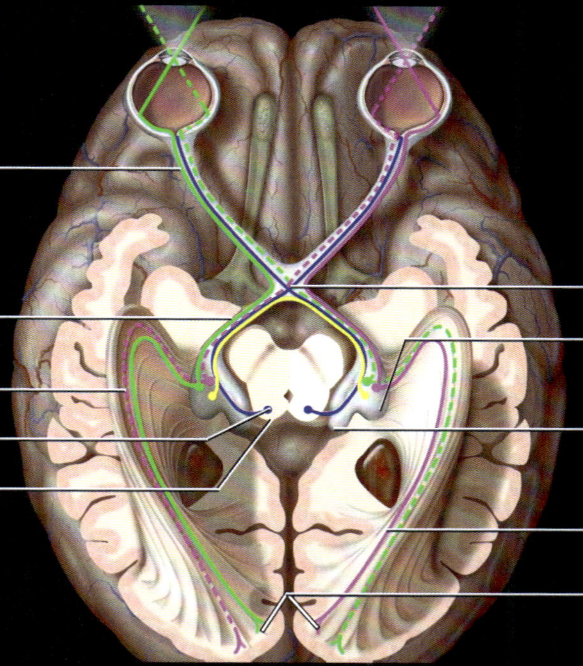

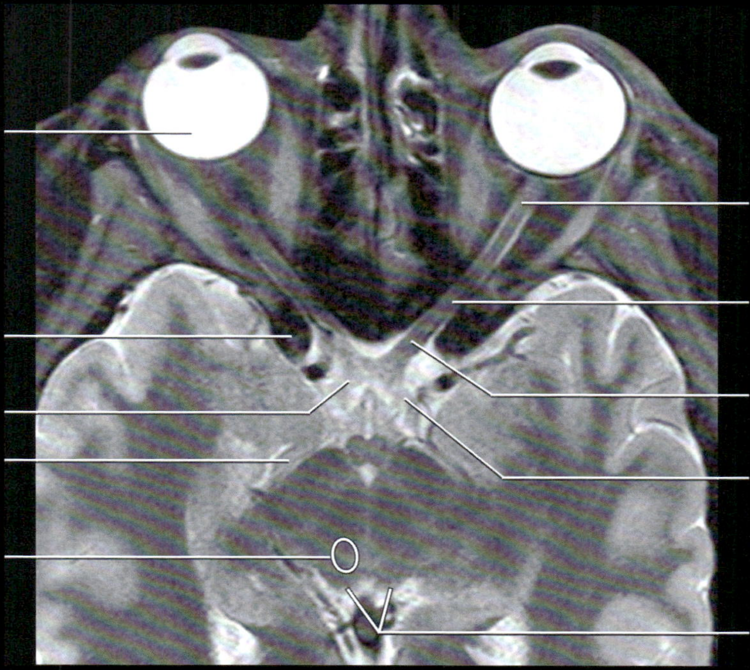

(Top) *Axial illustration depicts the visual pathway. Note how the axons originating from the nasal retina cross at the optic chiasm. Because of this, fibers from the left halves of both retinas course in the left optic tract, and fibers from the right halves of both retinas course in the right optic tract. The majority of retinal nerve fibers terminate in lateral geniculate bodies, where new neurons give rise to the optic radiation, which extends to the visual cortex. A few retinal nerve fibers (blue) involved in optic reflexes bypass the lateral geniculate bodies and terminate in pretectal nuclei.* ***(Bottom)*** *Axial STIR MRI shows many of the aspects of the visual pathway. Note the optic nerves leading to the optic chiasm with the beginnings of the optic tract extending posteriorly from the chiasm. The optic tracts eventually lead to the lateral geniculate bodies where they synapse with neurons that give rise to the optic radiations.*

VERTEBROBASILAR ARTERY INSUFFICIENCY

Key Facts

Introduction
- Neurological symptoms due to decreased blood flow in the brain's posterior circulation

Demographics
- Primarily caused by atherosclerotic changes that decrease the diameter of the blood vessel(s)
- Risk factors
  - Hypertension, diabetes, smoking, and dyslipidemia
  - Family history of heart disease, stroke; advanced age
- More common in men than women < 75 years of age
- More common in women than men > 75 years of age

Presentation
- Headaches, often accentuated by stooping or straining
- Drop attacks (sudden falls while standing, with rapid recovery)
- Binocular visual disturbance (blurring, dimming, diplopia, or complete loss of vision bilaterally)
- Focal neurologic deficits
  - Difficulty swallowing, vertigo, slurred speech, dizziness

Differential Diagnosis
- Transient ischemic attack
- Cardiac insufficiency
- Subarachnoid hemorrhage caused vasospasm

Evaluation/Work-Up
- Lipid and hypercoagulability panels
- EKG
- MRI/CT of vertebrobasilar distribution

Treatment
- If caused by ischemia, use anticoagulation/antiplatelet drugs
- Intracranial angioplasty
- Good prognosis if caught and treated early, before ischemic damage can develop

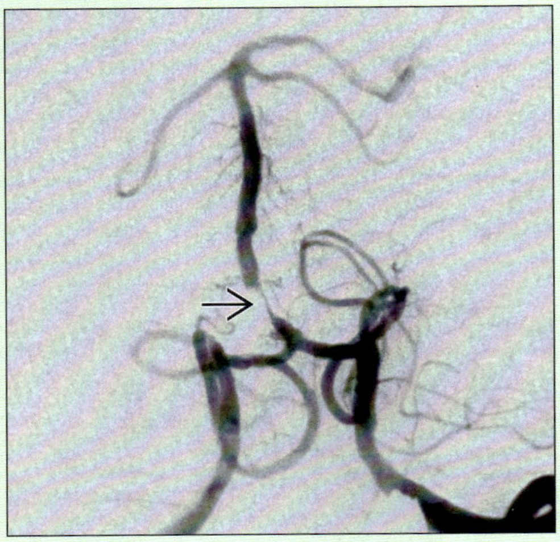

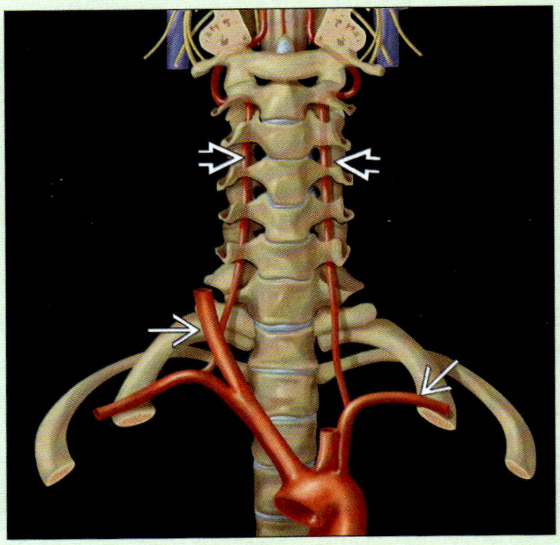

(Left) *Left vertebral artery DSA shows a short-segment pin-point stenosis of the proximal basilar artery ➙ in this patient presenting with episodic syncope.* ***(Right)*** *This graphic illustrates the location of the vertebral arteries ➙. The arteries originate off the subclavian arteries ➙ and then converge to form the basilar artery, which conveys blood to the posterior portion of the circle of Willis. Hypertension, diabetes, smoking, and dyslipidemia are risk factors for vascular disease.*

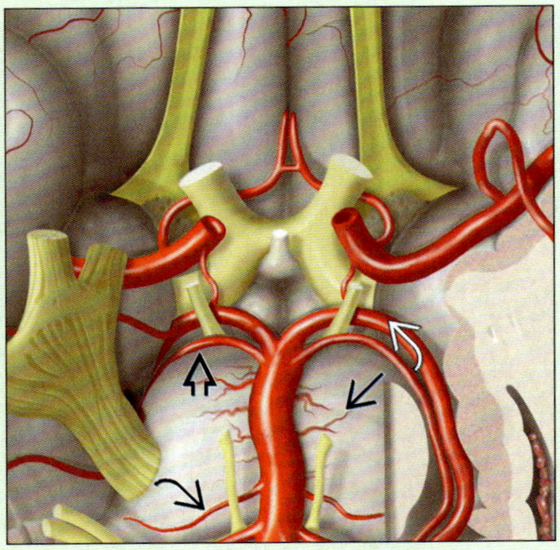

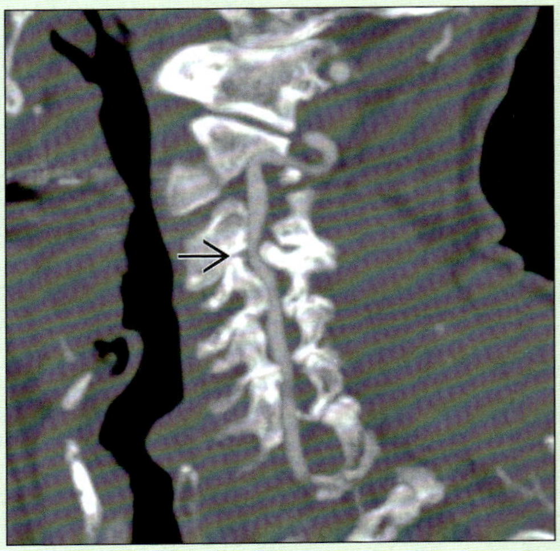

(Left) *This graphic illustrates the basilar artery originating at the confluence of the left and right vertebral arteries. Accessory arteries off the basilar include the pontine ➙, anterior inferior cerebellar ➙, superior cerebellar ➙, and the posterior cerebral ➙.* ***(Right)*** *Coronal CTA shows focal extrinsic narrowing of the left vertebral artery at the C3-C4 level due to facet degenerative hypertrophy and osteophyte formation ➙. Atherosclerosis is a more common cause of vertebrobasilar artery insufficiency disease.*

VERTEBROBASILAR ARTERY INSUFFICIENCY

INTRODUCTION

Abbreviations

- Vertebrobasilar artery insufficiency (VAI)

Definitions

- Neurological symptoms due to decreased blood flow in the brain's posterior circulation
  - Posterior circulation
    - Composed of the basilar and vertebral arteries feeding into the circle of Willis
    - Supplies blood to occipital cortex, midbrain, cerebellum, pons, medulla, and thalamus

DEMOGRAPHICS

Etiology/Risk Factors

- Primarily caused by atherosclerotic changes that decrease the diameter of the blood vessel(s)
- Risk factors
  - Hypertension, diabetes, smoking, and dyslipidemia
  - Family history of heart disease and stroke
  - Advanced age

Epidemiology

- More common in men than women < 75 years of age
- More common in women than men > 75 years of age

PRESENTATION

Symptoms

- Headaches, often accentuated by stooping or straining
- Drop attacks (sudden falls while standing with rapid recovery)
- Binocular visual disturbance (blurring, dimming, diplopia, or complete loss of vision)
- Dizziness, vertigo
- Weakness/sensory loss of the limbs or face
- Transient dysarthria

Exam Findings

- Decreased visual acuity
- Upper motor neurologic signs
- Abnormal cranial nerve exam, diplopia
- Focal neurologic deficits
  - Difficulty swallowing, vertigo, slurred speech, dizziness
- Reproducible symptoms with rotation of head

DIFFERENTIAL DIAGNOSIS

Transient Ischemic Attack

- Headaches are not as frequent or long-lasting as VAI
- Visual disturbance/loss is generally unilateral if anterior to the chiasm
  - May see hemifields bilaterally if posterior to chiasm
- Doppler imaging of carotid artery can detect vascular pathology

Cardiac Insufficiency

- Insufficiency can be caused by arrhythmia or heart failure
  - EKG and echocardiogram can detect these pathologies
- Will not have evidence of VAI on imaging
- Also look for dehydration and hypotension

Subarachnoid Hemorrhage-Caused Vasospasm

- Hemorrhage is commonly caused by bursting of aneurysm or traumatic brain injury
  - Can lead to spasm of vertebral or basilar arteries, mimicking VAI
- Vasospasm occurs no less than 3 days after hemorrhage begins
- CT perfusion imaging is highly sensitive for detection of subarachnoid hemorrhage
- Lumbar puncture with blood in the CSF is diagnostic
- Can be fatal or cause permanent damage if not immediately treated with vasodilator medication &/or angioplasty

EVALUATION/WORK-UP

Labs

- Lipid panel
- Test for hypercoagulation disorders
  - Protein C and S deficiency, factor V Leiden deficiency, antithrombin III, homocysteine, PT/PTT, antiphospholipid panel
- EKG

Imaging

- In area of vertebrobasilar distribution
  - CT angiography or CT perfusion imaging looking for active hemorrhage
  - Magnetic resonance angiography
  - MRI without contrast looking for areas of ischemia
  - Digital subtraction angiography
- Echocardiogram
- Doppler imaging of carotid artery

TREATMENT

Medical

- If caused by ischemia
  - If imaging rules out intracranial hemorrhage, use anticoagulation/antiplatelet drugs such as aspirin, clopidogrel, or warfarin to decrease chances of subsequent clots

Surgical

- Intracranial angioplasty
- Microsurgical removal of the stenotic lesion(s)

Follow-Up

- For worsening of symptoms after treatment initiation

Prognosis

- Good prognosis if caught and treated early, before ischemic damage can develop

SELECTED REFERENCES

1. Velat GJ et al: Vasospasm after aneurysmal subarachnoid hemorrhage: review of randomized controlled trials and meta-analyses in the literature. World Neurosurg. 76(5):446-54, 2011

CORTICAL BLINDNESS

Key Facts

Introduction

- Cortical blindness or cortical visual impairment refers to loss of vision in otherwise healthy eye(s) due to a lesion in the brain's occipital cortex
- Subtypes
  - Congenital
  - Acquired

Presentation

- Partial or complete blindness
- Visual hallucinations
- Occasionally, patient may preserve ability to perceive light
- Pupils remain reactive to light, does not cause afferent pupillary defect
- Macular sparing of vision may occur
- Funduscopy is normal
- Anton syndrome
- Blindsight
  - V1 cortex is damaged so there is not visual consciousness, but retina is presumably communicating to some other part of brain, enabling visually guided behavior and responses

Differential Diagnosis

- Differentiate from cortical blindness by the following
  - Cortical blindness will demonstrate normal pupillary response
  - Optic nerve will appear normal in cortical blindness

Evaluation/Work-Up

- CT or MRI of brain, MRA, CTA

Treatment

- Largely dependent upon underlying etiology
- Permanent complete loss of vision due to cortical blindness is rare
- Some patients may regain visual function completely

*(**Left**) Graphic of the lateral surface of the brain depicts major gyri and sulci. The occipital lobes ➔, which contain the primary visual cortex, are defined by the area of brain underlying the occipital bone. (**Right**) Axial MRI section shows occipital cortices ➔, responsible for primary visual processing. Injury to the occipital cortex, usually from ischemia, can lead to visual deficits though the eyes that may appear perfectly healthy.*

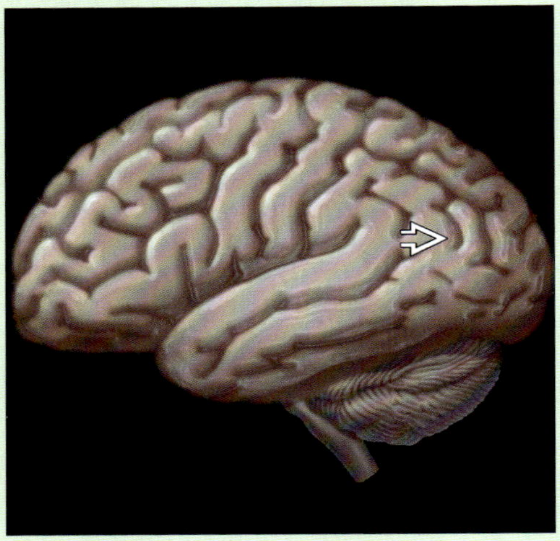

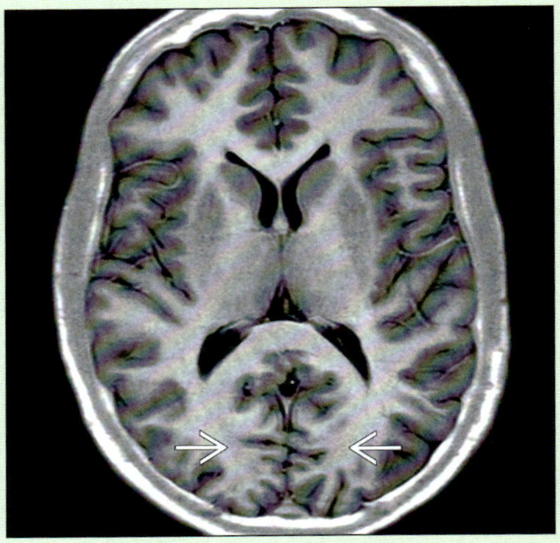

*(**Left**) Axial DWI MRI shows diffusion restriction in the right thalamus ➔ and medial occipital lobe ➔ related to an acute infarct of the posterior cerebral artery (PCA). The occipital lobe is the region most commonly affected in PCA ischemia. (**Right**) Axial FLAIR MRI shows hyperintensity in the medial temporal and occipital lobes related to an acute PCA infarct. Though ischemic injury is the most common cause of cortical blindness, other potential causes include trauma, infection, or eclampsia.*

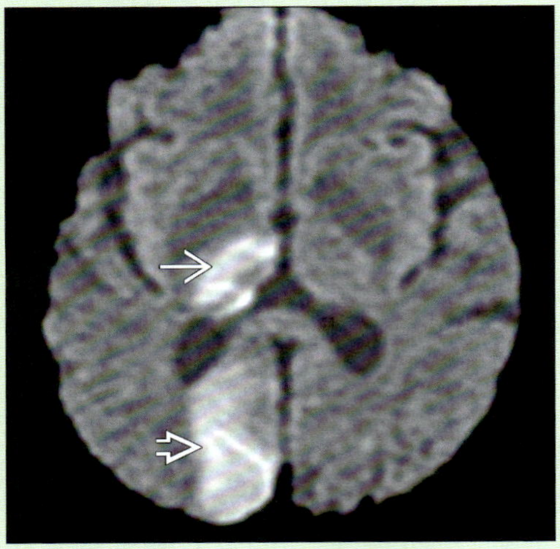

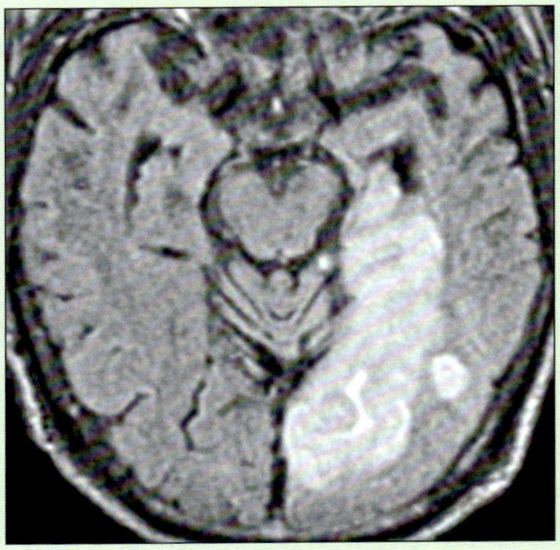

CORTICAL BLINDNESS

INTRODUCTION

Definitions

- Cortical blindness or cortical visual impairment refers to loss of vision in otherwise healthy eye(s) due to a lesion in the brain's occipital cortex
- Complete blindness is much less common than partial blindness (cortical visual impairment)

Subtypes

- Congenital
  - Congenital malformation of the occipital lobe
  - Perinatal trauma, ischemia, hemorrhage, meningitis, encephalitis, or congenital toxoplasmosis
  - Antenatal use of cocaine and amphetamines by mother
  - Metabolic disorders
- Acquired
  - Vascular
    - Ischemic
      - Hypoxic-ischemic injury is most common cause of cortical blindness
      - Occurs when posterior circulation of the brain is compromised
      - Blockage of 1 or both posterior cerebral arteries (PCAs)
    - Hemorrhagic
      - PCA distribution
    - Transient ischemic attack
  - Infectious
    - Meningitis
    - Encephalitis
    - Subacute sclerosing panencephalitis
    - Creutzfeldt-Jakob disease
  - Neoplastic
    - Tumors of occipital lobe and visual cortex
  - Traumatic
  - Eclampsia and (rarely) preeclampsia
    - Posterior reversible encephalopathy syndrome
  - Toxic
    - Hyperammonemia
  - Iatrogenic
    - Postcardiac surgery
    - Cerebral angiography
    - Antiepileptic medications

PRESENTATION

Symptoms

- Partial or complete blindness
- Visual hallucinations
- Riddoch phenomenon
  - Preservation of the ability to perceive moving but not static objects
- Occasionally, patient may preserve ability to perceive light

Exam Findings

- Pupils remain reactive to light, does not cause afferent pupillary defect
- Absent visual fixation and tracking
- Macular sparing of vision may occur
- Funduscopy and slit-lamp exam are normal

Associated Manifestations

- Anton syndrome
  - Occurs when the patient has complete denial or unawareness of their visual loss
  - Hallucinate and confabulate visual images
  - Most common with bilateral occipital infarctions
- Blindsight
  - Occurs when patient who lacks visual awareness exhibits visually guided behavior

DIFFERENTIAL DIAGNOSIS

Ocular Visual Impairment

- Differentiate from cortical blindness by the following
  - Cortical blindness will demonstrate normal pupillary response
  - Optic nerve will appear normal in cortical blindness
  - MRI/CT brain imaging

EVALUATION/WORK-UP

Imaging

- CT or MRI of brain, MRA, CTA
  - Evaluate occipital cortex

TREATMENT

Medical

- Visual stimulation activities over a long period of time
  - Most helpful in pediatric populations

Prognosis

- Largely dependent upon underlying etiology
- Permanent complete loss of vision due to cortical blindness is rare
  - Development of complete cortical blindness to a milder cortical visual impairment is more common outcome
  - Prognosis is best in patients < 40 years of age
  - Bilateral occipital lobe lesions have poorer prognosis
  - Prognosis is particularly poor when caused by stroke
- Some patients may regain visual function completely
  - Cortical blindness secondary to transient ischemic attacks, eclampsia, or antiepileptic drug use have better visual prognosis

SELECTED REFERENCES

1. Cereda C et al: Posterior cerebral artery territory infarctions. Front Neurol Neurosci. 30:128-31, 2012
2. Leopold DA: Primary visual cortex: awareness and blindsight. Annu Rev Neurosci. 35:91-109, 2012
3. Stasheff SF et al: Deficits in cortical visual function. Ophthalmol Clin North Am. 14(1):217-42, x, 2001
4. Good WV et al: Cortical visual impairment in children. Surv Ophthalmol. 38(4):351-64, 1994
5. Aldrich MS et al: Cortical blindness: etiology, diagnosis, and prognosis. Ann Neurol. 21(2):149-58, 1987

MIGRAINE

Key Facts

Introduction
- Chronic neurological disorder featuring moderate to severe headaches and often autonomic nervous system symptoms

Demographics
- Cause of migraines is not entirely understood
  - Headache pain is transmitted through trigeminal nerve
- Affects women > men

Presentation
- Usually unilateral but may be bilateral
- Photophobia, phonophobia, nausea/vomiting
- 15% have transient neurological symptoms
- No papilledema

Differential Diagnosis
- Retinal migraine
- Temporal arteritis
- Cluster headache

Evaluation/Work-Up
- Erythrocyte sedimentation rate and C-reactive protein
- Complete blood count, chem 10, liver function test
- Lumbar puncture
- Complete physical and neurological examination
- Head MRI &/or CT

Treatment
- Acute treatment: NSAIDs, acetaminophen, triptans, caffeine, ergot
- Prophylactic treatments: β-blockers, calcium channel blockers, triptans
- Migraine trigger site surgery; removal of trigger factors
- Occipital nerve block
- With treatment, headaches will usually decrease or cease completely
- Botulism toxin injections

*(**Left**) Coronal T2I MRI shows small punctate foci of increased signal intensity in the bilateral centrum semiovale → in this patient with chronic recurrent severe throbbing headaches. (**Right**) Axial T2 MRI FLAIR (same patient) more easily demonstrates bilateral centrum semiovale foci of increased signal intensity → secondary to presumed migraine-induced chronic ischemia.*

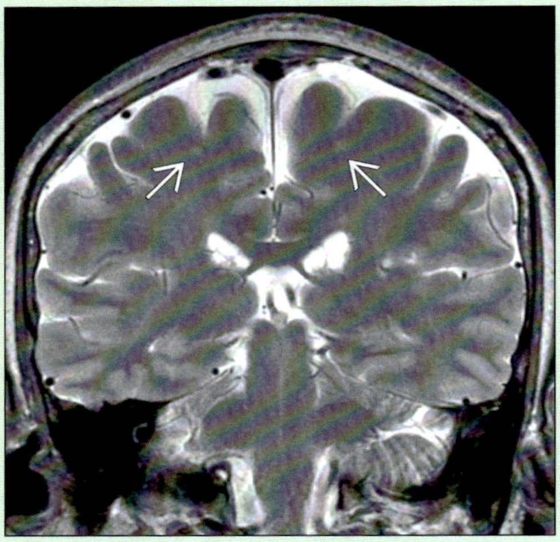

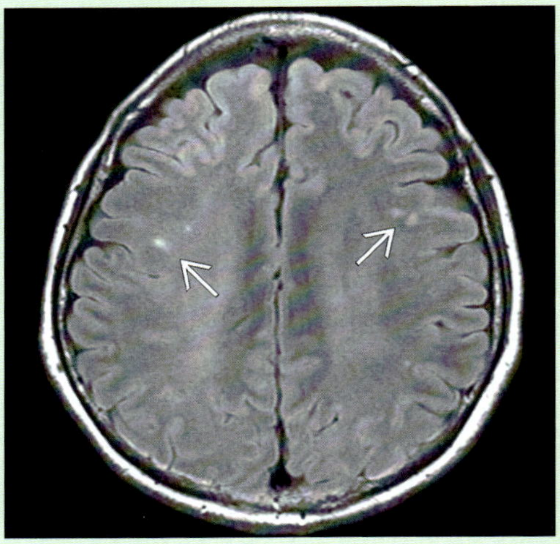

*(**Left**) Axial CECT shows diffuse SAH in the basal cisterns, anterior interhemispheric fissure →, and sylvian fissures → in a patient with a ruptured ACoA aneurysm. Note hydrocephalus of the lateral and 4th ventricles as well as intraventricular hemorrhage within the 4th ventricle →. (**Right**) Coronal oblique graphic shows vasculitis with medium vessel changes →, and parenchymal changes seen as multifocal areas of edema, infarction, and scattered hemorrhages within the basal ganglia and at the gray-white junction.*

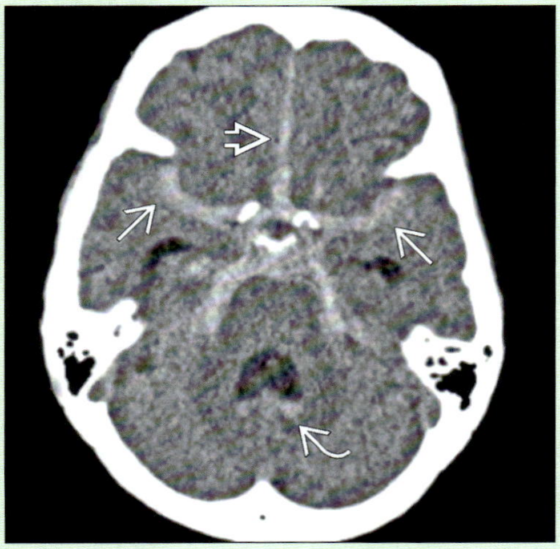

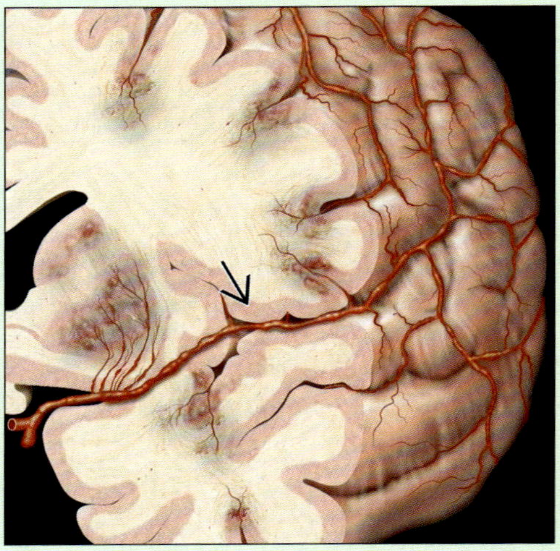

MIGRAINE

INTRODUCTION

Definitions

- Chronic neurological disorder featuring moderate to severe headaches and autonomic symptoms

Subtypes

- Familial hemiplegic migraine
- Retinal migraine

DEMOGRAPHICS

Etiology/Risk Factors

- Cause of migraines is not entirely understood but is thought to be polygenetic and influenced by environmental factors
  - Pain is transmitted through the trigeminal nerve
  - Triggers: Stress, diet (chocolate, certain cheeses, caffeine use/withdrawal), poor sleep, hormonal imbalance

Epidemiology

- In general population, migraines occur in
  - 6-7% of men and 18% of women

PRESENTATION

Symptoms

- Usually unilateral head pain
- Photophobia and phonophobia
- Nausea and vomiting
- Loss of vision/disturbance (e.g., fortification spectra)
- Transient focal neurologic symptoms
- Aura: Visual or other sensory disturbance that forewarns of a headache

Exam Findings

- No signs of papilledema
- Normal deep tendon reflexes
- No focal neurological deficits: Cranial nerves 1-12 intact

DIFFERENTIAL DIAGNOSIS

Retinal Migraine

- Ocular features including temporary monocular loss of vision associated with migraines
  - Headaches may or may not accompany vision loss
  - Vision loss may become irreversible over time
- Treatment does not differ from other migraines

Temporal (Giant Cell) Arteritis

- Most commonly occurs in 7th decade
- Symptoms include severe unilateral headache, vision loss, fatigue, weight loss, and fever
- Labs: Elevated erythrocyte sedimentation rate and elevated C-reactive protein
- If suspected, begin high-dose prednisone followed by artery biopsy

Cluster Headaches

- Characterized by excruciating pain; headaches have rapid onset without warning
- Unilateral; often accompanied by ipsilateral lacrimation and rhinorrhea
- Treated with 100% oxygen and verapamil

Tension-Type Headache

- Most common headache, generally triggered by stress
- Usually bilateral, band-like pressure around head lasting from 30 minutes to 1 week
- Treat by decreasing stress and with nonsteroidal anti-inflammatories or aspirin

EVALUATION/WORK-UP

Labs

- Erythrocyte sedimentation rate
- C-reactive protein
- Lumbar puncture if intracranial hemorrhage, infection, or neoplasm is suspected

Pathology

- Temporal artery biopsy if temporal arteritis is suspected

Imaging

- Consider head MRI &/or CT if patient has red flag headache symptoms such as
  - Previous history of cancer
  - Human immunodeficiency virus
  - Recent onset cranial nerve palsy
  - Accelerating pattern of pain or "worst headache of life"
  - Papilledema, focal weakness, loss of consciousness

TREATMENT

Medical

- Rest in a dark room
- Lifestyle modifications: Stress reduction, smoking cessation, diet and exercise
- 1st line: Aspirin, nonsteroidal anti-inflammatories, and caffeine-acetaminophen-aspirin pills
- 2nd line: Dihydroergotamine and triptans
- Propranolol is good for prophylaxis
- FL-41 glasses help reduce attack
- Botulism toxin injections

Surgical

- Trigger site surgery
  - Surgery can include avulsion of zygomaticotemporal branch of trigeminal nerve, corrugator muscle group removal, septoplasty, turbinectomy
- Occipital nerve block: Using steroids or local anesthetic

Follow-Up

- Instruct patients to follow-up immediately if they experience seizures, sensorimotor deficits, or rapidly worsening headaches

Prognosis

- With treatment, headaches will usually greatly decrease in frequency/intensity or cease completely

SELECTED REFERENCES

1. Kirbas S et al: Evaluation of the retinal changes in patients with chronic migraine. Acta Neurol Belg. 113(2):167-72, 2013

Key Facts

Introduction

- Visual impairment not explained by a structural abnormality or organic disease process
- Malingering
  - Claim of visual disability without actual symptoms
  - Secondary gain (i.e., financial gain)
- Functional disorder
  - Subconscious change
  - Linked to visual or emotional stress

Demographics

- May be precipitated by psychosocial stressors
  - Children often have stressors at home or school
  - Adults often have history of physical trauma or chronic pain
- Common in pediatrics (as high as 1 per 100 children)
- Female predominance
- May have secondary gain motivation

Presentation

- Often vague
- Blurry vision, monocular or binocular blindness
- Diplopia
- Metamorphopsia
- Patient may be unconcerned
- Visual field restriction
- Absence of pathology

Treatment

- Reassurance alone may be most effective
- Social support, confrontation rarely productive
  - Family, counseling, church group, etc.
- Accommodative/convergence therapy
- "Retinal rest," avoidance of activities
- Psychiatric evaluation
  - If part of syndrome with somatic complaints
- Regular ophthalmologic examinations
- Excellent long-term prognosis

*(**Left**) This fundus photo shows enlarged peripapillary vessels ➡ and slight optic disc pallor ⇨ in a patient with Leber hereditary optic neuropathy. This is a possible differential diagnosis for nonphysiologic vision loss. (Courtesy P. Bernstein, MD.) (**Right**) This fundus photo shows the round, sharply delineated "sunny-side up egg yolk" macular lesion characteristic of Best vitelliform dystrophy. This disease could possibly be confused with nonphysiologic vision loss.*

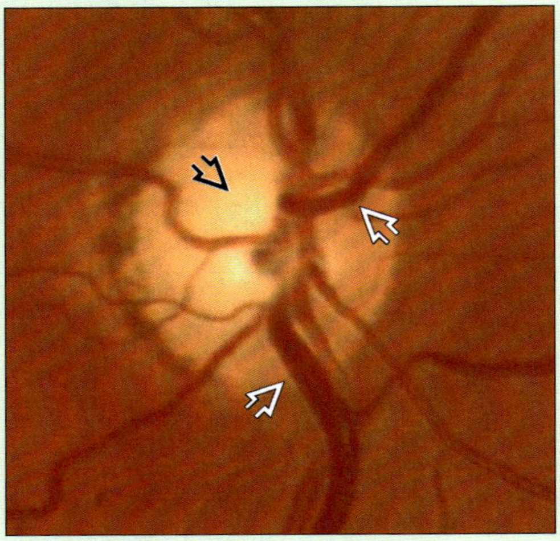

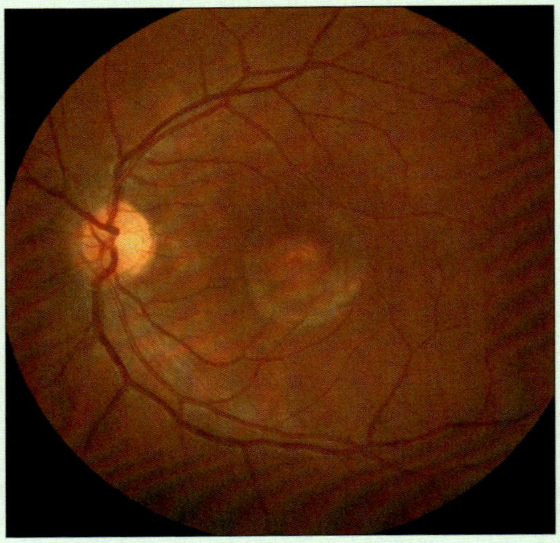

*(**Left**) This fundus photo shows Stargardt disease, which should be ruled out in cases of suspected nonphysiologic vision loss in patients 10-20 years of age. Exam findings may be normal initially or may include nonspecific mottling. (**Right**) This fundus photo shows a round detachment of sensory retina at the macula from central serous chorioretinopathy. As exam findings may be subtle early, this disease should be ruled out in adults with suspected nonphysiologic vision loss.*

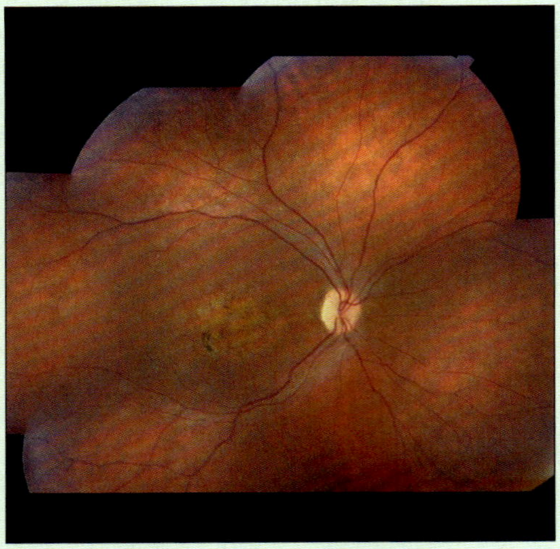

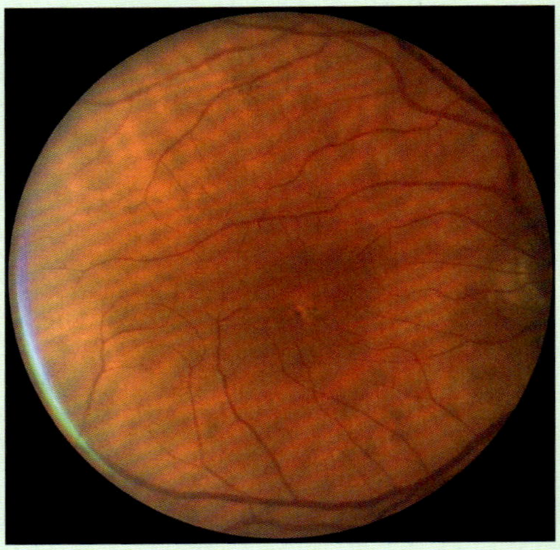

NONPHYSIOLOGIC VISUAL LOSS

INTRODUCTION

Definitions

- Visual impairment not explained by a structural abnormality or organic disease process
- Also known as functional visual loss
  - Avoids distinguishing the intentional feigning of symptoms from those outside patient consciousness

Subtypes

- Malingering
  - Claim of visual disability without actual symptoms
  - Secondary gain (i.e., financial gain)
- Functional disorder
  - Subconscious
  - Patient actually experiences symptoms
  - Often pediatric functional bilateral amblyopia
  - Linked to visual or emotional stress

DEMOGRAPHICS

Etiology/Risk Factors

- May be precipitated by psychosocial stressors
  - Children often have stressors at home or school
    - Possibility of abuse **must** be explored
  - Adults often have history of physical trauma or chronic pain
    - Secondary gain may be present

Epidemiology

- Common in pediatrics (as high as 1 per 100 children)
- Female predominance

PRESENTATION

Symptoms

- Often vague
- Blurry vision, monocular or binocular blindness
- Diplopia
- Metamorphopsia
- Visual field restriction
- Patient may be unconcerned

Exam Findings

- Absence of pathology
  - Fundus
  - Pupil responses
  - Refractive error by retinoscopy
  - Keratometry
- Visual acuity
  - Variable
  - Pinhole may reduce acuity
  - Clinical manipulation (e.g., with phoropter) may result in normal acuity
  - Optokinetic nystagmus reflex indicates ≥ 20/200 acuity
- Visual field/color vision
  - Nonorganic in nature
  - Confrontation → tubular fields
  - Kinetic visual fields → spiral or tubular
  - Static fields → isolated relative defect without pattern
- Accommodative/convergence excess/insufficiency
- Blepharospasm
- Eye-movement abnormalities

DIFFERENTIAL DIAGNOSIS

Leber Hereditary Optic Neuropathy

- May spare pupillary fibers despite severe vision loss

Other Suspected Pathologies

- Should be guided by patient history/symptoms
  - Macular dystrophies, retinitis pigmentosa sine pigmento, amblyopia, Stargardt disease, X-linked juvenile retinoschisis, central serous retinopathy, Best vitelliform dystrophy, retinal detachment, paraneoplastic optic neuropathy/retinopathy, chiasmal compressive lesion, retrobulbar optic neuropathy, keratoconus, acute zonal occult outer retinopathy, occipital infarct
  - Retinal diseases may be missed early in disease course due to minimal changes on retina exam

EVALUATION/WORK-UP

Imaging

- Fluorescein angiography or electrophysiological testing
  - Indicated if macular disease or dystrophy suspected
- Magnetic resonance imaging
  - Indicated if intracranial lesion suspected
- Visual fields can show spiral fields
- Fogging and phoropter "tricks"

Diagnosis

- Primarily a diagnosis of exclusion
- Reduced vision with otherwise normal ocular health necessitates exclusion of all other pathologies

TREATMENT

Medical

- Reassurance alone may be most effective
  - Social support: Family, friends, faith, counseling
- Accommodative/convergence therapy
- Refractive correction
- Psychiatric evaluation
  - Comanagement with psychiatrist may be most effective, especially if somatic complaints are present

Follow-Up

- Regular ophthalmologic examinations
- Consider neurology/psychiatry consultation
  - Coexisting organic disease is common

Prognosis

- Excellent long-term prognosis

SELECTED REFERENCES

1. Pula J: Functional vision loss. Curr Opin Ophthalmol. 23(6):460-5, 2012
2. Bruce BB et al: Functional visual loss. Neurol Clin. 28(3):789-802, 2010
3. Villegas RB et al: Functional vision loss: a diagnosis of exclusion. Optometry. 78(10):523-33, 2007
4. Lim SA et al: Functional visual loss in adults and children patient characteristics, management, and outcomes. Ophthalmology. 112(10):1821-8, 2005

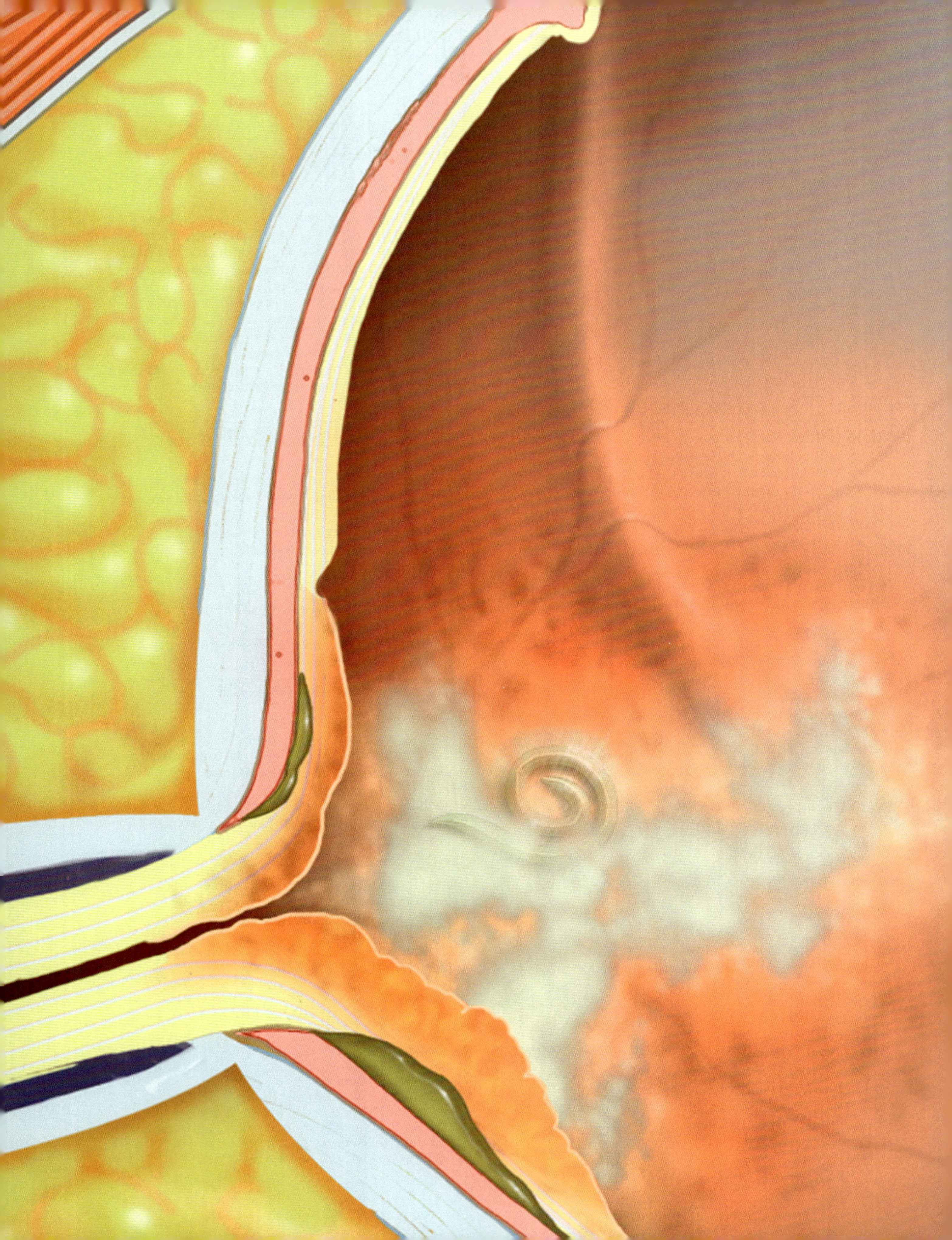

SECTION 1
Congenital Anomalies

MAJOR CLINICAL STUDIES: CONGENITAL ANOMALIES

SUPPLEMENTAL THERAPEUTIC OXYGEN FOR PRETHRESHOLD ROP (STOP-ROP MULTICENTER TRIAL)

Objective and Principal Conclusions
- Determine the efficacy, safety, and costs of providing supplemental oxygen in moderately severe (prethreshold) retinopathy of prematurity (ROP)
- Use of supplemental oxygen did not result in progression of prethreshold ROP but did increase risk of pulmonary adverse effects

Inclusion Criteria
- Newborns with prethreshold ROP in 1 or both eyes

Randomization Method
- Infants randomized to oxygen administration with continuous saturation monitoring at 1 of 2 oxygen saturation levels
  - Target pulse oximetry of 89-94% saturation
  - Target pulse oximetry of 96-99% saturation

Results
- Use of supplemental oxygen did not:
  - Cause additional progression of prethreshold ROP
  - Significantly reduce the number of infants requiring peripheral retinal ablative surgery following progression to threshold ROP
- Supplemental oxygen increased the risk of
  - Pneumonia, chronic lung disease exacerbaions
  - Need for oxygen, diuretics & hospitalization at 3 months of corrected age

CRYOTHERAPY FOR ROP (CRYO-ROP)

Objective and Principal Conclusions
- Determine if transscleral cryotherapy to the peripheral avascular region in severe ROP prevents cicatricial changes, reduces blindness, and decreases risk of retinal detachment (RD)
- Cryotherapy is recommended for both eyes whenever stage 3+ ROP involves ~ 1/2 the circumference in either zone I or zone II

Inclusion Criteria
- Birth weight: ≤ 1250 grams
- Age: ≥ 28 days
- No major ocular or systemic congenital anomalies
- Patients with threshold ROP on exam qualified for cryotherapy trial

Randomization Method
- Eyes with threshold ROP were randomized to transscleral cryotherapy or observation
  - Of the 9,751 infants identified with birth weights < 1,251 grams, 4,099 were systemically examined
  - Threshold ROP developed in 291 infants and cryotherapy was performed in 1/2 of these infants
  - Cryotherapy was performed to avascular retina 360° contiguously

Results
- Fundus photographs of the posterior pole showed abnormalities in 25.7% of eyes that received cryotherapy and in 47.4% of untreated eyes
- Abnormal visual acuity based on Teller Acuity Card testing was seen in 35% of the treated eyes compared to 56.3% in untreated eyes
- Cryotherapy reduces the risk of unfavorable retinal and functional outcome from threshold ROP
- When the entire cohort had 3-month follow-up, reduction in unfavorable structural outcome was 40% (31% [treated] vs. 51% [observed])
- Outcomes, 1 year: 46% reduction in unfavorable structural, 38% reduction in unfavorable functional
  - Unfavorable structural outcome
    - Retinal fold involving the macula, RD involving zone I, retrolental tissue or mass
  - Unfavorable functional outcome
    - If visual acuity was < 0.8 cycles per degree, per acuity card procedure; blind or low vision
- At 5.5 years, 40% reduction in unfavorable structural outcome and 24% reduction in unfavorable Snellen visual acuity functional outcome (visual acuity > 20/200) in treated eyes vs. untreated eyes
- Unexpected finding at 5.5 years: Treated eyes were less likely to have ≥ 20.40 visual acuity compared to controls but was not statistically significant (13% treated vs. 17% control)

BEVACIZUMAB ELIMINATES THE ANGIOGENIC THREAT OF ROP (BEAT-ROP)

Objective and Principal Conclusions
- Determine the efficacy of intravitreal bevacizumab vs. laser therapy in preventing ROP recurrence before 54 weeks postmenstrual age in infants with stage 3+ ROP
- Intravitreal bevacizumab vs. laser therapy in infants with stage 3+ ROP showed a significant benefit in zone I but not in zone II disease

Inclusion Criteria
- Infants with stage 3+ ROP in zone I or II posterior in each eye
- Excluded for stage 4 or 5 ROP in either eye

Randomization Method
- Infants (both eyes) were randomly assigned to treatment with intravitreal bevacizumab 0.625 mg in 0.025 mL of solution or peripheral retinal ablation with confluent laser therapy

Results
- In the bevacizumab group, 6 of 140 eyes (4 of 70 infants) had recurrent ROP vs. 32 of 146 eyes (19 of 73 infants) in the laser-therapy group (odds ratio with bevacizumab, 0.17; 95% confidence interval [CI], 0.05 to 0.53; $P = .002$)
- ROP recurrence in 2 of 31 infants with zone I disease in the bevacizumab group compared to 14 of 33 infants in the laser-therapy group (odds ratio with bevacizumab, 0.09; 95% CI, 0.02 to 0.43; $P = .003$)
- ROP recurrence in 5 of 40 infants with zone II disease in the bevacizumab group compared to 2 of 39 infants in the laser-therapy group (odds ratio with bevacizumab, 0.39; 95% CI, 0.07 to 2.11; $P = .027$)
- Mean (± SD) time to recurrence was 16.0 ± 4.6 weeks for the 6 eyes treated with intravitreal bevacizumab and 6.2 ± 5.7 weeks for the 32 eyes treated with laser therapy

- Complications included corneal opacity (1 case) and lens opacity (3 cases) seen after laser therapy in zone II posterior disease
- Number of infants intubated as part of treatment was greater in the laser-therapy group ($P < .001$)

CLINICAL TRIAL OF EYE PROPHYLAXIS IN NEWBORN

Objective and Principal Conclusions

- Compare effectiveness of silver nitrate drops, erythromycin ointment, or no medication in preventing neonatal conjunctivitis caused by *Chlamydia trachomatis* and other eye infections
- Compare side effects of silver nitrate drops and erythromycin ointment
- Both silver nitrate drops and erythromycin ointment are effective at preventing neonatal conjunctivitis, and both had minimal side effects

Inclusion Criteria

- Infants delivered vaginally or by cesarean section
- Staying at hospital ≥ 48 hrs following delivery
- Exclusion criteria
  - Siblings of infants enrolled in the study
  - Women who were culture positive for gonorrhea
  - Infants receiving systemic antimicrobials for reasons other than conjunctivitis
  - Women receiving antimicrobials at time of delivery
  - Families not available for follow-up after delivery

Randomization Method

- Randomized, double-masked trial
- Subjects were randomly assigned to receive silver nitrate drops, erythromycin ointment, or no treatment

Results

- 17% of patients developed mild conjunctivitis
  - Of those, 63% occurred during 1st 2 weeks of life
  - No significant difference in conjunctivitis rates in newborns delivered vaginally vs. cesarean section
  - Etiology included: *Haemophilus influenzae*, *Streptococcus pneumoniae*, *Neisseria cinerea*, *Klebsiella pneumoniae*, and *Chlamydia trachom*atis
  - Study suggests that bacteria were transmitted to the infants' eyes after birth and not from the birth canal
- Newborns randomized to silver nitrate drops had a 39% lower rate of conjunctivitis compared to those receiving no prophylaxis
  - Silver nitrate eye prophylaxis caused no sustained adverse effects
- Newborns randomized to erythromycin ointment had a 31% lower rate of conjunctivitis compared to those receiving no prophylaxis

COMPARISON OF TONO-PEN AND GOLDMANN APPLANATION TONOMETERS FOR MEASUREMENT OF IOP IN HEALTHY CHILDREN

Objective and Principal Conclusions

- Determine differences in IOP measured with Tono-Pen and Goldmann applanation tonometer (GAT) in normal children and adolescents
- Measurements of IOP did not differ significantly between that measured with Tono-Pen vs. GAT
- Younger age and higher IOP in the office setting was associated with a greater average difference

Inclusion Criteria

- Age < 18 years
- Cycloplegic refraction performed upon enrollment or within 6 months prior to enrollment
- Healthy corneas without structural abnormalities or microphthalmia
- No systemic conditions that would influence CCT or IOP
- No uveitis, glaucoma, or anterior segment anomalies
- No periocular steroid use within 3 months of entering study or current steroid use
- No Marfan syndrome
- No history of refractive or intraocular surgery
- No optic nerve abnormality

Randomization Method

- Patients had their IOP measured with the 2 instruments by separate, masked examiners in the office or under general anesthesia

Results

- Tono-Pen measured values slightly lower than the GAT for IOP < 11 mm Hg and slightly higher than the GAT for IOP > 11 mm Hg in the office setting
- Average difference (GAT) was 0.4 mm Hg at IOP of 10 mm Hg and -3.0 mm Hg at IOP of 20 mm Hg
- Larger differences between instruments were seen with younger age
- Standard error of measurement with Tono-Pen was 1.44 mm Hg and 1.82 mm Hg for the office and anesthesia settings respectively
- Thicker corneas were associated with higher IOP with both GAT and Tono-Pen

RELATED REFERENCES

1. National Institutes of Health, National Eye Institute: Clinical Trial of Eye Prophylaxis in the Newborn. http://www.nei.nih.gov/neitrials/static/study19.asp. Updated September 23, 1999. Accessed September 9, 2013
2. National Institutes of Health, National Eye Institute: Cryotherapy for Retinopathy of Prematurity (CRYO-ROP) - Outcome Study of Cryotherapy for Retinopathy of Prematurity. http://www.nei.nih.gov/neitrials/static/study32.asp. Updated November 4, 2003. Accessed September 9, 2013
3. National Institutes of Health, National Eye Institute: Supplemental Therapeutic Oxygen for Prethreshold Retinopathy of Prematurity (the STOP-ROP Multicenter Trial). http://www.nei.nih.gov/neitrials/static/study40.asp. Updated February 10, 2000. Accessed September 9, 2013
4. Bradfield YS et al: Comparison of Tono-Pen and Goldmann applanation tonometers for measurement of intraocular pressure in healthy children. J AAPOS. 16(3):242-8, 2012
5. Mintz-Hittner HA et al: Efficacy of intravitreal bevacizumab for stage 3+ retinopathy of prematurity. N Engl J Med. 364(7):603-15, 2011

AICARDI SYNDROME

Key Facts

Introduction
- Typically classified by a triad involving
  - Chorioretinal lacunae
  - Seizures, usually infantile spasms
  - Agenesis of corpus callosum

Demographics
- Affects females; lethal in males

Presentation
- Seizures
- Mental retardation
- Vertebral & costal malformations
- Chorioretinal lacunae
  - Pathognomonic for Aicardi syndrome
  - Yellow to white round, flat lesions found on retina
  - Typically do not affect vision unless on central foveal area
  - Often bilateral
  - Will often find multiple lacunae
- Optic nerve coloboma

Evaluation/Work-Up
- MRI
  - Central nervous system abnormalities
  - Agenesis of corpus callosum (partial or complete)
- EEG
  - Hypsarrhythmia
  - Intermittent bursts of high-amplitude slow and sharp waves in between low-amplitude waves

Treatment
- No standard course of treatment exists; treatment is usually supportive
- Total blindness is rare
- Antiepileptic medication often needed for focal seizures and spasms

__(Left)__ Fundus photo from a patient with Aicardi syndrome shows the typical appearance of chorioretinal lacunae ➔ and optic nerve head coloboma ➔ in this condition. __(Right)__ This fundus photograph shows a coloboma of the optic nerve ➔. Coloboma of the optic nerve is associated with Aicardi syndrome.

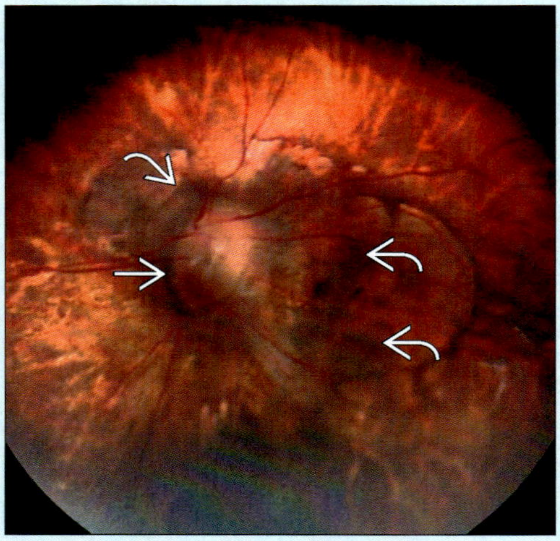

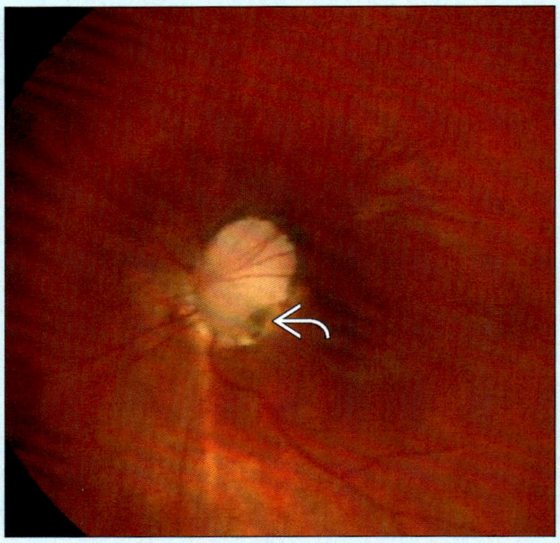

__(Left)__ Axial graphic of a classic optic disc coloboma shows a focal defect in the posterior globe ➔ at the site of the optic nerve head insertion. __(Right)__ Axial CECT shows a unilateral optic disc coloboma. There is a dehiscence of the posterior globe through a broad defect ➔ centered on the upper margin of the optic disc.

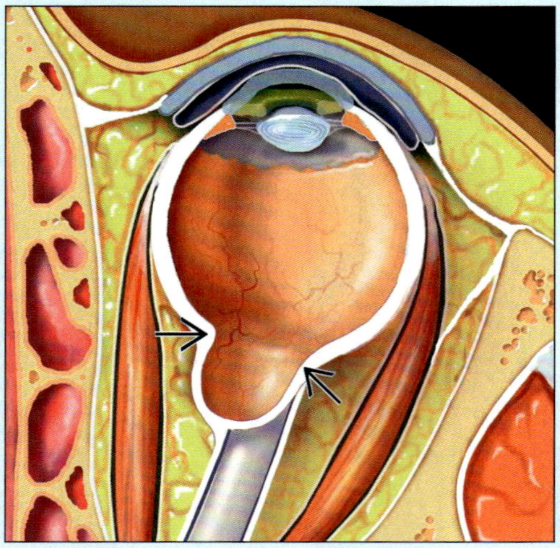

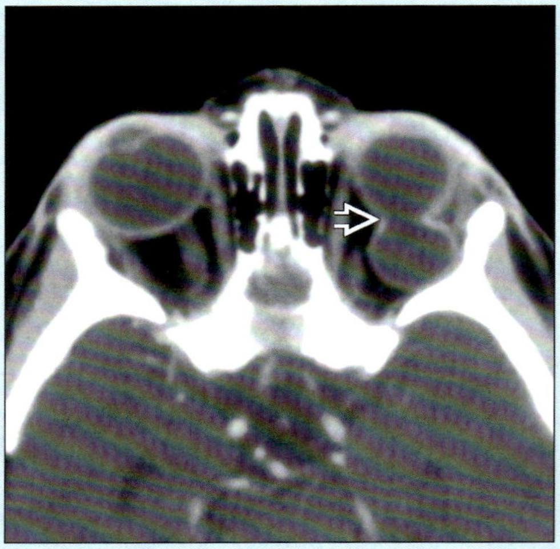

AICARDI SYNDROME

INTRODUCTION

Definitions

- Typically classified by a triad involving
  - Chorioretinal lacunae
  - Seizures, usually infantile spasms
  - Agenesis of corpus callosum

DEMOGRAPHICS

Etiology/Risk Factors

- Probable X-linked dominant inheritance

Epidemiology

- Prevalence of 1 per 100,000 people worldwide
- Affects females except those with Klinefelter syndrome, who have XXY karyotypes
- Lethal in males

PRESENTATION

Symptoms

- Seizures, usually infantile spasms
  - Most common age at 1st appearance is 3-4 months
- Mental retardation
  - Often profound
  - Most have difficulty learning components needed for language production
- Developmental delay
- Spastic hemiplegia
- Vision impairment

Exam Findings

- Ocular
  - Chorioretinal lacunae
    - Pathognomonic for Aicardi syndrome
    - Yellow/pink to white, round, flat lesions found on retina
    - Typically do not affect vision unless located in central foveal area
    - Often bilateral
    - Will usually find multiple lacunae
    - Size of lacunae rarely changes upon serial examinations
  - Optic nerve coloboma
  - Microphthalmos
    - Often unilateral or more pronounced on 1 side
- Systemic
  - Vertebral malformations
    - Fused vertebrae
    - Scoliosis
  - Costal malformations
    - Missing ribs
    - Bifurcated ribs
  - Microcephaly

DIFFERENTIAL DIAGNOSIS

Congenital Toxoplasmosis

- Presentation
  - Classic triad: Chorioretinitis, hydrocephalus, intracranial calcifications
  - Seizures
  - Mental retardation
  - Vision impairment
- May test positive for *Toxoplasma gondii* antibodies

Oculocerebrocutaneous Syndrome

- Presentation
  - Central nervous system malformations
  - Orbital cysts
  - Microphthalmia
  - Skin appendages

EVALUATION/WORK-UP

Imaging

- Central nervous system abnormalities
  - Agenesis of corpus callosum (partial or complete)
  - Pachygyria
  - Polymicrogyria
  - Cystic formations, such as arachnoid or choroid plexus cysts
  - Choroid plexus papilloma
  - Central nervous system malformations
    - Dandy-Walker malformation

Electroencephalogram (EEG)

- Hypsarrhythmia
- Intermittent bursts of high-amplitude slow and sharp waves in between low-amplitude waves

TREATMENT

Medical

- No standard course of treatment exists; treatment is usually supportive
  - Antiepileptic medication often needed for focal seizures and spasms

Surgical

- Orthopedic consultation &/or surgery may be necessary to correct scoliosis and other vertebral abnormalities

Prognosis

- ~ 76% survival rate at 6 years of age; however, most will have some degree of developmental delay
  - Few patients develop skills necessary to produce language, and many will only be able to function at a level of 12 months or younger
- Total blindness is rare

SELECTED REFERENCES

1. Fruhman G et al: Ophthalmologic findings in Aicardi syndrome. J AAPOS. 16(3):238-41, 2012
2. Kaye A: Toxoplasmosis: diagnosis, treatment, and prevention in congenitally exposed infants. J Pediatr Health Care. 25(6):355-64, 2011
3. Aicardi J: Aicardi syndrome. Brain Dev. 27(3):164-71, 2005
4. Moog U et al: Oculocerebrocutaneous syndrome: the brain malformation defines a core phenotype. J Med Genet. 42(12):913-21, 2005
5. Rosser T: Aicardi syndrome. Arch Neurol. 60(10):1471-3, 2003

COATS DISEASE

Key Facts

Introduction

- Congenital vascular disease of retina with abnormal retinal telangiectasias, aneurysms, and exudates

Demographics

- Associated with *NDP* gene mutation (chromosome Xp11.2)
- Typically presents between 0-20 years
- Male to female ratio = 3:1
- Average age at diagnosis is 6-10 years

Presentation

- Discrete zones of dilated retinal aneurysms, telangiectasias, lipid deposition, and subretinal exudate
- Superotemporal retina involvement seen in children and paramacular involvement in adult-onset disease
- Absence of identifiable posterior segment tumor

Evaluation/Work-Up

- CT scan identifies intraocular & intracranial abnormalities
- Fluorescein angiography detects aneurysms, leakage, and capillary nonperfusion
- Ocular coherence tomography (OCT) monitors subretinal exudate and fluid

Treatment

- Goal is to eliminate abnormal vessels
- Laser photocoagulation, cryotherapy, vitrectomy, enucleation
- Progressively worsening course is the norm with acute, stepwise deterioration intermixed with quiescent periods
- Visual acuity 20/200 or worse in 80% of cases, despite treatment
- Follow-up every 6 months to look for recurrence

*(**Left**) This image shows characteristic telangiectasias and dilated aneurysmal bulbs seen in a case of Coats disease. The telangiectasias here have a corkscrew appearance but may also appear kinked, looped, or beading. Perivascular sheathing, seen superiorly, is also a common finding. (**Right**) This image shows characteristic subretinal exudate and macular scaring in a case of Coats disease. The exudate acts as a stimulus for neovascularization and fibrous scar formation.*

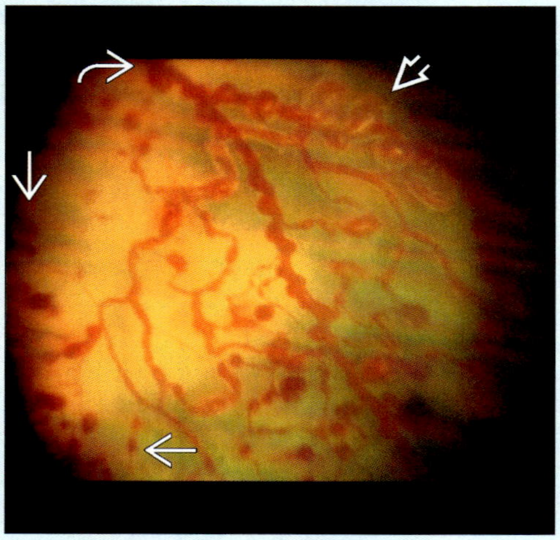

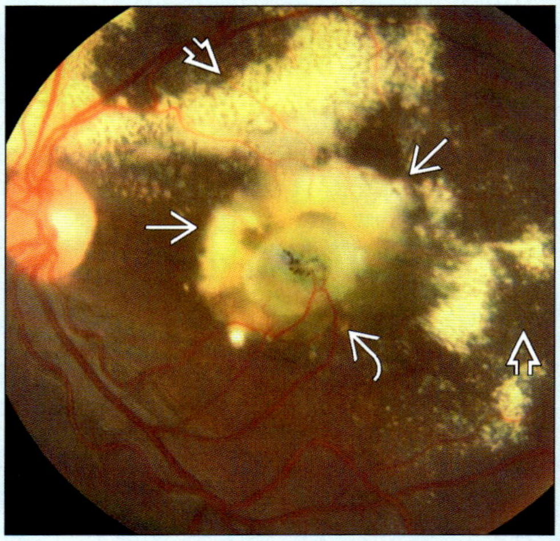

*(**Left**) This image demonstrates a retinal detachment in a patient with Coats disease. The retina is directly posterior to the lens with characteristic vascular changes, including dilated aneurysms and corkscrew telangiectasias. (**Right**) This fluorescein angiogram shows hyperfluorescent, light bulb-shaped, dilated aneurysms and tortuous telangiectatic vessels adjacent to an area of capillary nonperfusion located superotemporal to the macula.*

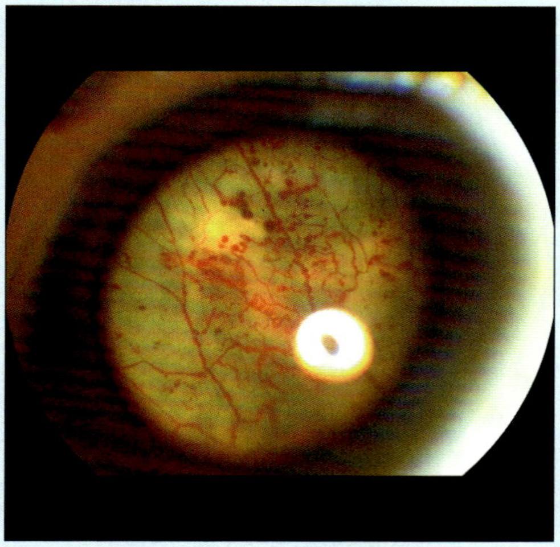

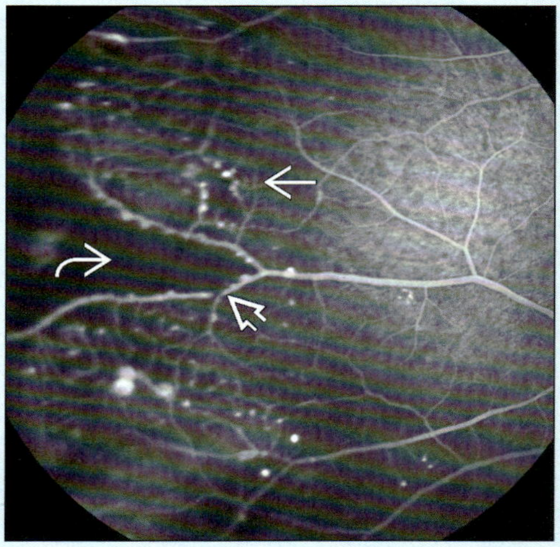

COATS DISEASE

INTRODUCTION

Definitions
- Congenital vascular disease of retina with abnormal retinal telangiectasias, aneurysms, and exudates
  - Loss of vascular endothelium leads to weakening of blood vessels, dilation → aneurysm formation and leakage → exudative retinopathy
  - Retinal telangiectasias appear as tortuous vessels
  - Fusiform aneurysms resemble light bulbs and are located near nonperfused fundus
  - Retinal exudates consist of lipid deposits, which leak from dilated capillaries

Subtypes
- Childhood disease
  - Vascular changes located in far periphery between equator and ora serrata
  - Widespread and dense lipid deposition
  - Hemorrhage is less common
- Adult disease
  - Vascular changes in parafoveal area
  - Localized and limited lipid deposition
  - Hemorrhage is common finding

DEMOGRAPHICS

Etiology/Risk Factors
- Associated with *NDP* gene mutation (chromosome Xp11.2)
  - Other genetic associations include *CRB1* gene mutation and deficiency of norrin retinal protein

Epidemiology
- Typically presents between 0-20 years
  - Average age at diagnosis is 6-10 years
  - Adult onset is associated with slower disease progression but perifoveal involvement
- Male to female ratio = 3:1

PRESENTATION

Symptoms
- 80-90% of cases are unilateral
  - Bilateral cases typically show asymmetric severity

Exam Findings
- Discrete zones of dilated retinal aneurysms, telangiectasias, lipid deposition, and subretinal exudate
  - Leaky capillaries release green-yellow exudates that settle in posterior pole
    - Subretinal fluid and exudate cause ↓ visual acuity
    - After subretinal fluid is resorbed, a lipid-rich exudate remains → retinal neovascularization and subretinal fibrous scar formation
  - Fusiform aneurysmal dilated blood vessels
    - Involving retinal veins, arteries, or capillaries
    - Large and grape-like, small and clustered, or light bulb shaped
    - Adjacent to areas of capillary nonperfusion
  - Telangiectasias
    - Retinal vasculature may appear tortuous, kinked, looped, or beading ± perivascular sheathing
- Superotemporal retina involvement seen in children and paramacular involvement in adult-onset disease
- Leukocoria and strabismus may be presenting complaint in nonverbal children
- Absence of identifiable posterior segment tumor
- Optic nerve neovascularization is rare
- Iris neovascularization can be seen

DIFFERENTIAL DIAGNOSIS

Retinal Angiomatosis (von Hippel-Lindau Disease)
- Autosomal dominant disorder consisting of vascular tumors of retina, central nervous system, and cerebellum
  - Visceral cysts and tumors (renal cell carcinoma)
- AV shunting is hallmark feature
- Retinal capillary hemangioblastoma ± subretinal exudates
  - Small, round tumor fed by large, dilated blood vessels
  - Subretinal exudates and fluid may lead to exudative retinal detachment (RD)
- Epiretinal membrane and macular traction
- Patients present at age 10-35 years with retinal findings

Retinoblastoma (RB)
- Telangiectatic vessels overlying retinal tumor surface branching from vessels feeding tumor
  - In Coats disease, surface vessels are not continuous with subretinal vessels, and intraocular calcification is absent
- Intraocular calcification seen on ultrasound or CT scan

Familial Exudative Vitreoretinopathy
- Bilateral disease of abnormal retinal vasculature with exudates and retinal traction
- Most commonly in temporal periphery

Retinopathy of Prematurity
- Altered development of retinal vasculature seen in newborns
- Risk factors include gestational age < 30 weeks, birth weight < 1.5 kg, supplemental oxygen therapy, or unstable course following delivery
- Immature vasculature categorized by location and presence of demarcation line separating normal and abnormal retina
  - ± elevated ridge, fibrovascular proliferation, and RD
  - Plus disease: Dilated veins and tortuous arteries with AV shunting

Persistent Fetal Vasculature
- Most common cause of unilateral cataract
  - Retrolental plaque with central opacity containing fibrovascular tissue
- Prominent hyaloid vessel remnant extends from optic nerve to posterior lens
  - Mittendorf dots: Anterior attachment site of hyaloid vessel remnant onto posterior lens capsule creating a central white opacity
  - Bergmeister papillae: Hyaloid vessel remnant seen in the inner optic disc
- Elongated ciliary processes seen through dilated pupil
- Radially oriented blood vessels on iris surface

COATS DISEASE

Shields Classification of Coats Disease		
Disease Stage	*Exam Findings*	*Treatment*
Stage 1	Telangiectasia	Laser photocoagulation
Stage 2A	Telangiectasia + extrafoveal exudation	Cryotherapy
Stage 2B	Telangiectasia + foveal exudation	Cryotherapy
Stage 3A	Subtotal exudative retinal detachment	Cryotherapy
Stage 3B	Total exudative retinal detachment	Surgical management
Stage 4	Total retinal detachment + secondary glaucoma	Surgical management; consider enucleation if pain, nausea, & vomiting
Stage 5	Advanced end-stage disease	Surgical management or enucleation

Shields JA et al: Classification and management of Coats disease: the 2000 Proctor Lecture. Am J Ophthalmol. 131(5):572-83, 2001.

EVALUATION/WORK-UP

Labs

- Subretinal aspirate
  - Cholesterol crystals and pigment-laden macrophages
  - Absence of tumor cells
    - Rule out RB 1st to prevent tumor seeding

Imaging

- CT scan
  - Identifies intraocular and intracranial abnormalities
  - Determines quality of retinal density
  - Exposes young patients to radiation
- Fluorescein angiography
  - Detects aneurysms, leakage, & capillary nonperfusion
  - Early and persistent leakage at sites of exudation and hemorrhage
- Ocular coherence tomography (OCT)
  - Monitors subretinal exudate and fluid
- Ultrasound
  - Identifies subretinal calcification to differentiate between Coats disease and RB
    - Calcification is rare in Coats disease

TREATMENT

Medical

- Intravitreal VEGF inhibitors (bevacizumab) are under study
  - Assists in subretinal fluid resorption, allowing for laser treatment
  - Used ± triamcinolone acetonide injection

Surgical

- Treatment goal is to eliminate abnormal vessels
  - Laser photocoagulation
    - Indicated for small lesions without subretinal fluid and with minimal exudate
    - Unable to treat if subretinal fluid is present, as retina must be flat to treat
    - May result in temporary increase in retinal exudate after destruction of abnormal vessels
  - Cryotherapy
    - Peripheral lesions, large exudates or exudative RD
    - Often used to treat childhood disease
    - May result in inflammation and poor vision
- May take up to 1 year for exudate to clear
- Multiple treatments needed if > 2 quadrants involved
- Surgical drainage of subretinal fluid with scleral buckle
  - Exudative RD
- Vitrectomy with injection of expandable gas bubble
  - Tractional RD
- Enucleation
  - Considered if intraocular pressure elevated or iris neovascularization

Follow-Up

- Laser photocoagulation or cryotherapy may require multiple treatments at 4-6 week intervals
- Follow-up every 6 months to look for recurrence
  - Seen up to 5 years after successful treatment

Prognosis

- Progressively worsening course is the norm with acute, step wise deterioration intermixed with quiescent periods
  - Visual acuity 20/200 or worse in 80% of cases, despite treatment
    - Seen in all patients with stage 4 or 5 disease
  - Poor prognostic factors: Persistent subretinal fluid following treatment, retinal macrocysts, involvement posterior to equator, diffuse or superior retinal involvement
- Disease may recur many years after treatment
- Complications
  - Leaky capillaries → retinal edema ± exudative RD
  - Macular involvement may leave exudate in fovea → permanent central vision loss
  - Vitreous hemorrhage or cells
  - Choroidal neovascularization
  - Phthisis bulbi
  - Anterior segment findings are indicative of severe disease
    - Cataract, rubeosis iridis, neovascular or angle-closure glaucoma

SELECTED REFERENCES

1. Wang KY et al: A combination of intravitreal bevacizumab injection with tunable argon yellow laser photocoagulation as a treatment for adult-onset Coats' disease. J Ocul Pharmacol Ther. 27(5):525-30, 2011

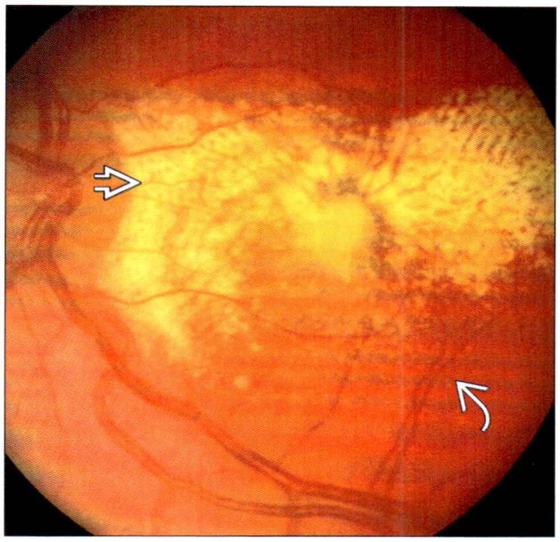

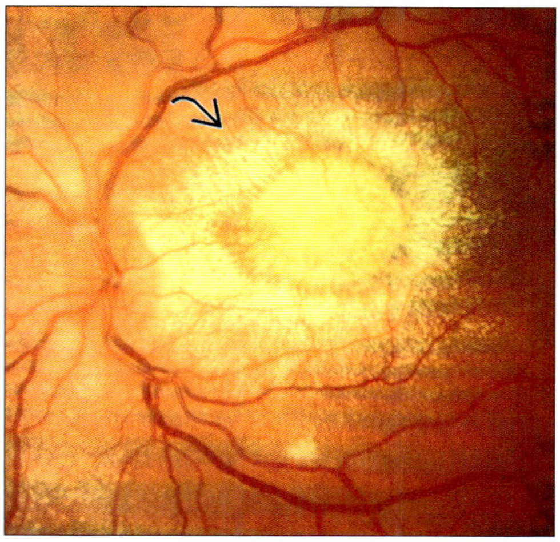

*(**Left**) This fundus photograph shows diffuse, yellow exudate ➡ in the posterior pole in a patient with Coats disease. The exudates consist of lipid deposition, which stimulates the growth of new blood vessels ➡ and fibrovascular membranes. (**Right**) This fundus photograph shows yellow exudate ➡ in the macula of a patient with Coats disease. Exudate in the posterior pole is challenging to treat because laser photocoagulation cannot be done if exudates are present and cryotherapy cannot be applied to the posterior pole.*

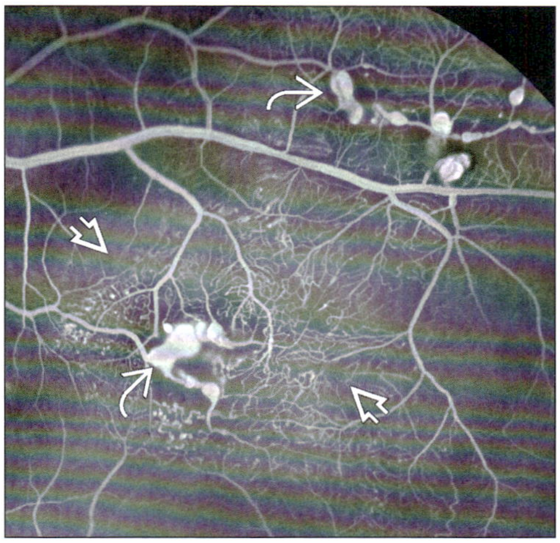

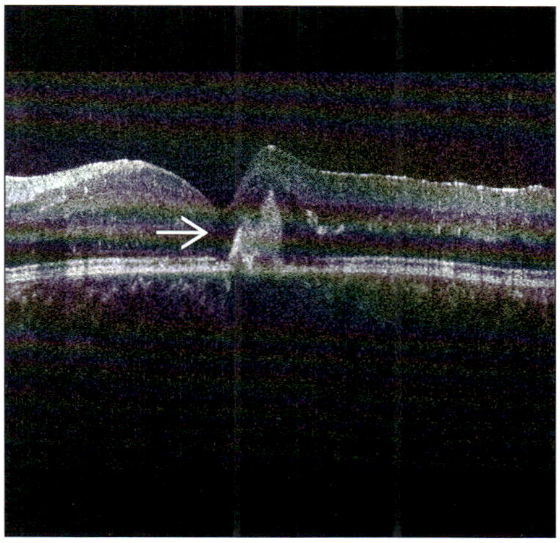

*(**Left**) This fluorescein angiogram shows hyperfluorescent dilated aneurysms ➡ and neovascularization ➡ in a patient with Coats disease. (**Right**) This OCT of the macula shows subretinal exudate ➡ in a case of Coats disease. OCT is used to monitor the progression of exudate or fluid and to monitor for resolution after therapy. For minimal subretinal fluid and no exudates, laser photocoagulation is preferred, whereas if exudate is present, cryotherapy can be done.*

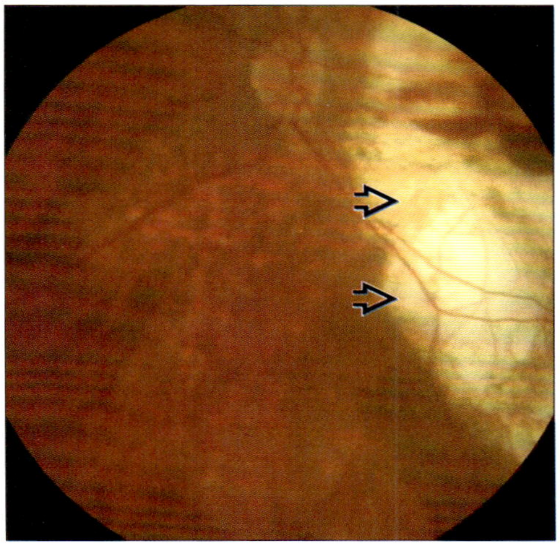

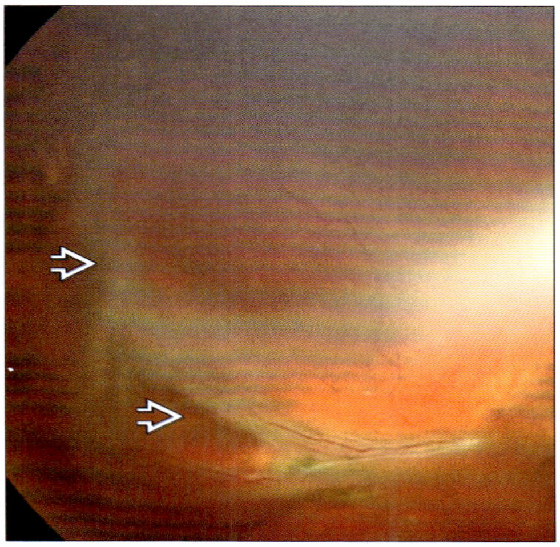

*(**Left**) This fundus photo shows an exophytic retinoblastoma growing outward and separating the retina from the choroid ➡. Fundus exam of an exophytic retinoblastoma appears similar to an exudative retinal detachment. Exophytic retinoblastoma is a differential diagnosis for Coats disease. (**Right**) This fundus photo shows a retinal fold ➡ with macular involvement in a patient with familial exudative vitreoretinopathy (FEVR). FEVR can occasionally be confused with Coats disease.*

CONGENITAL CATARACT

Key Facts

Introduction
- Lens opacity visible in the 1st year of life
- Classification based on anatomic location of opacity
  - Zonular, lamellar, nuclear, sutural, or polar

Demographics
- Frequency in developed countries is 1.2 to 6 per 10,000 births

Symptoms
- Milky, hazy, gray or white cloudiness of pupil
- Absence of red reflex normally seen in photos
- Unusual rapid eye movements (nystagmus)
- Family history of congenital cataract, maternal illness or drug ingestion during pregnancy, systemic or ocular symptoms suggesting syndromic or genetic etiology

Exam Findings
- White pupillary opacity (leukocoria) seen by direct visualization or slit-lamp exam
- Inability to visualize optic nerve or macula by direct ophthalmoscopy

Treatment
- Indications for cataract extraction and IOL implantation include visually significant central cataracts with diameter > 3 mm, dense nuclear cataracts, obstruction of visualization of fundus, and association with strabismus
- Timing of surgery dependent on degree of obscuration of visual axis and unilateral vs. bilateral involvement
  - Unilateral congenital cataract considered surgical emergency and should be extracted immediately
  - Bilateral congenital cataract may be removed up to 3 months of age

Follow-Up
- Treatment of amblyopia postoperatively with correction of refractive error and patching

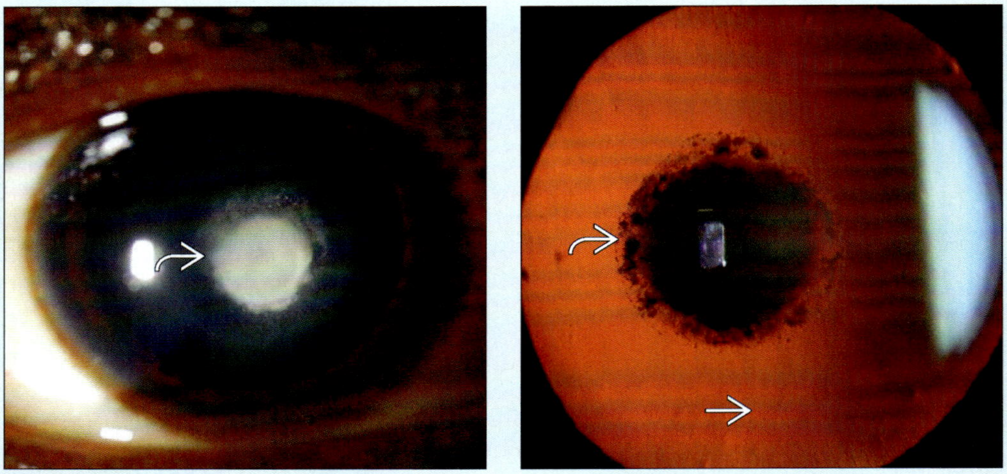

***(Left)** This slit-lamp photo shows a centrally located and whitish-gray congenital nuclear cataract ➔, representing an opacity of the fetal or embryonic lens nucleus. Note the clear lens cortex surrounding the cataract. **(Right)** This slit-lamp photo of a different patient shows retroillumination of a congenital nuclear cataract ➔. Note the clear lens cortex surrounding the cataract ➔.*

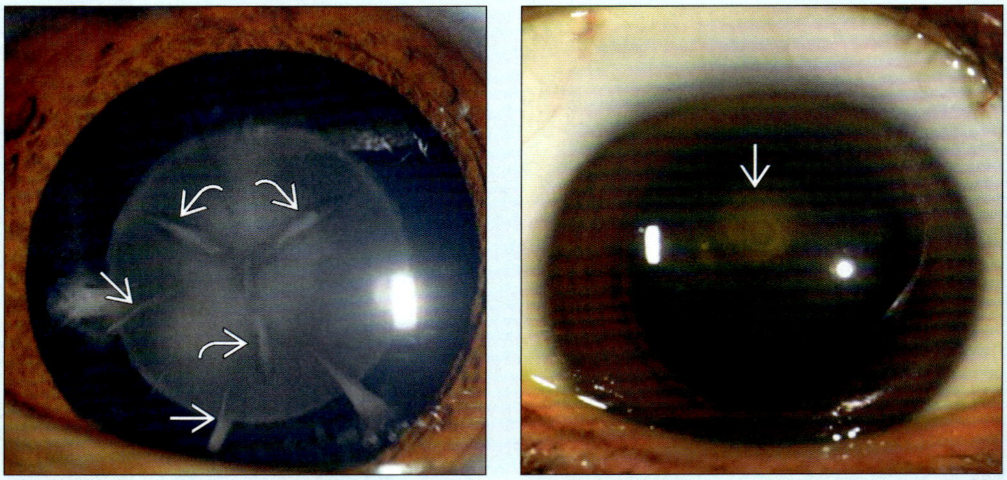

***(Left)** This slit-lamp photo shows a zonular cataract with prominent sutural opacities ➔ and peripheral radial opacities termed "riders" ➔. **(Right)** This slit-lamp photo shows a polar cataract affecting the posterior lens pole ➔. This subtype of cataract is stationary unlike the progressive nature of posterior subcapsular cataracts.*

CONGENITAL CATARACT

INTRODUCTION

Definitions

- Lens opacity visible in the 1st year of life
- Also called an infantile cataract

Subtypes

- Classification based on anatomic location of opacity
  - Zonular
    - Lamellar
      - Most common type of congenital cataract
      - Affects lens fibers formed at same time, creating a shell-like opacity
      - Often has arcuate opacities termed "riders"
    - Nuclear
      - Centrally located opacity ranging from dense to layering or dusty appearing
    - Sutural (stellate)
      - Affects regions where the lens fibers converge (sutures) and appears as a "Y"
  - Polar
    - Anterior
      - May be inherited as autosomal dominant trait or associated with microphthalmos, persistent pupillary membrane, or anterior lenticonus
      - Usually small, bilateral, nonprogressive, and does not significantly impair vision
    - Posterior subcapsular
      - Opacity on anterior surface of posterior capsule
      - Most common form of secondary cataract
    - Bipolar
      - Involves both anterior and posterior poles

DEMOGRAPHICS

Etiology/Risk Factors

- Caused by improper lens development
- Maternal rubella infection prior to 20 weeks gestation
- Low birth weight associated with increased risk of bilateral congenital cataract

Epidemiology

- 1/3 cases associated with other disease syndromes, 1/3 inherited, 1/3 idiopathic
- Frequency in developed countries is 1.2 to 6 per 10,000 births

PRESENTATION

Symptoms

- Milky, hazy, gray or white cloudiness of pupil
- Absence of red reflex normally seen in photos
- Unusual rapid eye movements (nystagmus)
- Family history of congenital cataract, maternal illness or drug ingestion during pregnancy, systemic or ocular symptoms suggesting syndromic or genetic etiology

Exam Findings

- White pupillary opacity (leukocoria) seen by direct visualization or slit-lamp exam
- Inability to visualize optic nerve or macula by direct ophthalmoscopy
- Abnormal visual evoked potentials testing

DIFFERENTIAL DIAGNOSIS

Retinoblastoma

- Malignant tumor of retina primarily affecting children

Persistent Fetal Vasculature (PFV)

- Retrolenticular fibrovascular tissue may induce cataract

Retinal Detachment

- May be associated with ocular toxocariasis, ROP, FEVR, and PFV

EVALUATION/WORK-UP

Labs

- Galactokinase activity level to rule out galactosemia
- Rubella antibody titer

Imaging

- Consider B-scan ultrasound if unable to adequately visualize fundus by direct or indirect ophthalmoscopy and to rule out retinoblastoma or retinal detachment
- Electroretinogram and visual evoked potentials to assess for possible deprivation amblyopia

TREATMENT

Medical

- If due to galactosemia, prompt removal of lactose and galactose from diet will remove lens opacity

Surgical

- Indications include visually significant central cataracts with diameter > 3 mm, dense nuclear cataracts, obstruction of visualization of fundus, and association with strabismus
- Timing of cataract extraction is largely dependent on degree of obscuration of visual axis and unilateral vs. bilateral involvement
  - Unilateral deprivation amblyopia results in greater visual impairment than bilateral deprivation
    - Unilateral congenital cataract considered surgical emergency and should be extracted immediately
    - Bilateral congenital cataract may be removed up to 3 months of age
  - Surgery involves cataract extraction, primary posterior capsulotomy, and limited anterior vitrectomy
    - Bag should be preserved to degree possible to enable placement of sulcus IOL at 2 years of age or later

Follow-Up

- Routine monitoring throughout life for development of glaucoma due to disruption of angle from lensectomy
- Treatment of amblyopia postoperatively with correction of refractive error (glasses or contacts) and patching; needs great parental involvement

Prognosis

- Better prognosis for bilateral vs. unilateral cases and for less dense cataracts

SELECTED REFERENCES

1. Trumler AA: Evaluation of pediatric cataracts and systemic disorders. Curr Opin Ophthalmol. 22(5):365-79, 2011

CONGENITAL GLAUCOMA

Key Facts

Introduction

- Occurs secondary to trabecular meshwork obstruction, resulting in elevated IOP and potentially irreversible visual field changes
- 2 different types: Primary glaucoma and secondary glaucoma, where latter is associated with other ocular and systemic anomalies

Demographics

- Very low incidence and prevalence
- Increased incidence in Saudi Arabia, South India, and Slovakia
- Bilateral disease in majority of cases
- Preponderance towards males

Presentation

- Classic triad of photophobia, epiphora, and blepharospasm
- Corneal edema
- Buphthalmos late

Differential Diagnosis

- Iridocorneal dysgenesis syndromes (Axenfeld-Rieder, Peters anomaly, and aniridia) and phacomatoses (Sturge-Weber syndrome and neurofibromatosis)

Evaluation/Work-Up

- Exam under anesthesia paramount to evaluation
- Findings of optic nerve changes, corneal enlargement, and buphthalmos highly suggestive of glaucoma

Treatment

- Mainly a surgical disease; goniotomy and trabeculotomy are first-line treatments, and trabeculectomy is a second-line treatment

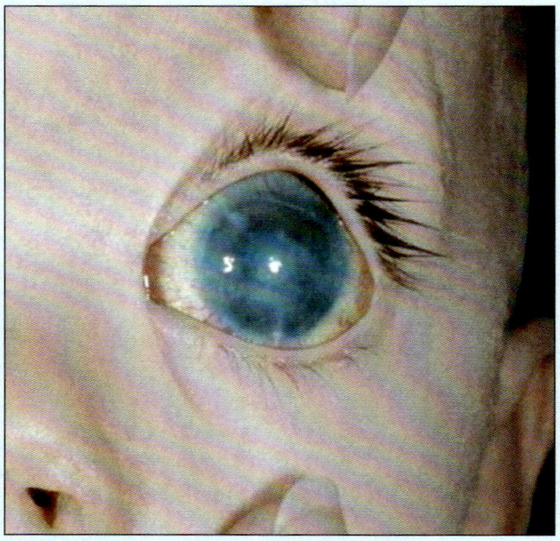

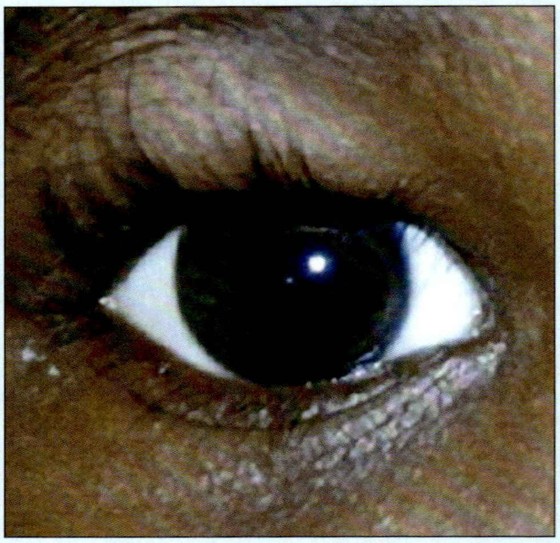

(Left) *This external photograph shows the eye of a child with congenital glaucoma. This patient, with the eyelids retracted, has easily visible buphthalmos (enlarged globe). (Courtesy G. Morshedi, MD.)* ***(Right)*** *This external photograph of a patient with congenital glaucoma demonstrates less obvious buphthalmos. Often, eyelid retraction and measurements of the eye are needed to reveal an enlarged globe. (Courtesy G. Morshedi, MD.)*

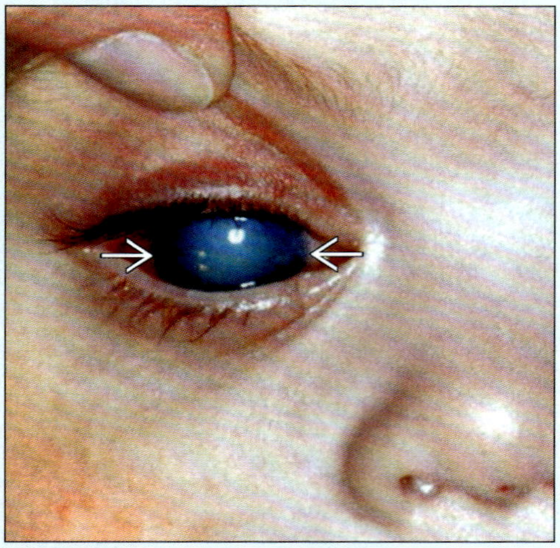

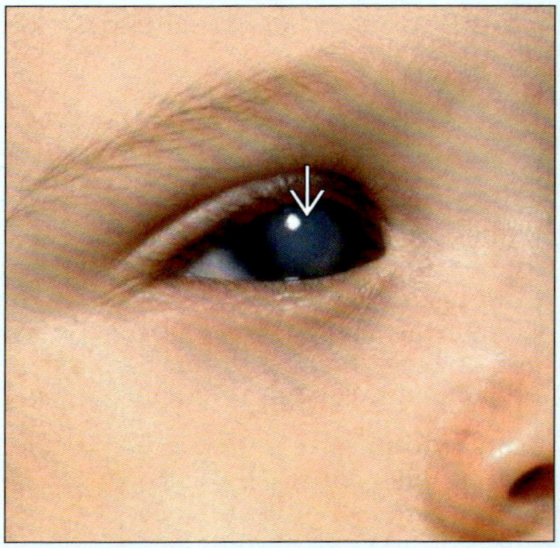

(Left) *This external photograph depicts an infant with congenital glaucoma. An enlarged corneal diameter is easily visible* ➔*. (Courtesy G. Morshedi, MD.)* ***(Right)*** *This external photograph is another example of congenital glaucoma. Corneal edema with accompanying corneal clouding* ➔ *is a typical finding in congenital glaucoma. The corneal edema is often accompanied by Haab stria, which are linear tears in the Descemet membrane. (Courtesy G. Morshedi, MD.)*

CONGENITAL GLAUCOMA

INTRODUCTION

Definitions

- Congenital form of glaucoma that occurs secondary to maldevelopment of anterior chamber angle, leading to elevated IOP and eventually to irreversible vision loss

Subtypes

- Primary: Results from isolated maldevelopment of trabecular meshwork and is not associated with other developmental ocular anomalies
- Secondary: Damage to aqueous outflow tract due to maldevelopment of another portion of eye; can be associated with systemic anomalies

DEMOGRAPHICS

Etiology/Risk Factors

- Higher risk in Slovakia, Saudi Arabia, and South India

Epidemiology

- Incidence: 1 per 10,000 births
- Prevalence: 8 per 100,000 children
- Bilateral disease in almost 80% of cases
- Nearly 70% of cases occur in males
- Evident hereditary pattern (often autosomal recessive); genes include *Glc3A*, *Glc3B*, *Glc3C*

PRESENTATION

Symptoms

- Generally manifests by 1 year of age
- Triad: Photophobia, epiphora, and blepharospasm

Exam Findings

- Increased IOP > 21 mm Hg, corneal edema, Haab striae, megalocornea, buphthalmos, optic nerve cupping

DIFFERENTIAL DIAGNOSIS

Iridocorneal Dysgenesis

- Axenfeld-Rieger syndrome: Posterior embryotoxon, iris stromal hypoplasia, corectopia, pseudopolycoria, and ectropion uveae are possible
  - Systemic malformations may include hypodontia, microdontia, maxillary hypoplasia, telecanthus, and hypertelorism
- Peters anomaly: Central cornea leukoma, microcornea, microphthalmia, missing endothelium, iris strands attached to cornea
- Aniridia: Absent or small iris remnant, lens subluxation, foveal hypoplasia, cataract, nystagmus, choroidal coloboma, and optic nerve hypoplasia
  - Also associated with Wilms tumor, genitourinary anomalies, and cerebellar ataxia

Phacomatoses

- Sturge-Weber syndrome: Hemangiomas of face, choroidal hemangioma, and meningeal angioma
  - Difficult to treat as elevated episcleral venous pressure reduces outflow; needs aqueous suppressants
- Neurofibromatosis: Tumor-like formations (neurofibromas), which can occur in CNS, skin, and mucous membranes

EVALUATION/WORK-UP

Imaging

- A-scan ultrasound

Exam Under Anesthesia

- Mainstay of evaluation
  - Corneal diameter (> 12 mm is highly suggestive of glaucoma
  - Increased IOP (> 21 mm Hg highly suggestive of glaucoma
  - Gonioscopy
  - Ophthalmoscopy (infant glaucomatous cup is commonly round, steep-walled, and central, surrounded by a pink rim)

TREATMENT

Medical

- β-blockers (timolol), topical carbonic anhydrase inhibitors (dorzolamide), prostaglandin analogues (latanoprost), α-2 agonists (brimonidine), other drugs (mannitol)
- Brimonidine is contraindicated in small children

Surgical

- Goniotomy: First-line treatment if angle can be visualized and corneal diameter < 14 mm
- Trabeculotomy: May be necessary if angle cannot be visualized
- Trabeculectomy ± mitomycin C (antifibrotic agent): May be useful when previous goniotomies or trabeculotomies have failed
- Emerging alternatives: Aqueous drainage surgical device (e.g., Ahmed valve), canaloplasty, mini shunts

Follow-Up

- Every 3-6 months indefinitely: IOP checks, nerve exam, and visual fields

Prognosis

- Excellent if IOP is well controlled long term; poor if IOP is uncontrolled after 1 or 2 surgical procedures
- Trabeculotomy: 80-90% success rate with low incidence of complications
- Trabeculectomy: 50-60% success rate in long-term studies; higher success rate if mitomycin C is part of treatment regimen, though this is associated with more complications

SELECTED REFERENCES

1. Alanazi FF et al: Primary and secondary congenital glaucoma: baseline features from a registry at King Khaled Eye Specialist Hospital, Riyadh, Saudi Arabia. Am J Ophthalmol. 155(5):882-9, 2013
2. Morales J et al: Current surgical options for the management of pediatric glaucoma. J Ophthalmol. 2013:763735, 2013
3. Mandal AK et al: Update on congenital glaucoma. Indian J Ophthalmol. 59 Suppl:S148-57, 2011

Key Facts

Introduction

- Obstruction of nasolacrimal duct (NLD) anywhere from puncta to distal duct at valve of Hasner (most common)

Demographics

- Seen in 20% of all normal newborns
- Resolves in 90% of affected infants by 12 months

Presentation

- Epiphora, ocular discharge, eyelash debris, injected conjunctiva, enlarged tear meniscus
- Palpation of lacrimal sac causes retrograde release of tears or mucous discharge through puncta
- Drop of fluorescein dye remains in lower eyelid or overflows onto cheek

Treatment

- Spontaneous resolution by 12 months of age in 75-90% of cases
- < 1% of cases resolve after 12 months
- Untreated NLD obstruction often becomes infected
- Lacrimal duct massage is first-line therapy
- Treat with antibiotics if dacryocystocele is suspected
- Lacrimal duct probing in office (6-9 months old) or operating room (> 12 months old)
  - If done in operating room, ± stenting with silicone tubing or balloon dilation of NLD
- Dacryocystorhinostomy: Surgical passageway between lacrimal sac and nasal cavity
- Conjunctivodacryocystorhinostomy: Placement of glass tube between caruncle and nasal cavity
- Acute dacryocystitis can develop and is a medical emergency in a newborn
- Chronic dacryocystitis occurs due to overgrowth of bacteria in NLD
- Nasal mucocele can develop when mucosal lining of NLD becomes distended with tears and protrudes into nasal cavity

*(**Left**) This graphic demonstrates the lacrimal drainage system including (1) the canaliculi, (3) nasolacrimal sac, nasolacrimal duct, and valve of Hasner, which is often the location of obstruction in congenital nasolacrimal duct obstructions. Mucus and pus backs up and accumulates around the caruncle (2). (**Right**) This drawing shows dilation of the left nasolacrimal sac secondary to obstruction at the level of the mid nasolacrimal duct →. The right nasolacrimal apparatus shows normal structures.*

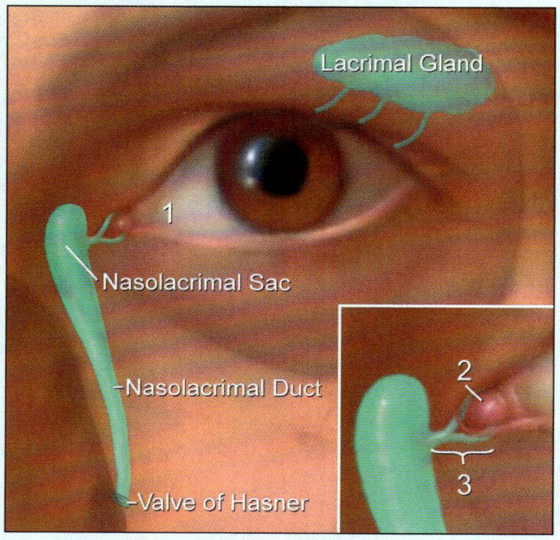

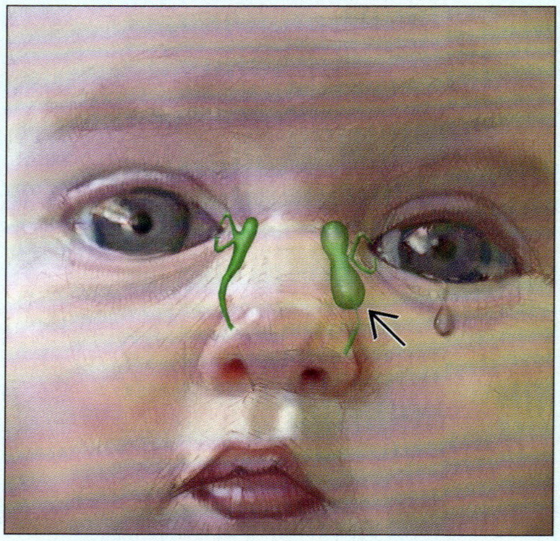

*(**Left**) This external photo shows a child with nasolacrimal duct obstruction. Note the enlarged tear meniscus and mucoid discharge on the eyelid margin →. (**Right**) The differential for nasolacrimal duct obstruction includes dacryocystocele. This coronal T2 MRI shows bilateral dacryocystocele with smooth bulbous dilation of the left nasolacrimal sac and proximal duct ➔. The right nasolacrimal sac ↪ is also mildly dilated.*

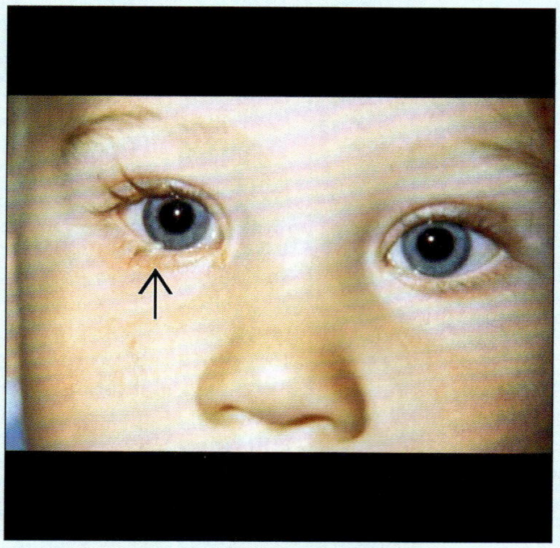

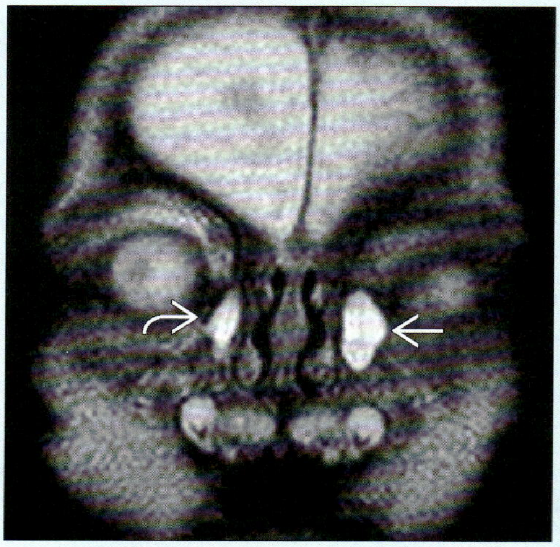

CONGENITAL NASOLACRIMAL DUCT OBSTRUCTION

INTRODUCTION

Definitions

- Obstruction of nasolacrimal duct (NLD) anywhere from puncta to distal duct at valve of Hasner (most common)

DEMOGRAPHICS

Epidemiology

- Seen in 20% of all normal newborns
- Resolves in 75-90% of affected infants by 12 months

PRESENTATION

Exam Findings

- Persistent epiphora
- Ocular discharge
- Debris on eyelashes
- Injected conjunctiva
- Enlarged tear meniscus
- Palpation of lacrimal sac causes retrograde release of tears or mucous discharge through puncta
- Dye disappearance test shows fluorescein dye remaining in lower eyelid or overflow onto cheek

DIFFERENTIAL DIAGNOSIS

Dacryocystocele/Dacryocele

- Obstruction to both proximal and distal ends of nasolacrimal system, creating a cyst
- Noticed soon after birth
- Skin overlaying cyst appears blue
- Medial canthal tendon displaced superiorly

Malposition of Puncta

- Normal positioning of puncta allows proper entry of tears into NLD drainage system
- Confirm normal positioning of puncta prior to diagnosing or treating NLD obstruction

TREATMENT

Medical

- Spontaneous resolution
  - Occurs by 12 months of age in 75-90% of cases
  - < 1% of cases resolve after 12 months
    - Lower resolution rate due to chronic infection
- Lacrimal duct massage (warm compresses)
  - First-line therapy
  - Apply pressure over lacrimal sac and course downward
  - Performed 2-3x per day
  - Empties lacrimal sac and may permanently open NLD
- Antibiotic therapy if dacryocystocele is suspected
  - Broad-spectrum topical treatment for 1-2 weeks
  - Does not eliminate source of NLD obstruction

Surgical

- Lacrimal duct probing
  - Can be done in office (6-9 months old) or operating room (> 12 months old)
  - Indicated for children > 12 months and children < 12 months with recurrent infections, lid irritation, or who undergo anesthesia for another procedure
  - If done in operating room, ± stenting with silicone tubing or balloon dilation of NLD
    - Stents are removed after 2-6 months, in office
- Dacryocystorhinostomy
  - Surgically create a passageway between lacrimal sac and nasal cavity
  - Reserved for NLD obstruction refractory to probing
  - Often required in children with abnormal anatomy
- Conjunctivodacryocystorhinostomy
  - Placement of a Pyrex glass tube between caruncle and nasal cavity
  - Reserved for children with severe anatomical abnormalities proximal to lacrimal sac, preventing other procedures
- Avoid decompression of an infected dacryocele through a skin incision to avoid creating a fistula

Prognosis

- Untreated NLD obstruction often becomes infected
- Acute dacryocystitis can develop and is a medical emergency in newborn
  - Erythema, warmth, swelling, and tenderness of lacrimal sac
  - Caused by *Staphylococcus epidermidis* or *Staphylococcus aureus*
  - Systemic antibiotics ± probing to prevent preseptal or orbital cellulitis, sepsis, meningitis, or brain abscess
    - Infection can spread to newborn's ethmoid sinuses and into orbit or CNS
    - If swelling does not resolve after a few days of antibiotic therapy, proceed to probing to decompress lacrimal sac
  - If probing, give preoperative antibiotics and culture any mucopurulent drainage
- Chronic dacryocystitis
  - Bacterial overgrowth in stagnant pool of tears in lacrimal sac
  - Caused by *Streptococcus pneumoniae, Haemophilus influenzae, Pseudomonas aeruginosa, Streptococcus viridans*
  - Retrograde mucopurulent drainage through puncta
  - Treat with topical antibiotics
- Nasal mucocele can develop when mucosal lining of NLD becomes distended with tears and protrudes into nasal cavity
  - May result in nasal obstruction and respiratory distress in obligate nose-breathers
  - Often leads to infection within a few weeks if condition does not resolve spontaneously
- Recurrence following surgical probing typically occurs within first 8 weeks

SELECTED REFERENCES

1. Pediatric Eye Disease Investigator Group: a randomized trial comparing the cost-effectiveness of 2 approaches for treating unilateral nasolacrimal duct obstruction. Arch Ophthalmol. 130(12):1525-33, 2012
2. Pediatric Eye Disease Investigator Group: Resolution of congenital nasolacrimal duct obstruction with nonsurgical management. Arch Ophthalmol. 130(6):730-4, 2012

CONGENITAL PTOSIS

Key Facts

Introduction
- Downward displacement of upper eyelid evident in early infancy

Subtypes
- Myogenic ptosis
- Aponeurotic ptosis
- Neurogenic ptosis
  - Jaw-winking syndrome (Marcus-Gunn jaw-winking), 3rd nerve palsy, congenital Horner syndrome

Presentation
- Droopy eyelid(s)
- Inability to close eyelid completely on downgaze
- Observe patient for compensating head/frontalis movements or efforts to hide ptosis (e.g., hair, hands)

Exam Findings
- Ptosis with or without lagophthalmos

Differential Diagnosis
- Mechanical ptosis, pseudoptosis, blepharochalasis, blepharophimosis syndrome

Evaluation/Work-Up
- Ptosis severity
- Levator muscle function
- Eyelid crease and superior sulcus
- Eyelid position at downgaze
- Visual field testing
- Acuity, manifest, and cycloplegic refraction

Treatment
- Frontalis suspension
  - Eyelid suspension to the frontalis muscle using autogenous fascia lata from thigh or temporal fascia
- Levator aponeurosis resection
  - Amount of resection based on severity
- Conjunctival müllerectomy

__(Left)__ This graphic depicts a normal eyelid. The levator palpebrae superioris is the most commonly affected muscle in myogenic ptosis. Aponeurotic ptosis is due to separation from anterior tarsus or failure of levator aponeurosis to insert at correct position. __(Right)__ This external photograph shows a patient with congenital Horner syndrome. This is an important cause of neurogenic congenital ptosis. Note the narrowed interpalpebral fissure on the right and the difference in pupil size.

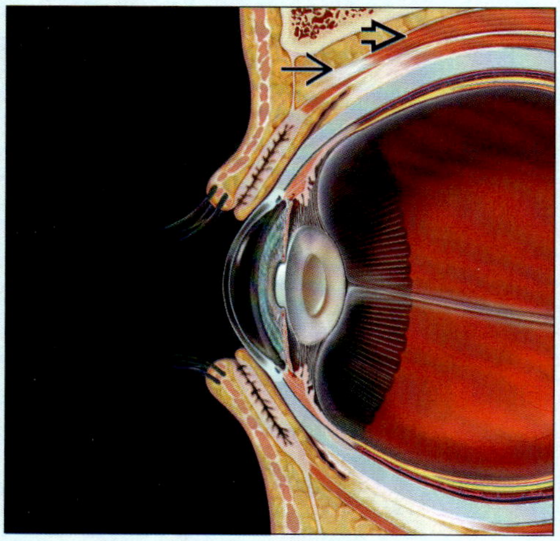

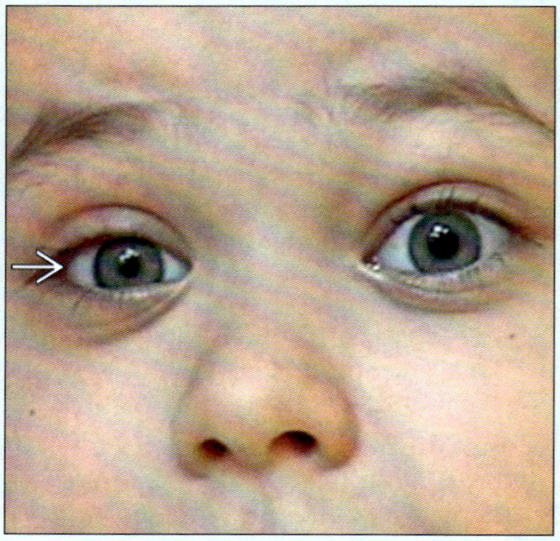

__(Left)__ This external photograph shows a patient with congenital 3rd nerve palsy. Third nerve palsy is an important cause of neurogenic congenital ptosis. __(Right)__ This external photograph depicts a patient with congenital ptosis. Patients with congenital ptosis should be evaluated for jaw-winking syndrome. In this syndrome, multiple retractions of the eyelid follow jaw movements due to aberrant connection between oculomotor (CN3) and trigeminal (CN5) nerves.

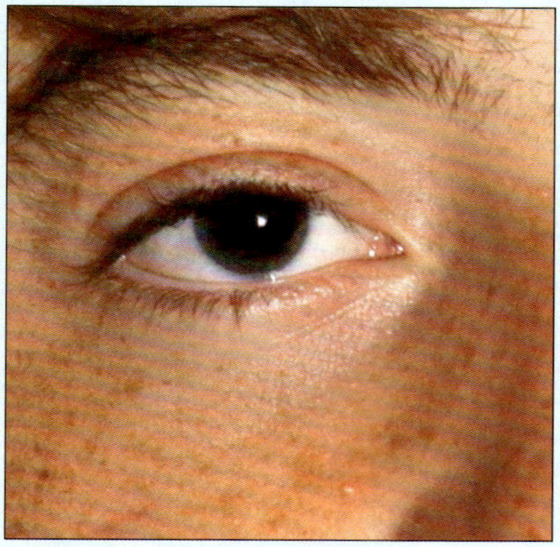

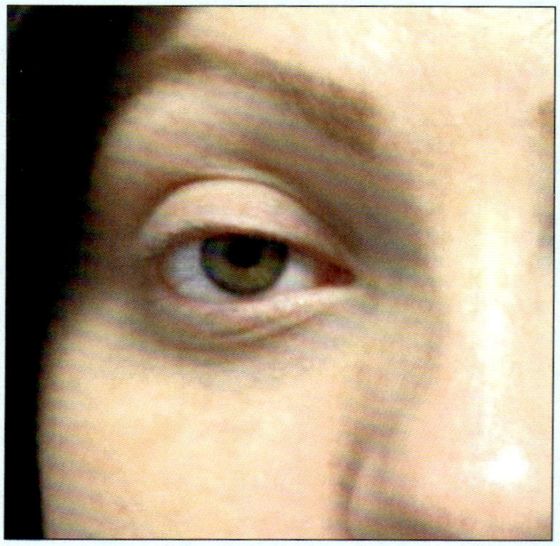

CONGENITAL PTOSIS

INTRODUCTION

Definitions
- Downward displacement of upper eyelid
- 75% of cases are unilateral
- Typically presents in first few weeks of life

Subtypes
- Myogenic ptosis
  - Most common type of congenital ptosis
  - Eyelid lag on downgaze, weak levator palpebrae superioris (LPS) function, and absent or indistinguishable eyelid crease
  - Caused by abnormal development in LPS and replacement of skeletal muscle fibers with fibroadipose tissue, causing weak muscle contraction and poor relaxation
    - Myotonic dystrophy (X-linked) or chronic progressive ophthalmoplegia (mitochondrial inheritance)
- Aponeurotic ptosis
  - Due to separation from anterior tarsus or failure of levator aponeurosis to insert at correct position
  - Possibly from birth trauma due to forceps delivery
- Neurogenic ptosis
  - Jaw-winking syndrome (Marcus-Gunn jaw-winking)
    - Multiple retractions of eyelid following jaw movements due to aberrant connection between oculomotor (CN3) and trigeminal nerves (CN5)
    - Abnormal eyelid movements typically decrease after puberty, possibly due to avoidance of behaviors that induce movements
  - CN3 Palsy
    - Presents with severe ptosis, deficits in adduction, elevation, depression, and mydriasis
    - Compressive form due to neoplasm or aneurysm
  - Congenital Horner syndrome
    - May result from labor trauma and brachial plexus injury or tumors (neuroblastoma) involving sympathetic chain
    - Presents with ptosis, anhidrosis, and miosis due to decreased function of sympathetically innervated Müller muscle of upper eyelid
    - Can cause iris heterochromia

PRESENTATION

Symptoms
- Droopy eyelid(s)
- Inability to close eyelid completely on downgaze
- Other symptoms depending on subtype

Exam Findings
- Ptosis with or without lagophthalmos
- Observe patient for compensating head/frontalis movements or efforts to hide ptosis (e.g., hair, hands)

DIFFERENTIAL DIAGNOSIS

Mechanical Ptosis
- Due to conjunctival scars or other lesion causing downward traction of eyelid

Pseudoptosis
- Resembles ptosis but is due to blepharophimosis, blepharochalasis, or other abnormality

Blepharochalasis
- Relaxation of skin of eyelid, due to atrophy of connective tissue

Blepharophimosis Syndrome
- Characterized by blepharophimosis, ptosis, epicanthus inversus, and telecanthus
- Autosomal dominant inheritance

EVALUATION/WORK-UP

Imaging
- Photographic documentation of primary eye position, compensatory head position, and aberrant movements

Evaluate
- Ptosis severity
  - Mild (≤ 2 mm), moderate (3 mm), or severe (≥ 4 mm)
- Levator muscle function
  - Good (8-12 mm), fair (5-7 mm), or absent
- Eyelid crease and superior sulcus
- Eyelid position at downgaze
- Visual field testing
- Acuity, manifest, and cycloplegic refraction

TREATMENT

Medical
- If considering conjunctival müllerectomy, patient must demonstrate appropriate function of Müller muscle with positive phenylephrine test
  - Positive test if ≥ 1.5 mm increase in margin-reflex-distance following 2 drops of 10% phenylephrine

Surgical
- Frontalis suspension
  - Eyelid suspension to the frontalis muscle using autogenous fascia lata from thigh or temporal fascia
  - Performed in cases of poor levator function or severe ptosis and in children < 3 or 4 years in whom levator function is difficult to measure
  - Should be bilateral for Marcus-Gunn jaw-winking
- Levator aponeurosis resection
  - Amount of resection based on severity
- Conjunctival müllerectomy
  - May be performed in all cases that have positive response to phenylephrine test

Prognosis
- Amblyopia occurs in 20% of patients

SELECTED REFERENCES

1. Griepentrog GJ et al: Amblyopia in childhood eyelid ptosis. Am J Ophthalmol. 155(6):1125-1128, 2013
2. de Figueiredo AR: Blepharoptosis. Semin Ophthalmol. 25(3):39-51, 2010
3. McMullan TF et al: Towards an understanding of congenital ptosis. Orbit. 25(3):179-84, 2006
4. Baroody M et al: Advances in the diagnosis and treatment of ptosis. Curr Opin Ophthalmol. 16(6):351-5, 2005

FAMILIAL EXUDATIVE VITREORETINOPATHY

Key Facts

Introduction

- Inherited disorder of abnormal retinal blood vessel development; most commonly presents in childhood but may progress at any age and is characterized by
  - Absence of vascular development in peripheral retina
  - Vitreoretinal traction, subretinal exudation, or retinal neovascularization occurring at any age
  - Birth at full term with timeline of disease progression not consistent with retinopathy of prematurity (ROP)

Demographics

- Family history positive for variable manifestations of familial exudative vitreoretinopathy in 37% of individuals
- Mean age at presentation: 6 years

Presentation

- Decreased or blurred vision, central or peripheral scotoma
- Often asymptomatic but may present with symptoms of retinal detachment
  - Flashes or floaters, shadow or curtain over portion of visual field

Exam Findings

- Macular dragging, temporal retinal folds, retinal neovascularization, vitreous hemorrhage, subretinal exudation, tractional retinal detachment

Evaluation/Work-Up

- Scleral depression under anesthesia may reveal findings easily missed on exam of young or uncooperative child
- Fluorescein angiography may reveal subtle vascular abnormalities in posterior pole and periphery not easily seen on clinical examination

Treatment

- Based on stage of disease progression

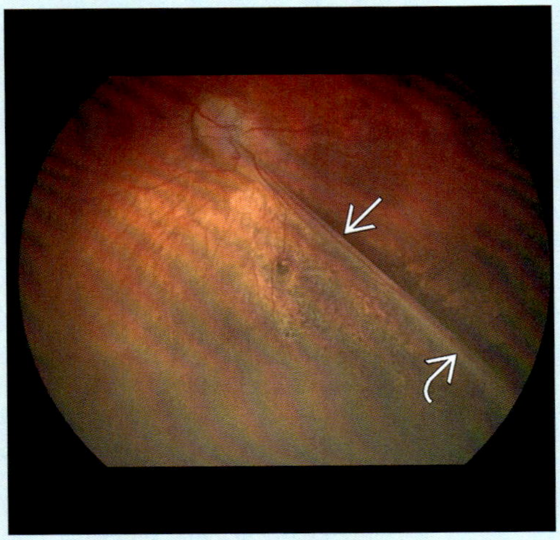

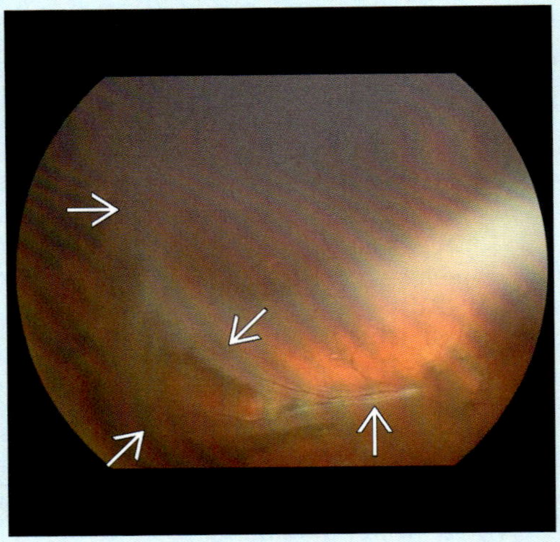

(Left) *This fundus photo shows a retinal fold with macular vasculature pulled toward the fold.* ***(Right)*** *This fundus photo shows a retinal fold with macular involvement. The retinal folds of FEVR are similar to those in ROP. Remember, however, that FEVR occurs in children with a positive family history of exudative vitreoretinopathy, non-premature birth, normal gestational age and birth weight, and absence of neonatal oxygen therapy and follows a variable time-course of disease progression.*

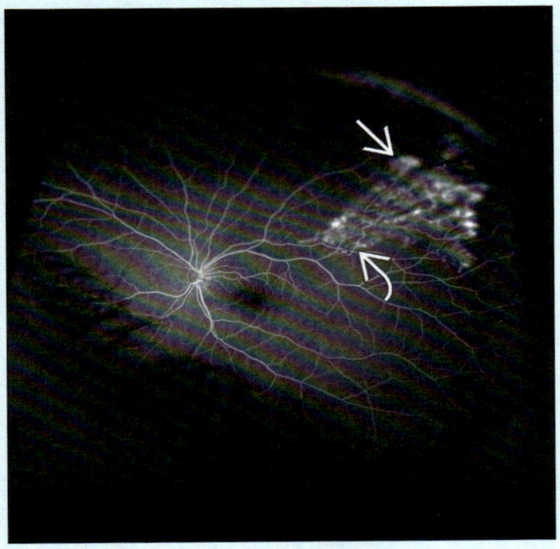

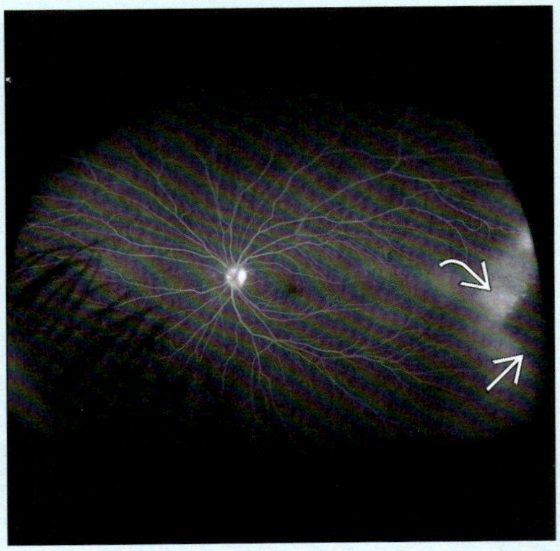

(Left) *This image using fluorescein angiography shows retinal vascular leakage and increasingly tortuous vasculature at the site of neovascularization of the peripheral retina. These exudative regions of neovascularization may benefit from laser photocoagulation.* ***(Right)*** *This image using fluorescein angiography again shows peripheral avascularity and vascular exudative leakage at the vascular-avascular junction.*

FAMILIAL EXUDATIVE VITREORETINOPATHY

INTRODUCTION

Abbreviations
- Familial exudative vitreoretinopathy (FEVR)

Definitions
- Inherited disorder of abnormal retinal blood vessel development
  - Most commonly presents in childhood but may progress at any age and is characterized by
    - Absence of vascular development in peripheral retina
    - Variable degrees of vitreoretinal traction, subretinal exudation, or retinal neovascularization at any age
    - Birth at full term with timeline of disease progression not consistent with retinopathy of prematurity (ROP)

Subtypes
- Disease progression based on similar staging system used for ROP
  - Stage 1: Avascular peripheral retina
  - Stage 2: Retinal neovascularization
    - With (2A) or without (2B) exudate
  - Stage 3: Extramacular retinal detachment
    - With (3A) or without (3B) exudate
  - Stage 4: Macula-involving retinal detachment
    - With (4A) or without (4B) exudate
  - Stage 5: Total retinal detachment

DEMOGRAPHICS

Etiology/Risk Factors
- Family history positive for variable manifestations of FEVR in 37% of individuals
- Multiple modes of inheritance with variable penetrance and associations with several genes, including
  - *FZD4* (autosomal dominant)
  - *LRP5* (autosomal dominant and recessive)
  - *NDP* (X-linked recessive)

Epidemiology
- Mean age at presentation: 6 years

PRESENTATION

Symptoms
- Decreased or blurred vision
- Often asymptomatic but may present with symptoms of retinal detachment
  - Central or peripheral scotoma
  - Flashes or floaters
  - Shadow or curtain over portion of visual field

Exam Findings
- Macular dragging
- Retinal folds
  - Radial retinal folds most often run temporally, with macular retinal vasculature pulled toward the fold
- Retinal neovascularization
- Vitreous hemorrhage
- Subretinal exudation
- Tractional retinal detachment

DIFFERENTIAL DIAGNOSIS

Retinopathy of Prematurity (ROP)
- While both ROP and FEVR may display avascularity of peripheral retina, individuals with ROP tend to be born prematurely with low birth weight and experience predictable timeline of disease progression

Persistent Fetal Vasculature (PFV)
- Retinal stalk seen in PFV may appear similar to retinal fold of FEVR, though PFV is rarely inherited and does not display avascularity of peripheral retina

EVALUATION/WORK-UP

Exam Under Anesthesia
- Scleral depression under anesthesia may reveal findings easily missed on exam of young or uncooperative child

Imaging
- FA may reveal subtle vascular abnormalities in posterior pole and periphery not easily seen on clinical examination

TREATMENT

Surgical
- Stage 1
  - No therapy required; periodic monitoring recommended
- Stage 2
  - Laser ablation to exudative regions of neovascularization
- Stages 3, 4, and 5
  - Scleral buckling or vitrectomy depending on extent of retinal detachment and location and degree of vitreoretinal traction
- Early surgical intervention recommended to prevent disease progression

Follow-Up
- Monitoring throughout life necessary due to unpredictable timeline of disease progression in which neovascular, tractional, or exudative activity may occur throughout childhood and adulthood

Prognosis
- Older age at presentation associated with improved prognosis, likely due to slowly progressive asymmetric retinal deterioration
- Poor visual prognosis for infants with FEVR

SELECTED REFERENCES

1. Ranchod TM et al: Clinical presentation of familial exudative vitreoretinopathy. Ophthalmology. 118(10):2070-5, 2011
2. Boonstra FN et al: Clinical and molecular evaluation of probands and family members with familial exudative vitreoretinopathy. Invest Ophthalmol Vis Sci. 50(9):4379-85, 2009
3. Pendergast SD et al: Familial exudative vitreoretinopathy. Results of surgical management. Ophthalmology. 105(6):1015-23, 1998
4. Benson WE: Familial exudative vitreoretinopathy. Trans Am Ophthalmol Soc. 93:473-521, 1995

MORNING GLORY SYNDROME

Key Facts

Introduction

- Congenital defect in formation of distal optic stalk resulting in a funnel-shaped, enlarged optic disc

Demographics

- Female to male ratio is 2:1
- Age at diagnosis depends on severity of vision loss
- Unilateral disease is more common than bilateral

Presentation

- Typically presents in childhood with strabismus and nonprogressive vision loss
- Optic disc resembles a morning glory flower and may be pink or orange in color
- Leukocoria
- Enlargement of optic disc with a central white tuft of glial tissue
- Afferent pupillary defect in affected eye

Evaluation/Work-Up

- CT of brain to rule out intracranial abnormalities associated with basal encephalocele
  - CT scan shows a dilated, funnel-shaped optic nerve as it merges with globe
- B-scan ultrasound: Posterior excavation of central optic nerve, optic nerve calcifications, central glial tuft
- CTA/MRA of internal carotid circulation to rule out moyamoya disease

Treatment

- Decreased visual acuity is not progressive and can be treated by correcting refractive error
- Strabismus surgery may be required
- Visual acuity ranges between 20/20 and no light perception
- Serous retinal detachment occurs in 30-35% of cases
- Contraction is rare and causes transient vision loss

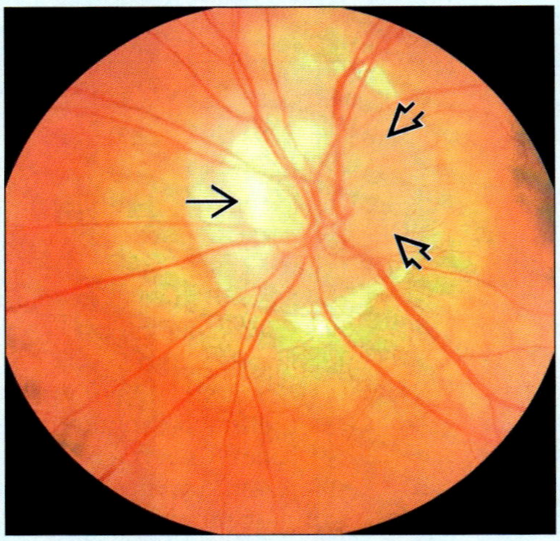

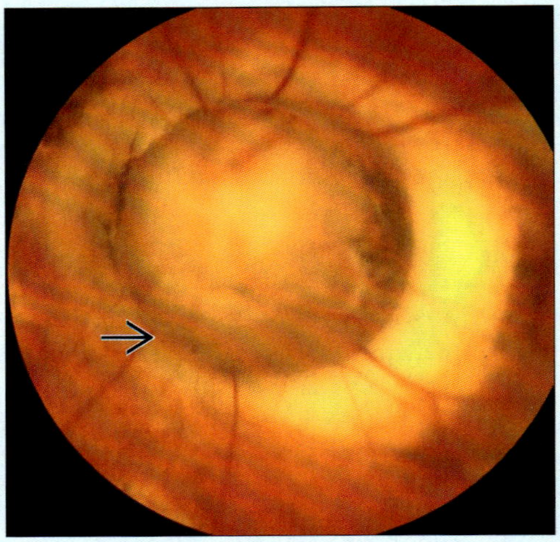

(Left) *Funduscopy shows an enlarged funnel-shaped optic disc → with central glial tissue as well as annular pigmentation ⇨, resulting in an appearance that resembles a morning glory flower.* ***(Right)*** *This fundus photograph shows the optic disc of a patient with morning glory syndrome. Note the enlarged disc with an orange hue →.*

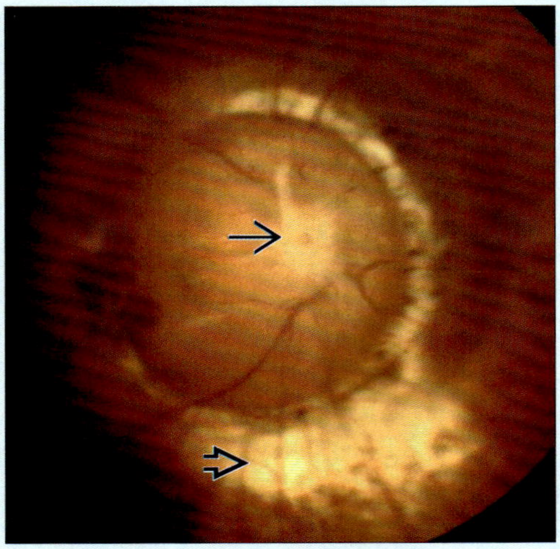

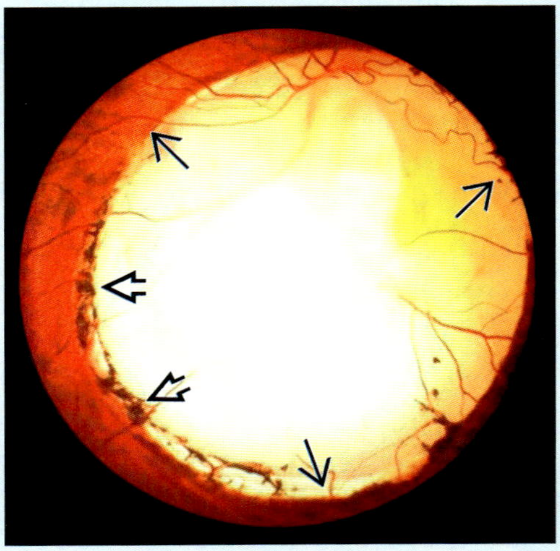

(Left) *This fundus photograph shows the optic disc of a patient with morning glory syndrome. The disc is enlarged, with an orange color. A central white tuft of glial tissue is visible →. Peripapillary pigment changes are also present ⇨.* ***(Right)*** *Funduscopy shows a large posterior coloboma centered at the optic nerve head →, with marginal pigmentation ⇨, suggesting chorioretinal involvement. Coloboma is an important differential diagnosis for morning glory syndrome.*

MORNING GLORY SYNDROME

INTRODUCTION

Definitions

- Funnel-shaped excavation of the posterior fundus, involving the optic disc

DEMOGRAPHICS

Etiology/Risk Factors

- Multiple proposed etiologies
  - Primary mesenchymal disorder or abnormal relative growth between mesoderm and ectoderm
  - Congenital defect in formation of distal optic stalk
  - Failed closure of embryonic fissure during development
- Associated with transsphenoidal basal encephalocele
  - Midline malformation in which the meninges ± hypothalamic tissue herniate inferiorly through a round defect in sphenoid bone
  - Discrete "V"- or "U"-shaped depigmentation of the fundus directly inferior to optic disc
  - ± duplication of pituitary stalk
- Associated with narrowing (moyamoya disease) or hypoplasia of the cerebral arteries
- Associated with midline CNS defects (absence of corpus callosum)

Epidemiology

- Female to male ratio is 2:1
- Age at diagnosis depends on severity of vision loss
- Rare in blacks
- Unilateral disease more common than bilateral

PRESENTATION

Symptoms

- Typically presents in childhood with strabismus
- Nonprogressive decrease in vision

Exam Findings

- Leukocoria
- Afferent pupillary defect in affected eye
- Optic disc findings
  - Enlargement
  - Orange or pink color
  - Center of disc can appear raised or depressed with funnel-shaped peripheral excavation
  - Central white tuft of glial tissue
  - Peripapillary pigmentary changes of the choroid and retina
  - Increased number of retinal blood vessels that follow an abnormally straight course across fundus
    - Extend radially from area of excavation with acutely angled branches
    - Multiple arteriovenous anastomoses
- Macular capture: Excavation extending temporally to involve macula
- Decreased visual acuity
  - Depends on presence of subretinal fluid and retinal detachment
- Enlarged blind spot, central scotoma, or hemianopia

DIFFERENTIAL DIAGNOSIS

Coloboma

- Optic nerve hypoplasia with thinning and excavation of inferior optic disc
  - Unilateral or bilateral disease
  - Minimal peripapillary pigmentary changes
  - Normal retinal blood vessels
  - Associated with iris, ciliary, or retinal colobomas
- Enlargement of affected disc(s)
- Superior visual field loss

Optic Pit

- Retinal tissue herniates through lamina cribrosa
  - Involves any portion of optic disc
  - Pit appears gray, yellow, or white
- Unilateral disease
- Enlarged blind spot with paracentral arcuate scotoma

Papillorenal Syndrome

- Renal hypoplasia and insufficiency with bilateral central optic disc cavitation
- Optic discs are normal in size
- Retinal vessels course over peripheral disc margin and are absent from central cavitation
- Associated with *PAX2* gene mutation

EVALUATION/WORK-UP

Imaging

- CT of brain to rule out intracranial abnormalities
  - CT scan shows a dilated, funnel-shaped optic nerve as it merges with the globe
- Fluorescein angiogram: Late hyperfluorescence ± rare arteriovenous or artery-to-artery malformations
- B-scan ultrasound: Posterior excavation of central optic nerve, optic nerve calcifications, central glial tuft
- MRI to rule out basal or transsphenoidal encephalocele
- CTA/MRA of the internal carotid circulation to rule out moyamoya disease

TREATMENT

Medical

- Decreased visual acuity does not progress and can be treated by correcting refractive error
- For amblyopia, occlusive therapy trial

Prognosis

- Visual acuity
  - Typically 20/200 to hand motion
  - Can range from 20/20 to no light perception
  - Worsened visual prognosis with macular involvement
- Retinal detachment (RD)
  - 30-35% of cases complicated by serous RD
- Contraction is rare and causes transient vision loss
- Functional amblyopia may cause severe vision loss

SELECTED REFERENCES

1. Knape RM et al: Morning glory disc anomaly and optic nerve coloboma. Clin Pediatr (Phila). 51(10):991-3, 2012
2. Golnik KC: Cavitary anomalies of the optic disc: neurologic significance. Curr Neurol Neurosci Rep. 8(5):409-13, 2008

PERSISTENT FETAL VASCULATURE

Key Facts

Introduction

- Persistent fetal vasculature (PFV)
  - Congenital disorder in which remnants of fetal hyaloid system persist and grow into a variable-sized fibrovascular mass, leading to abnormal retinal development and complications resulting from the effect of the mass on surrounding structures
- Anterior PFV
  - Retrolenticular fibrovascular tissue attached to ciliary bodies contracts, causing anterior segment to be reshaped, leading to secondary angle-closure glaucoma and cataract formation
- Posterior
  - Distinguished by an elevated vitreous membrane or stalk from optic nerve and retinal folds/detachment and optic nerve hypoplasia

Demographics

- Majority of cases are unilateral and present in infancy

Presentation

- White pupillary reflex (leukocoria)
- Small, crossed eyes

Exam Findings

- Cataract
- Microphthalmia
- Elongation of ciliary processes and angle-closure glaucoma
- Retinal traction, folds, dysplasia, detachments
- Strabismus

Treatment

- Lensectomy with membranectomy-vitrectomy to provide clear visual axis and prevent traction on ciliary bodies, retina, and other structures
  - Recommended if associated with progressive retinal detachment, angle-closure glaucoma, and recurrent intraocular hemorrhage

__(Left)__ This ultrasound image depicts a hyaloid vessel that has failed to regress in utero →, extending from the optic disc toward the posterior lens capsule. __(Right)__ This OCT image depicts a cross-sectional view of the retina with apparent elevation of the vitreous membrane → from the optic nerve. Seventy percent of cases of posterior PFV involve retinal folds or dysplasia and may lead to retinal detachment. Persistent fetal vasculature (PFV) may be associated with optic nerve hypoplasia.

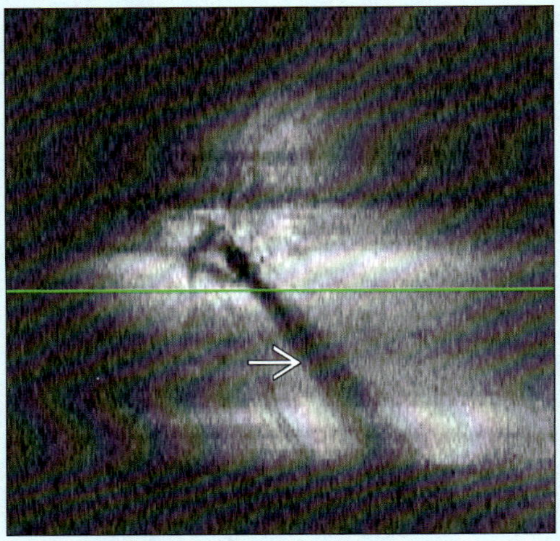

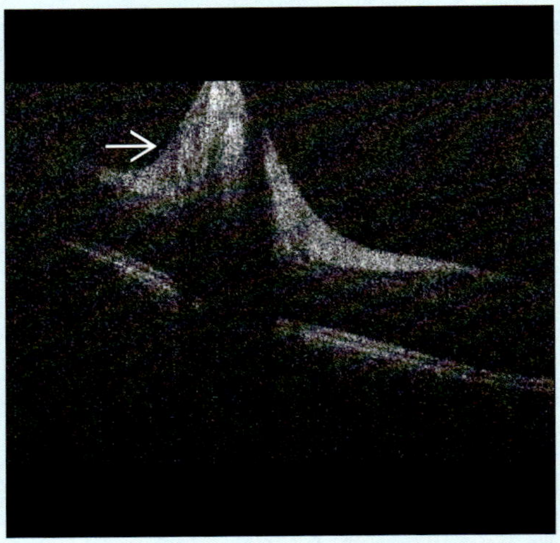

__(Left)__ This slit-lamp photo shows a congenital cataract → affecting the posterior lens pole, which may occur as a complication of PFV. __(Right)__ This slit-lamp photo displays a tractional retinal detachment →, a common complication of PFV, caused by contraction of the fibrovascular band that extends from the posterior lens to the retina due to failure of the fetal vasculature to regress.

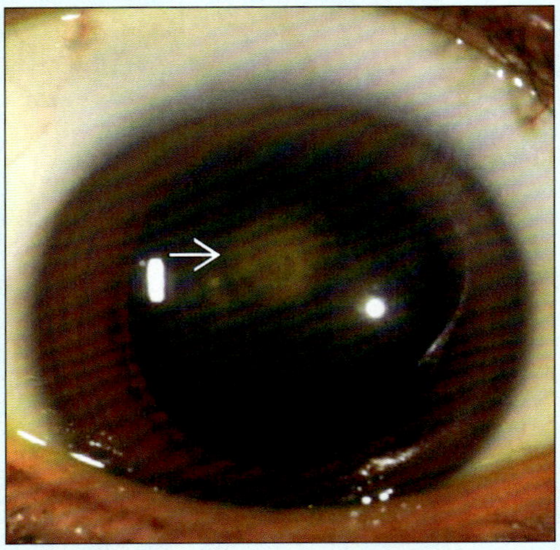

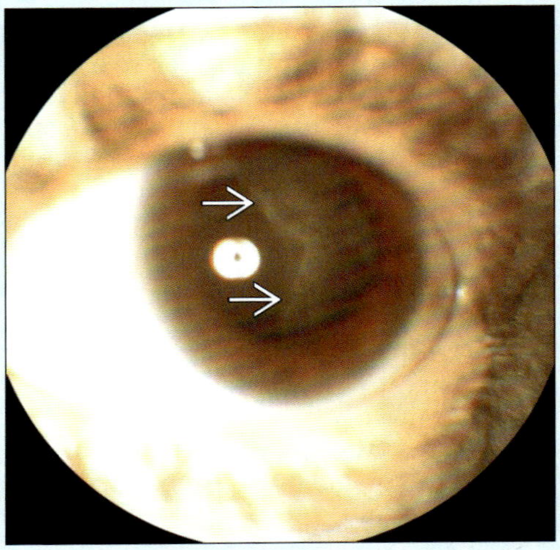

PERSISTENT FETAL VASCULATURE

INTRODUCTION

Abbreviations

- Persistent fetal vasculature (PFV); formerly termed persistent hyperplastic primary vitreous (PHPV)

Definitions

- Congenital disorder in which remnants of fetal hyaloid system persist and grow into a variable-sized fibrovascular mass, leading to abnormal retinal development and complications resulting from the effect of the mass on surrounding structures

Subtypes

- Anterior PFV
  - Also termed persistent tunica vasculosa lentis and persistent posterior fetal fibrovascular sheath of lens
  - Retrolenticular fibrovascular tissue attached to ciliary body contracts, causing anterior segment to be reshaped, leading to secondary angle-closure glaucoma and cataract formation
    - Distinguished by presence of retrolental opacity, elongated ciliary processes, or cataract on clinical examination
- Posterior PFV
  - Also termed falciform retinal septum and ablatio falciformis congenita
    - Distinguished by an elevated vitreous membrane or stalk from optic nerve and any of the following
      - Retinal fold or dysplasia (70% of cases of posterior PFV)
      - Retinal detachment
      - Optic nerve hypoplasia
- Most common subtype of PFV involves both anterior and posterior segments

DEMOGRAPHICS

Etiology/Risk Factors

- Prematurity &/or low birth weight

Epidemiology

- 80% of cases present before 1 year of age
- 90% of cases are unilateral

PRESENTATION

Symptoms

- White pupillary reflex (leukocoria) is most common presenting complaint
- Small, crossed eyes

Exam Findings

- Cataract
- Microphthalmia
- Elongation of ciliary body with angle-closure glaucoma
- Retinal traction, folds, dysplasia, detachments
- Lens subluxation
- Strabismus
- Normal remnants include Mittendorf dot (on back of lens) and Bergmeister papilla (on optic nerve)

Potential Complications

- Angle-closure glaucoma due to microphthalmia
- Vitreous hemorrhage
- Retinal or ciliary body detachment due to contraction of fibrovascular membranes
- Amblyopia
- Phthisis bulbi

DIFFERENTIAL DIAGNOSIS

Retinoblastoma

- Distinguished by absence of cataract and microphthalmia

Norrie Disease

- Retinal dysplasia with systemic manifestations such as mental retardation and hearing deficits

Ocular Toxocariasis

- May also include retinal folds and glial mass but typically presents between ages 4 and 6

EVALUATION/WORK-UP

Imaging

- Orbital CT to rule out retinoblastoma (with contrast to accentuate persistent fibrovascular membranes)
- B-scan ultrasound may help distinguish retrolental and vitreous components not seen on CT
- Consider preoperative electroretinography and visual evoked potential to assess visual potential following surgery

TREATMENT

Surgical

- Lensectomy with membranectomy-vitrectomy to provide clear visual axis and relieve traction on ciliary bodies, retina, and other structures
  - Recommended if associated with progressive retinal detachment, angle-closure glaucoma, and recurrent intraocular hemorrhage

Follow-Up

- Postoperative amblyopia therapy

Prognosis

- Worse prognosis in posterior PFV due to coexisting retinal and optic nerve abnormalities
- Early surgical intervention associated with improved postoperative visual outcomes

SELECTED REFERENCES

1. Zhao YE et al: Bilateral persistent fetal vasculature in an adult: Clinical manifestations and surgical outcomes. J Cataract Refract Surg. 36(8):1421-6, 2010
2. Müllner-Eidenböck A et al: Persistent fetal vasculature and minimal fetal vascular remnants: a frequent cause of unilateral congenital cataracts. Ophthalmology. 111(5):906-13, 2004
3. Silbert M et al: Persistent hyperplastic primary vitreous. Clin Eye Vis Care. 12(3-4):131-137, 2000

OCULAR SYPHILIS

Key Facts

Introduction
- Ocular infection caused by *Treponema pallidum*
  - Congenital or acquired transmission
- Often called the "great imitator" due to its similar presentation with other ocular disorders
- Ocular involvement rare and may occur at any stage

Demographics
- 1-2% of uveitis cases due to ocular syphilis
- Occurs in 10% of secondary syphilis cases

Presentation
- Most common symptoms: Visual changes (42%), headache (42%), and altered mental status (23%)

Exam Findings and Differential Diagnosis
- Uveitis, interstitial keratitis, chorioretinitis, optic atrophy, Argyll Robertson pupils, cataract, elevated IOP, CN palsies, conjunctivitis, scleritis

Evaluation/Work-Up
- Testing for syphilis recommended if history is highly suggestive or inflammation is severe, has unusual characteristics, or is refractory to corticosteroids
  - Preferred treponemal diagnostic tests include FTA-ABS, microhemagglutinin assay, or treponema pallidum particle agglutination assay
- All patients with ocular syphilis should undergo CSF and HIV testing

Treatment
- Treated like neurosyphilis along with management of associated ocular complications
  - Intravenous penicillin G or intramuscular procaine penicillin with probenecid for 10-14 days

Follow-Up
- CSF evaluation should be repeated every 6 months until cell counts normalize

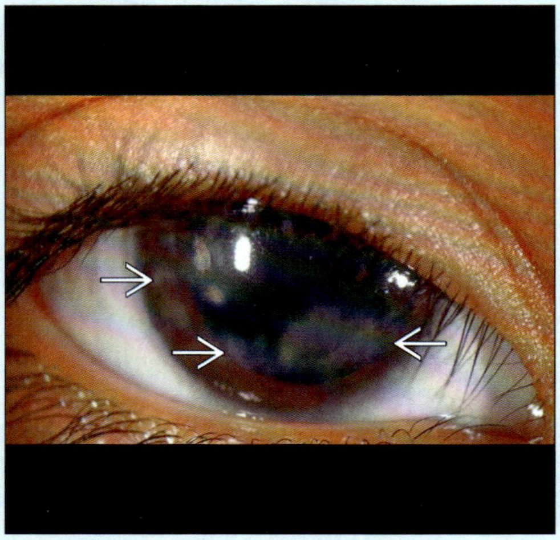
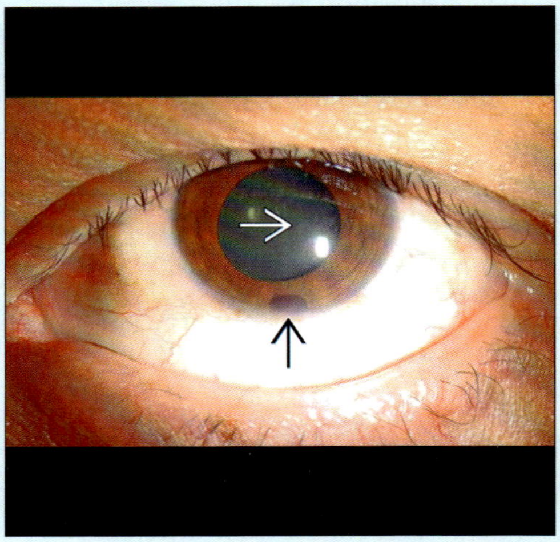

***(Left)** This external photo shows nonulcerative interstitial keratitis, the most common finding in untreated congenital syphilis. Observe the several areas of corneal opacification ➔. **(Right)** This external photo shows a patient with an iris cyst → and anterior uveitis ➔, both of which are common findings in congenital and ocular syphilis.*

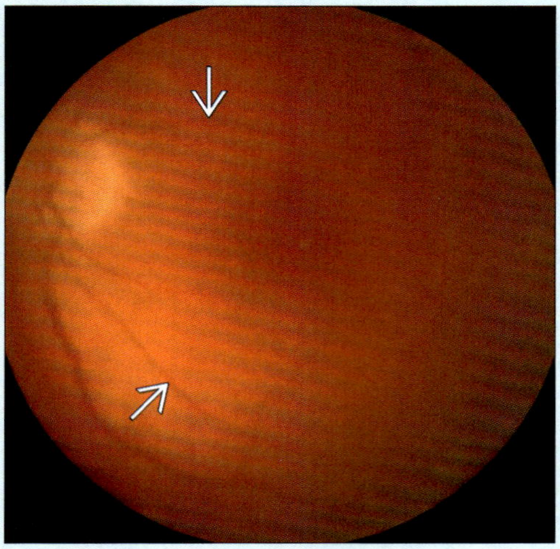
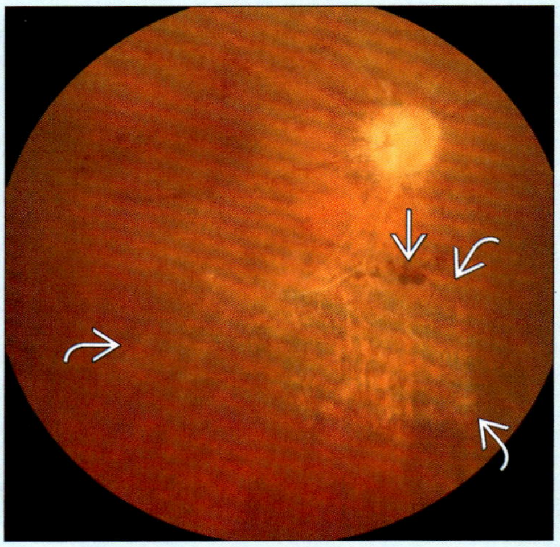

***(Left)** This fundus photo shows diffuse panuveitis throughout the image as evidenced by haziness and lack of details ➔ normally seen in the vasculature due to diffuse vitreous inflammation. **(Right)** This fundus photo shows a large area of choroidal and retinal atrophy seen in the retinal sector bordered by ➔ and retinal hemorrhage ➔ due to ocular syphilis.*

OCULAR SYPHILIS

INTRODUCTION

Definitions

- Ocular infection caused by *Treponema pallidum*
- Does not have pathognomonic features and is often called the "great imitator" due to its similar presentation with other ocular disorders
- Ocular involvement rare and may occur at any stage

Subtypes

- Congenital: Transplacental transmission after 10th week of gestation
- Acquired: Postnatal transmission by sexual activity

DEMOGRAPHICS

Etiology/Risk Factors

- Unprotected sexual activity

Epidemiology

- 1-2% of uveitis cases due to ocular syphilis
- Occurs in up to 10% of secondary syphilis cases

PRESENTATION

Symptoms

- Most common presenting symptoms include
  - Visual changes (42%)
  - Headache (42%)
  - Altered mental status (23%)
- 67% of cases have symptoms of secondary syphilis
  - Fever, malaise, pharyngitis, skin rashes, lymphadenopathy, anterior uveitis

Exam Findings

- Uveal tract
  - Uveitis is most common ocular finding of syphilis, occurring as early as 6 weeks following infection
  - Acute inflammation suggests early disease; chronic, insidious inflammation suggests late disease
  - Inflammation may be granulomatous or nongranulomatous, may occur unilaterally or bilaterally, and may involve anterior segment, posterior segment, or both
  - Syphilitic anterior uveitis may include iris nodules, dilated iris vessels (roseolae), iris atrophy, posterior synechiae, and ectopia lentis
  - Secondary cataract or glaucoma
  - Ground-glass chorioretinitis with retinal vasculitis
  - Acute syphilitic posterior placoid chorioretinopathy: Large, placoid, macular or peripapillary lesions and hypofluorescent, yellow spots (leopard spots) seen on fluorescein angiography
- Retina
  - Retinal vasculitis
  - Serous and exudative vitreous detachments
- Cornea
  - Localized or diffuse interstitial keratitis, unilateral or bilateral, and iritis ± keratic precipitates
- Optic nerve (ON)
  - Retrobulbar optic neuritis, papillitis ± retinal vasculitis, and vision loss due to nerve atrophy
  - Inflammatory disc edema
- Pupils
  - Argyll Robertson pupils; unequal, irregular, and miotic pupils with light-near dissociation
  - Most commonly seen late in disease progression
- Lens
  - Congenital or uveitic cataract
- Intraocular pressure
  - Ocular hypertension or uveitic glaucoma
- Extraocular motility
  - Various cranial nerve palsies
- Conjunctiva
  - Mucous patches, papillary conjunctivitis, or granulomatous conjunctivitis
- Sclera
  - Scleritis and episcleritis

DIFFERENTIAL DIAGNOSIS

Infectious Uveitis

- Viral, fungal, or bacterial uveitis with negative syphilis serologic testing (RPR, VDRL, FTA-ABS)

Inflammatory Uveitis

- Sarcoid uveitis (elevated angiotensin-converting enzyme level and abnormal chest x-ray); systemic lupus erythematosus uveitis (positive antinuclear antibody)

EVALUATION/WORK-UP

Laboratory Tests

- Testing for syphilis recommended if history is highly suggestive or inflammation is severe, has unusual characteristics, or is refractory to corticosteroids
  - Nontreponemal screening tests (RPR or VDRL) are insufficiently sensitive in late-stage syphilis when ocular disease primarily occurs
  - Preferred treponemal diagnostic tests include FTA-ABS, microhemagglutinin assay, or treponema pallidum particle agglutination assay
- All patients should undergo CSF and HIV testing

TREATMENT

Medical

- Ocular syphilis should be treated like neurosyphilis along with management of ocular complications
  - Intravenous penicillin G or intramuscular procaine penicillin with probenecid for 10-14 days

Follow-Up

- CSF evaluation should be repeated every 6 months until cell counts normalize

SELECTED REFERENCES

1. Chao JR et al: Syphilis: reemergence of an old adversary. Ophthalmology. 113(11):2074-9, 2006
2. Gaudio PA: Update on ocular syphilis. Curr Opin Ophthalmol. 17(6):562-6, 2006
3. Kiss S et al: Ocular manifestations and treatment of syphilis. Semin Ophthalmol. 20(3):161-7, 2005
4. Hariprasad SM et al: Keratopathy from congenital syphilis. Cornea. 21(6):608-9, 2002
5. Aldave AJ et al: Ocular syphilis. Curr Opin Ophthalmol. 12(6):433-41, 2001

OPHTHALMIA NEONATORUM

Key Facts

Introduction
- Conjunctivitis presenting in 1st month of life
  - Chemical conjunctivitis, chlamydial conjunctivitis, gonococcal conjunctivitis, HSV conjunctivitis

Etiology
- Due to contamination from mother during delivery

Presentation
- Chemical conjunctivitis usually presents with mild, purulent conjunctivitis within 24 hours after silver nitrate
- Chlamydial conjunctivitis presentation varies from mild to moderate eyelid swelling and scant, mucoid discharge to copious, purulent discharge 5-14 days after birth
- Gonococcal conjunctivitis often presents with sudden, severe, purulent conjunctivitis 3-5 days after birth
- HSV conjunctivitis often presents 6-14 days after birth

Exam Findings
- Findings of all subtypes include conjunctival hyperemia, chemosis, eyelid edema, purulent discharge

Evaluation/Work-Up
- Gram stain, PCR for chlamydia and HSV, viral and bacterial cultures with antibiotic sensitivities

Treatment
- Chemical: No treatment required; typically improves within 48 hours
- Chlamydial: Oral erythromycin for 14 days
- Gonococcal: Ceftriaxone IV or IM and hospitalization
- HSV: Topical antivirals, acyclovir for 14 days, and hospitalization
- Pediatrician follow-up for chlamydial pneumonia, disseminated gonococcal, systemic HSV infection, or syphilis

*(**Left**) This external photo demonstrates eyelid edema and purulent discharge ➡, frequently seen in ophthalmia neonatorum. (**Right**) This slit-lamp photograph demonstrates the significant conjunctival injection, chemosis, and discharge seen in gonococcal conjunctivitis.*

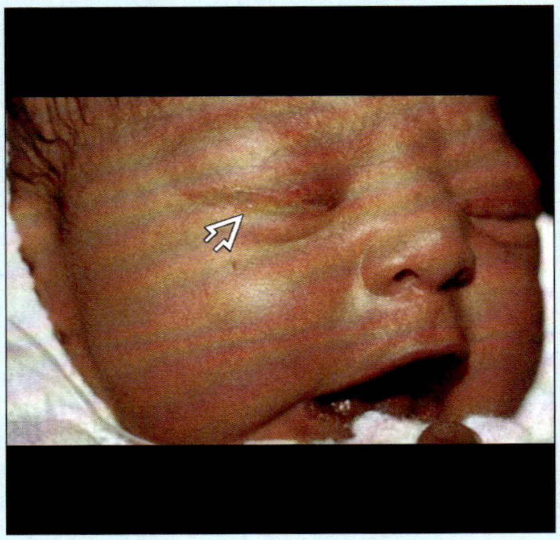

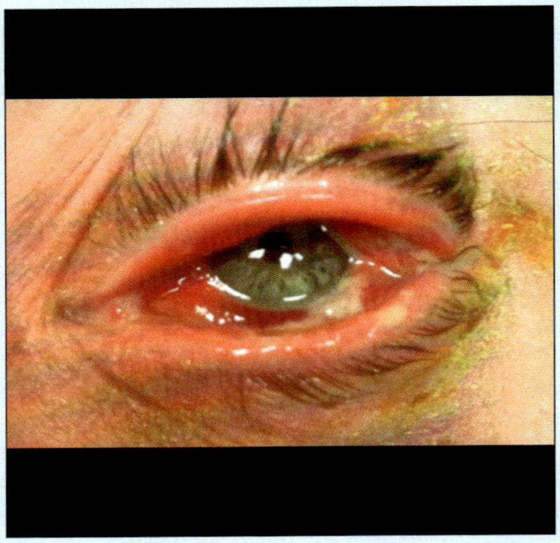

*(**Left**) This anteroposterior radiograph shows perihilar coarse lung markings and more focal opacities within the lingula and left lower lobe in this patient who presented with conjunctivitis and tachypnea and was found to have chlamydial conjunctivitis. (**Right**) This lateral radiograph shows the diffuse coarse lung opacities. The radiographic findings are nonspecific. Cultures were positive for chlamydia.*

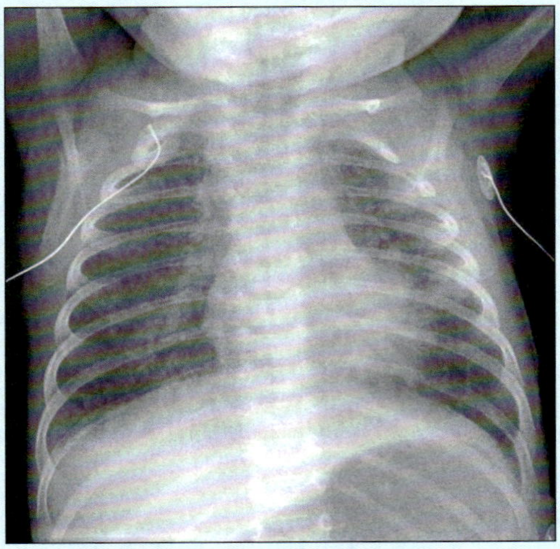

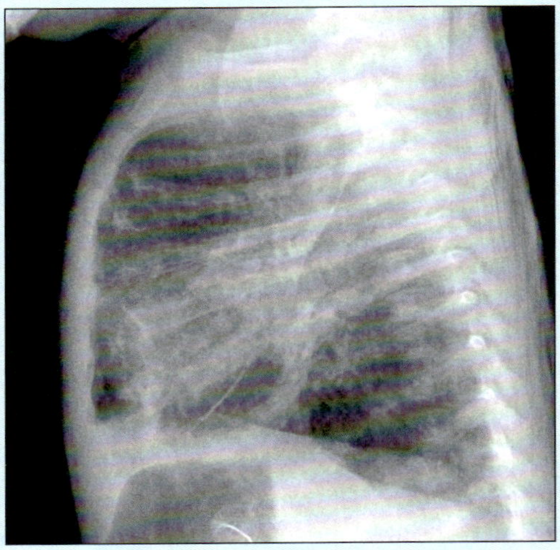

OPHTHALMIA NEONATORUM

INTRODUCTION

Synonyms
- Neonatal conjunctivitis

Definitions
- Conjunctivitis presenting in 1st month of life

Subtypes
- Noninfectious (chemical conjunctivitis)
  - Most common cause, typically following treatment with prophylactic topical silver nitrate
    - Prevents gonococcal conjunctivitis but ineffective in preventing chlamydial conjunctivitis
- Infectious
  - Chlamydial conjunctivitis (most common cause of infectious ophthalmia neonatorum)
    - Caused by infection with *Chlamydia trachomatis*
    - Conjunctival and corneal scarring, corneal infiltrates, and chlamydia pneumonia may result
  - Gonococcal conjunctivitis
    - Caused by infection with *Neisseria gonorrhoeae*
    - Corneal ulcers, perforation, conjunctival scarring, sepsis, and blindness may result
  - Herpes simplex virus
    - Less common than chlamydial or gonococcal conjunctivitis; may involve skin, eyes, and mouth

DEMOGRAPHICS

Etiology/Risk Factors
- Infectious ophthalmia neonatorum due to contamination during passage through mother's cervix and vagina during delivery
- Infant born vaginally to mother with active chlamydial infection has ~ 50% risk of infection

Epidemiology
- 30% of cases caused by *C. trachomatis*
- 25-50% of infants infected with chlamydia develop chlamydial conjunctivitis

PRESENTATION

Symptoms
- Chemical conjunctivitis
  - Typically presents within first 24 hours with mild, purulent conjunctivitis
- Chlamydial conjunctivitis
  - Presentation varies from mild to moderate eyelid swelling and scant, mucoid discharge to copious, purulent discharge, typically 5-14 days after birth
- Gonococcal conjunctivitis
  - Sudden, severe, grossly purulent conjunctivitis typically 3-5 days after birth
  - May be more mild or occur later in atypical cases
- HSV conjunctivitis
  - Typically presents 6-14 days after birth

Exam Findings
- Findings of all subtypes include conjunctival hyperemia, chemosis, eyelid edema, purulent discharge
- Findings unique to chlamydial conjunctivitis include pseudomembranes and mucopurulent discharge
- Findings unique to HSV conjunctivitis include serous discharge with dendritic keratitis or geographic ulcers

DIFFERENTIAL DIAGNOSIS

Dacryocystitis
- Inflammation of the lacrimal sac, often seen in infants and accompanied by pain, redness, and discharge

Congenital Nasolacrimal Duct Obstruction
- Excessive tearing and possible infectious conjunctivitis due to failure of tear duct canalization

EVALUATION/WORK-UP

Labs
- Conjunctival scrapings
  - Gram stain, PCR for chlamydia and HSV, viral and bacterial cultures with antibiotic sensitivities
- Gonococcal conjunctivitis should include work-up for disseminated infection (i.e., sepsis, meningitis)

TREATMENT

Medical
- Acute ophthalmia neonatorum should be treated as gonococcal conjunctivitis until culture results are available and then adjusted accordingly
  - Mother and sexual partners should be treated
- Chemical conjunctivitis
  - Requires no treatment; improves within 48 hours
  - Povidone iodine less commonly causes chemical conjunctivitis compared to other agents
- Chlamydial conjunctivitis
  - Prophylaxis with 1% silver nitrate drops, 0.5% erythromycin ophthalmic ointment, 1% tetracycline ointment, or povidone iodine 2.5% solution
    - All have comparable efficacy but do not prevent chlamydial pneumonia
  - Treat with oral erythromycin, 50 mg/kg/day divided into 4 daily doses for 14 days
- Gonococcal conjunctivitis
  - Ceftriaxone, 25 to 50 mg/kg IV or IM in single dose
  - Hospitalization and frequent saline irrigation until purulence subsides
- HSV conjunctivitis
  - Requires hospitalization due to frequent disseminated disease with potential neurologic or systemic manifestations and treatment with topical antivirals and acyclovir, 30 mg/kg/day in 3 divided doses for 14 days

Follow-Up
- Pediatrician follow-up for chlamydial pneumonia, disseminated gonococcal, syphilis systemic HSV infection
- Prognosis depends on infectious agent and time until starting appropriate treatment

SELECTED REFERENCES

1. Mayor MT et al: Diagnosis and management of gonococcal infections. Am Fam Physician. 86(10):931-8, 2012

TOXOCARIASIS

Key Facts

Demographics
- Usually caused by *Toxocara canis*, a helminth (parasitic worm) that typically infects dogs
- Infection typically results from ingestion of *Toxocara* ova from contaminated soil, food, or fecal material

Presentation
- Decreased visual acuity
- Ocular larva migrans syndrome
  - Typically unilateral
  - Leukocoria (especially in children)
  - Posterior uveitis
  - Retinal detachment
  - Temporal macular dragging with pseudoexotropia

Differential Diagnosis
- Retinoblastoma
  - Exam findings: Leukocoria (typically unilateral), strabismus
- Coats disease
  - Exam findings: Leukocoria (typically unilateral), strabismus, retinal telangiectasias, yellow-green exudates, subretinal fluid leakage
- Toxoplasmosis
  - Exam findings: Necrotizing retinitis with white retinal lesions, vitreitis, ± chorioretinal scarring

Evaluation/Work-Up
- Enzyme-linked immunosorbent assay

Treatment
- Steroids: Topical or systemic to reduce inflammation and complications of inflammation
- Vitrectomy or scleral buckle may be necessary to repair retinal detachment
- Albendazole

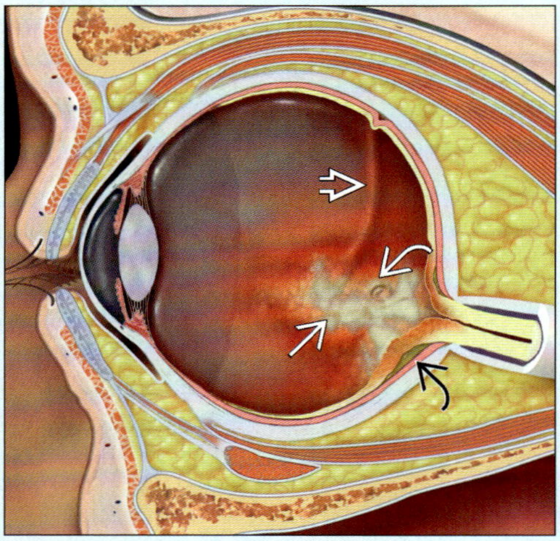

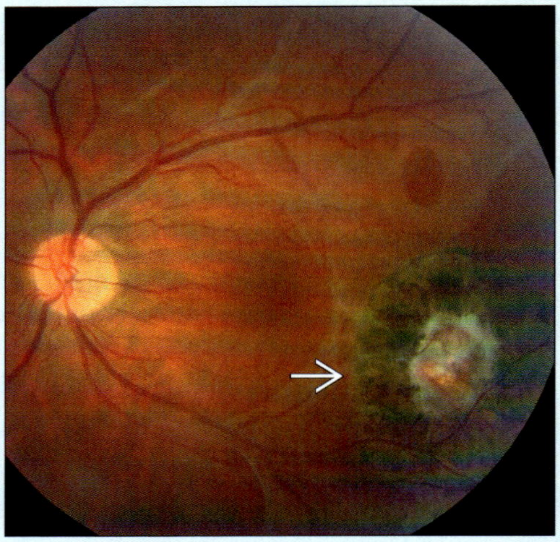

(Left) *This sagittal graphic demonstrates a granulomatous reaction ➔ secondary to an expired Toxocara larva ➔. A retinal fold ➔ is present due to postinflammatory changes and traction, as well as a small subretinal fluid collection ➔.* ***(Right)*** *This fundus photograph demonstrates a peripheral granuloma in a patient with positive enzyme-linked immunosorbent assay for toxocariasis ➔.*

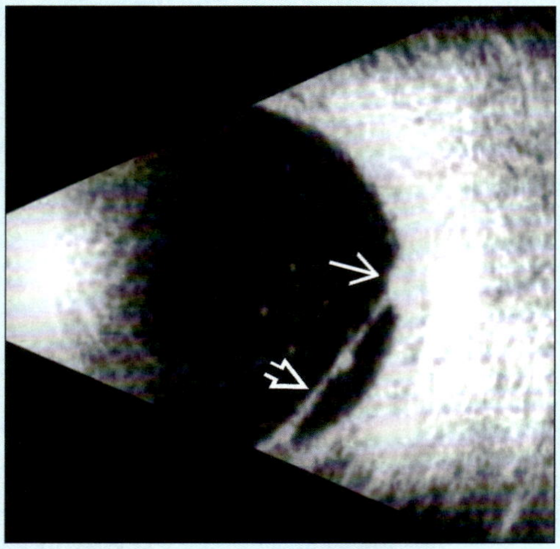

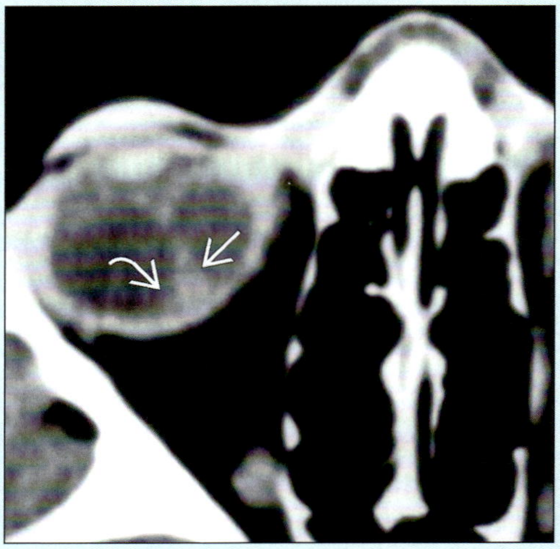

(Left) *B-scan ultrasound shows an echoic nodule at the posterior pole of the globe ➔, corresponding to a Toxocara granuloma. An intravitreal membrane ➔ is seen extending from the nodule. (Courtesy R. Harrie, MD.)* ***(Right)*** *Axial CECT shows a mildly enhancing nodule posteriorly in the right eye ➔. Adjacent chorioretinal thickening ➔ represents inflammatory changes, postinflammatory membranes, retinal folds, &/or subretinal fluid collection.*

TOXOCARIASIS

INTRODUCTION

Definitions

- Infection caused by the parasite *Toxocara canis* or *Toxocara cati*, classically resulting in uveitis or systemic symptoms

Subtypes

- Ocular larva migrans syndrome
- Visceral larva migrans syndrome (systemic)
  - Typically considered a distinct entity from ocular larva migrans syndrome
  - Characterized by fever, general malaise, rash, and hepatosplenomegaly
- Covert toxocariasis: Nonspecific with behavior changes

DEMOGRAPHICS

Etiology/Risk Factors

- Usually caused by *T. canis*, a helminth (parasitic worm) that typically infects dogs
  - Can also be caused by *T. cati*, a helminth that typically infects cats
- Infected animals deliver ova into their feces, which is deposited into soil
- Larvae mature and become infectious within soil
- Human infection typically results from ingestion of *Toxocara* ova in contaminated soil, undercooked food, or fecal material
  - Humans are accidental hosts
    - Larvae cannot mature into adult worms within humans
  - Larvae migrate through blood vessels to reach the eye, usually posterior segment
- Dog ownership has been found to be a risk factor

Epidemiology

- Typically infects children
- Higher prevalence in warm climates, although very low prevalence of the disease overall

PRESENTATION

Symptoms

- Ocular larva migrans syndrome
  - Decreased visual acuity
  - Redness &/or pain
  - Photophobia
  - Floaters

Exam Findings

- Ocular larva migrans syndrome
  - Typically unilateral
  - Leukocoria (especially in children)
  - Uveitis, usually posterior
  - Retinal detachment (tractional or rhegmatogenous)
  - Endophthalmitis
  - Posterior pole or peripheral granuloma
  - Temporal dragging of macula can cause pseudoexotropia (eye appears turned out but cover testing does not show misalignment)

DIFFERENTIAL DIAGNOSIS

Retinoblastoma

- Exam findings: Leukocoria (typically unilateral), strabismus
- May find calcium on B-scan ultrasound or CT scan, which is not found in toxocariasis
- Histopathologic examination may reveal presence of rosettes &/or fluorettes

Coats Disease

- Exam findings: Leukocoria (typically unilateral), strabismus, retinal telangiectasias, yellow-green exudates, subretinal fluid leakage
- May find evidence of cholesterol deposits on ultrasound, which is not found in toxocariasis

Toxoplasmosis

- Infection by *Toxoplasma gondii*, typically causing posterior uveitis
- Exam findings: Necrotizing retinitis with white retinal lesions, vitreitis, ± chorioretinal scarring

EVALUATION/WORK-UP

Labs

- Enzyme-linked immunosorbent assay better for visceral larva migrans

Imaging

- Fundus photography: Can show temporal dragging, cysts, or scars

TREATMENT

Medical

- Steroids: Topical or systemic to prevent membranes
  - If anterior inflammation, use cycloplegic
- Anti-helminth therapy (albendazole)
  - Current therapies directed more toward reducing inflammation
  - Some have had success using albendazole with visceral larva migrans syndrome

Surgical

- Vitrectomy or scleral buckle used to repair retinal detachment

Prognosis

- Vitreoretinal surgery can improve visual outcomes

SELECTED REFERENCES

1. Woodhall D et al: Ocular toxocariasis: epidemiologic, anatomic, and therapeutic variations based on a survey of ophthalmic subspecialists. Ophthalmology. 119(6):1211-7, 2012
2. Schneier AJ et al: Ocular toxocariasis: advances in diagnosis and treatment. Int Ophthalmol Clin. 51(4):135-44, 2011
3. Stewart JM et al: Prevalence, clinical features, and causes of vision loss among patients with ocular toxocariasis. Retina. 25(8):1005-13, 2005
4. Taylor MR: The epidemiology of ocular toxocariasis. J Helminthol. 75(2):109-18, 2001

NONACCIDENTAL TRAUMA (CHILD ABUSE)

Key Facts

Introduction
- Shaken baby syndrome (SBS) is a common form of nonaccidental head trauma (NAHT)
  - Classically characterized by bilateral retinal hemorrhages, subdural hemorrhage, and possible encephalopathy, without outward signs of direct trauma
  - Acceleration-deceleration forces produced from shaking cause tearing of bridging veins, resulting in subdural hemorrhage

Demographics
- Typically found in children < 2 years of age

Presentation
- Bilateral retinal hemorrhages (any layer)
- Optic nerve sheath hemorrhage
- Vitreous hemorrhage
- Perimacular folds

Differential Diagnosis
- Birthing trauma (association with vacuum delivery)
- Terson syndrome
  - Spontaneous or traumatic acute intracranial hemorrhage, usually subarachnoid
- Accidental head trauma
  - Examples include crush injuries, trauma due to motor vehicle collisions, etc.

Evaluation/Work-Up
- Funduscopic & full physical exam
- Head CT to detect presence of intracranial hemorrhage, usually subdural and cerebral edema
- Skeletal series of x-rays
- Refer to social services and alert pediatrician

Treatment
- Mortality of up to 30%
- No standard treatment exists

__(Left)__ This fundus photo demonstrates multiple hemorrhages at different levels within the posterior pole, consistent with nonaccidental trauma. __(Right)__ This is an external photo of a scleral cap from an enucleated globe, removed post mortem in a patient with nonaccidental trauma. Notice the diffuse retinal hemorrhages →.

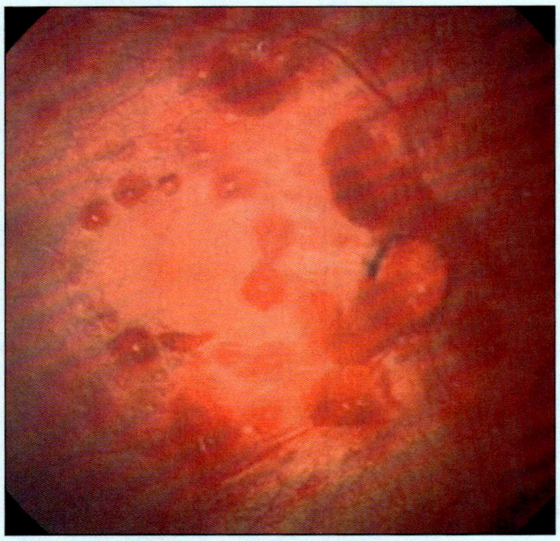

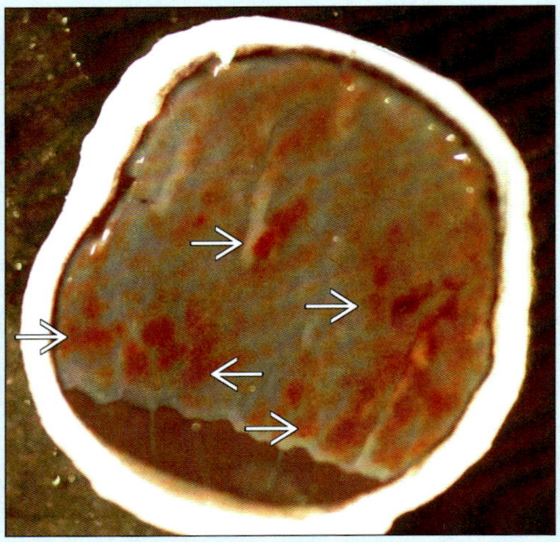

__(Left)__ This is an external photo of the optic nerve from an enucleated globe, removed post mortem in a patient with nonaccidental trauma. Note the blood → surrounding the optic nerve →. __(Right)__ Axial CT in this 12 week old with rib, skull, and humerus fractures and a duodenal hematoma shows a moderate subdural hematoma over the right cerebral hemisphere →, with a small amount of subdural blood on the left, causing a pseudo "empty delta" sign of the sagittal sinus →. These findings are seen in nonaccidental trauma.

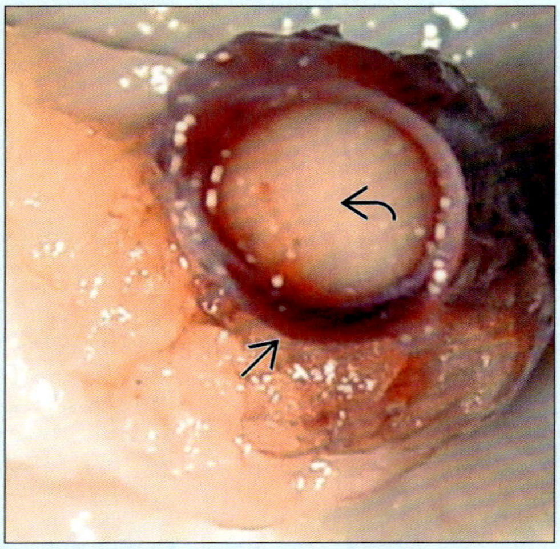

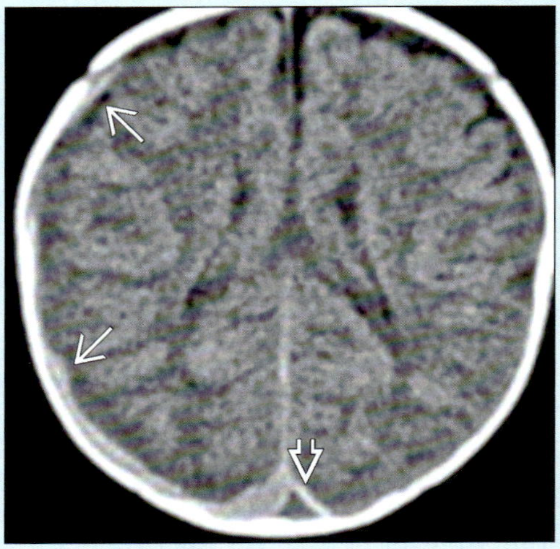

NONACCIDENTAL TRAUMA (CHILD ABUSE)

INTRODUCTION

Abbreviations
- Nonaccidental head trauma (NAHT)

Subtypes
- Shaken baby syndrome (SBS) is a common form of NAHT
  - Classically characterized by bilateral retinal hemorrhages, subdural hemorrhage, and possible encephalopathy, without outward signs of direct trauma
  - Acceleration-deceleration forces produced from shaking cause tearing of bridging veins, resulting in subdural hemorrhage

DEMOGRAPHICS

Etiology/Risk Factors
- Higher rates of NAHT/SBS found in
  - Children born to mothers < 21 years of age
    - However, fathers are more likely to commit abuse than mothers
  - Male children
  - Crying children, who are found to be inconsolable

Epidemiology
- Typically found in children < 2 years of age
- ~ 1,400 children per year affected by SBS in United States

PRESENTATION

Symptoms
- Spectrum of neurologic symptoms ranging from asymptomatic to irritable and lethargic with vomiting and seizures
- Irregular bruise pattern
- Evidence of direct ocular trauma is often absent in SBS

Exam Findings
- Bilateral retinal hemorrhages, usually located around posterior pole, can also be pre-, intra-, or subretinal
  - Flame-like, dot-and-blot, or white-centered hemorrhages
  - Unilateral hemorrhage can occur but is rare
- Optic nerve sheath hemorrhage
- Vitreous hemorrhage
- Perimacular folds
- Macular retinoschisis
- Retinal detachment

DIFFERENTIAL DIAGNOSIS

Birthing Trauma
- Retinal hemorrhage
  - Very rare in age > 1 month
- Typically associated with vacuum delivery

Terson Syndrome
- Spontaneous or traumatic acute intracranial hemorrhage, usually subarachnoid (vs. subdural in SBS)
  - Ruptured anterior communicating artery aneurysm is most common cause of hemorrhage
- Bilateral retinal hemorrhage, located in posterior pole
  - ~ 20-40% of patients with subarachnoid hemorrhage also have intraocular hemorrhage
- As blood clears, vision typically returns
- Rare in children

Accidental Head Trauma
- Examples include crush injuries, trauma due to motor vehicle collisions, etc.
- Retinal and optic nerve sheath hemorrhages may be found in severe cases but are very rare and far less common findings than in SBS
- Other injuries as a result of direct trauma present

EVALUATION/WORK-UP

Labs
- Cerebrospinal fluid analysis may reveal evidence of xanthochromia, suggesting history of intracranial bleeding

Pathology
- Bilateral retinal hemorrhages
- Optic nerve sheath hemorrhage
- Vitreous hemorrhage

Imaging
- Systemic
  - Head CT to detect presence of intracranial hemorrhage, usually subdural and cerebral edema
  - Skeletal survey to detect presence of suspicious fractures (e.g., broken ribs, spiral fracture of humerus, multiple fractures of long bones or fractures of different ages)

TREATMENT

Medical
- No standard treatment exists

Surgical
- Vitrectomy can be of use in appropriate candidates to clear vitreous hemorrhage

Prognosis
- Mortality of up to 30%
  - Degree of ocular hemorrhage often corresponds to degree of brain injury
- Most experience some permanent vision loss

SELECTED REFERENCES

1. Matschke J et al: Ocular pathology in shaken baby syndrome and other forms of infantile non-accidental head injury. Int J Legal Med. 123(3):189-97, 2009
2. Mungan NK: Update on shaken baby syndrome: ophthalmology. Curr Opin Ophthalmol. 18(5):392-7, 2007
3. Wygnanski-Jaffe T et al: Postmortem orbital findings in shaken baby syndrome. Am J Ophthalmol. 142(2):233-40, 2006
4. Keenan HT et al: A population-based study of inflicted traumatic brain injury in young children. JAMA. 290(5):621-6, 2003
5. Garfinkle AM et al: Terson's syndrome: a reversible cause of blindness following subarachnoid hemorrhage. J Neurosurg. 76(5):766-71, 1992

RETINOPATHY OF PREMATURITY

Key Facts

Introduction
- Developmental proliferative vascular disease seen in retina of premature infants
- Common cause of blindness in USA

Demographics
- Risk factors include gestational age, low birth weight (BW), and oxygen toxicity
- Incidence increasing in USA as more premature infants survive their stay in the NICU

Presentation
- Typically begins around 34 weeks postmenstrual age but may be evident as early as 30-32 weeks

Screening Guidelines
- Screen all infants with gestational age (GA) < 30 weeks or BW < 1,500 grams and those with BW 1,500-2,000 g or GA > 30 weeks who have increased risk of ROP based on complicated clinical course or supplemental O_2

Evaluation/Work-Up
- Dilated funduscopic exam with scleral depression
- Digital imaging may be useful as an adjunct
- Must document extent and severity of disease based on 4 standardized features: Zone, stage, extent, and presence or absence of plus disease

Treatment
- Indicated for infants with high-risk prethreshold disease (zone I ROP = stage 3 without plus disease or any stage with plus disease; zone II ROP = stage 2 or 3 with plus disease) and those with evidence of retinal detachment
- First-line treatment: Laser photocoagulation to peripheral avascular retina
- Avastin may be useful treatment for severe ROP, but long-term outcomes are unknown
- Aggressive follow-up necessary after treatment

__(Left)__ This fundus photograph shows an eye with stage 3 retinopathy of prematurity. Note the visible ridge with extraretinal vascular proliferation ➡. __(Right)__ This fundus photograph depicts an eye that has previously been treated with laser photocoagulation ➡. The demarcation line and ridge are visible ➡.

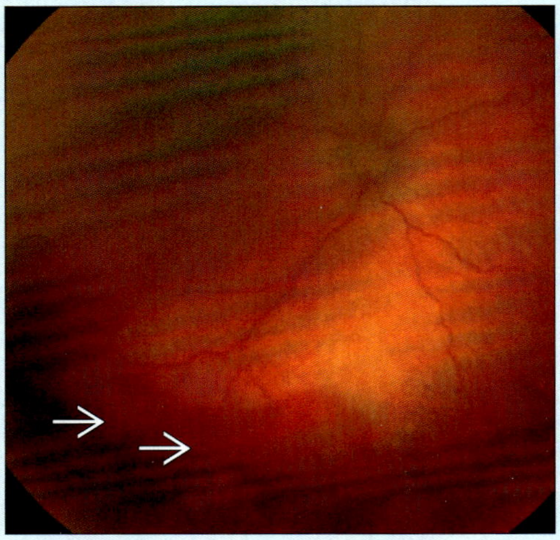

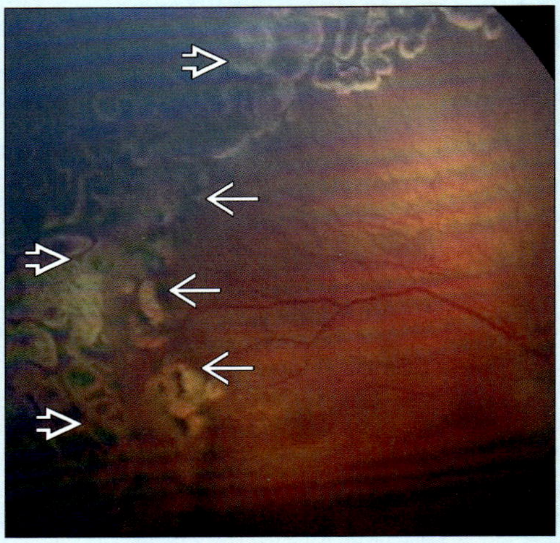

__(Left)__ This fundus photograph shows stage 1 retinopathy of prematurity. The demarcation line is visible ➡. __(Right)__ This fundus photograph shows retinopathy of prematurity with associated intraretinal hemorrhage ➡.

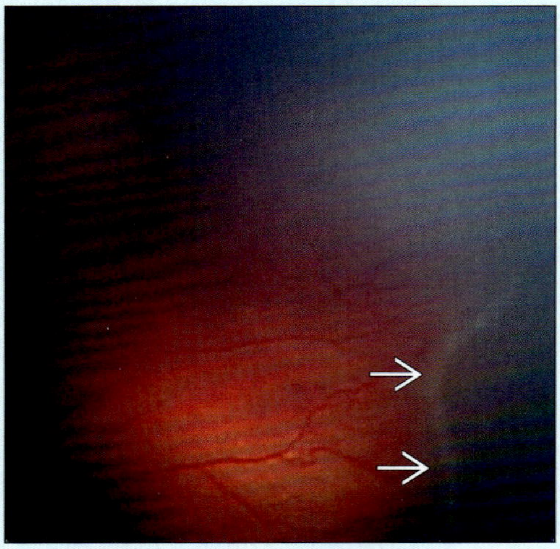

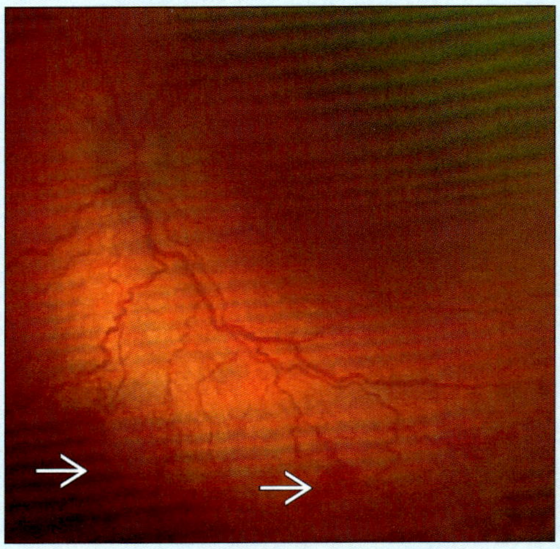

RETINOPATHY OF PREMATURITY

INTRODUCTION

Abbreviations

- Retinopathy of prematurity (ROP)

Definitions

- Proliferative vascular disorder that occurs in retina of premature infants, predisposing the infant to retinal detachment and blindness if untreated

DEMOGRAPHICS

Etiology/Risk Factors

- Gestational age < 32 weeks
- Low birth weight < 1,500 grams
- Supplemental oxygen exposure in NICU or complicated course

Epidemiology

- Incidence is increasing in USA because of increasing premature infant survivability

PRESENTATION

Exam Findings

- Mainstay of exam is indirect ophthalmoscopy with a lid speculum and scleral depression

Disease Classification

- Based on The International Classification of Retinopathy of Prematurity (2005)
- Location: Retina divided into 3 concentric zones centered around optic disc
  - Zone I = innermost (posterior pole); zone II = middle (area around zone I centered on macula, reaching to nasal ora serrata); zone III = outermost temporal crescent (ROP reaches ora serrata)
- Staging
  - 0 = no clear demarcation between avascular and vascular areas; 1 = clear demarcation between avascular and vascular areas; 2 = demarcation line gains height and depth; 3 = neovascularization protrudes into the vitreous; 4 = partial retinal detachment (4A does not involve fovea, 4B does); 5 = total retinal detachment
- Extent: Retina divided into clock hours; involvement expressed as # of clock hours affected
- Plus and pre-plus disease
  - Plus: Increased venous dilatation and arteriolar tortuosity of posterior retinal vessels in at least 2 quadrants with associated iris vascular engorgement, vitreous hemorrhage, iris neovascularization, or poor pupillary dilatation
  - Pre-plus: More arterial tortuosity and venous dilatation than normal but insufficient for the diagnosis of plus disease
- Aggressive posterior ROP (AP-ROP): Also called rush disease
  - Characteristics include posterior location, plus disease, and ill-defined retinopathy; progresses to total retinal detachment if untreated

DIFFERENTIAL DIAGNOSIS

Familial Exudative Vitreoretinopathy

- Genetic disease that occurs in full-term infants

Persistent Fetal Vascular Syndrome

- Typically unilateral with no correlation to prematurity

TREATMENT

Surgical

- Laser photocoagulation (transscleral vs. transpupillary approach): Now the mainstay of ROP treatment
- Thresholds for laser photocoagulation: Zone I ROP = stage 3 without plus disease or any stage with plus disease; zone II ROP = stages 2 or 3 with plus disease
- Stages 4 and 5 disease (partial or total RD): Vitrectomy or scleral buckle depending on surgeon's preferences

Follow-Up

- In short term (American Academy of Pediatrics 2013 guidelines)
  - 1 week or less follow-up: Zone I = stages 1 or 2 ROP or immature vascularization without ROP; zone II = stage 3 ROP or immature retina extending to the boundary of zone I; AP-ROP or suspicious AP-ROP
  - 1-2 week follow-up: Zone I = unequivocally regressing ROP; zone II = stage 2 ROP or immature vascularization
  - 2-week follow-up: Zone II = stage 1 ROP, regressing ROP, or immature vascularization
  - 2-3 week follow-up: Zone III = stage 1 or 2 ROP or regressing ROP
- In long term
  - If stages 1 or 2 ROP: Annual vision screening
  - If surgical treatment was necessitated: Every 1-2 weeks for 1-2 months, then less frequently depending on clinical course

Prognosis

- Stages 1-2 ROP: Outcomes similar to those in preterm infants without ROP
- Stage 3 or higher: Prognosis varies depending on zone (zone I worse than zone II, which is worse than zone III)
- Prognosis worse with plus disease, AP-ROP, and retinal detachment

Complications From ROP

- Myopia most common (laser-treated eyes less myopic than cryo-treated eyes in long-term studies), strabismus, amblyopia, anisometropia, tractional retinal detachment, retinal folds, dragging macula, glaucoma, microphthalmos, cataract, phthisis bulbi

SELECTED REFERENCES

1. Fierson WM; American Academy of Pediatrics Section on Ophthalmology; American Academy of Ophthalmology; American Association for Pediatric Ophthalmology and Strabismus; American Association of Certified Orthoptists: Screening examination of premature infants for retinopathy of prematurity. Pediatrics. 131(1):189-95, 2013

CHOROIDAL OSTEOMA

Key Facts

Introduction
- Benign tumor affecting choroid; made of bone

Demographics
- Unknown etiology
- Most often found in women in their 20s-30s

Presentation
- Can be asymptomatic
- Blurred vision
- Visual field defects, central scotoma possible
- Most often unilateral (75% of cases)
- Found in juxtapapillary or peripapillary region
- Yellow-white to pale-orange in color
- Vascular tufts with a spider-like appearance on tumor surface

Differential Diagnosis
- Circumscribed choroidal hemangioma
  - Lesion is orange-red in color and round with possible pigmented rim, located close to optic disc
- Amelanotic choroidal melanoma (or nevus)
  - Lesion is yellow in with possible mushroom shape
- Metastatic carcinoma
  - Lesion is typically white to yellow in color
- Calcification: Phthisis bulbi

Evaluation/Work-Up
- Ultrasound B-scan: Tumor appears highly reflective with shadowing posteriorly

Treatment
- Serial fundus examinations to check for neovascularization of the choroid and growth
- Neovascularization can be treated with laser photocoagulation, photodynamic therapy, or more recently with anti-VEGF
- Lacks malignant potential

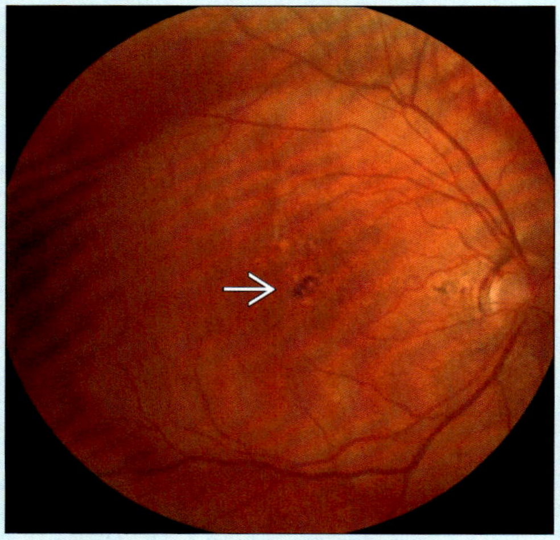
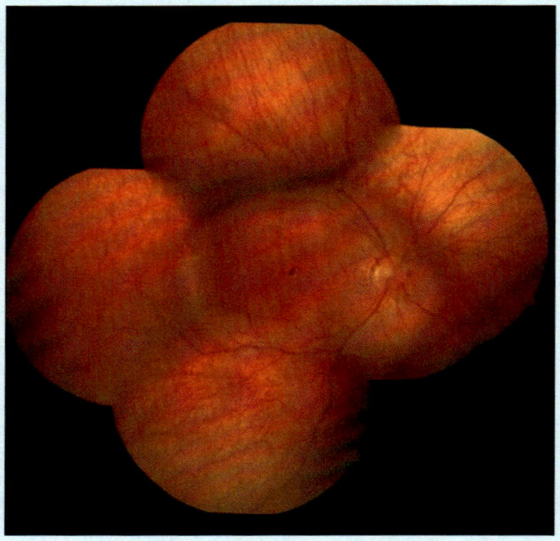

(Left) *Fundus photo demonstrates choroidal osteoma. This rare benign tumor is composed of bone and is usually unilateral. It most commonly presents in females during the 3rd to 4th decade of life. Note macular retinal pigment epithelial atrophy ➔.* ***(Right)*** *Fundus photo composite shows a well-circumscribed area of choroidal osteoma. This tumor contains osteocytes and osteoclasts, as well as mast cells and mesenchymal cells. Osteoma is highly reflective on B-scan ultrasound and appears bony on CT scan.*

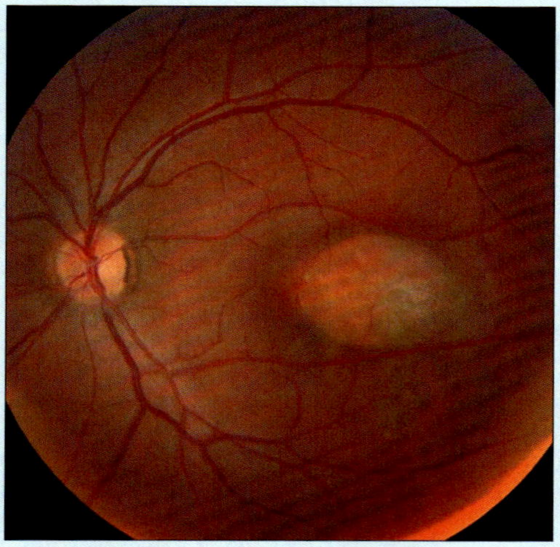
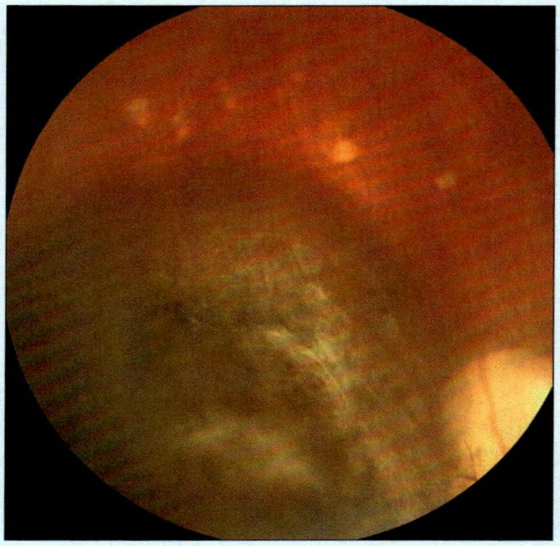

(Left) *Fundus photo shows choroidal hemangioma, which is a differential consideration when osteoma is suspected. Hemangioma is a benign vascular tumor that shows high internal reflectivity on A-scan ultrasound. Choroidal hemangioma can be associated with serous retinal detachment.* ***(Right)*** *Fundus photo shows choroidal melanoma, which is included in the differential diagnosis of osteoma. The amelanotic form of choroidal melanoma can be similar in appearance to choroidal osteoma.*

CHOROIDAL OSTEOMA

INTRODUCTION

Subtypes

- Choroidal osteoma
  - Benign tumor affecting choroid; made of bone
- Orbital osteoma
  - Extremely rare, more likely to originate from sinuses and extend into orbit

DEMOGRAPHICS

Etiology/Risk Factors

- Unknown etiology

Epidemiology

- Very rare
- Most often found in women in their 20s-30s

PRESENTATION

Symptoms

- Can be asymptomatic
- Blurred vision
- Visual field defects, central scotoma possible
- Metamorphopsia
- Photophobia

Exam Findings

- Fundus exam
  - Most often unilateral (75% of cases)
  - Found in juxtapapillary or peripapillary region
  - Yellow-white to pale-orange in color
  - Vascular tufts with a spider-like appearance on tumor surface

DIFFERENTIAL DIAGNOSIS

Circumscribed Choroidal Hemangioma

- Benign tumor of vascular origin, seen most often in ages ranging from 40s-60s
- Can be asymptomatic, or patients may have decreased visual acuity (VA)
- Lesion is orange-red in color and round, with possible pigmented rim, located close to optic disc
- Imaging
  - A-scan ultrasound: High internal reflectivity
  - Significant hyperfluorescence in early phase of indocyanine green angiography
- Common complication: Serous retinal detachment

Amelanotic Choroidal Melanoma (or Nevus)

- Lesion is yellow in color with possible mushroom shape
- Drusen

Metastatic Carcinoma

- Lesion is typically white to yellow in color
- Can be bilateral, may have multiple lesions

Calcification

- Phthisis bulbi
- Idiopathic sclerochoroidal calcification

EVALUATION/WORK-UP

Pathology

- Consists of mature bone with trabeculae in choroid
- Blood vessels, mast cells, mesenchymal cells in intratrabecular spaces
- Other cells include osteocytes and osteoclasts
- Retinal pigment epithelium may be atrophied

Imaging

- Ultrasound
  - B-scan: Tumor appears highly reflective with shadowing posteriorly
- CT scan with evidence of bone in location of choroid
- Fluorescein angiography
  - Early phase: Patchy hyperfluorescence
  - Late phase: Diffuse staining
- Indocyanine green angiography
  - Early phase: Hypofluorescence due to blockage by tumor
  - Late phase: Hyperfluorescence due to leakage

TREATMENT

Medical

- Neovascularization can be treated with laser photocoagulation or photodynamic therapy
- Current research into intravitreal injections of bevacizumab (anti-VEGF) for neovascularization treatment

Follow-Up

- No treatment for tumor
- Serial fundus examinations to check for neovascularization of choroid and growth
  - Growth occurs in ~ 40-64% of patients
    - Some can decalcify, which is associated with poorer visual outcomes

Prognosis

- Lacks malignant potential
- Poorer visual outcomes associated with choroidal neovascularization and decalcification
- 56-58% likelihood of VA deteriorating to 20/200 or worse within 10 years

SELECTED REFERENCES

1. Shields CL et al: Factors predictive of tumor growth, tumor decalcification, choroidal neovascularization, and visual outcome in 74 eyes with choroidal osteoma. Arch Ophthalmol. 123(12):1658-66, 2005
2. Singh AD et al: Choroidal hemangioma. Ophthalmol Clin North Am. 18(1):151-61, ix, 2005
3. Mashayekhi A et al: Circumscribed choroidal hemangioma. Curr Opin Ophthalmol. 14(3):142-9, 2003
4. Aylward GW et al: A long-term follow-up of choroidal osteoma. Arch Ophthalmol. 116(10):1337-41, 1998
5. Kadrmas EF et al: Choroidal osteoma. Int Ophthalmol Clin. 37(4):171-82, 1997

RETINOBLASTOMA

Key Facts

Introduction
- Aggressive eye cancer of infancy and childhood
  - Endophytic tumor originates in inner nuclear layer, extending into vitreous cavity
  - Exophytic tumor originates in outer nuclear layer, extending into subretinal space and potentially causing retinal detachment

Demographics
- Associated with *RB1* gene mutation
- Mortality ~ 70% in low- and middle-income countries where most affected children live
- 40% unilateral, 60% bilateral

Presentation
- White pupillary reflex present in 56% of cases
- Crossed eyes present in 23% of cases
- Red, painful eye
- Poor vision

Exam Findings
- Leukocoria
- Strabismus
- Exophthalmos
- Glaucoma

Treatment
- Ablative therapy with laser photocoagulation, cryotherapy, or transpupillary thermotherapy, possibly with local chemotherapy for small tumors
- Enucleation and adjuvant chemotherapy recommended in large, advanced tumors

Prognosis
- Improved prognosis with limited tumor seeding and small tumor size
- Poor prognosis with metastasis via hematogenous spread, tumor extension into CSF of subarachnoid space, or through lymphatic involvement

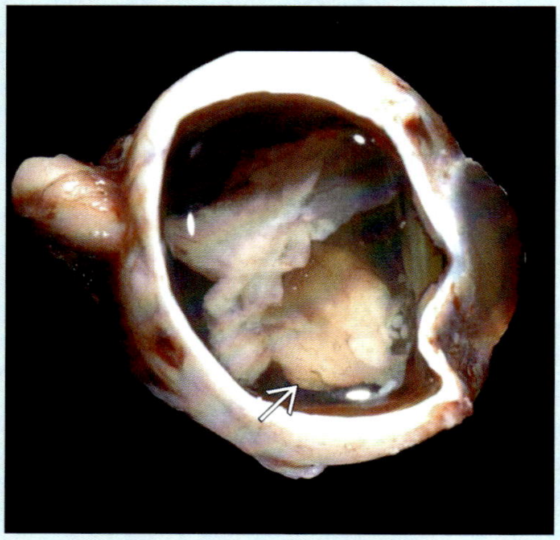
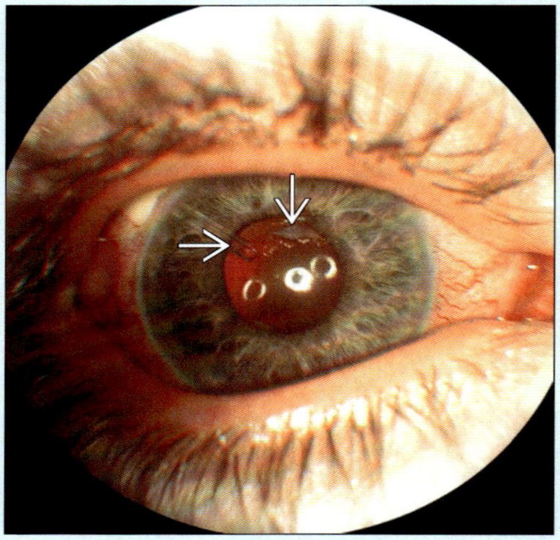

(Left) *This cross section of an enucleated globe shows a large endophytic retinoblastoma ➔ growing inward from the retina into the vitreous. Also notice that the mass is white or pearl colored and well circumscribed. When calcification is present, the tumor mass takes on a "cottage cheese" appearance.* ***(Right)*** *This external photo shows an endophytic retinoblastoma with floating, anteriorly displaced tumor seeds ➔.*

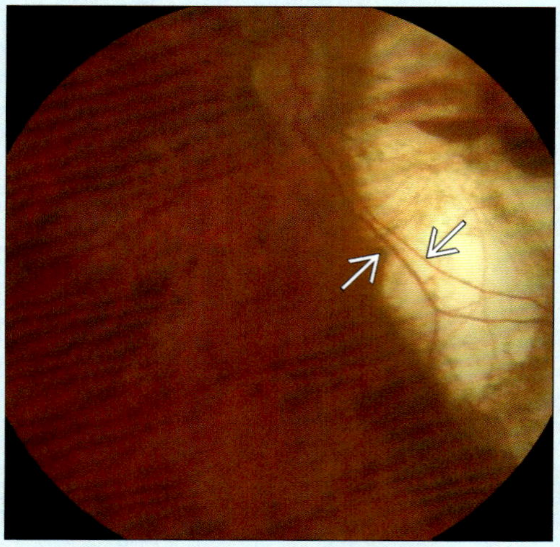
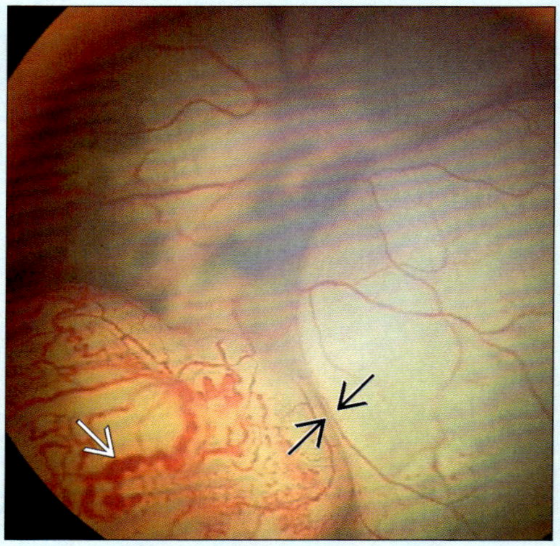

(Left) *This fundus photo shows an exophytic retinoblastoma growing outward and separating the retina from the choroid and slightly dilated feeding vessels, providing nutrients to the tumor ➔. Fundus exam of an exophytic retinoblastoma appears similar to an exudative retinal detachment.* ***(Right)*** *This fundus photo shows an exophytic retinoblastoma with prominent dilated and tortuous feeding vessels ➔ and nearly touching retinal to retinal detachments ➔.*

RETINOBLASTOMA

INTRODUCTION

Definitions
- Aggressive eye cancer of infancy and childhood

Subtypes
- Endophytic
  - Originates in inner nuclear layer of retina, extending into vitreous cavity
- Exophytic
  - Originates in outer nuclear layer, extending into subretinal space and potentially causing detachment

DEMOGRAPHICS

Etiology/Risk Factors
- Mutation in tumor-suppressor gene *RB1* gene
  - Constitutional loss of 1 RB1 allele predisposes to cancer development
  - Loss of both RB1 alleles from developing retinal cell initiates growth of retinoblastoma tumor

Epidemiology
- Mortality ~ 70% in low- and middle-income countries where most affected children live
- 1 case per 15,000-18,000 births
  - 40% unilateral; average age at diagnosis is 24 months
  - 60% bilateral (often hereditary); average age at diagnosis is 12 months

PRESENTATION

Symptoms
- White pupillary reflex present in 56% of cases
- Crossed eyes present in 23% of cases
- Red, painful eye; poor vision

Exam Findings
- Leukocoria
  - Macular tumors present earlier due to visualization of white reflex with direct gaze
    - Microaneurysms, neovascularization
  - Peripheral tumors have advanced, delayed presentation due to visualization only in peripheral gaze
  - Clear view of tumor may be impeded by vitreous hemorrhage, retinal detachment (RD), or inflammation
- Strabismus
- White spots on iris due to implantation growths on surface of iris or anteriorly displaced vitreous floaters
- Exophthalmos
- Glaucoma
- Trilateral retinoblastoma = bilateral retinoblastoma + pinealoblastoma (identified on MRI; very poor prognosis)

DIFFERENTIAL DIAGNOSIS

Persistent Fetal Vasculature
- May present with leukocoria and RD due to failure of primary vitreous to regress

Coats Disease
- Telangiectatic vessels with lipoproteinaceous leakage and subsequent RD with solid white or yellow material may simulate retinoblastoma

Endophthalmitis and Orbital Cellulitis
- Suggestive of spontaneous tumor necrosis and acute inflammation; prompt resolution without treatment suggests retinoblastoma

Cataract
- In eyes with dense cataracts obscuring view of fundus, consider US to rule out RD or intraocular tumor
- ROP, FEVR, and toxocariasis can also cause leukocoria

EVALUATION/WORK-UP

Labs
- Genetic testing for *RB1* gene mutation recommended when family history suggests cancer susceptibility

Pathology
- Fine-needle aspiration biopsy through cornea if imaging not possible or inconclusive

Imaging
- CT: Calcification and seeding of tumor into vitreous are both pathognomonic
- MRI: Useful in distinguishing tumor tissue density and to avoid external radiation of CT
- Ultrasound: Useful in distinguishing mixed, solid, cystic, and diffuse infiltrating tumor types

TREATMENT

Surgical
- Treatment individualized for each child based on International Classification of Retinoblastoma; other factors include laterality, size, risk for metastasis, seeding, and tumor relationship to surrounding tissues
  - Ablative therapy with laser photocoagulation, cryotherapy, or transpupillary thermotherapy, possibly with local chemotherapy (vincristine, carboplatin, VP-16) for small tumors < 3 mm in diameter
  - Enucleation with removal of large portion of optic nerve and adjuvant chemotherapy recommended in large, advanced tumors

Follow-Up
- Short-term follow-up for recurrence of primary tumor
- Long-term follow-up for individuals with heritable mutation to diagnose extraocular tumors

Prognosis
- Improved prognosis with limited tumor seeding and small tumor size
- Poor prognosis with metastasis via hematogenous spread, tumor extension into CSF of subarachnoid space, or through lymphatic involvement

SELECTED REFERENCES

1. Dimaras H et al: Retinoblastoma. Lancet. 379(9824):1436-46, 2012

AMBLYOPIA

Key Facts

Introduction
- Reduced visual acuity in excess of that explained by structural or visual pathway disease
- If treated while visual system is still maturing, amblyopia can usually be reversed and vision restored
  - Amblyopia is linked to abnormal visual experience (birth to age 8); commonly classified by etiology
  - Functional amblyopia: Decreased visual acuity without any observable organic defect; reversible
  - Organic amblyopia: Failure of visual pathway to develop due to a retinal or CNS lesion, toxic or metabolic disturbance; irreversible

Presentation
- Decreased vision, strabismus, ptosis seen in some patients

Exam Findings
- Strabismic amblyopia: Fixation defect
- Refractive amblyopia: Decreased visual acuity, anisometropia or ametropia, astigmatism of ≥ 1.00 D
- Stimulus deprivation: Cataract, ptosis, leukocoria

Treatment
- Refractive amblyopia: Correction of refractive error, occlusion therapy with 3+ hours of occlusion/day
- Strabismic and stimulus deprivation amblyopia: Surgical or refractive correction, occlusion therapy

Follow-up
- For full-time occlusions, follow-up at intervals of 1 week per year of age, but cannot stretch out follow-up longer than 4 weeks at any age
- Occlusion can be stopped when visual acuity is equal bilaterally or no progress after 3 months of occlusion

Prognosis
- Worse prognosis associated with early onset and delay in diagnosis and treatment

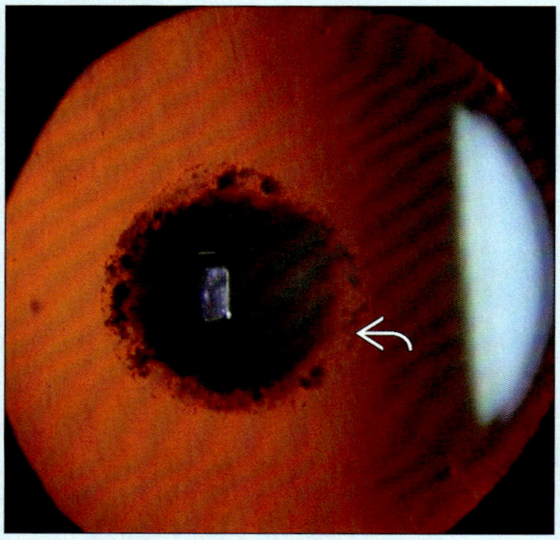
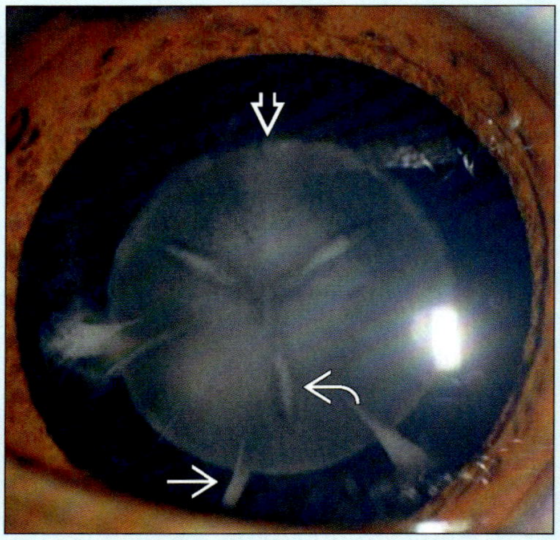

***(Left)** This slit-lamp photo shows retroillumination of a congenital nuclear cataract ➔. Close monitoring for amblyopia should be undertaken for patients with congenital cataracts, and extraction should occur if there is concern for poor visual development. **(Right)** This slit-lamp photo demonstrates a lamellar cataract ➔ with prominent sutural opacities ➔ and peripheral radial opacities ➔. Given the size of this cataract, there should be concern for amblyogenic potential.*

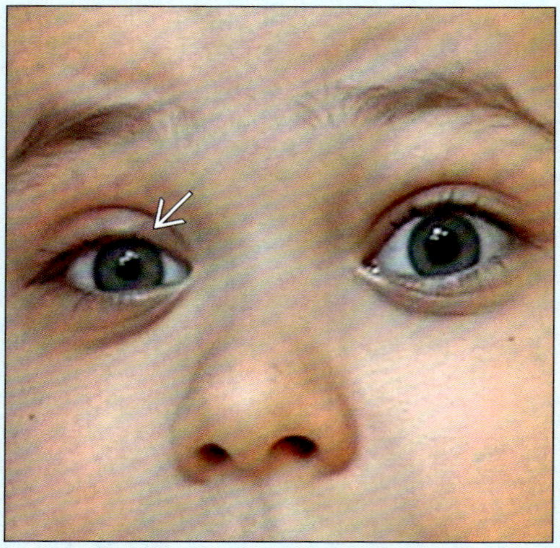
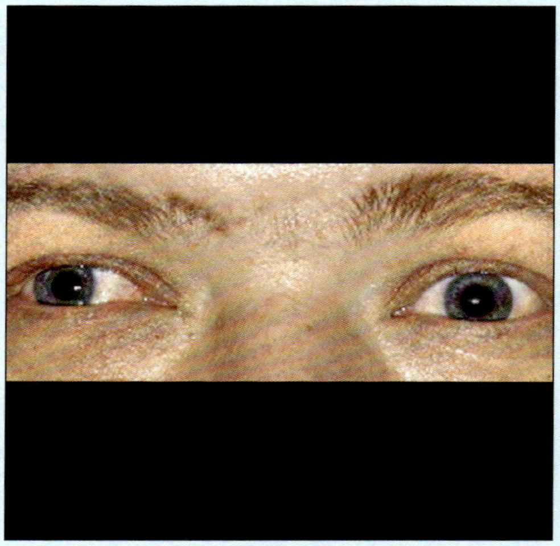

***(Left)** This external photo shows a patient with congenital ptosis ➔ caused by Horner syndrome. The patient's ptosis does not appear to interfere with her visual axis. It is important to monitor pediatric patients with ptosis for development of deprivation amblyopia. **(Right)** This external photograph shows the eyes of a patient with strabismus. The right eye is exotropic. Strabismus impairs binocular function and leads to amblyopia of the nonfixating eye in many cases.*

AMBLYOPIA

INTRODUCTION

Definitions
- Reduced visual acuity in excess of that explained by structural or visual pathway disease

Subtypes
- Amblyopia may occur due to prevention of normal visual experience from birth to age 8 and is commonly classified by etiology
- Strabismic amblyopia
  - Impairs binocular function by causing diplopia and visual confusion due to eye misalignment
  - Intermittent exotropia rarely causes amblyopia; esotropia greater risk of amblyopia than exotropia
- Stimulus deprivation amblyopia
  - Due to cataract, ptosis, or any visual axis opacity preventing clear image formation on retina
- Refractive amblyopia
  - Unilateral or bilateral refractive error due to anisometropia (unequal refractive error), ametropia (uncorrected refractive error), or meridional (due to high astigmatism in 1 or both eyes)
- Developmental amblyopia: Failure of visual pathway to develop due to a retinal or CNS lesion, toxic or metabolic disturbance; irreversible

DEMOGRAPHICS

Epidemiology
- Estimated incidence of 2-5%
- Stimulus deprivation causes < 3% of amblyopia

PRESENTATION

Symptoms
- Decreased vision, strabismus, ptosis occasionally seen
- In most cases, amblyopia only affects 1 eye, so even severe cases often go unnoticed by parents
- Anisometropic amblyopia may be asymptomatic due to absence of easily observable symptoms

Exam Findings
- Strabismic amblyopia
  - Fixation defect
- Refractive amblyopia
  - Decreased visual acuity, anisometropia, ametropia, or astigmatism of ≥ 1.00 D
- Stimulus deprivation amblyopia
  - Cataract, ptosis, absence of red reflex, leukocoria

EVALUATION/WORK-UP

Amblyopia Screening
- Cover-uncover test for eye misalignment
- Assessment of monocular visual acuity
- Refraction: Retinoscopy or autorefraction
- Examination of external structures, fundus, and media
- Rechecking visual acuity using refractive correction

TREATMENT

Refractive Amblyopia
- Correction of refractive error
  - If amblyopia ceases to improve, perform occlusion therapy to encourage use of amblyopic eye
- Occlusion therapy
  - Most cases benefit from 3-6 hours of occlusion daily
  - Conventional occlusion: Total deprivation of light and form vision (most common occlusion therapy)
- Penalization: Deprivation of form vision by blurring vision in good eye
  - Optical penalization: Undercorrecting refractive error in good eye
  - Pharmacological penalization: Blurring vision in good eye with atropine drops

Stimulus Deprivation Amblyopia
- Goal is to provide good 2nd eye, should better seeing eye be compromised, and to maximize stereopsis
  - Surgical correction of cause for stimulus deprivation
    - Cataract extraction, ptosis repair
  - Refractive correction to improve image quality
  - Occlusion therapy

Strabismic Amblyopia
- Refractive correction with occlusion more effective than refractive correction alone
- Occlusion therapy
- Disagreement exists whether to treat amblyopia and then correct strabismus or vice versa

Follow-Up
- For full-time occlusions, follow-up at intervals of 1 week per year of age, but cannot stretch out follow-up longer than 4 weeks at any age
- Occlusion can be stopped when visual acuity is equal bilaterally or no progress after 3 months of occlusion
  - Some experts advise gradually tapering occlusion therapy

Prognosis
- Worse prognosis associated with early onset and delay in diagnosis and treatment

SELECTED REFERENCES

1. Taylor K et al: Interventions for unilateral and bilateral refractive amblyopia. Cochrane Database Syst Rev. 4:CD005137, 2012
2. Schmucker C et al: Effectiveness of early in comparison to late(r) treatment in children with amblyopia or its risk factors: a systematic review. Ophthalmic Epidemiol. 17(1):7-17, 2010
3. Li T et al: Conventional occlusion versus pharmacologic penalization for amblyopia. Cochrane Database Syst Rev. (4):CD006460, 2009
4. Powell C et al: Vision screening for amblyopia in childhood. Cochrane Database Syst Rev. (3):CD005020, 2009
5. Hatt S et al: Interventions for stimulus deprivation amblyopia. Cochrane Database Syst Rev. (3):CD005136, 2006

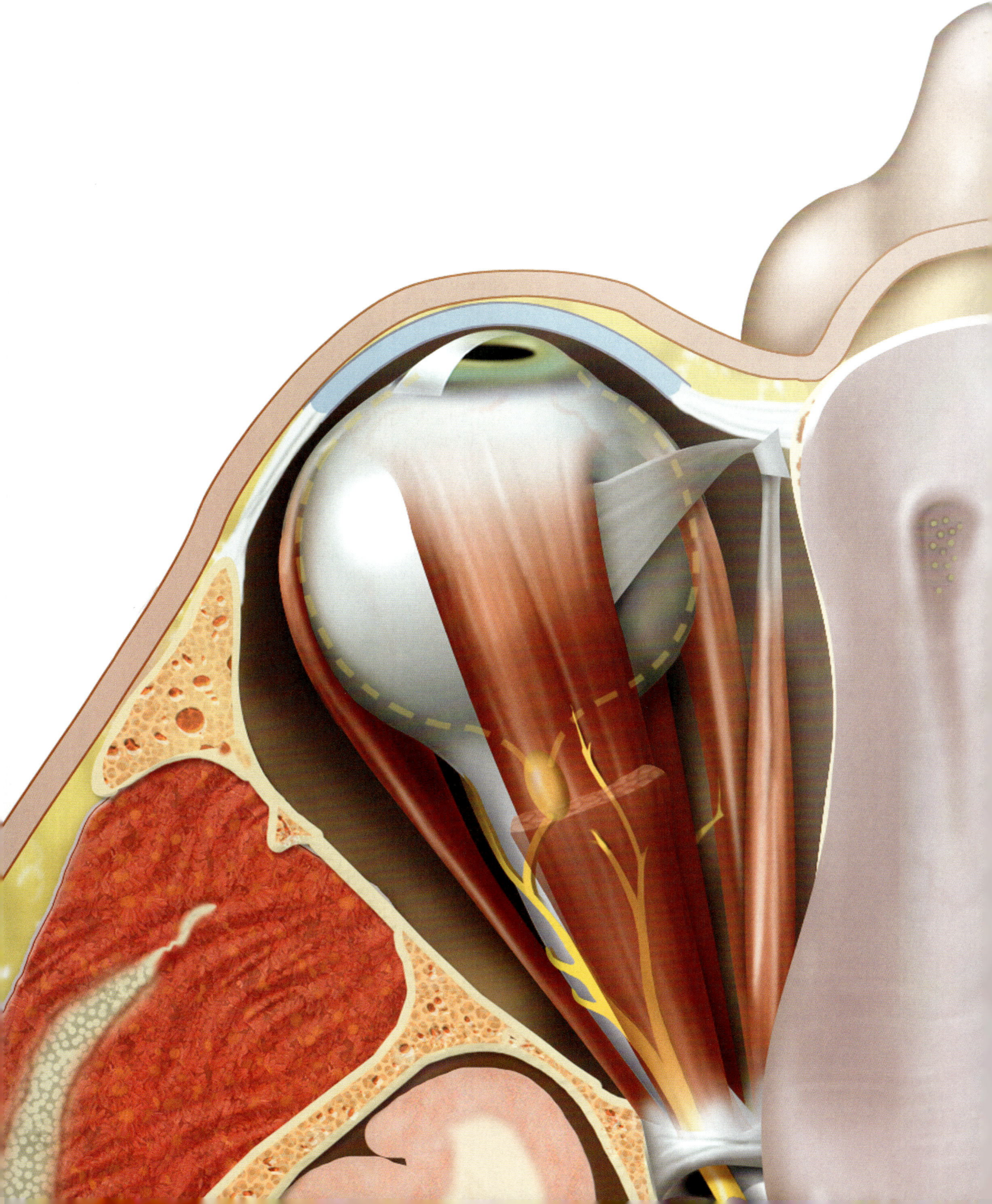

SECTION 2
Strabismus

Introduction and Overview

Congenital Disorders

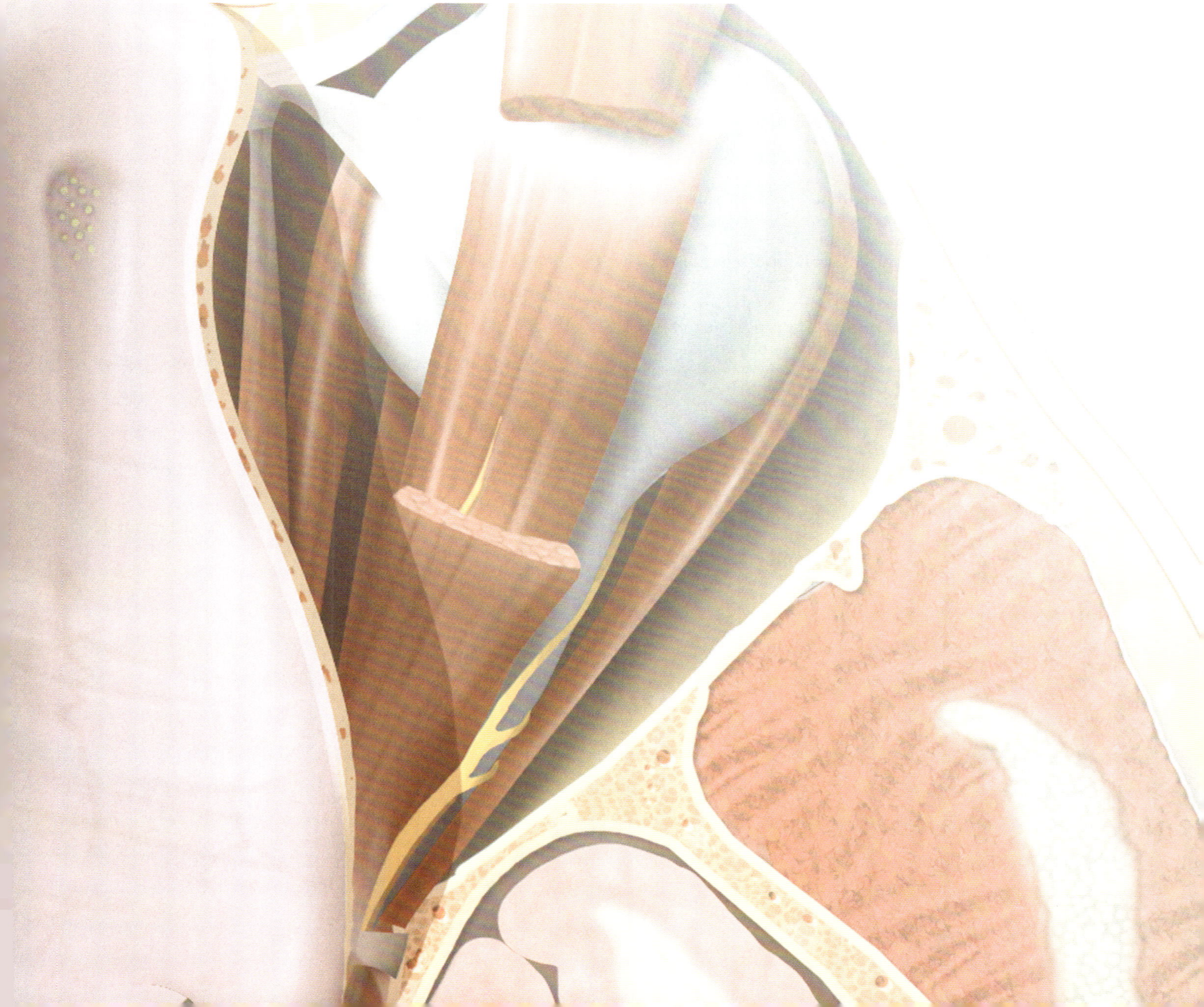

MAJOR CLINICAL STUDIES: AMBLYOPIA AND STRABISMUS

TERMINOLOGY

Abbreviations

- Best corrected visual acuity (BCVA)
- Early treatment for diabetic retinopathy study (ETDRS)

AMBLYOPIA TREATMENT STUDY: OCCLUSION VS. PHARMACOLOGIC TREATMENT FOR MODERATE AMBLYOPIA

Objective

- Compare outcomes of drug therapy with atropine to patching in successful treatment of amblyopia in patients ≤ 7 years
- Determine success rates of amblyopia
- Determine factors that may be considered in amblyopia treatment

Inclusion Criteria

- Age ≤ 7 years, visual acuity (VA) 20/40-20/100 in amblyopic eye, 20/40 or better in sound eye with ≥ 3 lines difference between eyes

Randomization Method

- Patients randomized into 2 groups
  - Patched 6-12 hours per day with increased patching time if no improvement in vision
  - 1 drop of atropine 1% per day in pharmacologic treatment group

Results

- Improvement in VA was initially faster in patching group, but after 6 months, there was no significant difference in VA between groups
- VA improved by ~ 3 lines in both groups with final VA 20/32 in patched group and $20/32^{-2}$ in atropine group
- Atropine was more accepted amongst parents
- Both patching and atropine are appropriate treatment choices in children with moderate amblyopia

PRISM ADAPTATION TRIAL

Objective and Principal Conclusion

- Determine if preoperative prism adaptation improves outcomes for acquired esotropia undergoing surgery for near deviation
- Determine factors that influence patient response to prism adaptation
- Improved surgical outcomes in patients with acquired esotropia

Inclusion Criteria

- Age ≥ 3 years, including adults
- Esotropia with onset at ≥ 6 months of age
- No history of previous eye muscle surgery

Randomization Method

- 60% of patients were randomly chosen to undergo prism adaptation prior to eye muscle surgery
  - Patients who responded to prism adaptation: 1/2 randomly selected to have surgery based on amount of prism required to correct deviation; other 1/2 had surgery based on amount of original esotropia
  - Patients who did not respond to prisms had surgery based on amount of esotropia measured
- 40% of patients were randomly assigned to forego prism adaptation and proceed with immediate surgery, which was based on amount of esotropia originally measured

Results

- No benefit in patients with hyperopic esotropia
- Patients showing fusion response to prisms had greatest benefit
- Predictors of successful fusion with prisms
  - Older age at onset of esotropia
  - Duration of esotropia < 1 year
  - Alternating fixation
  - Fusion on Worth 4-dot test when tested at near
  - Equal vision
- Augmented surgery was of greater benefit than conventional surgery
  - Augmented surgery is based on prism-adapted angle of deviation, rather than original amount of esotropia measured

TRIAL OF BIFOCALS IN MYOPIC CHILDREN WITH ESOPHORIA

Objective

- Determine if correction with bifocal lenses rather than single-vision lenses will slow ocular growth and progression of myopia in children with near-point esophoria
  - Axial length measured with ultrasound
  - Cycloplegic refraction measured with automated refractor
- Determine amount of close work performed by study participants
- Determine if parental myopia is a factor in myopia progression

Inclusion Criteria

- Boys age 6-12; girls age 6-11
- ≥ 0.5 diopters of myopia in both eyes
- Near-point esophoria with von Graefe prisms
- At least 20/25 VA in each eye
- 40 seconds of stereopsis
- No ocular disease or systemic disease that may alter refraction
- Willingness to wear bifocal spectacle lenses for 30 mo

Randomization Method

- Subjects were randomly assigned to wear either single-vision spectacle lenses or lenses with a +1.50 diopter add in a flat-top 28 mm segment
- Follow-up included automated refraction after cycloplegia with 1% tropicamide, biometry with A-scan, estimates of amount of study and other close work by questionnaires given to subjects and their parents, and amount of myopia in biologic parents

Results

- Myopia progression (difference between spherical equivalent at baseline and at 30-month follow-up exam, averaged over both eyes)
  - Avg 0.99 diopters for bifocals, 1.24 diopters for single vision (unadjusted $P = .106$, adjusted for age $P = .046$)
- Median progression rate for subjects: Bifocals = 0.92 diopters, single-vision = 1.24 diopters ($P = .047$)
- Myopia progressed more rapidly during school year than during summer vacation

- Difference in growth of vitreous chamber depth between 2 groups was significant (*P* = .046)

RANDOMIZED TRIAL OF TREATMENT OF AMBLYOPIA IN CHILDREN AGE 7-17

Objective and Principal Conclusions

- Study the effectiveness of treating amblyopia in children age 7-17
- In patients age 7-12 years, patching 2-6 hours a day + near visual activities + atropine can improve VA even if amblyopia has been previously treated
- In patients age 13-17, prescribing patching 2-6 hours a day + near visual activities may improve VA when amblyopia has not been previously treated but is of little benefit if amblyopia was previously treated with patching
- Most patients who are initially treated with optical correction alone will require additional treatment for amblyopia

Inclusion Criteria

- Age 7-17
- Unilateral amblyopia with a history of strabismus or an amblyogenic factor meeting study-specified criteria for strabismus &/or anisometropia on examination
- No amblyopia treatment (other than glasses) in past month and ≤ 1 month of amblyopia treatment in last 6 months
- BCVA of 20/40 to 20/400 in amblyopic eye
- BCVA of 20/25 or better in nonamblyopic eye
- No ocular cause for reduced VA
- ≤ 6 D of myopia in amblyopic eye
- If < 13 years, no more than 0.50 D of myopia in sound eye

Randomization Method

- Patients were randomized to either 2-6 hours per day of patching + near vision activities
  - + atropine sulfate for children aged 7-12 years
- Control group randomized to optical correction alone

Results

- 53% of patients aged 7-12 years in treatment group gained ≥ 10 letters ≥ 2 lines after 24 weeks vs. 25% of optical correction group (*P* < .001)
- 25% of patients aged 13-17 years in treatment group gained ≥10 letters ≥ 2 lines after 24 weeks vs. 23% of optical correction group (*P* = .22)
- Of patients who had been previously treated with patching &/or atropine, 47% of patients in treatment group gained ≥ 10 letters vs. 20% in optical correction group
- Most patients had a residual VA deficit

PILOT STUDY OF LEVODOPA DOSE AS TREATMENT FOR RESIDUAL AMBLYOPIA IN CHILDREN AGE 8-18 YEARS

Objective and Principal Conclusions

- Determine efficacy and safety of 2 doses of levodopa + daily ocular occlusion therapy of fellow eye in youth with residual amblyopia from strabismus, anisometropia, or both
- Levodopa for residual amblyopia was well tolerated and may improve VA
- Placebo-controlled trial is necessary

Inclusion Criteria

- Age 8-17 years
- BCVA between 67 and 18 letters on ETDRS chart in amblyopic eye (20/50 to 20/400)
- BCVA of 78 letters or better on ETDRS chart in fellow eye (20/25 or better)
- Undergoing treatment with patching for ≥ 2 hours per day
- < 5 letters or 1 LogMAR line of improvement since a previous visit ≥ 8 weeks prior while undergoing patching treatment

Randomization Method

- Patients continued patching for 2 hours per day and were randomized to receive 1 of 2 levodopa doses for 8 weeks, followed by a 1 week taper
  - Lower dose: 0.51 mg/kg 3x per day
  - Higher dose: 0.76 mg/kg 3x per day
- Levodopa was prepared in capsules combined with carbidopa 0.17 mg/kg 3x per day
  - To ↓ adverse effects from levodopa alone

Results

- Mean improvement in VA in amblyopic eye from baseline to 9 weeks was +4 (± 4) letters in lower dose group and +6 (± 6) letters in higher dose group
  - Mean difference between groups: -2 letters; 95% confidence interval: -6 to +1
- Improvement ≥ 10 letters seen in 13% of patients in lower dose group and 29% in higher dose group
- At 10 weeks after stopping levodopa treatment, mean change in VA in amblyopic eye from baseline was +5 (± 4) letters in lower dose group and +4 (± 5) letters in higher dose group
- Adverse events included headaches, upper respiratory tract infection, cough, rash, nausea, and vomiting

RELATED REFERENCES

1. National Institutes of Health, National Eye Institute: Amblyopia Treatment Study: Occlusion Versus Pharmacologic Therapy for Moderate Ablyopia. http://www.nei.nih.gov/neitrials/static/study73.asp. March 13, 2002. Accessed September 6, 2013
2. National Institutes of Health, National Eye Institute: Prism Adaptation Study. http://www.nei.nih.gov/neitrials/static/study20.asp. Updated September 23, 1999. Accessed September 6, 2013
3. National Institutes of Health, National Eye Institute: Trial of Bifocals in Myopic Children With Esophoria, A. http://www.nei.nih.gov/neitrials/static/study27.asp. Updated December 18, 2001. Accessed September 6, 2013
4. Repka MX et al: Pilot study of levodopa dose as treatment for residual amblyopia in children aged 8 years to younger than 18 years. Arch Ophthalmol. 128(9):1215-7, 2010
5. Scheiman MM et al: Randomized trial of treatment of amblyopia in children aged 7 to 17 years. Arch Ophthalmol. 123(4):437-47, 2005

STRABISMUS OVERVIEW

TERMINOLOGY

Definitions

- Esodeviation: Nasal eye deviation
- Exodeviation: Temporal eye deviation
- Hyperdeviation: Upward eye deviation
- Hypodeviation: Downward eye deviation
- -phoria: Suffix describing a deviation that is normally controlled by fusion (e.g., esophoria)
- -tropia: Suffix describing a deviation that exceeds the control of fusion (e.g., esotropia)

ESODEVIATIONS

Congenital (Infantile) Esotropia

- Esotropia occurring within 6 months of birth and often associated with neurological deficits
- Most common form of strabismus

Accommodative Acquired Esotropia

- Associated with accommodation due to uncorrected hyperopia causing excessive convergence
- Treatment with hyperopic correction, and surgery when refractive correction fails to improve deviation

Nonrefractive Accommodative Esotropia

- Also known as high AC/A ratio esotropia
- Due to abnormal relationships between accommodation and accommodative convergence
- Treatment options include bifocals, long-acting cholinesterase inhibitors, surgery, or observation

Nonaccommodative Acquired Esotropia

- Basic (acquired) esotropia starts after 6 months; not associated with accommodation

Incomitant Esodeviation

- Esodeviation varies with different gazes
- e.g., CN7 palsy, restrictive strabismus

EXODEVIATIONS

Intermittent Exotropia

- Most commonly occurring before age 5, deviation often appears during times of inattention, fatigue, or stress
- Associated amblyopia uncommon unless exotropia becomes constant or near constant

Constant Exotropia

- Often associated with neurologic/craniofacial disorders
- Sensory exotropia occurs in elderly due to refractive error, corneal/lens opacities, or macular lesions

OTHER FORMS OF STRABISMUS

Vertical Deviations

- May be incomitant and associated with over- or underaction of superior or inferior obliques
- May be treated with prisms to improve diplopia and cosmesis, though surgery typically recommended

A- and V-Pattern Strabismus

- A-pattern strabismus: Horizontal deviation that is increasingly convergent in upgaze &/or increasingly divergent in downgaze
- V-pattern strabismus: Horizontal deviation that is increasingly divergent in upgaze &/or increasingly convergent in downgaze

Duane Syndrome

- Limited unilateral or bilateral abduction and retraction due to aberrant innervation of lateral rectus muscles

Brown Syndrome

- Limited eye elevation in adduction due to congenitally shortened superior oblique muscle or tendon

Oculomotor Nerve Palsy

- Exotropia and possibly hypotropia due to palsy of oculomotor nerve from aneurysm congenital disorders, trauma, inflammation, infection, migraine, or neoplasm

Abducens Nerve Palsy

- Impaired abduction due to abducens nerve dysfunction, most commonly due to vascular disease

Thyroid (Graves) Ophthalmopathy

- Restrictive myopathy due to extraocular muscle edema, inflammation, and fibrosis
- Presentation may include strabismus, proptosis, lid retraction, and optic nerve compression

Chronic Progressive External Ophthalmoplegia

- Rare disease involving abnormalities in mitochondrial DNA, causing progressive paralysis of eyelids and extraocular muscles

Myasthenia Gravis

- Ptosis and strabismus due to fatigable weakness of extraocular muscles

Internuclear Ophthalmoplegia

- Impaired motility of adduction eye, classically with abducting nystagmus on lateral gaze, may be due to demyelinating disease, stroke, or brain tumor

TREATMENT

Surgery vs. Glasses

- Decision depends on risks to patient, potential for amblyopia/stereopsis/diplopia, and prior history

Main Treatment

- Surgical recession &/or resection of extraocular muscles to modify site of attachment
- If surgery is pursued, avoid anterior segment ischemia resulting from cutting > 3 anterior ciliary arteries
  - Each rectus has 2 ciliary arteries except for lateral rectus (which has only 1)
  - Ciliary-artery sparing surgery can be considered but is difficult
- Nonsurgical treatment involves use of prisms, orthoptics, &/or drugs to reduce accommodative convergence or provide temporary muscle paralysis

RELATED REFERENCES

1. Rowe FJ et al: Botulinum toxin for the treatment of strabismus. Cochrane Database Syst Rev. 2:CD006499, 2012

EXTRAOCULAR MUSCLE ANATOMY

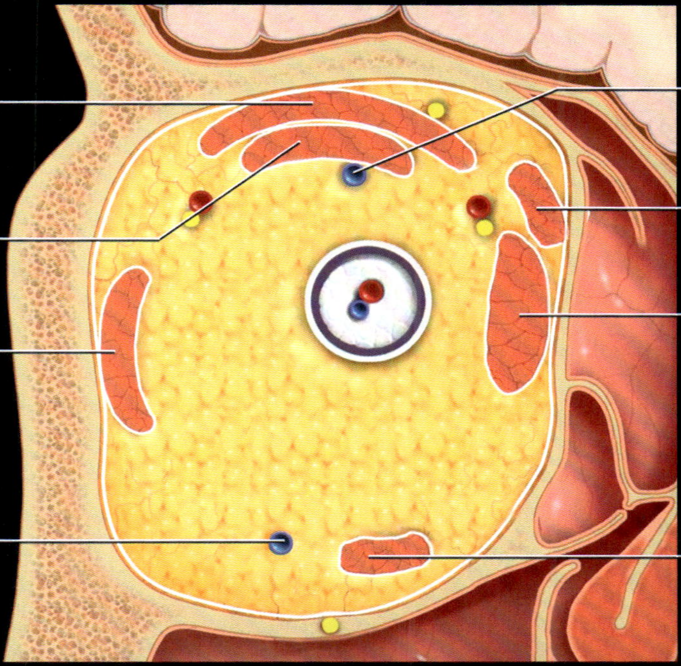

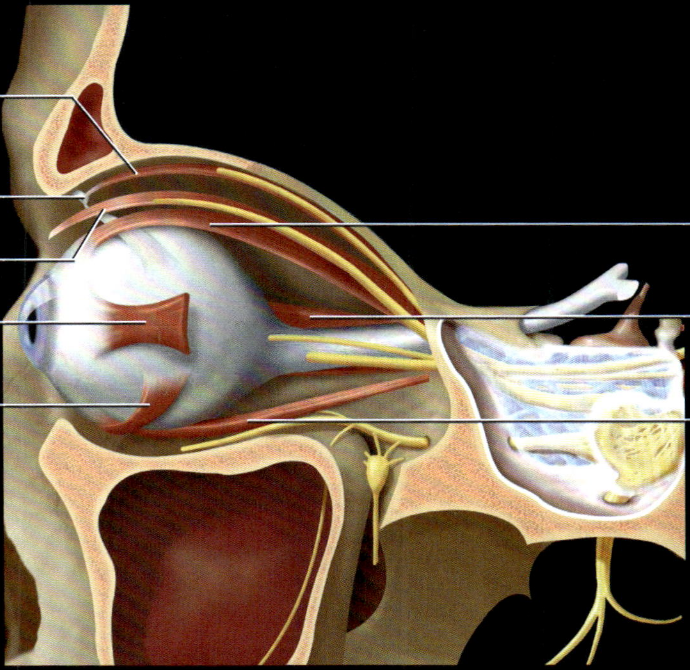

(Top) *This illustration depicts a coronal view of the right orbit. Understanding the anatomic location of each of the extraocular muscles is important in understanding strabismus.* ***(Bottom)*** *This illustration depicts a lateral view of the left orbit. The location of the origin and insertion of each extraocular muscle influences its effects on the globe.*

Key Facts

Introduction

- Short, tight superior oblique tendon or sheath
- Congenital causes
  - Inelastic superior oblique muscle tendon complex
  - Tight posterior tendon fibers prevent posterior eye from moving inferiorly during upgaze
  - Superior nasal orbital mass
  - Congenital inferior location of lateral rectus muscle
- Acquired etiology
  - Superior oblique tendon pathology
  - Trochlear pathology
  - Postoperative complications
  - Trauma
  - Inflammation

Presentation

- Inability to elevate eye in adduction
- Hypotropia in primary gaze possible
- Parents may notice 1 of their child's eyes drifting up under eyelid frequently (the normal eye)
- Patient often elevates chin and turns face away from affected eye which helps maintain binocular image fusion
- Exotropia in upgaze → "V" divergence in upgaze
- Positive forced duction test

Treatment

- May spontaneously improve
- Tenotomy or tenectomy of SO
- Wright silicon superior oblique tendon expander indicated if age > 4 years and hypodeviation in primary position
- Systemic anti-inflammatory medications if inflammatory etiology
- Monitor for recurrence of amblyopia, strabismus, and abnormal head positioning

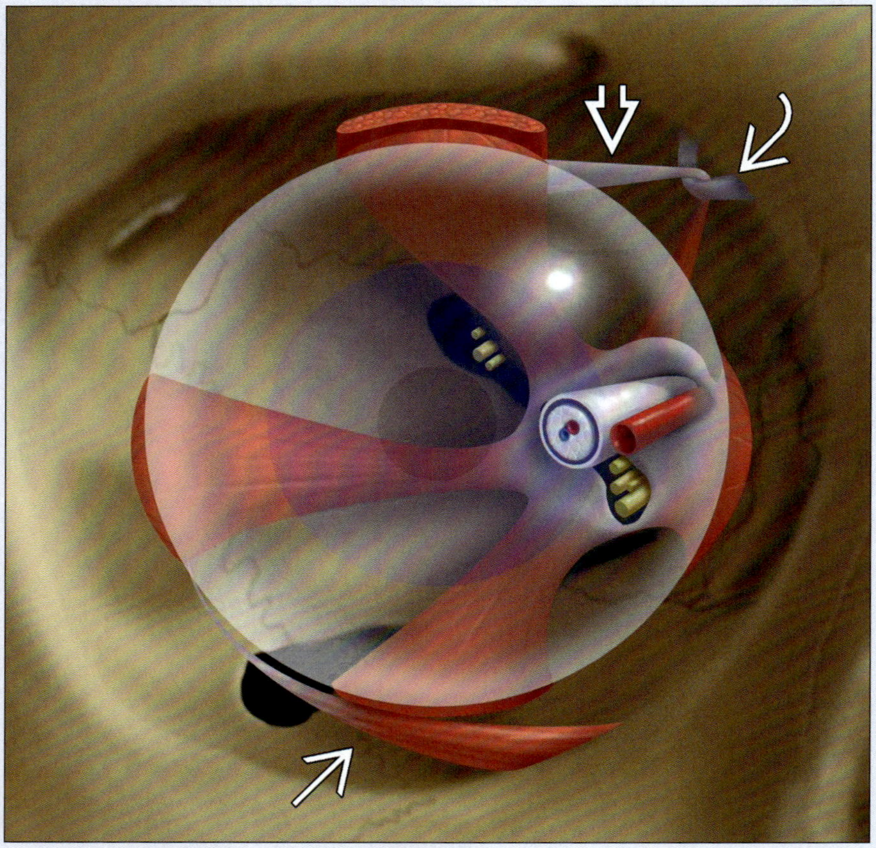

Brown syndrome is a condition caused by a short or tight superior oblique (SO) tendon or sheath ➡. Brown syndrome leads to a constant limitation in upgaze, particularly in adduction. The congenital subtype is typically related to an inelastic SO muscle tendon complex. Brown syndrome may also be acquired secondary to damage to the trochlea ➡ or the presence of a superior nasal mass. Inferior oblique ➡ paresis shares some features of Brown Syndrome, but may be differentiated by forced ductions and other testing. The eye is translucent in this graphic with muscles and tendons seen behind and around it.

BROWN SYNDROME

INTRODUCTION

Definitions

- Classically, a short, tight superior oblique (SO) tendon or sheath, which leads to constant limited upgaze and limited upgaze in adduction
- Abnormal movement of superior oblique tendon through the trochlea results in symptoms and abnormal findings on exam

Subtypes

- Congenital
  - Inelastic SO muscle tendon complex
  - Tight posterior SO tendon fibers preventing posterior eye from moving inferiorly during upgaze
  - Congenital inferior location of lateral rectus muscle
- Acquired
  - Tight or inelastic SO tendon
  - Superior nasal mass
    - Obstructs glide of SO tendon through trochlea
    - Orbital tumor, superior nasal glaucoma implant
  - Trochlear pathology
    - Sinusitis with peritrochlear inflammation
    - Idiopathic trochleitis
  - Postoperative complications
    - Surgical damage or scarring of trochlea
  - Inflammation
    - Inferior scarring of globe
    - Fibrosis of SO muscle associated with thyroid eye disease and Hurler-Scheie syndrome
    - SO click syndrome
  - Rheumatoid arthritis (rare)
  - Collagen disease with fibrosis and scarring

DEMOGRAPHICS

Etiology/Risk Factors

- Family history of amblyopia or strabismus
  - 35% of patients with congenital Brown syndrome

Epidemiology

- Rare cause of vertical strabismus
- Females (59%) more commonly affected than males (41%)
- Bilateral in 5-10% of cases

PRESENTATION

Symptoms

- Inability to elevate affected eye in adduction
- Hypotropia ± diplopia in primary gaze is possible
- Parents notice 1 of their child's eyes rolling up under eyelid frequently
  - When child looks superiorly, nonaffected eye raises while affected eye remains in primary position
- Elevated chin & face turn away from affected eye
  - Helps patient maintain binocular fusion of images
- Pain if inflammatory etiology

Exam Findings

- Chin-up posture with contralateral face turn
- Extraocular muscle testing
  - Limited upgaze worse in adduction
  - Exotropia in upgaze → "V" divergence in upgaze
- Positive forced duction test
  - Restricted elevation in adduction
- Widening of palpebral fissure on adduction
- May have downshoot in adduction

DIFFERENTIAL DIAGNOSIS

Double Elevator Palsy

- Congenital deficiency of elevation in 1 eye
- Restricted elevation in abduction and adduction
- Paretic or restrictive etiology
  - Superior rectus palsy (paretic)
  - Inferior rectus contraction (restrictive)

Inferior Oblique Paresis or Underaction

- Inability to elevate eye in adduction
- Forced duction testing normal
- Overaction of ipsilateral superior oblique

Thyroid Eye Disease

- Proptosis with eyelid retraction, eyelid fullness
- Diplopia secondary to extraocular muscle enlargement
- Pain and pressure behind the eyes
- + forced duction testing
- Systemic symptoms of hyperthyroidism

EVALUATION/WORK-UP

Imaging

- MRI of orbit indicated for acquired Brown syndrome associated with pain if patient has signs of inflammation or presents with atypical strabismus

TREATMENT

Medical

- Acquired causes may spontaneously improve
- Systemic anti-inflammatory medications
- Steroid injections near the trochlea

Surgical

- Consider surgery after 6-12 months of observation
- Wright silicon SO tendon expander
  - For patients with hypodeviation in primary position
  - Age > 4 years unless hypodeviation is so severe that it prevents fusion
- SO tenotomy
  - For patients with SO overaction
  - ± suture bridge between the ends of cut tendon
- SO recession
  - Undercorrection is common
- Exploratory surgery to locate and remove inflammatory nodules

Follow-Up

- Monitor patients for recurrence of amblyopia, strabismus, and abnormal head positioning

SELECTED REFERENCES

1. George JL et al: [Abnormal eyelid positions in Brown syndrome.] J Fr Ophtalmol. 27(6 Pt 1):579-87, 2004

CONGENITAL FIBROSIS SYNDROME

Key Facts

Demographics
- Defective innervation to the extraocular muscles (EOM) during development
- Replacement of contractile EOM tissue by fibrotic tissue
- Males = females
- ± family history

Presentation
- Restrictive ophthalmoplegia in 1 or more directions of gaze with sparing of lateral rectus muscle
- Eyes fixed in an infraducted position, 20-30° below midline
- ± Marcus Gunn jaw-winking phenomenon
- Compensatory backward head tilt is common
  - Due to more severe involvement of inferior rectus muscles
- Restricted motion during forced duction testing
  - Greatest restriction in abduction
- Jerking saccadic movements with upgaze
- Exotropia more common than esotropia

Evaluation/Work-Up
- MRI shows atrophy of involved muscles
- ± intracranial/orbit pathology or hypoplasia of CN3

Treatment
- EOM surgery to readjust globe alignment and lid ptosis
- Perform strabismus surgery before correcting ptosis
  - Eye muscle surgery can alter eyelid position
- Amblyopia is common
- Visual impairment secondary to ptosis and astigmatism
  - Visual acuity of 20/20 is rare
  - High refractive error with significant astigmatism

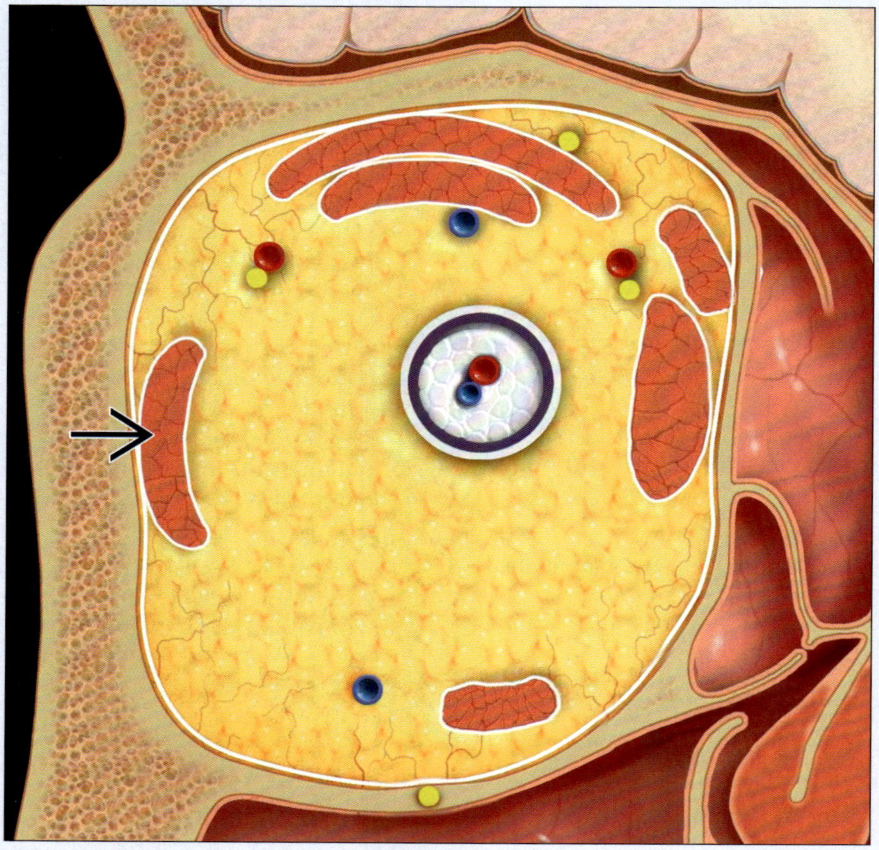

This illustration shows the extraocular muscles of eye movement. Congenital fibrosis syndrome is a result of defective innervation to these extraocular muscles. This results in replacement of the contractile extraocular muscle tissue by fibrotic tissue and presents as a restrictive ophthalmoplegia in 1 or more directions of gaze with sparing of the lateral rectus muscle ⇒. Congenital fibrosis syndrome is also notable for restricted motion during forced duction testing, which occurs as a result of the fibrotic tissue in the muscles.

CONGENITAL FIBROSIS SYNDROME

INTRODUCTION

Definitions

- Restriction of extraocular muscles (EOM)
  - Resulting in ophthalmoplegia and ptosis

Subtypes

- Type 1
  - Bilateral ptosis, hypotropia, miotic/nonreactive pupils
  - Horizontal strabismus, restricted horizontal gaze
  - Absent superior division of CN3 → abnormal levator palpebral superioris & superior rectus
  - Autosomal dominant, full penetrance, variable expression
  - Chromosome 12 (*KIF2A*)
- Type 2
  - Bilateral ptosis, exotropia, miotic/poorly reactive pupils
  - Severe horizontal and vertical restriction
  - Abnormal innervation to superior, medial, & inferior rectus and superior oblique
  - Autosomal recessive
  - Chromosome 11 (*PHOX2A*)
- Type 3
  - ± ptosis, bilateral or unilateral, reactive pupils
  - Hyper- or hypotropia
  - Horizontal and vertical restriction
  - Abnormal innervation to superior, medial, and inferior rectus
  - Autosomal dominant, incomplete penetrance, variable expression
  - Chromosome 12 (*KIF21A*), 13 (unknown), 16 (*TUBB3*)

DEMOGRAPHICS

Etiology/Risk Factors

- Defective innervation to extraocular muscles
- Replacement of contractile extraocular muscle tissue by fibrotic tissue
- Associated with facial dysmorphism, amblyopia, neurodevelopmental defects, coloboma, optic nerve dysplasia/hypoplasia, microphthalmia, oculocutaneous albinism, neural misdirection

Epidemiology

- Males = females
- ± family history

PRESENTATION

Exam Findings

- Restrictive ophthalmoplegia in 1 or more directions of gaze with sparing of lateral rectus muscle
- Backward head tilt compensates for infraduction
  - Due to severe involvement of inferior rectus muscles
  - Typically 20-30° of infraduction in primary gaze
- Restricted motion during forced duction testing
- ± Marcus Gunn jaw-winking syndrome
- Jerking saccadic movements with upgaze
- Exotropia more common than esotropia
- Visual impairment secondary to ptosis and astigmatism

DIFFERENTIAL DIAGNOSIS

Duane Syndrome

- Limited abduction, adduction, or both
- Globe retracts and eyelid fissure narrows on adduction

Brown Syndrome

- Short, tight superior oblique tendon or sheath
- Limited elevation in adduction
- Normal elevation in abduction
- Chin elevated and face turned away from affected eye

Moebius Syndrome

- Nonprogressive congenital disorder of the cranial nerves
  - → restricted elevation in adduction, V-pattern deviation, facial weakness

EVALUATION/WORK-UP

Pathology

- Electron microscopy
  - Collagen and dense fibrotic tissue replacing skeletal muscle fibers
  - Degeneration of skeletal muscle fibers

Imaging

- MRI shows atrophy of involved muscles
  - Use MRI to rule out intracranial or orbital pathology
  - ± hypoplasia of CN3

TREATMENT

Medical

- Correct refractive error, astigmatism, & treat amblyopia

Surgical

- EOM surgery to readjust globe alignment and lid ptosis
  - Perform strabismus surgery before correcting ptosis
    - Eye muscle surgery can alter eyelid position
  - Perform forced duction testing preoperatively and in the OR during surgery
- Ptosis surgery
  - Undercorrect ptosis to prevent unintentional overcorrection with exposure keratopathy

Prognosis

- Amblyopia is common
  - Patients seldom achieve binocularity
- Visual acuity of 20/20 is rare
  - High refractive error with significant astigmatism

SELECTED REFERENCES

1. Cooymans P et al: Congenital fibrosis of the extraocular muscles. Oman J Ophthalmol. 3(2):70-4, 2010
2. Lim KH et al: Abnormalities of the oculomotor nerve in congenital fibrosis of the extraocular muscles and congenital oculomotor palsy. Invest Ophthalmol Vis Sci. 48(4):1601-6, 2007
3. Traboulsi EI: Congenital abnormalities of cranial nerve development: overview, molecular mechanisms, and further evidence of heterogeneity and complexity of syndromes with congenital limitation of eye movements. Trans Am Ophthalmol Soc. 102:373-89, 2004

DOUBLE ELEVATOR PALSY

Key Facts

Introduction
- Inability to elevate 1 eye in all fields of gaze

Demographics
- 73% of cases due to a tight or contracted inferior rectus muscle
- Other causes include a weak or paretic superior rectus muscle or inferior oblique muscle, innervation abnormalities, and acquired mechanical and restrictive conditions of orbit
- Some cases are attributed to a combination of contracted and paretic muscles

Presentation
- Inability to elevate eye above primary position in all fields of horizontal gaze
- Hypotropia of affected eye in primary position
- Bell phenomenon may or may not be present
- Affected eye remains hypotropic or in primary position during upgaze, often mistaken as hypertropia of unaffected eye
- Forced duction testing
  - Positive if inferior rectus fibrosis/restriction
  - Negative if superior rectus and inferior oblique paresis
- Chin tilt often present when patient has a hypotropia of 10-20 prism diopters
- Ptosis (25%) or pseudoptosis (75%) of affected eye
- Prominent lower eyelid fold

Treatment
- Conservative treatment with base-up prism over affected eye
- Patching for amblyopia may be needed
- Surgery indicated if significant hypotropia in primary position and chin elevation
- Always perform forced duction testing prior to surgery
- Ptosis often corrects itself once hypotropia is corrected

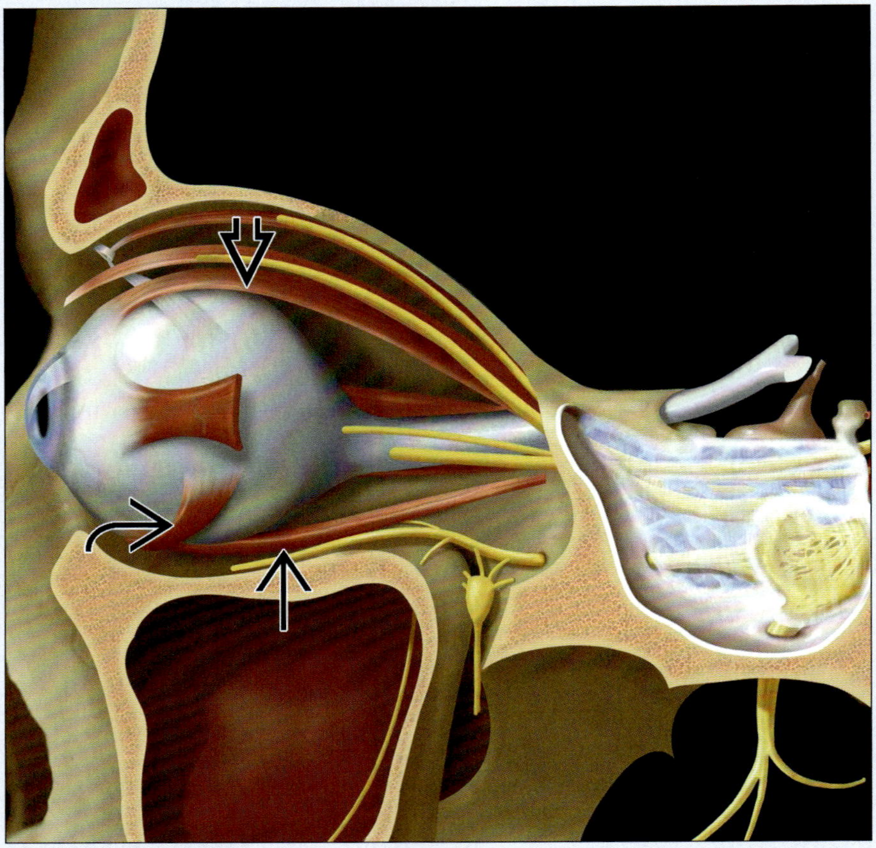

This illustration depicts a normal eye with the insertions of the muscles of eye movement. Double elevator palsy, also referred to as monocular elevation deficiency, is defined as the inability to elevate 1 eye in all fields of gaze. Most cases are congenital and are noticed in childhood, whereas some cases are acquired and occur later in life. 73% of cases are due to restriction of the inferior rectus muscle →. Other causes include a weak or paretic superior rectus muscle ⇨, a weak or paretic inferior oblique muscle ↪, or any combination of the 3.

DOUBLE ELEVATOR PALSY

INTRODUCTION

Definitions
- Congenital or acquired inability to elevate 1 eye in all fields of gaze
  - Neither superior rectus nor inferior oblique is able to elevate
  - Limitation of upgaze is equal in both abduction and adduction
- Also referred to as monocular elevation deficiency

DEMOGRAPHICS

Etiology/Risk Factors
- 73% of cases due to restriction of inferior rectus muscle
  - Tight, contracted inferior rectus muscle
- Other causes
  - Weak/paretic superior rectus muscle
  - Weak/paretic inferior oblique muscle
  - Innervation abnormalities
    - Supranuclear, nuclear, or infranuclear
  - Mechanical and restrictive conditions of orbit

PRESENTATION

Symptoms
- Inability to elevate affected eye above primary position
  - Occurs when looking medially, laterally, or forward
  - Complaint that eye (unaffected) disappears under upper eyelid
    - Chin-up head positioning

Exam Findings
- Hypotropia of affected eye in primary position
  - Minimal to no hypotropia in downgaze, slight to moderate hypotropia in primary position, and increased hypotropia in upgaze
- Forced duction testing
  - Positive if inferior rectus fibrosis/restriction
  - Negative if superior rectus and inferior oblique paresis
- ± Bell phenomenon
  - Is a normal upward and outward rolling of globe when patient attempts to close eyelid
  - Present if supranuclear innervation abnormality
  - Absent if tight inferior rectus muscle
- Upward chin tilt
  - Occurs if patient has a hypotropia of 10-20 prism diopters
  - Helps patient with binocularity and image fusion
- Ptosis or pseudoptosis of affected eye
  - Seen in primary gaze
  - Ptosis disappears with fixation of affected eye in pseudoptosis
  - Ptosis remaining during fixation indicates true ptosis
- Marcus-Gunn jaw-winking syndrome
  - Results in winking during chewing or sucking
- Prominent lower eyelid fold
  - Associated with restricted inferior rectus muscle
  - Can be due to attachments of inferior rectus tendon sheath to lower eyelid

DIFFERENTIAL DIAGNOSIS

Brown Syndrome
- Short, tight superior oblique tendon or tendon sheath
- Limited elevation of eye in adduction
- Restricted elevation in adduction during forced duction testing

Duane Syndrome
- Limited abduction, adduction, or both
- Globe retracts and eyelid fissure narrows on adduction
- Face turn toward lesioned eye in unilateral cases

Möbius Syndrome
- Nonprogressive congenital disorder of cranial nerves 6 and 7, and often others
- Results in facial diplegia, abduction deficit/paralysis, and severe esotropia

Infranuclear Palsy of Superior Rectus Muscle
- Bell phenomenon is absent

TREATMENT

Medical
- Conservative treatment with base-up prism over affected eye
- Patching for amblyopia may be needed

Surgical
- Not indicated if patient is orthophoric in primary position
- Surgery indicated if significant hypotropia in primary position, amblyopia, &/or chin elevation
  - Always perform forced duction testing prior to surgery
  - If positive, restriction to elevation requiring inferior rectus muscle recession
  - If negative, perform Hummelsheim transposition or Knapp procedure
    - Knapp procedure corrects up to 35 prism diopters
      - Transposition of medial and lateral rectus muscles up to superior rectus insertion site
      - Risk of anterior segment ischemia due to multiple muscle surgeries
- Ptosis often corrects itself once hypotropia is corrected
  - Reevaluate need for ptosis surgery after eye alignment is achieved
  - Treat ptosis with frontalis suspension or levator resection

Follow-Up
- Monitor ocular motility, head posture, pupillary function, visual acuity, cycloplegic refraction, and dilated fundus exam

SELECTED REFERENCES

1. Brodsky MC et al: Monocular elevation deficiency ("double elevator" palsy): a cautionary note. J Neuroophthalmol. 31(1):56-7, 2011
2. Samir A et al: A new approach for management of monocular elevation deficiency. J Clinic Experiment Ophthalmol. 2(3), 2011

DUANE RETRACTION SYNDROME

Key Facts

Introduction
- Duane retraction syndrome (DRS), also known as Stilling-Turk-Duane syndrome, is a congenital ocular motility disorder caused by aberrant innervation of the medial and lateral rectus muscles

Etiology
- Aberrant innervation of lateral rectus muscle by inferior division of CN3, the oculomotor nerve (normal innervation is by CN6, the abducens nerve)
- Most cases are sporadic, but autosomal dominant inheritance reported in 5-10% of cases

Presentation
- Strabismus
- Abnormal head position
- Double vision
- Patients with sporadic form of DRS have 10-20x greater risk of other congenital malformations
- Classification based on clinical findings
  - Type 1: Most common, occurs in 50-80% of cases; average age at presentation is 13 years
  - Type 2: Occurs in 14% of cases; average age at presentation is 23 years
  - Type 3: Occurs in 1% of cases; average age at presentation is 22 years

Treatment
- Medical
  - Treatment for refractive error and amblyopia should take place prior to surgical intervention
- Surgical
  - Indications for surgery include manifest deviation in primary gaze position, anomalous head position, up or downshoot in adduction, and painful globe retraction
- Follow-up
  - Surveillance important to prevent amblyopia

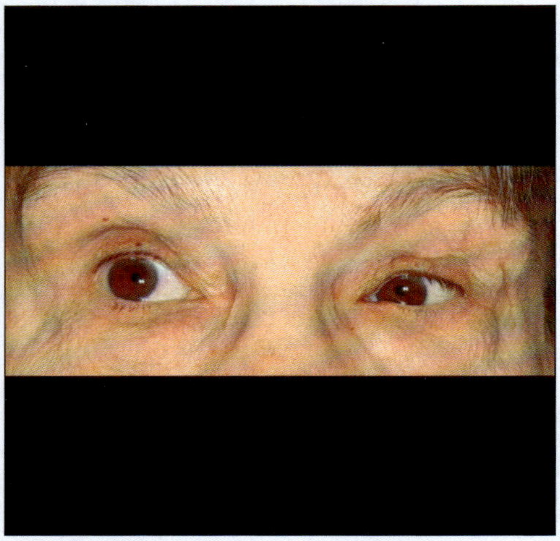
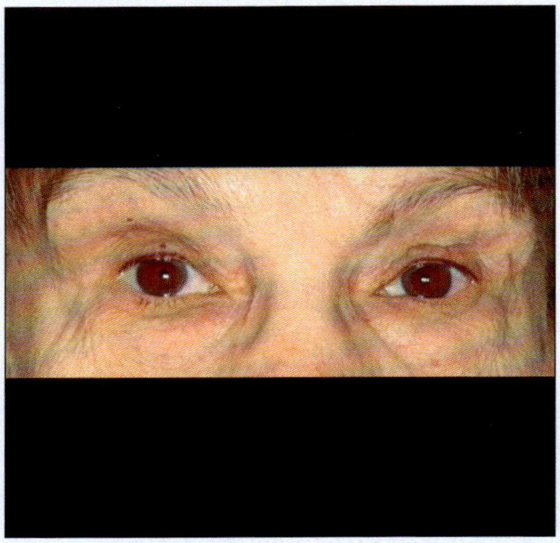

(Left) *This external photograph shows limited abduction of the right eye and palpebral fissure narrowing of the left eye, consistent with a diagnosis of type 1 Duane syndrome.* ***(Right)*** *This external photograph shows slight esotropia in primary gaze, consistent with a diagnosis of type 1 Duane syndrome.*

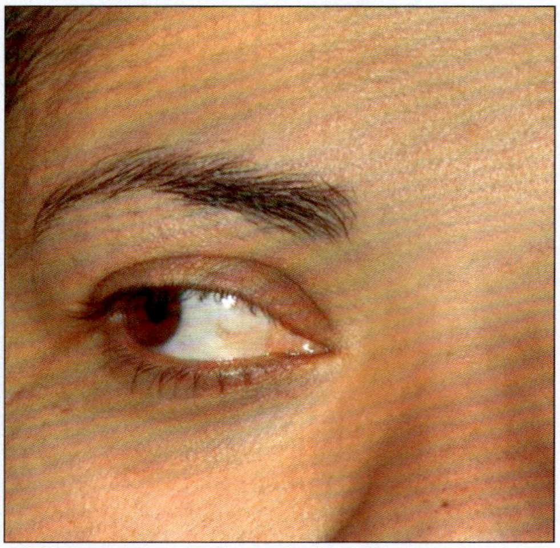
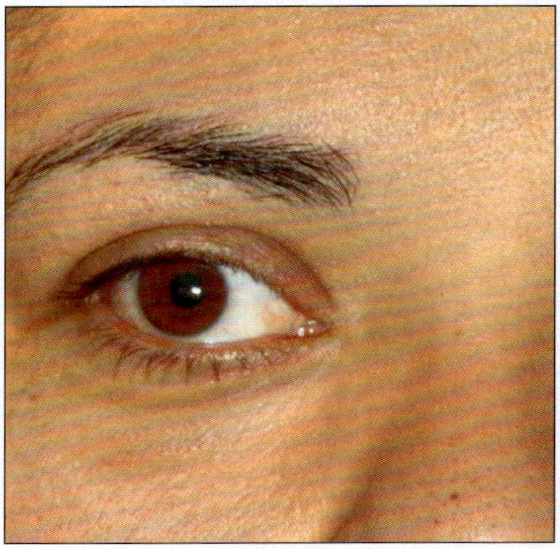

(Left) *This external photograph shows a patient with Duane syndrome in right gaze exhibiting intact abduction of the right eye.* ***(Right)*** *This external photograph shows the same patient attempting left gaze with impaired adduction of the right eye. This finding is consistent with a diagnosis of type 2 Duane syndrome.*

DUANE RETRACTION SYNDROME

INTRODUCTION

Abbreviations
- Duane retraction syndrome (DRS)

Synonyms
- Stilling-Turk-Duane syndrome

Definitions
- Congenital ocular motility disorder caused by aberrant innervation of the medial and lateral rectus muscles

DEMOGRAPHICS

Etiology/Risk Factors
- Aberrant innervation of lateral rectus muscle by inferior division of CN3, the oculomotor nerve (normal innervation is by CN6, the abducens nerve)
- Most cases are sporadic, but autosomal dominant inheritance reported in 5-10% of cases
  - Acquired cases may be due to mechanical or supranuclear etiologies

Epidemiology
- Incidence in general population is 0.1%
- Comprises ~ 1% of strabismus cases
- Female predominance (60%) in type 1 DRS
- Left eye involvement in 59%, right eye in 23%, and both eyes in 18% of cases

PRESENTATION

Symptoms
- Strabismus, abnormal head position, diplopia

Classification Based on Clinical Findings
- Type 1: Most common, occurs in 50-80% of cases; average age at presentation is 13 years
  - Frequent esotropia in primary gaze
  - Limited abduction and relatively normal adduction
- Type 2: Occurs in 14% of cases; average age at presentation is 23 years
  - Almost always exotropic in primary gaze
  - Limited or absent adduction with normal or slightly decreased abduction
- Type 3: Occurs in 1% of cases; average age at presentation is 22 years
  - Limited or absent abduction and adduction
  - Can be associated with primary gaze, esotropia, exotropia, or orthotropia
- All types involve globe retraction and narrowing of palpebral fissure on adduction
- When bilateral, may have different types in each eye

Associated Findings
- Patients with sporadic form of DRS have 10-20x greater risk of other congenital malformations
  - Associated syndromes include Holt-Oram syndrome, Okihiro syndrome, Wildervanck syndrome, morning glory syndrome, and Goldenhar syndrome
  - Systemic abnormalities include spina bifida, cleft palate, &/or congenital labyrinthine deafness
  - Ocular findings include iris dysplasia, cataracts, Marcus-Gunn jaw-winking syndrome, coloboma, hypermetropia, anisometropia, &/or amblyopia

DIFFERENTIAL DIAGNOSIS

Congenital 6th Nerve Palsy
- Results in large-angle esotropia in primary gaze

Brown Syndrome
- Limited eye elevation in adduction due to congenitally shortened superior oblique muscle or tendon

Strabismus
- Eye misalignment

EVALUATION/WORK-UP

Electromyogram (EMG) Findings
- Type 1
  - Reduced activity of lateral rectus muscle on abduction
  - Simultaneous contraction of lateral and medial rectus muscles on adduction
- Type 2
  - Innervational peaks of lateral rectus muscle on both attempted adduction and abduction
- Type 3
  - Electrical activity of both horizontal rectus muscles in primary gaze position, adduction, or abduction

TREATMENT

Medical
- Treatment for refractive error and amblyopia should take place prior to surgical intervention

Surgical
- Avoid rectus resections to avoid worsening globe retraction
- Indications for surgery include manifest deviation in primary gaze position, anomalous head position, up or downshoot in adduction, and painful globe retraction
- Types 1 and 3
  - Recession of medial rectus muscle or horizontal transposition of vertical rectus muscles
  - Recession of medial and lateral rectus muscles if up or downshoot in adduction or severe globe retraction
  - Y-splitting of lateral rectus muscle is another approach reported for treatment of upshoot/downshoot
- Type 2
  - If head turn is present, consider
    - Recession of ipsilateral lateral rectus if patient fixates with uninvolved eye
    - Recession of lateral rectus, possibly with Y-splitting, if upshoot or downshoot occurs in adduction

Follow-Up
- Surveillance important to prevent and treat amblyopia and should include routine visits every 3-6 months during 1st years of life and every 6-12 months in affected individuals ages 7-12 with binocular vision

SELECTED REFERENCES

1. Kekunnaya R et al: Duane retraction syndrome: series of 441 cases. J Pediatr Ophthalmol Strabismus. 49(3):164-9, 2012
2. Yüksel D et al: Review of the major findings about Duane retraction syndrome (DRS) leading to an updated form of classification. Vision Res. 50(23):2334-47, 2010

ESODEVIATIONS

Key Facts

Introduction
- Medial deviation of the eye
  - Congenital (infantile) esotropia
  - Accommodative esotropia
  - Nonaccommodative acquired (basic) esotropia
  - Incomitant esotropia

Presentation
- Constant or intermittently crossed eyes

Exam Findings
- Congenital esotropia
  - Constant esotropia > 30 prism diopters (PDs)
  - Versions may be limited but ductions and Doll's head are intact; often associated with > 3 diopters of hyperopia
- Accommodative esotropia
  - Angle of esotropia greater at near
  - Refractive: Moderate to high hyperopia; normal AC/A
  - Nonrefractive: Low hyperopia or myopia; high AC/A
- Nonaccommodative esotropia: Near deviation same as distance deviation; normal AC/A
- Incomitant esotropia: Increases in gaze toward paretic lateral rectus muscle; may be due to restrictive process

Treatment
- Congenital esotropia
  - Treatment of hyperopia and amblyopia; surgery if esodeviation remains
- Accommodative esotropia
  - Treatment of hyperopia with full hyperopic correction and treatment of amblyopia
- Nonaccommodative esotropia
  - Treatment of amblyopia and strabismus surgery for full prism-adapted deviation
- Incomitant esotropia
  - Strabismus surgery if spontaneous resolution does not occur within 6 months of follow-up

*(**Left**) External photo shows congenital esotropia. This condition affects up to 30% of children with neurologic deficits. Other expected exam findings may include cross-fixation, latent nystagmus, dissociated vertical deviation, and superior oblique overaction. (**Right**) External photo shows esotropia. Esotropia can be subdivided into 4 subtypes: Congenital, accommodative, nonaccommodative, and incomitant. Incomitant esotropia is frequently caused by abducens nerve (CN6) palsies.*

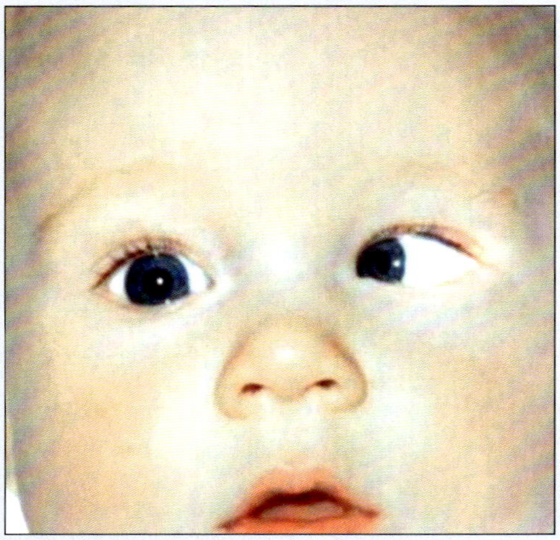

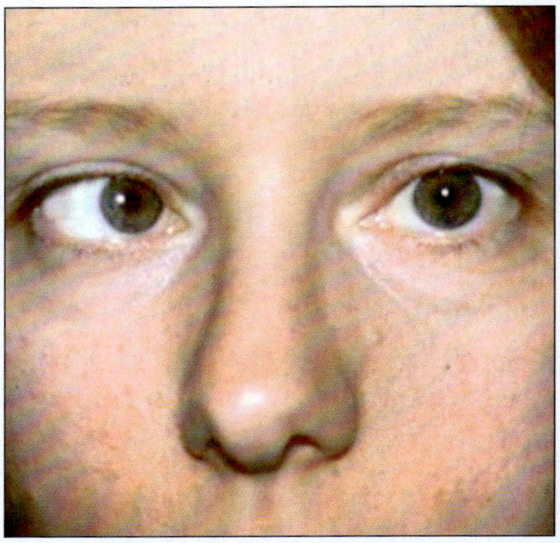

*(**Left**) External photo shows esotropia. Esotropia can be broadly defined as either concomitant (not varying with gaze direction) or incomitant (varying with gaze direction). Treatment options vary depending on the type of esotropia, but may include prism lenses, botulinum toxin injection, or surgical correction. (**Right**) Axial graphic shows the course of the abducens nerve (CN6) though the cavernous sinus ⇨ and annulus of Zinn ⇨. CN6 palsy is a common cause of acquired esodeviation.*

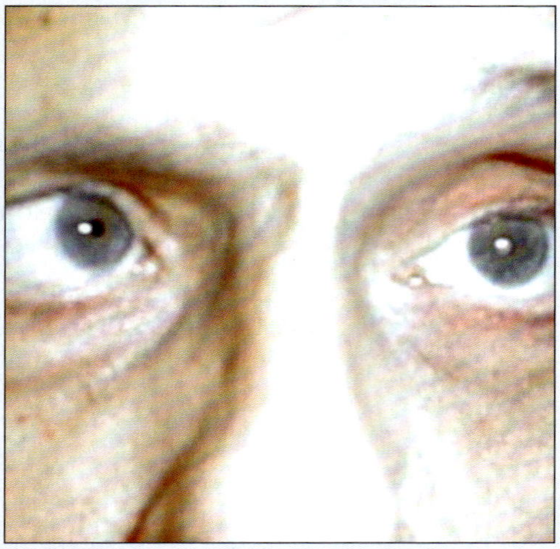

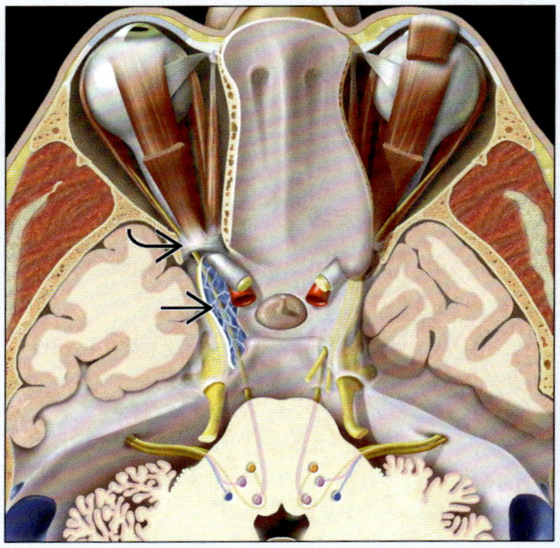

ESODEVIATIONS

INTRODUCTION

Definitions
- Medial eye deviation

Subtypes
- Congenital (infantile) esotropia
  - Presence of esotropia before 6 months of age
  - Occurs in up to 30% of children with neurologic deficits such as cerebral palsy and hydrocephalus
- Accommodative esotropia
  - Convergent deviation with accommodation
  - Onset 6 months to 7 years of age; average is 2.5 years
  - 2 types: Refractive and nonrefractive
- Nonaccommodative acquired (basic) esotropia
  - Develops after 6 months of age and not associated with accommodation
- Incomitant esotropia
  - Varies in different fields of gaze due to 6th nerve palsy from infection, immunologic process, or intracranial lesions; may also be secondary to restrictive process

DEMOGRAPHICS

Etiology/Risk Factors
- Accommodative esotropia may be inherited; 77% of cases have affected 1st- or 2nd-degree relatives

PRESENTATION

Symptoms
- Constantly crossed eyes or intermittently crossed eyes when fatigued or ill
- Deviation varies (incomitant) or does not vary with direction of gaze (concomitant)
- Double vision

Exam Findings
- Congenital esotropia
  - Constant esotropia > 30 prism diopters (PDs)
  - Doll's head shows intact abduction
  - Cross-fixation commonly seen, characterized by eye fixation in adduction with face turn toward fixing eye
  - Often associated with > 3 diopters of hyperopia
  - If amblyopia present, only better-seeing eye will fixate in all directions, making amblyopic eye appear to have abduction weakness
  - Persistent monocular smooth pursuit asymmetry
- Accommodative esotropia
  - Angle of esotropia greater at near due to excess convergence tone from accommodation
  - Misalignment may initially be intermittent; if untreated, may progress to constant deviation in weeks or months
  - Refractive
    - Moderate to high hyperopia with normal ratio of accommodative convergence to accommodation (AC/A)
  - Nonrefractive
    - Low hyperopia, or even myopia, with high AC/A
- Nonaccommodative esotropia
  - Near deviation same as distance deviation, without significant hyperopia, and normal AC/A
- Incomitant esotropia
  - Increases in gaze toward paretic lateral rectus muscle

DIFFERENTIAL DIAGNOSIS

Pseudoesotropia
- False appearance of congenital esotropia due to broad nasal bridge, prominent epicanthal folds, and narrow interpupillary distance

TREATMENT

Medical
- Congenital esotropia
  - Treatment of hyperopia and amblyopia; if esodeviation remains, surgery recommended for partially accommodative esotropia
- Accommodative esotropia
  - Treatment of hyperopia with full hyperopic correction and treatment of amblyopia
  - Gradually reduce hyperopic correction if alignment improves with spectacle use, visual acuity is equal, and high-grade binocularity is preserved
- Nonaccommodative esotropia
  - Treatment of amblyopia
- Incomitant esotropia
  - Spontaneous resolution in > 50% of traumatic palsies
  - Treatment of amblyopia
  - Consider injection of botulinum toxin into antagonist medial rectus to temporarily achieve alignment

Surgical
- Congenital esotropia
  - Timing of surgery is controversial though current trend suggests surgery at 3 months of age if deviation is constant, > 40 PDs, and stable or worsening
  - Most common surgical treatment includes bilateral medial rectus recession
- Accommodative esotropia
  - In older children and adults, refractive surgery is effective for correction of hyperopia and to achieve ocular alignment without spectacles
  - Strabismus surgery typically unnecessary, except in delayed spectacle correction, minimal improvement, or poor compliance, where surgery is required to correct nonaccommodative esotropia
- Nonaccommodative esotropia
  - Strabismus surgery for full prism-adapted deviation
- Incomitant esotropia
  - Strabismus surgery if spontaneous resolution does not occur within 6 months of follow-up
  - If incomplete 6th nerve palsy, recession of antagonist medial rectus and resection of lateral rectus muscles
  - If complete 6th nerve palsy, muscle transposition procedures may be required

SELECTED REFERENCES

1. Hutcheson KA: Childhood esotropia. Curr Opin Ophthalmol. 15(5):444-8, 2004
2. Guthrie ME et al: Congenital esotropia. Ophthalmol Clin North Am. 14(3):419-24, viii, 2001
3. Lambert SR: Accommodative esotropia. Ophthalmol Clin North Am. 14(3):425-32, 2001

EXODEVIATIONS

Key Facts

Introduction

- Outward eye deviation; may be unilateral or bilateral
- Subtypes of exodeviations
  - Exophoria
  - Divergence excess exotropia: Simulated and true divergence excess
  - Convergence insufficiency
  - Basic exotropia
  - Sensory exotropia
  - Congenital exotropia
  - Consecutive exotropia

Presentation

- Unilateral or bilateral exodeviation
  - Intermittent or constant
- Clinical exam should include prism and alternate cover testing at distances of 20 feet and 14 inches

Differential Diagnosis

- Pseudoexotropia
  - False appearance of exodeviation
  - May result from wide interpupillary distance or positive angle kappa

Treatment

- Intermittent exotropia
  - Medical treatment aimed at eliminating suppression using orthoptic exercises, part-time occlusion, minus lens, or prism therapy
  - Surgery if present ≥ 50% of waking hours
  - Unilateral lateral rectus recession with medial rectus resection or bilateral lateral rectus recession
- Constant exotropia
  - Early bilateral lateral rectus recession or unilateral lateral rectus recession with medial rectus resection
- Postoperative deviation is common and may require medical or surgical retreatment

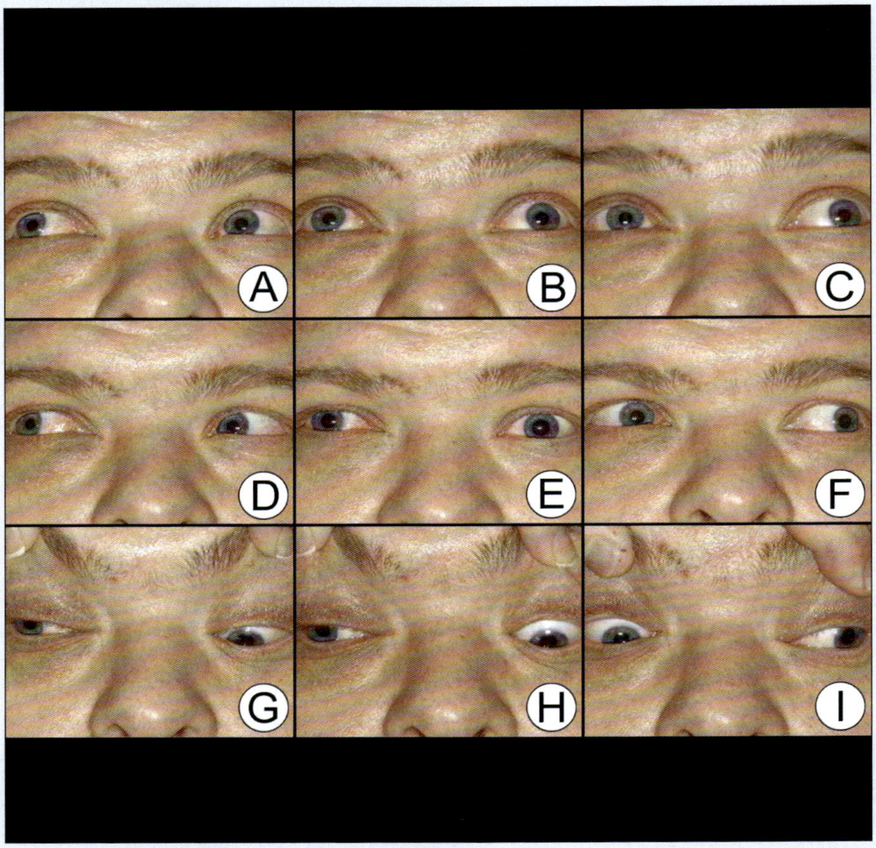

This 9-frame strabismus series shows a patient with constant exotropia in all fields of gaze and preferential fixation with the left eye. This large-angle manifest exotropia is most commonly secondary to decompensation of intermittent exotropia or sensory deprivation in adults.

EXODEVIATIONS

INTRODUCTION

Definitions
- Outward eye deviation; may be unilateral or bilateral

Subtypes
- Exophoria
  - Exodeviation controlled by fusion under conditions of normal binocular vision
- Intermittent exotropia is the most common type of exotropia
  - Basic exotropia
  - Divergence excess exotropia
    - Simulated divergence excess
    - True divergence excess
  - Convergence insufficiency
- Constant exotropia
  - Untreated intermittent exotropia often progresses to constant exotropia
    - Congenital exotropia
      - Uncommon in healthy infants; may have neurologic impairment or craniofacial disorders
    - Sensory exotropia
      - Caused by decreased unilateral visual acuity due to any condition, including anisometropia, corneal or lens opacities, optic atrophy or hypoplasia, macular lesions, and amblyopia
    - Consecutive exotropia
      - Caused by previous surgery for esotropia

DEMOGRAPHICS

Epidemiology
- 25% of strabismus due to exodeviations
- Intermittent exotropia is most common childhood exotropia; prevalence is 1% in children < age 11
- 2x as common in Asian populations and more common among females

PRESENTATION

Symptoms
- Intermittent exotropia
  - Onset usually before age 5 and as early as age 1
  - Unilateral exodeviation when viewing distant objects, when tired, or during periods of inattention
  - Closure of 1 eye or exodeviation in bright sunlight
  - Convergence insufficiency
    - Headaches, eye fatigue, difficulty with reading or near tasks, horizontal diplopia
- Constant exotropia
  - Outward eye deviation that is constantly present

Exam Findings
- Intermittent exotropia using prism cover test reveals
  - Basic exotropia: Deviation similar at distance and near fixation; within 10 prism diopters (PDs)
  - Divergence excess exotropia: Deviation larger at distance fixation than at near fixation; > 10 PD
    - Simulated divergence excess: Deviation at distance fixation and near < 10 PD after suspending accommodation or tenacious proximal fusion
    - True divergence excess: Near deviation less than distance despite focusing and fusion manipulation
- Convergence insufficiency: Near deviation larger than distance deviation
  - Remote near point of convergence
  - Decreased fusional convergence
  - Exophoria or even intermittent exotropia at near
- Constant exotropia: Large-angle constant exodeviation

DIFFERENTIAL DIAGNOSIS

Pseudoexotropia
- False appearance of exodeviation; may result from wide interpupillary distance or positive angle kappa

EVALUATION/WORK-UP

Clinical Exam
- Prism and alternate cover testing at distances of 20 feet and 14 inches with assessment of accommodative convergence/accommodation ratio (AC/A)

TREATMENT

Medical
- Intermittent exotropia
  - Eliminate suppression using orthoptic exercises, part-time occlusion, minus lens, or prism therapy
  - Convergence insufficiency
    - Orthoptic therapy and pencil push-ups

Surgical
- Intermittent exotropia: Surgery recommended if exotropia present for ≥ 50% of waking hours or deterioration of control for near fixation
  - Basic or simulated excess divergence exotropia should undergo unilateral lateral rectus recession with medial rectus resection; bilateral lateral rectus recession may also be appropriate for basic exotropia
  - Bilateral lateral rectus recession for true divergence excess
- Constant exotropia
  - Early bilateral lateral rectus recession or unilateral lateral rectus recession with medial rectus resection

Follow-Up
- Postoperative deviation is common and may be treated with observation, base-out prisms, occlusion to prevent amblyopia and relieve diplopia, botulinum toxin injections, or repeat surgery

SELECTED REFERENCES

1. Lavrich JB: Convergence insufficiency and its current treatment. Curr Opin Ophthalmol. 21(5):356-60, 2010
2. Clarke MP: Intermittent exotropia. J Pediatr Ophthalmol Strabismus. 44(3):153-7; quiz 178-9, 2007
3. Eibschitz-Tsimhoni M et al: Current concepts in the management of concomitant exodeviations. Compr Ophthalmol Update. 8(4):213-23, 2007
4. Richardson S et al: Interventions for intermittent distance exotropia. Cochrane Database Syst Rev. 2003; (2):CD003737. Review. Update in: Cochrane Database Syst Rev. (3):CD003737, 2006

CASE INDEX

CASE INDEX

CASE INDEX

INDEX

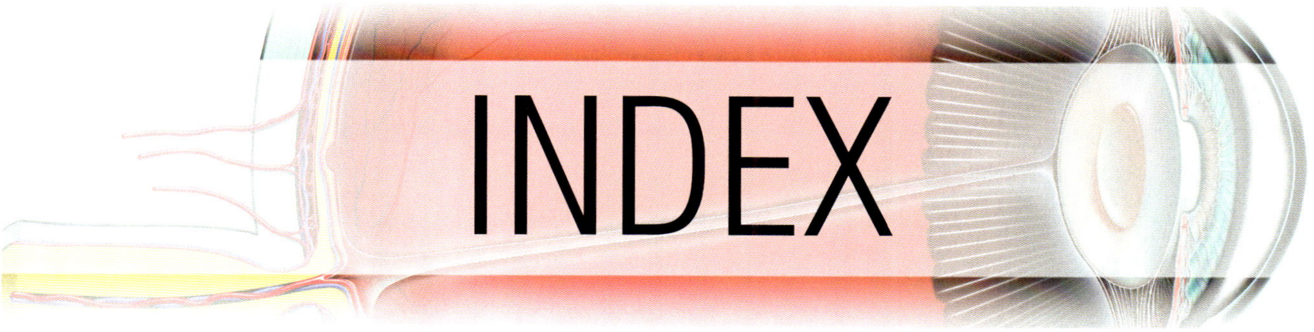

A

INDEX

INDEX

B

INDEX

C

INDEX

INDEX

INDEX

INDEX

INDEX

INDEX

INDEX

D

INDEX

INDEX

E

INDEX

INDEX

INDEX

INDEX

INDEX

INDEX

INDEX

INDEX

L

INDEX

M

INDEX

INDEX

INDEX

INDEX

INDEX

INDEX

INDEX

INDEX

INDEX

INDEX

INDEX

T

INDEX

INDEX

INDEX

W

X